KEY TOPICS

(continued)

Dermatologic and Cosmetic Procedures in Office Practice

Richard P. Usatine, MD
Professor, Dermatology and Cutaneous Surgery
Professor, Family and Community Medicine
Fellowship Director, Underserved Dermatology Fellowship
Medical Director, Skin Clinic, University Health System
University of Texas Health Science Center at San Antonio
San Antonio, Texas

John L. Pfenninger, MD
President and Director, Medical Procedures Center, PC
Private Practice
Midland, Michigan
Senior Consultant and Founder, National Procedures Institute
Austin, Texas
Clinical Professor, Michigan State University College of Human Medicine
East Lansing, Michigan

Daniel L. Stulberg, MD
Professor
Department of Family and Community Medicine
Director, Preceptorship Program
University of New Mexico
Albuquerque, New Mexico

Rebecca Small, MD
Assistant Clinical Professor, Department of Family and Community Medicine
University of California, San Francisco
San Francisco, California
Director, Medical Aesthetics Training, Natividad Medical Center
Family Medicine Residency Program
Salinas, California
Private Practice
Capitola, California

DERMATOLOGIC AND COSMETIC PROCEDURES IN OFFICE PRACTICE

ELSEVIER
SAUNDERS

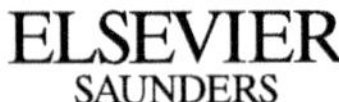

1600 John F. Kennedy Blvd.
Ste 1800
Philadelphia, PA 19103-2899

DERMATOLOGIC AND COSMETIC PROCEDURES IN OFFICE PRACTICE
ISBN: 978-1-4377-0580-5

Notices

Knowledge and best practice in this field are constantly changing. As new research and experience broaden our understanding, changes in research methods, professional practices, or medical treatment may become necessary.

Practitioners and researchers must always rely on their own experience and knowledge in evaluating and using any information, methods, compounds, or experiments described herein. In using such information or methods they should be mindful of their own safety and the safety of others, including parties for whom they have a professional responsibility.

With respect to any drug or pharmaceutical products identified, readers are advised to check the most current information provided (i) on procedures featured or (ii) by the manufacturer of each product to be administered, to verify the recommended dose or formula, the method and duration of administration, and contraindications. It is the responsibility of practitioners, relying on their own experience and knowledge of their patients, to make diagnoses, to determine dosages and the best treatment for each individual patient, and to take all appropriate safety precautions.

To the fullest extent of the law, neither the Publisher nor the authors, contributors, or editors, assume any liability for any injury and/or damage to persons or property as a matter of products liability, negligence or otherwise, or from any use or operation of any methods, products, instructions, or ideas contained in the material herein.

Library of Congress Cataloging-in-Publication Data

Dermatologic and cosmetic procedures in office practice / Richard Usatine ... [et al.].
p. ; cm.
Includes bibliographical references and index.
ISBN 978-1-4377-0580-5 (hardback : alk. paper)
1. Skin—Surgery. 2. Surgery, Plastic. 3. Medical offices. I. Usatine, Richard.
[DNLM: 1. Skin—surgery. 2. Skin Diseases—surgery. 3. Physicians' Offices. 4. Primary Health Care. 5. Reconstructive Surgical Procedures. WR 650]
RD520.D468 2012
617.4'77—dc23 2011021712

Acquisitions Editor: Kate Dimock
Developmental Editor: Julie Mirra
Publishing Services Manager: Pat Joiner-Myers
Senior Project Manager: Joy Moore
Design Manager: Ellen Zanolle

Printed in the United States of America

Last digit is the print number: 9 8 7 6 5 4

Contributors

Bret R. Baack, MD
Professor and Chief
Division of Plastic and Reconstructive Surgery
University of New Mexico
Albuquerque, New Mexico
Suture Material

Jimmy Chen, MD
Clinical Instructor
Department of Family and Community Medicine
Stanford University School of Medicine
Palo Alto, California
Hair Reduction with Lasers

Wendy C. Coates, MD
Professor
Department of Emergency Medicine
David Geffen School of Medicine at UCLA
Los Angeles, California
Laceration Repair

Lucia Diaz, MD
University of Texas Health Science Center at San Antonio
San Antonio, Texas
Wound Care

Robert Fawcett, MD
Associate Director
York Hospital Family Medicine Residency
York, Pennsylvania
Procedures to Treat Benign Conditions

Barbara Green, RPH, MS
Vice President, Clinical Affairs
NeoStrata Company, Inc.
Princeton, New Jersey
Skin Care Products

Dalano Hoang, DC
Clinic Director
Monterey Bay Laser Aesthetics
Capitola, California
Photorejuvenation with Lasers; Combination Cosmetic Treatments

Jonathan Karnes, MD
Assistant Professor and Clinical Family and Community Medicine Fellow
Underserved Dermatology Fellowship
University of Texas Health Science Center at San Antonio
San Antonio, Texas
Cysts and Lipomas

Francisca Kartono, DO
Resident
Botsford Hospital
Farmington Hills, Michigan
Tattoo Removal with Lasers

Nikki Kattalanos, PAC
Assistant Professor
Department of Family and Community Medicine
Director, Physician Assistant Program
University of New Mexico
Albuquerque, New Mexico
The Elliptical Excision

William Kirby, DO, FAOCD
Clinical Assistant Professor
Department of Dermatology
Western University of Health Sciences
Pomona, California
Tattoo Removal with Lasers

Jennifer Krejci-Manwaring, MD
Clinical Assistant Professor, Dermatology and Cutaneous Surgery
University of Texas Health Science Center at San Antonio
San Antonio, Texas
Preoperative Preparation

Corey Maas, MD
Associate Clinical Professor
Division of Facial Plastic and Reconstructive Surgery
Department of Otolaryngology–Head and Neck Surgery
University of California, San Francisco
San Francisco, California
Skin Resurfacing with Ablative Lasers

Ashfaq Marghoob, MD
Associate Professor, Dermatology
Memorial Sloan-Kettering Cancer Center
New York, New York
Dermoscopy

Patrick Moran, DO
Lincoln Avenue Family Medicine
Sunnyside, Washington
Incision and Drainage

Kathleen O'Hanlon, MD
Professor, Family and Community Health
Joan C. Edwards School of Medicine
Marshall University
Huntington, West Virginia
Chemical Peels

Ryan O'Quinn, MD
Medical Director
South Texas Skin Cancer Center
San Antonio, Texas
Flaps

John L. Pfenninger, MD
President and Director, Medical Procedures Center, PC
Private Practice
Midland, Michigan
Senior Consultant and Founder, National Procedures Institute
Austin, Texas
Clinical Professor, Michigan State University College of Human Medicine
East Lansing, Michigan
Choosing the Biopsy Type; Cysts and Lipomas; Electrosurgery; Intralesional Injections; When to Refer/Mohs Surgery; Surviving Financially

Racquel Quema, MD
Postgraduate Fellow, Clinical Dermatology
Queen Mary, University of London
London, United Kingdom
Microdermabrasion

Rebecca Small, MD
Assistant Clinical Professor, Department of Family and Community Medicine
University of California, San Francisco
San Francisco, California
Director, Medical Aesthetics Training, Natividad Medical Center
Family Medicine Residency Program
Salinas, California
Private Practice
Capitola, California
Aesthetic Principles and Consultation; Anesthesia for Cosmetic Procedures; Botulinum Toxin; Chemical Peels; Microdermabrasion; Skin Care Products; Dermal Fillers; Hair Reduction with Lasers; Photorejuvenation with Lasers; Wrinkle Reduction with Nonablative Lasers; Skin Resurfacing with Ablative Lasers; Tattoo Removal with Lasers; Combination Cosmetic Treatments; Procedures to Treat Benign Conditions; Surviving Financially

Daniel L. Stulberg, MD
Professor
Department of Family and Community Medicine
Director, Preceptorship Program
University of New Mexico
Albuquerque, New Mexico
Suture Material; Suturing Techniques; The Elliptical Excision; Cryosurgery; Incision and Drainage; Procedures to Treat Benign Conditions; Diagnosis and Treatment of Malignant and Premalignant Lesions

Richard P. Usatine, MD
Professor, Dermatology and Cutaneous Surgery
Professor, Family and Community Medicine
Fellowship Director, Underserved Dermatology Fellowship
Medical Director, Skin Clinic, University Health System
University of Texas Health Science Center at San Antonio
San Antonio, Texas
Preoperative Preparation; Setting Up Your Office: Facilities, Instruments, and Equipment; Anesthesia; Hemostasis; Suture Material; Suturing Techniques; Laceration Repair; Choosing the Biopsy Type; The Shave Biopsy; The Punch Biopsy; The Elliptical Excision; Cysts and Lipomas; Flaps; Electrosurgery; Cryosurgery; Intralesional Injections; Nail Procedures; Dermoscopy; Procedures to Treat Benign Conditions; Diagnosis and Treatment of Malignant and Premalignant Lesions; Wound Care; Complication: Postprocedural Adverse Effects and Their Prevention; When to Refer/Mohs Surgery

Ken Yu, MD
Chief, Division of Facial Plastic and Reconstructive Surgery
Department of Otolaryngology–Head and Neck Surgery
Wilford Hall Medical Center
Lackland Air Force Base
San Antonio, Texas
Skin Resurfacing with Ablative Lasers

Foreword

As a family physician educator who has a love of dermatology and skin procedures, it gives me great pleasure to write the Foreword for this book. As the author of *The Essential Guide to Primary Care Procedures*, I found Dr. Usatine's previous book on the subject, *Skin Surgery: A Practical Guide*, to be a strong influence on me as I developed my expertise in skin work. Since then, I have had the pleasure to work with all the lead authors of this volume. Dr. Richard Usatine and I have been involved in planning and teaching the American Academy of Family Physicians (AAFP) Skin Problems and Diseases Course for over 12 years. In the last 6 years, Dr. Usatine has chaired this course, and I have worked directly with him in the course design and implementation. Dr. Usatine is a true leader in dermatology education for primary care providers, and especially for family physicians. Not only does he teach dermatology procedures in lectures and workshops, but also he regularly publishes his work and photographs in the *American Family Physician* and *The Journal of Family Practice*. I also worked with Dr. Usatine on *The Color Atlas of Family Medicine* and know the quality of his clinical photographs. With his permission, I regularly use his photos in my own teaching of dermatology topics and procedures. Dr. Usatine's photographic images have now been published in primary care books around the world, including a new edition of a general practice book in Australia. He has written the dermatology chapters for a number of the best-selling family medicine textbooks. Dr. Usatine has been the dermatology editor for Essential Evidence Plus and Elsevier's First Consult. His photographs are now published in internal medicine textbooks and infectious disease books. I know of no finer teacher in Family Medicine in this area.

Dr. John Pfenninger is a world leader in procedural medicine for family physicians. He founded the National Procedures Institute, which has trained thousands of primary care physicians and providers in many types of procedural medicine. His best-selling *Procedures for Primary Care* is currently in its third edition. Dr. Pfenninger's own practice is predominately focused on procedural dermatology. He is a highly regarded expert in dermatology procedures. He is sought after as a speaker and mentor for primary care providers wanting to learn dermatologic procedures.

Drs. Stulberg and Small have also taught in the AAFP Skin Course. Dr. Stulberg has been teaching cryosurgery for years in the AAFP Scientific Assembly and the AAFP Skin Course. His dermatology photographs and writings have been widely published in the *American Family Physician*. He maintains a strong interest in dermatology, procedural medicine, and residency education. For many years Dr. Stulberg has been teaching dermatologic procedures to family medicine residents. Because of his skills in procedural dermatology, I asked him to contribute chapters to my book.

Dr. Small runs a medical aesthetics and family medicine practice in California and teaches aesthetics procedures nationwide. She is the director of medical aesthetics training for the residents at the University of California, San Francisco, family medicine residency program in the Natividad Medical Center. Her writing and photographs have appeared in the *American Family Physician* and my *Essential Guide to Primary Care Procedures*. She is an excellent teacher and writer about cosmetic procedures. She has a thriving practice focused on cosmetic procedures and knows the business of medicine as a physician in solo practice. After her family medicine residency, Dr. Small worked and trained with a plastic surgeon to develop her cosmetic skills. For the last 7 years Dr. Small has been integral to the California Youth Delinquency Program, providing complimentary laser tattoo removal for at-risk youth seeking a new start.

All the lead authors continue to work as family physicians in addition to their work in dermatology. Although Dr. Usatine spends 80% of his time in practicing dermatology, he still gives back to his community through primary care work in student-run free clinics for homeless individuals and families. He also leads medical missions to Ethiopia and Central America in which he supervises medical students interested in global health and caring for people living in extreme poverty.

Together these four experts in dermatologic procedures have created a book and DVD that will be an invaluable guide for primary care providers worldwide. The photographs are excellent and the videos are a great way to learn or hone skills in these procedures. The skills you will learn from this book and DVD will help your patients and make your practice of medicine more enjoyable and rewarding.

E.J. Mayeaux, MD

Preface

It is a great pleasure to release this book, DVD, and mobile application. The work on this book began in the 1990s when I had the great fortune of collaborating with leaders in dermatologic surgery to produce *Skin Surgery: A Practical Guide*. As a family physician, I was enthusiastic to learn these dermatologic procedures so that I could perform them well for my patients and teach them to other clinicians through photographs, writing, lectures, and workshops. Over the following 15 years, my additional experiences have allowed us to produce a book and a mobile application that have better photographs, new chapters and procedures, and high-definition video. This new work also includes a new section on cosmetic procedures.

The book begins with a section entitled "Getting Started" then follows with sections on basic procedures, cosmetic procedures, and a final section "Putting it all Together." The book, DVD, and mobile application are especially directed toward family physicians and other primary care providers. Nurse practitioners and physician assistants practicing dermatology or primary care will also find the material useful. In addition, the set of resources has a lot to offer to dermatology residents and dermatologists in their early stages of training.

The video segments on the DVD have been developed over the past 2 years mostly from surgeries performed in the University Health Systems' Skin Clinic in San Antonio. It is a unique clinic in which we train family medicine residents and senior medical students to perform dermatologic procedures. We also established the first family medicine–based underserved dermatology fellowship in the country in this clinic. Two fellows have completed the program and both have contributed to the video segments. Dr. Jonathan Karnes (current fellow) has contributed to the book and extensively to the video. We have included surgery from a talented Mohs surgeon to demonstrate how Mohs surgery is performed and how a flap is used to repair a large defect on the face. For clinicians interested in performing cosmetic procedures, there are videos demonstrating botulinum toxin injections and fillers.

Whatever your current level of procedural skills, these videos, photographs, and text will take you to the next level. You and your patients will benefit greatly from the material presented. Start by reading the initial section on "Getting Started." Then learn to master all the "Basic Procedures" by providing these procedures for your patients as needed. If you are inclined to learn aesthetic procedures, start with a few at a time and learn them well. Finally, use the "Putting it all Together" section to round out your procedural skills.

Richard P. Usatine, MD

Acknowledgments

I would like to acknowledge the support of my family. My children, Rebecca and Jeremy, are now grown adults, but when I first began to write about dermatologic procedures they were small children. In those years my photographs were 35mm slides often spread out on our dining room table. At the start of this book, my children still lived at home and would see my photographs displayed on the computer monitors within my study. Despite having to look at these surgical photographs, my daughter has become a biology teacher. My son is a physics major and will probably stay far away from dermatologic photos for his career. My wife of 28 years, Janna Lesser, has supported me throughout my career through her love and understanding.

I would like to acknowledge three dermatologists in San Antonio who have helped me grow into the clinician I am today. Dr. Eric Kraus has been the dermatology residency director at the University of Texas Health Science Center at San Antonio since the year I started with the university. He welcomed me to work with the dermatology division and shared dermatology consults with me from the start. Dr. Kraus supported my faculty appointment in dermatology and has always welcomed me as a colleague. He supported the development of the first Underserved Family Medicine Dermatology Fellowship in the nation. Dr. Kraus also welcomes my Fellows to train alongside the dermatology residents for their didactics and dermatopathology training.

I also want to thank Dr. Jennifer Krejci-Manwaring, who has been a wonderful colleague and friend throughout the years we have worked on this book. She co-authored the first chapter of the book and teaches family physicians and primary care providers in the AAFP Skin Course. She is just one of many supportive friends and colleagues in my dermatology division who has made my work in dermatology so much more enjoyable.

Dr. Ryan O'Quinn opened his Mohs surgery office to me to help me advance my surgical skills throughout my years in San Antonio. He also allowed the first filming for DVD to be performed in his private office with his private patients. He is the lead author on the flap chapter, and it is through Dr. O'Quinn that I best understand the practice and value of Mohs surgery.

I want to thank Dr. Ash Marghoob for his mentorship in dermoscopy. I have studied dermoscopy with Dr. Marghoob for the past 4 years. Dr. Marghoob is a world leader in dermoscopy research and education. He has co-authored books and many articles on dermoscopy. Dr. Marghoob began his career as a family physician and then became a board-certified dermatologist. He has taught dermoscopy at our AAFP Skin Course for years and is a strong advocate for teaching dermoscopy to all primary care physicians. Together we now teach dermoscopy workshops at the AAFP Scientific Assembly on a yearly basis. His work on our dermoscopy chapter has made this chapter into a great introduction to the science and practice of dermoscopy.

Finally I would like to thank all of my patients who have generously given of themselves to the creation of this book, mobile application, and DVD. They have allowed me to photograph their procedures knowing that these photographs and videos will be used to train doctors and providers caring for people with skin diseases. It is only through their generosity that we have this resource today.

Richard P. Usatine, MD

A special thanks to my wife, Kay, who helped with incorporating photos in the text and who also put up with me during yet "another project." I'd also like to acknowledge the co-editors of this text. They were super to work with, and Richard really did a great job keeping us all focused on the task of completing this book. It was fun!

John L. Pfenninger, MD

I would like to thank The Utah Valley Family Medicine Residency and Intermountain Healthcare for my first digital cameras complete with floppy disks and giving me the wings to fly into the arena of teaching dermatology to family physicians and clinicians. I would also like to thank my wife, Sandy, for her understanding of my long hours of work and time to teach at conferences.

Daniel L. Stulberg, MD

The University of California, San Francisco, and the Natividad Medical Center family medicine residents deserve special recognition. Their interest and enthusiasm for aesthetic procedures led me to develop the first family medicine residency aesthetics training curriculum in 2008. A special thanks to my Capitola office staff for the logistical and administrative support that made it possible to work on this book. I am indebted to my husband and my son. Their unwavering encouragement and support made my contribution to this book possible.

Rebecca Small, MD

We all want to thank the folks at Elsevier, especially Kate Dimock and Julie Mirra, for their belief in us and for their hard work on the book.

Contents

Video Contents

We acknowledge Robert D. Long, Jr., Lester Rosebrook, Bob Merill and the UTHSCSA video production department. I especially thank Robb Long for all the long hours of shooting and editing.

SECTION ONE

Getting Started

1 Preoperative Preparation

RICHARD P. USATINE, MD • JENNIFER KREJCI-MANWARING, MD

The practice of skin surgery in the office requires careful planning and a team of well-instructed support personnel. Other keys to success are thorough patient education and informed consent, preoperative screening, good surgical technique, and sterile surgical instruments. The use of universal precautions to prevent the transmission of infectious diseases is paramount to protecting the clinician, the medical staff, and the patient.

SURGICAL PLANNING

Surgical planning should consist of the following:

- Office scheduling
- Preoperative medical evaluation
- Informed consent
- Universal precautions
- Preoperative medications
- Standby medications and equipment
- Preoperative patient preparation (skin, hair, drapes)
- Sterilization of instruments
- Sterile technique.

SCHEDULING OF COMPLEX SURGERIES

Simple surgical procedures, such as shave or punch biopsies, need no special scheduling. These procedures can be done rapidly as the need arises. However, clinicians contemplating performing more complex surgical procedures in the office will benefit from careful, deliberate consideration of how best to integrate the surgeries into the office schedule. Proper scheduling is critical to producing the efficient, unhurried surgical atmosphere that is reassuring to both the patient and the staff.

Some offices schedule more complex surgeries at the end of the morning or the end of the afternoon to avoid being rushed by other patient responsibilities. This allows the clinician to approach surgery in an unhurried manner. Another strategy is to designate certain half-days for surgical procedures only.

Surgeons may also choose to perform more complex surgeries early in the week and avoid surgery on Friday so patients can be seen the day after surgery for a postoperative check. This type of schedule helps prevent weekend calls or unneeded trips to the emergency center if a patient develops a hematoma or other complication that can be easily handled in the office.

PREOPERATIVE MEDICAL EVALUATION

Medical History

A complete medical history and review of systems before minor surgery may not be necessary. Before a more complex skin procedure, however, the following information should be taken during the medical history:

- Current medications, especially anticoagulants, aspirin, and other nonsteroidal anti-inflammatory drugs (NSAIDs), cardiac drugs.
- Allergies, especially to antibiotics, tapes/adhesives, iodine, anesthetics (lidocaine).
- Cardiac disease (e.g., any condition requiring endocarditis prophylaxis such as a prosthetic heart valve), uncontrolled hypertension, epinephrine sensitivity, angina. The presence of a pacemaker or implantable defibrillator has implications for electrosurgery (see Chapter 14, *Electrosurgery*).
- Other illnesses and medical conditions (e.g., diabetes, seizure disorder, hematologic disorder or bleeding diathesis, joint replacement [positioning of grounding pad with electrosurgical device], high-risk groups for infectious diseases [e.g., injection drug users]).
- Pregnancy, lactation.
- Keloids or hypertrophic scars.
- Infectious diseases (e.g., hepatitis B or C, HIV/AIDS, methicillin-resistant staphylococcus aureus, tuberculosis).

For minor skin surgery under local anesthesia, blood pressure should be measured but does not need to be monitored unless the patient has a history of hypertension that is not controlled. Uncontrolled hypertension may lead to increased bleeding during surgery. If the blood pressure is significantly elevated, consider postponing the procedure or giving a dose of an appropriate antihypertensive agent prior to the start of the procedure. It is prudent to be more careful with fragile patients, such as the elderly, and to be particularly careful with the use of epinephrine-containing anesthetics in patients with a history of angina, cardiac disease, or sensitivity to epinephrine. It may help to warn these patients that they may develop an increased heart rate or a feeling of anxiety after injection of lidocaine with epinephrine.

Medical Contraindications

Skin surgery is not recommended on patients who have unstable angina because the epinephrine in the local anesthetic can precipitate angina. Although this is unlikely, it is worth having nitroglycerin in the office to deal with this potential situation. Patients who have uncontrolled diabetes mellitus may experience impaired wound healing. Closer follow-up after surgery may help avoid potential problems with these patients.

Informed Consent

Thorough discussion with patients regarding the benefits and risks of any planned surgical procedure and the alternatives to surgery is essential before surgery. It is always best to devote adequate time for this discussion so that all of the patient's questions can be answered in an unhurried manner. Although the optimal situation is to have the clinician who will perform the procedure provide the informed consent, a well-trained assistant can start the process and the clinician can answer any questions beyond the skills of the assistant. Risks include pain, bleeding, infection, scarring, change in pigmentation, regrowth, slow healing, change in anatomic appearance, skin indentation, skin protrusion, local nerve damage/numbness, loss of muscle function, and need for further treatment. A complete list of risks is listed in Appendix A on the sample consent form titled *Disclosure and Consent: Medical and Surgical Procedures*.

For many routine minor procedures, such as cryotherapy, a written consent may not be needed. However, clinicians may want to consider obtaining a written consent for any procedure, even as small as cryotherapy, if the procedure is to be performed on a cosmetically sensitive area such as the face or on those for whom scarring may be more of a concern. Written consent is always obtained for procedures that may have more significant adverse consequences, such as scarring or functional effects. Feel free to use or modify the form supplied in Appendix A for your own office.

For larger surgeries, show patients the planned excision before you begin the surgery. You can show the patient and any family in attendance your surgical markings before you start. Keep a handheld mirror nearby for excisions on the face so that your patient knows what you plan to do. This is a helpful method to make sure you truly have informed consent.

UNIVERSAL PRECAUTIONS

With the identification of AIDS in the 1980s, measures to prevent the transmission of contagious diseases to medical personnel have come to be known as *universal precautions*, and their use has been incorporated into every medical clinic, surgical center, or hospital. Diseases of chief concern are hepatitis B, hepatitis C, and HIV/AIDS. However, other contagious diseases, such as tuberculosis and syphilis, also present some potential risk to medical personnel.

The basics of universal precautions include the use of surgical gloves and the use of barrier clothing such as gowns, face masks, and eye protection; proper disposal of sharp, disposable surgical instruments, such as needles and scalpel blades, in special puncture-proof containers; disposal of all contaminated drapes and other soft items in specially marked biohazard containers; and collection and disposal of this material by professional hazardous-waste removal companies.

For skin surgery we have found it especially helpful to practice choreographed surgery, with particular attention paid to any sharp instruments. We handle only one sharp instrument at a time and are aware of its position at all times. All sharps should be counted as they are placed on and removed from the surgical tray. Avoid recapping needles that have been used with a patient. If a recap must be done, use the one-handed recap technique in which the needle sheath is positioned against an inanimate object. When suturing, use an instrument such as Adson forceps to load the needle onto the needle driver rather than your fingers. We take particular care to avoid rushing when performing surgery and also attempt to have extra help available—within earshot—at all times.

MEDICATIONS

Anticoagulation/Antiplatelet Therapy

The clinician needs to find out which medications the patient is taking in order to determine if there will be an increased risk of bleeding in the intraoperative or postoperative period. This includes warfarin, aspirin, NSAIDs, clopidogrel, and low-molecular-weight heparin. For larger surgeries, one might query patients about their use of any vitamin, herbal, or other over-the-counter supplements because some of these can alter the coagulation profile (see Box 1-1).

The issue of whether to stop anticoagulation/antiplatelet therapy before surgery has been controversial, but the best evidence now points toward continuing these medications. One large study of 2394 patients with 5950 lesions found four independent risk factors for postoperative bleeding:

- Age 67 years or older (odds ratio [OR] 4.7)
- Warfarin therapy (OR 2.9)
- Surgery on or around the ear (OR 2.6)
- Closure with a skin flap or graft (OR 2.7).[1]

Aspirin therapy was not an independent risk factor for bleeding. The researchers concluded that "most postoperative bleeds were inconvenient but not life threatening, unlike the potential risk of thromboembolism after stopping warfarin or aspirin." They recommended not to discontinue aspirin before skin surgery.[1]

In a meta-analysis of complications attributed to anticoagulation among patients following cutaneous surgery, a total of six studies representing 1373 patients met criteria for inclusion. Among patients taking aspirin or warfarin, 1.3% and 5.7%, respectively, experienced a severe postoperative complication. Patients taking warfarin were nearly seven times as likely to have a moderate-to-severe complication compared to controls.

BOX 1-1 *Supplements That Alter Coagulation*

Dietary Supplements with Anticoagulant Activity

Bilberry
Black currant
Bladderwrack
Cayenne fruit
Celery plant
Da huang
Danshen
Devil's claw
Dong quai
Evening primrose seed oil
Feverfew
Garlic
German chamomile
Ginger
Gingko
Ginseng, Panax
Horse chestnut
Kava kava root
Licorice
Meadowsweet
Papaya
Poplar
Red clover
Sweet clover
Tamarind
Vitamin E
Willow bark

Herbal Supplements with Coagulant Activity

Alfalfa
Goldenseal
Green tea

Source: Adapted from Dinehart SM. Dietary supplements: Altered coagulation and effects on bruising. *Dermatol Surg.* 2005;31:819–826.

Patients taking aspirin or NSAIDs were more than twice as likely to have a moderate-to-severe complication compared to controls.[2]

In 2326 patients operated on by a single surgeon, warfarin was used by 28 patients, 228 took aspirin, and the remainder took neither. There was no difference in the complication rate among the three groups. Researchers concluded that patients taking aspirin or warfarin do not need to discontinue these medications before minor dermatologic procedures.[3]

In a prospective study of 51 patients undergoing a range of minor cutaneous surgical procedures including excision biopsies, local flaps, and skin grafts, patients continued their normal warfarin regimen. The international normalized ratio (INR) was checked on the day of surgery and it ranged from 1.1 to 4.0. No problems were encountered during surgery, but two patients presented with bleeding postoperatively a few days later. The study concluded that it is not necessary to modify warfarin regimens for minor cutaneous surgery.[4]

In a prospective controlled observational study, 65 patients on warfarin underwent excision of 70 cutaneous tumors. There was no increase in bleeding tendency during surgery with those on warfarin when compared with controls. Five patients on warfarin (8%) reported moderate or severe postoperative bleeding. All patients on warfarin with bleeding complications had an INR of <2.6 at the time of surgery.[5] Bleeding risk could not be correlated with INR. The researchers suggested that it is crucial to observe meticulous hemostasis in all patients on warfarin regardless of INR.[5]

Warfarin and medically necessary aspirin should be continued as well as clopidogrel and low-molecular-weight heparin.[6] Exceptional care must be taken to prevent bleeding by using electrosurgery, tying off vessels, and applying handheld pressure for hemostasis. Pressure dressings can also help minimize the risk of hematoma. Lastly, patients should be made aware of the small but increased risk of postoperative bleeding and given verbal and written postoperative instructions.

Antibiotic Prophylaxis

Preoperative antibiotics such as oral cephalexin, dicloxacillin, or clindamycin may be recommended for use with patients who have a higher risk of infection.[7] These situations might include a patient who has a contaminated or infected lesion; a lesion in an area of increased bacteria, such as the axilla, ear, or mouth; a lesion on a hand or foot, especially in patients with peripheral vascular disease; a situation in which the operation might take more than 1 hour or if the wound was open for more than 1 hour; a patient for whom complete sterile technique was not optimal; or any situation in which an infection would have serious consequences, such as in a patient with diabetes or neutropenia. See Table 1-1 for classification of wound infection risk and the need for antibiotic prophylaxis. The 2008 Advisory Statement from the American Academy of

TABLE 1-1 Classification of Wound Infection Risk

Class	Antibiotic Prophylaxis Needed?
Clean: noncontaminated skin, sterile technique = 5% infection	No
Clean contaminated: wounds in oral cavity, respiratory tract, axilla/perineum; breaks in aseptic technique = 10% infection rate	Consider
Contaminated: trauma, acute nonpurulent inflammation, major breaks in aseptic technique (intact, inflamed cysts; tumors with clinical inflammation) = 20% to 30% infection rate	Yes
Infected: gross contamination with foreign bodies, devitalized tissue (ruptured cysts; tumors with purulent, necrotic material) = 30% to 40% infection rate	Yes

Source: From Haas AF, Grekin RC. Antibiotic prophylaxis in dermatologic surgery. *J Am Acad Dermatol.* 1995;32:155–176.

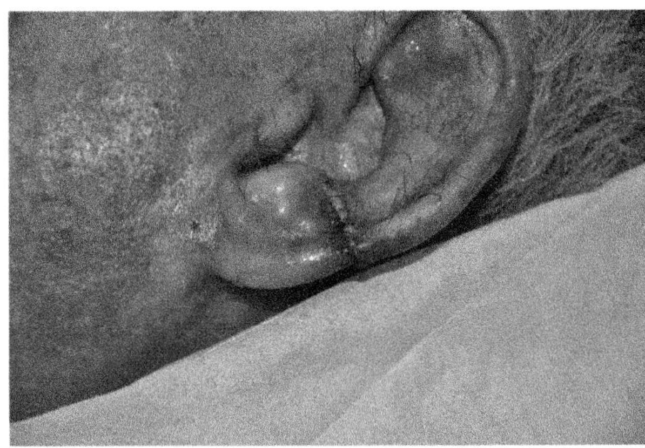

FIGURE 1-1 Completed repair of a wedge excision to remove a squamous cell carcinoma from the ear. Consider using prophylactic antibiotics with such a surgery because there is a higher risk of infection after a wedge excision of the ear. *(Copyright Richard P. Usatine, MD.)*

Dermatology (AAD) on antibiotic prophylaxis in dermatologic surgery stated that antibiotics may be indicated for the prevention of surgical-site infections for:

- Procedures on the lower extremities or groin
- Wedge excisions of the lip and ear (Figure 1-1)
- Skin flaps on the nose
- Skin grafts
- Patients with extensive inflammatory skin disease.[7]

Table 1-2 provides recommendations for antibiotic prophylaxis in patients at increased risk of surgical-site infection.

In a 5-year prospective observational study, infection incidence was significantly higher in patients with diabetes (4.2%, 23/551) than in those without (2.0%, 135/6673) ($p < .001$).[8] Noninfective complications were similar. Although this study demonstrates the increased risk, it does not prove that antibiotic prophylaxis will decrease this risk. However, the choice to use antibiotic prophylaxis is a complicated decision that should be made based on all available data and known patient risks.

Endocarditis Prophylaxis

The recommendations of the American Heart Association (AHA) for the prevention of bacterial endocarditis were last published in 2007.[9] Endocarditis prophylaxis is not needed for incision or biopsy of noninfected surgically scrubbed skin no matter what endocarditis risk factors are present. The 2007 guidelines state that antibiotic prophylaxis is indicated for patients undergoing dermatologic surgery on *infected skin* or surgery that involves breach of oral mucosa for patients with underlying cardiac conditions associated with the highest risk of an adverse outcome from infective endocarditis.

For individuals at highest risk for endocarditis who undergo a surgical procedure that involves infected skin or skin structures, it is reasonable for the therapeutic regimen administered for treatment of the infection to contain an agent active against staphylococci and beta-hemolytic streptococci, such as an antistaphylococcal penicillin or a cephalosporin (SOR C).[9] Vancomycin or clindamycin may be administered to patients unable to tolerate a beta-lactam antibiotic or who are known or suspected to have an infection caused by

TABLE 1-2 Antibiotic Prophylaxis for Patients at Increased Risk of Surgical-Site Infection

Surgical Site	Medication	Dose*
Wedge on lip or ear, flap on nose, all grafts	Cephalexin **or** dicloxacillin	2 g
Groin or lower extremity	Cephalexin **or** TMP-SMX-DS **or** Levofloxacin	2 g 1 tablet 500 mg
Allergic to PCN		
Lip, ear, flap on nose, all grafts	Clindamycin, **or**	600 mg
Groin or lower extremity	Azithromycin, clarithromycin **or** TMP-SMX-DS **or** Levofloxacin	500 mg 1 tablet 500 mg
Unable to Take Oral Medication		
Lip, ear, flap on nose, all grafts	Cefazolin, ceftriaxone	1 g IM/IV
Groin or lower extremity	Ceftriaxone	1–2 g IV
Unable to Take Oral Medication and Allergic to PCN		
Lip, ear, flap on nose, all grafts	Clindamycin	600 mg IM/IV
Groin or lower extremity	Clindamycin + gentamicin	600 mg, 2 mg/kg IV

*Give one hour before surgery.
IM, intramuscular; IV, intravenous; PCN, penicillin; TMP-SMX-DS, trimethoprim-sulfamethoxazole double strength.
Source: Adapted from Wright TI, Baddour LM, Berbari EF, *et al.* Antibiotic prophylaxis in dermatologic surgery: advisory statement 2008. *J Am Acad Dermatol.* 2008;59:464–473.

TABLE 1-3 Regimens to Prevent Infective Endocarditis in a Dermatologic Procedure[a]

Single dose given 30 to 60 min before procedure.

Situation	Agent	Adults	Children
Oral	Amoxicillin	2 g	50 mg/kg
Unable to take oral medication	Ampicillin **or** Cefazolin **or** ceftriaxone	2 g IM or IV 1 g IM or IV	50 mg/kg IM or IV 50 mg/kg IM or IV
Allergic to penicillins or ampicillin (oral)	Cephalexin[b,c] **or** Clindamycin **or** Azithromycin, clarithromycin	2 g 600 mg 500 mg	50 mg/kg 20 mg/kg 15 mg/kg
Allergic to penicillins or ampicillin **and** unable to take oral medication	Cefazolin **or** ceftriaxone[c] Clindamycin	1 g IM or IV 600 mg IM or IV	50 mg/kg IM or IV 20 mg/kg IM or IV

IM, intramuscular; IV, intravenous.
[a]Antibiotic prophylaxis is indicated for patients undergoing dermatologic surgery on infected skin or that involves breach of oral mucosa for patients with underlying cardiac conditions associated with the highest risk of adverse outcome from infective endocarditis. See Box 1-2.
[b]Or other first- or second-generation oral cephalosporin in equivalent adult or pediatric dosage.
[c]Cephalosporins should not be used in an individual with a history of anaphylaxis, angioedema, or urticaria with penicillins or ampicillin.
Source: From Wilson W, Taubert KA, Gewitz M, *et al.* Prevention of infective endocarditis: guidelines from the American Heart Association: a guideline from the American Heart Association Rheumatic Fever, Endocarditis, and Kawasaki Disease Committee, Council on Cardiovascular Disease in the Young, and the Council on Clinical Cardiology, Council on Cardiovascular Surgery and Anesthesia, and the Quality of Care and Outcomes Research Interdisciplinary Working Group. *Circulation.* 2007;116:1736–1754.

methicillin-resistant *Staphylococcus aureus.*[9] Suggested antibiotic prophylaxis regimens for dermatologic surgical procedures that breach the oral mucosa or involve infected skin in patients at high risk for infective endocarditis or hematogenous total joint infection are recommended in Table 1-3.[7]

One published mnemonic to help remember when and how to use prophylactic antibiotics in skin surgery is *I PREVENT.* This represents Immunosuppressed patients; patients with a Prosthetic valve; some patients with a joint Replacement; a history of infective Endocarditis; a Valvulopathy in cardiac transplant recipients; Endocrine disorders such as uncontrolled diabetes mellitus; Neonatal disorders including unrepaired cyanotic heart disorders (CHDs), repaired CHD with prosthetic material, or repaired CHD with residual defects; and the Tetrad of antibiotics: amoxicillin, cephalexin, clindamycin, and ciprofloxacin.[10]

BOX 1-2 *High-Risk Cardiac Conditions for Which Antibiotic Prophylaxis Is Indicated with Infected Skin or Breach of Oral Mucosa*

- Prosthetic cardiac valve
- Previous infective endocarditis
- Congenital heart disease (CHD)
  - Unrepaired cyanotic CHD, including palliative shunts and conduits
  - Completely repaired congenital heart defects with prosthetic material or device, whether placed by a surgical or catheter intervention, during the first 6 months after procedure
  - Repaired CHD with residual defects at site or adjacent to site of prosthetic patch or prosthetic device (which inhibits endothelialization)
- Cardiac transplantation recipients who develop cardiac valvulopathy[9]

Anxiolytics at Time of Surgery

Antianxiety medications such as alprazolam, diazepam, or lorazepam can be useful in the very anxious patient who does not respond to nonpharmacologic methods of relaxation (such as slow abdominal breathing). If these medications are administered sublingually, the onset of action can be quicker than when they are administered orally. These medications should not be given to a patient who will be driving home. All patients given intraoperative or preoperative sedatives must be accompanied by an adult, must be counseled not to drive on the day of the surgery, must be observed postoperatively until the sedative effect has sufficiently diminished, and must be counseled that their mental capacities may be diminished for a prolonged period after surgery.

STANDBY MEDICATIONS AND EQUIPMENT

It is helpful to have injectable diphenhydramine and epinephrine available for subcutaneous injection in case of an anaphylactic reaction to anesthesia, latex, or other medication. It may also be helpful to have an Ambubag, an insertable airway, oxygen, a cardiac monitor, and a defibrillator in your office, but these items are not absolutely necessary.

PREOPERATIVE PATIENT PREPARATION

Preparation of the Skin

The most common preoperative preparations to be used on the skin include alcohol, Betadine (povidone-iodine), and Hibiclens (chlorhexidine). The main advantages of using chlorhexidine are that it has a longer lasting antibacterial effect than povidone-iodine and the risk of contact sensitivity may be less. One disadvantage of using chlorhexidine, however, is that it is more toxic to the eye if it accidentally drops into it. However, if the eye is flushed immediately, no damage may be done. Caution must be taken when using alcohol to be sure that all of the alcohol has evaporated before any electrosurgery is performed in the area.

The most important part of the preoperative preparation of the skin is the mechanical rubbing of the antiseptic onto the skin with the gauze. Although the gauze may not need to be sterile for the first prep, it might help to use sterile gauze in the last prep. It is actually impossible to sterilize the skin because bacteria can extend into hair follicles. The goal of the preoperative preparation of the skin is to reduce the bacteria on the skin surface by scrubbing the skin with a good antiseptic such as povidone-iodine or chlorhexidine. Povidone-iodine must be allowed to dry on the skin for its effect to be optimal. Chlorhexidine has the advantage of not staining the skin and being easy to wash off. Povidone-iodine has the advantage of being easy to see where it was applied but should be avoided in persons with iodine allergies. However, Darouiche *et al.* found a greater than 40% reduction in total surgical-site infections among patients undergoing clean-contaminated surgery who had received a single chlorhexidine-alcohol scrub as compared with a povidone-iodine scrub.[11]

An 8-oz pump bottle of chlorhexidine can be kept in each examination/procedure room and can be used repeatedly by pumping the solution onto clean or sterile gauze. Povidone-iodine swab sticks are convenient, but a bit more expensive than povidone-iodine in a bottle applied with gauze.

Preparation of Hair

The best method of hair removal over a surgical site is to use scissors to cut the hair. Using scissors to clip hair is now the preferred method for preoperative hair removal because a close shave with a razor causes minute abrasions of the skin that can increase the chance of infection.[12] A depilatory cream may also be used but this is messy and more time consuming. A chemical depilatory could be used by the patient the day before surgery if desired. The scalp is the area of the body in which the hairs can most interfere with surgery. Plastering down the hair with petrolatum or other ointment can decrease the number of hairs that interfere with surgery without causing a noticeable loss of hair during the postoperative period. Hair ties and bobby pins are invaluable items to have in the office (Figure 1-2).

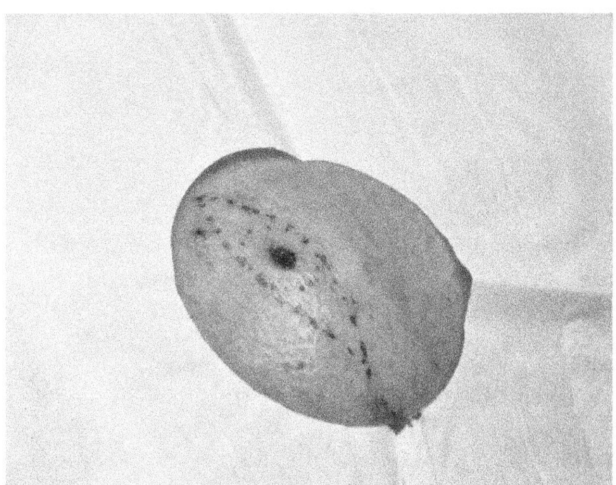

FIGURE 1-2 A fenestrated drape is used to produce a sterile field for the surgical removal of a basal cell carcinoma. *(Copyright Richard P. Usatine, MD.)*

Drapes

The use of sterile fenestrated aperture drapes (drapes with a hole) is recommended when suturing is performed so that the sutures do not drag over nonsterile skin (Figure 1-3). Sterile drapes are not necessary for small procedures, such as a shave biopsy, where suturing is not performed. Disposable or linen-quality sterile drapes are adequate for the procedures described in this book. You can create your own aperture drapes by cutting a hole in a sterile disposable drape. This allows you to customize the size of the hole you need. This should be done with sterile suture scissors and not tissue scissors to avoid dulling your more expensive instruments. You can also use the paper that is used to wrap surgical trays before sterilization for this purpose to save money. Drapes can be cut in a variety of sizes with a variety of holes and then sterilized alone or as part of a packet. Some prepackaged disposable sterile drapes come with adhesive around the aperture to stabilize the drape and isolate the field.

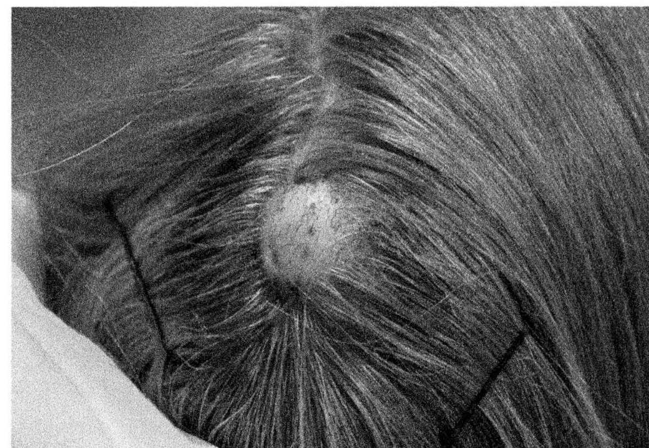

FIGURE 1-3 Hair on the scalp was cut short with clean scissors to make it easier to excise this ellipse over a pilar cyst. Note how the hairs surrounding the surgical site are held down with bobby pins. Petrolatum ointment can also be used to keep the surrounding hair out of the surgical field. *(Copyright Richard P. Usatine, MD.)*

STERILE TECHNIQUE

Absolute sterile technique is not necessary for most minor skin surgical procedures. This is true for cryosurgery and electrosurgery, but also for shave biopsy of the skin, curettage, incision and drainage, and other small surgical procedures in which the wounds are left open to heal without suturing. Although all instruments must be sterile before use for these procedures, the clinician may use nonsterile gloves. Sterile drapes are not needed for these procedures. Of course it is standard policy to use razor blades, scalpel blades, and needles that are disposed of at the end of the procedure.

Sterile technique is necessary when performing surgery in which the wound will be closed, such as with suturing or staples. Careful instruction of ancillary surgical personnel in sterile technique is necessary.

Sterilization of Instruments

Before sterilization, instruments must be cleaned of blood and debris. This can be done manually with a soft toothbrush, an ultrasonic cleaner, or a combination of these procedures.

A steam sterilizer (autoclave) is necessary to sterilize instruments and ensure that diseases such as viral hepatitis or HIV are not transmitted from patient to patient. Holding solutions should not be used to sterilize instruments. They are inadequate for proper sterilization and can only be used to temporarily hold or clean instruments. The instruments should be placed in sterilization bags with indicator strips to ensure the sterilization process is effective. These bags come in a variety of sizes to accommodate different instrument sets. Self-sealing bags cost a bit more than those that must be taped, but the convenience outweighs the cost.

Instruments can be packaged in sets for specific procedures such as punch biopsies, elliptical excisions, or nail surgery. Instruments can also be sterilized separately, but they need to be moved in a sterile manner onto the sterile surgical stand. It can be helpful to create surgical packs that contain a number of cotton-tipped applicators and gauze or just include these in the sets of instruments. This can save one the time of opening individually sterilized packets and can save money by allowing one to buy applicators and gauze in bulk.

TIME-OUT

With the encouragement of the Joint Commission (previously JCAHO, the Joint Commission on Accreditation of Healthcare Organizations), most hospitals are now mandating *surgical time-outs* prior to all surgery to reduce errors. This consists of identifying the patient by two forms of identification and confirming that the consent has been obtained, any required studies have been done, required equipment and required staff are present, and the surgical site has been identified prior to proceeding with the surgery. This is typically documented in writing or the electronic medical record (EMR) by the clinician or another member of the team present and prior to the start of the procedure. At any time or with any concern, any member of the team or staff may request a time-out to confirm that all is in order.

CONCLUSION

Outpatient skin surgery requires careful preparation to ensure the safety of the patient and medical personnel and optimal results. Strict adherence to universal precautions to prevent the transmission of contagious disease is now standard operating procedure. Brief medical evaluation by the clinician before performing procedures is recommended and preoperative medications including antibiotic prophylaxis should be reviewed. Informed patient consent, standby medications and equipment, preparation of the operative site, sterilization of equipment, and sterile technique are all areas that require preoperative consideration. Proper preoperative planning is essential for all successful office procedures.

References

1. Dixon AJ, Dixon MP, Dixon JB. Bleeding complications in skin cancer surgery are associated with warfarin but not aspirin therapy. *Br J Surg.* 2007;94:1356–1360.
2. Lewis KG, Dufresne Jr RG. A meta-analysis of complications attributed to anticoagulation among patients following cutaneous surgery. *Dermatol Surg.* 2008;34:160–164.
3. Shalom A, Klein D, Friedman T, Westreich M. Lack of complications in minor skin lesion excisions in patients taking aspirin or warfarin products. *Am Surg.* 2008;74:354–357.
4. Sugden P, Siddiqui H. Continuing warfarin during cutaneous surgery. *Surgeon.* 2008;6:148–150.
5. Blasdale C, Lawrence CM. Perioperative international normalized ratio level is a poor predictor of postoperative bleeding complications in dermatological surgery patients taking warfarin. *Br J Dermatol.* 2008;158:522–526.
6. Hurst EA, Yu SS, Grekin RC, Neuhaus IM. Bleeding complications in dermatologic surgery. *Semin Cutan Med Surg.* 2007;26:189–195.
7. Wright TI, Baddour LM, Berbari EF, *et al.* Antibiotic prophylaxis in dermatologic surgery: advisory statement 2008. *J Am Acad Dermatol.* 2008;59:464–473.
8. Dixon AJ, Dixon MP, Dixon JB. Prospective study of skin surgery in patients with and without known diabetes. *Dermatol Surg.* 2009;35:1035–1040.
9. Wilson W, Taubert KA, Gewitz M, *et al.* Prevention of infective endocarditis: guidelines from the American Heart Association: a guideline from the American Heart Association Rheumatic Fever, Endocarditis, and Kawasaki Disease Committee, Council on Cardiovascular Disease in the Young, and the Council on Clinical Cardiology, Council on Cardiovascular Surgery and Anesthesia, and the Quality of Care and Outcomes Research Interdisciplinary Working Group. *Circulation.* 2007;116:1736–1754.
10. Moorhead C, Torres A. I PREVENT bacterial resistance. An update on the use of antibiotics in dermatologic surgery. *Dermatol Surg.* 2009;35:1532–1538.
11. Darouiche RO, Wall Jr MJ, Itani KMF, *et al.* Chlorhexidine-alcohol versus povidone-iodine for surgical-site antisepsis. *N Engl J Med.* 2010;362:18–26.
12. Tanner J, Woodings D, Moncaster K. Preoperative hair removal to reduce surgical site infection. *Cochrane Database Syst Rev.* 2006;CD004122.

2 Setting Up Your Office: Facilities, Instruments, and Equipment

RICHARD P. USATINE, MD

A lot of time, thought, and money go into setting up any medical office. If you already have a running medical office and you just want to improve the setting for dermatologic and cosmetic procedures, you are more than halfway there. If you are starting with a concept or an empty space, you will have many choices to make but you will have the advantage of doing things correctly from the start. Initial choices about office flow and layout are crucial to creating an efficient and effective office practice. We start our discussion with lighting and surgical/exam tables.

LIGHTING

Simple surgical procedures can be performed in almost any office if the lighting is adequate. Standard office lighting is often too dim to allow proper visualization of the operative field. When setting up a new facility, it is worth spending time to research the ceiling lights. Consider doubling the number of fixtures to have clear lighting. For many clinicians, this will provide adequate lighting for performing simple surgical procedures.

Headlamps can also be used to illuminate the operative area. When used in conjunction with loupes, headlamps are valuable when performing finely detailed procedures. A good penlight or otoscope can be helpful to illuminate a specific area during an exam.

Surgical Lamps

Adequate lighting is best achieved by using surgical lamps that are either ceiling mounted or on a rolling base. There are many lamps from which to choose. We are pleased with the Burton Outpatient II light in our main procedure room (Figure 2-1A). It is very bright but does not get hot. This is Burton's number one surgical light and is shadow free, can be focused, and is guaranteed to have a no-drift arm. We have found the light to be too bright at times so we have taped photo diffuser sheets over the lights. Another option is to put in a dimmer so you can control the light output. This light focuses with a central handle. The central handle can be covered with a sterile cover, but we just ask our medical assistant to reposition the light when needed. Many other lights are available, but it is worth getting a good one.

If you get a better quality light in your main procedure room, it will be easier to see for more complex surgeries. A floor lamp may be used in your other exam rooms, but if you count on it in your procedure room, you may have lower quality light and need to deal with the inconvenience of the stand taking up floor space.

Floor Lamps

You should have at least one good-quality movable floor lamp for your exam rooms. One per room is optimal but one good movable lamp is a good start. Look for a lamp that provides excellent illumination, ease of movement, and stability in a small exam light for the floor. The Burton SuperNova exam light (Figure 2-1B) is one lamp that works well for us, but many other floor lamps are available that provide similar features. A gooseneck lamp with a bare incandescent light bulb gets hot and the light is not optimal for skin procedures.

Woods Lamp

The Woods lamp (Figure 2-2) uses an ultraviolet light and is useful for diagnosing or evaluating fungal infections including *Microsporum canis* and *Malassezia furfur*. It is also helpful for identifying the coral red fluorescence of erythrasma. It can be used for accentuating the hypopigmentation of vitiligo. In melasma, it is used to see if the hyperpigmentation is within the epidermal or dermal layer. Outside of dermatology the Woods lamp helps to diagnose corneal abrasions.

We use the Burton ultraviolet light. It uses fluorescent bulbs that produce UV-A at an approximately 360-nm wavelength. This is not harmful to the eyes or skin. It has a magnifier lens with three power magnifications and a focal length of 8 in.

SURGICAL TABLE, STOOLS, AND MAYO STANDS

It is essential to have at least one good surgical table with a height adjustment. The best tables have preset positions that move the table to the optimal height for your work. Also, make sure that you find a table that allows the back and foot adjustments to move simultaneously. If not, it can take a long time to get the patient in the proper position for procedures. It may also help to have a table that spins on a center axis for positioning the patient at the best angle in the room. Make sure that the table has stirrups. Even if you do not do gynecologic exams, stirrups can be helpful for skin procedures performed in the inguinal or genital area. Consider obstetrical knee supports (crutches) with the table if you will be doing colposcopy or long procedures in which patients remain in the lithotomy position.

Individual preferences will determine if a clinician performs most procedures while sitting or standing. It is best to avoid bending over the surgical table for the

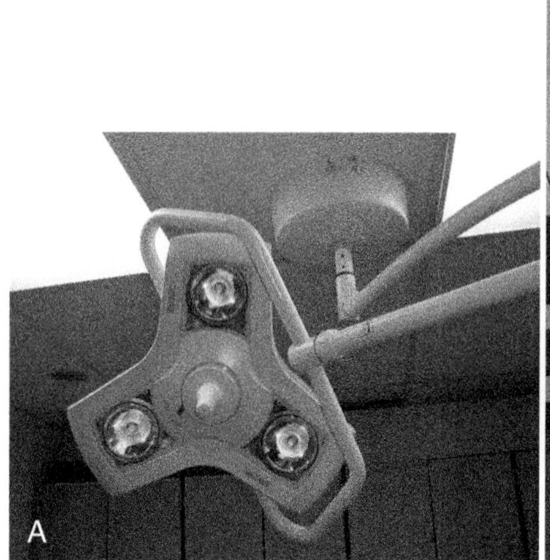

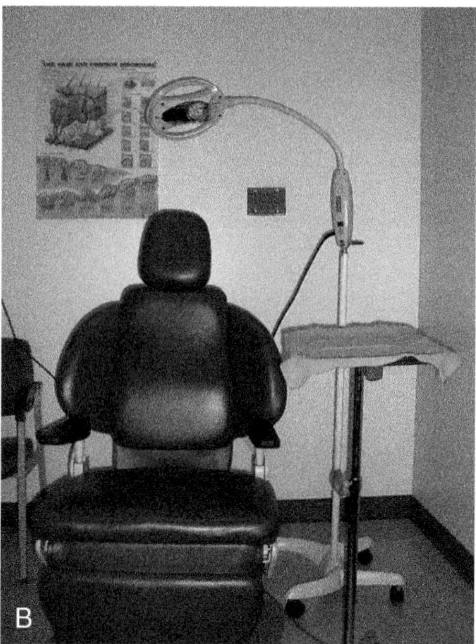

FIGURE 2-1 (A) Ceiling-mounted surgical light. (B) Exam room with Mayo stand, lift chair, Burton SuperNova exam light, and poster of the skin. *(Copyright Richard P. Usatine, MD.)*

health of your back and neck. It helps to adjust your table and stool for good body ergonomics. An easily adjustable pneumatic stool is advantageous. Ideally, the stool has foot-actuated controls that allow you to change the height while you are scrubbed in. Otherwise a large hand control for the height adjustment is better than a small one.

Each room should have a Mayo stand to hold surgical instruments during surgery (Figure 2-1B). Make sure these stands are stable and that the height can be adjusted. We prefer the ones with four or five wheels, rather than those with only two wheels.

Elaborate operating room facilities are not necessary to do any of the procedures described in this book, although one might wish to perform most procedures in a "clean" room that is not also being used for "dirty" procedures such as sigmoidoscopies.

FIGURE 2-2 Woods lamp. Ultraviolet light for the diagnosis of fungal infections, erythrasma, vitiligo, and melasma. *(Copyright Richard P. Usatine, MD.)*

HAND INSTRUMENTS

Small surgical instruments can be categorized by their purpose in surgery, such as the following:

- *Cutting:* scalpels, razor blades, scissors, punches, curettes
- *Tissue holding:* forceps, skin hooks
- *Undermining:* scissors
- *Hemostasis:* hemostats or mosquitos
- *Suturing and wound closure:* needle holders, scissors, staplers.

Instruments used to perform excisions include scalpel handles with blades, forceps, skin hooks, hemostats, scissors, and a needle holder. High-quality instruments that will last and perform well during surgical procedures should be purchased. A high-quality needle holder is important because a poorly manufactured one will not hold needles properly. The best surgical instruments are often made in Germany, England, and the United States. Some of the less expensive surgical instruments are manufactured in Pakistan, and the quality is comparable to the cost. Poorly made disposable hand instruments should be avoided.

Cutting

Scalpels

A scalpel has two parts, the handle and blade. The four most useful blades (Figure 2-3A) for skin surgery are:

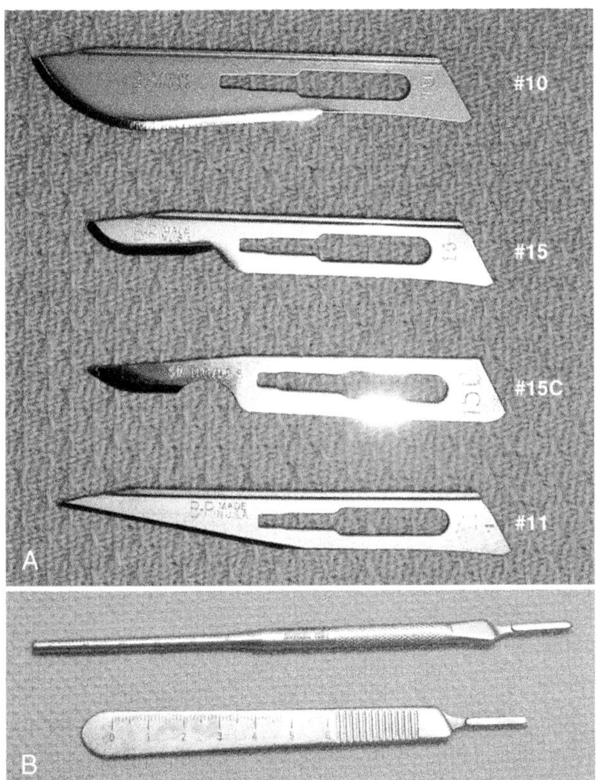

FIGURE 2-3 (A) Scalpel blades used in skin surgery. (B) Scalpel handles with ruler markings. Note the round handle was designed by a surgeon for increased dexterity during more challenging surgeries (Siegel handle). *(Copyright Richard P. Usatine, MD.)*

- *No. 15 blade:* most commonly used blade for skin surgery.
- *No. 15C blade:* shorter and thinner blade with a finer point than the traditional No. 15 blade. It is useful for fine plastics work on the face.
- *No. 11 blade:* sharply pointed with a cutting blade on both sides, making it useful for incision and drainage of an abscess or cyst.
- *No. 10 blade:* larger than a No. 15 blade with the same shape. It is useful for doing a shave biopsy of a large lesion or for cutting a thick callus on the foot. Some surgeons prefer it for large skin excisions on the back because the skin is so thick in this location.

Blades are disposable and can be purchased separately or preattached to disposable plastic handles. The advantage of a totally disposable scalpel is that it eliminates the risk of being cut while attaching or removing a disposable blade from a nondisposable metal handle. The risk of being cut is low with good dexterity and experience. A needle holder or hemostat is helpful when placing a blade on the handle or taking it off. Blade-removal instruments can also be purchased. Although disposable scalpels are convenient, they are not as stable or as sharp as a metal scalpel handle with a disposable blade. For elliptical excisions and flaps, I prefer the sharp blades on a nondisposable metal handle. Special scalpel handles have been designed by surgeons for increased dexterity during more challenging surgeries (Figure 2-3B). Most metal scalpel handles come with

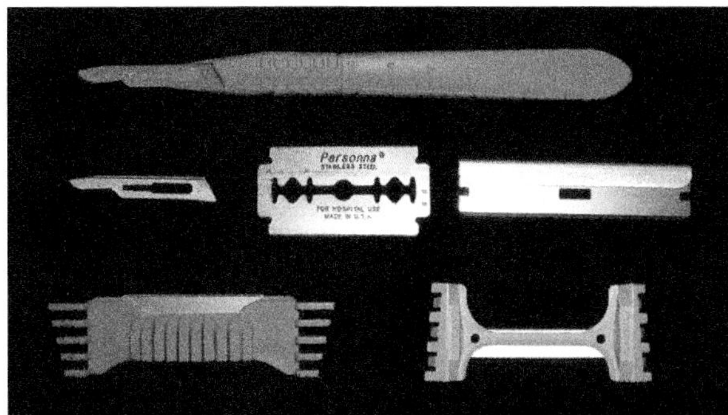

FIGURE 2-4 Razors and scalpels for shave biopsies. The DermaBlade is the blue-handled blade in the bottom right corner. *(Copyright Richard P. Usatine, MD.)*

a ruler marking for measuring the size of your surgical cuts (Figure 2-3B).

Personna Plus Microcoat blades are particularly sharp Teflon-coated blades. However, sharp disposable blades are also available from Bard-Parker, Cincinnati Surgical, and Swann-Morton. It may be worthwhile to try out more than one type to determine which one meets your personal needs and budget.

Razor Blades

The full range of razor blades (Figure 2-4) is discussed in detail in Chapter 9, *The Shave Biopsy*. The DermaBlade is a particularly easy and sharp blade to use for the novice and the expert. The Personna super double-edge blade is very sharp and can be broken in half for easy use. Although these do not come in sterile packaging, they can be used for shave biopsies without putting them through the autoclave. At pennies a blade, these are the most cost-effective tool for shave biopsies. They can be broken in half within their paper container to avoid cutting your hand prior to use.

Scissors

Figure 2-5 shows different types of scissors used in skin surgery. The most versatile and affordable scissor for snip excisions and cutting the base of a punch biopsy is the iris scissor, a small, sharp-tipped scissor that may be straight or curved. Use of the straight or curved iris is a

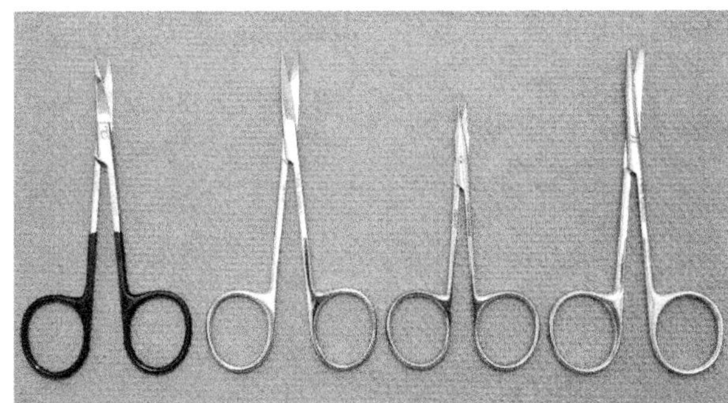

FIGURE 2-5 Assorted scissors for skin surgery: Supercut iris scissor, gold-handled iris scissor, Gradle scissor, and a tissue undermining scissor. *(Copyright Richard P. Usatine, MD.)*

matter of personal preference. The curved scissor is a bit more expensive and may allow the operator to get under a punch biopsy specimen with some ease. Scissor length varies from 3 to 5 in. The iris scissor can be used for suture removal and cutting sutures, but the ones used for this purpose should be kept separate from tissue-cutting scissors to avoid dulling your best surgical scissors. The iris scissor can also be used for blunt dissection and undermining. Scissors need periodic sharpening, but properly cleaned and treated instruments will generally last a long time and are worth the investment.

Gradle scissors have very small blades for fine cutting and undermining. These scissors can be invaluable with a punch biopsy of the nail matrix in which the tissue is friable and would be easy to crush if a less fine pair of scissors were used. Gradle scissors are more expensive than standard iris scissors.

Many companies make specific undermining scissors with sharp or blunt tips and sharp blades. Some of these are tenotomy scissors or Metzenbaum scissors. These could be used instead of the all-purpose iris scissor. New technologies are being used to make the blades of scissors sharper. For a premium price you can now buy scissors that are as sharp as a scalpel (e.g., Supercut scissors). Endarterectomy scissors, which have a longer handle with blunt tips, also provide excellent control and precision for delicate work, but at a somewhat higher price.[1]

Punches

Punches come in sizes ranging from 2 to 10 mm. Clinicians may choose between disposable, one-use punches and reusable steel punches (Figure 2-6). Disposable punches are presterilized and need no maintenance. Reusable punches require cleaning and sterilization between procedures and must be sharpened periodically. We use disposable punches only because they are always sharp and convenient.

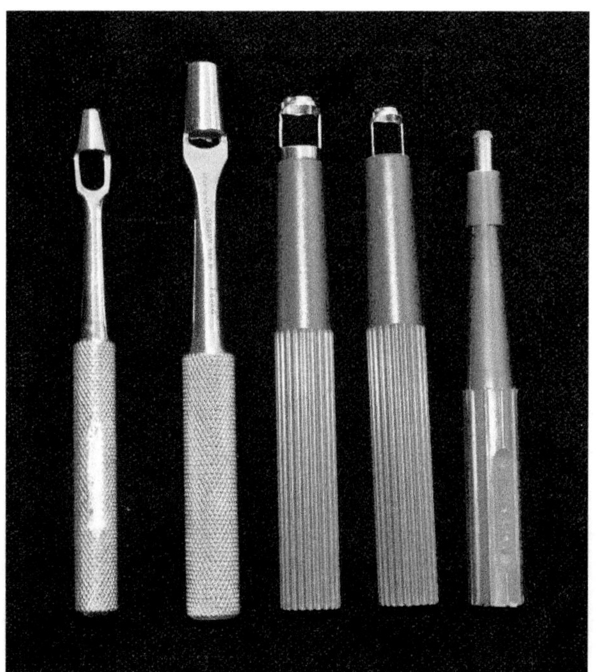

FIGURE 2-6 Assortment of punch types, including two nondisposable punches, two open punches, and one closed punch. *(Copyright Richard P. Usatine, MD.)*

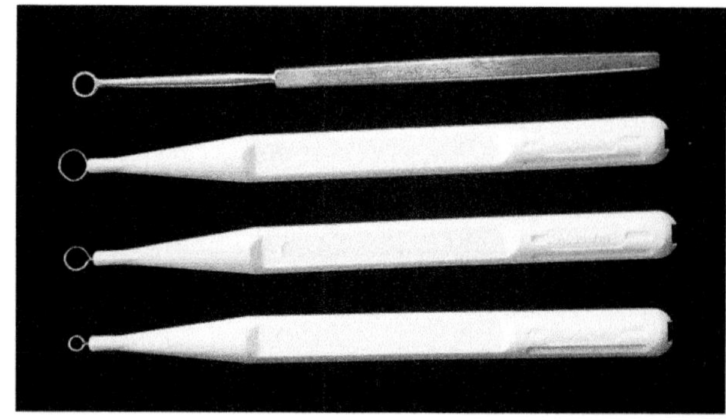

FIGURE 2-7 One reusable curette and three disposable curettes ranging from 7, 5 to 3 mm. *(Copyright Richard P. Usatine, MD.)*

The new Huot VisiPunch has the wonderful advantage of allowing the clinician to see through the punch instrument while performing the procedure. This allows you to place the punch on the skin and make sure the whole lesion is within the punch before starting the cut. Also, you can see the depth better and have a better idea of when the punch core releases from the dermis below. These come in the full range of sizes between 2 and 10 mm. Although a wide range of punch instruments is produced by many manufacturers from 2 to 10 mm, the most useful punch biopsy instruments range from 3 to 6 mm. See Chapter 10, *The Punch Biopsy*, for more information on this surgical tool.

Curettes

Dermal curettes (Figure 2-7) are useful for treating pyogenic granulomas, molluscum contagiosum, seborrheic keratoses, basal cell carcinomas, and squamous cell carcinomas. The head of the curette may be round (Fox curette) or oval (Piffard curette). One side of the curette head is dull. The other side has a sharp blade that is designed to cut through friable or soft tissue but is not so sharp as to cut normal skin. This allows the curette to distinguish between abnormal and normal tissue and to selectively remove the abnormal tissue.

Curettes range in size from 2 to 7.5 mm. Nondisposable and disposable curettes are available. The size and shape of the curette used are in part determined by personal preference. Larger curettes allow for removal of larger lesions with fewer strokes. Smaller curettes are more precise and can be used on smaller lesions and for curettage of small pockets of tumor that are more difficult to reach with larger curettes. A range of curettes should be available in the office. Disposable curettes that range from 2 to 7 mm can be purchased. We keep 3-, 5-, and 7-mm curettes in our office and find that this covers our needs (Figure 2-7). Currently we are using the Acu-Dispo-Curette by Acuderm, but other companies also produce excellent disposable curettes.

Tissue Holding

A large variety of forceps and skin hooks are available that enable a clinician to handle skin in a means that facilitates cutting, undermining, and suturing. The goal of tissue holding is to provide the most stability during these procedures while minimizing skin trauma and scarring.

Forceps

Basic types of forceps include tissue forceps, dressing forceps, and splinter forceps. To aid in removing splinters, splinter forceps have sharp tips and no teeth. Dressing and tissue forceps are available with and without teeth. Opinions vary about the value of teeth on forceps. Some clinicians believe that they can handle skin more atraumatically when forceps have teeth, whereas others believe there is less tissue trauma without teeth. This is an issue that may be determined by personal preference.

The most commonly used type of forceps in skin surgery is the Adson forceps, which has a broad handle and a long narrow tip (Figure 2-8). One common configuration is one tooth on one tip fitting into two teeth on the other tip. Many variations of this configuration exist. We suggest you start with the basic 4¾-in. Adson forceps, with and without teeth, and experiment with others as needed. I personally prefer the teeth for suturing and the forceps without teeth when lifting the punch specimen up to cut the base. Adson forceps without teeth may tend to crush healthy tissue if one is applying a strong force to hold skin under tension.

The use of good-quality forceps with small teeth and accurate apposition is important. This allows you to pass the suture needle back and forth between the forceps and needle holder without touching the needle with your fingers, thereby decreasing your risks for a needlestick. Most cheap disposable forceps do not hold suture needles well at all.

Skin Hooks

Skin hooks are capable of holding tissue in the least traumatic manner. They are better than forceps for reflecting skin while undermining without crushing skin edges. Skin hooks are especially useful for holding skin while undermining and while placing deep sutures (Figure 2-9). Skin hooks are available with single- or double-pronged hooks and with sharp or blunt prongs (Figure 2-8). Single, sharp-pronged hooks are the most versatile type of skin hook. The double-pronged skin hook can be useful in retracting the proximal nail fold and in office gynecologic surgery.

Skin hooks may be used for many of the same purposes as forceps and for additional procedures such as the following:

- Holding a wound edge while undermining the skin.
- Retracting a skin edge to expose bleeding sites and to obtain hemostasis.
- Pulling together the edges of an ellipse to see if there was sufficient undermining to allow for closure.
- Moving a flap into place while placing the key suture.

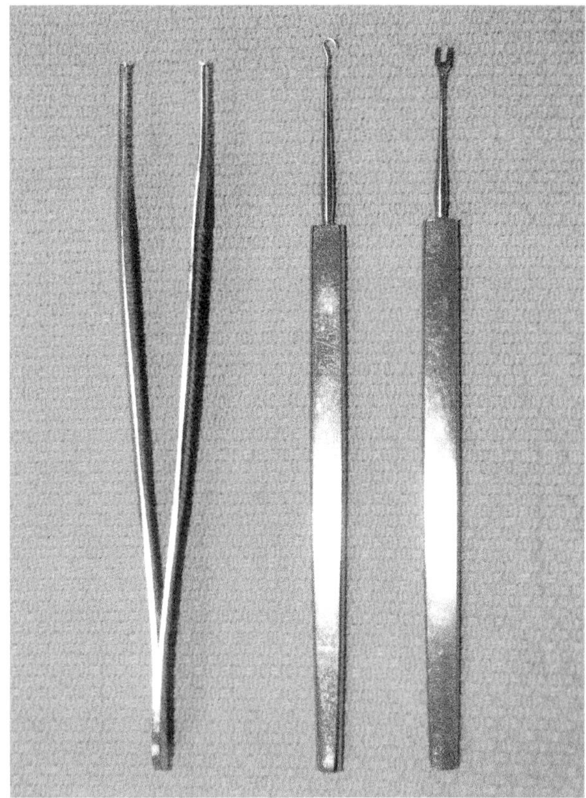

FIGURE 2-8 Instruments for holding skin: Adson forceps with microfine teeth, one single-pronged skin hook and one double-pronged skin hook. *(Copyright Richard P. Usatine, MD.)*

- Determining the degree of skin redundancy while treating dog ears (standing cones).
- Holding traction on the corners of an ellipse while placing sutures or staples.

Undermining

The skin may be undermined with any type of sharp tissue scissor. Blunt dissection will cause less trauma to the tissue and displace vessels and nerves rather than

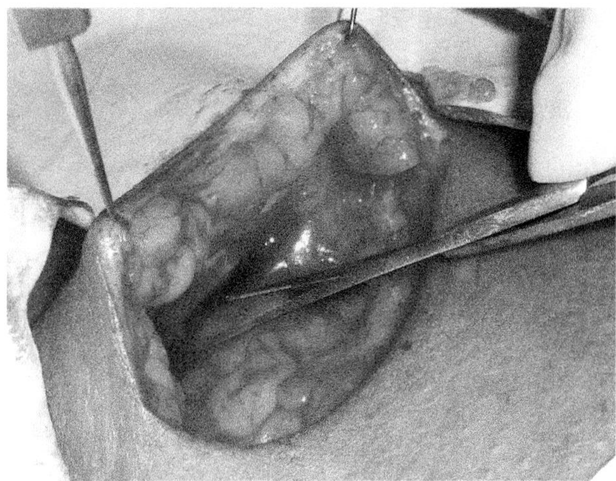

FIGURE 2-9 Skin hooks being used to hold up skin atraumatically while providing visualization for undermining tissue. *(Copyright Richard P. Usatine, MD.)*

cut through them. Undermining with a scalpel is more likely to cut vessels and nerves, but can be done. A sharp iris scissor is a good affordable choice for blunt dissection and cutting tissue while undermining. Other options include tenotomy scissors, Gradle scissors, Metzenbaum scissors, endarterectomy scissors, and specific undermining scissors (Figure 2-5).

Hemostasis

Hemostats are useful to clamp bleeding vessels selected for electrocoagulation or ligation. Hemostats may also be used to break up loculations after opening an abscess or for blunt dissection around cysts and lipomas. Hemostats may be curved or straight and are useful for clamping and tying bleeding vessels and tissue. These come in sizes between 3.5 and 5 in. Larger hemostats are known as Kelly clamps and smaller hemostats are called mosquitos. Personal preference determines the size and shape used. Curved hemostats are particularly useful for blunt dissection around subcutaneous masses and for reaching inside an abscess to break up loculations. Straight heavy-duty hemostats can be useful in partial and full toenail removal.

Wound Closure

Needle Holders

Needle holders for skin surgery should be relatively short because the suturing is not being done in a deep cavity. A short handle allows for more precise needle handling. Smooth rather than serrated jaws are less likely to fray sutures while doing instrument ties. The Webster needle holder with smooth jaws is commonly used in skin surgery and is available in 4¾- and 5-in. sizes. Larger and heavier needle holders may be helpful when suturing tougher, thicker skin (e.g., on the back). Small, fine-needle holders are useful for fine work on the face and other delicate areas. It is important to have good-quality needle holders. Needle holders with gold-plated finger rings and tungsten carbide inserts are worth the price if you do skin surgery on a regular basis (Figure 2-10).The gold-plated handle is not crucial but it is often a sign that the needle holder is of excellent quality.

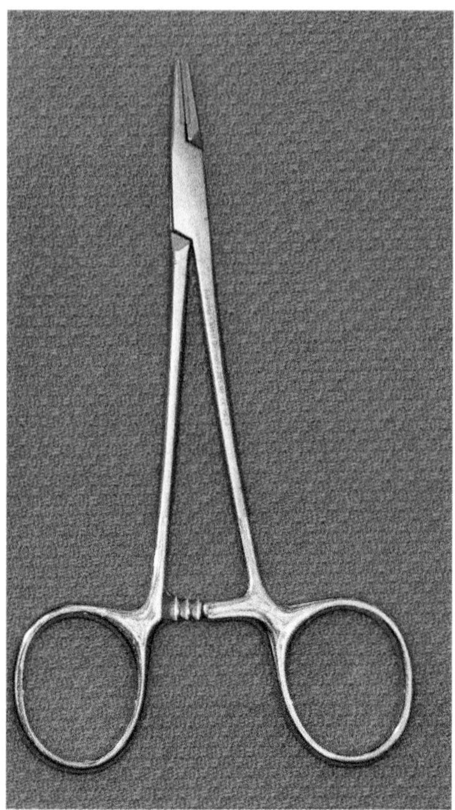

FIGURE 2-10 High quality needle holder with gold-plated finger rings and tungsten carbide inserts for stable needle holding. *(Copyright Richard P. Usatine, MD.)*

Suture-Cutting Scissors

Virtually any type of scissor may be used to cut sutures during surgery or remove sutures after some wound healing has occurred. There may be an advantage to using a designated pair of scissors for suture cutting because tissue-cutting scissors will become dull if often used to cut sutures. Iris scissors work well to cut sutures during surgery or to remove sutures postoperatively. These fine, sharp-tipped scissors can easily go under the suture to cut it for removal. Special suture-removal scissors have a hook on the end of one blade that is designed to slip under the suture and cut it without traumatizing the underlying skin. Examples of suture-cutting scissors include the Spencer, Shortbent, and Littauer stitch scissors.

Staplers

Staples are more expensive for wound closure than sutures and are generally not used in cosmetically sensitive areas. Staples are best applied to long incisions on the scalp, trunk, or extremities. In these areas, wounds can be closed more rapidly with staples than sutures. Staplers may be reusable or disposable. Reusable staplers are autoclavable and are used with sterile staple cartridges. This is not an essential item for the office.

Small Instrument Sets

To save time and expense, it helps to establish standard instrument sets for use in the office. Suggested sets for different surgical needs include the following:

Punch or Small Excision Set *(Figure 2-11)*

- Iris scissors
- Adson forceps (with and without teeth)
- Webster needle holder (smooth)
- Cotton-tipped applicators and gauze (may be added before autoclaving).

Ellipse or Large Excision Set *(Figure 2-12)*

- Blade handle
- Two hemostats
- Adson forceps (with and without teeth)

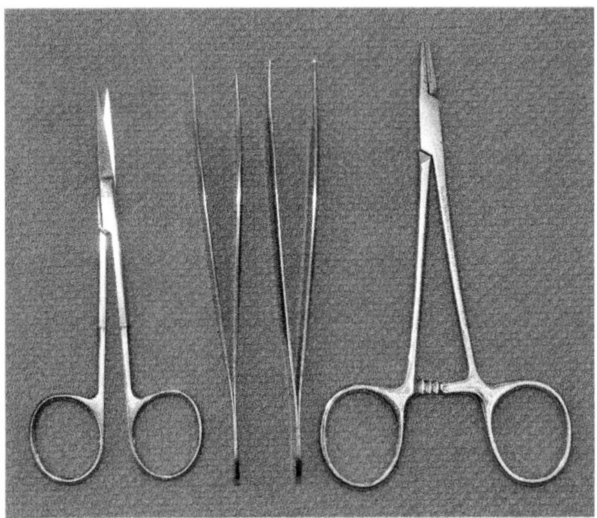

FIGURE 2-11 Punch instrument set. *(Copyright Richard P. Usatine, MD.)*

- Two skin hooks (single, sharp prong)
- Webster needle holder
- Iris scissors (or another scissor for undermining)
- Designated suture scissors (optional)
- Metal basin (optional, used for cleaning and irrigating with sterile saline)
- Cotton-tipped applicators and gauze (may be added before autoclaving).

Adding clean cotton-tipped applicators (CTAs) and clean cotton gauze (purchased in bulk packs) to be autoclaved in surgical sets is an efficient way to prepare for surgery and save money. This saves setup time and money over individually packaged sterile gauze and CTAs. It also avoids wasting of the paper that covers individually wrapped sterile gauze and CTAs, making for a greener office.

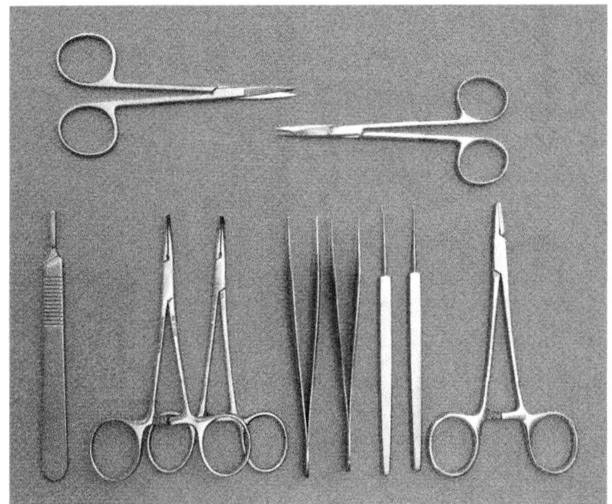

FIGURE 2-12 Elliptical excision set. *(Copyright Richard P. Usatine, MD.)*

Information on nail surgery equipment is found in Chapter 18, *Nail Procedures*.

Surgical Skin Markers

It is extremely helpful to draw lines where you intend to cut. This is true for all types of biopsies and excisions and not just for large ellipses and flaps. It is best to mark the skin before administering anesthesia because the anesthesia may distort the lesion or make it less visible.

A number of various types of surgical markers are available. The standard markers use gentian violet and are nontoxic. Preoperative prepping with alcohol will rub off the gentian violet, but povidone-iodine and chlorhexidine will not. These markers can be purchased in sterile packages for single use in a sterile procedure. However, for procedures such as shave biopsies and snip excisions that will not be sutured, the marker need not be sterile. A fine-point marker is most useful. Twin-tipped markers are available that have a broad tip on one end and a fine tip on the other. A sterile marker costs approximately $1 to $2. A nonsterile marker is less expensive. A sterile marker can be used over again as long as it has not touched body fluids and the patient is prepped after marking. These markers do not tattoo the skin.

MAGNIFICATION DEVICES

It is helpful to have at least one device available to magnify lesions. A wide range of magnifying lenses is available, from inexpensive handheld magnifying lenses to expensive binocular loupes. Good-quality magnification with good lighting will allow the clinician to see small features, such as telangiectasias, that may not be visible to the naked eye. Keeping a small magnifying glass in your office or pocket is a great way to start. A small handheld lighted magnifying loupe (5× to 10×) is a compact and inexpensive option available in most hobby or electronic stores.

The advantage of loupes that are mounted to eyeglasses or a headband is that the clinician is able to use both hands in a procedure while getting the benefit of magnification. Magnification levels range from 1.5× to 6×. Two times magnification should be sufficient for most skin lesion diagnoses and procedures and provides a comfortable working distance from the lesion in focus (about 10 in.). The OptiVISOR is a good starting device and various clip-on lights can be added to this product (Figure 2-13). Customized binocular loupes are expensive, high-quality optical instruments that are used by oral surgeons and in the operating room.

A dermatoscope provides magnification, light, and the ability to see patterns below the skin. These devices are most helpful in the diagnosis of skin cancers and other benign tumors. Dermatoscopes come in polarized and nonpolarized modes with some new hybrid dermatoscopes that have both modes available. See Chapter 32, *Dermoscopy*, for further information.

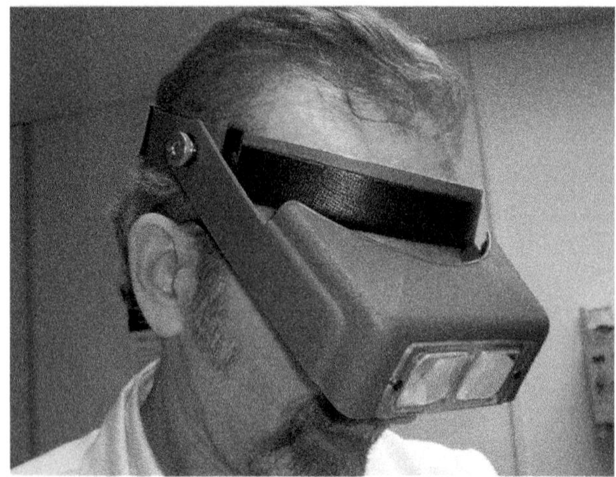

FIGURE 2-13 OptiVISOR loop providing 2x magnification and some eye protection. *(Copyright Richard P. Usatine, MD.)*

PROTECTIVE GEAR

To be protected from blood and fluids during surgery, clinicians must wear surgical gloves and eye protection. Surgical masks and eye protection are especially important for surgeries on known high-risk individuals or for surgeries in which the risk of exposure to blood or fluid is greatest. One particularly well-designed protective device is the Splash Shield, which covers the full face with clear plastic on a comfortable head band (Figure 2-14). Although eyeglasses offer some protection, a face shield provides the best coverage. If you use a laser, special eye shields will be needed. (See Chapters 26 through 30 and Appendix B for information on laser eye shields.)

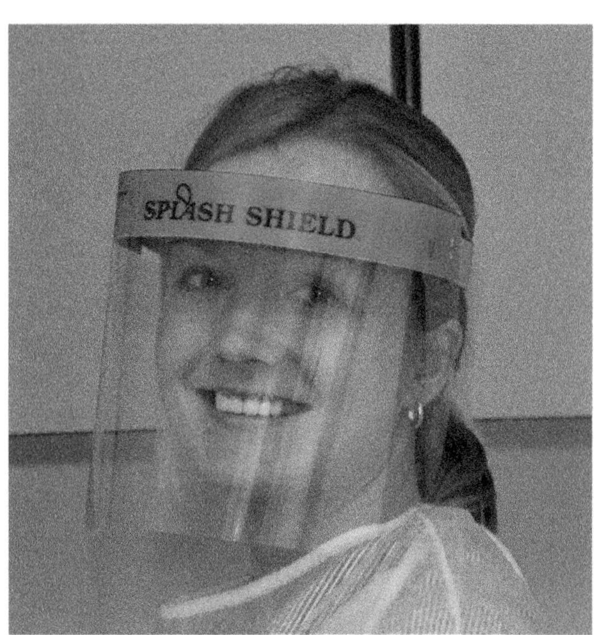

FIGURE 2-14 Splash Shield to prevent splash exposures. *(Copyright Richard P. Usatine, MD.)*

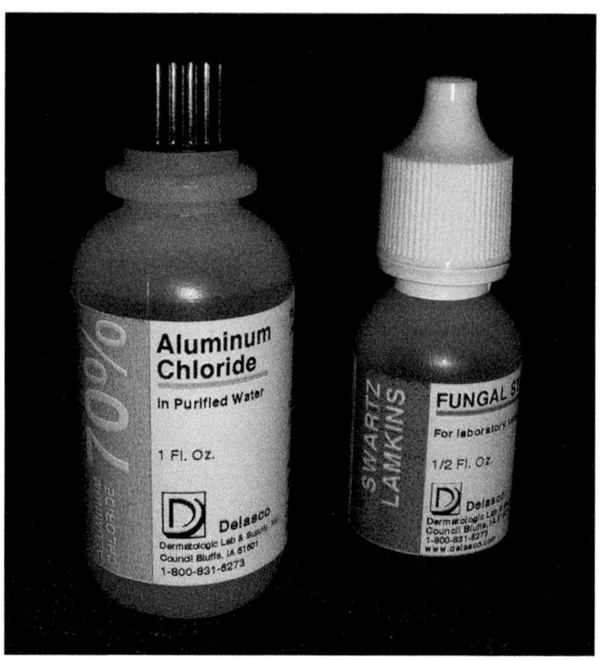

FIGURE 2-15 Aluminum chloride bottle and fungal stain bottle. *(Copyright Richard P. Usatine, MD.)*

MEDICATIONS AND CHEMICALS

Medical offices should keep the following medications and chemicals on hand:

Anesthetics

- Lidocaine with and without epinephrine (1% and 2%)
- Topical lidocaine jelly
- EMLA and other topical anesthetics as needed (see Chapters 3 and 20 for more information).

Chemicals *(Figure 2-15)*

- Aluminum chloride (70% in water) (see Chapter 4, *Hemostasis*)
- Fungal stain (Swartz-Lamkins stain) helps for doing KOH preps looking for fungal infections.

Injectables *(Figure 2-16)*

- Bicarbonate (for buffering lidocaine) (see Chapter 3, *Anesthesia*)
- Sterile saline (for diluting injectable triamcinolone)
- Triamcinolone for injection (Kenalog), 10 and 40 mg/mL (see Chapter 16, *Intralesional Injections*).

EQUIPMENT

Cryotherapy Equipment

Cryotherapy equipment for liquid nitrogen includes the following:

- Storage tank (Dewar) with method to remove liquid nitrogen (Figure 2-17)

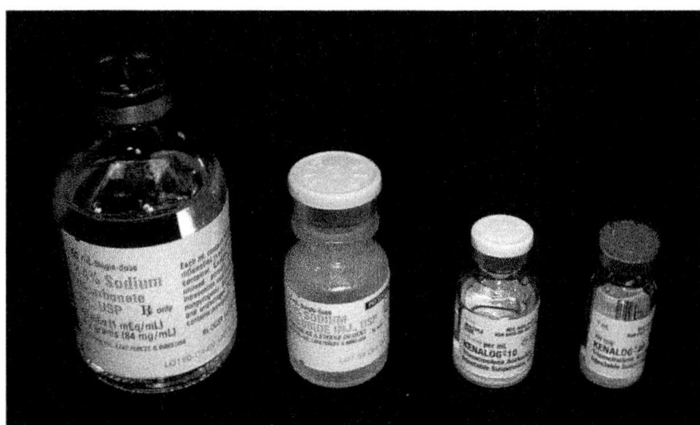

FIGURE 2-16 Injectables: bicarbonate, sterile saline, and triamcinolone. *(Copyright Richard P. Usatine, MD.)*

- Cryogun (Figure 2-18)
- Cryo Tweezers (Figure 2-19) are great for easy treatment of skin tags, especially those around the eyelids.

Although this equipment can cost from $500 to $1000, it will pay for itself many times over and allow you to treat actinic keratoses, warts, condyloma, seborrheic keratoses, and other benign lesions. See Chapter 15, *Cryosurgery*, for more on this topic.

Electrosurgery Equipment

Having at least one electrosurgical instrument is essential before performing elliptical excisions (see Chapter 14, *Electrosurgery*). While the bleeding of shave biopsies can easily be stopped with chemicals, deeper excisions will often require electrocoagulation to obtain adequate hemostasis.

The least expensive way to begin is to get one single electrosurgical unit that is capable of electrocoagulation and electrodestruction but is not a cutting device. These can be obtained for about $1000 and if on wheels can be easily moved from one exam room to another. The next step up is to have multiple units of this type mounted in each exam room (Figure 2-20). For many thousands of dollars an electrosurgical unit with cutting capability can be purchased. Generally one unit per office practice is sufficient and this is usually kept in the principal surgical/procedural room. A smoke evacuator is especially important if a cutting unit is used because cutting produces more smoke (plume).

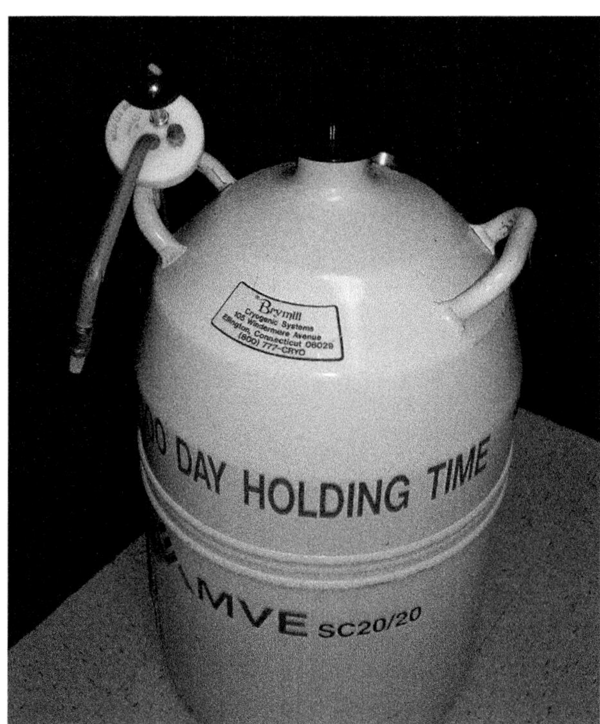

FIGURE 2-17 Storage tank (Dewar) with method to remove liquid nitrogen. *(Copyright Richard P. Usatine, MD.)*

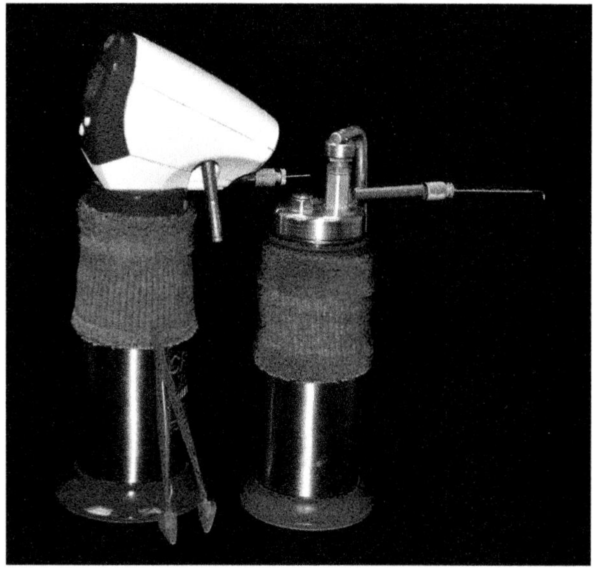

FIGURE 2-18 Methods for cryosurgery: Cryo-Tracker, Cryo Tweezer, and Cry-Ac. *(Copyright Richard P. Usatine, MD.)*

Electrosurgery without Cutting

- Bovie Aaron 900 (www.boviemed.com)
- ConMed Hyfrecator Plus (www.conmed.com/electrosurgery_home955.php)

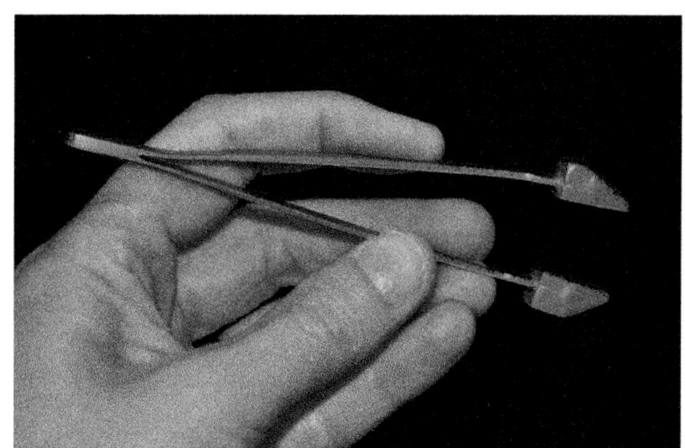

FIGURE 2-19 Cryo Tweezer for skin tags. *(Copyright Richard P. Usatine, MD.)*

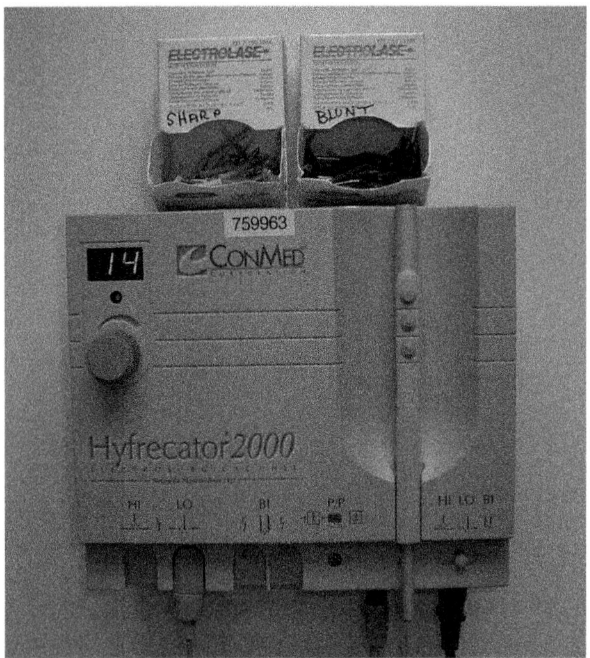

FIGURE 2-20 Electrosurgical instrument mounted on the wall. *(Copyright Richard P. Usatine, MD.)*

Electrosurgery with Cutting

- Bovie Aaron 950 (www.boviemed.com)
- Ellman Surgitron radio-frequency units (www.ellman.com)
- Wallach units (www.wallachsurgical.com/Electrosurgical.htm)

Smoke evacuators are made by all of the companies listed above. The equipment for cosmetic procedures will be covered in Chapters 19 through 31.

DISPOSABLE ITEMS

- Needles (18 to 30 gauge, including 27 gauge)
- Syringes (1, 3, 5 or 6, 10 or 12 mL, Luer-Lok preferable so the needle does not come off during injections)
- Nu-Gauze ¼- and ½-inch, noniodinated for packing wounds
- Alcohol wipes, gauze, gloves, fenestrated drapes, slides, cover-slips, adhesive bandages, cotton-tipped applicators, petrolatum, and antibiotic ointments
- Sutures (see Chapter 5, *Suture Material*)
- Tape. Durapore tape (Figure 2-21) and cloth tape work well but there are many other types from which to choose.

PHOTOGRAPHIC EQUIPMENT

A digital camera is essential for all dermatologic procedures, not just cosmetic procedures. It is best to choose a digital camera that has a good macro function for close-up photographs. It also helps to have the ability to adjust the light so that one can avoid creating photos that are too bleached out by a flash that is too powerful at short distances. When shopping for a camera, consider more than just the number of megapixels. Look also for a camera that fits your photographic needs as a clinician. Consider the size and whether you want to carry it on you or leave a large single-lens reflex (SLR) camera in one place and get it as needed. I prefer to have one small camera on my belt (or white coat pocket) and then keep a larger SLR in the office for those photos that will be improved by this larger format.

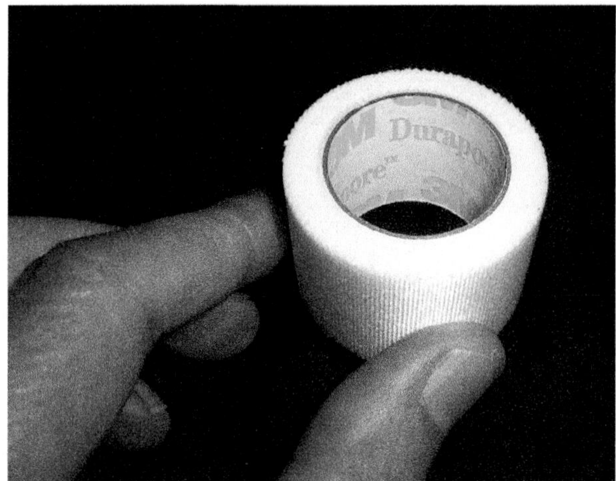

FIGURE 2-21 Durapore tape is one type of tape that has good holding power and is easy to work with. *(Copyright Richard P. Usatine, MD.)*

Photograph all lesions prior to excision or biopsy and create a system to be able to return to those photos as needed. I place all my photos in folders by the day on which they were taken, so I can retrieve them using the dates in the patients' charts. Other methods involve photographing the patients' label after completing the clinical photos. While this method helps to identify the patient, care must be taken to keep your photos securely protected so as to avoid HIPAA violations.

The camera is an excellent way to communicate with your patients to provide education and informed consent. Taking a photograph of a lesion on the back or top of the scalp can allow you to show the patient the lesion that you are concerned about on the digital screen of your camera. This creates a better informed patient in a discussion of the choices for diagnosis or treatment. The camera is also a good way to engage a child in a positive caring relationship. Of course, you must ask parents for permission before shooting photographs of children. Most children are delighted to have their picture taken and want to see the result on your camera. Use your camera creatively and this will add to the fun and quality of your practice.

WHAT TO HAVE IN EACH EXAM ROOM

- Alcohol wipes, gauze, tape, gloves, slides, adhesive bandages, cotton-tip applicators, petrolatum

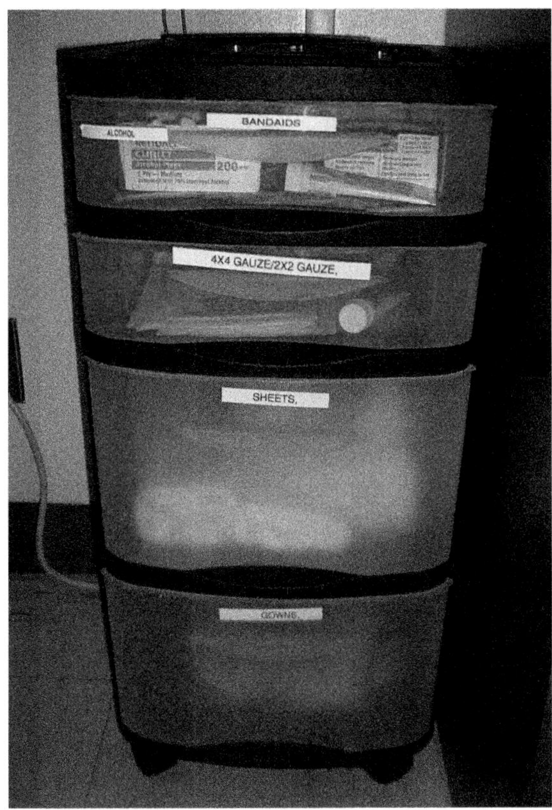

FIGURE 2-22 Plastic drawers help augment storage space in exam rooms so everything you need is right at your fingertips. *(Copyright Richard P. Usatine, MD.)*

- Small, easy-to-access portable plastic drawers to keep the above items in one place (Figure 2-22). Well-stocked built-in cabinets are an acceptable alternative.
- Mayo stands (Figure 2-1B), preferably with four or five wheels
- Inexpensive hand mirrors, which are great to have for communication with patients. If the mirror disappears, it can be easily replaced.

CONCLUSION

To do skin surgery well, it is important to have the appropriate instruments and equipment for the procedure. Good instruments and equipment that are well maintained will facilitate the diagnosis and treatment of skin disorders. The resource list below provides sources for the best instruments, supplies, and equipment.

Resources

Acuderm (800-327-0015; www.acuderm.com)
Delasco Dermatologic Buying Guide, a comprehensive selection of dermatologic supplies and equipment (800-831-6273; www.delasco.com)
Ethicon (www.ethicon.com)
George Tiemann & Co. (www.georgetiemann.com)
Henry Schein (800-772-4346; www.henryschein.com)
Huot Instruments, including VisiPunch (866-212-8466; www.huotinstruments.com)
Miltex (800-645-8000; www.miltex.com)
Moore Medical (800-234-1464; www.mooremedical.com)
Sklar Surgical Instruments (www.sklarcorp.com/HomeUS.aspx)
Splash Shield, covers the full face with clear plastic on a comfortable headband (800-536-6686; splashshield@aol.com).

Reference

1. Kannler C, Jellinek N, Maloney ME. Surgical pearl: The use of endarterectomy scissors in dermatologic surgery. *J Am Acad Dermatol.* 2005;53:873–874.

3 Anesthesia

RICHARD P. USATINE, MD

Local anesthesia is the reversible loss of sensation to a localized area achieved by the injection or topical application of anesthetic agents. Regional anesthesia involves larger areas and is achieved by nerve block and/or field blocks through the use of injectable anesthetic agents. Local anesthetics block the pain fibers of a nerve better than those fibers that carry sensations of pressure, touch, and temperature. Therefore, if the patient feels pressure or pulling but no pain, the patient should be reassured that this is not unusual. Many anesthetic agents can be injected or applied topically.

TOPICAL ANESTHETICS

Common anesthetics include the following:

- EMLA (eutectic mixture of local anesthetics; 2.5% lidocaine and 2.5% prilocaine cream) (Rx) (Figure 3-1)
- LMX 4 and LMX 5 (4% liposome-encapsulated lidocaine and 5% cream) (OTC)
- Topical lidocaine (2% and 4% gel or viscous solution, 5% ointment, 10% spray)
- Tridocaine gel (20% benzocaine, 6% lidocaine, 4% tetracaine) (available from Canada).

Table 3-1 shows the onset of action for the most commonly used topical anesthetics in skin procedures. EMLA (eutectic mixture of local anesthetics) cream consists of 2.5% lidocaine and 2.5% prilocaine in an oil-in-water emulsion. This anesthetic cream works best if applied for 30 minutes under occlusion or 60 minutes without occlusion before anesthesia is needed. It can be useful in treating children or a patient of any age who is afraid of needles. EMLA cream is used for some laser procedures, superficial light electrodesiccation of benign growths, and curettage of molluscum contagiosum. In Figure 3-1B the EMLA has been applied to the lower eyelids before electrodesiccation of syringomas. EMLA is available in 5-g tubes with occlusive dressings or in 30-g tubes without dressings. EMLA should not be used in infants younger than 3 months because the metabolites of prilocaine form methemoglobin. In one randomized control trial, EMLA and LMX 4 provided comparable levels of anesthesia after a single 30-minute application under occlusion prior to electrodesiccation of dermatosis papulosa nigra.[1]

Topical lidocaine is available as a 2% and 4% gel or viscous solution, a 5% ointment, or a 10% spray. Regardless of the vehicle, topical lidocaine takes 15 to 30 minutes to produce anesthesia on mucosal surfaces. The degree of anesthesia is not comparable to injectable lidocaine, and unless it is combined with another agent such as phenylephrine, it has no vasoconstrictive action. Therefore, for mucosal surgery in the mouth, it is best to inject 1% lidocaine with epinephrine after the topical lidocaine has numbed the surface. For this purpose, it is easy to put topical lidocaine gel on a cotton swab and have the patient hold it against the mucous membrane before the subsequent injection. This technique might be used to anesthetize a mucocele or fibroma on the lip.

Tridocaine (20% benzocaine, 6% lidocaine, 4% tetracaine) is a local analgesic, anesthetic, and antipruritic. It is used to prevent pain associated with laser surgery, superficial skin surgery, needle insertion, and intravenous cannulation. It is indicated for intact skin only and anesthesia is obtained in 10 to 15 minutes. It can be purchased online from Canadian sources or be created by a compounding pharmacy.

EMLA Technique for Intact Skin

1. Use alcohol wipes to remove oil from the area of skin to be anesthetized.
2. Apply EMLA in a thick layer to skin then apply occlusive dressing (Tegaderm, OpSite, or plastic wrap) for 30 to 60 minutes. Thicker skin may take more than 1 hour to achieve anesthesia.
3. Remove EMLA with alcohol or with a tissue.
4. Perform the procedure or additional anesthesia without delay. Topical anesthesia will last only minutes after the EMLA is removed.

TOPICAL REFRIGERANTS/ CRYOANESTHESIA

- Ethyl chloride spray
- Medi-Frig (tetrafluoroethane) (Ellman International, Inc.)
- Liquid nitrogen.

Topical refrigerants make the skin cold and provide some anesthesia for the removal of small superficial skin lesions such as skin tags and molluscum. These agents provide some cryoanesthesia before snip excisions of skin tags or curettage of molluscum. Cryoanesthesia does not provide adequate anesthesia for the removal of larger lesions. These agents are sprayed on the skin until a white frost develops. The numbing effect is partial at best and disappears in seconds. Refrigerant sprays may be used before injecting local anesthesia with a needle in a needle-phobic patient. While these sprays are probably less effective than EMLA, they work faster and are therefore more convenient if the patient can tolerate the subsequent procedure.

Ethyl chloride is the only one of the refrigerants listed that is flammable, so it must not be used before electrosurgery. Medi-Frig can be safely used before

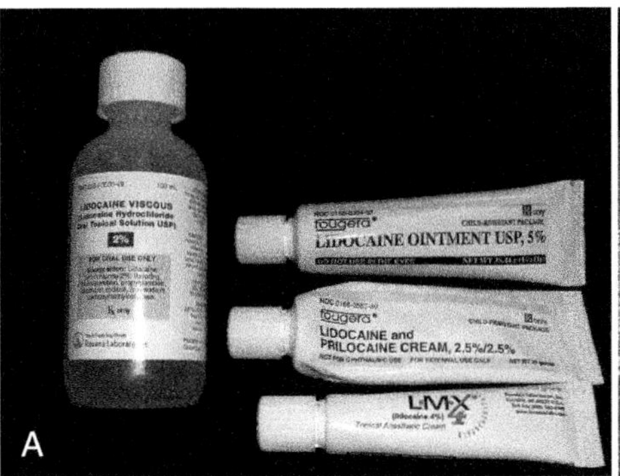

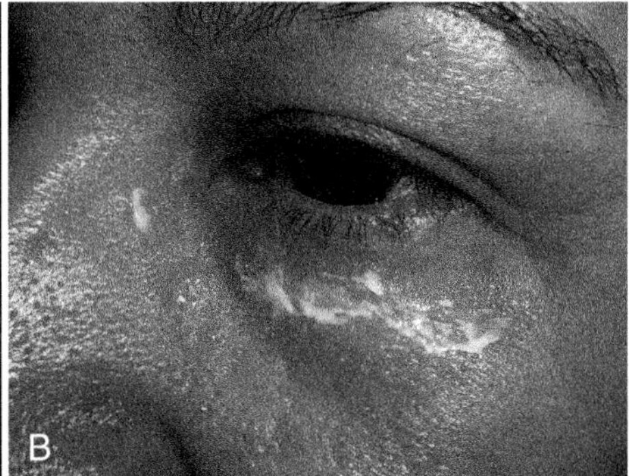

FIGURE 3-1 (A) An assortment of topical anesthetics for skin surgery. (B) EMLA was applied to the lower eyelids prior to electrosurgery of syringomas.

electrosurgery for small skin tags and molluscum contagiosum. The manufacturers of Medi-Frig claim that it is nontoxic and ozone safe, whereas the label on ethyl chloride warns against inhaling too much of the product.

Liquid nitrogen can freeze the skin to cause a numbing effect; however, its use causes immediate pain and little real anesthesia. Rather than using liquid nitrogen for local anesthesia for skin tag excision, it is easier and less painful to use the liquid nitrogen with a Cryo Tweezer to treat the skin tags directly (see Chapter 15, *Cryosurgery*). Also, liquid nitrogen can be sprayed or directly applied to skin tags or molluscum rather than using it as anesthesia. This also avoids the need to deal with blood and hemostasis issues.

Contact cooling devices and assistive external devices are frequently used in laser treatments and are covered in Chapter 20, *Anesthesia for Cosmetic Procedures*.

LOCAL ANESTHESIA BY INJECTION

Lidocaine is the most widely used local anesthetic for injection in skin surgery. Bupivacaine (Marcaine) is used occasionally when long-lasting anesthesia is desired. Lidocaine has the advantage of having a more rapid onset (within 1 minute) and shorter duration of anesthesia than bupivacaine. This shorter duration is sufficient and preferable for most skin surgery. When lidocaine is mixed with epinephrine, it lasts almost as long as bupivacaine and hurts less.[2] See Table 3-2 for a comparison of amide local anesthetics.

Epinephrine

Epinephrine is a vasoconstrictor, whereas lidocaine alone is a vasodilator. Epinephrine with lidocaine decreases bleeding during surgery. Also, the vasoconstriction of epinephrine keeps the lidocaine in the area where it was injected, thereby decreasing immediate systemic absorption and toxicity while increasing the duration of anesthesia. This allows greater amounts of lidocaine to be used safely for local anesthesia by reducing systemic absorption and increasing the local action of the lidocaine.

1% Lidocaine with Epinephrine

For most skin surgery procedures, the recommended anesthetic is 1% lidocaine with epinephrine. Its advantages include almost immediate anesthesia, adequate duration of anesthesia, and decreased bleeding because of the epinephrine. The incidence of true allergies is negligible. Lidocaine without epinephrine has a duration of 1.5 to 2 hours, whereas lidocaine with epinephrine has a duration of 2 to 6 hours.[3] The most common commercial preparation contains 1% lidocaine (10 mg/mL) with 1:100,000 of epinephrine. In a study that measured the effect of subdermal injection of lidocaine combined with epinephrine on cutaneous blood flow,

TABLE 3-1 Topical Anesthetics

Topical Anesthetic	Ingredients	Vehicle	Onset of Action (min)
EMLA	2.5% lidocaine and 2.5% prilocaine	Cream	60–120
LMX 4 LMX 5	Liposome-encapsulated lidocaine 4% and 5% cream	Liposome-encapsulated cream	30–60
Topical lidocaine	2% and 4% gel or viscous solution, 5% ointment, 10% spray	Viscous solution, ointment, spray	30–60
Tridocaine gel (available from Canada) (aka BLT)	20% benzocaine, 6% lidocaine, 4% tetracaine	Gel	30–60

TABLE 3-2 Local Anesthetics for Injection

Generic Name	Brand Name	Onset (min)	Duration Plain (h)	Duration with Epinephrine (h)	Maximum Dose Plain (mg/kg) for Adults	Maximum Dose with Epinephrine (mg/kg) for Adults
Lidocaine	Xylocaine	Rapid	1–2	2–4	5	7
Bupivacaine	Marcaine	2–10	2–4	4–8	2.5	3

laser Doppler imaging demonstrated an immediate decrease in cutaneous blood flow, which was maximal at 10 minutes in the forearm and 8 minutes in the face.[4]

Note that the initial skin blanching with injection is due to hydrostatic pressure along with the effect of epinephrine. When hemostasis is critical to the procedure, it is best to wait 8 to 10 minutes for the epinephrine to produce maximal vasoconstriction. Waiting is less important for shave biopsies of lesions that are not very vascular in patients who are not anticoagulated (Figure 3-2). Injecting enough anesthetic so that the skin is firm can limit the amount of bleeding because small blood vessels become compressed by the anesthetic fluid (Figure 3-3).

Maximal Doses

Maximal safe doses of 1% lidocaine with or without epinephrine are found in Table 3-3. Above these doses the risk of neurotoxicity and seizures is increased. In most adults (over 50 kg) up to 35 mL of 1% lidocaine with epinephrine is safe. Use of 1% lidocaine is preferable to 2% in most cases because a larger volume of anesthesia produces greater hemostasis and makes most cutaneous surgery easier to perform. Two percent lidocaine without epinephrine is useful in various nerve blocks including digital blocks when less volume is needed. Some clinicians prefer 2% lidocaine with epinephrine when they want to avoid tissue distortion from too much anesthetic volume. In this case, toxicity is not an issue because less than 5 mL of anesthesia are being used.

Decreasing the Pain of Local Anesthesia

Techniques to decrease the pain caused by injection of local anesthesia include the following:

- Inject very slowly because tissue distention hurts.
- Use a small-gauge needle (27 or 30 gauge).
- Pinch or vibrate the skin as the needle enters (based on the gate theory of pain).
- Distract the patient in conversation or with music.
- Add sodium bicarbonate to the lidocaine.
- Warm anesthesia to 40°C.
- Use only one injection site if possible and place subsequent injections into areas already anesthetized.

The main technique for decreasing the pain of injection is to inject the local anesthetic very slowly using a small-gauge needle (27 or 30 gauge). The larger the gauge number, the smaller the needle diameter and the less painful the injection. Use 30-gauge needles on the most sensitive areas including the face, the ears, the

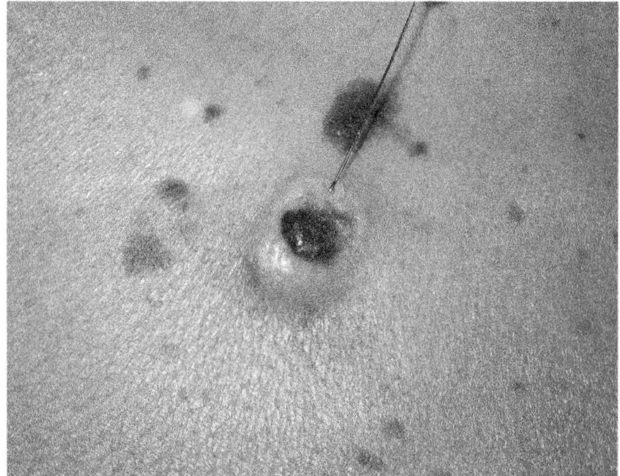

FIGURE 3-2 Local anesthetic injected under and around a seborrheic keratosis prior to shave biopsy to confirm that this highly pigmented lesion is benign. The elevation of the tissue makes the shave easier to perform.

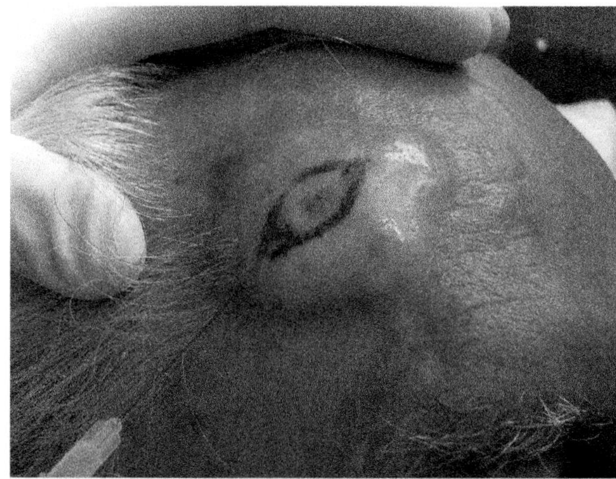

FIGURE 3-3 Local anesthesia before excising a basal cell carcinoma on the forehead. Note how the tissue distends in this location to improve hemostasis as well as ensure adequate anesthesia.

TABLE 3-3 Maximum Doses of 1% Lidocaine (10 mg/mL)

Type of Lidocaine	Maximum Adult Dose (mg/kg)	Maximum Child Dose (mg/kg)	Maximum mL for 50-kg Adult	Maximum mL for 70-kg Adult	Maximum mL for 30-kg Child
1% Lidocaine without epinephrine	5	1.5–2	25	28	4.5–6
1% Lidocaine with epinephrine	7	3–4	35	49	9–12

fingers, and the genitals. When injecting anesthesia for a laceration repair, injecting from within a laceration is less painful than injecting into intact skin.[5]

It may be helpful to pinch or vibrate the skin as the needle enters and distract the patient with conversation. Although the needle should be inserted quickly, the injection will be less painful if the volume of anesthesia is injected slowly. The more superficial the injection, the more painful it is. For example, an injection bleb similar to that of a tuberculin skin test is more painful than a deeper subcutaneous injection. It is usually less painful if the injection is done slowly and deeply at first, followed by redirecting the needle for a more superficial, dermal, blanching type of injection. In this manner, a volume of 5 mL or more can be given slowly through one injection site. Skin blanching and visible tissue distention help determine the area that has been anesthetized. Also, tissue induration can be palpated to determine the distribution of the anesthesia. If need be, this area can be extended by reinjecting through another site that has already been anesthetized.

Adding sodium bicarbonate (8.4% for injection) in a 1:10 dilution to the lidocaine and epinephrine anesthetic solution markedly decreases the pain caused by injection (e.g., 1 mL of sodium bicarbonate can be added to 9 mL of lidocaine). The addition of sodium bicarbonate neutralizes the commercially available lidocaine-epinephrine solutions that have a pH of 4 to 6. Although this takes more time, your patients will appreciate that the injection is less painful. The lidocaine-bicarbonate syringes need to be made at the time of use or may be kept for 1 week at room temperature and up to 2 weeks with refrigeration.[6] In our office we make the following syringes each morning:

- 3-mL syringes with 2.25 mL of lidocaine and 0.25 mL bicarbonate.
- 5- or 6-mL syringes with 4.5 mL of lidocaine and 0.5 mL bicarbonate.
- 10- or 12-mL syringes with 9 mL of lidocaine and 1 mL bicarbonate.

A warm (40°C) and neutral (pH 7.35) anesthetic preparation has been found to be less painful on injection than room-temperature nonneutral preparations.[7–9] One study suggests that warming and buffering have a synergistic effect.[8] Skin infiltration with warm buffered lidocaine was significantly less painful than infiltration with room-temperature unbuffered lidocaine, warm lidocaine, or buffered lidocaine.[8] In another study, the mean pain scores for the four solutions were 44.2 for plain lidocaine, 42.2 for warmed lidocaine, 36.7 for buffered lidocaine, and 29.2 for warmed buffered lidocaine (lower numbers equal less pain).[9] In one study, to reduce the pain of lidocaine infiltration, buffering was more effective than warming (warming was only to 38.9°C).[10]

Injection Technique

See video on the DVD for further learning. 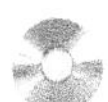

The skin surface can be cleaned adequately with an alcohol wipe. Gloves should be clean, but need not be sterile for the injections. When performing a biopsy or excision, it is helpful to mark the planned lines of incision with a surgical marker before doing the injection. This prevents losing sight of a nonpigmented lesion when the swelling and blanching occur from the anesthesia. The lines and circles drawn provide a guide to the biopsy or excision. Start anesthesia by inserting the needle into one site of the circumference of the circle of anesthesia needed around the lesion—typically 5 mm back for a shave or punch biopsy. Most anesthesia for a shave or punch biopsy can be done with one injection.

For shave and punch biopsies, the tip of the needle should reach the deep dermis so that an elevation and blanching of the tissue occurs (Figures 3-2 and 3-3). If the anesthetic is injected too deep into the subcutaneous tissue, no elevation will occur. When an injection is superficial in the dermis, you may see an accentuation of the follicles called peau d'orange. This skin distention is more painful than the pain that occurs with a deeper dermis injection. However, if you intend to do a shave biopsy, you can start with a deeper dermis injection and finish with a more superficial injection to raise the lesion for biopsy. Starting deeper and adjusting the needle to a more superficial level is an effective technique (this can be done without removing the needle from the original injection site).

If the lesion to be removed is large, a second insertion site may be needed. When injecting subcutaneously, it is important to pull back on the plunger before injecting at any one site to avoid injecting into a vessel. Advancing the needle and injecting simultaneously can be done in the dermis but should be avoided in the subcutaneous tissue because of the presence of larger blood vessels.

Preloading a number of syringes at the start of each day can save time if several procedures are to be done that day. A smaller syringe requires less force for injections. Three-milliliter and 5-mL (or 6-mL) syringes are a good compromise between cost and comfort. These hold enough anesthetic for most small procedures and will be comfortable for the injector.

ADVERSE REACTIONS

Adverse reactions to lidocaine and epinephrine and the needle used for injections include the following:

Lidocaine

- Allergy to lidocaine
- Central nervous system (CNS) effects from too much lidocaine (light-headedness, tinnitus, perioral tingling, metallic taste, tremors, slurred speech, and seizures)[1]
- Cardiovascular effects from too much lidocaine (myocardial depression, arrhythmias).

Epinephrine

- Tachycardia
- Anxiety
- Tremulousness
- Decreased peripheral circulation.

Needle

- Laceration of nerve (rare but more likely during a nerve block)
- Infection or abscess from lack of sterile technique.

For patients with normal circulation, it is safe to use epinephrine for local anesthesia in areas such as the tip of the nose, the fingers and toes, the ears, or the penis despite old dogma that epinephrine should not be used in these areas (Figure 3-4). However, epinephrine is generally not recommended for digital ring blocks, full ring blocks around the ear, penile nerve blocks, and other regional or field blocks in these areas. Furthermore, epinephrine should not be used in the very distal extremities of a patient with poor circulation such as patients with peripheral vascular disease or Raynaud's phenomenon.

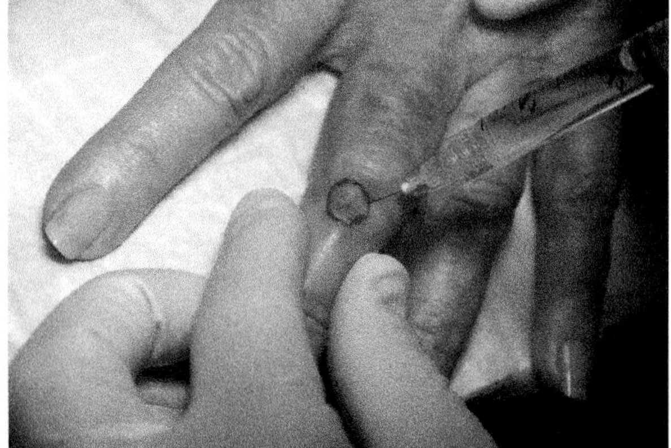

FIGURE 3-4 Local anesthetic with epinephrine is safe to use on the digits, nose, ears, and penis in a patient with normal circulation about to undergo a local excision. In this case, a squamous cell carcinoma was about to be excised from the finger using Mohs surgery. While a digital block without epinephrine is another option, local anesthetic used at the site of surgery with epinephrine allows for better hemostasis during the excision. *(Copyright Richard P. Usatine, MD.)*

A number of studies have even provided evidence to dispute the dogma that using epinephrine in a digital block produces digital necrosis.[11–13] Proper injection technique and adequate selection of patients (absence of thrombotic, vasospastic conditions, or uncontrolled hypertension) are mandatory to minimize complications. The addition of epinephrine, in fact, reduced the need for the use of tourniquets and large volumes of anesthetic and provided better and longer pain control during digital procedures.[11–13] We still choose to use 2% lidocaine without epinephrine for digital blocks but do use epinephrine in wing blocks when a matrix biopsy is planned (see Chapter 18, *Nail Procedures*).

Some patients ask that no epinephrine be used because it makes them anxious. It is true that some patients may get tachycardia for a few minutes along with a feeling of anxiousness shortly after the injection. This can usually be handled by warning the patient about this and reassuring him or her that the feeling will pass in a few minutes. For most patients, this may have occurred in the past during a dental procedure (reason enough for anxiety in many people).

Rare adverse effects associated with too large a systemic dose of injectable anesthetics (injection into a vein or too large a dose of the anesthetic) include myocardial depression and CNS effects such as light-headedness, tinnitus, perioral tingling, metallic taste, tremors, slurred speech, and seizures.[1]

Lidocaine Allergies

Lidocaine allergies are extremely rare. Almost all patients who report an allergy actually have had a vasovagal reaction with lidocaine injections or sensitivity to the epinephrine effects. Other patients are actually allergic to the paraben preservative in the multidose vials of lidocaine or they had an allergic reaction to a local anesthetic ester such as Novocain (procaine, novocaine). Because the paraben is not added to the single-use vials, it may be helpful to try these vials when the patient reports an allergy.

The ester forms of local anesthetics, such as novocaine, produce more allergic reactions. Fortunately, there is no cross-reactivity between novocaine and lidocaine. Therefore, lidocaine use is safe in a patient with a true novocaine allergy. Most dentists currently use lidocaine. Patients may think they are receiving novocaine in the dentist's office, but they are most likely receiving lidocaine or articaine, which has increased perfusion in bone.

The approach to a patient who reports a specific allergy to lidocaine is to take a careful history to determine if a vasovagal or epinephrine reaction may be the actual cause of the patient's adverse experience. Referral to an allergist is rarely indicated, except for someone with a history consistent with a life-threatening type of allergic reaction. It is reasonable to try a test injection of a small amount of lidocaine (from a single-use vial), because true systemic lidocaine reactions are so rare.

BOX 3-1 *Nerve Blocks*

Advantages

- Anesthetizes the nerve before it reaches the operative site.
- Affects a large area with small amount of anesthetic.
- No distortion of operative site.

Disadvantages

- No vasoconstriction.
- Longer onset.
- Shorter duration.
- Risk of nerve laceration.

Technique: General Principles

- Use lidocaine and/or longer acting anesthetic.
- Use a 5-mL syringe.
- Use a 27- or 30-gauge ½-inch needle.
- Inject slowly into subcutaneous plane in vicinity of nerve.
- Avoid directly hitting the nerve (back off if sharp pain when inserting needle).
- Do not inject directly into the foramen.
- Pull back on the plunger before infiltrating.
- Wait 10 to 15 minutes for the full effect.

Source: Adapted from Vidimos A, Ammirati C, Pobleti-Lopez C. *Dermatologic Surgery*. Philadelphia: Elsevier; 2009.

An alternative to lidocaine is injectable diphenhydramine (Benadryl) or normal saline. Diphenhydramine provides adequate short-term anesthesia, but it may cause the patient to become drowsy. When normal saline is injected to induce a firm wheal, it provides a few minutes of anesthesia as well.

NERVE BLOCKS

See video on the DVD for further learning. 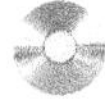

Digital blocks and regional blocks are examples of nerve blocks (see Boxes 3-1 to 3-5). The advantages of a nerve block are that it provides a longer duration of anesthesia and does not distort the anatomic landmarks.

BOX 3-2 *Supraorbital/Supratrochlear Nerve Block (V1)*

Provides sensation to forehead.

Indications

- Laser resurfacing.
- Large surgical defects.

Location

- Supraorbital nerve—midpupillary line along superior bony orbit.
- Supratrochlear nerve—superior/medial corner of bony orbit.

Technique: General Principles

- Inject about 1 mL lidocaine (±epinephrine) in subcutaneous fat overlying supraorbital foramen.
- Inject about 1 mL at root of nose/medial border of orbit.

Source: Adapted from Vidimos A, Ammirati C, Pobleti-Lopez C. *Dermatologic Surgery*. Philadelphia: Elsevier; 2009.

BOX 3-3 *Infraorbital Block (V2)*

Provides sensation to lower eyelid, medial cheek, nose, and upper lip.

Indications

- Fillers.
- Laser resurfacing.
- Large surgical defects.

Location

- Foramen is 1 cm inferior to the infraorbital ridge along the midpupillary line.

Technique: General Principles

- Approach through the oral cavity.
- The nerve is 0.5 to 1 cm above superior labial sulcus.
- Anesthetize oral mucosa with topical benzocaine first.
- Enter at apex of first bicuspid and direct needle toward estimated location of foramen.
- Inject 1 to 2 mL with a ½-inch needle (27 or 30 gauge).

Source: Adapted from Vidimos A, Ammirati C, Pobleti-Lopez C. *Dermatologic Surgery*. Philadelphia: Elsevier; 2009.

BOX 3-4 *Mental Nerve Block (V3)*

Sensation to lower lip, chin, and mucous membranes.

Indications

- Fillers.
- Laser resurfacing.
- Large surgical defects.

Location

- Midway between upper and lower edge of mandible below second bicuspid (midpupillary line).

Technique: General Principles

- Approach through the oral cavity.
- Anesthetize oral mucosa with topical benzocaine first.
- 27- or 30-gauge ½-inch needle.
- Enter inferior labial sulcus between first and second bicuspids.
- Inject 1 to 2 mL around mental foramen.

Source: Adapted from Vidimos A, Ammirati C, Pobleti-Lopez C. *Dermatologic Surgery*. Philadelphia: Elsevier; 2009.

BOX 3-5 *Digital Block*

Paired dorsal and medial digital nerves.

Indications

- Nail plate avulsion.
- Nail unit biopsy.
- Distal digit surgery.
- Periungual warts.

Technique: General Principles

- Use *plain* lidocaine 1% or 2%.
- Use a 5-mL syringe.
- Use a 27- or 30-gauge needle.
- Apply topical anesthesia or ice prior to injecting.
- Use no more than 5 mL total volume.

Source: Adapted from Vidimos A, Ammirati C, Pobleti-Lopez C. *Dermatologic Surgery*. Philadelphia: Elsevier; 2009.

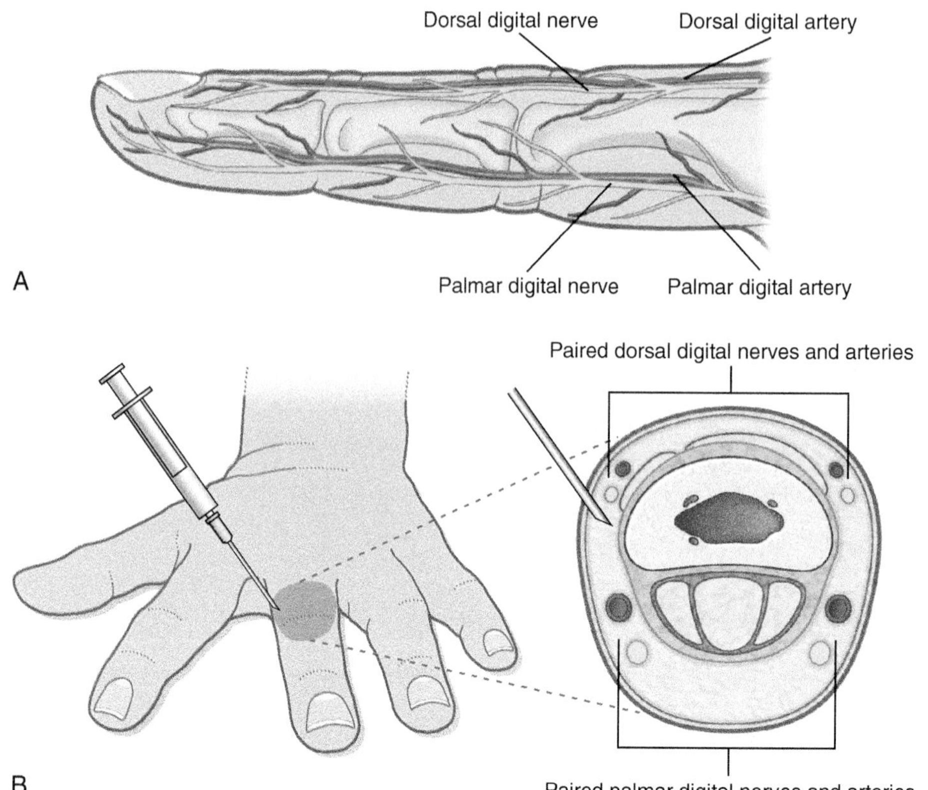

FIGURE 3-5 Digital innervation and nerve block. **(A)** Dorsal and palmar digital arteries and nerves run together. **(B)** A dorsal approach for administration of a digital nerve block allows anesthesia of dorsal and palmar bundles with one puncture. *(From Robinson J, Hanke CW, Siegel D, Fratila A.* Surgery of the Skin. *London: Mosby; 2010.)*

The digital block can be more effective than a local injection on the digit especially for surgery around the nail. Anesthetizing the digital nerves with lidocaine will almost always provide good anesthesia. Injection on each side of the digit with lidocaine will anesthetize both dorsal and ventral nerves on either side of the digit (Figure 3-5). A 3- to 5-mL syringe may be used with 1% or 2% lidocaine, delivering 1.0 to 1.5 mL on each side of the digit and 1.0 mL on the top (Figure 3-6).

A wing block is an alterative for surgery on any part of the nail unit (Figure 3-7). The main advantage over a digital block is that it provides better hemostasis at the site of surgery regardless of whether or not epinephrine is used. Some clinicians will use half-strength epinephrine by mixing 2% lidocaine with 1% lidocaine with epinephrine in a 1 : 1 solution. Wing blocks work faster than a digital block, but the injection usually hurts more at first. A wing block can be performed after a digital block to help with hemostasis and to ensure excellent anesthesia (see Chapter 18, *Nail Procedures*).

Regional blocks (i.e., infraorbital, supraorbital, or mental nerve blocks) are helpful when a larger area of the face is to be anesthetized and anatomic distortion is to be avoided. For that reason, facial regional blocks are very helpful for cosmetic procedures involving fillers and ablative lasers. These blocks can be done with a small amount of 1% or 2% lidocaine (0.5 to 1.0 mL) without epinephrine. See Figure 3-8 for a guide on where to inject for these blocks. The clinician should be aware that these blocks do not assist in hemostasis so

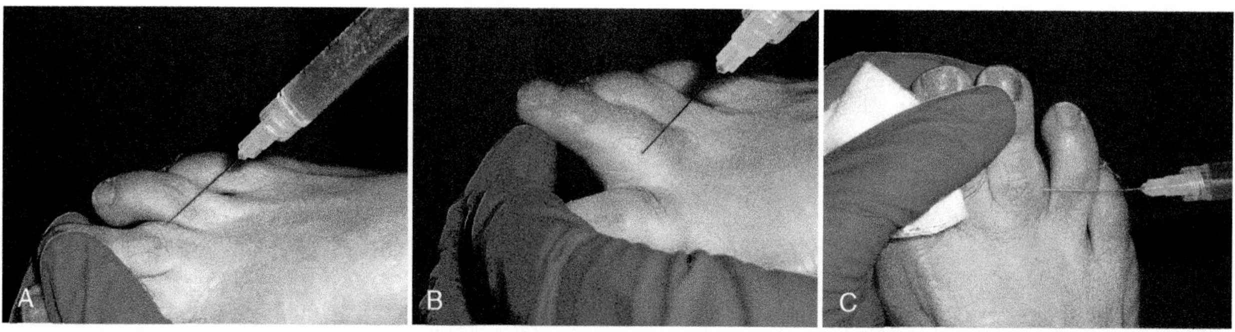

FIGURE 3-6 Three steps of a digital block prior to nail matrix biopsy for longitudinal melanonychia. **(A)** Injection into the affected side. **(B)** Injection into the other side of the digit. **(C)** Anesthetizing the nerves that run on the dorsum of the toe.

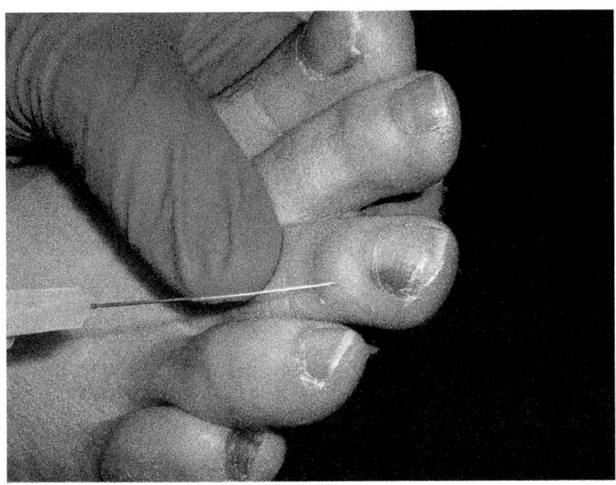

FIGURE 3-7 Prior to a nail matrix biopsy, a wing block ensures that the procedure is painless and minimizes bleeding during the procedure. Lidocaine with half-strength epinephrine is used.

some lidocaine with epinephrine may still be useful at the local area as an adjunct to the regional block. Regional blocks can be done through the skin as in Figure 3-8 or using an intraoral approach as in Figure 3-9. Oral surgeons regularly use the intraoral approach (Figure 3-10). See Chapter 20, *Anesthesia for Cosmetic Procedures,* for more additional information on these blocks.

Field or Ring Block

See video on the DVD for further learning. 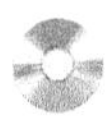

A field block creates a "wall" of anesthesia around an area to be anesthetized. Rather than injecting the anesthetic directly into the area to be numbed, the anesthetic is injected around it to affect the nerves that normally transmit sensations of pain and touch (Figure 3-11). A field block is useful when it is necessary to avoid distorting the tissue to be cut, in cases of infection, and in locations where local anesthesia may not work adequately. Epinephrine is used with lidocaine to decrease bleeding.

The ring block is especially useful before draining an abscess or removing a deep epidermal cyst. The acid environment of the abscess can hydrolyze the anesthetic. The field block allows the anesthetic to work on normal surrounding tissue and avoids the problem of distending the abscess further by keeping the anesthetic out of the abscess cavity. A 27-gauge, 1½-inch needle is useful for administering a field block. In Figure 3-11, the ring block injections are marked on the skin. Each subsequent injection goes into an area that was previously anesthetized. This method also minimizes the chance that you will be sprayed by the contents of a distended abscess or cyst.

Pregnancy and Lactation

Local anesthetics can cross the placental membrane by passive diffusion. Shave and punch biopsies involve such a small amount of local anesthetic that there is little risk to the fetus. Lidocaine is pregnancy category B and epinephrine is pregnancy category C. Epinephrine should be used conservatively, because large doses can cause decreased placental perfusion. Elective and large procedures are best delayed until after delivery.[14]

Lidocaine and epinephrine are excreted in breast milk and should be used with caution in women who

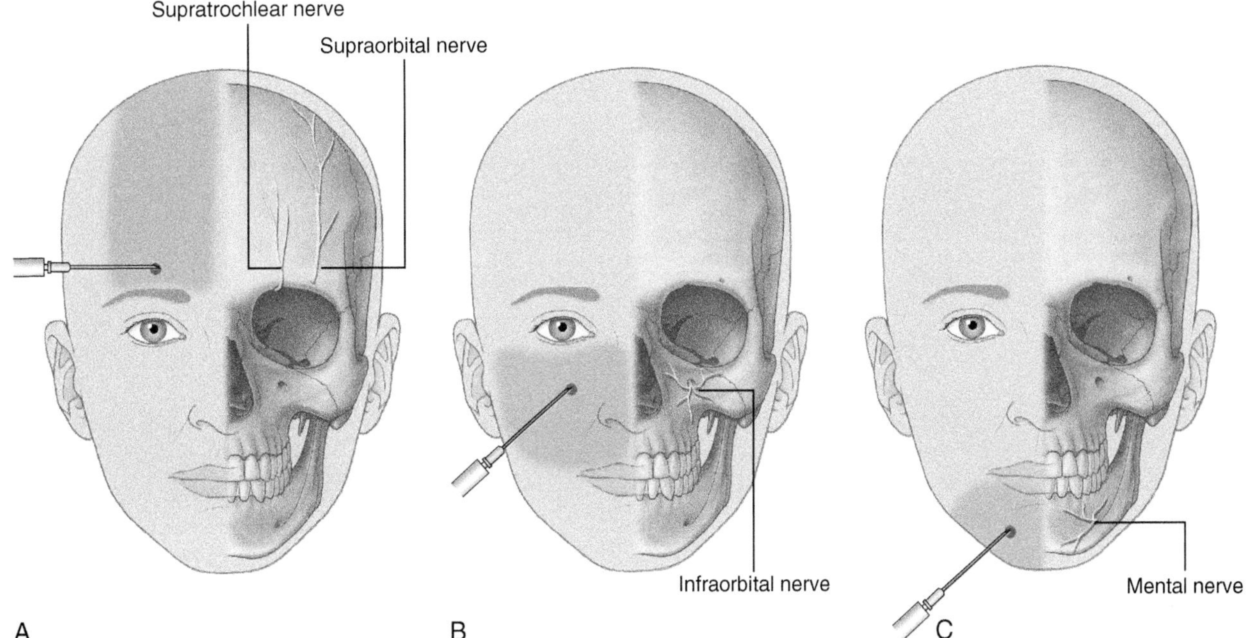

FIGURE 3-8 Location and sensory distribution for nerve blocks. (A) Supraorbital and supratrochlear nerve block. (B) Infraorbital nerve block (follow the midpupillary line). (C) Mental nerve block. *(From Robinson J, Hanke CW, Siegel D, Fratila A.* Surgery of the Skin. *London: Mosby; 2010.)*

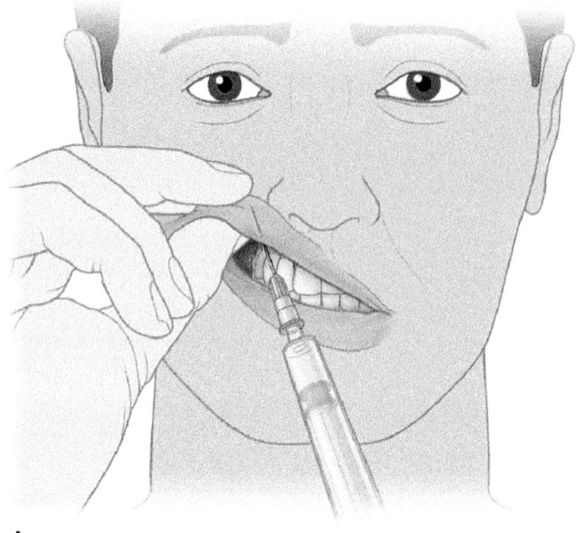

A

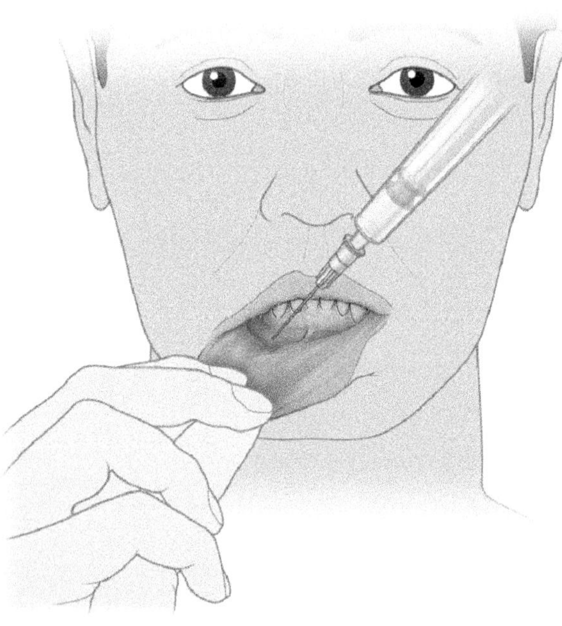

B

FIGURE 3-9 Intraoral route for blocking infraorbital and mental nerves. *(From Robinson J, Hanke CW, Siegel D, Fratila A. Surgery of the Skin. London: Mosby; 2010.)*

are nursing. If a procedure with local anesthesia is needed, the woman may pump her breast milk several hours after the procedure and discard the expressed milk.[14]

SUMMARY OF MATERIALS

Most Useful Anesthetics

- Topical anesthetics: EMLA, topical lidocaine gel.
- Injectable anesthetics, especially 1% lidocaine with epinephrine and 2% lidocaine without epinephrine for digital blocks.

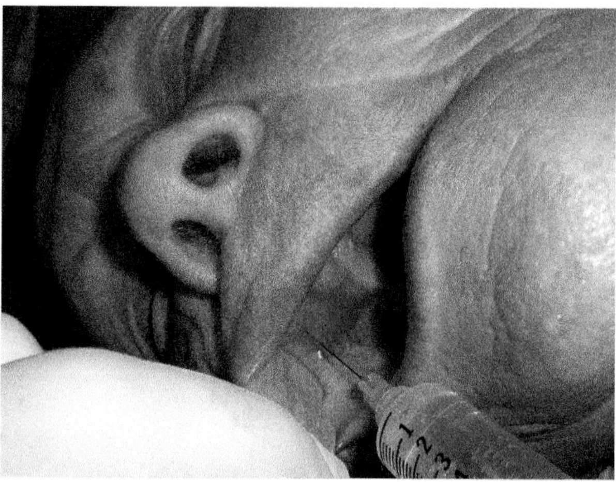

FIGURE 3-10 An intraoral infraorbital block performed using 2% lidocaine. Note that this patient is edentulous. The amount of anesthetic needed is only 1 mL.

Needles

- An 18- to 22-gauge needle is useful for drawing up anesthetic from a vial.
- The 27- and 30-gauge needles are optimal for most local injections, digital blocks, and field blocks (27-gauge × 1.25 inch and 30-gauge × 1 inch are excellent). We use the 30-gauge needles on the face, genitalia, and for any small procedure and reserve the 27-gauge needles for the trunk and extremities when larger volumes need to be injected.

Syringes

- A 3-mL syringe is optimal for most shave biopsies.
- A 5-mL or 6-mL syringe is adequate for most punch biopsies.
- A 10-mL or 12-mL syringe may be helpful with elliptical excisions.

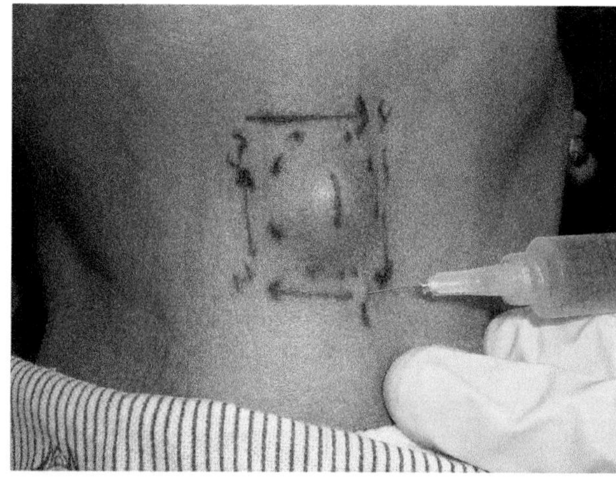

FIGURE 3-11 A ring block around an epidermal inclusion cyst. Arrows are marked to see where each of the four injections will take place to create a circumferential block. This method helps to anesthetize the whole area and avoids injecting lidocaine directly into the cyst—which is not needed and increases the chance that the cyst will squirt fluid at the surgeon doing the procedure.

See Chapter 2 for a list of distributors of surgical and anesthetic supplies.

CONCLUSION

A thorough understanding of the techniques for administering local anesthesia is essential for the performance of painless skin surgery. A safely and properly anesthetized patient will allow for the most controlled and highest quality surgery. Keeping the patient comfortable will create a happy customer and help to establish a good relationship with the health care provider.

References

1. Carter EL, Coppola CA, Barsanti FA. A randomized, double-blind comparison of two topical anesthetic formulations prior to electrodesiccation of dermatosis papulosa nigra. *Dermatol Surg.* 2006;32:1–6.
2. Howe NR, Williams JM. Pain of injection and duration of anesthesia for intradermal infiltration of lidocaine, bupivacaine, and etidocaine. *J Dermatol Surg Oncol.* 1994;20:459–464.
3. Achar S, Kundu S. Principles of office anesthesia: part I. Infiltrative anesthesia. *Am Fam Physician.* 2002;66:91–94.
4. Ghali S, Knox KR, Verbesey J, *et al.* Effects of lidocaine and epinephrine on cutaneous blood flow. *J Plast Reconstr Aesthet Surg.* 2008;61:1226–1231.
5. Bartfield JM, Sokaris SJ, Raccio-Robak N. Local anesthesia for lacerations: pain of infiltration inside vs outside the wound. *Acad Emerg Med.* 1998;5:100–104.
6. Bartfield JM, Homer PJ, Ford DT, Sternklar P. Buffered lidocaine as a local anesthetic: an investigation of shelf life. *Ann Emerg Med.* 1992;21:16–19.
7. Yang CH, Hsu HC, Shen SC, *et al.* Warm and neutral tumescent anesthetic solutions are essential factors for a less painful injection. *Dermatol Surg.* 2006;32:1119–1122.
8. Mader TJ, Playe SJ, Garb JL. Reducing the pain of local anesthetic infiltration: warming and buffering have a synergistic effect. *Ann Emerg Med.* 1994;23:550–554.
9. Colaric KB, Overton DT, Moore K. Pain reduction in lidocaine administration through buffering and warming. *Am J Emerg Med.* 1998;16:353–356.
10. Bartfield JM, Crisafulli KM, Raccio-Robak N, Salluzzo RF. The effects of warming and buffering on pain of infiltration of lidocaine. *Acad Emerg Med.* 1995;2:254–258.
11. Krunic AL, Wang LC, Soltani K, *et al.* Digital anesthesia with epinephrine: an old myth revisited. *J Am Acad Dermatol.* 2004; 51:755–759.
12. Thomson CJ, Lalonde DH, Denkler KA, Feicht AJ. A critical look at the evidence for and against elective epinephrine use in the finger. *Plast Reconstr Surg.* 2007;119:260–266.
13. Lalonde D, Bell M, Benoit P, *et al.* A multicenter prospective study of 3,110 consecutive cases of elective epinephrine use in the fingers and hand: the Dalhousie Project clinical phase. *J Hand Surg [Am].* 2005;30:1061–1067.
14. Vidimos A, Ammirati C, Pobleti-Lopez C. Dermatologic Surgery. Philadelphia: Elsevier; 2009.

4 Hemostasis

RICHARD P. USATINE, MD

Achieving hemostasis is an essential component of all surgery. The goal of hemostasis in surgery is to control bleeding while avoiding unnecessary tissue destruction. It is important to understand the advantages and disadvantages of all methods of hemostasis to be able to choose the appropriate methods for each surgical situation. Hemostasis can be achieved by chemical agents that produce superficial hemostasis or by electrocoagulation for deeper hemostasis. Hemostasis may also be achieved by physical methods that involve pressure, sutures, or gelatin sponges.

TYPES OF HEMOSTASIS

- Chemical/topical
- Electrocoagulation
- Direct pressure or pressure dressing
- Sutures and ties
- Physical agents (gelatin sponge).

CHEMICAL HEMOSTATIC AGENTS

- Aluminum chloride (preferred agent)
- Monsel's solution (ferric subsulfate).
- Silver nitrate sticks (not recommended; see discussion in text).

General Principles of Chemical Hemostasis

Chemical hemostatic agents work by causing protein precipitation, which stops the bleeding. These agents work best in a dry field, allowing the chemical to go directly to the bleeding tissue without being diluted by pooled blood. Chemical agents are useful after a shave biopsy or a small punch biopsy. Chemical agents should not be used in deep wounds that will be closed with sutures.

All of the hemostatic chemicals can be damaging to the eye. Exercise great caution when using chemical agents after a shave or snip (scissors) biopsy on the eyelids or near the eye. The chemical from a dripping cotton-tipped applicator can run into the eye when the biopsy is close to the globe. The Cryo Tweezer described in Chapter 15 is a preferred method for treating skin tags or warts around the eye to avoid chemical exposures. Using electrosurgery for hemostasis can also keep chemicals away from the eye. If aluminum chloride is to be used in this location, dry off the chemical agent on the cotton-tipped applicator with a gauze pad before carefully touching the cotton-tipped applicator to the eyelid or periocular skin. If any chemical does get into the eye, the eye should be flushed immediately.

Aluminum Chloride

See video on the DVD for further learning. 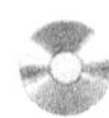

Aluminum chloride comes in strengths from 20% to 70% available in water- or alcohol-based solutions (Figure 4-1). Alcohol alone (anhydrous alcohol) will support a solution of up to 20%, so the stronger concentrations are either in water or a mixture of water and alcohol. I prefer to use aluminum chloride in an aqueous solution because it can be used safely with electrosurgery and comes in higher concentrations. With an alcohol-based solution, it is possible to ignite the alcohol when electrosurgery is performed in the same field. However, drying the field after applying the alcohol-based solution makes it safe to use with electrosurgery.

Aqueous aluminum chloride can be ordered as a 35% or 70% solution from Delasco (see the *Resources* section at the end of the chapter for ordering information). Both are inexpensive and excellent for hemostasis. No studies are available to determine whether one percentage is better than another. I use 70% with good results. These solutions have a 3-year shelf life. Drysol, the brand name of 20% aluminum chloride in anhydrous ethyl alcohol that is sold by prescription to treat hyperhidrosis, also produces hemostasis but is more expensive to purchase and messier to use.

The major advantage of aluminum chloride is that it is a clear solution that does not stain or tattoo the tissue. It does not cause tissue necrosis and does not damage the normal skin surrounding the wound. Aluminum chloride should not be used in deep wounds that will be sutured because it can delay healing and increase scarring.[1]

When using aluminum chloride after a shave or punch biopsy, first dry the field with a cotton-tipped applicator or gauze. The aluminum chloride should then be applied to the dry field by rolling or twisting the moist applicator against the open wound (Figure 4-2). Although light pressure may work, it often helps to use heavier pressure while twisting the applicator clockwise and counterclockwise against the area. After a 2- to 4-mm punch biopsy, a dry cotton-tipped applicator can be held with downward pressure against the open hole to dry the field. If sutures are not to be used, the aluminum chloride should be applied with downward pressure and held against the wound until hemostasis is achieved (Figure 4-3).

Monsel's Solution

Monsel's solution consists of 20% ferric subsulfate. It is used to produce hemostasis after biopsies of the skin and cervix. It is applied to the skin in the same manner

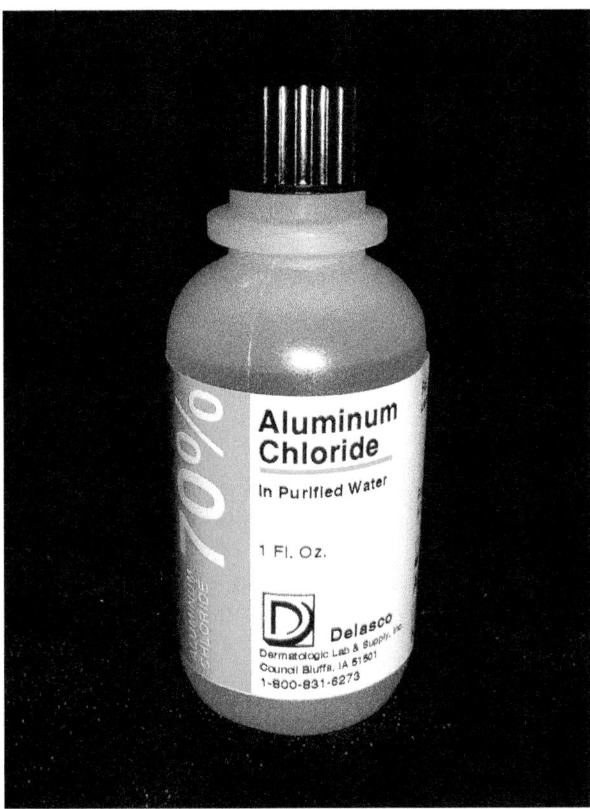

FIGURE 4-1 70% aluminum chloride in purified water is a useful topical hemostatic agent. *(Copyright Richard P. Usatine, MD.)*

as aluminum chloride. There is a small risk of tattooing the skin through iron deposition. One major nuisance in using Monsel's solution is that the iron precipitates around the top of the container, making it difficult to open. Aluminum chloride containers are always easy to open.

Monsel's solution can leave a histologic artifact in the skin. Therefore, when a repeat biopsy is performed in an area where Monsel's solution was previously used, it helps to warn the pathologist.[1]

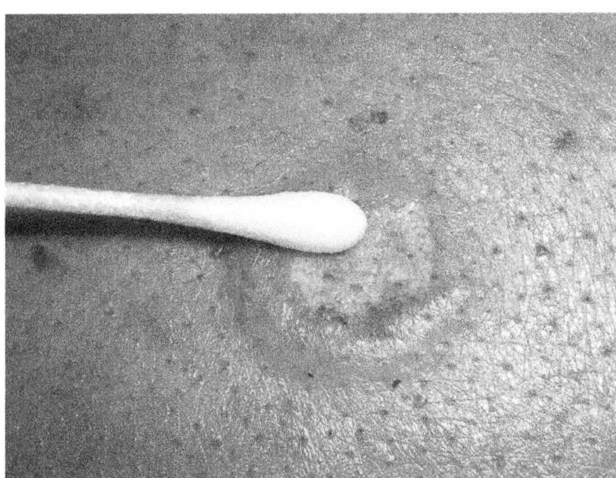

FIGURE 4-2 Clear aluminum chloride on a cotton-tipped applicator being used to stop bleeding after shave excision of a seborrheic keratosis. *(Copyright Richard P. Usatine, MD.)*

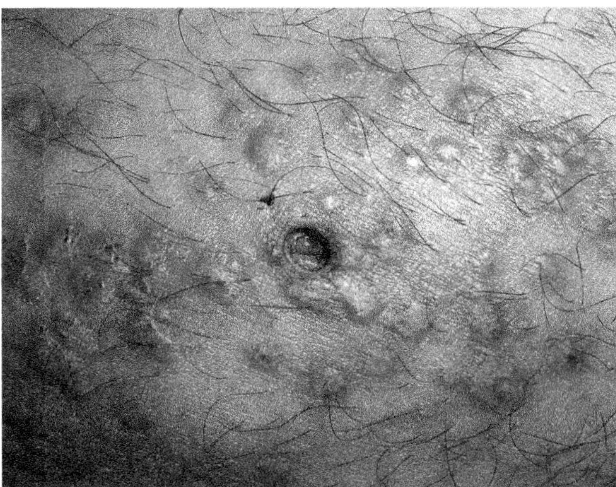

FIGURE 4-3 A 4-mm punch biopsy being left open to heal by secondary intention. Hemostasis was achieved using aluminum chloride. *(Copyright Richard P. Usatine, MD.)*

Silver Nitrate

Silver nitrate comes in easy-to-use sticks. Its hemostatic action is slower and the response to it is more variable. Silver nitrate may tattoo the skin black with silver. Silver nitrate has been used to treat umbilical granulomas in infants, but there are better and safer options.[2]

ELECTROCOAGULATION

See video on the DVD for further learning. 

Electrocoagulation is an ideal method for controlling bleeding during surgery. This is especially true with an excision that will be closed with sutures. Electrocoagulation is essential in most elliptical excisions and all flaps. During surgery, electrocoagulation helps to produce a relatively bloodless field (Figure 4-4). This helps to see the landmarks for placing both deep and superficial sutures. Electrocoagulation can prevent

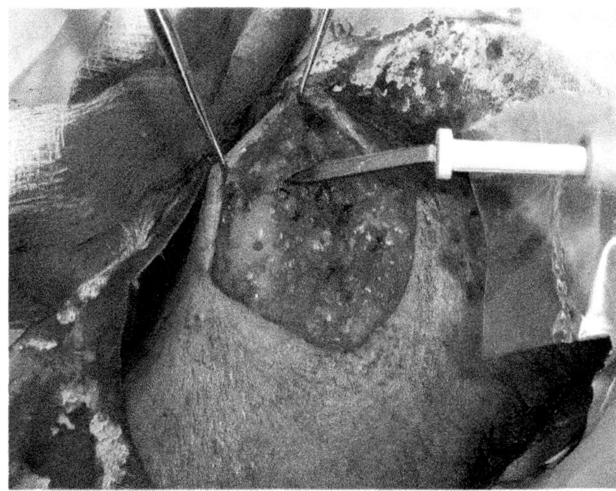

FIGURE 4-4 An electrosurgical instrument is being used to stop bleeders after undermining the wound edges. Note that the surgical assistant is using two skin hooks to hold open the undermined skin while the clinician is using the Hyfrecator to stop the bleeding. *(Copyright Richard P. Usatine, MD.)*

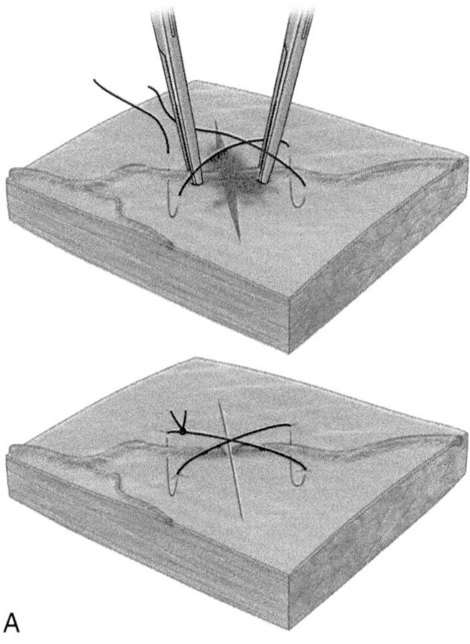

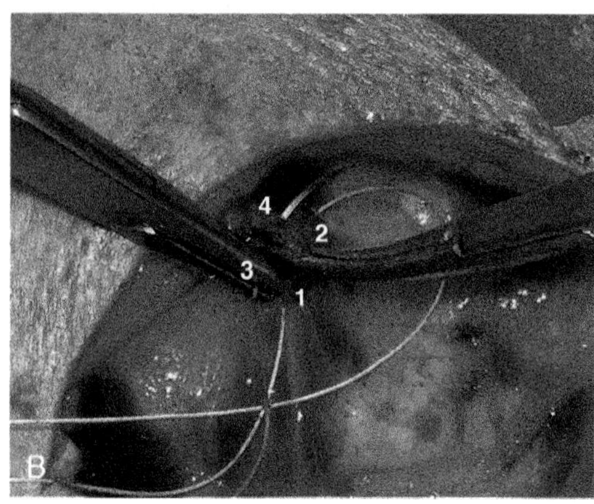

FIGURE 4-5 The figure-of-eight suture can be used to stop bleeding with absorbable suture below the epidermis or nonabsorbable suture on the surface. **(A)** A figure-of-eight suture pulls tissue together to tamponade bleeding vessels. **(B)** Start the figure-of-eight suture by clamping the bleeding vessel or tissue with one or two hemostats. The bleeding should stop before proceeding with the suture. Insert the needle with absorbable suture at #1 going under the hemostat and exiting the tissue at #2. Reload the needle and insert the needle at #3 and exit at #4 with the second stitch parallel to the first. Then tie the suture between points #1 and #4, creating the crossover figure-of-eight suture. The hemostat may be released once the first or second tie is in place. *(**A:** From Robinson J, Hanke W, Sengelmann R, Siegel D.* Surgery of the Skin: Procedural Dermatology, *2nd ed. Philadelphia: Mosby; 2010;* ***B:*** *Copyright Richard P. Usatine, MD.)*

See video on the DVD for further learning.

postoperative bleeding and hematoma formation. Patients should, however, still be given information on what to do if postoperative bleeding occurs and a number to call if help is needed.

Electrosurgery is an alternative method of hemostasis after a shave biopsy. It can also be used as a backup in the rare instance in which chemical agents fail to provide hemostasis after a shave. First dry the surgical field with a cotton-tipped applicator or gauze before using electrosurgery, especially after a chemical agent in an alcohol solution has been used.

Electrosurgery is an ideal method for hemostasis when tissue destruction is desired. This is true when shaving off a pyogenic granuloma or hemangioma. The electrodestruction diminishes the likelihood of regrowth of vascular tissue while achieving hemostasis. Another example of this is during electrodesiccation and curettage of a basal cell carcinoma (BCC). The electrodesiccation simultaneously destroys malignant tissue and produces hemostasis. (See Chapter 14, *Electrosurgery*, for further information on this procedure.)

In surgical wounds that need closure, it is important not to use so much electrocoagulation that it produces large areas of char and tissue necrosis. This can increase the risk of wound infection. When a vessel is not responding to electrocoagulation, use a suture. One easy method is to use an absorbable suture with a small figure-of-eight suture around the vessel (Figure 4-5). For example, if you are already using Vicryl for your deep sutures, just use this for the hemostatic stitch. The U-suture (square suture) is another method of obtaining hemostasis with a deep absorbable suture (Figure 4-6).

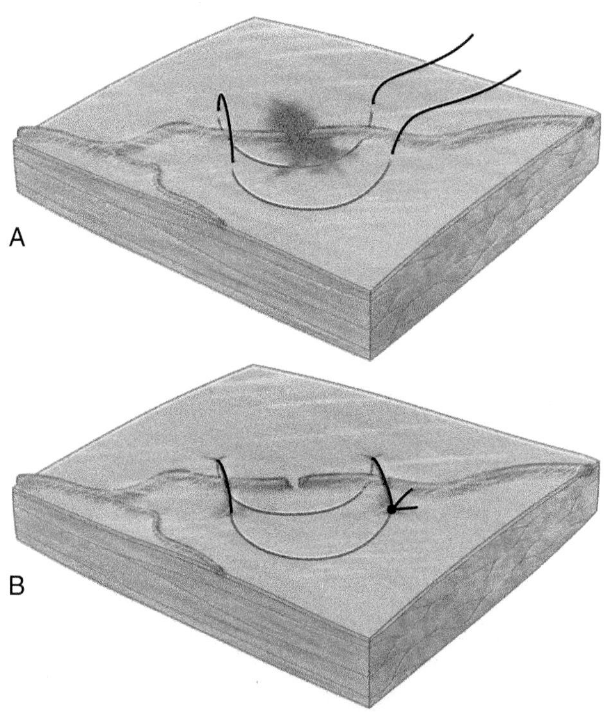

FIGURE 4-6 The U-suture (square suture) is one way to stop bleeding at the edge of an incision similar to the horizontal mattress suture. It can also be placed deep with an absorbable suture. *(From Robinson J, Hanke W, Sengelmann R, Siegel D.* Surgery of the Skin: Procedural Dermatology, *2nd ed. Philadelphia: Mosby; 2010.)*

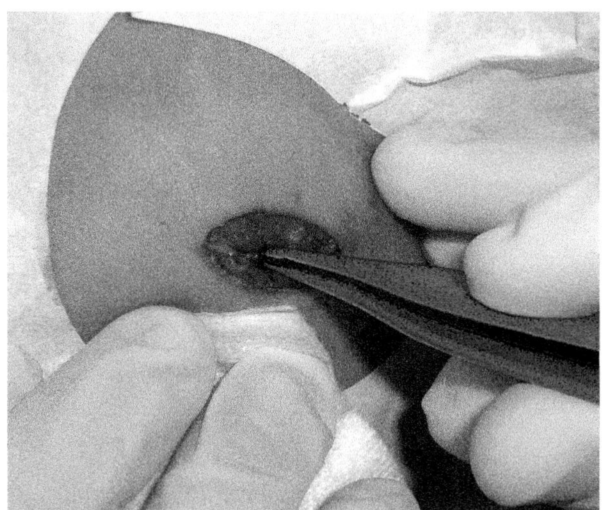

FIGURE 4-7 Bipolar forceps are useful for focused hemostasis and safer when the patient has a pacemaker. *(Copyright Richard P. Usatine, MD.)*

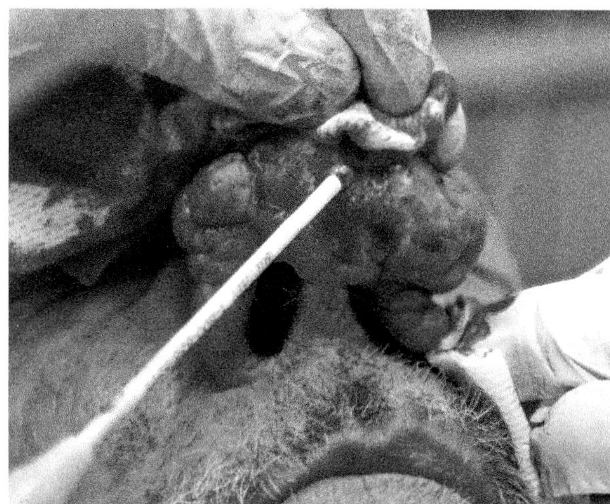

FIGURE 4-8 Ball electrode used on a radio-frequency electrosurgery device for electrocoagulation in a wet field. *(Copyright Richard P. Usatine, MD.)*

Electrosurgical Equipment and Its Use

Modern electrosurgical equipment uses an alternating current transferred to the patient through cold electrodes. The tissue is heated through tissue resistance to the current. The current used can range from 0.5 to 4 MHz (radio-frequency). The various types of electrosurgical units are covered in detail in Chapter 14.

Regardless of the type of unit used, there are four major ways to produce electrocoagulation:

1. The electrode comes in direct contact with the bleeding site or vessel.
2. The electrode is touched to a hemostat or forceps that is grasping the bleeding tissue or vessel and then activated.
3. Special bipolar forceps are used to grasp the tissue and are activated with a foot peddle (Figure 4-7).
4. Use "cut and coagulation" with an electrosurgical unit that can cut tissue and produce hemostasis simultaneously (see Chapter 14).

Working in a Bloody Field

Bipolar forceps have the advantage of working in a bloody field that is not entirely dry (Figure 4-7). It is still best to dry the field as much as possible, but the current can still pass through the bleeding tissue despite the presence of blood. The ball electrode on the Surgitron can also work in a bloody field (Figure 4-8). When a standard electrode is not working because the field has too much blood, it may help to grasp the bleeding tissue with a hemostat or forceps and direct the current through the instrument to stop the bleeding. The bipolar forceps is the safest method to use in a patient with a pacemaker or implantable defibrillator (see Chapter 14, *Electrosurgery*).

In Figure 4-9, a pyogenic granuloma was just shaved off the lip of a postpartum woman. A dry cotton-tipped applicator was rolled ahead of the electrode with pressure to dry the field for electrocoagulation with a Hyfrecator electrode. Because this was a very vascular lesion, the electrocoagulation was applied as the cotton-tipped applicator was lifted from the bleeding site.

Because a shave excision does not need to be a sterile procedure, the handpiece and the electrode should be clean but do not have to be sterile. However, when doing an excision in which sutures will be placed, the electrode must be sterile and the handpiece needs to be sterile or covered in a sterile sheath. Most cutting units have a handpiece that can be sterilized in an autoclave. Con-Med, which manufactures the Hyfrecator Plus, produces sterile handpiece sheaths to be used in sterile surgical procedures. A sterile surgical glove may also be used as a sterile sheath. Just drop the handpiece through one of the longer fingers on the glove.

To summarize, electrocoagulation should be used in the following situations:

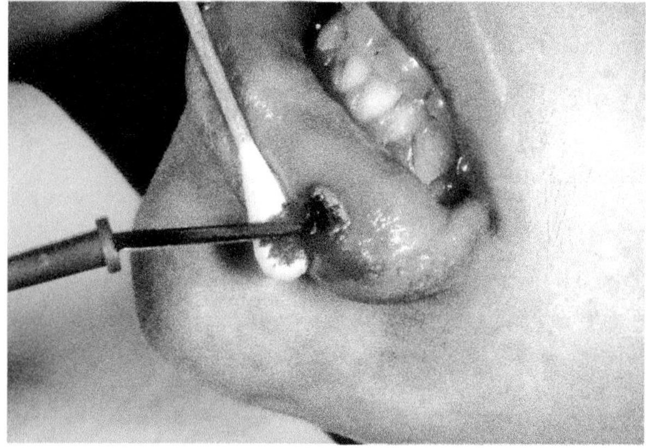

FIGURE 4-9 After excising a pyogenic granuloma from the lip, a Hyfrecator is used to destroy any remaining abnormal tissue and to achieve hemostasis. Note that the cotton-tipped applicator is being rolled just ahead of the electrosurgical electrode. *(Copyright Richard P. Usatine, MD.)*

- In a wound that will be closed with sutures
- To obtain a bloodless field during surgery
- To prevent postoperative bleeding and hematomas
- When the chemical hemostatic agent fails after a shave or punch biopsy
- When tissue destruction is desired (e.g., with removal of a BCC or a pyogenic granuloma).

When using electrocoagulation near the eye, the physician should be aware that the spark will arc to the area closest to the electrode. Make sure that the treatment area is closer to the electrode than the globe. A spark to the globe is potentially damaging to the eye.

MECHANICAL HEMOSTASIS: PRESSURE AND SUTURES

The direct application of pressure works to slow and stop bleeding in many surgical procedures. A large blood vessel that does not stop bleeding with electrocoagulation can be ligated. Suturing a wound is a form of pressure application that brings the two open sides in direct opposition to each other. Packing an open wound (such as a drained abscess) also is a form of direct application of internal pressure.

After suturing an elliptical excision, it is wise to apply a pressure dressing to decrease the risk of hematoma formation. This can be left in place for 24 hours and is described further in Chapter 35, *Wound Care*. We recommend that patients apply direct pressure for 5 to 10 minutes by the clock if postoperative bleeding occurs at home. Increasingly longer periods of time can be attempted as needed. Of course, if the bleeding continues patients will need to access direct care.

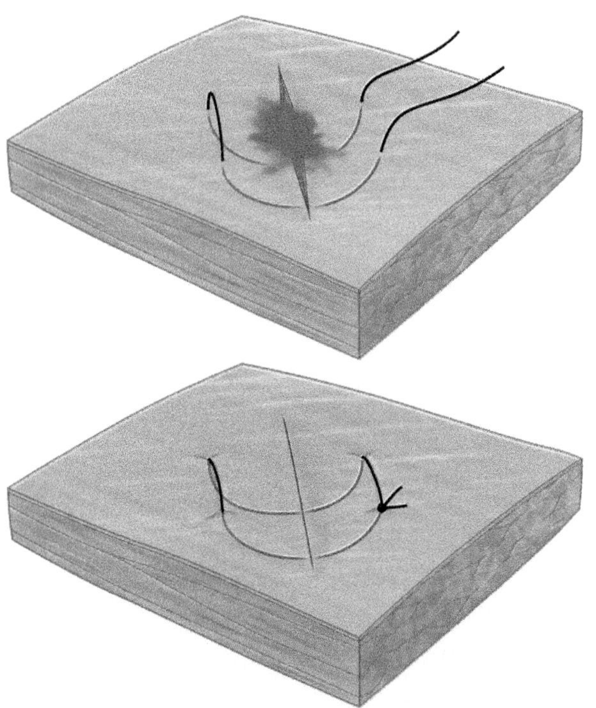

FIGURE 4-10 A horizontal mattress suture can be used to minimize oozing at the cut edges. *(From Robinson J, Hanke W, Sengelmann R, Siegel D.* Surgery of the Skin: Procedural Dermatology, *2nd ed. Philadelphia: Mosby; 2010.)*

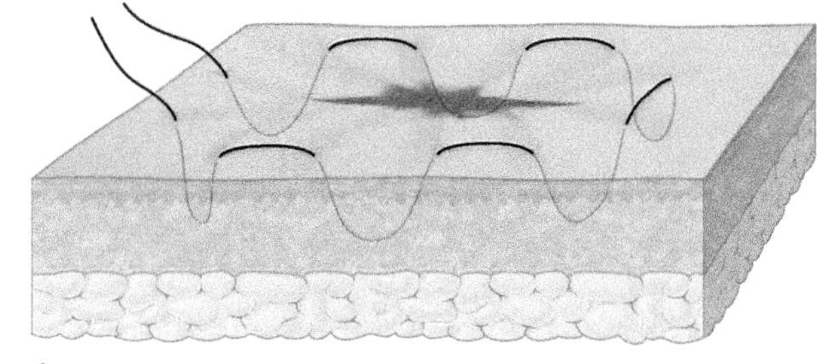

A

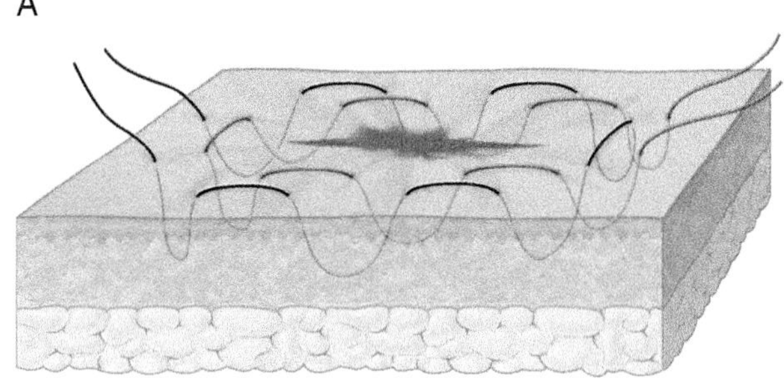

B

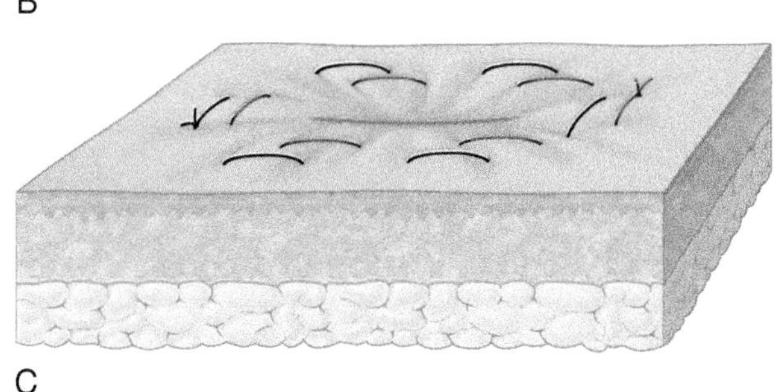

C

FIGURE 4-11 A double purse-string suture can be used when other methods fail. A 3-0 or 4-0 Prolene suture with PS-2 needle is useful for this technique. **(A)** The first purse string is placed around the central lesion, with both ends of suture terminating on one side of the lesion. **(B)** The second purse string is begun on the opposite end of the first suture and placed around the central lesion. **(C)** Hemostasis is achieved as both purse-string ends are cinched tight, tamponading the vessels peripheral to the centrally excised lesion. *(From Robinson J, Hanke W, Sengelmann R, Siegel D.* Surgery of the Skin: Procedural Dermatology, *2nd ed. Philadelphia: Mosby; 2010.)*

In skin surgery, blood vessels may require tying off. It is usually quicker to use the electrosurgery unit for small blood vessels, with the exception of superficial large arteries such as labial or temporal arteries. These vessels can be clamped with a small hemostat and tied off with absorbable sutures. The figure-of-eight suture and U-shaped suture are useful in this setting (Figures 4-5 and 4-6). Horizontal mattress sutures can be used to stop oozing on the edges of the wound and achieve wound eversion (Figure 4-10).

Purse String Stitch

The purse string stitch is depicted in Figure 4-11. A single purse-string suture may be tried at first. A double purse-string suture can be used when other methods fail (Figure 4-11). A 3-0 or 4-0 Prolene suture with at

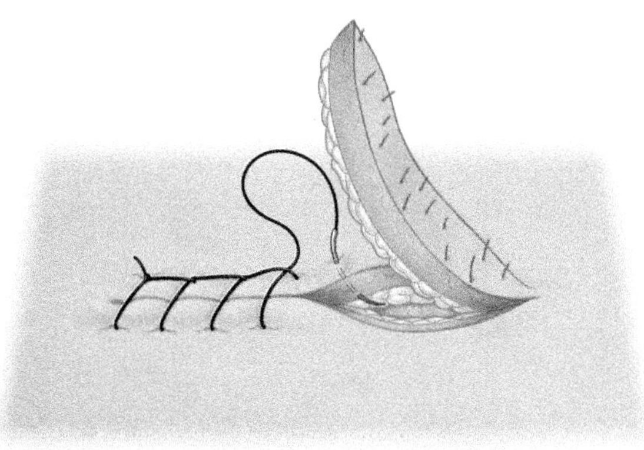

FIGURE 4-12 A running locked suture provides more hemostasis than a running suture that is not locked. *(From Robinson J, Hanke W, Sengelmann R, Siegel D.* Surgery of the Skin: Procedural Dermatology, *2nd ed. Philadelphia: Mosby; 2010.)*

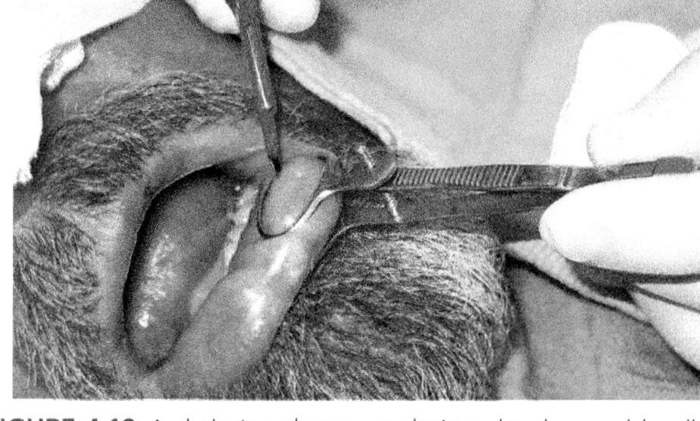

FIGURE 4-13 A chalazion clamp was designed to keep a bloodless field on the eyelid when removing a chalazion. It also can be used on the lip to provide hemostasis during surgery. *(From Robinson J, Hanke W, Sengelmann R, Siegel D.* Surgery of the Skin: Procedural Dermatology, *2nd ed. Philadelphia: Mosby; 2010.)*

least a 16-mm needle is useful for this technique. The first purse string is placed around the central lesion, with both ends of the suture terminating on one side of the lesion. The second purse string is begun on the opposite end of the first suture and placed around the central lesion. Hemostasis is achieved as both purse-string ends are cinched tight, tamponading the vessels peripheral to the centrally excised lesion.[3]

Locked Stitch

A running locked suture (Figure 4-12) provides more hemostasis than a running suture that is not locked. In most skin surgery the locking is not needed and increases the risk of necrosis of the wound edges. When bleeding is continuing despite other methods, the benefits outweigh the risks of locking the sutures.

Using Tourniquets and Clamps to Prevent Bleeding

A chalazion clamp was designed to keep a bloodless field on the eyelid when removing a chalazion. It also can be used on the lip to provide hemostasis during surgery (Figure 4-13). A finger tourniquet can be made with a surgical glove to create a bloodless field for finger surgery (Figure 4-14).

PHYSICAL AGENTS (GELATING SPONGE)

A number of gelatin sponges are sold to produce hemostasis. These include Gelfoam, Helistat, Oxycel, and Avitene. A piece of Gelfoam can be placed into the hole of a punch biopsy that is not sutured. Absorbable hemostats (e.g., Surgicel, Collastat, and Instat) are also available. All of these products are expensive and have no proven advantage over the less expensive chemical agents.

CONCLUSION

Many techniques are available to control bleeding during and after surgery. Judicious application of these hemostatic methods can save time, minimize complications, and maximize the cosmetic outcome of surgery

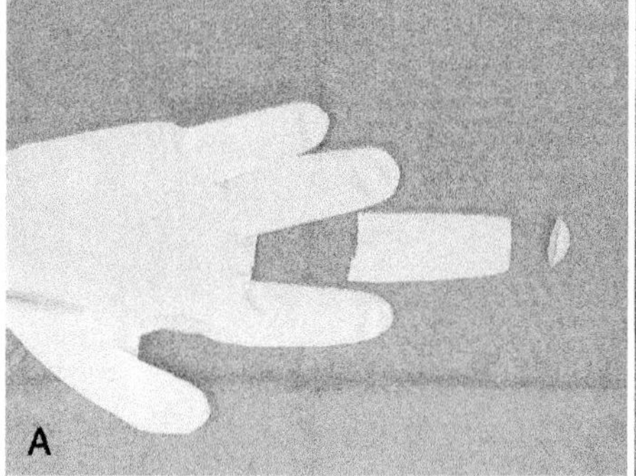

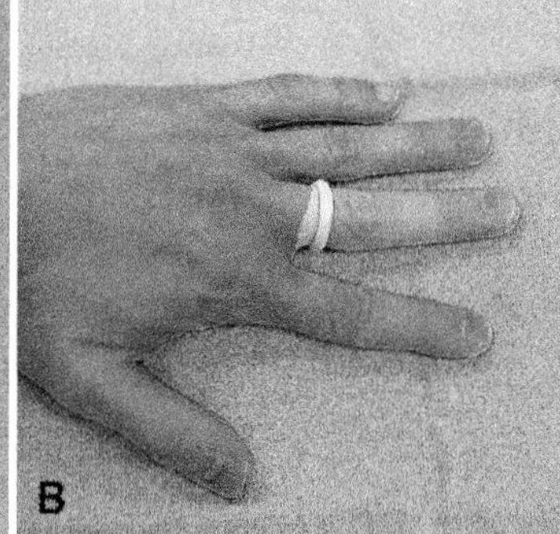

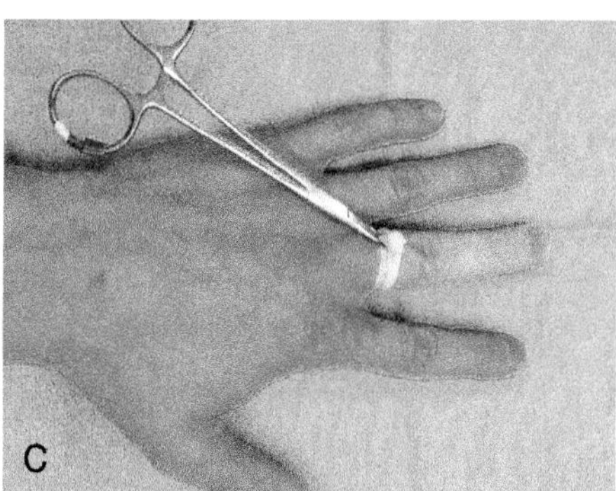

FIGURE 4-14 A finger tourniquet can be made with a surgical glove to create a bloodless field for finger surgery. (A) The middle finger from a surgical glove is severed at both its base and its tip. (B) The finger glove is placed over the treated digit and rolled back proximally, forming the tourniquet. (C) A curved hemostat grasps the ring tourniquet with the loops facing away from the surgical field (optional step—provides additional compression and ensures tourniquet is not forgotten and left in place). *(From Robinson J, Hanke W, Sengelmann R, Siegel D.* Surgery of the Skin: Procedural Dermatology, *2nd ed. Philadelphia: Mosby; 2010.)*

TABLE 4-1 Recommended Hemostasis Methods for Various Procedures

Procedure	Hemostasis Method
Shave biopsy	Aluminum chloride; light electrocoagulation if this fails.
Punch biopsy	If sutured: suturing usually stops bleeding but pressure and/or electrocoagulation may also be needed.
Elliptical excision	If not sutured: pressure, aluminum chloride, and electrosurgery if needed. External pressure and electrocoagulation to produce dry field. Tying off of vessels and bleeding areas as needed. Closing with sutures. Applying external pressure dressing. *Note:* Chemical agents should not be used.
Curettage	Aluminum chloride or electrocoagulation.
Scissor surgery	Aluminum chloride or electrocoagulation (snip surgery).
Incision and drainage	Packing of the wound, which produces hemostasis by pressure.

by reducing unnecessary tissue destruction. A summary of recommended hemostasis methods for various procedures is given in Table 4-1.

Resources

Chemical agents and electrosurgery equipment can be ordered from the Delasco Dermatologic Buying Guide (800-831-6273; www.delasco.com) and from some of the other resources listed in Chapter 2.

References

1. Olmstead PM, Lund HZ, Leonard DD. Monsel's solution: a histologic nuisance. *J Am Acad Dermatol.* 1980;3:492–498.
2. Daniels J. Is silver nitrate the best agent for management of umbilical granulomas? *Arch Dis Child.* 2001;85(5):432.
3. Nguyen T. Hemostasis. In: Robinson J, Hanke W, Sengelmann R, Siegel D, eds. *Surgery of the Skin: Procedural Dermatology*. Philadelphia: Elsevier; 2005:245–258.

5 Suture Material

BRET R. BAACK, MD • DANIEL L. STULBERG, MD •
RICHARD P. USATINE, MD

Many types of sutures are available, each with its own material properties, performance, and uses. The most useful sutures for skin surgery are described in detail in Tables 5-1 and 5-2.

HISTORY

The use of sutures to close wounds is certainly not limited to the modern era. Ancient civilizations developed innovative methods to close wounds based on the materials then available. Horsetail hair threaded onto eyed needles made from bone was utilized by the Greeks as early as 5000 to 3000 B.C. An Egyptian scroll dating back to 3000 B.C. describes the use of linen as suture material.[1] South American Indians essentially created the first surgical "stapler" by using the heads of pincher ants to close wounds. The Roman physician Galen described the use of absorbable suture, specifically catgut, in 175 A.D.[2] Sterile suture material was formally introduced by Lister in 1869 by treating catgut with chromic acid.[3] Interestingly, the benefit of using sterile sutures was discovered during the American Civil War a few years earlier (1861–1865). Due to a lack of available suture material, Confederate surgeons were reduced to using horsetail hair, which they boiled to make more pliable. This inadvertent sterilization of the suture material most likely led to the lower wound infection rate they experienced as compared to their Union colleagues.[4]

WOUND HEALING AND SUTURES

All sutures are foreign bodies and may increase the risk of wound infection if not used properly or left in place too long. The goal is to use the minimum suture required to keep the wound together until it heals. Deep (buried) or subcuticular sutures are beneficial in keeping wounds closed without leaving marks on the skin. External sutures are left in place just long enough to keep the wound closed because each extra day increases the risk of "railroad track" skin marking. Smaller sutures generally leave fewer skin marks and can lead to a better cosmetic result.

Wound healing is described by tensile strength, the force per unit area required to pull a wound apart. Studies show that a wound does not begin to gain significant tensile strength until about 3 weeks after closure at which point it has only 10% of its final tensile strength. Tensile strength increases more quickly after 3 weeks and reaches its maximum strength at around 60 days. It never returns to more than 80% of normal skin.[5] Thus, wounds subject to any tension should usually be closed in two layers: a deeper dermal layer with suture material that will maintain significant strength for 6 to 8 weeks, and a second superficial skin suture that can be removed in 7 days or less without fear of wound disruption. A suture or staple left in the skin for more than 10 days will often allow epithelial cells to grow from the surface down into the dermis along the suture or staple tract, resulting in permanent scar tissue on each side of the incision scar itself and detracting from the final appearance of the healed wound. In addition, a suture that is tied too tight will cause necrosis and subsequent scarring of the enclosed tissue within the loop, resulting in cross-hatch marks, or "railroad tracks." The goal of the superficial suture layer is to carefully approximate the epidermis, not to add significant strength to the closure. The deeper dermal sutures should take nearly all tension off the epidermal closure.

SUTURE MATERIAL PROPERTIES

Suture material is judged by several characteristics:

- Ease of handling and knot-holding ability
- Absorbability
- Breaking strength
- Visibility
- Tissue reactivity.

Ease of Handling and Knot-Holding Ability

These characteristics are generally determined by whether the suture is monofilamentous or multifilamentous. Monofilament sutures are smooth, synthetic in nature, and usually are stiffer and retain a high memory of their original shape within the package. Thus, they have a tendency to partially retain their packaging loop shape, which gets in the way of suturing and can sometimes lead to the dreaded "knot" that forms in the middle of the suture while performing a running stitch. In addition, their "slickness" makes it necessary to tie square knots (at least four ties) or use an extra tie when securing a surgical knot. However, they also tend to slide easily through tissues, cause very little tissue reaction, and do not tend to harbor bacteria on their surface. For these reasons monofilament sutures are preferred for external skin sutures. Multifilamentous sutures are twisted or braided to make them easier to tie and to improve their knot-holding ability, but the trade-off is that they have the potential to harbor bacteria between the strands, leading to an increased wound infection rate.

TABLE 5-1 Characteristics of Absorbable Sutures

Suture	Composition	Color	Absorption + (slow) to ++++ (rapid)	Breaking Strength + (weak) to ++++ (strong)	Tissue Reaction + (low) to ++++ (high)	Uses	Caveats
Braided synthetic Vicryl (Ethicon) Polysorb and Dexon (Syneture)	Copolymer of glycolide and lactide (Vicryl and Polysorb) or homopolymer of glycolic acid (Dexon)	Undyed (white) or dyed (violet or green)	++	+++	++	Interrupted deep dermal closure, oral mucosa, vessel ligation	Use as interrupted rather than running subcuticular suture.
Braided synthetic Vicryl Rapide (Ethicon)	Copolymer of glycolide and lactide	Undyed (white) or dyed (violet or green)	++++	+++	++	Interrupted deep dermal closure, oral mucosa, vessel ligation	Use as interrupted rather than running subcuticular suture. Can be substituted for plain gut due to fast absorption.
Monofilament synthetic PDS II and Monocryl (Ethicon) Maxon, Biosyn, and Caprosyn (Syneture)	Various polymers	Undyed (clear) or dyed (violet)	+ (PDS II, Maxon); ++ (Monocryl, Biosyn); ++++ (Caprosyn)	+ (Caprosyn); ++ (Monocryl, Biosyn); +++ (Maxon)	++	Subcuticular closure, fascia	Causes less tissue reaction, but requires four to five ties for secure knot. Leave knot on outside of skin for subcuticular closure (see text).
Plain gut	Serosa of beef intestine or submucosa of sheep intestine	Light tan	++++	+	++++	Eyelid close to lid margin (where suture removal would be difficult)	Use five ties, because it tends to untie when wet.
Chromic gut	Same as above, but treated with chromic salts to delay absorption	Brown	+++	+	+++	Oral and nasal mucosa	When used inside the mouth, it is usually gone within 1 to 2 weeks.
Fast-absorbing gut	Plain gut treated with heat to facilitate more rapid absorption	Light tan	++++	+	++++	Facial wounds under low tension	Maintains strength for 5 to 7 days and is completely absorbed within 2 to 4 weeks.

TABLE 5-2 Nonabsorbable Sutures

Suture	Composition	Color	Breaking Strength + (weak) to ++++ (strong)	Construction	Caveats
Nylon Ethilon and Nurolon (Ethicon) Dermalon, Monosof, and Surgilon (Syneture)	Synthetic polymer of Nylon 6	Undyed (clear) or dyed (black or blue)	+++	Ethilon and Monosof: black monofilament Dermalon: blue monofilament Nurolon and Surgilon: black braided	Is ideal for epidermal closure.
Polypropylene Prolene (Ethicon) Surgipro (Syneture)	Synthetic polymer of polypropylene (Prolene) or polypropylene and polyethylene (Surgipro)	Undyed (clear) or dyed (blue)	+++	Monofilament	Is ideal for epidermal closure and subcuticular pull-out suture (slides out easier than nylon); also useful in hair-bearing scalp.
Silk	Protein-rich thread spun by silkworms	Black or white	++	Braided	Can be used for closure of oral mucosa, but requires removal. Used mainly for vessel ligation and bowel anastomoses.

Absorbability and Breaking Strength

These terms are somewhat interrelated, as the absorbability of the suture correlates with the breaking strength of the suture with time. The United States Pharmacopeia (USP) officially defines absorbable sutures as those that lose breaking strength within 60 days, whereas nonabsorbable sutures retain their breaking strength beyond 60 days. See Table 5-3 for the details of strength retention and absorption in absorbable sutures. Breaking strength relates to the material used for construction of the suture as well as its diameter. The USP also defines the diameter of sutures. Sutures used for the skin usually range from 3-0 (relatively thick) to 6-0 (relatively thin). The smallest suture now available is 11-0 (about one-third the diameter of a human hair) and is utilized for the microsurgical repair of small blood vessels.

Visibility

Sutures range in visibility from clear, white, or light tan in color, to highly visible sutures that are blue, purple, green, or black. In general, lighter colored sutures are used as buried absorbable sutures in the dermis because a darker color could potentially be seen through the skin. Darker colored nonabsorbable sutures are used for the epidermal closure because their visibility aids in later removal. When suturing a wound in the hair-bearing scalp in an individual with dark hair, use a blue rather than a black suture to assist in suture removal. Once it was discovered that the practice of shaving hair for surgery actually increases the risk of wound infection, it became helpful to use sutures that can be distinguished from the surrounding hair. Of course, black or blue sutures will work equally well in a patient with blond hair.

Tissue Reactivity

This characteristic refers to the inflammatory response that suture material elicits in the body. Sutures derived from animal sources such as catgut and silk tend to elicit intense inflammatory reactions, whereas synthetic materials generate less of a response.

ABSORBABLE SUTURES

The absorbable sutures available in the United States are described in Table 5-1. Ethicon, a division of Johnson & Johnson, and Syneture, a division of Covidien, control 99% of the U.S. market (Ethicon, ~80%; Syneture, ~20%).[6] Although absorbable suture is defined by its loss of strength within 60 days, the suture is not completely gone at that time. Even quickly absorbing sutures such as catgut can be found in the tissues for up to two years.[7]

Surgical Gut

Gut sutures have been used since 175 A.D. In addition to sutures, gut was also used for violin strings and bowstrings and, more recently, tennis racket strings. Gut sutures, also referred to as *catgut*, are derived from the intimal layer of the small intestines of sheep or cattle,

TABLE 5-3 Absorbable Sutures—Strength Retention and Absorption Profile

Ethicon Sutures	Material	Construction	Color	Strength Retention Profile	Absorption Profile
Coated Vicryl Plus Antibacterial (polyglactin 910) suture	Polyglactin 910	Braided/ monofilament	Violet/undyed (natural)	75% at 2 weeks 50% at 3 weeks 25% at 4 weeks (5-0 and larger)	56–70 days (63 days average)
Monocryl Plus Antibacterial (poliglecaprone 25) suture	Poliglecaprone 25 Irgacare MP	Monofilament	Undyed and dyed (violet)	Undyed/dyed: 50%–60%/60%–70% at 1 week 20%–30%/30%–40% at 2 weeks	91–119 days
PDS Plus Antibacterial (polydioxanone) suture	Polydioxanone Polydioxanone and Irgacare MP	Monofilament	Violet /undyed (clear)	4-0 smaller 3-0 larger 60% 80% at 2 weeks 40% 70% at 4 weeks 35% 60% at 6 weeks	183–238 days
Vicryl Rapide (polyglactin 910) suture	Polyglactin 910	Braided	Undyed (natural)	50% at 5 days 0% at 10–14 days	42 days
Coated Vicryl (polyglactin 910) suture	Polyglactin 910	Braided/ monofilament	Violet/undyed (natural)	75% at 2 weeks 50% at 3 weeks 25% at 4 weeks (6-0 and larger)	56–70 days (63 days average)
Monocryl (poliglecaprone 25) suture	Poliglecaprone 25	Monofilament	Undyed and dyed (violet)	Undyed/dyed 50%–60%/60%–70% at 1 week 20%–30%/30%–40% at 2 weeks	91–119 days
PDS II (polydioxanone) suture	Polydioxanone Polydioxanone and Irgacare MP	Monofilament	Violet/undyed (clear)	4-0 smaller 3-0 larger 60% 80% at 2 weeks 40% 70% at 4 weeks 35% 60% at 6 weeks	183–238 days
Surgical gut suture–chromic	Beef serosa or sheep submucosa	Monofilament (virtual)	Brown/blue dyed	21–28 days	90 days
Surgical cut suture–plain	Beef serosa or sheep submucosa	Monofilament (virtual)	Yellowish-tan	7–10 days	70 days

Source: Courtesy of Ethicon, Somerville, NJ.

and have nothing to do with cats. The origin of the name is unknown, but is thought to be derived from the word *kitgut* (fiddle string) with *kit* being the name of an Arabian fiddle with strings made from sheep intestine.[8] Due to its heterogeneic derivation, it is highly inflammatory and is broken down quickly *in vivo*. Plain gut retains significant strength for only 4 to 5 days. Gut can be treated with chromic salts to essentially double its resistance to absorption. It is useful for closing oral, nasal, or vaginal mucosa where significant strength is not required beyond a week. Plain gut can be used in areas where suture removal may be difficult, such as near the lash line of the eyelids, but should not be used if the wound is under any tension. When using plain gut, five knots are necessary because it has a tendency to untie spontaneously when wetted.

As early as 1894 concerns were raised that the use of gut suture could potentially transmit anthrax bacilli and spores or other infectious material in the sheep.[8] In the 1990s, the use of gut diminished significantly in Europe due to concerns about possible transmission of bovine spongiform encephalopathy ("mad-cow disease"), although there has never been a documented case of this occurring. Currently, the raw material is derived from herds certified free of the disease, and is highly processed. However, synthetic sutures are available that have comparable absorption profiles and handling characteristics and are less reactive, such as Vicryl Rapide™ (Ethicon) and Caprosyn™ (Syneture), that can be substituted for plain and chromic gut (see Table 5-1).

Synthetic Braided and Monofilament Sutures

These types of sutures are manufactured utilizing various polymer combinations to provide a suture with:

- Uniform chemical composition with predictable absorption patterns
- Less tissue reaction by avoiding naturally occurring organic material.

The first of these was Dexon™ (Syneture), which became commercially available in 1971.[2,9] It is a synthetic braided homopolymer of glycolic acid. In 1974 Vicryl™ (Ethicon) was introduced. Vicryl (polyglactin 910) is a synthetic braided copolymer of glycolide and L-lactide. These sutures are absorbed by gradual hydrolysis rather than by the host inflammatory response caused by gut. Their braided surfaces allow for easy handling and secure knots. However, the larger surface area and interstices of braided material can lead to entrapment of bacteria and possibly lead to a localized inflammation ("spitting" of the suture) (Figure 5-1) or more generalized wound infection.

In an attempt to decrease this risk of infection while maintaining prolonged tensile strength, synthetic monofilament sutures were developed. Their smooth surfaces diminish bacterial adherence compared to braided absorbable sutures. Examples are Monocryl™ (Ethicon) and Biosyn™ (Syneture), as well as somewhat more rapidly dissolving sutures such as PDS™ (Ethicon) and Maxon™ (Syneture). Vicryl or Dexon is recommended for interrupted deep dermal closure due to their superior knot-holding abilities and maintenance of significant tensile strength for at least 3 weeks. The absorbable monofilament sutures such as Monocryl or Biosyn are recommended for running subcuticular closures due to their lesser tendency to harbor bacteria.

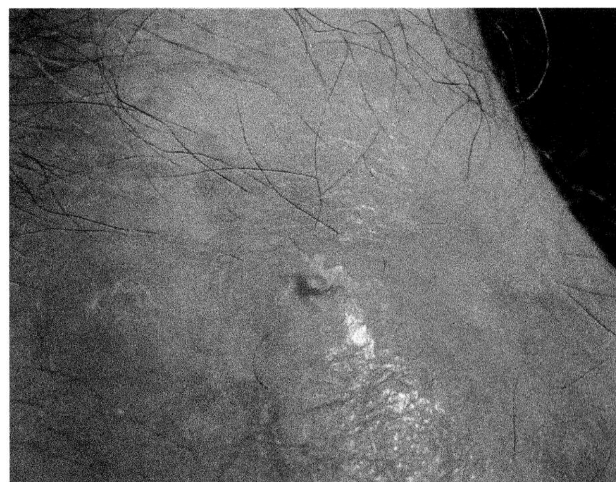

FIGURE 5-1 Spitting suture. *(Copyright Richard P. Usatine, MD.)*

When using absorbable monofilament sutures for running subcuticular closures, it is best to tie the end knots on the outside of the skin rather than burying them. This will avoid tissue inflammation and localized scarring as a result of placing a bulky knot with four to five throws below the skin. Taping down the ends with tissue tapes is another alternative. It is easy to clip off the knots at around 10 to 14 days, leaving the subcuticular portion of the suture intact.

Bioactive Sutures

In 2002, Ethicon released Coated Vicryl Plus™, an absorbable braided suture coated with triclosan, a broad-spectrum biocide used for more than 30 years in products such as toothpaste and soap. Its efficacy has been demonstrated in vivo and in animal models in which *S. aureus* is introduced into the wound during closure.[10] Preliminary results suggest a reduction in sternal wound infections when used for closure of the sternal incision, and a reduction in shunt-infection rates when the suture is used for skin closure following the insertion of cerebrospinal fluid (CSF) shunts.[11,12] This is the first "bioactive" suture to serve the dual purpose of closing a defect as well as decreasing the wound infection rate.

NONABSORBABLE SUTURES

Nonabsorbable sutures are typically used to close the epidermal layer of skin due to their low tissue reactivity and superior strength compared to absorbable sutures.

They are also used for closure of fascia as well as hernia or tendon repair because they lose very little tensile strength with time. See Table 5-2 for an overview of the nonabsorbable sutures and their relevant properties.

Silk

Prior to the introduction of synthetic sutures, silk (nonabsorbable) and gut were the two sutures most commonly in use. Although classified by the USP as a nonabsorbable suture, silk does undergo phagocytosis as well as enzymatic degradation and is usually nonexistent after 2 years. Surgical silk is derived from the domesticated silkworm thread that is processed, dyed black, braided, and coated with wax or silicone to diminish tissue friction. Due to its derivation from organic substances, it is highly inflammatory, second only to gut. It is easy to handle and knots tie securely, but has low tensile strength compared to most sutures. These properties and the introduction of better synthetic sutures have made silk sutures less useful. It can be useful for the closure of oral mucosa because it is softer in the mouth than other sutures. Silk, however, needs to be removed, so chromic or plain gut is often used in the mouth as an alternative.

Nylon

The synthetic polymer Nylon 6 (Ethilon™ [Ethicon]) or Nylon 6,6 (Monosof and Dermalon™ [Syneture]) is an offshoot of synthetic materials that were developed for clothing and other commercial uses. It is uniform in consistency, and as a nonorganic substance generates much less tissue reaction than silk. It is available as either a monofilament or braided into a multifilament that feels and handles much like silk. The monofilament strand has low tissue friction, and is ideal for epidermal closure, although four to five throws are generally required for a secure knot.

Polypropylene

Polypropylene (Prolene™ [Ethicon] and Surgipro™ [Syneture]) is a synthetic monofilament suture developed in the 1970s to improve on the properties of nylon. Compared to nylon, it has greater tensile strength and less tissue adherence, making it ideal for a pull-out subcuticular suture. Even so, it is a good idea when closing a long incision with a subcuticular Prolene suture to bring out a loop of suture every 5 to 6 cm to make later removal easier. Another consideration would be to use a synthetic absorbable monofilament suture in that circumstance to avoid suture removal altogether. Polypropylene is excellent for running sutures on the face after a deep closure with buried absorbable sutures.

NEEDLES

Surgical needles are available in a dizzying array of choices. Unfortunately, the nomenclature of needles is not standardized and depends on the manufacturer. Needles differ in shape, size, and point characteristics.

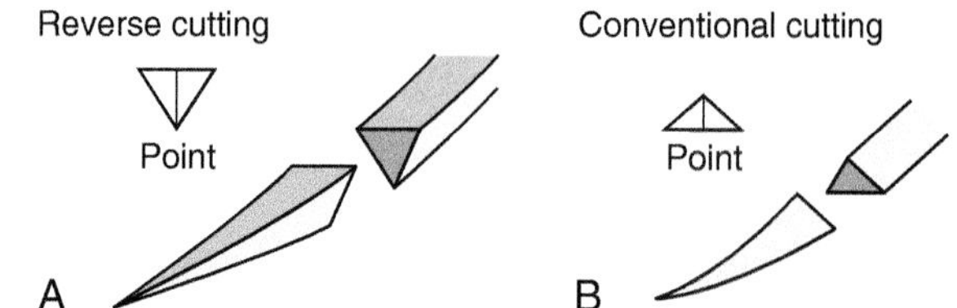

FIGURE 5-2 (A) Reverse-cutting needles. (B) Conventional cutting needles. *(Redrawn from and courtesy of Ethicon product catalog Sutures/Adhesives/Drains/Hernia Repair.)*

The *shape* of the needle can be straight, three-eighths, half circle, five-eighths, or J-hooked. The most popular skin needle is the three-eighths curved, as it is easy to manipulate in skin and superficial wounds with a slight supination of the wrist. A half circle or five-eighths curved needle is useful in confined spaces such as deep in the mouth.

Needle sizes for skin surgery usually range from 13 to 19 mm. Useful needles for skin surgery are those that are three-eighths of a circle and come in lengths of 13, 16, and 19 mm.

Needle points can be blunt, tapered, cutting, or spatulated. A cutting needle is preferred for skin surgery. Its cross section is triangular rather than round, and thus stronger and more resistant to bending. The conventional cutting needle has one pointed edge along the inside of the curve of the needle, and thus can potentially cut tissue along a wound edge. To avoid this problem, the reverse-cutting needle was created so that the third cutting edge is on the outside curve of the needle, away from the edge of the wound (Figure 5-2).

Needles from Ethicon used in skin surgery are named with the following nomenclature:

- **P** or **PS** (plastic): fine reverse-cutting plastics needle
- **PC** (precision cosmetic): fine conventional cutting plastics needle
- **FS** (for skin): basic reverse-cutting skin needle—not as sharp as the plastics needles.

See Figure 5-3 for a comparison of the many types of three-eighths needles made by Ethicon that are used in skin surgery.

Needles from Syneture used in skin surgery are named with the following nomenclature:

- **P** (plastic): fine reverse-cutting plastics needle
- **DX** (= **PC**): conventional cutting plastics needle
- **C** (cutaneous) (= **FS**): reverse-cutting skin needle.

See Tables 5-4 and 5-5 for more details about needles and sutures. Personal preferences for needles develop through experience and help clinicians choose their preferred needle in each surgical situation.

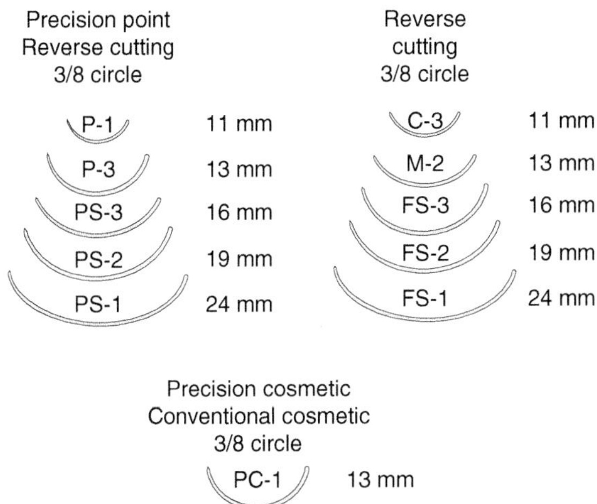

FIGURE 5-3 Needles for skin surgery. *(Adapted from Ethicon product catalog* Sutures/Adhesives/Drains/Hernia Repair.*)*

SUTURE AND NEEDLE SELECTION

Suture Selection

The ideal suture would hold tissues together until they have gained enough tensile strength to heal without the risk of dehiscence. After that time, the suture material would disappear, leaving no sign that it was ever there. Although no such suture currently exists, some sutures are more appropriate for certain circumstances than others. For tissues that heal slowly such as fascia and tendon, a nonabsorbable suture is preferred. For skin, a two-layered closure is preferred, with suture size varying depending on the area of the body. Extremity and trunk skin tends to be thicker and under more tension than facial skin, and therefore larger needles and sutures are preferred. Table 5-6 is a listing of preferred suture by location. The sutures listed are manufactured by Ethicon, as they currently provide 80% of sutures in the United States. We have no ties (pun intended) to Ethicon and have found both Ethicon and Syneture sutures to be equal in performance.

Needle Type

A vast array of needles are available to the surgeon depending on the intended usage of the suture. Plastics needles are preferred because these are sharper than standard skin needles. Reverse-cutting needles avoid inadvertently slicing through the skin at the edge of the wound while passing the needle through the tissue. A three-eighths curvature is recommended unless one is working deep in the mouth where a half-curved needle may be easier to manipulate.

Needle Length

Needle length is chosen based on the skin thickness and the desired length of the placed sutures. When closing thin skin on the face or genital area, a 13-mm needle length is a good choice for both the absorbable and nonabsorbable sutures. When suturing the back it helps to have a longer needle such as one that is 19 mm in length. For other areas of intermediate skin thickness, a 16-mm needle length should be adequate.

Keep in mind that a larger needle allows for larger and fewer stitches when running a suture whether it is external or subcuticular. A 16-mm needle is a good length for closing a punch biopsy regardless of the location. With experience your choices may vary and be different based on personal preference.

Length of Suture

Most sutures for the skin will be 18 inches in length. One way to save money on sutures used for closing punch biopsies is to purchase a suture that is only 9 inches in length. This is adequate for one to three interrupted sutures and can be half the price of the full-length suture. Delasco sells this in 4-0 and 5-0 nylon on a plastics reverse-cutting needle of 16-mm length with three-eighths of a circle configuration.

CONCLUSION

The large variety of sutures available makes it difficult to decide which products are going to be right for you and your patients. Table 5-5 contains detailed information about the commonly stocked skin sutures in an office practice. To do the procedures in this book, you will need at least one type of absorbable and one type

TABLE 5-4 High-Quality Needles for Skin

Ethicon	Syneture	Needle Size (mm)	Needle Type	Geometry
P3	P-13	13	Reverse cutting	3/8 circle
PS-3	P-11	16	Reverse cutting	3/8 circle
PS-2	P-12	19	Reverse cutting	3/8 circle
PC-1	DX-13	13	Conventional cutting	3/8 circle
PC-3	DX-16	16	Conventional cutting	3/8 circle

TABLE 5-5 Details of Recommended Sutures

Suture	Needle	Needle Size (mm)	Needle Type	Order #	Color
Coated Vicryl (Polyglactin)					
5-0	P-3	13	Reverse cutting	J493G	Undyed
4-0	P-3	13	Reverse cutting	J494G	Undyed
5-0	PS-3	16	Reverse cutting	J500G	Undyed
3-0	PS-2	19	Reverse cutting	J427H	Undyed
Prolene (Polypropylene)					
6-0	P-3	13	Reverse cutting	8695G	Blue
5-0	P-3	13	Reverse cutting	8698G	Blue
6-0	PS-3	16	Reverse cutting	8680G	Blue
5-0	PS-3	16	Reverse cutting	8681G	Blue
4-0	PS-2	19	Reverse cutting	8682G	Blue
Nylon					
5-0	PS-3	16	Reverse cutting	1668G	Black
4-0	PS-2	19	Reverse cutting	1667G	Black
Biopsy Suture for Punch Biopsies with 9-inch Length Suture (Delasco Brand)					
Nylon					
5-0	PS-3	16	Reverse cutting	BDL-50B	Black
4-0	PS-3	16	Reverse cutting	BDL-40B	Black

of nonabsorbable suture. The minimum starting set should probably include:

Work on Face

- Polyglactin (Vicryl), 4-0 and 5-0 with 13- and 16-mm needles (Dexon is an alternative)
- Polypropylene (Prolene or Surgipro), 5-0 and 6-0 with 13- and 16-mm needles.

Work on the Neck and Below

- Polyglactin (Vicryl), 4-0 with 16-mm needle (Dexon is an alternative)
- Nylon and/or polypropylene 4-0 and 5-0 with 16-mm needle.

Work in Deeper Wounds or Areas That Will Be Stretched with Activity or Are under Tension (Back, Shoulders, Legs)

- Polyglactin (Vicryl), 3-0 with 16- or 19-mm needle
- Nylon and/or Prolene 4-0 with 19-mm needle.

Reverse cutting is probably the best starting needle type because it will be less likely to inadvertently cut tissue. Then consider trying conventional cutting needles to see what works best in your hands.

Consider carrying some silk if you work on mucosal membranes. Silk is softer inside the mouth. Fast-absorbing sutures such as fast-absorbing gut, Vicryl Rapide, or Caprosyn can be used for patients who may not be able to return easily for suture removal and can also be used inside the mouth.

Add a monofilament absorbable suture if you will be doing subcuticular closures in which the suture will remain in place to dissolve over time. Do not buy too many sutures at first until you settle on the sutures that will be best in your practice.

Resources

Delasco, for ordering sutures, especially for the special punch biopsy suture (www.delasco.com)

Ethicon, for an excellent online catalog of all Ethicon sutures, which can be searched by suture type or needle type (http://ecatalog.ethicon.com)

Ethicon Wound Closure Manual, full 229-page comprehensive manual (www.pilonidal.org/pdfs/wound_closure.pdf)

Ethicon Wound Closure Manual, a 127-page version with book layout design (www.uphs.upenn.edu/surgery/dse/simulation/Wound_Closure_Manual.pdf)

Syneture (www.syneture.com).

TABLE 5-6 Recommendation of Suture by Location

Location	Suture	Comments	Suture Removal*
Scalp	Galea: 3-0 Vicryl Skin: interrupted or running 3-0 or 4-0 Prolene or Nylon	Suturing galea will alleviate tension on the skin–avoid dermal sutures as these may injure hair follicles. Blue color of Prolene will allow easier suture removal, especially in the midst of dark hair. For extensive scalp lacerations consider the use of a surgical stapler.	7–10 days
Face	Dermis: interrupted 5-0 Vicryl Skin: interrupted or running 5-0 or 6-0 Prolene or Nylon	Closure of the dermis with absorbable suture allows early skin suture removal and avoids cross-hatch marks	5–7 days
Nose	Skin: interrupted 5-0 or 6-0 Prolene or Nylon	Use deep sutures on the nose sparingly if at all–the sebaceous nature of the nasal tip skin frequently results in suture abscesses if sutures are buried	5–7 days
Ear	Skin: interrupted 5-0 or 6-0 Prolene or Nylon	There is no need to suture ear cartilage for routine through and through ear lacerations–closing the skin on both the anterior and posterior surface of the ear is sufficient to re-establish stability	5–7 days
Lip	Orbicularis muscle: 4-0 Vicryl Dermis: 4-0 or 5-0 Vicryl Skin: interrupted or running 5-0 or 6-0 Prolene or Nylon Oral mucosa: interrupted 5-0 chromic	Mark the vermilion border prior to infiltration of local anesthetic–the first dermal stitch should be at this point	5–7 days for the skin sutures
Intra-oral	3-0, 4-0, or 5-0 chromic gut (silk is an alternative that will require suture removal)	Size of chromic used is dependent on the tension of the closure	None
Neck	Dermis: 4-0 Vicryl Skin: interrupted or running 5-0 Prolene or Nylon, or 4-0 Monocryl or Prolene subcuticular	For small wounds or lacerations in elderly individuals with thin anterior neck skin, a single layer closure is acceptable. In this case, remove sutures in 7 days and tape wound for additional 1–2 weeks	7 days
Trunk, arms, legs	Dermis: interrupted 3-0 or 4-0 Vicryl Skin: 4-0 Monocryl or Prolene subcuticular or running	If using Monocryl, can leave the end knots on the outside of the skin and clip in 10–14 days to avoid excessive foreign body reaction at these spots	10–14 days for Prolene or Monocryl knots
Digits	Skin: interrupted 4-0 Nylon or Prolene	Usually a single-layer closure is preferred due to the thick epidermal layer	10–14 days

*Increased time may be necessary for patients on chronic corticosteroids or in high-tension areas such as the soles or palms.

References

1. Stroumtsos O. *Perspectives on Sutures*. Pearl River, NY: Davis and Geck; 1978:1–90.
2. Katz AR, Turner RJ. Evaluation of tensile and absorption properties of polyglycolic acid sutures. *Surg Gynecol Obstet*. 1970; 131:701–716.
3. Goldenberg I. Catgut, silk, and silver—the story of surgical sutures. *Surgery*. 1959;46:908–912.
4. McCallum JE. *Military Medicine: From Ancient Times to the 21st Century*. Santa Barbara, CA: ABC-CLIO; 2008:383–313.
5. Levenson SM, Geever EF, Crowley LV, *et al*. The healing of rat skin wounds. *Ann Surg*. 1965;161:293–308.
6. Sluggish demand keeps suture pricing relatively flat. *Hosp Mater Manage*. 2009;34(1):6–8.
7. Bennett RG. Selection of wound closure materials. *J Am Acad Dermatol*. 1988;18:619–637.
8. Booth AW. The preparation of surgical catgut. *Therapeut Gazette*. 1894;18:810–819.
9. Herrmann JB, Kelly RJ, Higgins GA. Polyglycolic acid sutures. Laboratory and clinical evaluation of a new absorbable suture material. *Arch Surg*. 1970;100:486–490.
10. Storch ML, Rothenburger SJ, Jacinto G. Experimental efficacy study of coated Vicryl plus antibacterial suture in guinea pigs challenged with *Staphylococcus aureus*. *Surg Infect (Larchmt)*. 2004;5:281–288.
11. Fleck T, Moidl R, Blacky A, *et al*. Triclosan-coated sutures for the reduction of sternal wound infections: economic considerations. *Ann Thorac Surg*. 2007;84:232–236.
12. Rozzelle CJ, Leonardo J, Li V. Antimicrobial suture wound closure for cerebrospinal fluid shunt surgery: a prospective, double-blinded, randomized controlled trial. *J Neurosurg Pediatr*. 2008; 2:111–117.

6 Suturing Techniques

DANIEL L. STULBERG, MD • RICHARD P. USATINE, MD

Suturing techniques should be considered as a part of the global picture of removing lesions and being able to skillfully repair the defect to obtain good healing and cosmetic results. In most procedures, prior to starting the incision, the clinician will assess the lesion to be excised and consider the margin required and the area of the body. After this inspection, the provider will plan the excision and the anticipated repair and then select the appropriate suture to place on the surgical tray before cutting. Small punch excisions can be repaired by one or more simple interrupted sutures or a figure-of-eight suture. Larger wounds may be optimally closed with a combination of buried deep sutures, mattress sutures, and simple interrupted or simple running sutures.

A good closure result depends on multiple steps. In general, the first aspect in a large excision is to make sure that there is enough stretch in the skin to close the skin edges with minimal tension. After adequate undermining, close the deep tissues with absorbable sutures to help approximate the skin edges, reduce the dead space, help with hemostasis, and reduce the risk of hematoma formation. If the skin edges are fragile or there is some tension, mattress sutures can help close the wound successfully. The final closure is then performed most commonly with interrupted sutures, running simple, running horizontal mattress sutures, or running subcuticular sutures.

BASIC SKILLS

See video on the DVD for further learning. 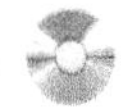

The clinician must acquire certain basic suturing skills as discussed next.

Loading the Needle Holder (Driver)

1. Even though a needle holder has holes in the handle for the thumb and a finger, it is often easier to place sutures at the correct angle by placing the needle holder in the palm of your hand instead of putting your thumb and finger in the holes (Figure 6-1).
2. Grasp the needle two-thirds of the way from the point to the swaged-on thread. In most cases the needle will be loaded perpendicular to the needle holder, but for some techniques it helps to use another angle.
3. Needles used for skin surgery are curved in the arc of a circle. Work with the curve of the needle and follow the arc to prevent bending the needle.

Using Forceps in the Nondominant Hand

Learn to suture with a good pair of Adson forceps in the nondominant hand (Figure 6-2). The forceps can be used to:

1. Hold the skin edge gently when inserting the suture needle.
2. Provide some stability of the skin on the opposite side while pushing the needle through and out of the skin.
3. Grasp the needle once it is pushed through the skin (this is a better method than holding the needle with the fingers).
4. Hold the needle when reloading the needle holder.

Although some of these techniques can be performed with a skin hook, these are advanced skills that are optional.

Performing an Instrument Tie

See video on the DVD for further learning. 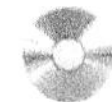

To perform an instrument tie (Figure 6-3):

1. Wrap the first throw of the knot twice around the needle as a surgeon's or friction knot (especially if the suture is monofilament) to hold the skin edge together better.
2. Pull the suture with enough tension for the skin edges to just meet and not cause any puckering.
3. Place the second throw and pull until it meets the first throw squarely, but do not tighten yet. Leaving a loop in the second throw will avoid too much tension on the skin margins. Tension can cause a railroad or cross-hatch pattern of scarring perpendicular to the suture line. Leaving the loop loose will also allow for a bit of swelling of the skin that is normal.
4. Place the third throw and now tighten to cinch the knot.

In general, place four throws for your knots. Five throws are a good idea at the beginning and end of a running suture because if this opens the whole length of the suture can be lost.

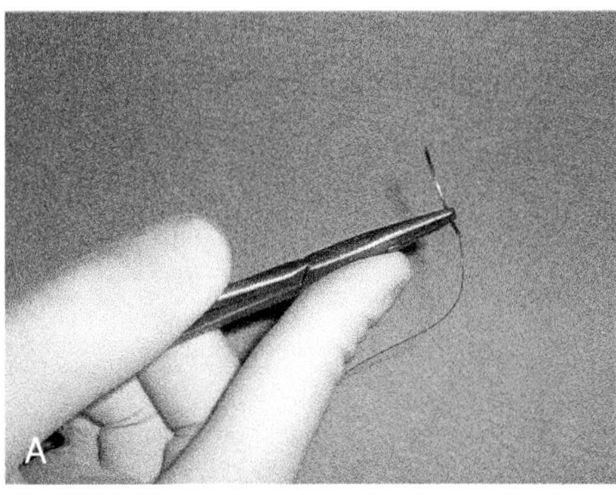

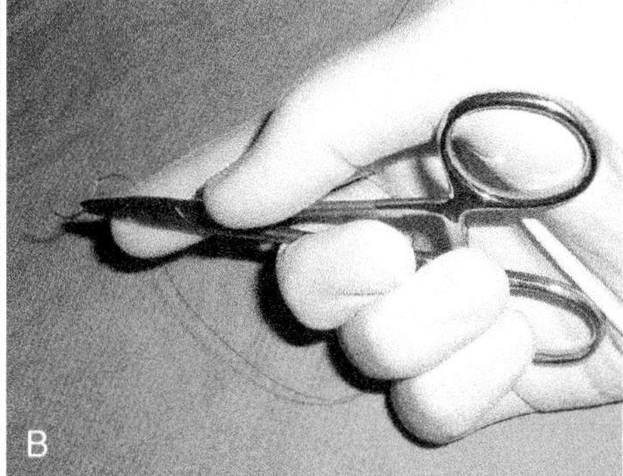

FIGURE 6-1 A, B. Needle holder in the palm of the hand with the needle correctly loaded. Although some surgeons prefer to put their fingers in the loops, this method offers maximum dexterity. *(Copyright Richard P. Usatine, MD.)*

SPECIFIC SUTURING TECHNIQUES

See video on the DVD for further learning. 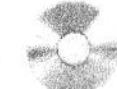

Simple Interrupted Suture

The simple interrupted suture (Figure 6-4) is the most basic suturing technique to master and is used to close anything from small incisions under little tension to a large excision under tension in conjunction with deep sutures. Pronate the wrist to place the point of the needle perpendicular (or even 10° more than perpendicular) to the skin, and then rotate the needle through the skin. The needle should enter and exit the skin at the same depth from the skin surface on both sides to maintain good apposition. Also the needle should enter and exit the epidermis equidistant from the wound margin on each side.

The reason for creating a flask shape path is to promote eversion of the wound edge. Eversion will heal in a flat scar when the fibrosis of healing pulls the skin edges downward. Without wound eversion the scar may be depressed (Figure 6-5). Methods of obtaining eversion include the following (Figure 6-6):

- Overaccentuating the arc of the needle's path to point slightly away from the skin edge and then rotating it through the skin
- Indenting the skin lateral to the wound with the forceps to deflect the skin edge upward while suturing
- Gently elevating the edge of the wound with a forceps or skin hook while placing the sutures.

If the skin edges are uneven, this can be corrected by keeping the depth from the surface equal on both sides (Figure 6-7).

Simple interrupted sutures are useful for small wounds as well as for excellent control and placement along larger wounds. The rule of halves is to place the first suture at the midpoint of the wound and then to place subsequent sutures halfway between the first suture and the end of the wound and then proceed in a similar fashion until the wound is closed (see Figure 11-23 in Chapter 11, *The Elliptical Excision*). This technique is useful to avoid standing cones (dog ears) at the ends from uneven suturing and can also be used to even out an asymmetrical defect where one side is longer than the other.

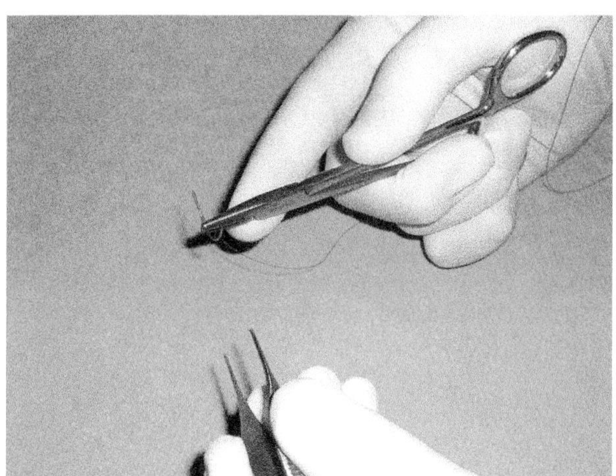

FIGURE 6-2 Using Adson forceps in the nondominant hand while suturing. *(Copyright Richard P. Usatine, MD.)*

Deep or Buried Sutures

Deep or buried sutures are placed using absorbable suture materials. Most deep sutures are placed vertically, but deep horizontal mattress sutures may also be used.

Deep sutures perform five important functions:

1. Relieve tension.
2. Close dead space.
3. Provide hemostasis.
4. Oppose dermis.
5. Produce eversion.

Deep Vertical Sutures (Figure 6-8)

The path of a deep or buried suture (Figure 6-8) is designed to bury the knot and keep it from poking through the skin. Insert the needle point in the undermined area at the base of the wound. Then pass the

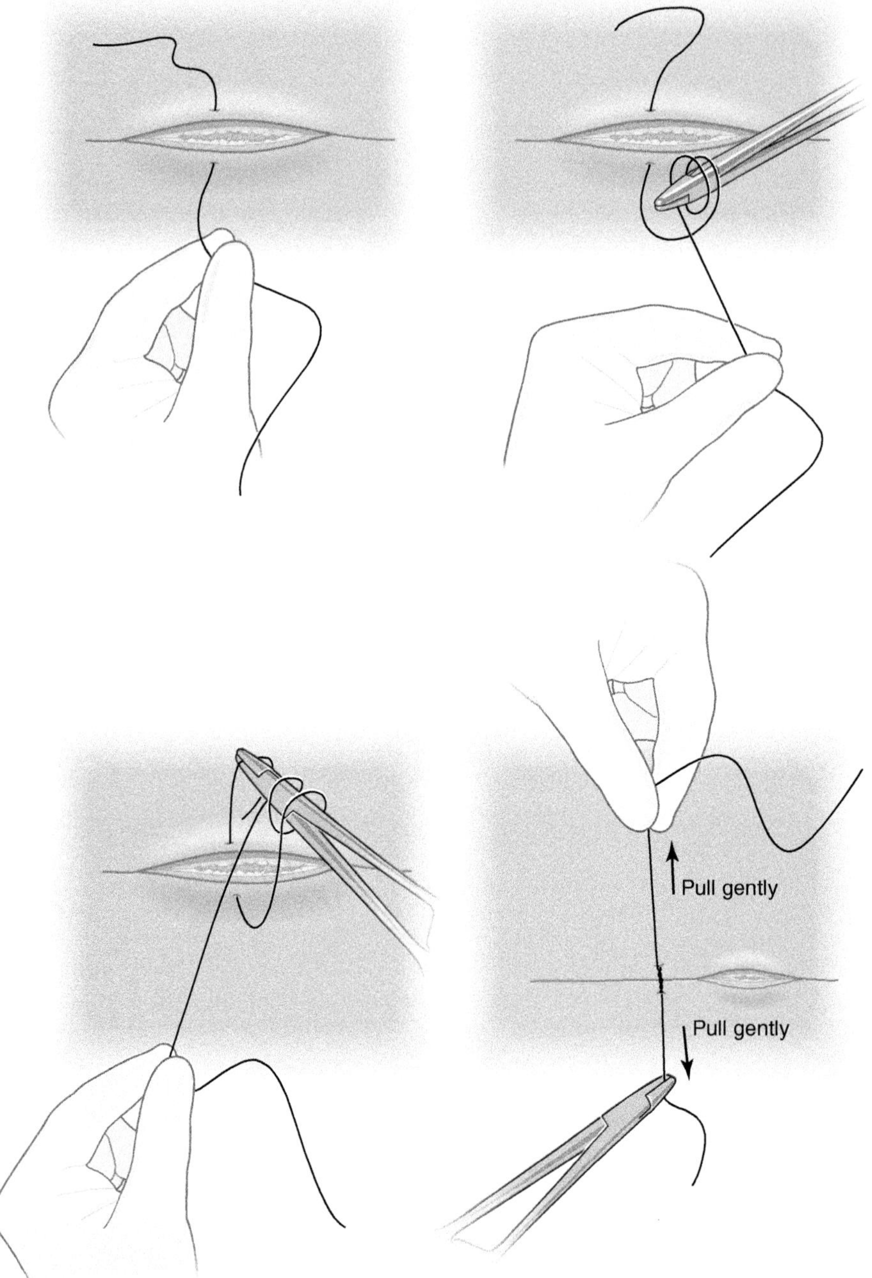

FIGURE 6-3 The start of an instrument tie. Loop the suture twice around the tip of the holder and open the needle holder to grasp the short end of the suture. Cross or reverse your hands to pull the suture down. *(From Vidimos A, Ammirati C, Poblete-Lopez C.* Dermatologic Surgery. *London: Saunders; 2008.)*

needle through the tissue away from the midline of the wound and come up in the superficial dermis. Hold the needle with your forceps and let go of the needle with your needle holder. Then pass the needle back to the needle holder in the direction needed for the second half of the stitch. Pull the suture through, leaving a short end in the middle of the wound and reload the needle.

Insert the needle at the same depth in the dermis on the opposite side of the wound and rotate the needle through the tissue coming out at the base of the wound in the undermined area at the same depth as the first suture. Tie this off with square-knot throws and cut the ends short so the knot stays deep within the wound.

When tying the knot it helps to have both ends of the suture on the same side and to start with a surgeon's knot of two throws. Pull the suture parallel to the wound rather than perpendicular to it. Cinch the knot down tightly before starting the second throw. If the wound is under tension and the knot is slipping, a surgical assistant may help by holding the tissue together between the first and second knot.

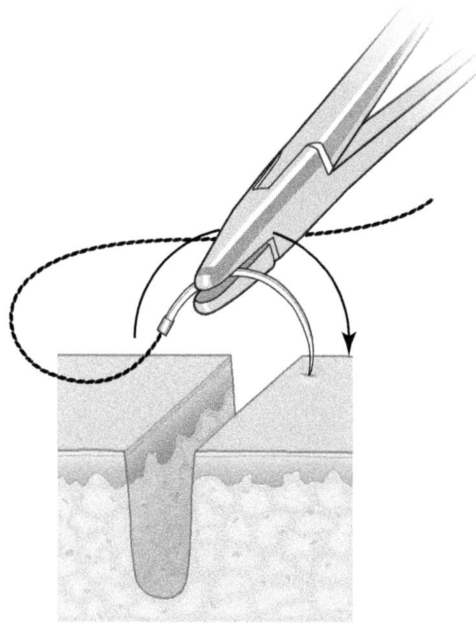

FIGURE 6-4 Inserting the needle perpendicular to the skin while initiating a simple interrupted suture. *(From Vidimos A, Ammirati C, Poblete-Lopez C.* Dermatologic Surgery. *London: Saunders; 2008.)*

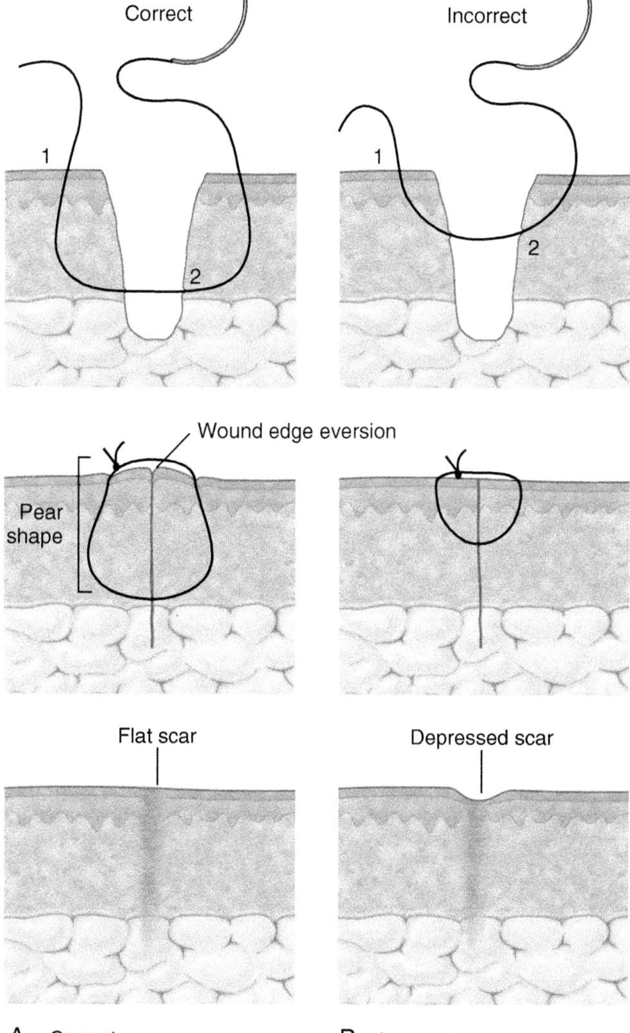

FIGURE 6-5 Proper placement of epidermal sutures involves looping a larger portion of the dermis and/or subcutis than the epidermis. This creates a pear-shaped suture which everts wound edges **(A)**. Failure of wound edge eversion often leads to a more depressed, noticeable scar **(B)**. Numbers indicate entry points of the needle. *(Adapted from Taylor RS. Needles, sutures, and suturing.* Atlas Office Proced. *1999;2:53–74.) (From Robinson J, Hanke W, Sengelmann R, Siegel D.* Surgery of the Skin: Procedural Dermatology, *2nd ed. Philadelphia: Mosby; 2010.)*

Buried Vertical Mattress Sutures

See video on the DVD for further learning. 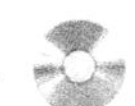

The buried vertical mattress suture (Figure 6-9) is created using a special technique that produces a heart-shaped pattern in the deep tissue to improve wound eversion. The needle is placed as described above but will go up to dermal-epidermal junction (DEJ) then come out 2 mm below the DEJ. If you merely make a circle with the deep stitch, the tension vectors may pull the edges down and invert the wound.

Deep Horizontal Mattress Suture

See video on the DVD for further learning. 

The deep or buried horizontal mattress suture (Figure 6-10) can be useful when it is desirable to take tension off the wound but the skin is not very thick, such as that on the face. The absorbable suture is placed through

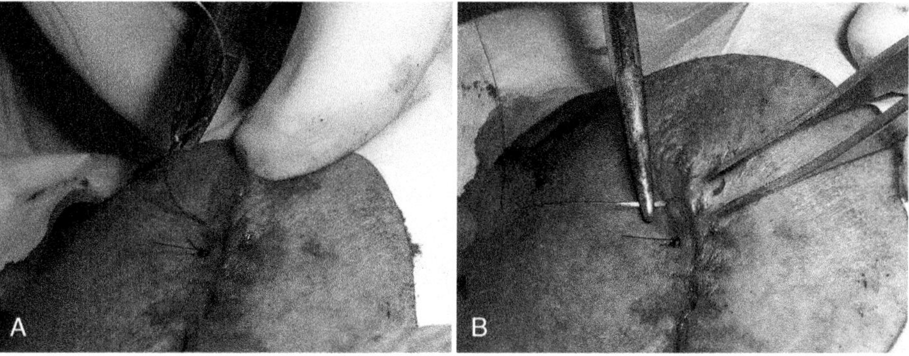

FIGURE 6-6 Methods for obtaining eversion. **(A)** Note how the needle is entering the skin at a 90-degree angle. **(B)** The forceps are being used to push against the skin and ensure that the needle leaves the skin at a 90-degree angle. *(Copyright Richard P. Usatine, MD.)*

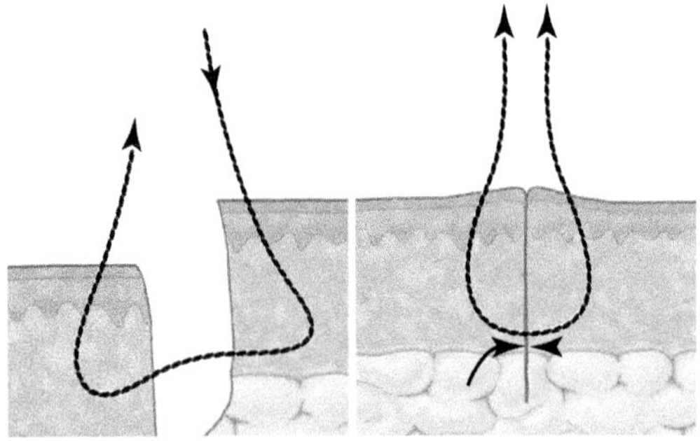

FIGURE 6-7 Using a simple interrupted suture to make even any skin edges that are uneven. Place the suture deep on the low side and shallow on the high side. *(From Vidimos A, Ammirati C, Poblete-Lopez C.* Dermatologic Surgery. *London: Saunders; 2008.)*

the dermis at the same level on both sides and tied in the same manner as the deep vertical mattress suture. This suture does not close dead space as well as the deep vertical mattress suture, but it can be easier to place when the skin is thin and not much undermining is needed.

Buried Dermal Sutures

A

B

C

FIGURE 6-8 Buried dermal sutures. **(A)** Conventional buried suture placement results in mild wound eversion. **(B)** Buried vertical mattress suture placement results in moderate to significant wound eversion. **(C)** Buried butterfly suture placement results in the greatest degree of wound eversion. Numbers indicate entry points of the needle. *(From Robinson J, Hanke W, Sengelmann R, Siegel D.* Surgery of the Skin: Procedural Dermatology, *2nd ed. Philadelphia: Mosby; 2010.)*

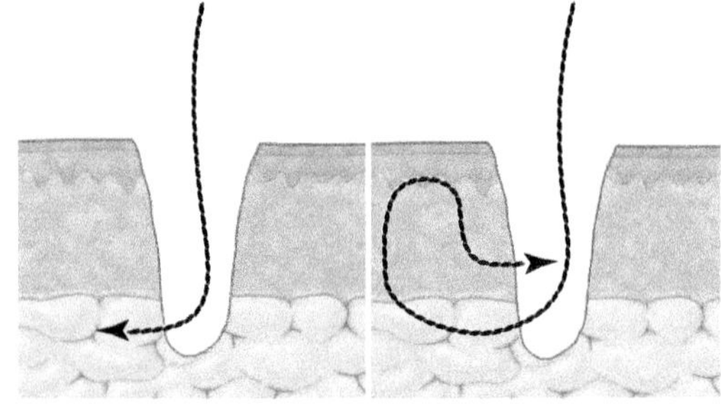

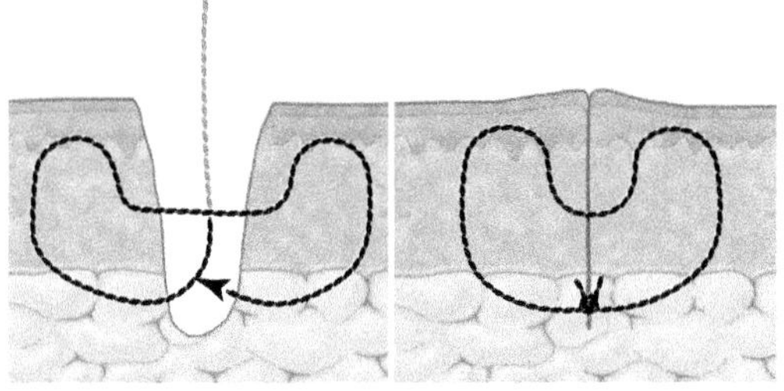

FIGURE 6-9 The buried vertical mattress suture is a variation of the simple buried suture with the intent of increasing wound eversion. The path of the suture creates a heart shape. *(From Vidimos A, Ammirati C, Poblete-Lopez C.* Dermatologic Surgery. *London: Saunders; 2008.)*

Removing a Deep Suture

If any deep suture does not come out as planned, it is better to remove it and start over than to allow the suture to cause anatomic distortion or inadequate closure. Even the best skin surgeons need to remove poorly executed deep sutures on a regular to daily basis. Practice will help but no surgeon should be ashamed to remove a suture that does not perform its duty well.

Running Simple Sutures

See video on the DVD for further learning. 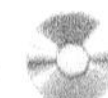

A running simple suture (Figure 6-11) is an efficient way to close long repairs that are not under tension or no longer under tension after the deep sutures were

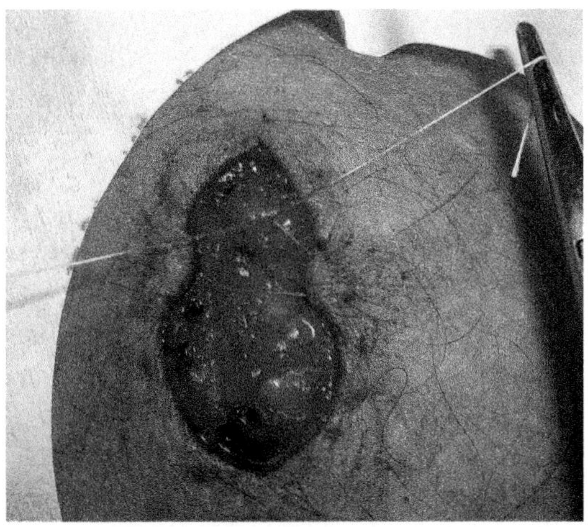

FIGURE 6-10 Buried (deep) horizontal mattress suture.

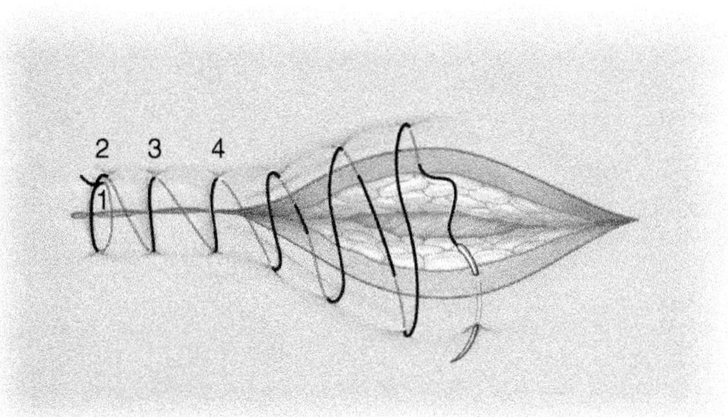

FIGURE 6-11 Running simple suture (running cuticular suture). Multiple simple sutures are placed in succession, allowing for rapid closure of wounds. Numbers indicate entry points of the needle. *(Adapted from Taylor RS. Needles, sutures, and suturing.* Atlas Office Proced. *1999;2:53–74.) (From Robinson J, Hanke W, Sengelmann R, Siegel D.* Surgery of the Skin: Procedural Dermatology, *2nd ed. Philadelphia: Mosby; 2010.)*

placed. Start by placing a simple interrupted suture at one end of the wound and tie it with at least four to five throws. Instead of cutting both ends of the suture, cut only the short end and preserve the length of the suture with the needle attached. Continue the repair by placing the next stitch further along the wound and passing the needle through the skin on both sides and repeating the process along the length of the surgical defect. Insert the needle perpendicular to the skin to promote wound eversion. Once the end of the wound is reached and the wound is closed, instead of pulling the last loop tight, leave it long enough to use it as an end to tie. Tie the suture to this loop and then cut the loop and the needle end of the suture.

Vertical Mattress Sutures

Vertical mattress sutures (Figure 6-12) distribute some of the stress and cutting force of the suture over a broader area. The vertical mattress suture shifts much of the tension away from the skin edge. The suture is placed similarly to a simple interrupted suture, but it is started further from the skin margin and emerges equidistant on the other side of the wound often referred to as *far-far*. The course of the needle is then reversed and the needle is placed closer to the skin edge on the same side where the needle just emerged. The needle is then advanced to come out equidistant from the wound on the opposite side of the wound and back toward the first insertion of the needle. These are placed close to the skin edge, *near-near*, and the two ends are tied with the knot lying away from the skin edge. This allows the skin edges to evert while placing the greatest amount of tension between the far and near entrance points of the suture instead of directly on the skin margin. To learn the sequence of steps in this technique it may be helpful to remember the saying *far-far-near-near*. Additional vertical mattress sutures may be placed along the wound to complete the repair.

Alternatively, once the tension is managed by strategically placed vertical mattress sutures, the repair of the intervening spaces may be completed with simple interrupted sutures or a running simple suture to approximate the skin edges. Use care to not inadvertently cut the previously placed sutures when placing the needle of the running suture past them. Be careful to not use tightly pulled thin suture in fragile skin because it can cut through the skin just like a cheese wire cuts through cheese.

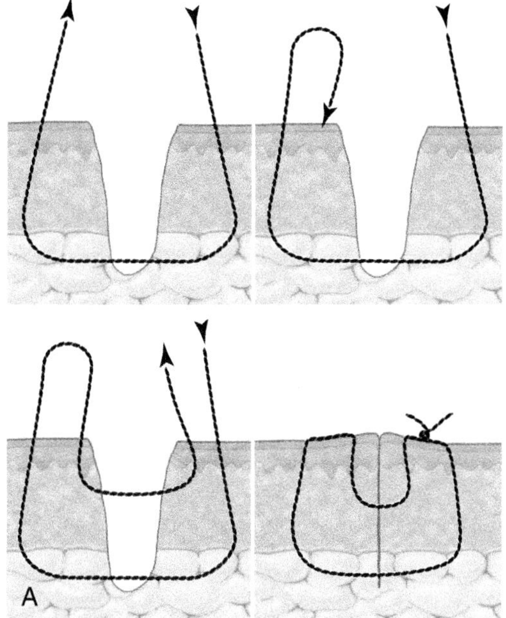

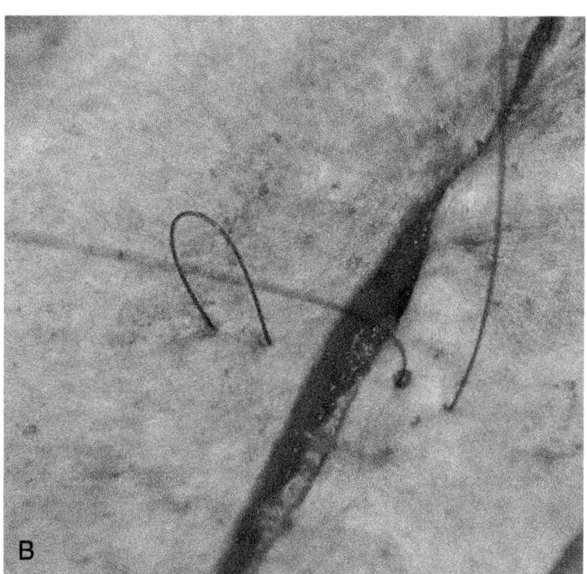

FIGURE 6-12 **(A)** The vertical mattress suture. **(B)** The vertical mattress suture prior to tying the knot. *(A: From Vidimos A, Ammirati C, Poblete-Lopez C.* Dermatologic Surgery. *London: Saunders; 2008; B: Copyright Richard P. Usatine, MD.)*

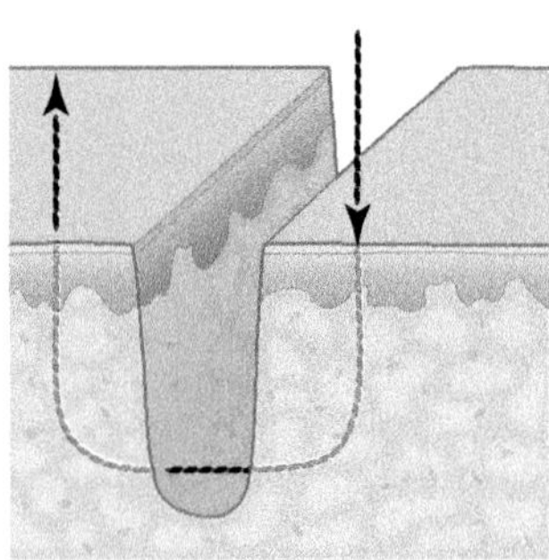
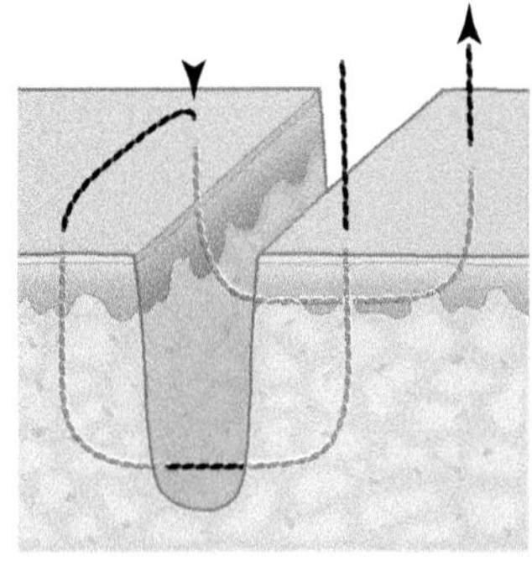
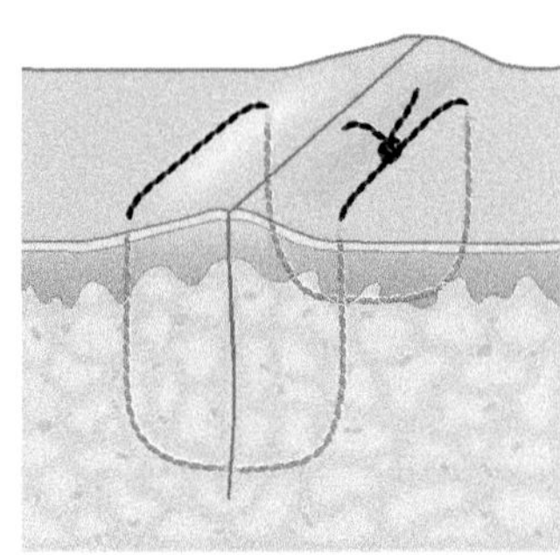

FIGURE 6-13 The horizontal mattress suture. *(From Vidimos A, Ammirati C, Poblete-Lopez C.* Dermatologic Surgery. *London: Saunders; 2008.)*

Horizontal Mattress Sutures

Horizontal mattress sutures (Figure 6-13) are another option for placing tension away from the skin edges. Instead of placing the suture *far-far-near-near*, the four entrance/exit sites are equidistant from the wound margin, but the two lines of suture crossing the wound margin are parallel in a horizontal plane in contrast to the two lines of suture in the vertical mattress, which are in a vertical plane. Start the horizontal mattress suture on one side of the wound as in a simple interrupted suture and exit on the opposite side of the wound equidistant from the wound. Reverse the needle and insert it equidistant from the wound edge several millimeters lateral to the exit site and then emerge equidistant on the opposite side of the wound. Finally, tie the suture on the side of initial needle entry. This places the tension mostly along the section of the suture where the open loop is and the segment with the knot that is parallel to the wound margin. As above, the repair can be completed with additional horizontal mattress sutures or simple interrupted sutures or a running simple suture to approximate the skin edges.

Running Horizontal Mattress Sutures

This variation combines the distribution of tension away from the wound edge possible with a traditional horizontal mattress suture with some of the speed of a running simple suture (Figure 6-14). The suture is started as a simple suture at the end of the incision or beyond the end of the incision where there is little or no tension and the suture is tied and the short non-needle end is cut. The needle is then moved parallel to the incision several millimeters away from the exit of the first suture and is placed through the skin and subcutaneous tissues across the incision to emerge equidistant on the other side of the incision. The needle is then placed several millimeters further along and parallel to the incision to repeat the process in the other direction. This will make a series of alternating dashes on either side of the incision, which will carry the tension of the suture instead of the tension being on the wound edges themselves. The suture material will be traversing the wound incision perpendicular and deep to the incision.

Once the end of the incision is reached in this fashion, the suture can be tied to itself as in the simple running suture above. If the repair is long, removal can be facilitated by occasionally placing a simple suture across and over the incision instead of under it.[1] This segment can be easier to cut in contrast to the segments parallel to the incision, which due to the tension on them may be difficult to elevate. This tension is also what helps to approximate the wound, evert the skin edges, and avoid undue tension at the skin edges. Because there are only two knots to tie (one at each end), it is relatively quick to place.

Corner (Tip) Stitch

The corner, or tip, stitch (Figure 6-15) is useful in more complex wounds, advancements, and Z-plasties where a point needs to be sutured into a corner. This suture is very similar to the horizontal mattress suture and it distributes tension away from the point of the flap or similar tissue. Start the needle on the side of the wound opposite the point but lateral to where the point of tissue is to reside. Pass it through the tissue in the dermis. Next, enter into the corresponding portion of the point of tissue in the same level of the dermis and travel through it, remaining in the dermis and coming out on the other side of the point. Return to the original side of the wound via the dermis and tie the initial and emerging suture ends on the wound edge opposite from the point of loose tissue. The suture never emerges through the epidermis of the point of tissue and the tension is distributed somewhat away from the fragile point of tissue and its blood supply.

Figure-of-Eight Sutures

The advantage of a figure-of-eight suture (Figure 6-16) is that it acts like two interrupted sutures, but only has one knot to tie. It is useful for medium-sized punch biopsies 4 to 6 mm in diameter that can be closed with a single figure-of-eight suture. Start the needle on one side of the wound and emerge equidistant on the other side of the wound. Without tying, return the needle to the original side of the wound, insert it further along the wound and equidistant from the wound margin as the first site and emerge equidistant on the other side.

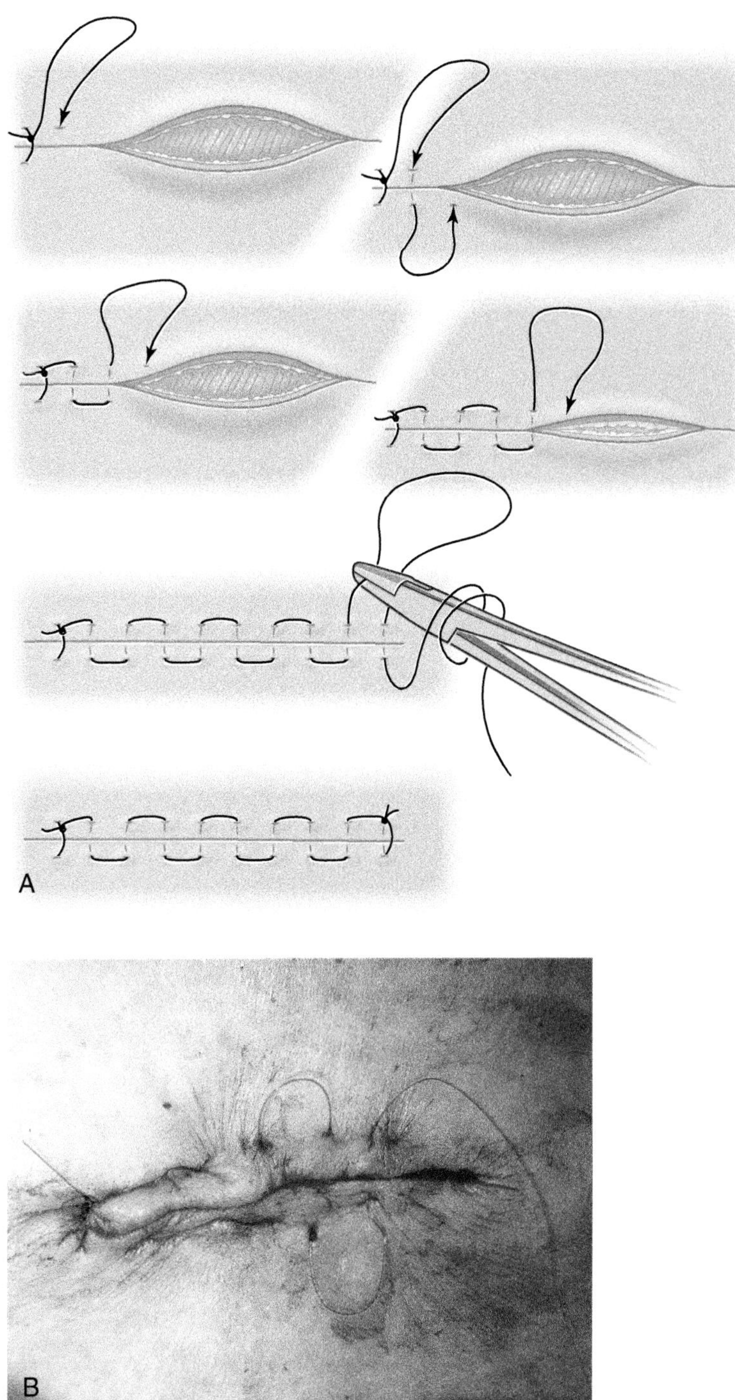

FIGURE 6-14 (A) The running horizontal mattress suture. (B) The running horizontal mattress suture causes eversion of the skin. (*A: From Vidimos A, Ammirati C, Poblete-Lopez C.* Dermatologic Surgery. *London: Saunders; 2008; B: Copyright Richard P. Usatine, MD.*)

Tying the suture from the entry point to the final point will pull the wound together and the suture will cross over itself in an X or figure-eight pattern. This technique does not provide as much control as two simple interrupted sutures, but is quicker and adequate for medium-sized punch biopsies. Alternatively, the figure-of-eight process can be reversed by placing the suture diagonally across the wound, then returning the needle to the original side opposite the exit point to place the next suture diagonally crossing the first suture under the skin to the opposite side. This will place the X deep and two parallel lines of suture over the skin (Figure 6-16).

Running Subcuticular Sutures

A running subcuticular stitch (Figure 6-17) is used to avoid making punctures through the epidermis and may leave less scarring. It can be performed with absorbable suture remaining in the tissues or can have nonabsorbable suture knots at both ends above the skin that are removed at a later time. If it is completely buried, then one advantage is that there is no need for suture removal. Before placing this suture the wound should be approximated with deep sutures as described above to reduce any tension on the skin edges because

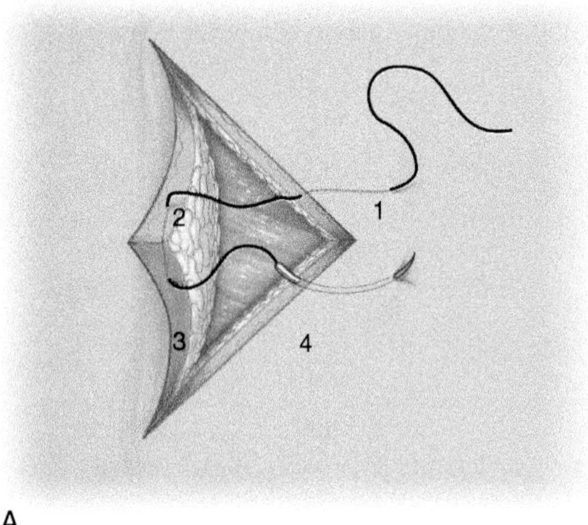

A

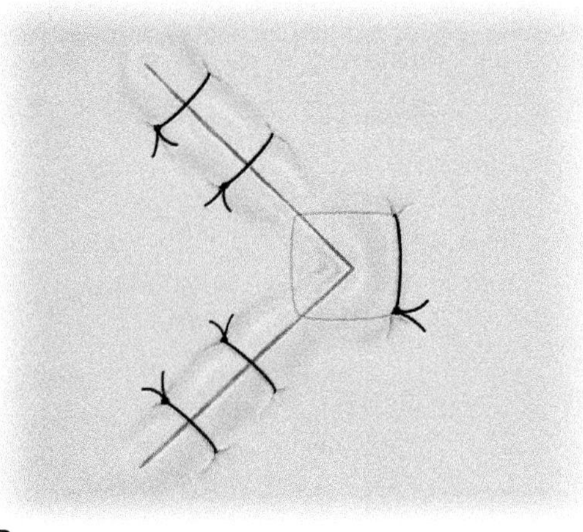

B

FIGURE 6-15 The three-point corner (tip) suture (half-buried horizontal mattress tip stitch). **(A)** This suture is started as an interrupted suture (1) on the V portion of the wound crossing over to the tip of the flap (2). A horizontal bite is made through the dermis of the tip (3). The needle is then directed back across the wound and tied (4). **(B)** Final appearance of this suture after placement. Numbers indicate entry points of the needle. *(Adapted with permission from Robinson JK. Technique of suture placement. In Robinson J, Hanke W, Sengelmann R, Siegel D.* Surgery of the Skin: Procedural Dermatology, *2nd ed. Philadelphia: Mosby; 2010.)*

control of wound approximation is reduced with this technique.

With absorbable suture, anchor one end by a small suture deep in the dermis near the end of the wound to make a knot at that point around a small amount of dermis. Cut the short end and then place the needle through the subcutaneous tissue to bury the knot and emerge at the apex. Start from this point and rotate the needle in a plane parallel to the skin surface through the dermis on one side and then the other side of the wound with the entry point directly opposite the emerging point. The suture should be placed at the same level in the dermis to maintain the skin repair level. Proceed to the other end of the wound until it is closed and tie the suture back to the last loop as described in the simple running suture. Cut the loop and then—being careful not to cut the newly placed suture—place the needle deep through the wound and emerge through the skin outside the wound. This will bury the knot deeply and the suture can be cut at the skin surface so that the end will drop under the skin.

To make a running subcuticular suture completely removable, approximate the wound as above. Next start the skin repair by placing a nonabsorbable monofilament suture beyond the end of the surgical wound and emerging at the apex of the wound. No knot is made at this time, so be careful not to inadvertently pull the loose end into the wound. The loose end can be clamped with a hemostat to avoid losing it. Proceed as above, suturing along the length of the wound. If the wound is long, it can be helpful to create a loop that can be cut so that the entire length of the suture does not need to be pulled only from one end. To make a loop, place a suture from the dermis on one side up through the dermis across from it, then up through the epidermis and across to the other side. Place the needle through the epidermis to emerge back to the level of the dermis to resume the subcuticular suture to the opposite end of the wound. To complete the suture, place the last suture through the apex of the wound and emerge beyond the apex. Loop the suture around the needle holder several times and then grasp the suture at the skin surface to create a knot at the skin to hold it in place. Repeat for several throws to hold it in place. Repeat at the original apex.

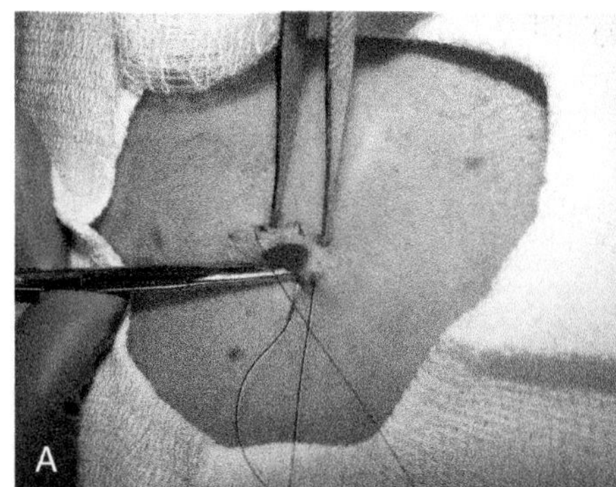

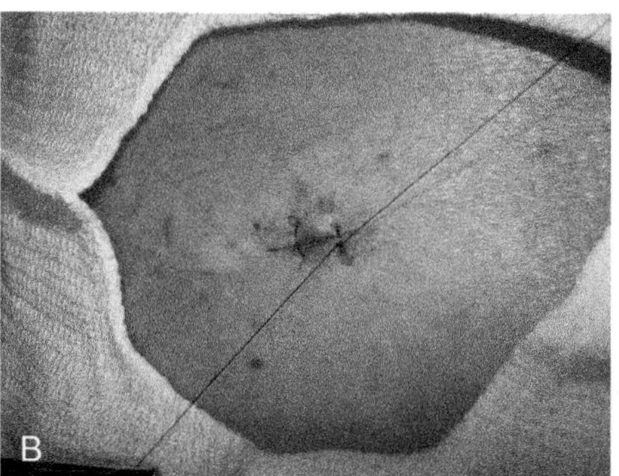

FIGURE 6-16 **(A)** A figure-of-eight suture is being used to close a punch biopsy. In this case the suture is being crossed below the skin. **(B)** This produces two parallel sutures above the skin with the convenience of only one knot to tie. *(Copyright Daniel L. Stulberg, MD.)*

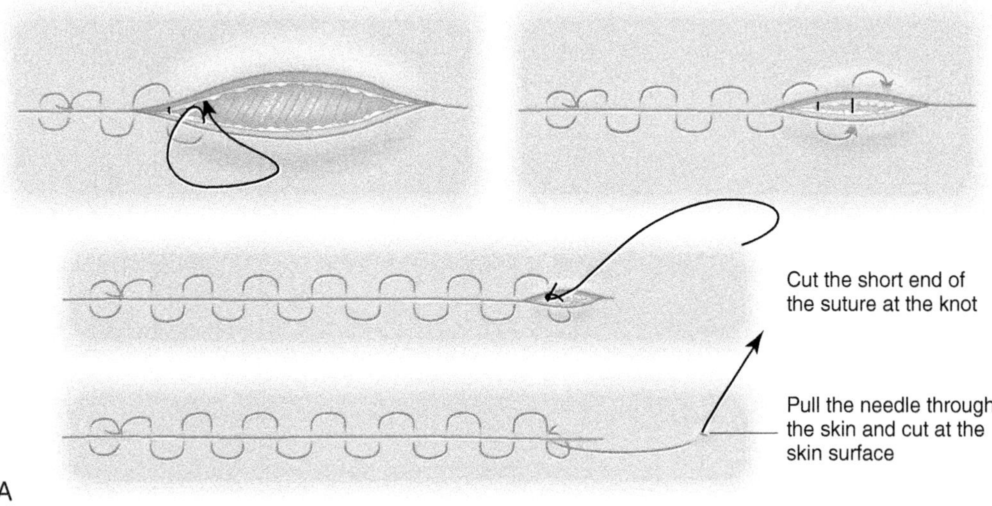

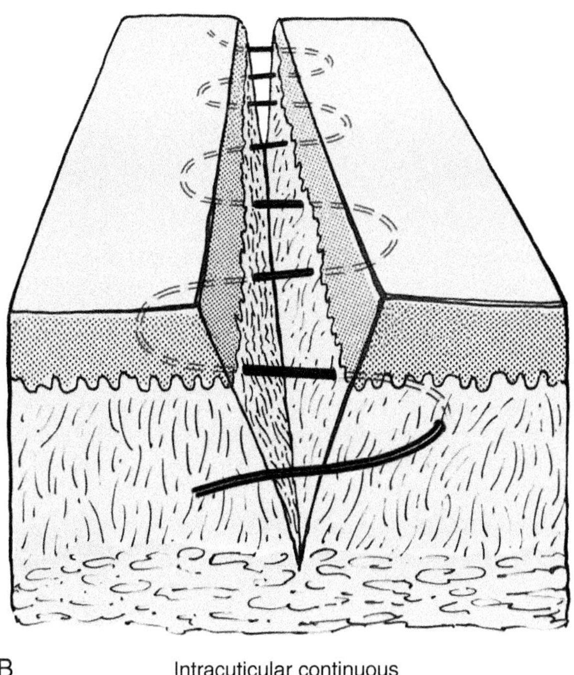

FIGURE 6-17 **(A)** Running subcuticular suture performed with absorbable suture. In this case the knots on both ends are buried. The suture is initiated with a simple dermal interrupted suture. Cut only the short end after tying the knot. After completing the running subcuticular suture, the suture end is tied off with another dermal interrupted suture. Cut only the short end. The needle end is then passed through the end of the incision and exited distal to the incision. The needle is pulled with tension. This pulls the knot deeper into the wound. The suture is then cut at the skin surface. **(B)** Running subcuticular suture is placed at the level of the upper dermis. *(A: From Vidimos A, Ammirati C, Poblete-Lopez C.* Dermatologic Surgery. *London: Saunders; 2008; B: Baker SR.* Local Flaps in Facial Reconstruction, *2nd ed. London: Mosby; 2007.)*

Two-Layer Closure

After excising a skin cancer with margins, a two-layer closure (Figure 6-18) is often required. This is the strongest closure for skin surgery because the buried absorbable suture will take more than 1 month to dissolve. So whenever the superficial sutures are removed, the deep sutures go on working to prevent dehiscence and unattractive scar widening. This method also is the best at preventing hematomas because it effectively closes the dead space. Learn to use the two-layer closure because it should be the workhorse for performing skin surgery.

Additionally, the two-layer closure automatically can be billed as an intermediate closure (see Chapter 38, *Surviving Financially*). Billing for an intermediate closure will approximately double what is paid for the surgical procedure. Many insurance companies will require prior approval so keep this in mind when scheduling an excision that will require a two-layer closure. Most

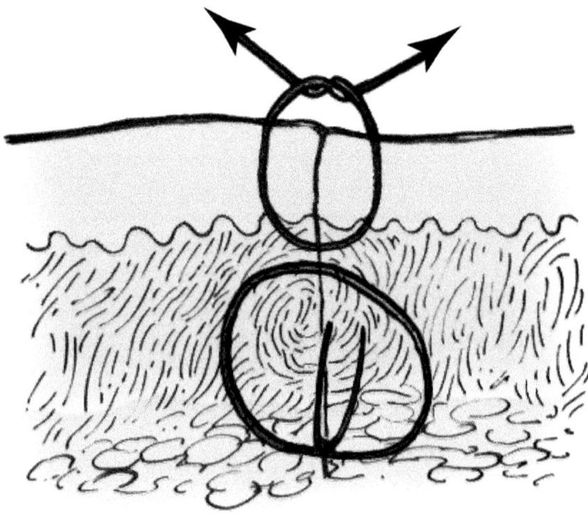

FIGURE 6-18 The two-layer closure consists of a deep absorbable suture with a more superficial nonabsorbable suture. *(From Baker SR. Local Flaps in Facial Reconstruction, 2nd ed. London: Mosby; 2007.)*

importantly this closure provides the best result for many skin excisions.

SUTURE REMOVAL

Nonabsorbable cutaneous sutures can be safely removed early on when good deep sutures have been placed. The typical time periods used are 5 to 6 days on the face and 7 to 10 days for the trunk and extremities. There is a balance between the risk of dehiscence if the sutures are removed too soon and scarring at the site of the sutures if they are left in too long. At removal, wound closure tapes may be placed across the wound for protection and to provide a small amount of support to the wound closure. The patient can remove these a week or two later if they have not spontaneously fallen off by then.

ALTERNATIVE SUTURING TECHNIQUES

Wound Closure Tapes

Wound closure tapes may be used as an adjunct for skin closure in addition to deep sutures and skin sutures. Some clinicians will use wound closure tapes alone for linear excisions of lipomas or cysts when there is no tension on the wound edges. For elliptical excisions it is important to close the dermis and relieve wound tension if wound closure tapes are to be the only epidermal closure used.

It helps to apply a liquid adhesive (tincture of benzoin or Mastisol) to facilitate adherence of the wound closure tapes. Wound closure tapes, which come in ⅛-, ¼-, and ½-inch widths, can be cut in half so they are not as long for small wounds typical in the office setting.

Wound closure tapes also provide an occlusive dressing and a moist healing environment. This is convenient because the patient does not need to change any dressings at all. The disadvantage is that if there is any bleeding or drainage, the tapes will get discolored and may dislodge. If the edges start to curl up or are nonadherent, they can be trimmed with nail clippers or scissors to reduce the likelihood of them getting inadvertently pulled off.

Glues

Cyanoacrylate glues (2-octylcyanoacrylate, Dermabond) have been used for years for closure of wounds due to lacerations when there is no tension on the skin edges. A review of their use in the operating room found no increased rate of infection or dehiscence, but the studies excluded wounds under high tension.[2] If a surgical wound of an excision is approximated with no significant tension due to well-placed deep sutures, then skin glue is an option for the final skin closure[3] (see Chapter 7, *Laceration Repair*).

LEARNING THE TECHNIQUES: SUGGESTIONS ON HOW TO PRACTICE

Pigs' feet (fresh or previously frozen) and artificial skin pads provide a good medium for practice (Figure 6-19). Nectarines can be sutured to practice a deft touch because their skin is fragile and care is needed to follow the curve of the needle and avoid tension or it will tear (similar to the fragile skin of the elderly).

CONCLUSION

Skin can be sutured in various ways to achieve good healing and cosmesis. Clinicians should be familiar

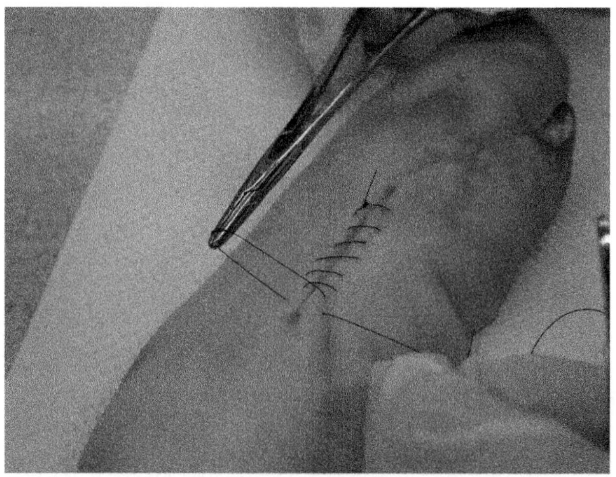

FIGURE 6-19 Using a pig's foot to practice a simple running suture. This figure is demonstrating how the final knot will be tied to a loop of suture material. *(Copyright Richard P. Usatine, MD.)*

TABLE 6-1 Advantages and Disadvantages of Suturing Techniques

Suture Technique	Advantage for Clinician	Disadvantage for Clinician	Advantage for Patient	Disadvantage for Patient	Well Suited for
Simple interrupted	Accurate control of depth, placement, and tension.	Time consuming, each one needs to be tied.	Can line up wounds better when there is a mismatch in height or length of the two sides.	Potential for "railroad track" scarring.	Small wounds and to line up larger wounds.
Simple deep or buried vertical mattress	Relieves tension, closes dead space, provides hemostasis, opposes dermis, produces eversion.	Takes more skill and experience to do well.	Decreased chance of dehiscence and hematoma.	Suture material retained in tissues can cause spitting sutures or suture granulomas.	Closing wounds that have some tension and/or dead space.
Deep horizontal mattress	Opposes dermis in areas where skin is thin. Less undermining is needed.	Takes more skill and experience to do well, does not close dead space as well as buried vertical mattress.	Decreased chance of dehiscence.	Spitting sutures or suture granulomas.	Closing wounds under tension that are not very deep.
Vertical mattress	Excellent wound eversion, decreased wound tension. Adds support to wounds under stress.	Requires more time to place than simple interrupted suture—not as good as deep sutures for relieving tension.	Wound eversion can prevent depressed scarring.	Potential for "railroad track" scarring but not as obvious as with simple interrupted sutures.	Closing wounds under tension when not using deep sutures or in addition to deep sutures when extra eversion is desired.
Horizontal mattress	Distributes tension away from skin edge.	Suture removed is more difficult.	Wound eversion can prevent depressed scarring.	Risk of ischemia at wound edge if too tight.	Closing short wounds or part of a long wound under tension with good eversion.
Running horizontal mattress	Faster than individual horizontal mattress sutures and achieves good wound eversion.	Requires more time to place than simple running suture.	Wound eversion can prevent depressed scarring.	Suture can sink into the skin, which can be uncomfortable to remove.	Closing long wounds under tension with good eversion.
Figure-of-eight	Ideal suture to stop bleeding during skin surgery.	Is more time consuming than electrocoagulation.	Effective way to get hemostasis.	Can produce scarring if used after punch biopsy.	Hemostasis, alternative for closing punch biopsies.
Running subcuticular—absorbable	Can produce a very good cosmetic result.	Takes more time and skill to place. Not for wounds under tension.	No "railroad track" scars. No suture removal.	Suture material retained in tissues as possible nidus of inflammation or infection.	Cosmetically sensitive areas or if suture removal is an issue.
Running subcuticular—nonabsorbable	Can produce a very good cosmetic result.	Takes more time and skill to place. Not for wounds under tension.	No "railroad track" scars.	Requires suture removal.	Cosmetically sensitive areas.
Staples	Quick to place.	Less control than sutures, higher cost.	Quick to place.	Multiple entry points, hard material in skin, can leave ugly scarring.	Large scalp wounds where cosmesis is not an issue.

with several techniques so they can use them—or often a combination of them—as the situation requires to achieve good approximation of the deep tissues, reduction or distribution of tension, and apposition of the dermis with slight eversion of the skin to reduce the risk of dehiscence and unnecessary scarring. Table 6-1 summarizes the advantages and disadvantages of the suturing techniques discussed in this chapter.

References

1. Wang SQ, Goldberg LH. Surgical pearl: Running horizontal mattress suture with intermittent simple loops. *J Am Acad Dermatol.* 2006;55:870–871.
2. Coulthard P, Esposito M, Worthington HV, *et al.* Tissue adhesives for closure of surgical incisions. *Cochrane Database Syst Rev.* 2002;3:CD004287. DOI:10.1002/14651858.CD004287.pub2.
3. Toriumi DM, Bagal AA. Cyanoacrylate tissue adhesives for skin closure in the outpatient setting. *Otolaryngol Clin North Am.* 2002;35(1).

SECTION TWO

Basic Procedures

7 Laceration Repair

RICHARD P. USATINE, MD • WENDY C. COATES, MD

When lacerations require intervention, they may be repaired with sutures, surgical adhesive strips, tissue adhesives, or staples. The goals of laceration repair are as follows:

1. Achieve hemostasis.
2. Prevent infection.
3. Preserve function.
4. Restore appearance
5. Minimize patient discomfort.

In repairing skin, it is helpful to understand the three phases of wound healing:

- Phase 1: Initial Lag Phase (Days 0 to 5)
  - No gain in wound strength.
- Phase 2: Fibroplasia Phase (Days 5 to 14)
  - Increase in wound strength occurs.
  - At 2 weeks, the wound has achieved only 7% of its final strength.
- Phase 3: Final Maturation Phase (Day 14 Until Healing Is Complete)
  - Further connective tissue remodeling.
  - Up to 80% of normal skin strength.

Nonabsorbable skin sutures or staples are used to give the wound strength during the first two phases. After the nonabsorbable skin sutures or staples are removed, surgical adhesive strips or previously placed deep absorbable sutures play an important role in the final phases of wound healing.

Patients should be asked about their tetanus immune status and prophylaxis should be considered. Analgesic medication may need to be provided in the acute setting and for a few days thereafter depending on the extent of the trauma and patient preferences. For most patients, acetaminophen or ibuprofen should be sufficient, but in selected patients, prescription narcotics may be indicated.

INDICATIONS FOR REPAIR

- Lacerations that are open and less than 12 hours old (less than 24 hours old on the face)
- Some bite wounds in cosmetically important areas (close follow-up recommended).

CONTRAINDICATIONS FOR REPAIR

- Wounds more than 12 hours old (more than 24 hours old on the face)
- Animal and human bite wounds (exceptions: facial wounds, dog bite wounds)
- Puncture wounds.

SUPPLIES AND EQUIPMENT

- Surgical prep: povidone-iodine (Betadine) or chlorhexidine (Hibiclens).
- Ruler marked in units of centimeters.
- Irrigation device for contaminated wounds: 30-mL syringe with 18-gauge angiocatheter or commercially manufactured splash shield device (Figure 7-1) and sterile saline.
- 1% or 2% lidocaine with or without epinephrine (see Chapter 3, *Anesthesia*).
- Syringes and 27- or 30-gauge needle (small-gauge needles are preferred to administer anesthesia).
- Sterile drapes; fenestrated drape (applied so that the hole is over the laceration).
- 4- × 4-inch gauze sponges; cotton-tipped applicators are useful for hemostasis.
- Sterile instruments: 4½-inch needle holder; curved or straight Iris scissors; one mosquito hemostat; suture scissors; Adson forceps with teeth; skin hooks (*optional*).
- No. 15 blade for excisions with blade handle (single disposable unit also available).
- Sutures (see Chapter 5, *Suture Material*), surgical adhesive strips, staples, or tissue adhesive.
- Skin-marking pen (if wound revision is needed).
- Electrosurgical unit should be available for electrocoagulation.
- Protective mask with plastic shield for eyes or other types of personal protective equipment (see Chapter 2, Figure 2-14).

PREPROCEDURE PATIENT PREPARATION

The patient should be informed of the nature of his or her lacerations. If the laceration is in a cosmetically important area, consider offering the option of a specialist, such as a plastic surgeon or ophthalmologist, for the repair. Advise the patient about the risks of pain, bleeding, dehiscence, infection, and scarring. Inform the patient that most repairs cause some permanent scarring, although attempts will be made to optimize the appearance. Warn patients of the risks of hyperpigmentation or hypopigmentation, hypertrophic scars, keloids, nerve damage, alopecia, and distortion of the original anatomy. After a discussion of risks and benefits

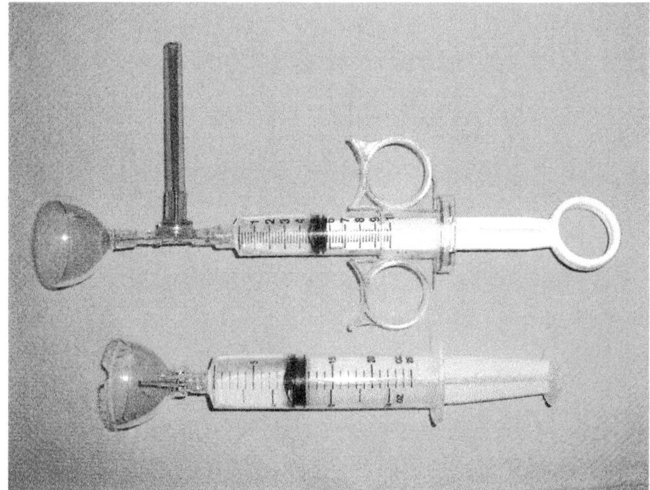

FIGURE 7-1 Many useful devices are available for irrigating dirty wounds, including the Zerowet Klenzalac system, which has a special syringe attached to a splash shield, and the more simple Zerowet Supershield for use on a standard syringe. *(Copyright Richard P. Usatine, MD.)*

have the patient sign a consent form before beginning the procedure (see Chapter 1, *Preoperative Preparation*).

Initial Assessment

The initial evaluation before anesthesia should include a history of how the wound was sustained, factors that might impair healing, tetanus immunization history, and an assessment of peripheral neurovascular status. See Table 7-1 for essentials of wound assessment. The clinician should consider the possibility of domestic violence in patients with traumatic wounds, especially if lacerations appear on the face or if multiple injuries of varying ages are noted.

In general, antibiotics are not needed for either wound or subacute bacterial endocarditis (SBE) prophylaxis for cutaneous procedures[1] (see Chapter 1). Consideration should be given to coverage for *Staphylococcus aureus* and MRSA infection in several situations.

TABLE 7-1 Essentials of Wound Assessment

Parameters	Factors to Consider
Mechanism of injury	Sharp vs. blunt trauma, bite
Dirty vs. clean	Outdoors vs. kitchen sink
Time since injury	Suture up to 12 h; 24 h on face
Foreign body	Explore and obtain radiograph for metal or glass
Functional examination	Neurovascular, muscular, tendons
Need for prophylactic antibiotics	If needed, give ASAP and cover *Staphylococcus aureus*; irrigate well

The following are major goals for prescribing antibiotics before or after skin surgery:

1. Prevention of a new wound infection
2. Prevention of the spread of an existing local infection
3. Treatment of an existing infection
4. Prevention of bacterial endocarditis.

The clinical decision-making process of whether or not to use antibiotics before or after skin surgery is complex. The physician must consider host factors, the anatomic location of the surgery, the sources that might contaminate the wound, and method of wound injury. The multiple factors to be considered when making a decision about antibiotic prophylaxis for skin procedures are:

Coexisting Conditions

- Diabetes mellitus
- Peripheral vascular disease
- Frail elderly patients
- Immunocompromised
- Previous radiation to the site
- Malnutrition (e.g., alcoholism, chemotherapy)
- History of previous infection or slow healing
- Chronic steroid use
- Morbid obesity.

Locations

- Axilla, mouth and anogenital areas have higher levels of bacterial colonization
- End arterial locations (fingers, toes) with diseases of vascular compromise
- Over joint spaces where there is a possibility of entering joint (e.g., metacarpal-phalangeal joints).

Contamination

- Dirty wounds, especially barnyards, meatpacking plants, etc.
- Less than optimal sterile technique (should be rare)
- Deep puncture wounds
- Bites (especially human and cat bites)
- Presence of a retained foreign body.

Method of Wound Injury

- Crush injury (10-fold increase in infection) with devitalized skin
- Penetrating injury.

The recommendations of the American Heart Association (AHA) for the prevention of bacterial endocarditis were last published in 2007 and are discussed in Chapter 1.[1] Endocarditis prophylaxis is not needed for incision or biopsy of surgically scrubbed noninfected skin no matter what endocarditis risk factors are present. The 2007 guidelines state that antibiotic prophylaxis is recommended for procedures on infected skin and skin structures for patients with underlying cardiac conditions associated with the highest risk of adverse outcome from infective endocarditis (see Chapter 1, Box 1-2 and Table 1-3).[1]

Cummings *et al.* performed a meta-analysis of randomized studies on the use of antibiotics to prevent infection of simple wounds.[2] They concluded that there is no evidence in published trials that prophylactic antibiotics offer protection against infection of nonbite wounds in patients treated in emergency departments. However, prophylactic antibiotics did reduce the incidence of infection in patients with dog-bite wounds in another meta-analysis.[3] The authors concluded that it may be reasonable to limit prophylactic antibiotics to patients with dog-bite wounds that are at highest risk for infection.[3]

Controversy exists over which bite injuries should be treated with prophylactic antibiotics. Cat- and dog-bite injuries carry the risk of infection with *Pasteurella multocida*, and human-bite injuries carry the risk of infection with *Eikenella corrodens* and *S. aureus*. Based on the microbiology of these wounds, amoxicillin/clavulanate provides good prophylactic coverage for the bacteria affecting most bite injuries. Alternatives include second-generation cephalosporins or clindamycin with a fluoroquinolone.

Antibiotics have a role in the treatment of many established skin infections. However, most skin abscesses are better treated with incision and drainage rather than with antibiotics. For skin procedures of infected skin, no specific evidence exists as to whether to give an antibiotic and the appropriate timing for its administration. Recommendations for timing before the procedure vary from 1 hour (which is typical timing for bacterial endocarditis prophylaxis) to within 30 minutes of the procedure. Whereas a single second dose 6 hours later was the standard in the past, it is no longer currently recommended for bacterial endocarditis prophylaxis but may be advocated for further treatment of the infection.

The best method for prevention of wound infections is to clean and irrigate traumatic wounds well, rather than relying on prophylactic antibiotics. The physician needs to weigh the benefits and the risks of antibiotic use based on the individual patient and the circumstances of the wound repair or skin surgery.

Local and Regional Anesthesia

In traumatic wounds, neurovascular integrity should be assessed prior to administration of anesthesia. The wound should then be fully anesthetized to allow for painless examination of the tissue damage, thorough irrigation, and adequate closure. Many wounds can be adequately anesthetized with 1% or 2% lidocaine. Consider using lidocaine with epinephrine to provide increased hemostasis if there are no contraindications to epinephrine use in the patient, the location, or the wound itself (see Chapter 3, *Anesthesia*). Topical anesthetics are effective for wounds that do not involve mucosal surfaces. A combination of lidocaine, epinephrine, and tetracaine (LET) applied with a saturated cotton ball or as a gel formulation directly into the wound provides adequate anesthesia for many wounds.[4,5]

Regional anesthesia may be desirable in cases where the volume of locally infiltrated anesthesia might exceed the safe maximum dosage (see Chapter 3, Table 3-3) or in cosmetically important areas where a local infiltration might distort the anatomy to impair a meticulous closure. If a regional anesthetic technique is employed, lidocaine without epinephrine is the optimal choice, because epinephrine's role as a vasoconstrictor is not needed at a site remote to the traumatic wound.

Follow these instructions to minimize the pain of injecting local anesthetic:

- Use a small-gauge needle (27 or 30 gauge).
- Inject slowly.
- Inject directly into the dermis through the open wound (not through intact skin).
- Warm anesthetic to body temperature (optional).
- Buffer the anesthetic with sodium bicarbonate (1 mL bicarbonate for .9 mL lidocaine) (*optional*).

Wound Preparation

After the initial assessment and administration of local or regional anesthetic, and antibiotics if indicated, wounds should be inspected thoroughly for foreign bodies, deep tissue layer damage, and injury to nerve, vessel, or tendon. Underlying bone or joint injury should be considered in wounds sustained as a result of traumatic force. A radiograph should be obtained to look for retained glass or metal in wounds sustained from broken glass or metal and to assess for joint integrity or fractures in traumatic injuries. Complex wounds or those in cosmetically important areas should be closed by a practitioner with the appropriate expertise.

Determine If the Wound Needs Intervention to Close

One study assessed the difference in clinical outcome between lacerations of the hand closed with sutures and those treated conservatively.[6] Consecutive patients with uncomplicated lacerations of the hand (full thickness < 2 cm; without tendon, joint, fracture, or nerve complications) who would normally require sutures were randomized to suturing or conservative treatment. The mean time to resume normal activities was the same in both groups (3.4 days). Patients treated conservatively had less pain and treatment time was 14 (10 to 18) minutes shorter. The groups did not differ significantly in the assessment of cosmetic appearance on the visual analogue scale. Conservative treatment was faster and less painful.[6]

Cleansing

After the wound is anesthetized, cleansing of the wound should be performed by irrigation with normal saline at 8 to 12 psi of pressure. This can be accomplished by attaching an 18-gauge angiocatheter or a commercially available splash shield to a 20- or 30-mL syringe. At least 200 mL of irrigation is recommended. Irrijet and Zerowet were superior to an angiocatheter in preventing splatter during wound model irrigation.[3] Zerowet was particularly effective in preventing splatter onto the irrigator's face (Figure 7-1).[3]

A multicenter comparison of tap water versus sterile saline for wound irrigation published in 2007 showed equivalent rates of wound infection in immunocompetent patients.[7] The tap water group irrigated their own wounds under the water tap for a minimum of 2 minutes after they had the wound anesthetized. Higher risk wounds were excluded from the study, indicating that tap water is a reasonable cleansing alternative for low-risk lacerations. In one randomized clinical trial, warmed saline was more comfortable and soothing than room-temperature saline as a wound irrigant among patients with linear lacerations.[8]

Chemical compounds such as hexachlorophene (pHisoHex), chlorhexidine gluconate (Hibiclens), or povidone-iodine (Betadine) should not be used inside wounds but may be applied to external, intact skin if desired. Greasy contaminants can be removed with any petroleum-based product, such as petrolatum or bacitracin ointment. To prevent a road rash tattoo, wrap petroleum gauze around the fingers and wipe off the asphalt and other foreign material embedded in the skin after anesthesia. Topical and regional anesthetic techniques are particularly effective in this situation.

Debridement

After the cleansing process, wounds should be examined for devitalized tissue that needs removal or debridement. This debridement may convert a jagged, contaminated wound into a clean surgical one and can be accomplished with a scalpel or sharp tissue scissors. As much tissue as possible should be preserved in case future scar revision is necessary. After debridement, wound edges should be held together to see if they are under any tension. Wounds under significant tension are best repaired by a two-layer closure. In dirty wounds, however, this may increase the incidence of infection.

Undermining

Undermining can significantly reduce skin tension when there is a gap to be closed. Undermining may increase the risk of infection and thus should be avoided in dirty wounds. Care should be taken to minimize the use of this technique in areas with poor blood supply, because the process of undermining reduces it further. Extreme care is also needed when undermining around vital structures. Approximately one-third to one-half of the undermined tissue is freed up to be brought into the defect. When needed and if possible, undermine bilaterally as far back as the wound is wide.

CLOSURE TECHNIQUE

Ideally, four principles should be incorporated in the process of closing any wound:

1. *Control all bleeding before closure.* This can be accomplished by applying direct pressure for at least 5 minutes, applying an ice pack, adding epinephrine to the local anesthetic when appropriate, with electrocoagulation, or by tying off bleeders with absorbable sutures.
2. *Eliminate "dead space."* Eliminate areas where tissue fluid and blood can accumulate.
3. *Accurately approximate tissue layers to each other.* Scars are most visible when shadows are created by depressed or elevated tissue. Also be sure that anatomic areas match on each side in critical areas such as the vermilion border of the lip or the eyebrows.
4. *Approximate the wound with minimal skin tension.* If the amount of tension will be significant, undermining and/or deep, inverted, buried sutures are used to decrease the tension on the skin margin. Ideally, when the repair is completed the wound will be tented up slightly.

Choice of Sutures

Most lacerations will be closed with nylon. If a two-layer closure is needed, an absorbable suture such as polyglactin 910 (Vicryl) or a synthetic absorbable monofilament suture is a good choice for the deep layer. Silk sutures may be considered for closure in the mouth or other areas where the nylon ends will be bothersome. Alternately, rapidly absorbing Vicryl Rapide may be used in oral lacerations without the need for suture removal. In one study, otherwise healthy children with facial lacerations were randomized to repair using fast-absorbing catgut or nylon suture.[9] There were no significant differences in the rates of infection, wound dehiscence, keloid formation, and parental satisfaction between the absorbable catgut and the nylon suture.[9] Fast-absorbing catgut suture is not as easy to work with as nylon but does have the advantage of not requiring suture removal in children who may be very fearful of the suture removal process.

Suggested suture size and time of removal based on anatomic areas is found in Table 7-2.

Sutured Repairs

See video on the DVD for further learning. 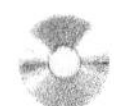

Lacerations are approximated with sutures using a variety of techniques (see Chapter 6, *Suturing Techniques*), as discussed in the following subsections.

Simple Interrupted Suture

On completion of a simple interrupted suture (Figure 7-2), the skin margins should be slightly everted. The needle should enter the skin surface at a 90-degree angle. The stitch should be as wide as it is deep. The suture on both sides of the wound should be equal distance from the wound margin and of equal depth. The final shape should appear like that of a pear (see Chapter 6, Figure 6-5). As a general rule, these sutures need to be no closer than 2 mm in a fine plastic closure and can be substantially farther apart in other types of closures. The distance between sutures should equal half the total distance of the sutures across the incision.

TABLE 7-2 Suture Size and Time of Removal

Anatomic Area	Days Until Removal	External Suture Size	Buried Absorbable Suture Size
Face	3-6	5-0 or 6-0	4-0 or 5-0
Scalp	10-14	4-0, staples	3-0 or 4-0
Upper body	7-10	4-0	4-0
Hand	7-10	4-0 or 5-0	4-0
Lower body	10-14	4-0	3-0 or 4-0
Over joint (splint recommended)	14-21	4-0	3-0 or 4-0

Source: Adapted from Coates WC. Lacerations to the face. In Tintinalli JE, Kellen GD, Stapczynski JS. *Emergency Medicine, A Comprehensive Study Guide*, 6th ed. New York: McGraw-Hill; 2004.

The finer the suture, the closer the stitch needs to be. Avoid tying the knots too tightly. The knots should be lined up on the same side of the wound, usually the one with the best blood supply or least interference with comfort (e.g., away from eyelid).

Simple Running Stitch

The advantages of the simple running stitch (Figure 7-3) in sterile wounds under little or no tension are that it is quick, it distributes tension evenly, and it provides excellent cosmetic results. If there is significant gaping of the wound, interrupted suture methods should be used. Because the risk of contamination is increased with traumatic lacerations, the simple running stitch is less desirable in these wounds. In case of infection, the entire wound closure would need to be removed. The relative disadvantage of removing the entire stitch at one time also poses a problem in wounds under some increased tension. With interrupted techniques, some sutures may be removed early for better cosmesis, whereas a few remaining ones can be left for prevention of dehiscence and removed at a later date. The simple running stitch is ideal in the scalp and is often used in elliptical excision repairs.

Deep Suture with Inverted Knot or Buried Stitch

Deeper wounds or wounds under tension are best closed by providing structural support and not relying solely on nonabsorbable superficial sutures. Well-placed deep absorbable sutures (Figure 7-4 and Chapter 6, Figure 6-9) can do much to aid in closing a wound, remove tension from the superficial skin sutures, and decrease scarring by providing increased wound support long after the epidermal sutures have been removed. Deep sutures also close dead space, which decreases the risk of hematomas and dehiscence.

The inverted knot technique places the knot as far below the skin margins as possible to avoid suture spitting (migration of deep sutures to the skin surface). It also keeps the ends of the cut suture from protruding through the wound margin. To start the stitch, begin at the bottom of the wound (in the undermined area if undermining was used) and come up usually just below the epidermal-dermal junction (remember, "Bottoms up!"). Go straight across the incision, enter at the same level at the opposite side, then go down to the base at the same depth once again and tie. Care should be

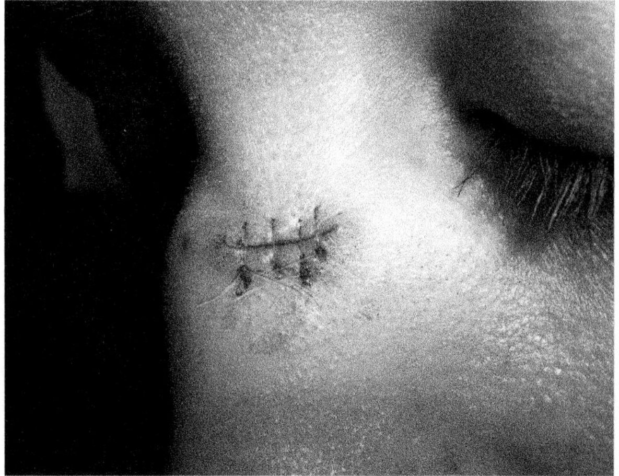

FIGURE 7-2 Simple interrupted suture of a small nose laceration. *(Copyright Richard P. Usatine, MD.)*

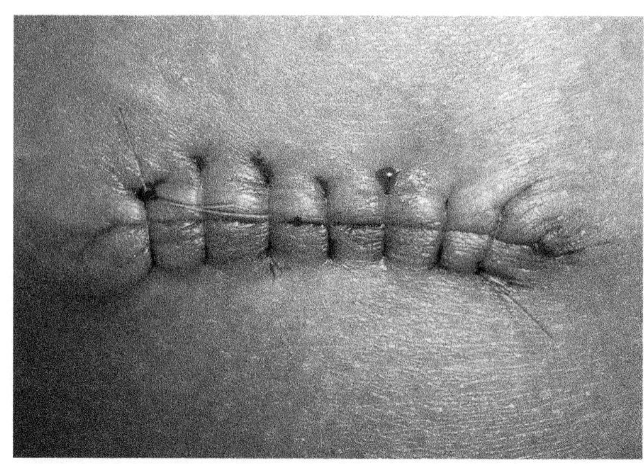

FIGURE 7-3 Running stitch. Always keep the depth of the suture placement the same on each side. *(Copyright Richard P. Usatine, MD.)*

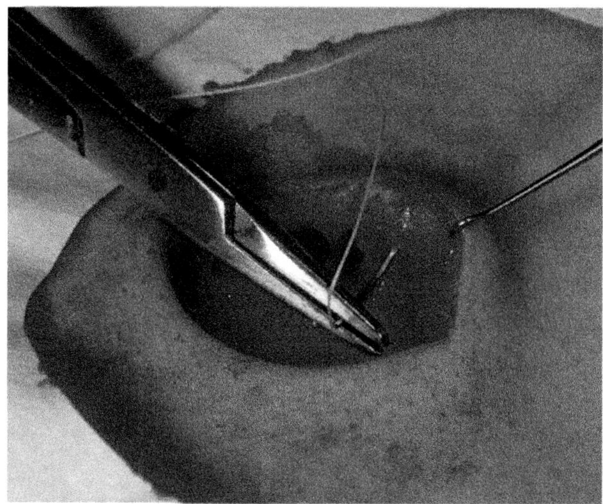

FIGURE 7-4 Deep stitch with absorbable suture material. The suture needle should enter deep in the skin below the dermis where the undermining was accomplished and exit in the upper dermis. *(Copyright Richard P. Usatine, MD.)*

taken to achieve symmetry of depth and width on both sides of the laceration. For a more detailed discussion of the deep vertical mattress suture, see Chapter 6. The epidermis is then fully closed with a closure of choice (nonabsorbable suture, wound closure strips, or tissue adhesive).

Vertical Mattress Suture

The vertical mattress suture (Figure 7-5 and Chapter 6, Figure 6-12) promotes eversion of the wound edges of the skin. It is also useful when the natural tendency of loose skin is to create inversion of the wound margins, which should be avoided. A good example is the loose, flabby skin under the triceps muscle and thin skin in older people. The stitch is also appropriate when the skin is very thin and interrupted sutures have a tendency to pull through.

Horizontal Mattress Suture

The horizontal mattress suture (see Chapter 6, Figure 6-13) is helpful in wounds under a moderate amount of tension and also promotes wound edge eversion. It is especially useful on the palms or soles and in patients who are poor candidates for deep sutures because of susceptibility to wound infections. It is not recommended in wounds that are located in cosmetically important areas.

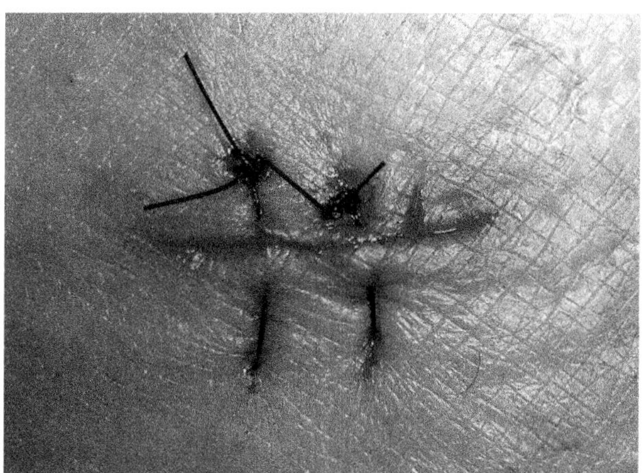

FIGURE 7-5 Vertical mattress suture. *(Copyright Richard P. Usatine, MD.)*

Subcuticular Running Suture (Figure 7-6 and Chapter 6, Figure 6-17)

The subcuticular running suture (Figure 7-6 and Chapter 6, Figure 6-17) is used to close linear wounds that are under minimal tension; it yields an excellent cosmetic result. It is advantageous in patients who tend to form hypertrophic scars or keloids, because it minimizes the number of times the skin's surface must be perforated with the suture needle. Meticulous alignment of each stitch is critical to prevent gaps in the linear wound. The ends of the suture do not need to be tied; taping under slight tension preserves approximation. If desired, the two ends can be tied over the wound, or a knot can be placed at each end to prevent slippage. Usually a polypropylene-coated nylon works best. Steri-Strips, strips, or tissue glue can be used to supplement this type of stitch. Special care must be taken to avoid pressure on the wound, since this stitch separates easily.

Three-Point or Half-Buried Mattress Suture (Chapter 6, Figure 6-15)

The three-point or half-buried mattress suture (see Chapter 6, Figure 6-15) is designed to permit closure of

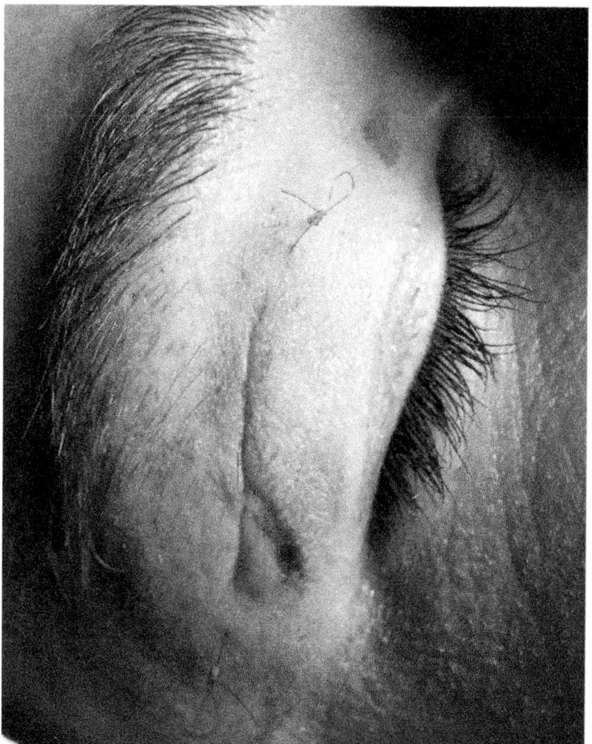

FIGURE 7-6 Subcuticular running suture. *(Courtesy of Joe Deng, MD.)*

the acute corner tip of a laceration without impairing blood flow to the tip. It is an intradermal stitch in which the needle is inserted initially into the intact skin on the nonflap portion of the wound and passed through the skin at the mid-dermis level; at the same level, the suture is then passed transversely through the tip of the flap, returned on the opposite side of the wound, and brought through the skin, paralleling the point of entrance. The suture is tied by drawing the tip snugly into place in good approximation. Care should be taken not to have the knot tied over the point of the flap. This same approach can be used in closing a stellate laceration, drawing the tips together in a purse-string fashion. The resulting knot should be placed over the segment of the stellate laceration with the best blood supply. Repair of a "T" laceration also uses this technique.

Surgical Adhesive Strips (Steri-Strips)

Surgical adhesive strips may be used alone for small, superficial wounds (especially in young children).[10,11] When these strips suffice to close a wound, they are more easily placed without physical or psychological trauma to the child. Wounds closed with adhesive strips are more resistant to infection than are sutured wounds. However, surgical adhesive strips are not appropriate for deep lacerations because they do not provide adequate deep-tissue approximation or skin-edge eversion when used alone. Surgical adhesive strips with or without gum mastic did not provide any additional strength to wounds closed by subcuticular continuous suture.[12] Surgical adhesive strips are especially helpful after suture removal to prevent dehiscence and may be left on until they fall off. Patients may shower with them on after the initial 24 hours.

Surgical adhesive strips adhere better to the skin when a sticky substance is applied to the skin first. Tincture of benzoin and gum mastic (Mastisol) are both helpful. Studies have shown that gum mastic offers superior adhesive qualities compared with benzoin and has a lower incidence of postoperative contact dermatitis and subsequent skin discoloration.[13,14]

Tissue Adhesives

Tissue adhesives may be used to close certain wounds that are not under any tension and are not at risk for infection. These can be purchased as octylcyanoacrylate (Dermabond) and butylcyanoacrylate (SkinStitch). A Cochrane systematic review provides evidence that tissue adhesives are an option to sutures, staples, and adhesive strips for the management of simple traumatic lacerations that are not under tension nor prone to wound infection.[15] Overall, no significant differences were found in cosmetic scores at the reported assessment periods between tissue adhesives and these other methods. At 1 to 3 months, a subgroup analysis significantly favored butylcyanoacrylate over all other skin closure methods. Tissue adhesives significantly lowered the time to complete the procedure, the levels of pain, and the incidence of erythema. However, the data revealed a significant increase in the rate of dehiscence with the use of tissue adhesives when compared with the other methods of skin closure.[16]

Tissue adhesives and surgical adhesive strips are both excellent "no needle" alternatives for the closure of suitable pediatric lacerations.[10] These two techniques are similar in efficacy, parental acceptability, and cosmetic outcome.[10] Appropriate wound preparation techniques, such as irrigation under local or topical anesthesia, are still necessary. Nail bed repair performed using tissue adhesives is significantly faster than suture repair.[17] Tissue adhesives provide similar cosmetic and functional results in the management of acute nail bed lacerations.[17]

Tissue adhesives should be avoided on any wound that has any tension. They should not be used on any area that can be flexed (i.e., a knuckle or wrist). If it is necessary to use on a jointed area, immobilize the joint with a splint. Cover eyes with gauze when working on the forehead or near the eye. Consider using petrolatum to create a barrier between the cut and the eyes to minimize the chance of the product running into the eye. If the product enters the eye, it may be removed by applying an ophthalmic ointment, which will eventually dissolve the adhesive. This can be followed by gentle irrigation, often performed several hours later by the patient at home using water in their hands over a sink. Appropriate treatment for any resulting corneal abrasion should be followed.

Follow these guidelines, which are adapted from SkinStitch information, when using tissue adhesives (Figure 7-7):

1. Tap glue down into the bottom bulb of the applicator.
2. Holding the applicator tip upright, snip the tip as close to the end as possible.
3. Never put the glue in the wound.
4. Apply a thin layer of adhesive along the edge of the area to be treated, or use the multiple dot technique.
5. Pull the adhesive across to the other side of the wound, using the applicator as a hockey stick. In effect, you are building a bridge over the minor cut or wound.
6. Hold the wound edges together for 30 to 60 seconds.
7. Apply a second and third thin coat. Remember, two or three thin layers are actually stronger than one thick coat.
8. Some patients may experience mild burning; this is normal, but warn patients so they do not move and ruin the adhesion.
9. A Steri-Strip can be used for extra strength or to keep a child from picking at the wound.

Staples

Staples are most often used to repair scalp lacerations. In one randomized trial of children (ages 1 to 16 years) with simple scalp lacerations, patients were randomly assigned to either a stapling or suturing procedure.[18] Procedure time was significantly lower in the stapling

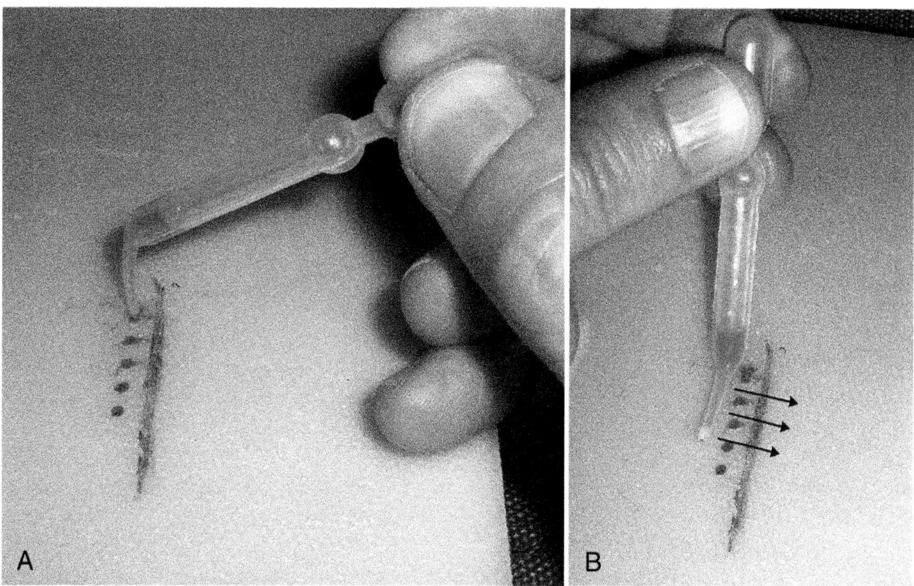

FIGURE 7-7 Use of tissue adhesive to close a laceration not under tension. **(A)** Better to apply 2 or 3 thin coats rather than one thick coat. Apply drops (approx. size as above) about ¼″ apart and next to the area to be covered. These small drops will prevent running and when spread will create thin coats and dry in about 30 minutes. **(B)** Then, twirl the applicator and use the spreader to spread the drops. *(Photographs courtesy of Richard P. Usatine, MD. Device courtesy of SkinStich Corp, Massena, NY.)*

group ($P = 0.001$). There were no significant differences in the final follow-up cosmetic score between the two groups.[18] Although staples are faster to apply to the scalp, the cost of the materials is greater. Scalp stapling should not be attempted in men who are already bald or in wounds that extend to the forehead.

Delayed Primary Closure (Tertiary Intention)

Primary closure is defined by the use of sutures, strips, or adhesives to close the wound at the time of initial surgery or evaluation. Healing by secondary intention occurs when no attempt is made to close the wound and the wound heals naturally by granulation. This method is used after a simple shave biopsy, in grossly contaminated or infected wounds, or in wounds that present far too late to consider closure.

Delayed primary closure is healing by tertiary intention. This technique is used for wounds that are greater than 12 hours old (24 hours for facial lacerations) but would cosmetically benefit from closure in a few days. After anesthetizing, evaluating, and irrigating the wound, insert a small piece of petroleum gauze between the wound edges and place the patient on an antibiotic, such as cephalexin, for 5 days. On the third day, the patient should return for definitive repair. If the wound appears clean and free of infection and has not started the granulation process, the repair can proceed. The wound is reanesthetized, reirrigated, and closed primarily with nonabsorbable sutures (i.e., no deep sutures because they increase the chance of infection). The patient continues the course of prescribed antibiotics and suture removal occurs at the interval beginning at the time of suturing (Table 7-2).

COMPLICATIONS

The complications of laceration repair are the same as when a biopsy or surgical excision is performed (bleeding, infection, dehiscence, etc.). The main differences relate to coexisting trauma such as crush injuries that can devitalize tissue around the laceration or lead to underlying injuries to tendons, vessels, bones, or joints. For discussion of complications and their treatment and prevention see Chapter 36, *Complications*.

POSTPROCEDURE PATIENT EDUCATION

Most wounds are best protected with some sort of dressing during the first 24 to 48 hours after closure. Continued oozing might be expected or pressure might be needed. For hemostasis, a pressure dressing should be applied. This could be a folded gauze over a thin strip of sterile ointment over the suture line with tape over it, or a nonstick type of gauze dressing covered with gauze and tape. Trade names for nonstick dressings include Xeroform, Adaptic, and Telfa. It is not usually necessary to keep a wound completely dry after 24 hours, because the epidermis has formed a seal by this time. Therefore, patients may shower after 24 hours and redress the wound after gently drying it. Immersion of the laceration should be avoided because the sutures provide an avenue to introduce into the wound the bacteria present in a body of water (e.g., bath, Jacuzzi, swimming pool, lake, ocean, kitchen sink).

Moist healing (application of petrolatum after gentle washing twice daily) aids in quicker healing. Although antibiotic ointments were traditionally used for dressings postsurgically, Smack et al. determined that clean wounds heal just as well when white petrolatum is applied.[19] Neomycin and bacitracin are frequent contact allergens and have not been proven to prevent infections after a laceration is repaired. Application of any of these products should be limited to the smallest possible area over the suture line. Extension over the wound edges may lead to maceration of the skin and reduce its ability to hold the sutures securely in place, thus causing them to pull through and lead to wound dehiscence.

Suggestions for the timing for skin suture removal are listed in Table 7-2.

Wounds on the face or scalp may be dressed with a thin layer of antibiotic ointment or petrolatum in lieu of a mechanical dressing. It is best to cover them at night to avoid drying. Instruct patients to return if signs of wound infection appear, including erythema, pus, lymphangitis, or fever. A routine wound check is not necessary for patients who understand the importance of monitoring the wound for signs of infection. All wounds should be covered with sunscreen for at least 6 months following the repair if they are located on areas exposed to the sun.

CONSIDERATIONS FOR SPECIFIC ANATOMIC REPAIRS

Lip

When evaluating a patient with a superficial lip laceration, it is important to note whether the laceration extends through the vermilion border. In this instance, the vermilion border should be approximated first with a 6-0 nylon (or polypropylene) suture. There is no room for error in this area, because even a 1-mm discrepancy is a cosmetic problem.

For lip lacerations that extend through multiple layers, a more complex repair must be performed. A through-and-through laceration is repaired in three steps. After ensuring the integrity of the teeth, the mucosal layer is gently irrigated and closed with a soft suture for comfort (4-0 silk or Vicryl Rapide). Next, the wound is reirrigated from the outside and the muscle layer closed with an absorbable suture. Finally, the skin is closed with simple interrupted sutures. It is reasonable to consider an infraorbital regional nerve block for an upper lip laceration or a mandibular regional nerve block for a lower lip laceration (see Chapter 3).

Eyelid

Lacerations around the eye require careful examination of ocular structures. The integrity of the globe should be carefully assessed, and a thorough eye exam is warranted. If a visual abnormality, lacrimal system defect, or globe rupture is suspected, immediate referral is indicated. Repair by an ophthalmologist or oculoplastic specialist is warranted in wounds that involve the lacrimal system, lid lacerations that extend through the tarsal plate, or wounds that cross the palpebral margins.

For an uncomplicated lid laceration, a small (6-0) suture is used. Care must be taken to place the suture through the skin only and to avoid penetration through the tarsal plate or globe (Figure 7-6). Regional anesthesia with a supraorbital nerve block for the upper lid or an infraorbital nerve block for the lower lid may be useful (see Chapter 3).

Nose

Nasal lacerations can be repaired using standard techniques after careful evaluation for underlying injury. In many cases an underlying nasal bone fracture or cartilage disruption is present. If the nasal bone is fractured and a laceration is present, it should be treated as an open fracture and appropriate antibiotics prescribed. Nasal cartilage rarely requires suturing, because it is held in place by surrounding anatomic structures and regains stability when the overlying skin is sutured. Lacerations to the alar margins must be aligned carefully. When a blunt force trauma causes a nasal laceration, a careful examination for a septal hematoma should be undertaken. Epistaxis should be controlled prior to the repair and may involve packing or referral to an ENT specialist.

Nail Bed

Nail bed lacerations are suspected when there has been blunt trauma to the nail area and a subungual hematoma occupies greater than 50% of the surface under the nail. If the nail is loose, it should be removed and the underlying nail bed laceration repaired. In addition, to preserve the natural smoothness of the nail bed when an underlying laceration has occurred, the practitioner can consider removing the nail of the patient who has a >50% subungual hematoma. The wound is repaired with a rapidly absorbing suture, such as Vicryl Rapide or with tissue adhesive.

Alternately, a patient with a nail bed laceration can have a partial nail removal on the distal side of the laceration. Using an 18-gauge needle, two or three holes are bored into the proximal end of the nail bed laceration. The sutures are directed through these holes on the proximal nail and into the soft tissue on the distal side of the nail bed.

Thorough anesthesia is required and is best achieved using a digital or metacarpal block. If the nail is removed, it can be used as the resulting dressing postprocedure. It can be reinserted into the eponychium to ensure that new nail growth can occur. In the event that the nail itself cannot be replaced, future nail growth can be promoted by inserting a small piece of nonadherent gauze into the eponychium. To protect the sensitive nail bed area, a bulky finger dressing can be applied over a single layer of nonadherent gauze. Alternately, a commercially available synthetic nail product can be placed over the area to afford protection against painful trauma.

CPT/BILLING CODES AND ICD-9-CM DIAGNOSTIC CODES

Coding and billing becomes very complex for laceration repair and excisions. Important factors to list for billing personnel are as follows:

- Location
- Length of closure
- Intermediate repair includes either undermining or placement of deep buried sutures. Intermediate repair increases the amount that can be billed significantly. Do not forget to bill for this portion if your repair is truly an intermediate one.

Suture removal is included in the initial charge if the original sutures were placed by the same group of physicians. Suture removal can be billed if performed by an unassociated physician or group. If a laceration is repaired in a simple fashion (no undermining, deep sutures or flaps), the fee includes suture removal.

CONCLUSION

In the treatment of lacerations, careful inspection, adequate irrigation, skilled closure, and appropriate wound care can produce the best functional and cosmetic results. See Box 7-1 for a list of suturing pearls for lacerations. The principles and steps covered in this chapter show how lacerations can be repaired with maximal skill and minimal discomfort to the patient.

Resources

Splash Shield, covers the full face with clear plastic on a comfortable headband (800-536-6686; splashshield@aol.com)

Zerowet Supershield and Zerowet Klenzalac irrigation system (www.zerowet.com; 800-438-0938).

The remainder of the equipment can be obtained from any medical supplier, including those listed in Chapter 2.

BOX 7-1 *Suturing Pearls for Lacerations*

- Use 27- to 30-gauge needle for anesthesia, using a slow injections into the open laceration.
- Use 1% lidocaine with epi (epinephrine is helpful to achieve hemostasis)
- Undermine only when needed.
- Eliminate dead space with deep sutures.
- Use deep inverted buried absorbable sutures to reduce skin tension ("Bottoms up!").
- Evert skin edges slightly ("Build pyramids, not ditches").
- Place interrupted sutures half to full as far apart as they are across. The more tension, the more sutures needed. Follow the Erlenmeyer flask (or pear) shape. The finer the suture, the more sutures needed, but the less scarring.
- Edema occurs after closure. Only approximate tissues; do not strangulate the skin.
- Begin gentle washing of wound after 12 to 24 h; if Steri-Strips and/or tissue glues are not used, apply an ointment to keep the wound moist to speed healing.
- Apply Steri-Strips after suture removal in wounds under tension.

References

1. Wilson W, Taubert KA, Gewitz M, *et al.* Prevention of infective endocarditis: guidelines from the American Heart Association: a guideline from the American Heart Association Rheumatic Fever, Endocarditis, and Kawasaki Disease Committee, Council on Cardiovascular Disease in the Young, and the Council on Clinical Cardiology, Council on Cardiovascular Surgery and Anesthesia, and the Quality of Care and Outcomes Research Interdisciplinary Working Group 3. *Circulation.* 2007;116:1736–1754.
2. Cummings P, Del Beccaro MA. Antibiotics to prevent infection of simple wounds: a meta-analysis of randomized studies. *Am J Emerg Med.* 1995;13:396–400.
3. Cummings P. Antibiotics to prevent infection in patients with dog bite wounds: a meta-analysis of randomized trials. *Ann Emerg Med.* 1994;23:535–540.
4. Adler AJ, Dubinisky I, Eisen J. Does the use of topical lidocaine, epinephrine, and tetracaine solution provide sufficient anesthesia for laceration repair? *Acad Emerg Med.* 1998;5:108–112.
5. Resch K, Schilling C, Borchert BD, *et al.* Topical anesthesia for pediatric lacerations: a randomized trial of lidocaine-epinephrine-tetracaine solution versus gel. *Ann Emerg Med.* 1998;32:693–697.
6. Quinn J, Cummings S, Callaham M, Sellers K. Suturing versus conservative management of lacerations of the hand: randomised controlled trial. *Br Med J.* 2002;325:299.
7. Moscati RM, Mayrose J, Reardon RF, *et al.* A multicenter comparison of tap water versus sterile saline for wound irrigation. *Acad Emerg Med.* 2007;14:404–409.
8. Ernst AA, Gershoff L, Miller P, *et al.* Warmed versus room temperature saline for laceration irrigation: a randomized clinical trial. *South Med J.* 2003;96:436–439.
9. Luck RP, Flood R, Eyal D, *et al.* Cosmetic outcomes of absorbable versus nonabsorbable sutures in pediatric facial lacerations. *Pediatr Emerg Care.* 2008;24:137–142.
10. Mattick A, Clegg G, Beattie T, Ahmad T. A randomised, controlled trial comparing a tissue adhesive (2-octylcyanoacrylate) with adhesive strips (Steristrips) for paediatric laceration repair. *Emerg Med J.* 2002;19:405–407.
11. Zempsky WT, Parrotti D, Grem C, Nichols J. Randomized controlled comparison of cosmetic outcomes of simple facial lacerations closed with Steri-Strip skin closures or Dermabond tissue adhesive. *Pediatr Emerg Care.* 2004;20:519–524.
12. Yavuzer R, Kelly C, Durrani N, *et al.* Reinforcement of subcuticular continuous suture closure with surgical adhesive strips and gum mastic: is there any additional strength provided? *Am J Surg.* 2005;189:315–318.
13. Mikhail GR, Selak L, Salo S. Reinforcement of surgical adhesive strips. *J Dermatol Surg Oncol.* 1986;12:904–905, 908.
14. Lesesne CB. The postoperative use of wound adhesives. Gum mastic versus benzoin, USP. *J Dermatol Surg Oncol.* 1992;18:990.
15. Farion K, Osmond MH, Hartling L, *et al.* Tissue adhesives for traumatic lacerations in children and adults. *Cochrane Database Syst Rev.* 2002;CD003326.
16. Beam JW. Tissue adhesives for simple traumatic lacerations. *J Athl Train.* 2008;43:222–224.
17. Strauss EJ, Weil WM, Jordan C, Paksima N. A prospective, randomized, controlled trial of 2-octylcyanoacrylate versus suture repair for nail bed injuries. *J Hand Surg [Am].* 2008;33:250–253.
18. Khan AN, Dayan PS, Miller S, *et al.* Cosmetic outcome of scalp wound closure with staples in the pediatric emergency department: a prospective, randomized trial. *Pediatr Emerg Care.* 2002;18:171–173.
19. Smack DP, Harrington AC, Dunn C, *et al.* Infection and allergy incidence in ambulatory surgery patients using white petrolatum vs bacitracin ointment. A randomized controlled trial. *JAMA.* 1996;276:972–977.

8 Choosing the Biopsy Type

JOHN L. PFENNINGER, MD • RICHARD P. USATINE, MD

A biopsy of the skin is performed to ascertain or confirm the diagnosis of skin lesions, both benign and malignant, and in many cases, to simultaneously remove them. Skin biopsies can be categorized into five types (Figure 8-1):

1. Shave
2. Punch
3. Curettement
4. Wedge (incisional)
5. Excisional (elliptical)

See video on the DVD for further learning. 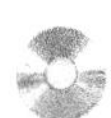

Choosing which type of biopsy to perform influences the diagnostic yield, the cosmetic result, and the cost and time required for the physician to perform the procedure. The clinician must also understand the parameters for selecting that portion of a lesion that will provide the most information to a pathologist.[1–3]

GENERAL PRINCIPLES

Shave Biopsy

See video on the DVD for further learning. 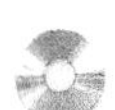

The choice of biopsy technique has much to do with the physician's initial assessment of the lesion. It is particularly important to consider the depth of involvement within the skin. The shave method is particularly suited to lesions confined to the epidermis and upper dermis, such as seborrheic or actinic keratoses, basal cell carcinomas (BCCs), squamous cell carcinomas (SCCs), and many benign nevi. Chapter 9, *The Shave Biopsy*, provides detailed information on this topic.

Advantages

- Minimal equipment is needed.
- The risk of bleeding is minimal, making the procedure suitable for patients on anticoagulants.
- It is a fast procedure because no sutures are required.
- It allows for rapid healing because a full-thickness wound is not created.
- Relatively large, raised lesions can be easily removed with the biopsy. With the entire lesion removed, there is much less risk of missing an abnormality as can happen with a punch or partial curettement biopsy, which does not remove the entire lesion. The pathology report will indicate whether the entire lesion has been removed or not.
- It is a particularly useful procedure in certain anatomic areas, such as the back and the shin, that are difficult to suture due to skin tension.
- Cosmetic results of a shave biopsy are generally excellent; in many cases, but not all, results will be superior to those achieved with a full-thickness excision biopsy with suture closure.

Disadvantages

- A possible indentation scar may result if a deep shave is performed.
- The lesion could recur.
- Transecting a melanoma can alter the interpretation of true depth, which is required for treatment. However, the type of biopsy does not appear to affect long-term outcomes.[4]
- The clinician may not shave deep enough for fear of scarring and thus not provide the pathologist with enough material for evaluation.

Punch Biopsy

See video on the DVD for further learning. 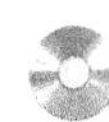

A punch biopsy is the method of choice for most inflammatory or infiltrative diseases and for other lesions in which the predominant pathology lies in the dermis, such as a dermatofibroma. A punch biopsy produces a full-thickness specimen of the skin that, when done properly, extends to the subcutaneous fat. Chapter 10, *The Punch Biopsy*, provides detailed information on this topic.

Advantages

- Minimal equipment is needed.
- The procedure is quick, easy, and simple.
- It provides a full-depth specimen.

Disadvantages

- Bleeding may be more of a problem than with a shave biopsy but usually is controlled with pressure, topical hemostatic agents, or a suture.
- Care must be taken not to penetrate too deeply over nerves, arteries, and thin skin.
- The most advanced area of the lesion may not be the site chosen for the biopsy. This sampling error can result in a missed diagnosis such as in a melanoma when only a portion of a pigmented lesion is cancer.

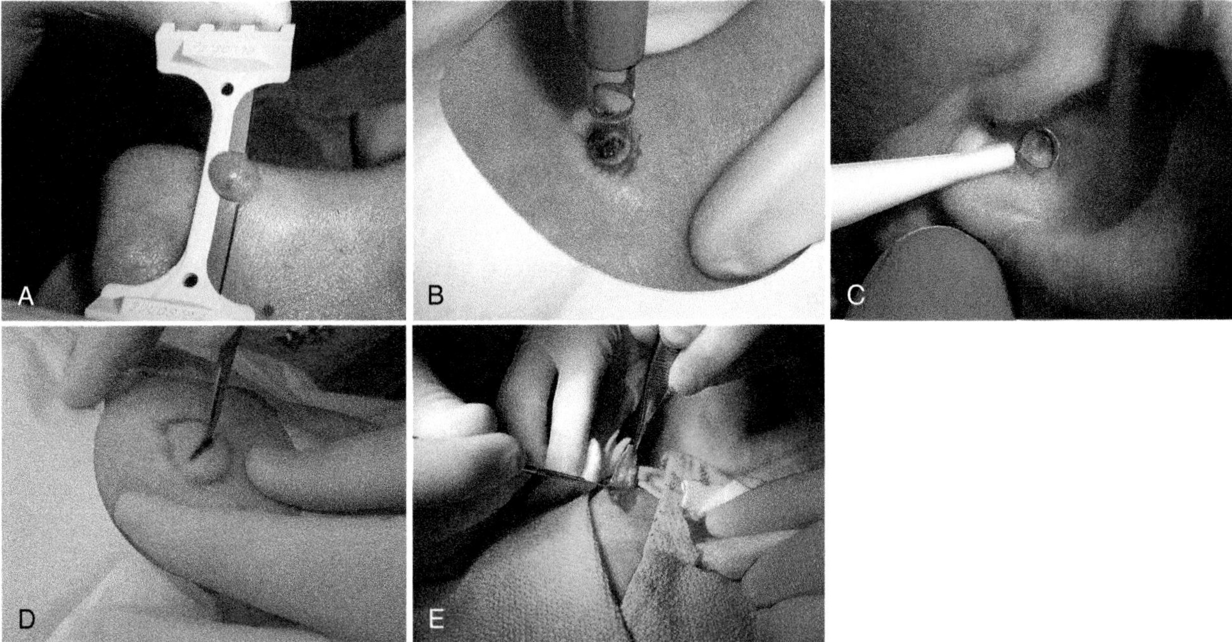

FIGURE 8-1 Five biopsy methods: (A) Shave; (B) punch; (C) curettement; (D) incision; (E) excision. *(Copyright Richard P. Usatine, MD.)*

Curettement Biopsy

Using a sharp curette is another method of biopsy. A disposable 3-mm curette is a good choice. This size of curette is best suited for difficult areas such as in the canthal folds where the skin is thin and mobile or in areas that are difficult to access such as an ear canal or nostril. Care must be taken not to go too deep and injure vital tissue. A small lesion can be curetted off and sent to pathology (Figure 8-2).

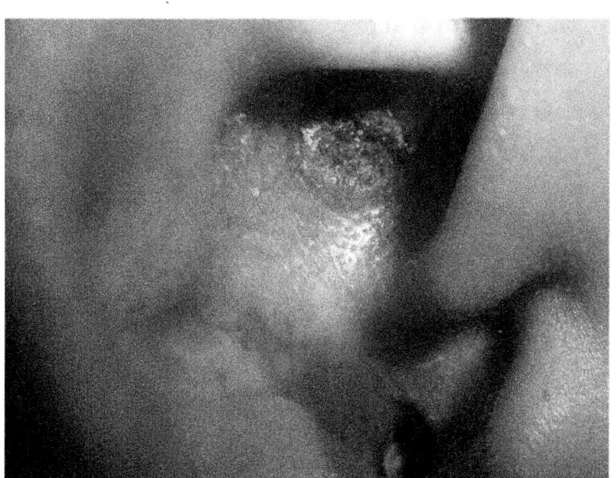

FIGURE 8-2 Squamous cell carcinoma in the upper pinna. A 3-0 curette is able to obtain tissue more easily than a scalpel, razor, or punch in this location. However, if the curette is not adequately sharp, a scalpel may obtain a better sample. *(Copyright Richard P. Usatine, MD.)*

Incisional and Excisional Biopsy

See video on the DVD for further learning. 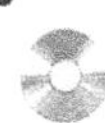

The term *incisional biopsy* refers to the process of excising a portion of a lesion using full-thickness excision techniques. It is used for obtaining a large sample of a large lesion, but not the entire lesion. The term *excisional* biopsy refers to full-thickness excision of the entire lesion. Both generally require some type of closure, which is usually done with sutures. See Chapter 11 for more detailed information about elliptical excisions.

Excision may be the biopsy method of choice for large potentially malignant lesions since a more focal biopsy may miss the malignant portion of the abnormality. Lesions highly suggestive of malignant melanoma (Figure 8-3) are often excised since the resulting specimen will provide a full-depth sample, which is needed for prognosis and treatment. The disadvantages of excising all "suspicious" lesions are that (1) it can lead to overtreatment for benign lesions and more tissue is removed than what is needed, which adds to the cost and increases scarring and other complications (e.g., excising a totally benign nevus or minimally atypical one), and (2) another surgery is often required because the initial ellipse is often performed with margins smaller than recommended for definitive treatment.

The excisional technique is also used to diagnose and remove dermal lesions, subcutaneous cysts and tumors (epidermal cysts and lipomas), and lesions that are too deep or too large to be removed by punch (generally greater than 5 mm in diameter) or shave. Cysts and especially lipomas may be removed with a deep linear

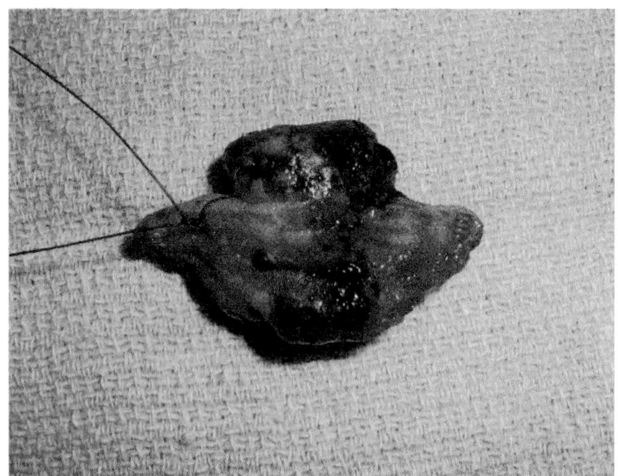

FIGURE 8-3 Full-thickness biopsy of a deep nodular melanoma. The nodular growth pattern predicted a deeper melanoma. *(Copyright Richard P. Usatine, MD.)*

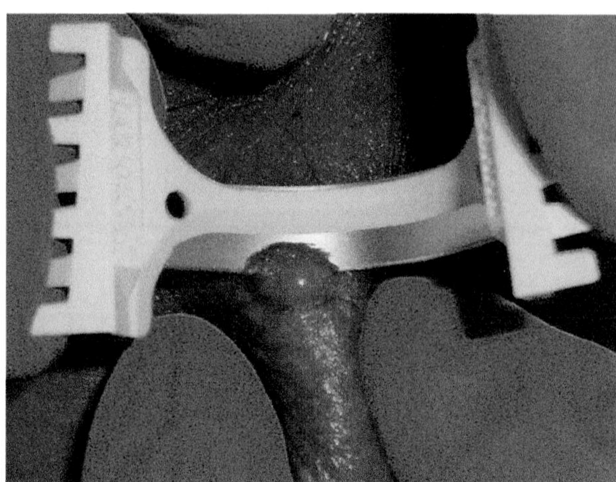

FIGURE 8-5 A shave biopsy of an intact blister in a patient with suspected bullous pemphigoid. *(Copyright Richard P. Usatine, MD.)*

incision rather than removing an elliptical portion of the skin (see Chapter 12, *Cysts and Lipomas*).

CHOICE OF SITE TO BIOPSY

When the decision has been made to biopsy a lesion, along with choosing the *method* of biopsy, the clinician must also choose the *site* (exact spot in the lesion) that will be biopsied.

If a "rash" or inflammatory process is present, select a "fresh" lesion that has recently appeared rather than one that has been present longer. Oftentimes, older lesions have been excoriated or secondarily infected, obscuring the primary pathology. Choose a lesion on the upper body rather than the lower body whenever possible (Figure 8-4). The histology may be easier to interpret and the healing should be more rapid. Biopsies of the lower legs are more likely to get infected or have delayed healing. Also avoid the axilla and groin if possible because these areas are more prone to infections.

If a vesicular-bullous reaction is present, it is best to biopsy an intact bulla with some normal tissue (Figure 8-5). It is helpful for the pathologist to examine the edge of the bulla to characterize the exact etiology of the disease process.

If lesions are scattered throughout the body, choose a site where aesthetic considerations are less of a concern (e.g., avoid the face) and where scarring is less likely. The sternum, shoulders, upper back, and areas of skin tension are more likely to scar. Also, choose a lesion on the upper body rather than the lower body whenever possible.

When direct immunofluorescence (DIF) testing is to be done, biopsies are usually taken from perilesional skin (Figure 8-6). That means the biopsy will not include

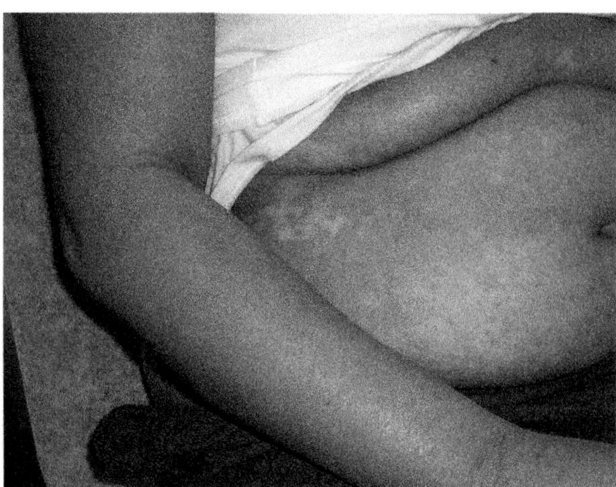

FIGURE 8-4 Erythroderma in a 19-year-old woman from head to toe. A 4-mm punch biopsy was performed on her arm rather than the leg. *(Copyright Richard P. Usatine, MD.)*

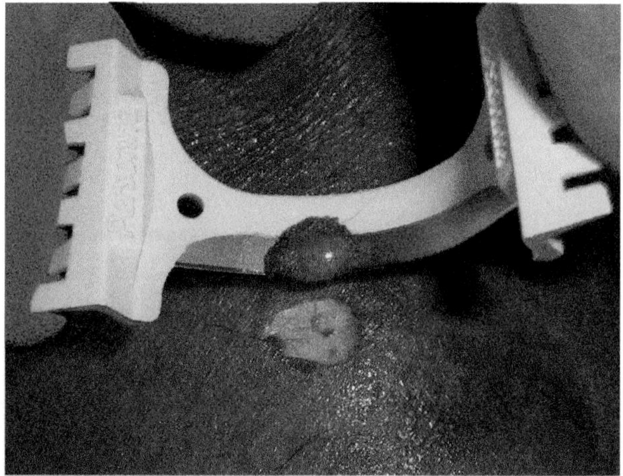

FIGURE 8-6 A shave biopsy was performed of an intact blister including perilesional skin in a patient with suspected bullous pemphigoid. The specimen shows that the blister remained intact and there is sufficient perilesional skin to the left of the blister to cut from the specimen and send separately for direct immunofluorescence. *(Copyright Richard P. Usatine, MD.)*

the bulla or erosion at all. The specimen is generally obtained with a shave or punch biopsy next to the visible pathology. DIF studies are especially helpful for autoimmune bullous diseases because antibodies will light up in the skin (Figure 8-7). They do not have to be done on the initial biopsy but may be performed to clarify and add data to a standard biopsy for hematoxylin and eosin (H&E) staining. There are only a few autoimmune diseases in which lesional skin is preferred (see Table 8-1). A 4-mm punch is adequate. It must be sent to the lab in special Michel's media (or on saline-soaked gauze). This media should be kept in the refrigerator and can expire. If the cap is on tight and the media has just expired, it is probably still usable. See Table 8-1 for more information on the DIF biopsy.

If a basal cell carcinoma is suspected, it is often easy to shave off the whole lesion. If the lesion is large, almost

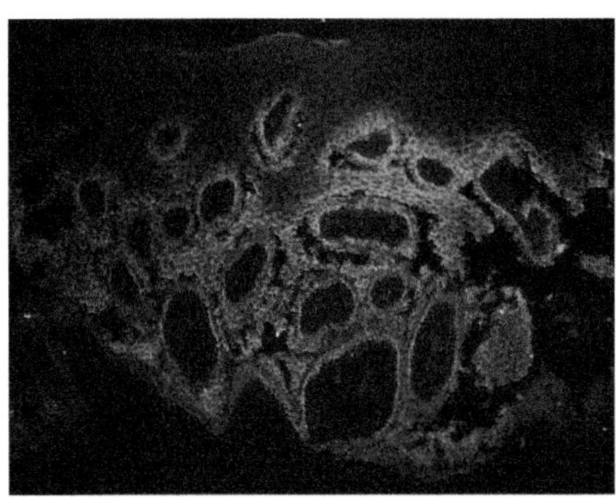

FIGURE 8-7 Immunofluorescence microscopy of a skin biopsy displays prominent intercellular "fish-net" deposition of C3 as well as a suprabasilar cleft within the epidermis. This confirms the diagnosis of pemphigus vulgaris. *(Courtesy of Robert Law, MD.)*

TABLE 8-1 Location for Direct Immunofluorescence Biopsies

Disease	Location of Biopsy	Findings
Pemphigus vulgaris	Perilesional	Intercellular deposition of IgG.
Pemphigus foliaceus	Perilesional	Intercellular deposition of IgG.
IgA pemphigus	Perilesional	Intercellular deposition of IgA.
Paraneoplastic pemphigus	Perilesional	Intercellular deposition of IgG. Antibodies also directed to simple or transitional epithelium (rat bladder).
Bullous pemphigoid	Perilesional	Linear basement membrane staining with IgG and/or C3. Salt split samples will localize to the epidermal side.
Cicatricial pemphigoid (MMP)	Perilesional skin, mucosa, or conjunctiva	Linear basement membrane staining with IgG and/or C3. Salt split samples show variable localization.
Herpes gestationis	Perilesional	Linear basement membrane staining with C3, IgG is generally less pronounced.
Epidermolysis bullosa acquisita	Perilesional	Heavy IgG and/or C3 along the basement membrane zone. Salt split samples will localize to the dermal side.
Dermatitis herpetiformis	Lesional or normal skin from disease-prone area	Granular IgA within dermal papillae.
Lichen planus	Inflamed, but nonulcerated mucosa or skin	Clumps of cytoid bodies and fibrinogen in the basement membrane zone.
Lupus band test	Normal skin	Granular IgG or IgM along the basement membrane zone.
Discoid lupus erythematosus	Lesional skin	Granular deposition of IgG, IgM, and/or IgA along the basement membrane zone in conjunction with cytoid bodies.
Systemic lupus erythematosus	Lesional skin	Same as for discoid lupus.
Bullous lupus erythematosus	Perilesional skin	Heavy IgG and/or C3 along the basement membrane zone.
Vasculitis	Early lesion	Perivascular IgA: Henoch Schoenlein purpura. Perivascular IgM/IgG/C3: other forms of vasculitis.
Linear IgA dermatitis	Perilesional skin	Linear IgA deposition at the basement membrane zone.
Porphyria/pseudoporphyria cutanea tarda	Perilesional	Linear IgG, IgM, and C3 around vessels and dermal-epidermal junction.

Source: Courtesy of Robert Law, MD.

any area can be biopsied but it is better to select a raised-up border rather than an ulcerated portion. Biopsying the latter may inaccurately provide a pathology specimen that shows only inflammation and reparative debris if not sampled deeply enough. Curettement and punch methods can also be used. An advantage with curettement is that if the tissue is necrotic, it feels "soft" with curetting and also has a classic appearance. The appearance and feel can confirm the initial impression, and treatment can be performed immediately (electrodesiccation and curettage ×3) (see Chapter 14, *Electrosurgery*).

If a squamous cell carcinoma is suspected, and the lesion is too large to shave off in its entirety, biopsy centrally and try to obtain a deep sample so the pathologist can determine the extent of invasion. Peripheral areas may only involve actinic change, missing the most advanced pathology. A broad deep shave is usually adequate for a biopsy. A second biopsy/excision may be needed if the pathologist reports that there is squamous dysplasia and a SCC cannot be ruled out.

If a melanoma is suspected, it is best to provide a specimen with adequate depth. Unfortunately choosing the darkest and most raised area does not guarantee the correct diagnosis. Although a full elliptical excision has been considered the gold standard, in some circumstances this is not desirable, for instance, in a large pigmented lesion on the face. In cases of suspected lentigo maligna melanoma on the face, a broad shave provides a better sample than a few punch biopsies and is less deforming that a large full-thickness biopsy. It is also just not practical to perform an elliptical excision on every potentially malignant pigmented lesion. It may be better in some instances to sample the whole lesion with a broad deep shave than to do one or more punch biopsies. Of course, sooner or later, an unsuspecting melanoma may be biopsied with a shave that misses the true depth of the lesion. Note, however, that it is far better to biopsy a lesion—regardless of the method—and find a melanoma early than to delay and procrastinate, thus missing an opportunity for early detection and treatment.[4] Suspected early thin melanomas can easily be biopsied with a deep shave technique. When sampling a suspected thick nodular melanoma, a deep sample will be needed to find the Breslow level and plan the definitive surgery. Dermoscopy (see Chapter 32) is a tool that can help you choose the most suspicious area to biopsy in a large lesion if it is impractical to biopsy the whole lesion. Fortunately, nonexcisional biopsies do not negatively influence melanoma patient survival and, in general, do closely correlate with the true depth of the lesion.[5,6]

Documentation of Biopsy Site

With all biopsies (especially if multiple lesions are obtained), record a detailed description of the biopsy site and, if possible, include a diagram or photo in the medical record. Biopsy sites may heal quickly and can be difficult to find later when definitive treatment is necessary. Photos can aid in identifying correct locations. If it is not easy to place photographs in the medical record, make sure the camera is set to record the correct date of the photo. Then the prebiopsy photo can be found by searching the electronic files by date. Some clinicians photograph the patient label at the same time to make it easier to locate a preop photo. Adequate privacy protection is necessary to ensure that photo storage options are HIPAA compliant (password protected and data encryption) if a computer is used.

IS IT CANCER?

Pigmented Lesions: Melanoma and Its Differential Diagnoses

Early detection and prompt removal of *melanoma* can be lifesaving. The early signs of melanoma are summarized as *ABCDE,* where *A* = asymmetry, *B* = borders (irregular), *C* = color (variegated), *D* = diameter (greater than 6 mm), and *E* = evolving and elevation (Figure 8-8).[7] Some have suggested adding an *F* for a change in *feeling* since some melanomas present with onset of pruritus in a nevus. However, not all melanomas show these signs and not all lesions with these signs are

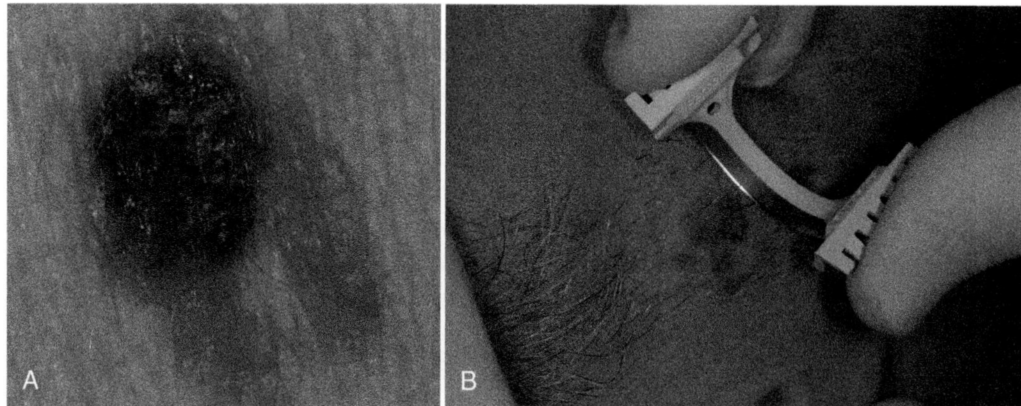

FIGURE 8-8 (A) Melanoma *in situ* on the arm showing asymmetry, irregular borders, variegated color, and a diameter of greater than 6 mm. (B) A broad shave biopsy of a melanoma *in situ* on the face of a 49-year-old man. A punch biopsy may have missed the melanoma and elliptical excision may have been too aggressive if this turned out to be a seborrheic keratosis or solar lentigo. *(Copyright Richard P. Usatine, MD.)*

melanomas. The dermatoscope can be used to increase your sensitivity and specificity for detecting melanoma (see Chapter 32, *Dermoscopy*). Whether or not a dermatoscope is used, it is incumbent on the clinician to biopsy any suspicious pigmented lesion. We cannot overemphasize that patient history is of utmost importance in the evaluation of any lesion and should never be taken lightly. If a patient is concerned that a pigmented lesion has changed, most often it deserves a biopsy/removal.

Pigmented lesions highly suggestive of melanoma should be biopsied for depth because treatment is primarily based on that parameter. Other considerations needed to select the proper treatment include whether there is neural or vascular involvement and whether ulceration is present. Some suggest that all suspected melanomas be biopsied using the excisional technique (full-thickness excision with suture closure). This practice presents several problems: (1) How much free margin should be obtained? Most commonly, a simple excision with a margin of 5 mm (melanoma *in situ*) to 1 cm (up to 1 mm of invasion with no other warning signs on pathology) is needed for treatment. If the invasion is greater than 1.5 mm, a 2-cm margin is recommended.[8,9] So, should the excisional biopsy always have a 1-cm margin? Most lesions will not be a melanoma. Should the excision then just remove the lesion with no free margins? Using excision as the primary approach for biopsying a suspicious lesion will not only cost more and, in many cases, remove an excess amount of normal tissue, but will most likely require that the patient have a second surgery if a melanoma is found. (2) Full surgical excision takes significant time and skills. Many primary care clinicians are not prepared to excise all suspicious lesions. Referral for a biopsy takes time, increases the cost, and may not be readily available. Patients also may not comply with seeing another physician. The optimal time to biopsy is when the lesion is first evaluated. A shave or a punch biopsy takes only a few minutes and then therapy can be based on the results. This approach saves time and limits costs, while reducing unnecessary scarring, infected wounds, and return visits to the office. Survival time does not appear to be influenced by the method of biopsy.[5]

If a melanoma is truly suspected, a deep shave biopsy may indeed be the ideal method of sampling (Figure 8-8B). A punch biopsy can have significant sampling errors and false-negative results unless the whole lesion is removed or multiple biopsies are obtained from larger lesions. The object is to detect melanoma early and save lives. If a larger lesion is atypical in appearance, the entire lesion will need to be removed but the initial biopsy will at least help determine required margins for excision, or if a referral is indicated. A punch biopsy may be used as long as a negative (nonmalignant) biopsy of a suspicious lesion larger than the initial punch is followed up with an excision in which all the remaining tissue is excised and examined (Figure 8-9).

Pigmented lesions that are unusual and are considered to have a low, but definite, possibility of malignancy or dysplasia (atypia) also require prompt biopsy. If these lesions are small (up to 6 to 7 mm), a saucer-type shave excision with narrow margins (1 to 2 mm) is the method of choice. Very small lesions, those less than 3 mm in diameter, can often be adequately excised by using the deep shave technique or a 4-mm punch to remove the entire lesion. Large lesions (those greater than 2 cm in diameter), with a low level of suspicion, may be investigated by doing a 4-mm punch biopsy in the area of highest suspicion (i.e., the blackest area or the area of greatest elevation) or with frank excision (Figure 8-10).

Lentigo Maligna

Lentigo maligna (LM) is one type of melanoma *in situ*. Flat, macular lesions suspected of being lentigo maligna (Figure 8-11) present a problem because many of these lesions are very large (often over 2 cm in diameter) and frequently are present on the face in 50 to 70 year olds. They are interesting because the radial growth phase may last for years and the vertical (invasive) phase may never develop. Excisional biopsy is preferred for small lesions, but this method may be impractical for large lesions. A broad shave biopsy of suspected LM or lentigo maligna melanoma (LMM) should provide a better tissue sample than one or more punch biopsies and will not cause the cosmetic deformities of a large full-thickness biopsy (Figure 8-11).

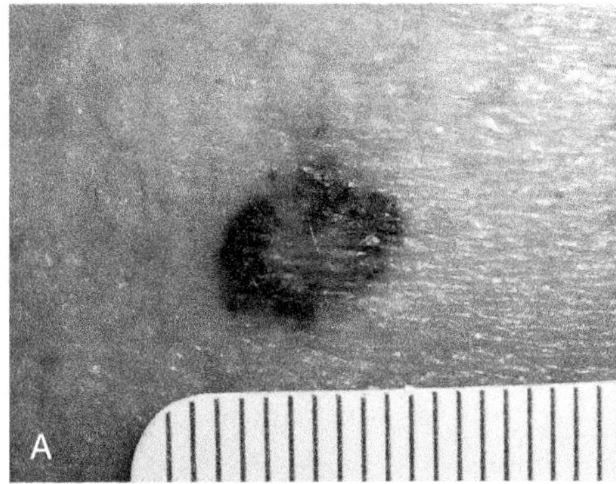

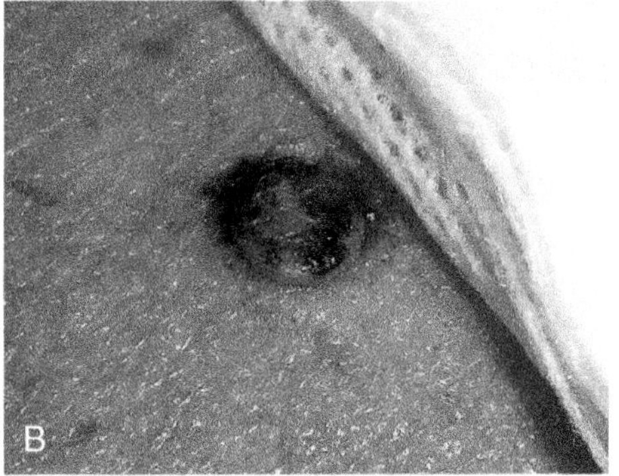

FIGURE 8-9 (A) Suspected melanoma with signs of regression in the center. (B) A 6-mm punch biopsy was performed of this 6- × 9-mm suspected melanoma and the dermatopathologist stated that she would have preferred a scoop shave of the whole lesion. Although the full depth of the lesion biopsied was seen, the lack of access to the remaining portion made it difficult to provide a Breslow depth with confidence. Because of the regression the full lesion was excised with 1-cm margins and only melanoma *in situ* was found. *(Copyright Richard P. Usatine, MD.)*

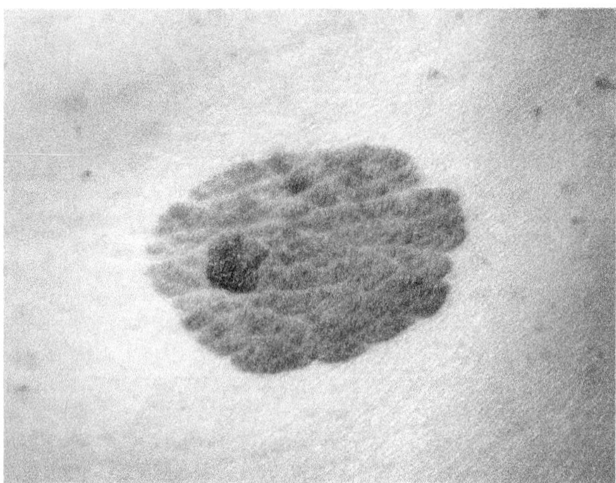

FIGURE 8-10 A seborrheic keratosis that has all five ABCDE criteria. A shave or punch biopsy should be adequate to confirm that this is benign. Dermoscopy would also be helpful and might prevent the need for a biopsy. *(Copyright Richard P. Usatine, MD.)*

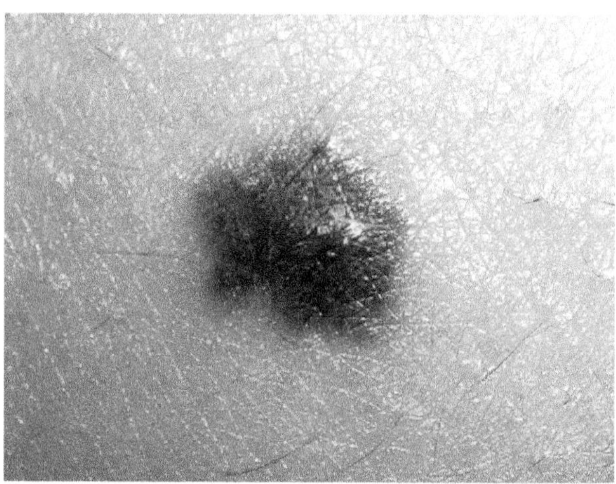

FIGURE 8-12 Compound dysplastic melanocytic nevus (nevus with architecture disorder). *(Copyright Richard P. Usatine, MD.)*

Atypical Moles (Dysplastic Nevi)

Terminology can be confusing. *Atypical* and *dysplastic* are often used interchangeably in dermatologic communication. The current recommended NIH nomenclature, however, is "nevus with architectural disorder" (Figure 8-12). See Box 8-1 for further clarification.

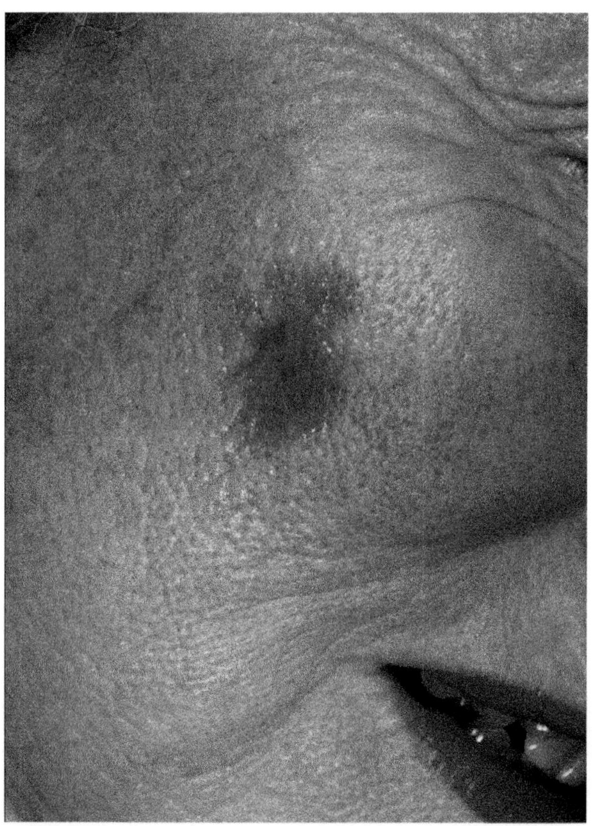

FIGURE 8-11 Lentigo maligna that is best biopsied with a broad shave of the whole pigmented area. *(Courtesy of the Skin Cancer Foundation, New York, NY.)*

Many benign lesions are so characteristic that a biopsy is not necessary. On the other hand, early melanoma can be exceedingly difficult to diagnose (some lesions are not even pigmented). Considering this, and also taking into consideration that the morphology of benign pigmented lesions can be remarkably varied, it is best to be cautious when dealing with atypical pigmented lesions. *Biopsies should be performed on all questionable pigmented lesions.* Another very basic premise that should be closely adhered to is that *any nevus that the patient reports to have changed should be considered for biopsy despite the clinical appearance.* Also keep in mind that normal benign nevi can go through an evolution over time.

Although benign, atypical nevi have clinical, histologic, and biologic behavior distinct from common nevocellular nevi. Two percent to 8% of the population have nevi that fit the definition of atypical moles. Clinically, these nevi are large (5 to 12 mm in diameter), are characteristically multicolored (with shades of brown, tan, or pink), and have irregular borders that tend to be indistinct (Figure 8-12). They usually have a flat macular component, are frequently multiple, and are most common on the trunk. In contrast to common nevi, atypical moles usually begin to appear during adolescence and continue to appear during young adult life.

The clinical approach to multiple atypical moles has evolved since their first description. There still remains a difference of opinion as to their proper management. Atypical moles may not all require biopsy, such as in patients with more than 100 of these moles. Any pigmented lesion that the physician is uncertain about or that has changed, however, should still undergo biopsy. One of the most common reasons for lawsuits is missing a melanoma.

Patients with a few atypical moles can also be divided into those with a personal history or a first-degree relative with a history of melanoma, and those without

BOX 8-1 *Nevus with Architectural Disorder (Dysplastic Nevus)*

We use the recommended NIH nomenclature of *nevus with architectural disorder*. If there is atypia, it is graded as either mild or severe (we do not use moderate). If there is severe atypia and the lesion has not been excised, a comment on the report will recommend conservative excision. There will also be a comment indicating that this lesion may be part of the familial mole melanoma syndrome.

Atypical Melanocytic Hyperplasia

Lesions that have intraepidermal spread that falls short of melanoma *in situ* are classified as *atypical melanocytic hyperplasia*. The atypia is not graded, because it is the pattern that is of concern. The report will include a comment that AMH may represent an evolutionary precursor to melanoma and recommend that the lesion be conservatively excised.

Atypical Compound Nevus

Lesions that have atypia in both the junctional and dermal components, but in the absence of diagnostic melanoma, are classified as *atypical compound nevi*. Often, we will perform immunomarkers to determine proliferative activity to exclude nevoid melanoma on these lesions. For lesions designated as atypical compound nevi (ACN), we recommend conservative excision. Please note that we do not use the terms *atypical compound nevus* and *nevus with architectural disorder (dysplastic nevus)* synonymously. Dysplastic nevi have atypia only at the junction, not ascending cells (AMH) and not dermal atypia (ACN).

Margin Assessment

Margin examination may be requested; however, only the Mohs technique allows examination of 100% of the margin. For all other types of biopsies and excisions, margins are sampled only. The greater the sampling, the higher the degree of confidence in the margin assessment. To increase the degree of sampling, larger specimens may be sectioned during grossing and then step sectioned to view multiple cuts on the slide. We report that the "examined margins are negative" or that the lesion extends to the deep or a lateral margin. Note, however, that while a positive margin is positive, a negative margin does not ensure that the lesion has been completely removed. For example, if you do a shave excision of a BCC, we will say on the report that the examined margins are negative. This means that on the two dimensions that can be examined on a slide, the margins are negative, not necessarily that the lesion has been fully removed. If a specimen is oriented (tagged), we will use color-coded inks. In the event a margin is positive, we will be able to describe which margin is positive.

Source: Courtesy of Terry L. Barrett, MD.

such a history (sporadic atypical moles). Patients with sporadic atypical moles are probably not at as great a risk for developing melanoma.[10,11]

Benign Nevi

Many will request *mole removal purely for cosmetic reasons*. Alternatively, the lesions may be in areas of repeated trauma (e.g., from shaving, combing, irritation from clothes or jewelry). Shave biopsy is the treatment of choice for most totally benign-appearing nevi, and the lesion should still be sent for histological examination. In Figure 8-13, the raised lesion could be a benign nevus or a BCC. If the history suggests a nevus, a shave biopsy would be the method of choice. Removal of some nevi on the face may yield a better cosmetic result when accomplished by punch or meticulous excision when large. Size, location, age of the patient, history, and type of skin all are factored into the decision. Nevi with a deeper intradermal component tend to recur or become pigmented after shave removal especially in younger patients. A shave can still be performed but the patient should be forewarned as a part of informed consent that regrowth or pigment changes may still require full-depth excision later. *For nevi with hair* a shave biopsy is often too superficial to remove the deeper root of the hair follicle. In this instance, to reduce potential scarring from an excision, a shave can be performed and if hair does regrow, simple epilation techniques can remove it. It is again important to inform the patient of the potential for hair growth.

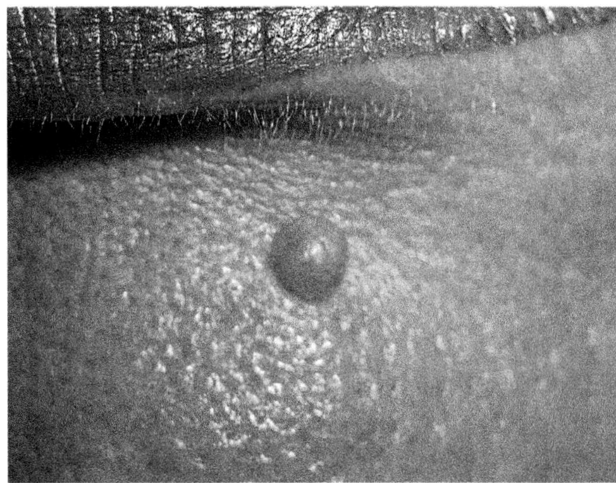

FIGURE 8-13 Intradermal nevus that is pearly with telangiectasias and spotty pigmentation. A shave biopsy was performed to rule out BCC and to obtain a good cosmetic result. *(Copyright Richard P. Usatine, MD.)*

Seborrheic Keratoses

Most seborrheic keratoses will not need a biopsy. However, because some of these lesions mimic malignant tumors such as melanomas when they are darkly pigmented, biopsy should be performed if any doubt exists (Figure 8-10). Dermoscopy (see Chapter 32) can help make this distinction and avoid a biopsy in many cases. When performing a biopsy on seborrheic keratoses, care should be taken to avoid unnecessarily deep or destructive techniques. Seborrheic keratoses are epidermal lesions. Shave biopsy is the biopsy technique of choice unless the suspicion of melanoma is high. Treatment with cryotherapy without biopsy is very acceptable for lesions in which the clinical diagnosis is certain. However, lesions that fail to resolve after 6 weeks should be evaluated and a biopsy considered.

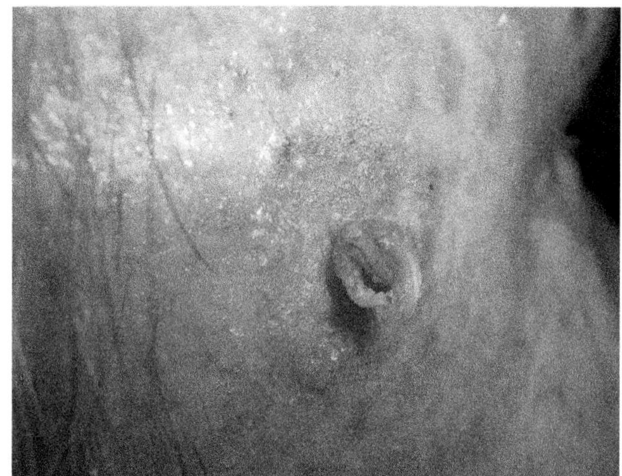

FIGURE 8-14 A cutaneous horn arising in a squamous cell carcinoma on the face. *(Copyright Richard P. Usatine, MD.)*

Nonpigmented Lesions Suspicious for Cancer

Actinic Keratoses

Actinic keratoses can be very superficial or hypertrophic. They are considered a precancerous lesion and as such, should be treated or biopsied. Thinner obvious lesions can be treated with topical agents, cryotherapy, or electrodesiccation without biopsy initially. If lesions persist after treatment, or if there is concern about a cancer at the base, then a shave biopsy or curettement is indicated. With high-risk lesions such as those with a *cutaneous horn,* a deeper saucer-type shave is best to provide the pathologist with enough tissue to discern invasion (Figure 8-14).

Keratoacanthomas

The history and clinical appearance of keratoacanthomas (KAs) are quite distinct. They grow rapidly in a matter of months and appear most like a BCC with central keratin plug (Figure 8-15). It is considered a variant of SCC. If suspected, smaller lesions (8 to 10 mm) can be removed with a deep saucer-type shave followed by electrodesiccation and curettage (×3). For larger lesions, full-thickness excision is the best method of biopsy/removal.

Basal Cell Carcinoma

The majority of BCCs are relatively small (less than 1 cm), raised tumors on the face, head, neck, or exposed parts of the trunk and extremities. Nearly any method can be used to biopsy these lesions if their exact nature is uncertain. With curettement, the typical soft necrotic tissue can be identified so treatment with electrodesiccation and curettage (ED&C) can be immediately performed (see Chapter 14, *Electrosurgery,* and Chapter 34, *Diagnosis and Treatment of Malignant and Premalignant Lesions*). Shave biopsy can be used for most of these tumors and has the advantage of not producing a deeper or full-thickness wound should the lesion prove not to be a cancer (Figure 8-16). A punch biopsy of the raised "pearly border" can also be performed. Although data on this issue is not available, some clinicians will not use ED&C on a BCC that was diagnosed with a punch biopsy. If an excisional biopsy is planned because the diagnosis of BCC is likely, then 3 to 5 mm of clear margin should be included in the specimen to reduce the likelihood that further excisions will be needed (see Chapter 11, *The Elliptical Excision*).

Sclerosing (morpheaform, aggressive) BCCs are flat and more difficult to diagnose clinically and histopathologically. Therefore, a punch specimen is usually preferred, although a deeper shave often will be adequate to make the diagnosis. However, as seen in Figure 8-17, these lesions are most often flat and difficult to biopsy with the shave technique. It is difficult to discern margins of the abnormality clinically and for all but the smallest of lesions, excision will be needed for treatment. These lesions are fibrotic and often do not lend themselves to curettement. They also have a higher recurrence rate.

Pigmented BCCs can appear very much like melanomas (Figure 8-18). In these instances, a biopsy for depth may be indicated.

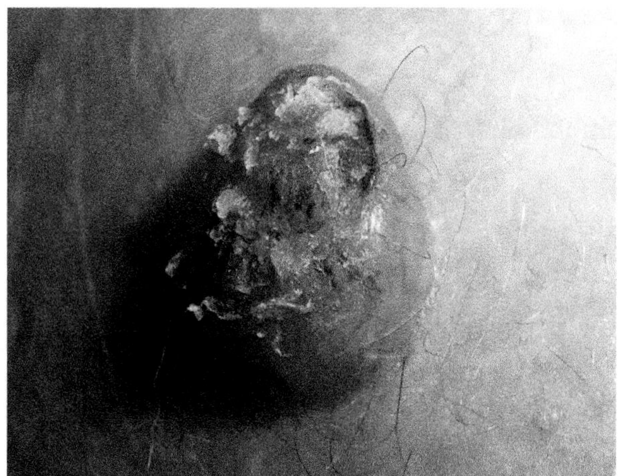

FIGURE 8-15 A keratoacanthoma with a pearly raised border and a keratin-like volcanic core. *(Copyright Richard P. Usatine, MD.)*

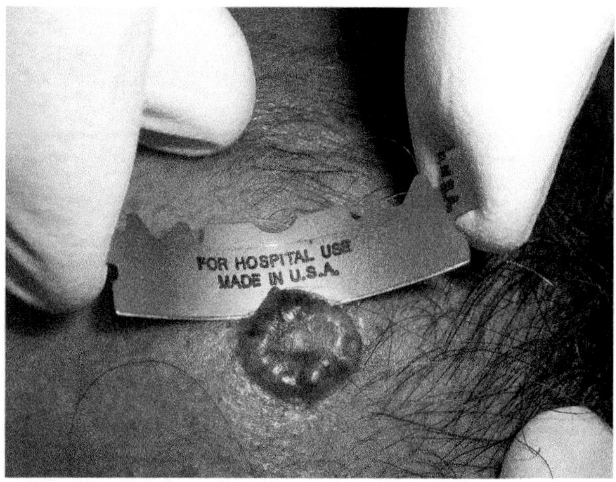

FIGURE 8-16 A razor blade being used for a shave biopsy of a nodular BCC. *(Copyright Richard P. Usatine, MD.)*

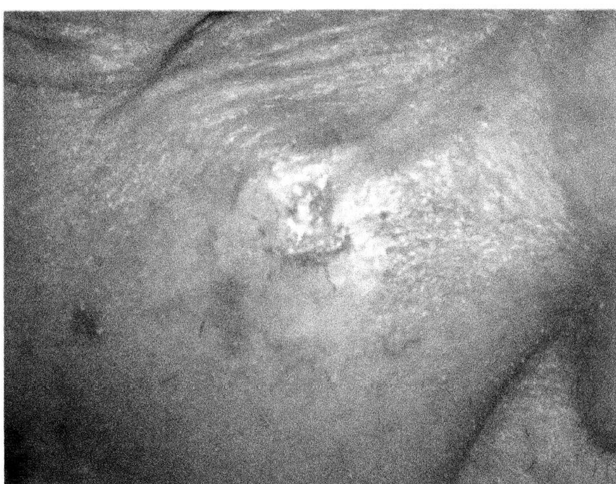

FIGURE 8-17 A morpheaform basal cell carcinoma on the face. The preferred biopsy type is a punch biopsy or a deep shave. *(Courtesy of the Skin Cancer Foundation, New York, NY.)*

Squamous Cell Carcinomas

Squamous cell carcinoma can be difficult to diagnose by histopathology. It can easily be mistaken by the pathologist for actinic keratosis, especially if the biopsy was made along the periphery of the lesion. If an SCC is suspected, sample the central portion of the lesion using a deep shave or a punch biopsy. When performing a shave biopsy, care must be taken to get a specimen with adequate depth to enable the pathologist to render an accurate opinion (Figure 8-19). As with BCC, the physician should carefully record the site of biopsy. For large lesions, particularly those in or around the oral cavity and ears, it is important to check for lymphadenopathy. Prompt treatment after diagnosis of SCC is essential because some of these lesions have the potential for metastasis (see Chapter 34).

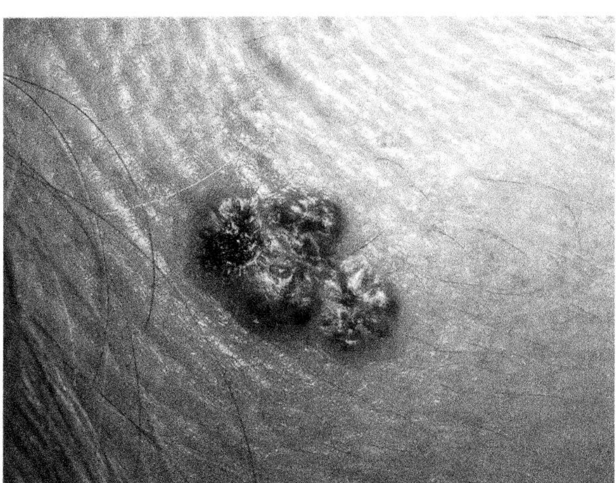

FIGURE 8-18 Pigmented BCC on the temple of an elderly woman. A deep shave biopsy was performed in case this turned out to be a melanoma. While doing the shave biopsy, the tissue below the lesion was viewed to make sure that the shave was below the pigment. With the similar morphology throughout, a punch biopsy should have provided adequate initial information whether or not this turned out to be a BCC or melanoma. *(Copyright Richard P. Usatine, MD.)*

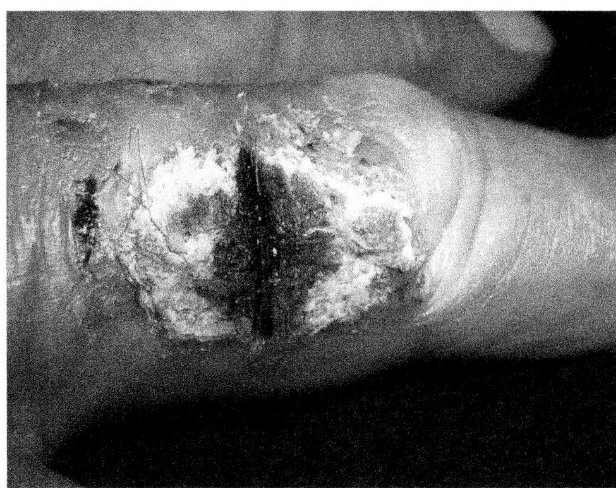

FIGURE 8-19 Squamous cell carcinoma on the finger. The first two shave biopsies did not reveal a squamous cell carcinoma. A third deeper and broader shave biopsy was adequate to make the diagnosis. The lesson here is not to believe a benign biopsy result if you believe the lesion is truly cancer. The thick keratin and the fear of damaging the finger's function prevented a correct diagnosis with the first two biopsies. *(Copyright Richard P. Usatine, MD.)*

Amelanotic Melanomas

Everyone is concerned about missing an amelanotic melanoma clinically. Rest assured that even the best specialist clinicians will misdiagnose these lesions clinically. It is far better to biopsy a lesion of uncertain etiology than to just observe it (Figure 8-20).

INFLAMMATORY DISORDERS

Various inflammatory disorders present as unknown rashes, and a punch biopsy will provide adequate tissue for diagnosis (e.g., lichen planus, psoriasis and cutaneous lupus erythematosus). The typical malar rash of *systemic lupus erythematosus* (SLE) in a patient with a strongly positive antinuclear antibody (ANA) does not

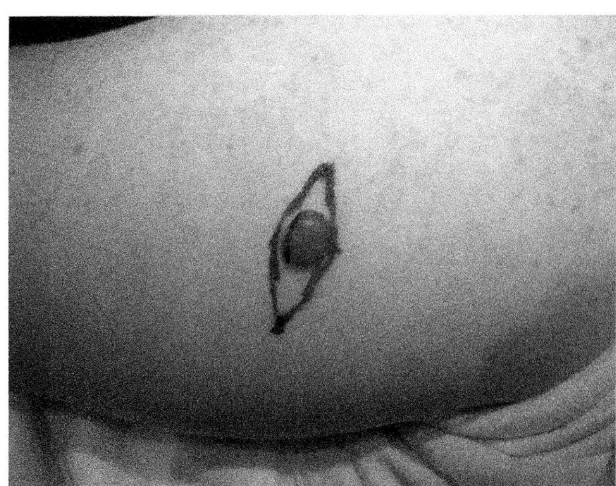

FIGURE 8-20 An amelanotic melanoma about to be excised. The diagnosis was not obvious but the elliptical excision provided great tissue for diagnosis. *(Courtesy of E. J. Mayeaux.)*

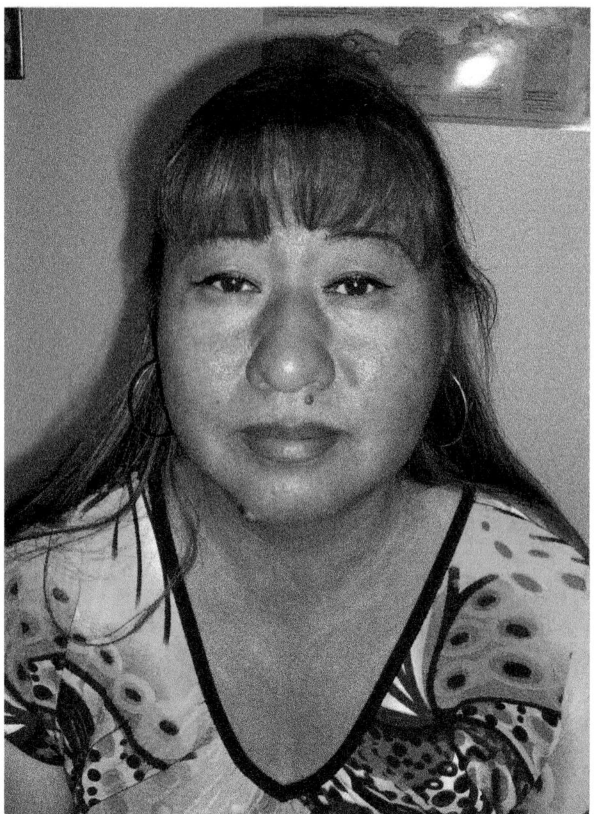

FIGURE 8-21 An erythematous eruption in photoexposed areas turned out to be subacute cutaneous lupus erythematosus proven by a 4-mm punch biopsy on the anterior chest. *(Copyright Richard P. Usatine, MD.)*

require a biopsy for diagnosis. However, some cases of cutaneous lupus may need a biopsy for diagnosis (Figure 8-21). *Lichen planus* presents with different morphologies from atrophic to hypertrophic, from solid to bullous. A punch biopsy is needed for definitive diagnosis (Figure 8-22). A 4-mm punch biopsy is usually preferred (see Chapter 10, *The Punch Biopsy*).

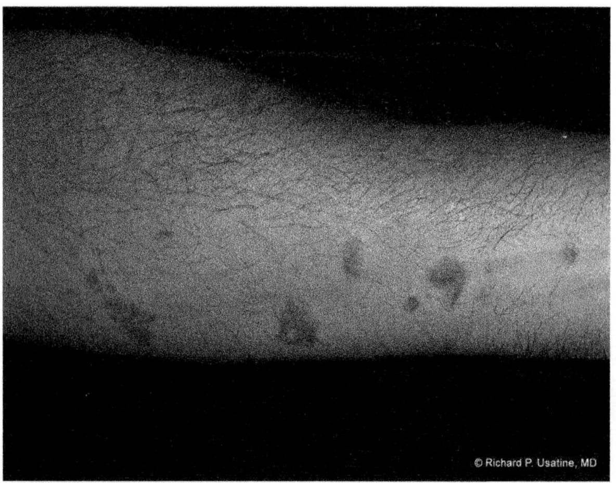

FIGURE 8-22 An atrophic variant of lichen planus in a 36-year-old man proven by a 4-mm punch biopsy. The biopsy was essential for diagnosis of this rare variant of lichen planus. *(Copyright Richard P. Usatine, MD.)*

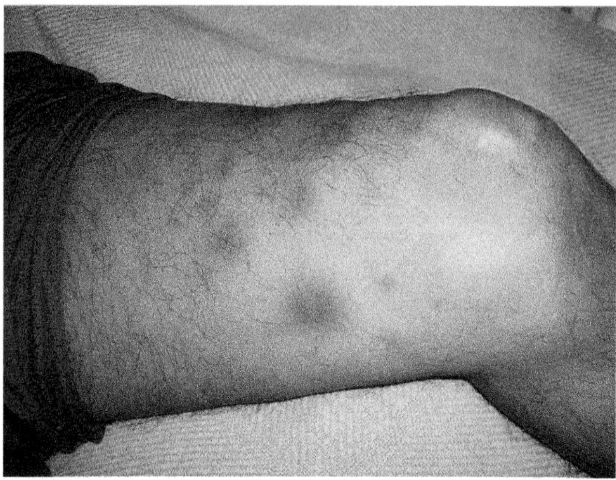

FIGURE 8-23 Erythema nodosum is a panniculitis. Therefore, a punch biopsy should be deep and obtain subcutaneous fat. This patient had erythema nodosum leprosum. *(Copyright Richard P. Usatine, MD.)*

Almost all inflammatory dermatoses have a dermal component. Punch biopsy is necessary to preserve the dermal architecture so the dermatopathologist can evaluate the cellular infiltrate, both as to its nature and its pattern. In most cases in which a punch biopsy is indicated, the biopsy need only go through the dermis, and the specimen is cut off at the top of the subcutaneous fat. However, to diagnose *erythema nodosum* (Figure 8-23), the punch specimen should include as much of the subcutaneous fat as possible. This is because erythema nodosum is really a panniculitis, with the overlying dermis secondarily involved.

INFILTRATIVE DISORDERS

Infiltrative disorders, such as *granulomas,* also require a punch rather than a shave biopsy to deliver a suitable specimen for dermatopathologic examination. Examples of infiltrative disorders include *sarcoidosis* (Figure 8-24), *cutaneous T-cell lymphoma* (Figure 8-25), and *granuloma annulare* (Figure 8-26). *Morphea* (Figure 8-27) and *lichen sclerosis* (Figure 8-28) are diagnosed with punch biopsies as well.

ERYTHRODERMA

Erythroderma is a dangerous dermatologic condition in which the skin becomes red and begins to peel off in flakes (Figure 8-29). The impaired skin barrier makes the person vulnerable to dehydration and infection. It is the dermatologic manifestation of a number of underlying disease processes, including various forms of dermatitis, drug reactions, and lymphoproliferative disorders. The key to proper diagnosis and treatment is contingent on a good biopsy.

A short differential diagnosis of erythroderma includes:

- Psoriasis
- Drug reaction

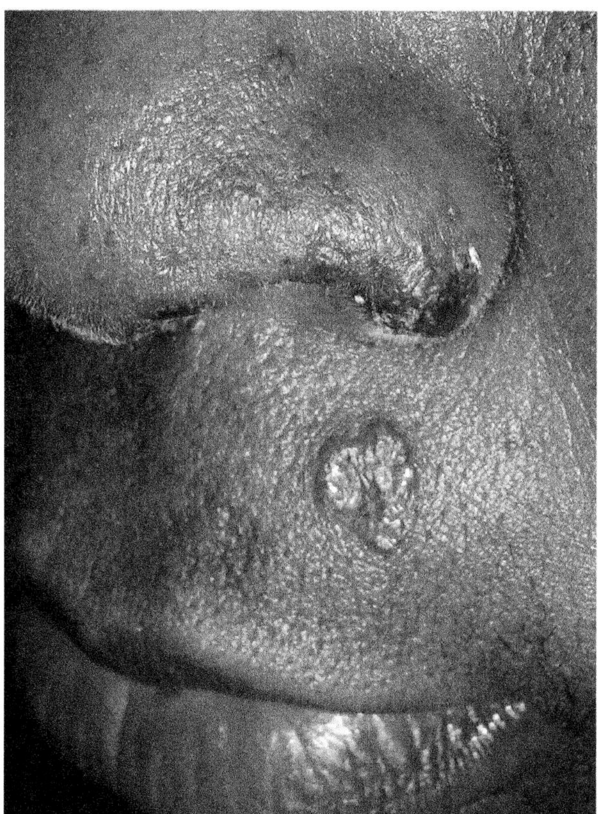

FIGURE 8-24 Sarcoidosis is an infiltrative disease found often on the face and nasal rim. Whereas the morphology and distribution in a black woman is highly suggestive of sarcoidosis, it is best to confirm the diagnosis with a biopsy. In this case it is best to biopsy the lesion below the nose rather than risk anatomic distortion of the nasal rim. A punch biopsy is generally preferred. *(Copyright Richard P. Usatine, MD.)*

- Atopic and contact dermatis
- Seborrheic dermatitis
- Dermatomyositis
- Cutaneous T-cell lymphoma (CTCL)
- Idiopathic.

Because erythroderma covers most of the body, there are many areas from which to choose for the biopsy.

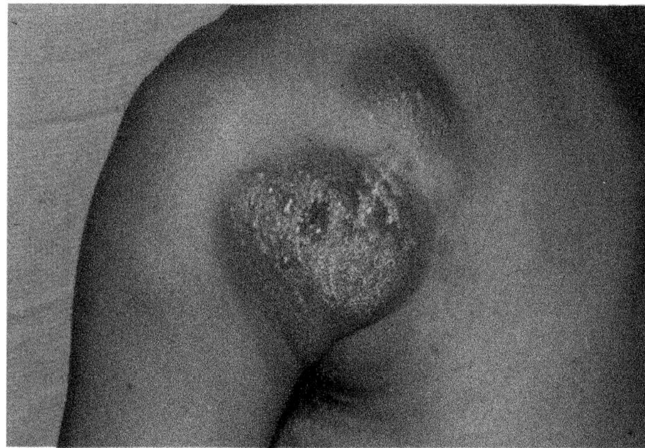

FIGURE 8-25 Cutaneous T-cell lymphoma in the more advanced tumor stage. A 4-mm punch biopsy was sufficient to make the diagnosis *(Courtesy of UTHSCSA Division of Dermatology.)*

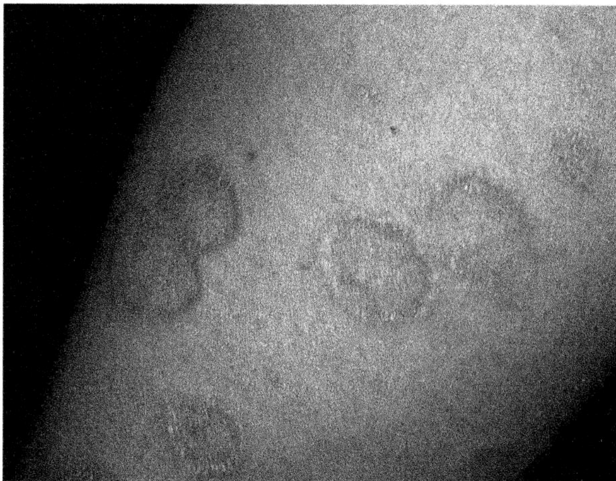

FIGURE 8-26 Disseminated granuloma annulare on the arm. A 4-mm punch biopsy of a granulomatous ring is recommended if the diagnosis is in question. *(Copyright Richard P. Usatine, MD.)*

Like most diagnostic challenges, the 4-mm punch biopsy is the standard method for obtaining tissue. Choose an area on the upper body such as the arm or trunk with significant skin involvement. If there are pustules as in possible pustular psoriasis, biopsy a pustule (Figure 8-30). Send this for a stat pathology consult while initiating treatment. Many patients will need hospitalization, but it is usually easiest to do the biopsy in the office before transferring the patient to the hospital.

BULLOUS LESIONS

Many bullous lesions are seen with *bullous impetigo* to *pemphigus* and *bullous pemphigoid* (Figure 8-31).

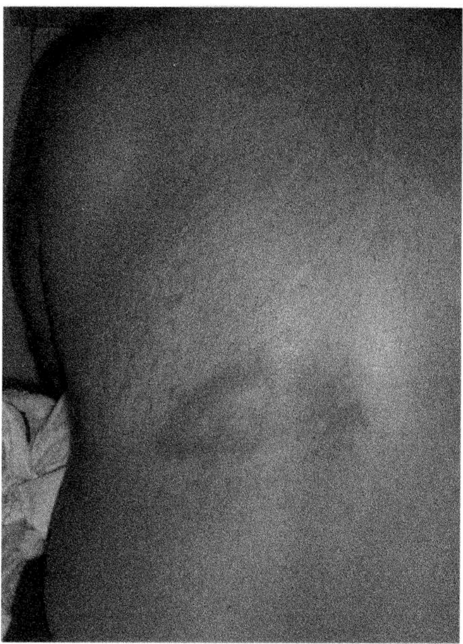

FIGURE 8-27 Morphea (localized scleroderma) on the back of a man. A 4-mm punch biopsy was used to make the diagnosis. *(Copyright Richard P. Usatine, MD.)*

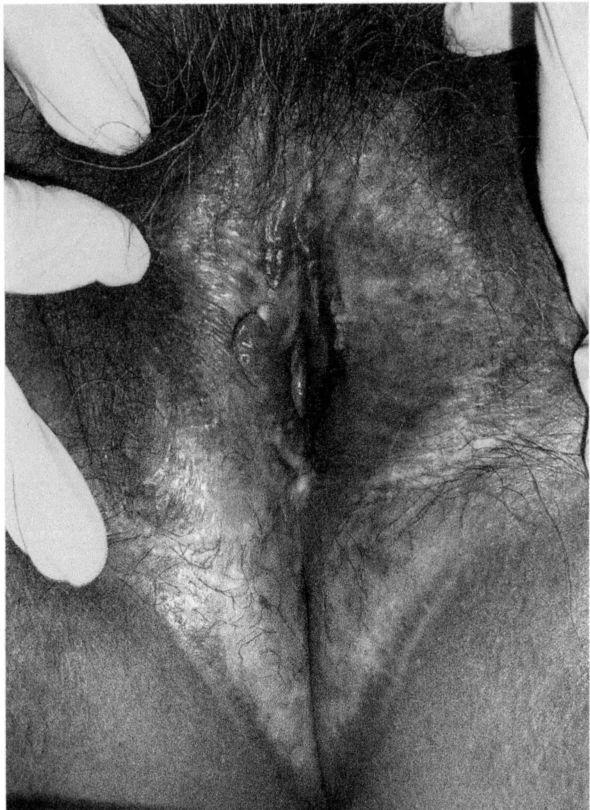

FIGURE 8-28 Lichen sclerosis at atrophicus on the vulva and perineum. The clinical impression was confirmed with a 3-mm punch biopsy that was left open to heal by second intention. Sutures in this area can be very uncomfortable and the tissue heals well without suturing. The whitest area was chosen to rule out vulvar intraepithelial neoplasia. *(Copyright Richard P. Usatine, MD.)*

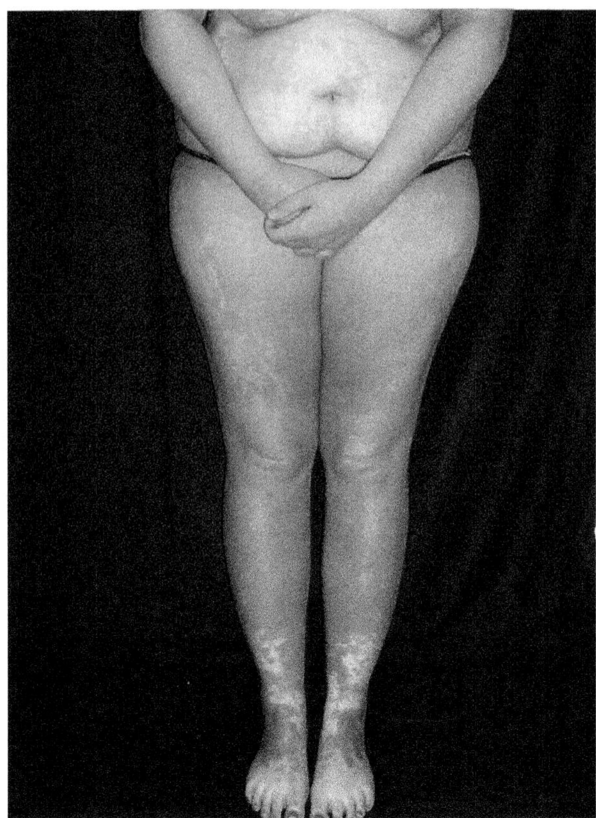

FIGURE 8-29 Erythroderma in a 19-year-old woman. A stat punch biopsy was done to obtain a diagnosis. *(Copyright Richard P. Usatine, MD.)*

Although bullous impetigo can be diagnosed and treated based on history and physical exam, the autoimmune forms of bullous diseases should be biopsied while initiating treatment. These diseases are often treated with prolonged courses of oral steroids and immunosuppressive medications, so it is essential to have the correct diagnosis from the start. Start with one 4-mm punch biopsy of an established lesion including the edge of the blister. A shave biopsy is an alternative as long as the epidermis of the blister stays attached to the specimen. If possible biopsy a new blister and remove the whole lesion. This is sent in formalin for H&E staining. Further information is obtained with a 4-mm punch biopsy for DIF. Biopsy the *perilesional* skin and send the specimen in Michel's media (see earlier discussion under *Choice of Site to Biopsy*). If this media is not available, send the specimen in a sterile urine cup on top of a sterile gauze soaked with sterile saline and alert the pathologist that the specimen is not in Michel's media. See Table 8-1 for more detailed information on where and how to biopsy tissue for DIF.

SUSPECTED INFECTIOUS RASH

In most cases of common infectious diseases the diagnosis can be made clinically, with a KOH preparation or with a culture. Sometimes a 4-mm punch biopsy may be needed for bacterial and fungal stains. Fungal infections are often diagnosed with periodic acid Schiff (PAS) stains. If the rash might have an infectious origin and standard biopsies in formalin are not providing the answer, send fresh tissue in a sterile urine cup on top of a sterile gauze soaked with sterile saline and ask for other studies including AFB stains and cultures.

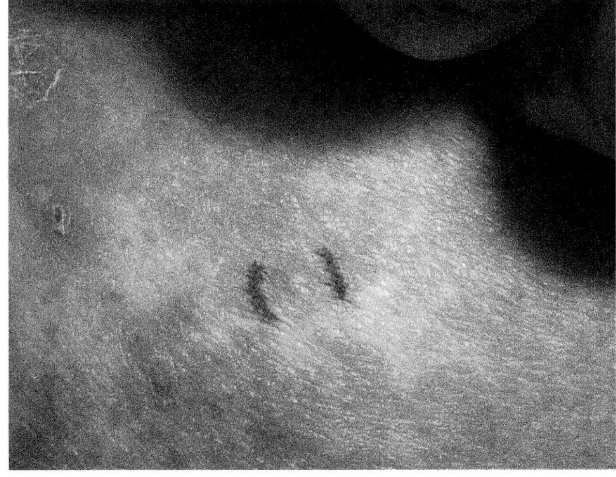

FIGURE 8-30 A close-up of a small pustule in a 67-year-old woman with erythroderma. A 4-mm punch biopsy of this site made the diagnosis of pustular psoriasis. *(Copyright Richard P. Usatine, MD.)*

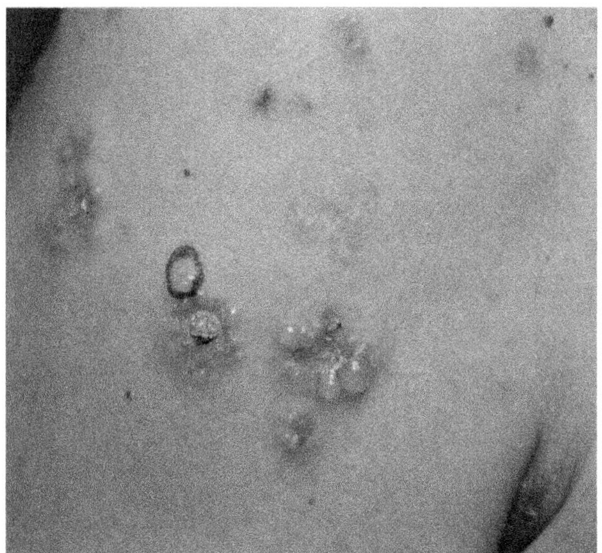

FIGURE 8-31 New onset bullous pemphigoid in a man with a previous history of psoriasis. A shave biopsy of an intact bulla on the arm was performed at the site marked by the surgical marker. Note how the oval marking is drawn around one intact bulla and some perilesional skin. This biopsy specimen is then transected with a blade so that the bulla is sent off in formalin and the perilesional skin is sent for direct immunofluorescence. *(Copyright Richard P. Usatine, MD.)*

Diagnosing a "Rash"

For most challenging rashes, a 4-mm punch biopsy will be helpful to make the diagnosis. However, in many instances it may be better to send the patient for a consultation rather than doing a "blind" biopsy because the histology can be very nonspecific.

CONSIDERATIONS FOR SPECIFIC ANATOMIC AREAS

Anterior Shin

The thin skin on the shin makes both excision and punch biopsy more complicated. Shave biopsy is preferred when it is a reasonable alternative.

Hands and Feet

Care must be taken when performing punch biopsies on the hands and feet because of proximity to vessels, tendons, bone, and nerves since the skin is so thin. The sensory nerves along the lateral sides of the fingers lie within reach of a biopsy punch. On the dorsum of the hand, tendons are vulnerable. When a punch biopsy is needed on the palm of the hand to distinguish between palmar psoriasis and hand dermatitis, it is best to choose an area that has sufficient soft tissue between the skin and the bones and tendons. The thenar eminence is a good choice if the rash involves this area.

Chest and Buttocks

The chest and buttocks may be considered cosmetic areas and may require particular care to avoid scarring. Keloidal or hypertrophic scarring is common in both of these areas. Large, deep shave biopsies should be avoided if possible.

Scalp (Alopecia)

Biopsy is almost always needed to diagnose the various forms of scarring alopecia (including lichen planopilaris and folliculitis decalvans) (Figure 8-32). Androgenic alopecia, telogen effluvium, and alopecia areata are not scarring and can often be diagnosed clinically without a biopsy. The type of inflammatory infiltrates seen on histology can vary and are used to classify the scarring alopecias:

- *Lymphocytic:* discoid lupus erythematosus, lichen planopilaris, and central centrifugal scarring alopecia
- *Neutrophilic:* folliculitis decalvans and dissecting folliculitis
- *Mixed:* acne keloidalis nuchae.

Usually two 4-mm punch biopsies are preferred so the pathologist can cut one specimen longitudinally and the other vertically. This gives additional information that may be needed for a firm diagnosis.

Ears, Eyelids, Nose, and Lips

Shave biopsies are often preferred on the ears, eyelids, nose, and lips. If a punch biopsy is indicated, use of a 3-mm punch will avoid most problems with dog ears (see Chapter 10). On the ears it is best to avoid cutting into the cartilage unless it is necessary for the diagnosis. On the eyelids, care must be taken to avoid the conjunctival margin and the lacrimal ducts to avoid scarring that will lead to eye dysfunction. On the nose, a

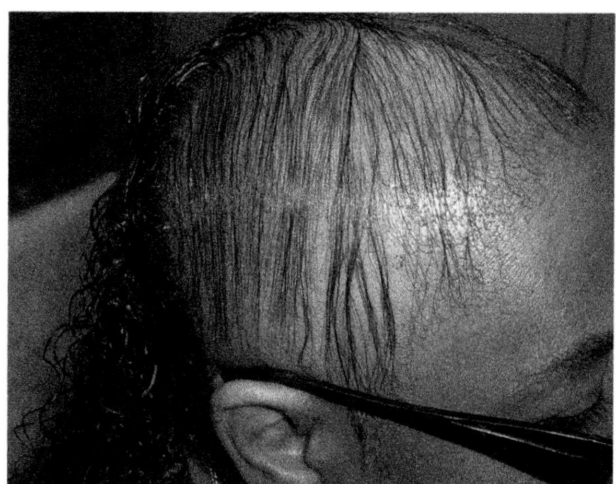

FIGURE 8-32 The patient presented with hair loss of unknown etiology. Two 4-mm punch biopsies were performed. Each biopsy site was marked with a surgical marker around remaining hair follicles. It is important to give the pathologist remaining hair follicles and not completely bald scalp. *(Copyright Richard P. Usatine, MD.)*

shave biopsy is often preferred if the lesion is not pigmented. A large punch biopsy can distort the anatomy of the nose. On the lips, care must be taken to align the vermilion border if any sutures are used.

HOW TO SUBMIT A SPECIMEN TO THE LAB

To obtain the most accurate diagnosis from the pathologist, it is important to provide all of the relevant information on the submission form that accompanies the specimen. Drs. Boyd and Neldner[12] have developed the "five D's" mnemonic to remember the essential information to include on the requisition form:

- Description
- Demographics
- Duration
- Diameter
- Diagnosis.

Description

The physician should write a description of the appearance of the lesion. Examples of common descriptive terms include *erythema, scale, pearly, raised, pigmented, ulcerating, crusted, nodular, papular, macular, vesicular,* and *bullous*.

Demographics

The age and sex of the patient should be noted as well as travel history, ethnicity, family history, etc. Even an occupational history (gardener) or other personal history (extensive tanning bed use) can be immensely helpful.

Duration

How long a lesion has been present will help define the possible diagnoses.

Diameter

Recording the size of the lesion is especially important if the physician has not excised the entire lesion. Pigmented lesions larger than 6 mm are more likely to be melanoma. Unless recorded, the pathologist will not know the size of an incompletely excised lesion. For eruptions, one can record the distribution of the eruption.

Diagnosis

A clinician should commit to the most likely diagnosis and record it on the lab requisition. In most cases alternative diagnoses should be included. It is not expected that the diagnoses recorded will be correct all of the time; if they were, the pathologist would not be needed. However, submitting the "best guess" of the differential diagnosis may be helpful to the pathologist. It also helps the clinician improve diagnostic acumen by obtaining the histologic feedback. Always go back to the differential diagnosis when looking at the final result. This can actually be fun.

Two additional "D's" to consider include:

Diseases

Knowing of other significant diseases the patient has such as SLE, RA, HIV, or immune suppression can certainly aid the pathologist in discerning the nature of some lesions.

Drugs

Medications (e.g., topical steroids) can alter the appearance of a lesion or be the cause of an inflammatory change (e.g., allergy to neomycin). It is important then to note both what the patient is using/taking (if pertinent) and what may have been used to treat the lesion.

Following the "seven D's" approach to submitting a specimen will improve communication with the pathologist and maximize the accuracy of the final histologic diagnosis.

CONCLUSION

The choice of biopsy technique can substantially affect the cosmetic result, the diagnostic information obtained, the time required to perform the procedure, and the cost. Shave, punch, curettage, incisional, and excisional biopsies each have advantages and disadvantages. (See Chapters 9, 10, and 11 for further information on these procedures.) Choosing among these biopsy techniques requires consideration of the size and morphology of the lesion in question, its anatomic location, the experience and skill of the physician, and the initial assessment of the diagnosis. It is of utmost importance that clinicians feel comfortable performing skin biopsies and, although it may not affect patient survival with a short delay between diagnostic biopsy and definitive treatment for melanoma, delaying the initial biopsy itself may have grave consequences.[13]

References

1. Bergfield WF, Pfenninger JL, Weinstock MA. Skin biopsy: selecting an optimal technique. *Patient Care*. 2001;(March 30):11.
2. Tran KT, Wright NA, Cockrell CJ. Biopsy of the pigmented lesion—when and how. *J Am Acad Dermatol*. 2008;59:852–871.
3. Achar S. Principles of skin biopsies for the primary care physician. *Am Fam Physician*. 1996;54:2411.
4. Oppenheim EB. Failure to biopsy skin lesions prompts litigation. *Medical Malpractice Prevention*. April 1990:5–6.
5. Molenkamp BG, Sluijter BJR, Oosterhof B, *et al*. Non-radical diagnostic biopsies do no negatively influence melanoma patient survival. *Ann Surg Oncol*. 2007;14(4):1424–1430.
6. Ng PCJ, Garzilai DA, Ismail SA, *et al*. Evaluating invasive cutaneous melanoma: Is the initial biopsy representative of the final depth? *Am Acad Dermatol*. 2003;48(3):420–424.
7. McGovern TW, Litaker MS. Clinical predictors of malignant pigmented lesions: a comparison of the Glasgow seven-point

checklist and the American Cancer Society's ABCDs of pigmented lesions. *J Dermatol Surg Oncol*. 1992;18:22–26.
8. Lens MB, Nathan P, Bataille V. Excision margins for primary cutaneous melanoma. Updated pooled analysis of randomized controlled trials. *Arch Surg*. 2007;142(9):885–891.
9. NIH Consensus Conference. Diagnosis and treatment of early melanoma. *JAMA*. 1992;268:10, 1314–1319.
10. Greene MH, Clark WH, Tucker MA, *et al*. High risk of malignant melanoma in melanoma-prone families with dysplastic nevi. *Ann Intern Med*. 1985;102:458–465.
11. Clark WH Jr. The dysplastic nevus syndrome. *Arch Dermatol*. 1988;124:1207–1210.
12. Boyd A, Neldner K. How to submit a specimen for cutaneous pathology analysis. *Arch Fam Med*. 1997;(6):64–66.
13. McKenna DB, Lee RJ, Prescott RJ, Doherty VR. The time from diagnostic excision biopsy to wide local excision for primary cutaneous malignant melanoma may not affect patient survival. *Br J Dermatol*. 2002;147(2):48–54.

Additional Reading

Garcia C. Skin biopsy techniques (Chap 14). *In*: Robinson JK, Hanks CW, Sengelmann RD, Siegel DM, eds. *Surgery of the Skin*. Philadelphia: Mosby/Elsevier; 2005.

Habif TP. Dermatologic surgical procedures (Chap 27). *In*: *Clinical Dermatology, A Color Guide to Diagnosis and Therapy*. 4th ed. Philadelphia: Mosby/Elsevier; 2004.

Pfenninger JL. Skin biopsy (Chap 32). *In*: Pfenninger JL, Fowler GC, eds. *Pfenninger and Fowler's Procedures for Primary Care*. Philadelphia: Mosby/Elsevier; 2011.

Videos

Pfenninger JL. How to Perform Skin Biopsy: A Guide for Clinicians. Creative Health Communications, www.creativehealthcommunications.com; 2005. Also available through the National Procedures Institute, www.npinstitute.com.

Pfenninger JL. Common Office Dermatologic Procedures. Creative Health Communications, www.creativehealthcommunications.com; 2005. Also available through the National Procedures Institute, www.npinstitute.com.

9 The Shave Biopsy

RICHARD P. USATINE, MD

The shave biopsy is one of the most useful approaches for obtaining tissue for diagnostic purposes and for the removal of benign surface neoplasms. It is especially fast, easy, and effective when the lesion is raised above the skin surface. The shave biopsy is also valuable for diagnosing many cutaneous malignancies, including basal cell carcinomas (BCCs) and squamous cell carcinomas (SCCs). It is also an effective tool for removing benign lesions such as intradermal nevi and seborrheic keratoses. After a shave biopsy, hemostasis is easily obtained with aluminum chloride. The surface is allowed to heal naturally, and no sutures are needed. The excision site usually heals well with a good cosmetic result.

INDICATIONS

The following lesions are among those that are frequently diagnosed by shave biopsy:

- BCC (Figure 9-1)
- SCC (Figure 9-2)
- Keratoacanthoma (KA) (Figure 9-3)
- Dysplastic nevus (Figure 9-4).

Shave excision can also be used to remove the following benign lesions:

- Benign melanocytic nevus
- Seborrheic keratosis (Figure 9-5)
- Sebaceous hyperplasia
- Pyogenic granuloma (PG) (Figure 9-6)
- Skin tag with a broad base
- Single large wart
- Neurofibroma.

When a pigmented lesion appears to be benign and its removal is for cosmetic reasons, it is acceptable to use a shave excision. However, it is essential to send biopsies of all potentially suspicious lesions for review by a pathologist. A typical skin tag does not need to be sent to pathology.

CONTRAINDICATIONS

There are no contraindications for shave biopsy based on location of the lesion. The use of a shave biopsy to diagnose a melanoma is controversial with a wide range of opinions. A superficial shave biopsy of a suspected melanoma runs the risk of losing important depth information used for staging and margin determination. However, if the melanoma is thin and the shave biopsy gets below the tumor, then nothing is lost. On the other hand, if a punch biopsy is performed of a large lesion and the punch misses the area with melanoma, this false-negative result can lead to missing the diagnosis of the melanoma. Although doing a complete full-thickness biopsy of a small suspected melanoma is optimal, this may be too deforming for a large superficial pigmented lesion on the face that might possibly be lentigo maligna melanoma (LMM) but appears more consistent with a solar lentigo (Figure 9-7). A broad scoop shave biopsy of LMM (Figure 9-8) may give a better tissue sample than one or more punch biopsies and will not cause the cosmetic deformities of a large full-thickness biopsy. It is also common practice to use a broad scoop shave to remove an atypical mole suspected of being a dysplastic nevus.

In reality, the biopsy type is based on suspected diagnosis, size, location, patient preferences, and time considerations. It is better to diagnose a melanoma by shave biopsy than to lose a patient with melanoma to follow-up because you did not have the time to do an elliptical biopsy.

ADVANTAGES OF A SHAVE BIOPSY

The advantages of a shave biopsy can be broken down into two categories: those that are related to the clinician and those that are related to the patient. Advantages of a shave biopsy for the clinician include the following:

- Can be performed rapidly.
- Sutures are not needed.
- Procedure is relatively easy to learn.
- Multiple lesions can be easily excised at one time.
- An assistant is not required.
- Strict sterile procedure is not required.

The following advantages of a shave biopsy benefit the patient:

- There are no sutures that need to be removed.
- Wound care is usually simple.
- Restriction of activities is not needed during wound healing.
- The risks of infection and bleeding are reduced.
- It may give a better cosmetic result than a full-thickness excision.
- Even if a change in pigmentation occurs, it is easily covered by cosmetics.

A number of studies have shown the shave biopsy to produce a better cosmetic result than the punch biopsy and the fusiform diagnostic excision.[1-3]

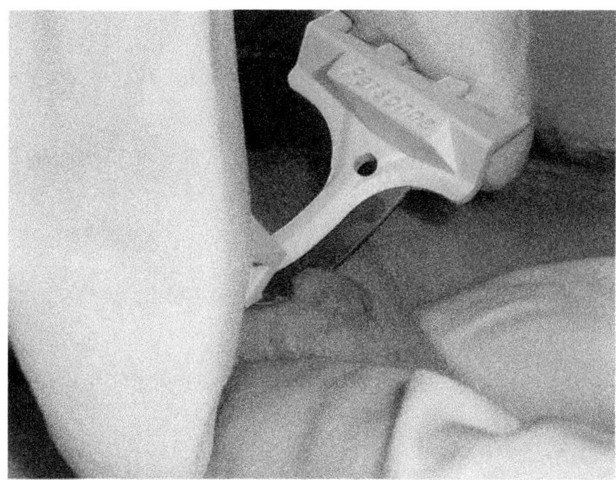

FIGURE 9-1 Elevated pearly lesion in the nasolabial fold with telangiectasias. A shave biopsy is performed to rule out a BCC. *(Copyright Richard P. Usatine, MD.)*

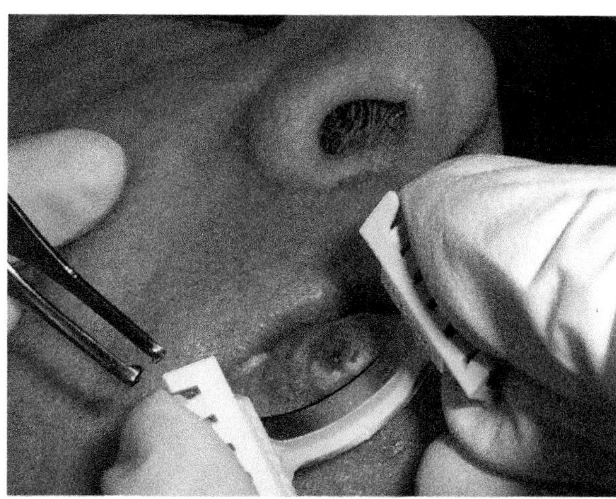

FIGURE 9-2 Shave biopsy of SCC on the lip. *(Copyright Richard P. Usatine, MD.)*

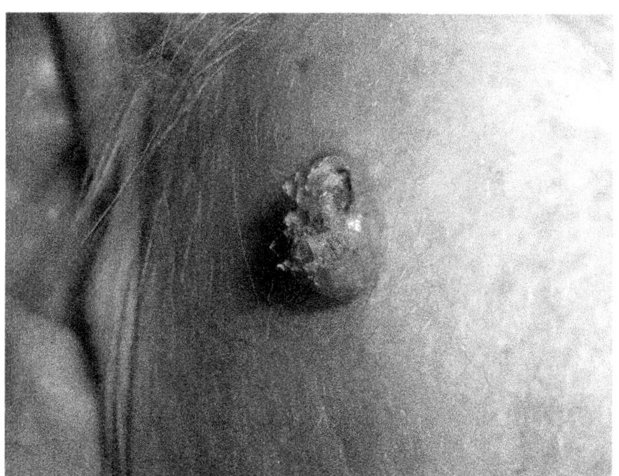

FIGURE 9-3 A keratoacanthoma on face is appropriate for a shave biopsy. *(Copyright Richard P. Usatine, MD.)*

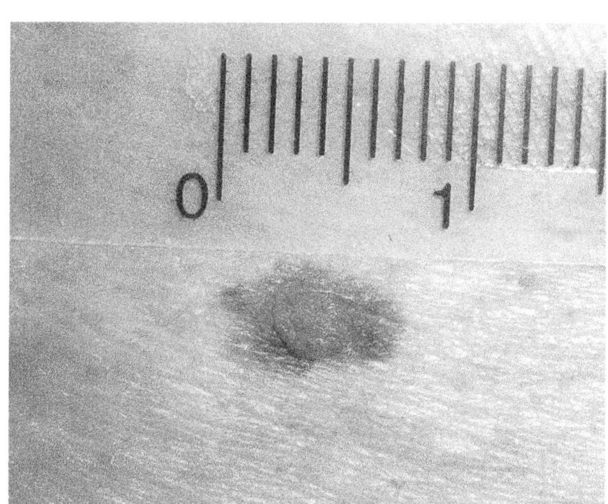

FIGURE 9-4 Dysplastic nevus can be shaved with a deep shave for diagnosis and treatment. *(Copyright Richard P. Usatine, MD.)*

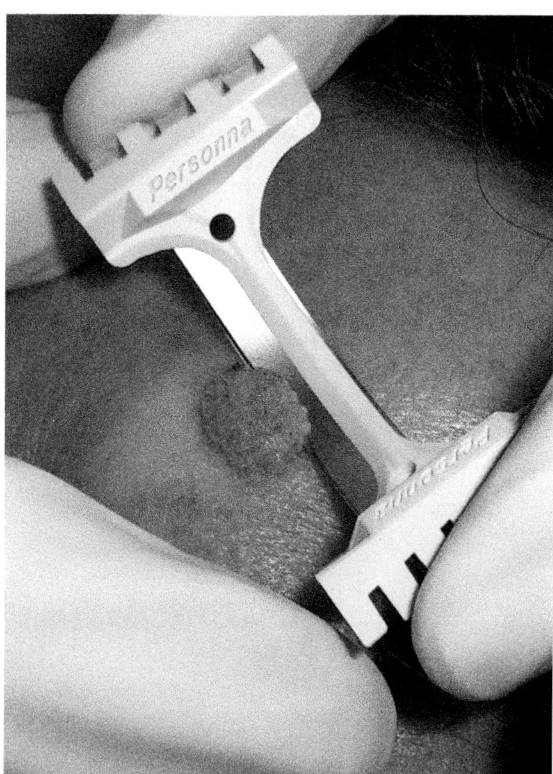

FIGURE 9-5 Shave excision of a verrucous-appearing seborrheic keratosis on the forehead. *(Copyright Richard P. Usatine, MD.)*

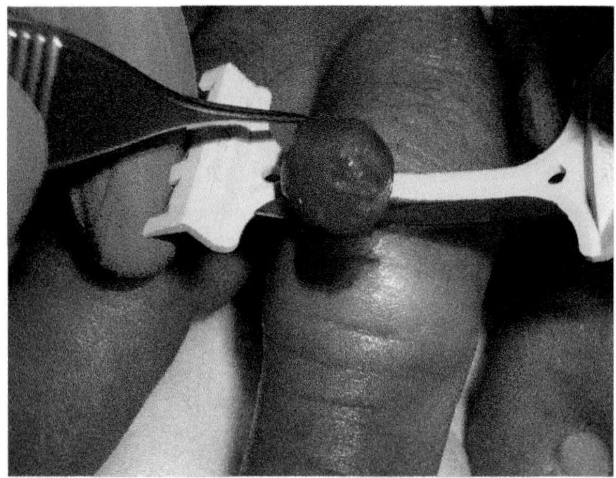

FIGURE 9-6 Shave biopsy of PG on finger. *(Copyright Richard P. Usatine, MD.)*

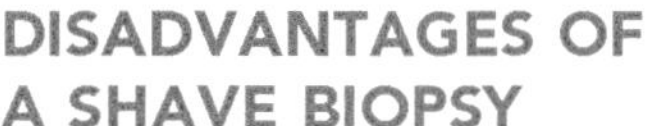

DISADVANTAGES OF A SHAVE BIOPSY

As with the advantages of the shave biopsy, the disadvantages can also be categorized into those for the clinician and those for the patient. Disadvantages for the clinician include the following:

- If the lesion turns out to be a melanoma, the shave may interfere with determining the depth of the lesion if the shave did not get below the tumor and the whole lesion was removed.
- Shave biopsies of flat lesions are more challenging than elevated lesions and a punch biopsy may be easier for an inexperienced clinician.

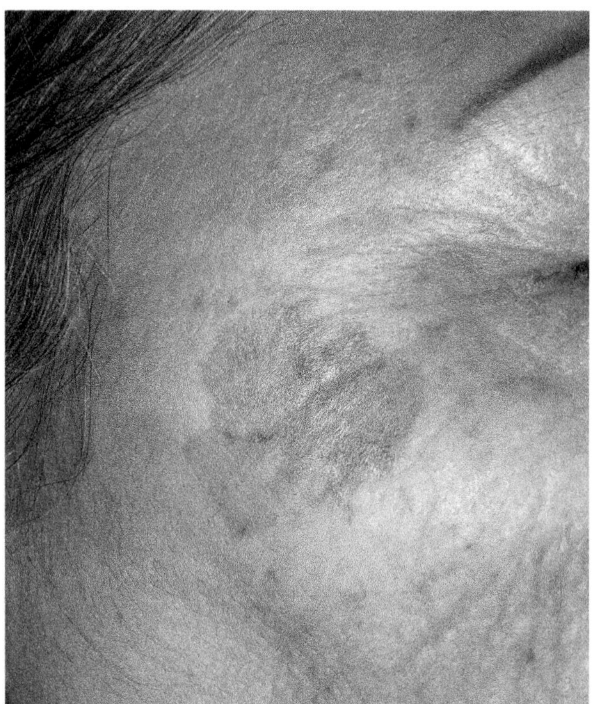

FIGURE 9-7 Solar lentigo. *(Copyright Richard P. Usatine, MD.)*

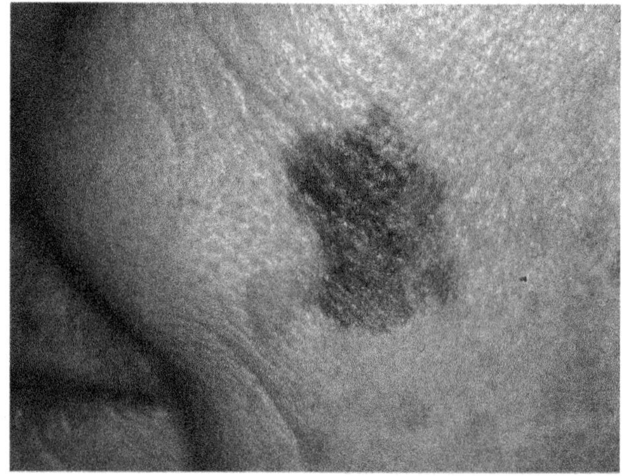

FIGURE 9-8 Lentigo maligna melanoma. *(Copyright Richard P. Usatine, MD.)*

For the patient, the disadvantages of shave biopsy include the following:

- An indentation (divot) may remain.
- Hypopigmentation or hyperpigmentation may result.
- Regrowth may occur.
- A second surgery may be needed if the whole lesion needs excision.
- Scarring may occur over the whole biopsy site.

A superficial shave biopsy should heal with little to no indentation of the skin.[4] Deep-shave biopsies are more likely to leave an indentation. Persistence rates of melanocytic lesions for shave biopsy range from approximately 13% to 28%.[5] Persistence does not always translate into regrowth. If regrowth does occur, it is important to have access to the original pathology report to avoid overdiagnosing a benign regrowth as a melanoma (pseudomelanoma). Methods useful to differentiate pseudomelanoma from melanoma include accurate clinical records of prior biopsy sites along with evidence of scarring within the current biopsy.[5]

EQUIPMENT

The minimum equipment necessary for a shave biopsy is a sharp blade (razor blade or No. 15 scalpel), a 3-mL syringe and needle for local anesthesia, and cotton-tipped applicators (CTAs) and aluminum chloride for hemostasis. It is handy to have a forceps to hold the lesion during the shave procedure or to transfer the tissue into the biopsy container. (The end of a CTA can also be used to do this transfer in many cases.) A surgical marking pen can be useful and is best used before administering the anesthesia.

The Personna DermaBlade is an excellent razor blade for shave biopsies. The blue plastic handle makes it easy and safe to grip the sharp razor blade and control the blade for an accurate and precise shave excision. The cost of the disposable DermaBlade is about the same as a standard disposable No. 15 scalpel. Other options

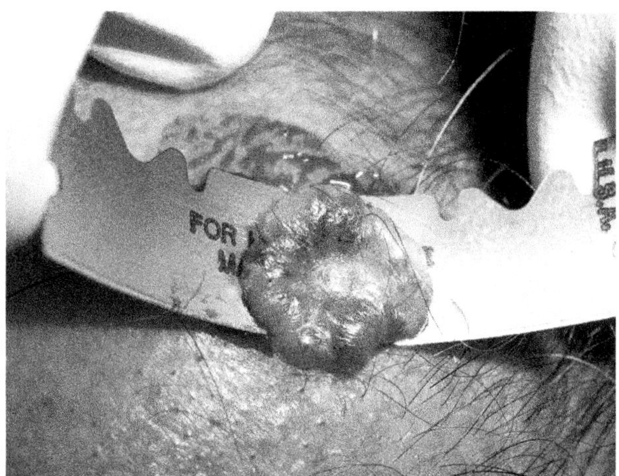

FIGURE 9-9 Shave biopsy with a double-edge Personna blade that was snapped in half before use. The blade easily cuts through this pigmented BCC. *(Copyright Richard P. Usatine, MD.)*

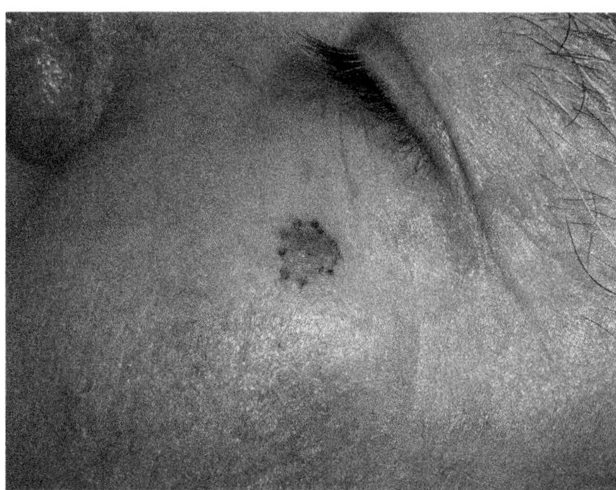

FIGURE 9-11 A nonpigmented growth on the cheek that could be an early nonmelanoma skin cancer. The subtle findings and lack of pigment make it a good candidate for preanesthesia marking with a surgical marker. *(Copyright Richard P. Usatine, MD.)*

include the Personna or Wilkinson double-edge razor blade. The Personna (or Personna Plus with Teflon coating) double-edge blade is very sharp and can be broken in half for easy use (Figure 9-9). Although these do not come in sterile packaging, they can be safely used for shave biopsies without using the autoclave. At approximately 15 cents per cutting blade (30 cents per two-sided blade), these are the most cost-effective tool for shave biopsies. They can be broken in half within their paper container to avoid cutting your hand prior to use. It might take some more time to get used to the bare blade, but once you have mastered its use, you will find this type of low-cost blade to be sharp and effective.

Miltex produces a BiopBlade flexible scalpel for shave biopsies. Its design is similar to that of the DermaBlade, using a single-edge razor blade with a plastic bendable handle. It is currently more expensive than the DermaBlade and has no advantages over the DermaBlade. The plastic handle can snap in half if the blade is bent incorrectly. The Personna single-edge razor blade is too rigid for shave biopsies. All of these blades (Figure 9-10) are available for purchase through Delasco (www.delasco.com) and some can be purchased through other suppliers.

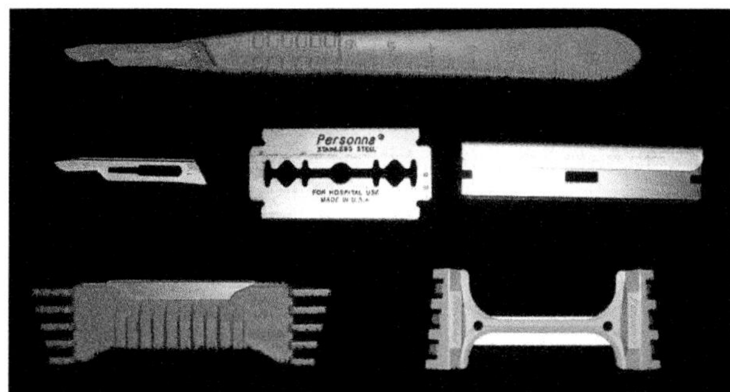

FIGURE 9-10 Equipment used to perform a shave biopsy. *(Copyright Richard P. Usatine, MD.)*

SHAVE BIOPSY: STEPS AND PRINCIPLES

See video on the DVD for further learning. 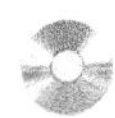

Three critical steps in the shave biopsy include:

- Using 1% lidocaine with epinephrine for anesthesia and hemostasis.
- Stabilizing the lesion to allow for controlled removal of the biopsy.
- Dealing with any residual tissue after the initial shave.

Preoperative Measures

- After determining that the shave technique is the best method for the patient, obtain informed consent. (See Appendix A for an informed consent form titled *Disclosure and Consent: Medical and Surgical Procedures.*) By visual inspection and palpation, determine the likely depth of the lesion and plan the depth of your biopsy based on the probable diagnosis and your physical exam.
- Lightly prep the area with alcohol or another antiseptic. There is no evidence that this preparation decreases the already extremely low infection rate, but it is easy to do.
- If it appears that the lesion will have fewer visible margins after the anesthesia, it helps to mark the area to be shaved with a surgical marker. It need not be a sterile marker. Consider marking the margins of nonpigmented relatively flat lesions that may only be actinic keratoses or sebaceous hyperplasia (but are somewhat suspicious for early skin cancer), because after injection the margins of these lesions may not be visible (Figure 9-11).
- Inject local anesthesia. Use a 30-gauge needle with approximately 2 to 3 mL of 1% lidocaine and

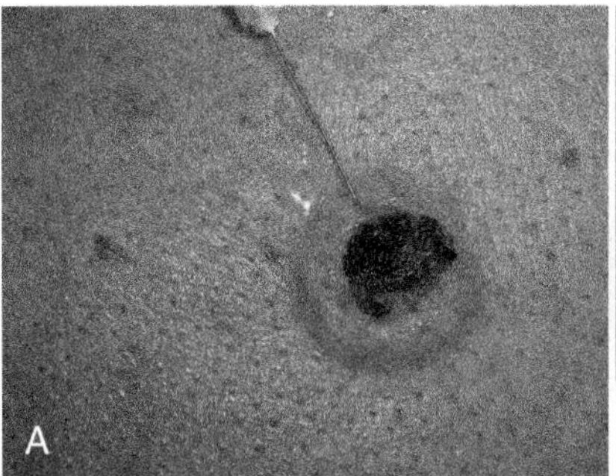

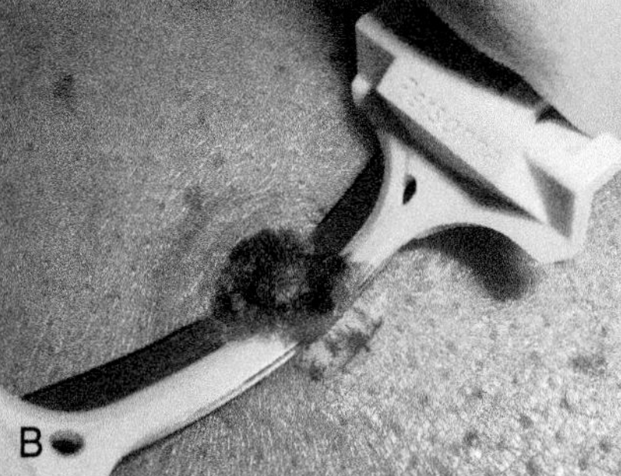

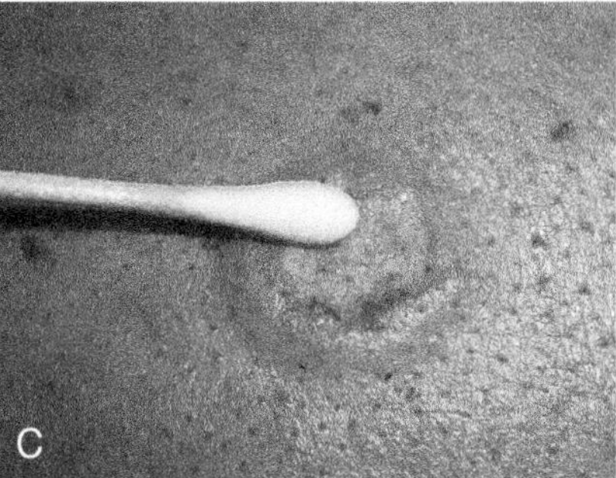

FIGURE 9-12 Pigmented lesion subjected to a shave biopsy to confirm clinical impression of seborrheic keratosis and rule out melanoma: **(A)** Anesthesia is given. **(B)** Shave is performed. **(C)** Aluminum chloride is used to stop any bleeding. *(Copyright Richard P. Usatine, MD.)*

epinephrine (buffer the lidocaine for less pain; see Chapter 3, *Anesthesia*). Start with the needle under the lesion (greater depth is less painful) and then give the last amount of anesthesia closer to the skin surface. If the lesion is flat, consider raising the lesion some with the anesthesia (Figure 9-12A).

CUTTING THE SHAVE BIOPSY

Using a Razor Blade

See video on the DVD for further learning. 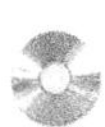

- Determine how you will use your forceps or other hand to stabilize the lesion to keep it from moving during the shave.
- Grasp one end of the razor blade between the thumb and the second and third fingers of your dominant hand, creating a gentle bend in the blade (Figure 9-12B). Place the blade on the skin surface and gently advance it into the lesion while moving the blade in a side-to-side fashion. Do not bend the blade too much to avoid causing an indentation in the middle of the shave. Ideally, the blade should be mostly flat in the area of the shave.
- Apply gentle forward pressure during this side-to-side sawing motion and allow the blade to move through the lesion without excess pressure. With the bare razor blade you may need to put one finger against the back of the blade to push it forward when the lesion is firm. Watch each side of the blade to make sure that it is cutting where you intend to cut.
- On some specimens, there is a tendency for the specimen to flip over at the end of the biopsy. If needed use the forceps or the stick-end of a CTA to stabilize the specimen for the final cut.
- Obtain hemostasis with aluminum chloride on a CTA (Figure 9-12C). Do not make the CTA too wet with aluminum chloride and use downward pressure with a twisting motion to get the best hemostasis. Occasionally a very vascular lesion will require electrocoagulation to obtain hemostasis.

Using a Scalpel Blade

See video on the DVD for further learning. 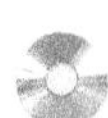

- Hold the No. 15 scalpel blade (on or off a blade handle) parallel to the surface of the skin (Figure 9-13).
- Use the middle of the blade while cutting. Watch the scalpel blade on both sides of the lesion so as to remove the lesion in its entirety without affecting normal skin around the lesion.
- Move the blade through the tissue using a minimal sawing movement. The slight sawing motion helps the blade move through the tissue, but too much sawing will produce scalloped edges.
- Use the forceps or stick-end of a CTA to stabilize the specimen for the final cut.

Snip Excision with Scissors

See video on the DVD for further learning. 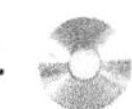

Another variation of the shave excision for small raised lesions is the snip excision performed with sharp scissors (Figure 9-14). Anesthesia and hemostasis are executed in the same manner as for the other types of shave excision. The only difference is that the lesion is snipped off with sharp scissors rather than shaved with a blade. Lesions particularly amenable to snip excision are skin tags, small warts, and polypoid nevi. We recommend using a good pair of sharp iris scissors (straight or curved). Small lesions may be snipped without anesthesia, but larger lesions should be anesthetized with 1% lidocaine and epinephrine. The lesion is grasped with forceps and cut at the base with the scissors. The crushing effect of the scissor on the soft tissue helps to prevent bleeding. Additional hemostasis can be achieved with aluminum chloride or electrosurgery.

Electrosurgical Shave

See video on the DVD for further learning. 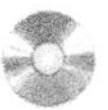

A loop electrode may be used to perform an electrosurgical shave (Figure 9-15). The loop electrode can be

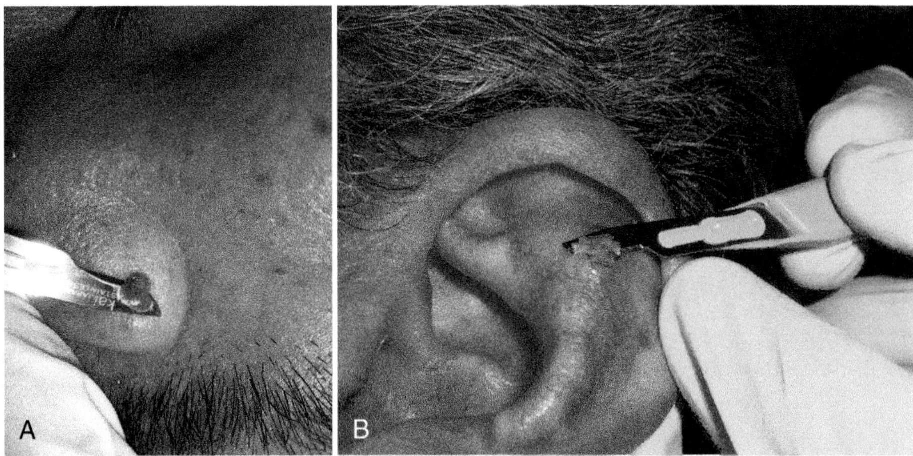

FIGURE 9-13 Shave biopsies with a scalpel in tight places where a small No. 15 scalpel blade is easier to maneuver than a larger razor blade: (**A**) Shave of pigmented lesion on nose. Path showed SK. (**B**) Shave of nonpigmented lesion in ear. Path showed an actinic keratosis. *(Copyright Richard P. Usatine, MD.)*

used to feather the remaining tissue and sculpt a nice result. One downside is that there will be burn artifact on the biopsy specimen. Also, if the lesion is caused by human papillomavirus (HPV), there is a very small risk of transmission of the HPV by the plume. Whether the instrument is set on cut only or cut and coag, it is important to not use too much power, which can result in unnecessary tissue destruction leading to increased scarring. (Also see Chapter 14, *Electrosurgery*.)

Scoop Shave (Deep-Shave Saucerization Technique)

A saucerization technique involves the removal of the lesion using a deep shave or scoop technique with 1 to 2 mm of surrounding normal skin laterally and extending into the deep dermis (Figure 9-16).[5] For thin and small-diameter melanocytic lesions, a scoop shave can remove the entire lesion.[5] The National Comprehensive Cancer Network (NCCN) recommendations suggest

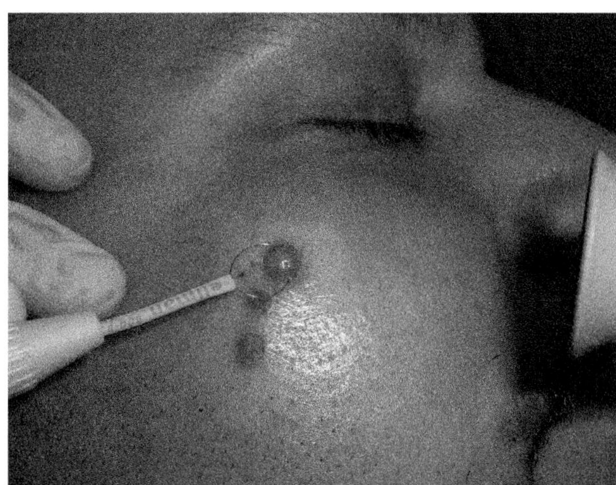

FIGURE 9-15 The use of a radio-frequency electrosurgical loop to perform a shave excision of a benign intradermal nevus. Note the two areas where two other nevi had been excised using this method with some mild feathering for an optimal cosmetic result. *(Copyright Richard P. Usatine, MD.)*

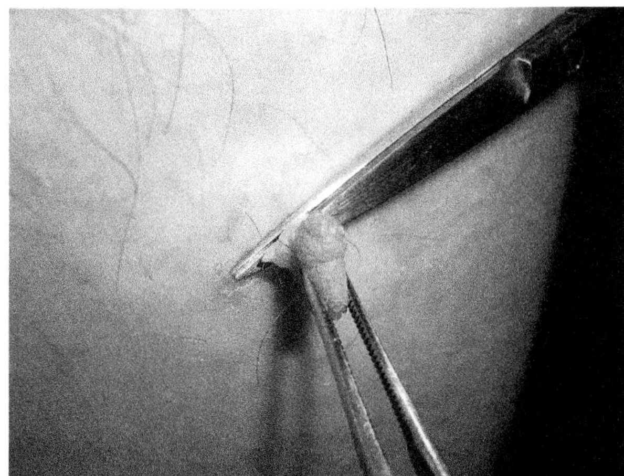

FIGURE 9-14 Snip excision of a skin tag. The scissor crushes the base and helps achieve quick hemostasis. *(Copyright Richard P. Usatine, MD.)*

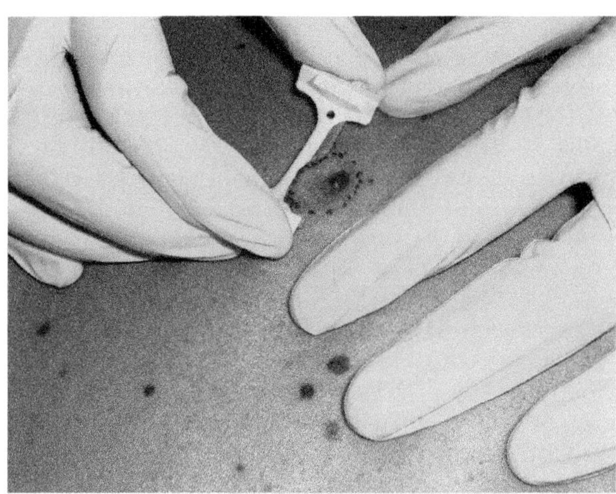

FIGURE 9-16 Scoop shave of a dysplastic nevus that was not fully excised with the initial shave. *(Copyright Richard P. Usatine, MD.)*

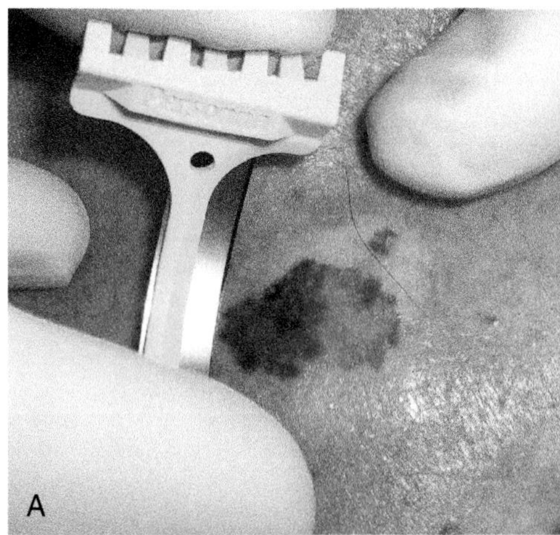

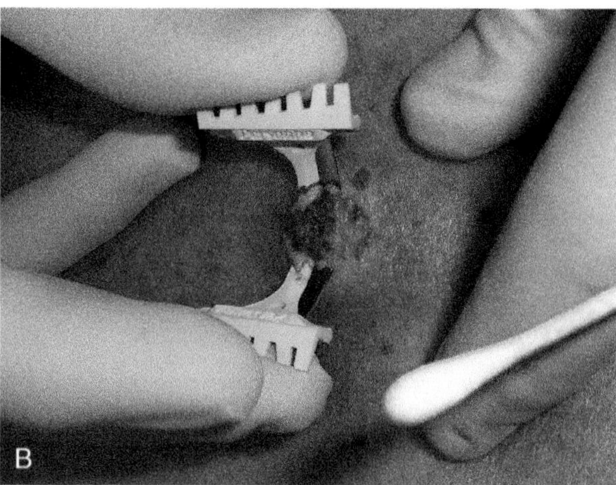

FIGURE 9-17 **(A)** Pigmented lesion on the back suspected to be a superficial spreading melanoma. **(B)** The scoop shave using a DermaBlade of most of the highly pigmented area produced a good specimen for diagnosis of melanoma (Breslow's thickness of 0.6 mm). Note how the shave went completely under the pigmented lesion and the depth information was not lost. If pigment were to be found below the shave, a deeper shave or full-thickness incisional biopsy could be performed of the remaining lesion. In most cases it is best to shave off the entire lesion to reduce the risk of sampling error. *(Copyright Richard P. Usatine, MD.)*

deep-shave biopsies be used when the index of suspicion for melanoma is low.[5] However, a deep-shave biopsy can also be performed for suspected melanoma in certain circumstances (see Chapter 8, *Choosing the Biopsy Type*).

It is easier to do a scoop shave with a DermaBlade or other razor blade than a scalpel. Start by marking the area to be cut, including the planned margin. If the lesion is suspected to be a dysplastic nevus, mark a 2-mm margin around the edge of the pigment. Direct the blade downward at an angle of 30 to 45 degrees with the skin to get underneath the pigment. Continue the shave straight across the base and come upward, leaving another 2 mm from the edge of the pigment. The scoop shave should go into the deep dermis. If a full-thickness biopsy is to be performed into the subcutaneous fat, it is suggested that this be performed with an elliptical excision and closed with sutures. If a few small fat globules are visible at the base of the shave, the area can heal well by second intention.

A pigmented lesion on the back suspected to be a superficial spreading melanoma can be easily and safely biopsied with a deep-shave approach (Figure 9-17). The scoop shave using a razor blade of the thickest pigmented area produces a good specimen for diagnosis of melanoma. (Breslow's thickness of 0.6 mm was obtained in Figure 9-7.) In Figure 9-17 note how the shave went completely under the pigment and the depth information was not lost. If pigment were to be found below the shave, a deeper shave or full-thickness incisional biopsy could be performed of the remaining lesion.

When performing a deep scoop shave to remove a nonmelanoma skin cancer, it is appropriate to cut down deep enough so that small fat globules will be visible (Figure 9-18). If all margins are clear this can serve as the definitive treatment for less aggressive nonmelanoma skin cancers such as superficial or nodular BCCs (not sclerosing) or SCC *in situ*. This method is not recommended for skin cancers larger than 2 cm or in danger areas around vital structures. Definitive treatment for invasive SCC and melanoma should include a full-thickness excision with appropriate margins. As with all skin cancers, regular examinations need to be done to investigate for recurrence and new cancers. A shave excision of any depth should never be the definitive surgery to treat a melanoma.

Landscape Shave

The landscape shave samples a narrow portion across a large pigmented lesion so that the pathologist is able to compare the symmetry of melanocyte nests in determining the diagnosis. Because this biopsy has a tendency to curl, it may be placed on a Telfa pad, the nonadherent portion of a Band-Aid, or a piece of cardboard before placing it in the formalin. Write that this is a landscape shave on the pathology consult and suggest that the specimen be processed with longitudinal slices rather than bread-loafing along the short axis.

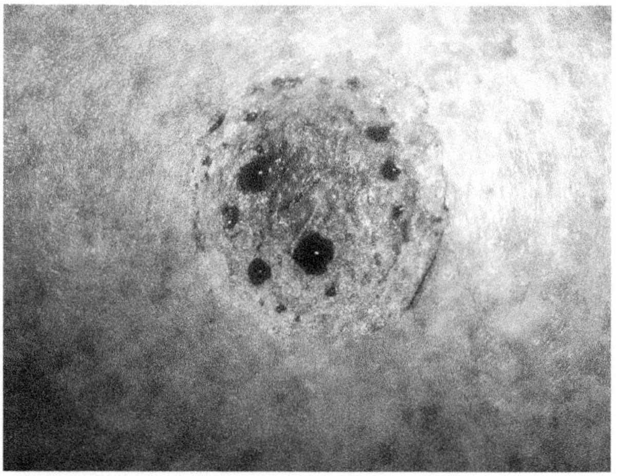

FIGURE 9-18 Deep shave showing a few glistening fat globules. *(Copyright Richard P. Usatine, MD.)*

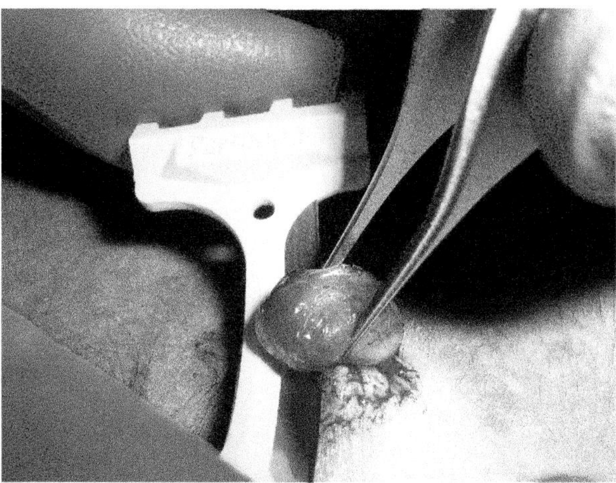

FIGURE 9-19 The forceps stabilize the raised lesion while the shave is performed. This pyogenic granuloma is being excised with a DermaBlade shave excision. *(Copyright Richard P. Usatine, MD.)*

Stabilization Techniques

Lesions should be stabilized during the shave biopsy to maximize the control during cutting. In Figure 9-19, forceps are used, and in Figure 9-20, the skin is pinched because the lesion is very flat. Note how the fingers of the nondominant hand are kept in the biopsy area to provide gentle countertraction and to stabilize the tissue. On certain areas of thin skin near vital structures such as the eye or hand, it may be necessary to pinch and elevate the surrounding skin with one hand while doing the biopsy with the other. The end of a CTA is useful for preventing the lesion from flipping over near the final portion of the cut (Figure 9-21). Raising a flat lesion with anesthetic just prior to excision can help stabilize the lesion but may increase the risk of indentation. Regardless of which method is used, it is important to not pull up on the lesion to avoid creating an unintended deep indentation.

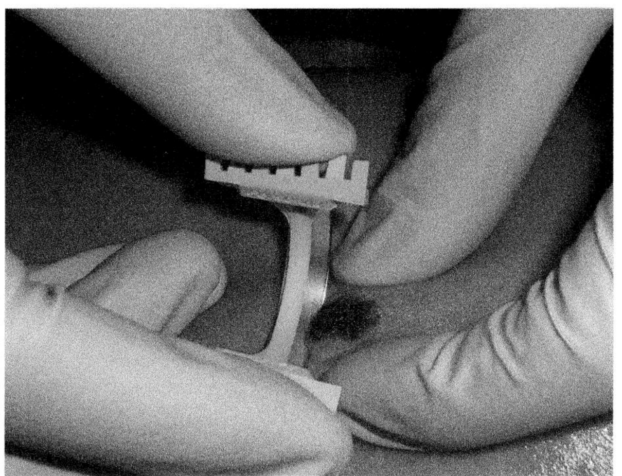

FIGURE 9-20 The start of this shave biopsy is stabilized by pinching the skin between the thumb and index finger of the nondominant hand. Once the shave is begun the fingers can be removed away from the blade. Care must be taken to avoid cutting oneself. *(Copyright Richard P. Usatine, MD.)*

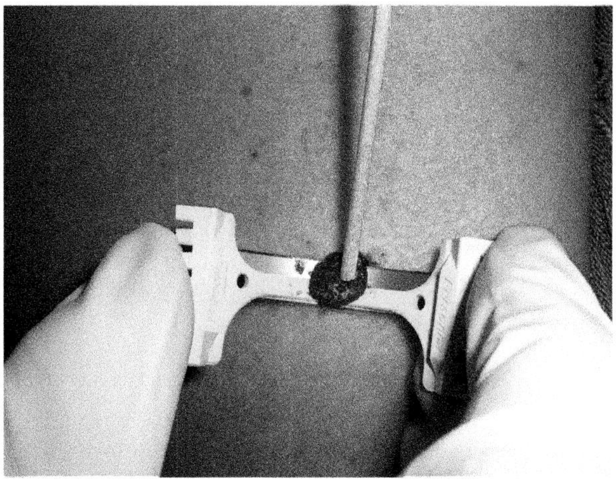

FIGURE 9-21 Shave biopsy with the end of a CTA stabilizing the lesion from flipping over, which can make it difficult to finish the final cut. *(Copyright Richard P. Usatine, MD.)*

Hemostasis

Many shave biopsies can be performed within a minute after the injection of lidocaine and epinephrine. If the lesion is a very vascular (pyogenic granuloma) or the biopsy site is very vascular (such as the lip), it is best to wait 10 minutes for the epinephrine to take full effect (9-2). If enough time has elapsed between the administration of anesthesia and the start of the biopsy, the procedure can be virtually bloodless.

After the biopsy, blot the site with a dry cotton-tipped applicator or gauze to remove any pooled blood. Then roll and twist another CTA that has been dipped in aluminum chloride back and forth over the site. Apply downward pressure with the twisting applicator to stop the bleeding (Figure 9-12C). It is important to not leave wet blood in the field because this will dilute the aluminum chloride and minimize its effectiveness. Monsel's solution (ferric subsulfate) may be used instead of aluminum chloride but it has a slight risk of tattooing the skin. If chemical hemostasis does not stop the bleeding or if it is desirable to destroy any remaining tissue then electrosurgery may be used (see Chapter 4, *Hemostasis*).

Remaining Tissue after Shave Biopsy

Remaining tissue is often found at the trailing edge of the lesion where the blade finished the shave. First obtain hemostasis and then cut the remaining tissue off with your blade. If the tissue is too small to stabilize for a second cut, options to remove the remaining tissue include scraping with the blade perpendicular to the skin or using a curette or electrodesiccation (Figure 9-22). If using electrodesiccation, the charred tissue may be left alone or wiped away with a moist gauze pad or a curette.

Aftercare

After the procedure is complete, place a small amount of clean petrolatum and an adhesive bandage over the

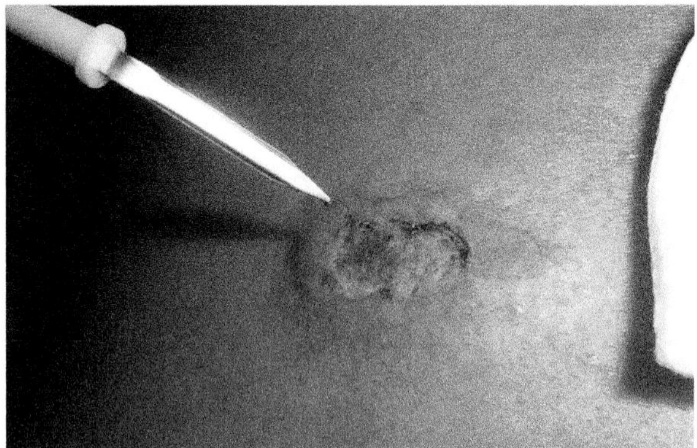

FIGURE 9-22 The Hyfrecator is used to destroy some remaining tissue on the edge of the excision. Note that the original hemostasis was obtained with aluminum chloride to minimize potential scarring that is more likely to occur with electrosurgery of the entire excision site. *(Copyright Richard P. Usatine, MD.)*

biopsy site and give the patient wound care instructions. See the patient handout titled *Care of Your Skin after a Shave Biopsy* in Appendix A.

Pathology and Follow-Up

Send all pigmented lesions and any lesion suspicious for cancer to the pathologist. Skin tags may not need to be sent if these are typical and benign in their appearance. If the pathologist reports that the lesion appears benign, does not have atypical features, but is incompletely excised, there is usually no need to do a further or deeper excision. However, if the pathologist recommends further excision because of suspicion for malignancy or there is a chance of malignant transformation, this recommendation must be followed.

If the lesion is premalignant (such as an actinic keratosis), it should be reexamined after it fully heals. If there is remaining scaling or evidence of the original lesion, it may be treated with cryotherapy instead of doing another excision.

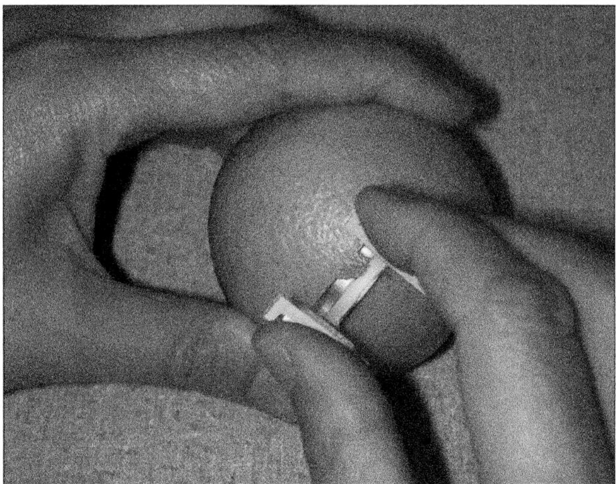

FIGURE 9-23 The skin of an orange provides a good practice medium for the shave biopsy. *(Copyright Richard P. Usatine, MD.)*

If the lesion turns out to be nonmelanoma skin cancer (NMSC), definitive treatment will be necessary unless the original biopsy was deep and the pathologist unambiguously states that there are clear margins. If you intend to remove a whole BCC or SCC *in situ* with a shave excision using a deeper and broader approach, and your pathologist reports clear margins, you may give the patient the choice to not have additional surgery. Always perform full-thickness excisions for sclerosing, micronodular or infiltrating BCCs and invasive SCC (see Chapter 34, *Diagnosis and Treatment of Malignant and Premalignant Lesions*).

SUGGESTION FOR LEARNING THE SHAVE BIOPSY TECHNIQUE

When learning the shave biopsy technique, it may be helpful to practice on an orange. Use a razor blade or No. 15 blade and attempt to remove portions of the outer skin without encroaching on the underlying pulp (Figure 9-23). Practice performing the shave at different depths and sizes.

LESS THAN OPTIMAL OUTCOMES

Infections are rare complications of shave biopsies.

Expected but less than optimal outcomes that often occur after shave biopsies include the following:

- Producing an indentation or divot in the skin. This is expected after a scoop shave. Also this is more common in a shave done on a convex surface such as the nose (Figure 9-24).
- Erythema that may last for months and often resolves.
- Slow healing for deeper shaves and areas such as the lower leg.

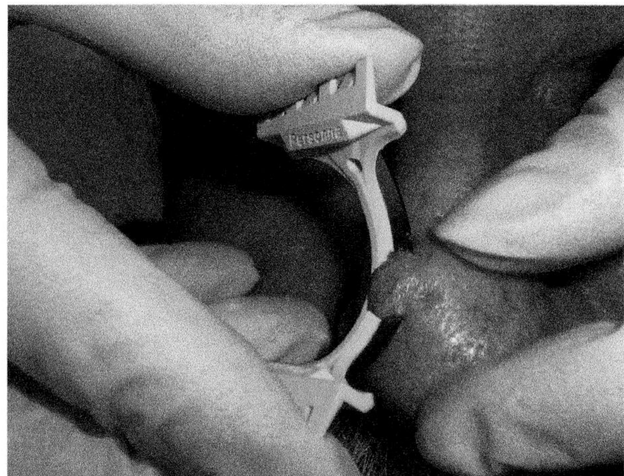

FIGURE 9-24 Shave biopsy of a suspected BCC on the nose. Note how the nose is held between the fingers to stabilize it for the shave biopsy. An indentation would be acceptable cosmetically because the likelihood of skin cancer was high and the patient would need a second procedure to eradicate the BCC. This patient received Mohs surgery after the biopsy proved the lesion to be a BCC. *(Copyright Richard P. Usatine, MD.)*

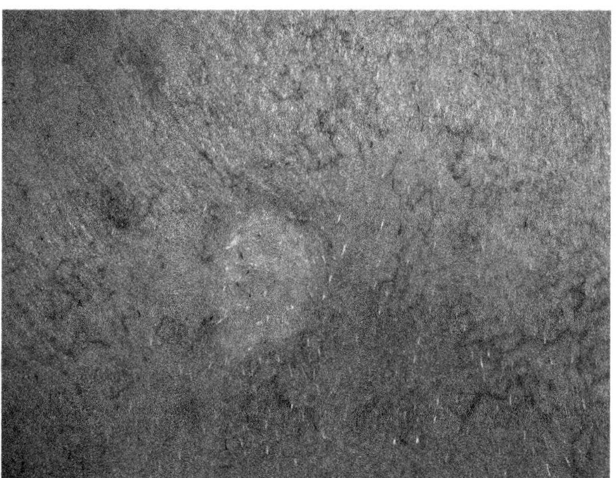

FIGURE 9-25 Hypopigmentation that occurred after a shave biopsy of a basal cell carcinoma on the face. The patient did not return for definitive surgery after the biopsy was made with a DermaBlade, but no further tumor growth occurred over the following year and the shave biopsy site was hypopigmented but appeared tumor free. The patient preferred watchful waiting and no further surgery. *(Copyright Richard P. Usatine, MD.)*

- Hypopigmentation or hyperpigmentation that can be permanent (Figure 9-25).
- Regrowth of incompletely excised lesion. Pigment developing at the site of a nevus removed by shave biopsy is common (Figure 9-26).

Serious complications are extremely rare after a shave biopsy.

After shave biopsy, erythema may persist for months, and hypopigmentation may be permanent in some individuals. In the case of melanocytic nevi some will regrow after removal by this technique. In nevi with hair, the hair may regrow if the nevus is excised with a shave biopsy alone. This type of nevus may be best removed with a deeper elliptical excision. Alternatively, the hair follicles remaining after a shave biopsy may be destroyed with electrosurgery.

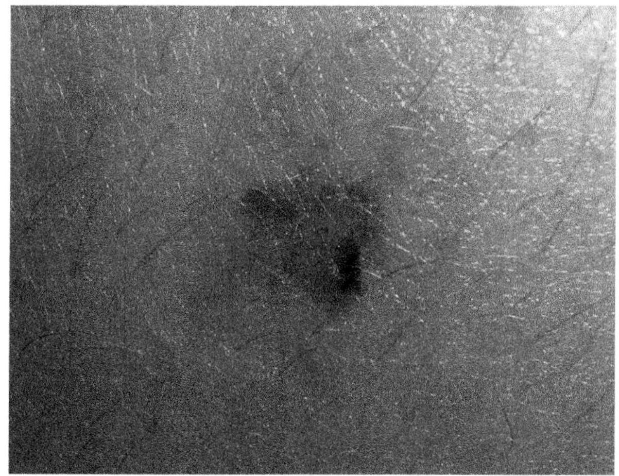

FIGURE 9-26 Pigment that returned after the shave biopsy of an intradermal nevus. *(Copyright Richard P. Usatine, MD.)*

Cosmetic Results

Gambichler et al.[4] examined the cosmetic outcome of macular melanocytic lesions utilizing the deep-shave biopsy technique with a razor blade followed by chemical hemostasis. During routine skin cancer screening 45 patients with 77 macular melanocytic nevi were prospectively recruited. Histologically, 88% of the melanocytic lesions were described as completely excised and 60% were diagnosed as atypical melanocytic nevi. At 6 months, 56 sites were available for evaluation and mild hypopigmentation was observed in 52%, hyperpigmentation in 32%, and erythema in 23%. Recurrent nevi occurred in 13% at 6 months. The evaluation of the cosmetic outcome by the patients was better than the evaluation by the physician.[4]

In another prospective study, shave excision of 204 common acquired melanocytic nevi was performed.[6] Mid-dermal shave biopsies were performed using a No. 15 blade followed by gentle electrocoagulation. Three months after surgery, cosmetically excellent results occurred in 33% of the patients, acceptable results in 59%, and poor results in 8% as assessed by two dermatologists. The likelihood of having an imperceptible scar was significantly greater in lesions excised from the face. Of 192 patients surveyed, 98% stated that "the scar looked better than the original mole" and would undergo the procedure again. Clinical and dermatoscopic recurrences were observed in 19.6% of the scars.[6]

Our experience is that shave excisions heal with less scarring than electrodesiccation and curettage (ED&C), which often leads to hypertrophic scarring.

MAKING A DIAGNOSIS

It helps to have a good idea of the differential diagnosis before choosing the biopsy type and location. For most shave biopsies, a clinician should excise the whole lesion or sample the portion of the lesion that appears to have the worst pathology. However, for bullous disorders such as pemphigus or pemphigoid, it is best to use a scoop shave under an intact bulla or at the border of a bulla. A punch biopsy at the border of the bulla may yield an equally good specimen. Both methods help to keep the epidermis attached to the dermis at the edge of the bulla.

ADDITIONAL EXAMPLES FOR SHAVE BIOPSY

Basal Cell Carcinomas

In Figure 9-27, a shave biopsy is preferred on the nasal ala rather than a punch biopsy. After the diagnosis was made, this patient was referred for Mohs surgery. One study showed that specimens from punch and shave biopsies of suspected BCCs produced equivalent diagnostic accuracy rates: 80.7% and 75.9%, respectively. Either biopsy technique is appropriate for a BCC.[7] The woman in Figure 9-28 has had multiple BCCs and had

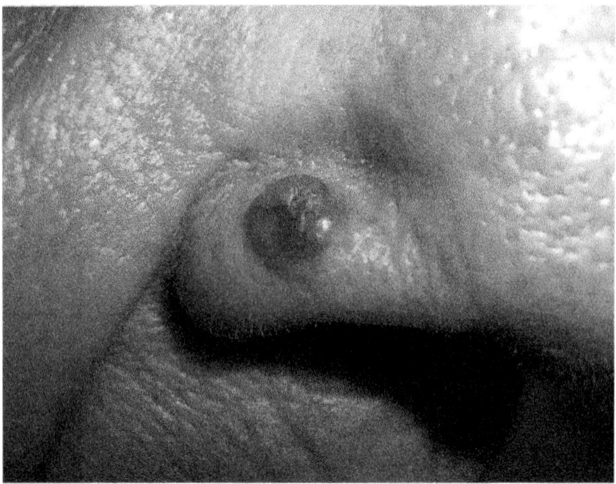

FIGURE 9-27 For a BCC on nasal ala, a shave biopsy is preferred over a punch biopsy. *(Copyright Richard P. Usatine, MD.)*

chosen to have a shave excision of a small BCC on her cheek. A previous biopsy had proven the diagnosis and she wanted less invasive surgery than a full elliptical excision. The margins were clear and the area healed with minimal scarring.

Pyogenic Granuloma

Most pyogenic granulomas are easy to distinguish based on their clinical appearance and behavior. The rare amelanotic melanoma can appear similar to a pyogenic granuloma. Thus, it is best to send all suspected pyogenic granulomas for histologic confirmation. The easiest way to do this is to do an initial shave excision before performing ED&C of the base of the pyogenic granuloma. In Figure 9-29 an electrosurgical loop is being used for the initial shave biopsy. This could easily be done with a razor blade. Most importantly the remaining tissue is curetted and the base is treated with electrodesiccation. See Chapter 33, *Procedures to Treat Benign Conditions*.

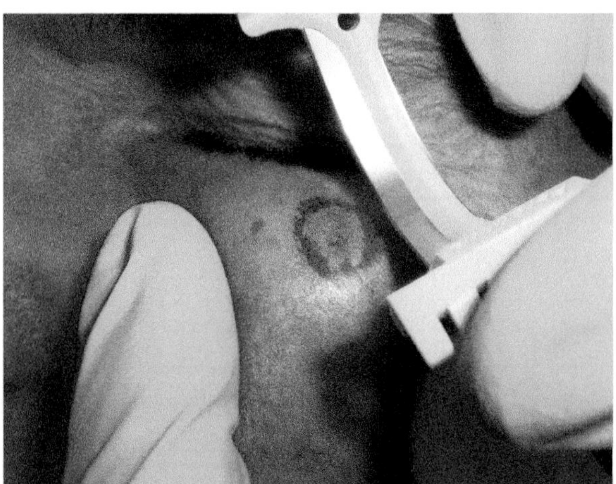

FIGURE 9-28 Shave excision of a small BCC on the cheek. A previous biopsy had proven the diagnosis and the patient wanted less invasive surgery than a full elliptical excision. The margins were clear and the area healed with minimal scarring. *(Copyright Richard P. Usatine, MD.)*

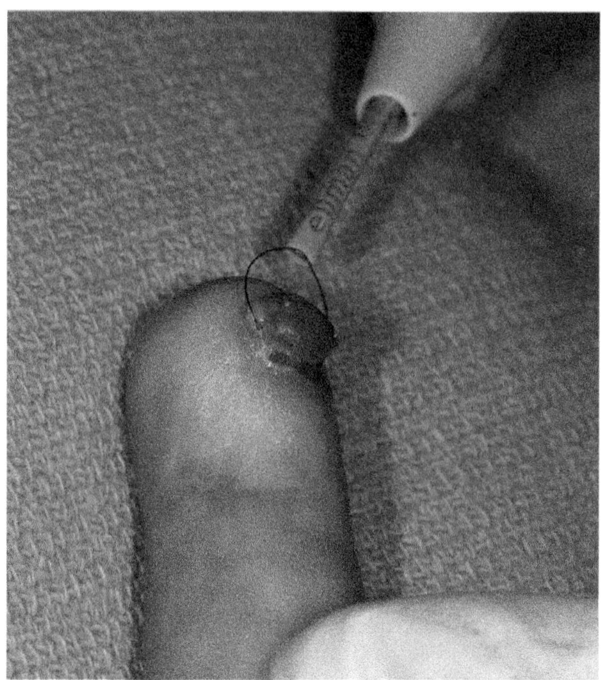

FIGURE 9-29 Electrosurgical shave of PG on a finger. This is followed by curettage and electrodesiccation of the base to stop bleeding and prevent regrowth. *(Copyright Richard P. Usatine, MD.)*

Psoriasis

Psoriasis is frequently a diagnosis made on clinical appearance and history only. Sometimes psoriasis presents in an atypical pattern and a biopsy is needed to make the diagnosis. The patient in Figure 9-30 developed a rash on his penis and had no other skin findings. A shave biopsy of the lesion allowed the diagnosis of psoriasis to be made. While a punch biopsy would have provided adequate tissue, greater risks are involved in a punch biopsy of the penis. Having a definitive diagnosis was helpful to guide treatment of this disturbing eruption.

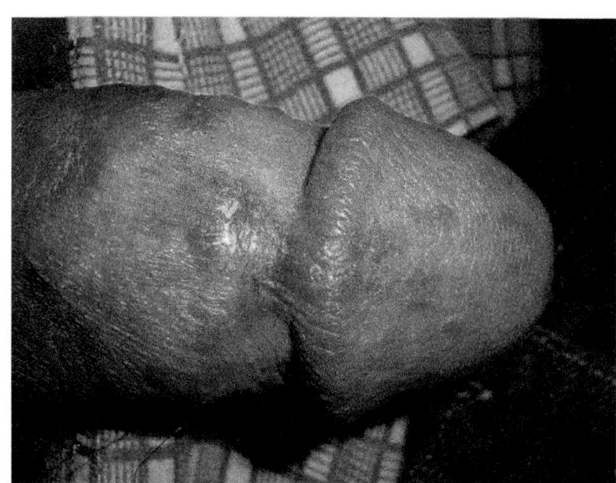

FIGURE 9-30 A shave biopsy of a plaque on this penis demonstrated psoriasis. *(Copyright Richard P. Usatine, MD.)*

CODING AND BILLING PEARLS

The shave procedure is either used as a form of biopsy and billed under the biopsy codes or used to fully excise a lesion that is benign and then billed under the shave excision codes. It can be confusing sometimes to decide whether the procedure is a "biopsy" or "excision." Clear-cut examples of shave biopsies include sampling a possible skin cancer or removing a piece of skin to determine the cause of an unknown rash. Shave excisions are those procedures that are used to remove a benign nevus, a seborrheic keratosis, or another benign lesion. The intent is to excise the whole lesion, and even though it is recommended that all pigmented lesions be sent for confirmatory pathologic diagnosis, the primary reason for the procedure was not a "biopsy" but a removal of the lesion itself. Make sure that the documentation is consistent with the procedure that is billed. If the shave is done as a biopsy, call it a shave biopsy, but if the shave is done as an excision, call it a shave excision or just an excision.

CPT codes and fees for shave biopsies are summarized in Table 38-7 of Chapter 38, *Surviving Financially*. Note that, although these codes cover shave biopsies, they also cover biopsies done by punch or curette. The codes are based on location only and not on the size of the biopsy or lesion. The codes are also independent of whether the lesion turns out to be benign or malignant, so there is no need to wait for the pathology result to submit the bill.

Selected CPT codes and fees for shave excisions are provided in Table 38-10 of Chapter 38. These codes are based on size and location, so it is crucial to measure the lesion before excising it. Do not estimate the size later because estimates are usually rounded to the nearest centimeter and the reimbursement goes up 0.1 cm above each rounded number (e.g., payment is greater for a shave excision of a 1.1-cm lesion than a 1.0-cm lesion). Location also matters but these codes are generally used for benign lesions rather than skin cancers. Most skin cancers will be excised deeply or destroyed and there are codes specific to these procedures on malignant lesions.

CONCLUSION

The shave biopsy is one of the most useful techniques in dermatologic surgery. It is widely applicable to many skin lesions and can be performed rapidly in the office setting with minimal equipment. Every clinician who performs skin surgery should master this technique.

References

1. Grabski WJ, Salasche SJ, Mulvaney MJ. Razor-blade surgery. *J Dermatol Surg Oncol.* 1990;16:1121–1126.
2. Harrison PV. Good results after shave excision of benign moles. *J Dermatol Surg Oncol.* 1985;11:668, 686.
3. Hudson-Peacock MJ, Bishop J, Lawrence CM. Shave excision of benign papular naevocytic naevi. *Br J Plast Surg.* 1995;48: 318–322.
4. Gambichler T, Senger E, Rapp S, *et al.* Deep shave excision of macular melanocytic nevi with the razor blade biopsy technique. *Dermatol Surg.* 2000;26:662–666.
5. Tran KT, Wright NA, Cockerell CJ. Biopsy of the pigmented lesion—when and how. *J Am Acad Dermatol.* 2008;59(5):852–871.
6. Ferrandiz L, Moreno-Ramirez D, Camacho FM. Shave excision of common acquired melanocytic nevi: cosmetic outcome, recurrences, and complications. *Dermatol Surg.* 2005;31:1112–1115.
7. Russell EB, Carrington PR, Smoller BR. Basal cell carcinoma: a comparison of shave biopsy versus punch biopsy techniques in subtype diagnosis. *J Am Acad Dermatol.* 1999;41:69–71.

10 The Punch Biopsy

RICHARD P. USATINE, MD

The punch biopsy is an easy method for removing a round full-thickness skin specimen. It is often used to diagnose skin lesions of uncertain etiology. The main advantage of the punch biopsy over the shave technique is that it yields deeper tissue with preserved architecture for pathologic evaluation. It is also easier to perform on flat lesions for clinicians who have not mastered the art of the shave biopsy for lesions that are not elevated.

Flat lesions that are amenable to punch biopsy include inflammatory skin conditions such as drug eruptions, dermatoses, psoriasis, and cutaneous lupus (Figure 10-1). Infiltrative skin conditions such as sarcoidosis and granuloma annulare also can be diagnosed with a punch biopsy (Figure 10-2). In addition, a punch biopsy may be used to diagnose all types of skin cancers including melanoma and cutaneous lymphomas (Figure 10-3).

A punch biopsy is one option in the diagnosis of melanoma if the entire lesion is large, making it too difficult to remove the whole lesion at the time of biopsy. In this case, the diagnostic yield will generally be best if a biopsy is performed on the darkest, most elevated, and/or most suspicious areas (Figure 10-4). Using a dermatoscope may help identify a suspicious area for the punch biopsy (see Chapter 32, *Dermoscopy*). If the suspicion for melanoma is high, excising the entire lesion is preferred, when possible, to improve the diagnostic yield. There are also times when a broad scoop shave may provide better tissue for the pathologist. The highest risk of using a punch biopsy to diagnose a melanoma is the risk of a false-negative result. If the lesion remains suspicious for melanoma and a punch biopsy was performed with a negative result, the remainder of the lesion should be excised for histology (see Chapter 8, *Choosing the Biopsy Type*).

INDICATIONS

Punch biopsy can be used to diagnose any skin condition or disease. The following are amenable to punch biopsy for diagnosis:

- Bullous diseases (Figure 10-5)
- Cicatricial alopecias (Figure 10-6)
- Inflammatory skin disease such as dermatoses, psoriasis, and vasculitis
- Infiltrative diseases such as cutaneous sarcoidosis and granuloma annulare
- Melanoma and cutaneous lymphomas (including nail melanoma)
- Oral lesions such as lichen planus (Figure 10-7)
- Vulvar diseases including vulvar intraepithelial neoplasia (VIN) (Figure 10-8).

The following types of conditions may be diagnosed with a shave biopsy, but a punch biopsy can be an acceptable alternative:

- All types of nonmelanoma skin cancers and precancers (Figure 10-9)
- All benign skin neoplasms.

Punch biopsy can be used to remove any small skin lesion. The following lesions are often removed using this technique:

- Small nevi
- Small dermatofibromas.

A punch instrument can be used to create an opening in an epidermal inclusion cyst for a minimally invasive cyst removal. Some clinicians use a punch incision to remove small lipomas (see Chapter 12, *Cysts and Lipomas*).

RELATIVE CONTRAINDICATIONS AND CAUTIONS

Punch biopsy is a more invasive biopsy technique than needed for most BCCs or SCCs, which can be diagnosed by shave biopsy. In one study there was no significant difference in the accuracy rate for histologic classification of BCCs with both the shave and the punch biopsy.[1] Punch biopsies generally bleed more than shave biopsies and the risk of infection is somewhat higher than for a shave biopsy.

A punch biopsy does have certain risks that are greater than those of a shave biopsy, including the possibility of cutting larger blood vessels and nerves. Therefore, clinicians must be familiar with the underlying anatomy. Fortunately, most major nerves and blood vessels are deeper than a punch instrument, but digital nerves and the temporal branch of the facial nerve are more superficial and care needs to be taken in these areas (Figure 11-2 of Chapter 11). Punch biopsies over the digits or the eyelid margins are generally to be avoided. When possible, it is also prudent to avoid doing a punch biopsy over superficial arteries such as digital or temporal arteries. Caution should also be exercised over areas where there is little soft tissue between the skin and the bone (over the tibia, digits, and ulna) because the punch can cut through the underlying bone.

ADVANTAGES OF A PUNCH BIOPSY

The advantages of a punch biopsy for the clinician include the following:

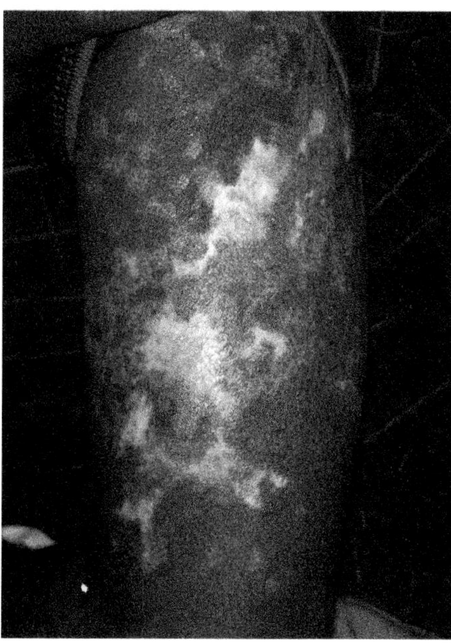

FIGURE 10-1 Cutaneous lupus (discoid lupus) with hypopigmentation and skin atrophy. The best method for diagnosis is a 4-mm punch biopsy. *(Copyright Richard P. Usatine, MD.)*

- A punch can be performed rapidly (faster than a freehand ellipse).
- It is relatively easy to learn.
- Sutures are not needed for smaller punch biopsies.
- Strict sterile procedure is not required if sutures are not to be placed.

The following advantages of a punch biopsy benefit the patient:

- Wound care is usually simple.
- Activities are not usually restricted during wound healing.
- The risks of infection and bleeding are reduced when the punch is small.

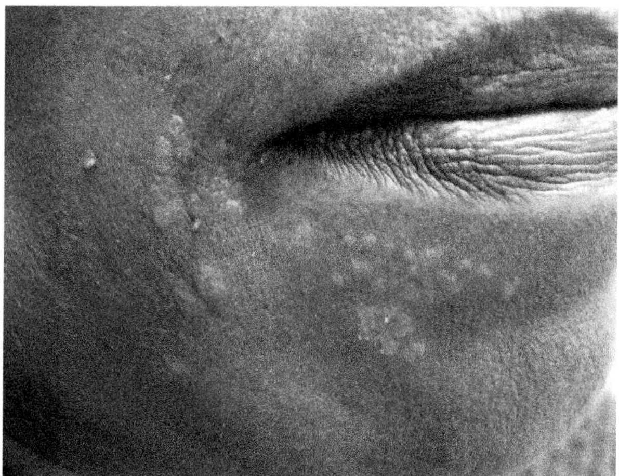

FIGURE 10-2 Cutaneous sarcoidosis on the face of a black woman. Although this is likely to be sarcoidosis by its appearance, a 4-mm punch biopsy was used to confirm the diagnosis. *(Copyright Richard P. Usatine, MD.)*

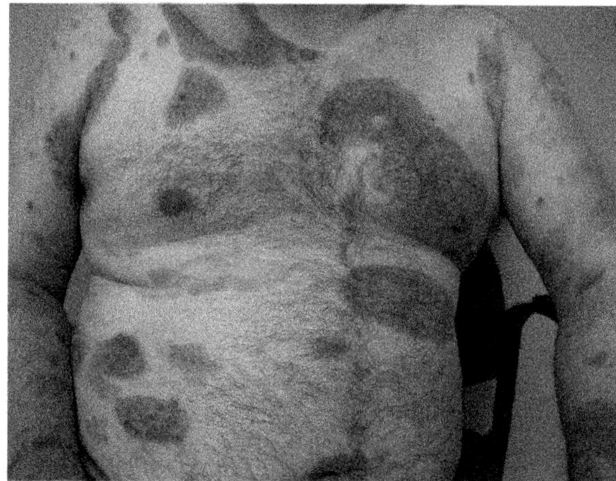

FIGURE 10-3 Mycosis fungoides. A previous biopsy years before was read as atopic dermatitis. When the skin disease did not respond to topical steroids and subsequently worsened, a new 4-mm punch biopsy detected cutaneous T-cell lymphoma. *(Courtesy of Debra Henderson, MD.)*

DISADVANTAGES OF A PUNCH BIOPSY

The disadvantages of a punch biopsy for the clinician include the following:

- Punch biopsies bleed more than shave biopsies so that it may take more time to achieve hemostasis.
- When sutures are placed, the procedure is a sterile one, requiring greater time and equipment costs than a shave biopsy.
- The clinician must schedule time for suture removal at a return visit.

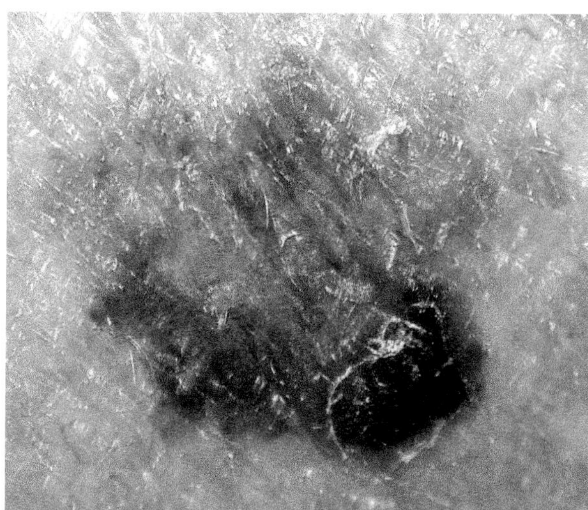

FIGURE 10-4 A lesion suspicious for melanoma on the arm. It was too large to be fully excised easily, so a punch biopsy was performed of the darkest most raised area and the lesion was determined to be a superficial spreading melanoma with a 0.25-mm depth. The full melanoma was excised with 1-cm margins and the depth was unchanged when the full lesion was evaluated histologically. *(Courtesy of Eric Kraus, MD.)*

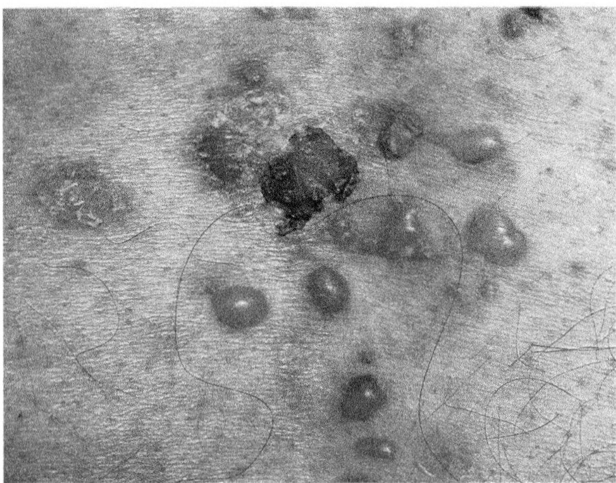

FIGURE 10-5 Bullous pemphigoid on the back of a 57-year-old man with many intact bullae. A 4-mm punch biopsy was performed on the edge of an intact bulla and the diagnosis was confirmed. *(Copyright Richard P. Usatine, MD.)*

- Punch biopsies of a melanoma may miss the malignancy if the sampling turns out to be a nonmelanoma part of the lesion.

For the patient, the disadvantages of a punch biopsy include the following:

- Scarring with a cross-hatch from a suture can occur.
- Dog ears that bulge above the surface of the skin might result.
- A second surgery may be needed if the whole lesion was not fully excised.

MAKING A DIAGNOSIS

It helps to have a good idea of the differential diagnosis before choosing the biopsy type and location. For most punch biopsies, a clinician should choose a punch size

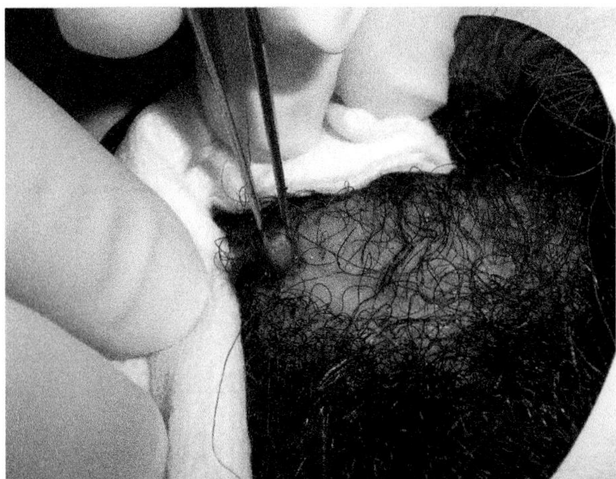

FIGURE 10-6 A 4-mm punch biopsy of the scalp is performed in this young woman with scarring alopecia. Subcutaneous fat is visible at the base of the biopsy. The patient was determined to have lichen planopilaris. *(Copyright Richard P. Usatine, MD.)*

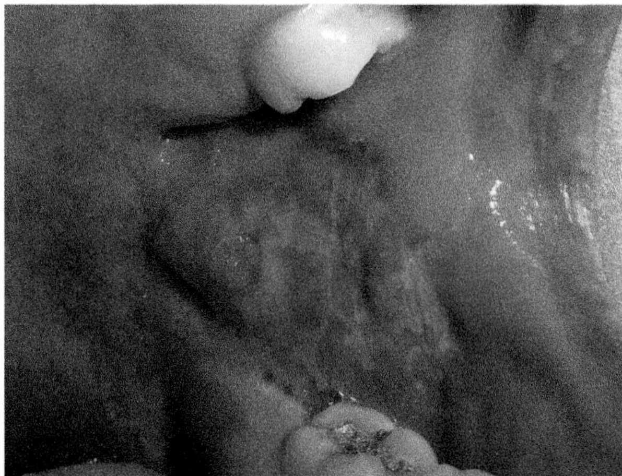

FIGURE 10-7 Lichen planus with a lacy white pattern on the buccal mucosa. The presence of Wickham's striae bilaterally in the mouth makes lichen planus likely. To establish a diagnosis histologically, a 4-mm punch biopsy of the buccal mucosa can be performed. Hemostasis can be achieved with aluminum chloride or electrocoagulation. A suture is rarely needed and is generally more uncomfortable for the patient. *(Copyright Richard P. Usatine, MD.)*

that will result in excision of the whole lesion or will provide a sample of the portion of the lesion that appears to have the worst pathology. However, for bullous disorders such as pemphigus or pemphigoid, it is best to punch the edge of the bulla to include the

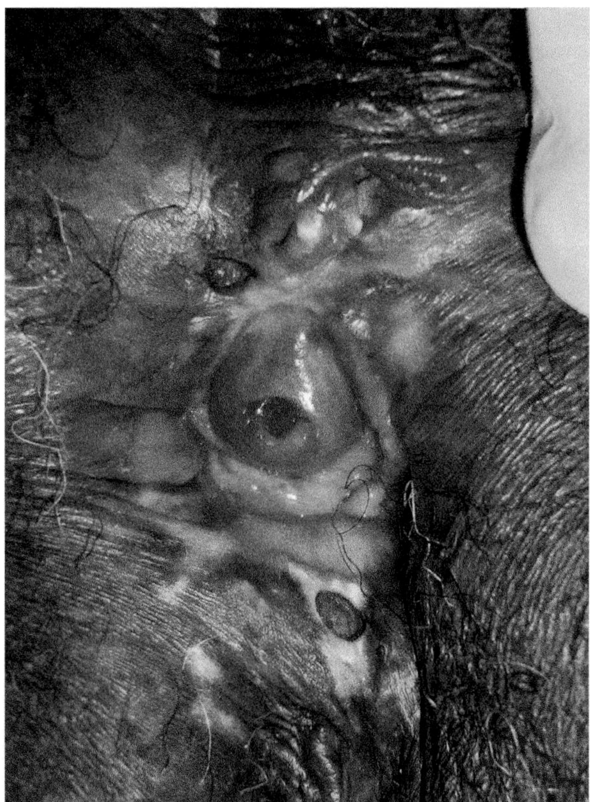

FIGURE 10-8 A 59-year-old woman with a long history of condyloma acuminata has suspicious areas of leukoplakia of the vulva. This photograph shows the vulva after two punch biopsies were performed. Both areas were found to have vulvar intraepithelial neoplasia 2 (VIN 2). *(Copyright Richard P. Usatine, MD.)*

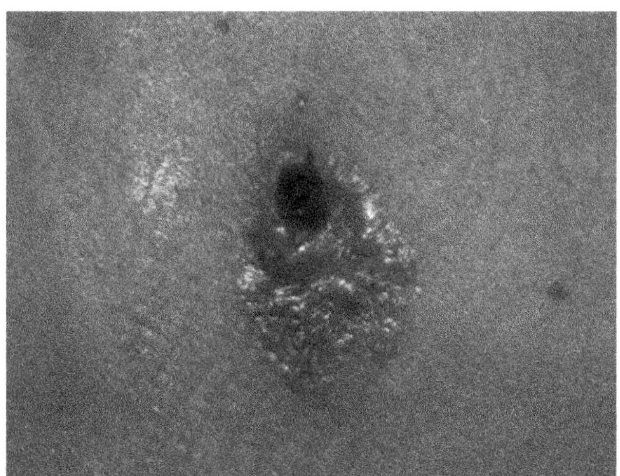

FIGURE 10-9 Nodular BCC on the back. A punch biopsy was used to establish the diagnosis. However, a shave biopsy would have been adequate and less invasive. *(Copyright Richard P. Usatine, MD.)*

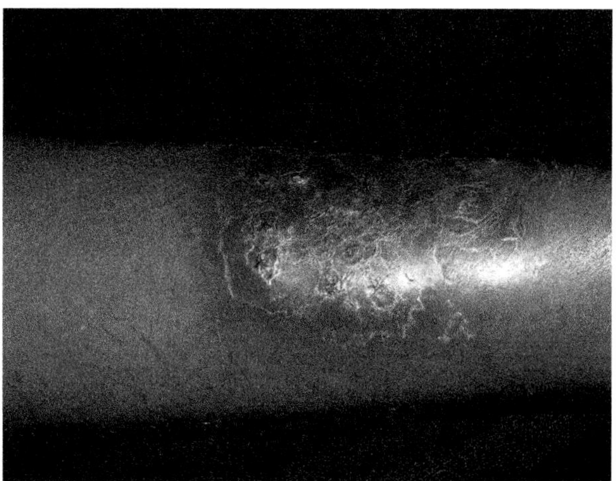

FIGURE 10-11 Pyoderma gangrenosum on the leg, with diagnosis confirmed by punch biopsy of an active edge. *(Copyright Richard P. Usatine, MD.)*

perilesional skin (Figure 10-10). A scoop shave under an intact bulla or at the border of a bulla may yield an equally good specimen. The goal is to keep the epidermis attached to the dermis at the edge of the bulla.

When performing a biopsy on an ulcerative lesion of unknown origin, it is helpful to remove tissue from the edge of the ulcer rather than the center portion. For example, if pyoderma gangrenosum is suspected, the biopsy should include the edge of the lesion, with some perilesional skin (Figure 10-11).

Additionally, before starting the biopsy the clinician should also have in mind whether the specimen will be sent for standard formalin-fixed hematoxylin and eosin (H&E) stain, direct immunofluorescence (DIF), or culture. For example, to diagnose bullous disorders, the specimen may be sent for both H&E and DIF. The biopsy for immunofluorescence is performed on perilesional skin not including the lesion itself. Suspected conditions for which a biopsy may be needed for DIF include the following:

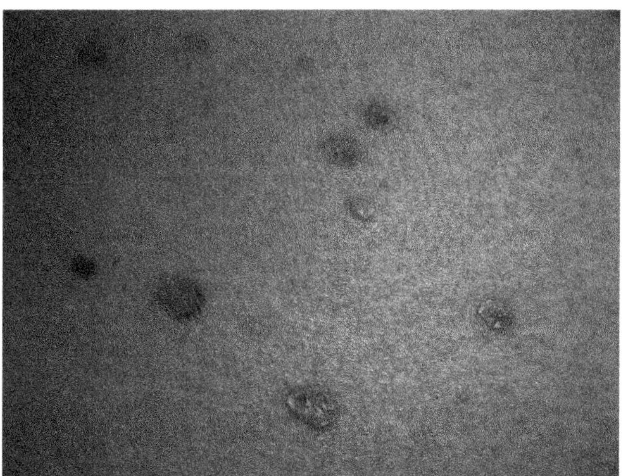

FIGURE 10-10 Bullous lichen planus on the back. A punch biopsy should include a whole intact bulla or the edge of a bulla. *(Copyright Richard P. Usatine, MD.)*

- Discoid lupus erythematosus and SLE (Figure 10-1)
- Pemphigus (Figure 10-12)
- Bullous pemphigoid (Figure 10-5)
- Lichen planus (Figure 10-13)
- Cicatricial alopecia (Figure 10-6)
- Epidermolysis bullosa acquisita (Figure 10-14).

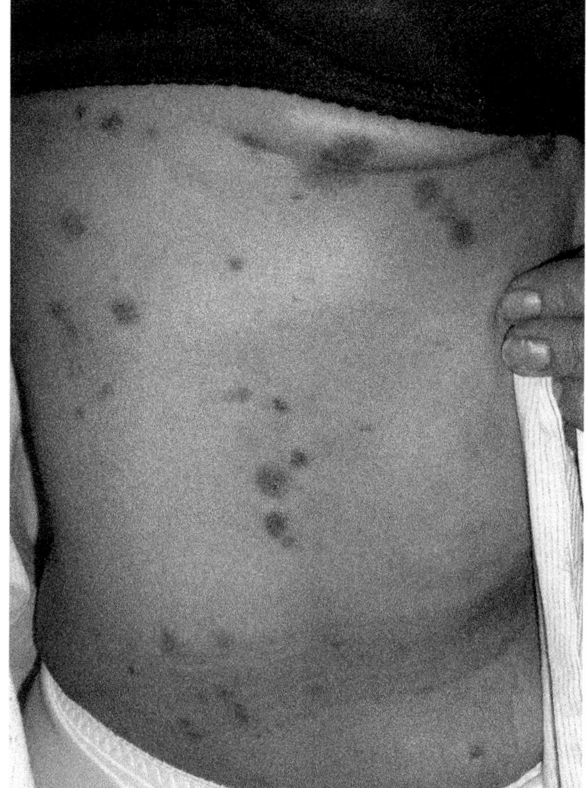

FIGURE 10-12 Pemphigus foliaceous on the trunk. A 4-mm punch biopsy was performed on the edge of a bulla. If direct immunofluorescence is needed, a second 4-mm punch biopsy should be performed on perilesional skin of a relatively fresh lesion. *(Copyright Richard P. Usatine, MD.)*

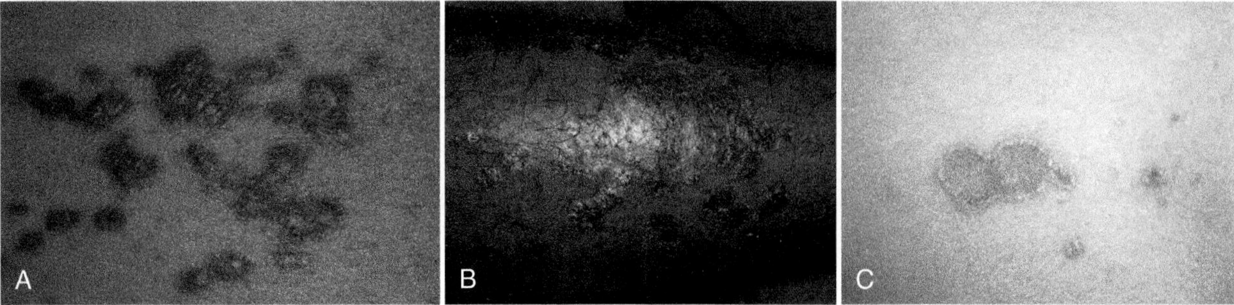

FIGURE 10-13 Three variations of lichen planus (LP): (A) LP on the back of a black woman. (B) Hypertrophic LP on the leg. (C) Annular LP on the breast. All three diagnoses were made with 4-mm punch biopsies sent for standard pathology. *(Copyright Richard P. Usatine, MD.)*

Some of these conditions may be diagnosed with standard histology only and the biopsy for DIF may be a second step only if needed. DIF requires Michel's media for transport and should not be put into standard formalin. Unfortunately, this medium needs refrigeration and has a short shelf-life so keeping it around the office is inconvenient. If two specimens are being sent simultaneously for DIF and standard pathology, two punch biopsies should be performed remembering that the DIF specimen is taken from perilesional skin.

If a fungal infection is suspected, periodic acid Schiff (PAS) stains are useful and can be done from the specimen in the formalin. If a culture is desired for a deep fungal infection such as sporotrichosis, the specimen can be sent on a sterile saline-soaked sterile gauze pad in a sterile urine container (Figure 10-15). This technique also works for suspected atypical mycobacterial infections (Figure 10-16).

EQUIPMENT

The following equipment is used to perform a punch biopsy (Figure 10-17):

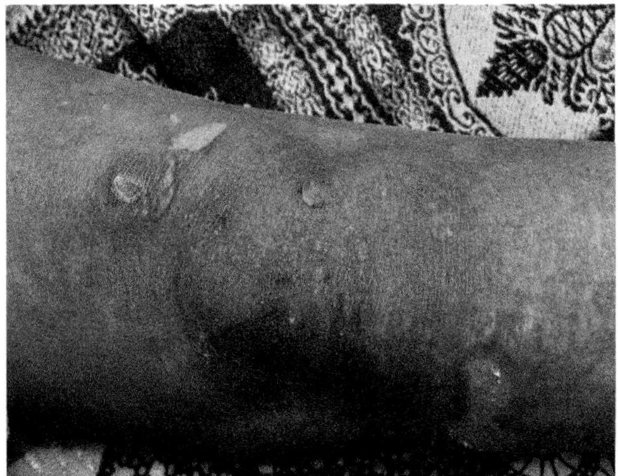

FIGURE 10-14 Epidermolysis bullosa acquisita seen with blisters and erosions on the leg. Because there are many disorders that can do this, a 4-mm punch biopsy of a blister or the edge of a blister should be performed for a definitive diagnosis. Additional information can be obtained with a second 4-mm punch biopsy for direct immunofluorescence on perilesional skin. *(Copyright Richard P. Usatine, MD.)*

- Punches (also called trephines) (2 to 10 mm are available; 3 to 6 mm are preferred)
- Iris scissors (curved or straight)
- Adson forceps without teeth for lifting the specimen gently
- Needle holder and sutures or hemostatic solution
- Adson forceps with teeth for suturing (optional).

Punches come in various sizes ranging from 2 to 10 mm and are available as reusable steel punches and disposable punches (Figure 10-18). Disposable punches have the advantage of being presterilized and there is no concern about them losing their sharp edge. Reusable punches are more expensive, require sterilization between procedures, and must be maintained by proper, skilled sharpening. We use disposable punches for quality and convenience.

The Huot VisiPunch has the wonderful advantage of allowing the clinician to see through the punch instrument while performing the procedure. This allows one to place the punch on the skin and make sure the whole lesion is within the punch before starting the cut. Also, one can see the depth better and have a better idea of when the punch core releases from the dermis below. (Fusiform punches are available and are described in Chapter 11, *The Elliptical Excision*).

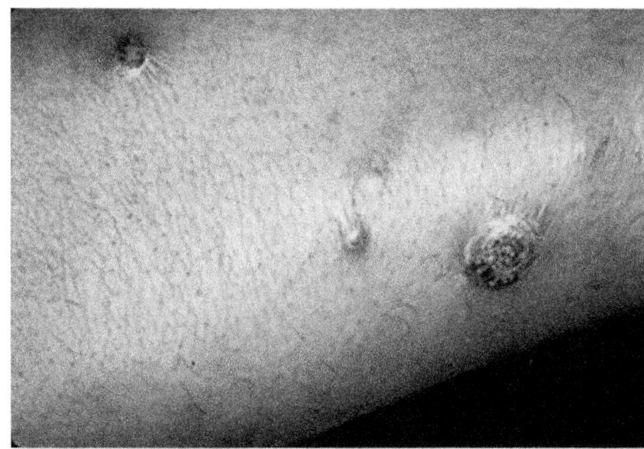

FIGURE 10-15 Disseminated sporotrichosis. A 4-mm punch biopsy was sent for standard histology and a second 4-mm punch was sent on sterile saline for fungal culture. *(Courtesy of Eric Kraus, MD.)*

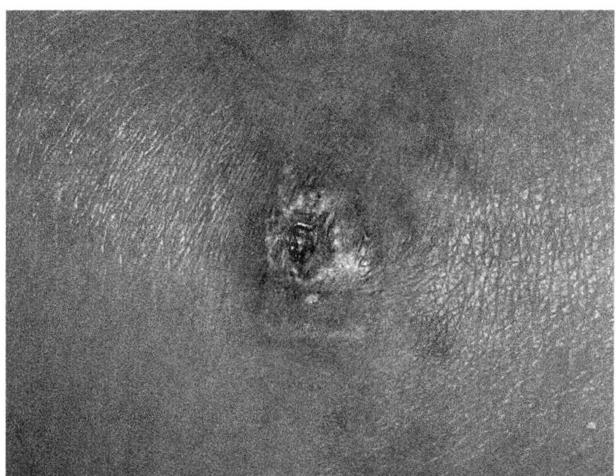

FIGURE 10-16 Mycobacterium abscessus infection on the leg diagnosed with a 4-mm punch biopsy sent for AFB stain and culture. *(Copyright Richard P. Usatine, MD.)*

CHOOSING THE PUNCH SIZE

A 4-mm punch is usually adequate to obtain sufficient tissue for pathology. When the lesion is smaller than 6 mm, the punch size can be determined by the diameter required to completely excise the tissue. Punch biopsies done with 10-mm punches may produce standing cones ("dog ears") when closure is attempted (see Chapter 12). If the lesion requires a punch of larger than 6 mm, it is best to do an elliptical excision (see Chapter 11). Punch biopsies between 3 and 6 mm should obtain adequate tissue and be easy to close with a good cosmetic result. A minimum of a 4-mm punch is generally preferred by the dermatopathologist to provide adequate tissue for diagnosis.

CHOOSING WHETHER TO SUTURE THE PUNCH DEFECT

- Punch defects 2 or 3 mm in size can be left to heal by secondary intention.

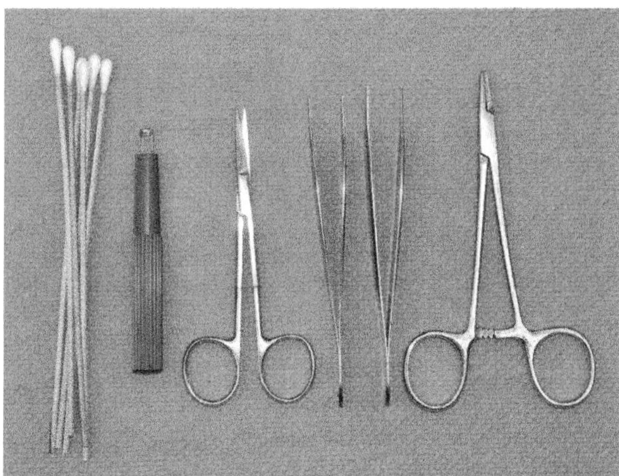

FIGURE 10-17 Punch biopsy instrument set. The needle holder and extra Adson forceps with teeth are useful when the punch defect is sutured. *(Copyright Richard P. Usatine, MD.)*

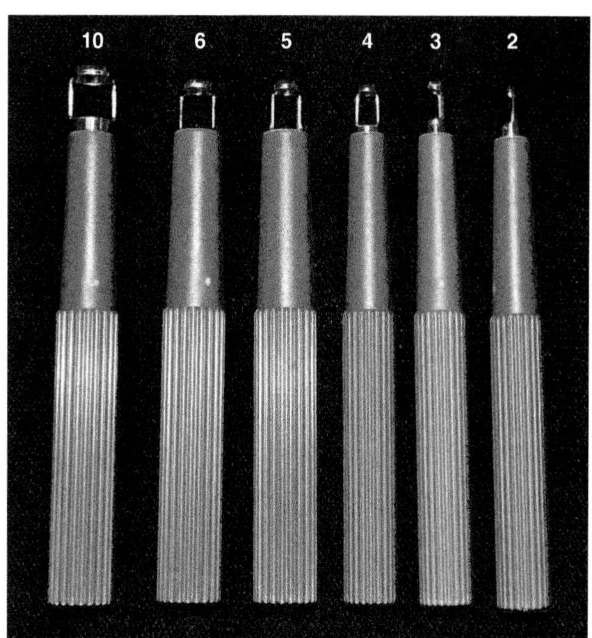

FIGURE 10-18 Punch biopsy instruments with visible window to improve the procedure (VisiPunch). Huot instruments makes these sharp and effective tools from 2 to 10 mm in diameter. *(Copyright Richard P. Usatine, MD.)*

- Punch defects of 4 mm in one study healed as well by secondary intention compared with suturing with one interrupted 4-0 nylon suture.[2] Blinded observers saw relatively little difference in the 4-mm punch results at 9 months. Note that no electrosurgery, aluminum chloride, or other hemostatic agents were applied to the biopsy sites, only Gelfoam was used for hemostasis in the nonsutured wounds. All wounds were dressed with petrolatum under gauze covered by an occlusive transparent dressing (Tegaderm). Dressings were left in place for 3 days, after which the Gelfoam was removed from the second-intention site and both biopsy sites were cleansed with water to remove any exudate. Tegaderm was reapplied at that visit and then weekly by the patient until the biopsy sites were completely healed or reepithelialized. Although these results are encouraging for the choice to leave 4-mm or less punch defects open to heal naturally, the use of Gelfoam and Tegaderm, both expensive materials, is not representative of standard punch aftercare. Also, this study required an additional visit 3 days postop. Also at 2 weeks, pain was reported more commonly for the site treated by second-intention healing and the pain lasted longer for the second-intention sites than for the primary closure sites.[2] Not surprisingly, unblinded patients preferred suture closer of the 8-mm punch biopsy sites.[2] With this data, I personally inform the patient of the risks and benefits of suturing and make a joint decision keeping many factors in mind.
- If a biopsy is being performed on an inflammatory lesion in which there may be a secondary bacterial infectious component, it is better not to suture the

wound, but rather to allow it to heal by secondary intention. Although the worsening or creation of an infection in a punch biopsy is extremely rare, it is even more rare to see an infection if the site has been left open.

PUNCH BIOPSY: STEPS AND PRINCIPLES

Critical steps in a punch biopsy procedure include the following:

- Using 1% lidocaine with epinephrine for anesthesia and hemostasis.
- Cutting the punch biopsy down to the correct depth (into subcutaneous fat)
- Not crushing the tissue while handling the specimen.
- Stopping the bleeding adequately
- Avoiding dog ears in the final repair.

Preoperative Measures

- Determine the size punch needed and consider the pros and cons for suturing the defect if the punch size is 4 mm or less.
- Discuss with the patient the biopsy options and pros and cons for suturing the defect if the punch size is 4 mm or less. Obtain informed consent in writing. (See Appendix A for a sample informed consent form titled *Disclosure and Consent: Medical and Surgical Procedures.*)
- If sutures are to be used, choose the type of suture and set up the sterile supplies and equipment for the procedure.
- If the punch site will become less visible after anesthesia is applied, it helps to mark the area to be punched with a surgical marker. It need not be a sterile marker if the skin is prepped after marking. If the punch will be taken from a large involved area, the marking helps to make sure that the anesthesia and cut are in the same area.
- Lightly prep the area with alcohol or another antiseptic.
- Inject local anesthesia. Use a 27- or 30-gauge needle with 1% lidocaine and epinephrine (buffer the lidocaine for less pain; see Chapter 3). Start with the needle under the lesion (greater depth is less painful) and then give the last amount of anesthesia closer to the skin surface. It is important to infiltrate the skin surface and the dermis to the full depth of the planned punch (Figure 10-19B). Wait 10 minutes for maximum vasoconstriction and hemostasis. This is a good time to complete your pathology consult.

CUTTING THE PUNCH BIOPSY

See video on the DVD for further learning. 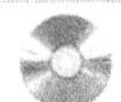

- Prep the area with iodine (Betadine) or chlorhexidine (Hibiclens).
- If sutures are to be placed, clean your hands and apply sterile gloves and use a sterile fenestrated drape.
- Avoiding dog ears can be done by stretching the skin perpendicular to skin lines before and during the punch (Figure 10-19D). This tension should be maintained throughout the punch procedure until the dermis is fully breached. This stretching perpendicular to relaxed skin tension lines will allow the resultant wound, circular under tension, to revert to an oval or fusiform shape when the retention is relaxed. The oval defect will be aligned with the relaxed skin tension line to facilitate closure and optimize cosmesis. This is more important with punch biopsies over 5 mm in diameter.
- In Figure 10-19A, a pigmented lesion is being biopsied with a 4-mm punch. The punch is held above the area and is brought down over the specimen so that the specimen is centered under the punch (Figure 10-19C).
- The punch is then held between the thumb and forefinger of the dominant hand.
- With downward pressure, the punch instrument is rapidly rotated back and forth between the fingers until it penetrates completely through the dermis. Feel for a sensation of getting through a firm substance and moving into the less firm subcutaneous (SQ) fat. Pull up the punch and look for signs that the depth is correct. The punch specimen often raises above the surrounding tissue when the tissue has been cut to the fat layer (the dermis holds it in place if the depth is not correct). The bleeding is often increased when the cut reaches the SQ fat, and if you pull up on the specimen you may see the yellow fat color below. If the cut was not deep enough, reinsert the punch and continue cutting until the depth is correct.
- The punch instrument is then removed, and the specimen remains in the center of the site. Rarely the specimen may shear off and pull away with the punch. If this happens, it can be removed from the punch with a needle. One advantage of the Visi-Punch is that the punch specimen never gets stuck in the metal tube of a sealed punch.
- If the specimen is not elevated, apply downward compression of the area around the specimen for elevation. The specimen can then be further elevated gently with a forceps (being careful not to crush the specimen) (Figure 10-19E) and cut from its base with a sharp iris scissor (Figure 10-19F). Variations on this method include putting a skin hook or small needle into one side of the specimen and elevating it.
- It is important to remember that every effort needs to be made to handle the specimen lightly and to resist the tendency to compress or crush the specimen with the teeth of the forceps. Crushed samples may result in distortion of nuclei or cell architecture.[3]
- Be prepared to handle bleeding that may drip down the skin by placing a gauze under the punch

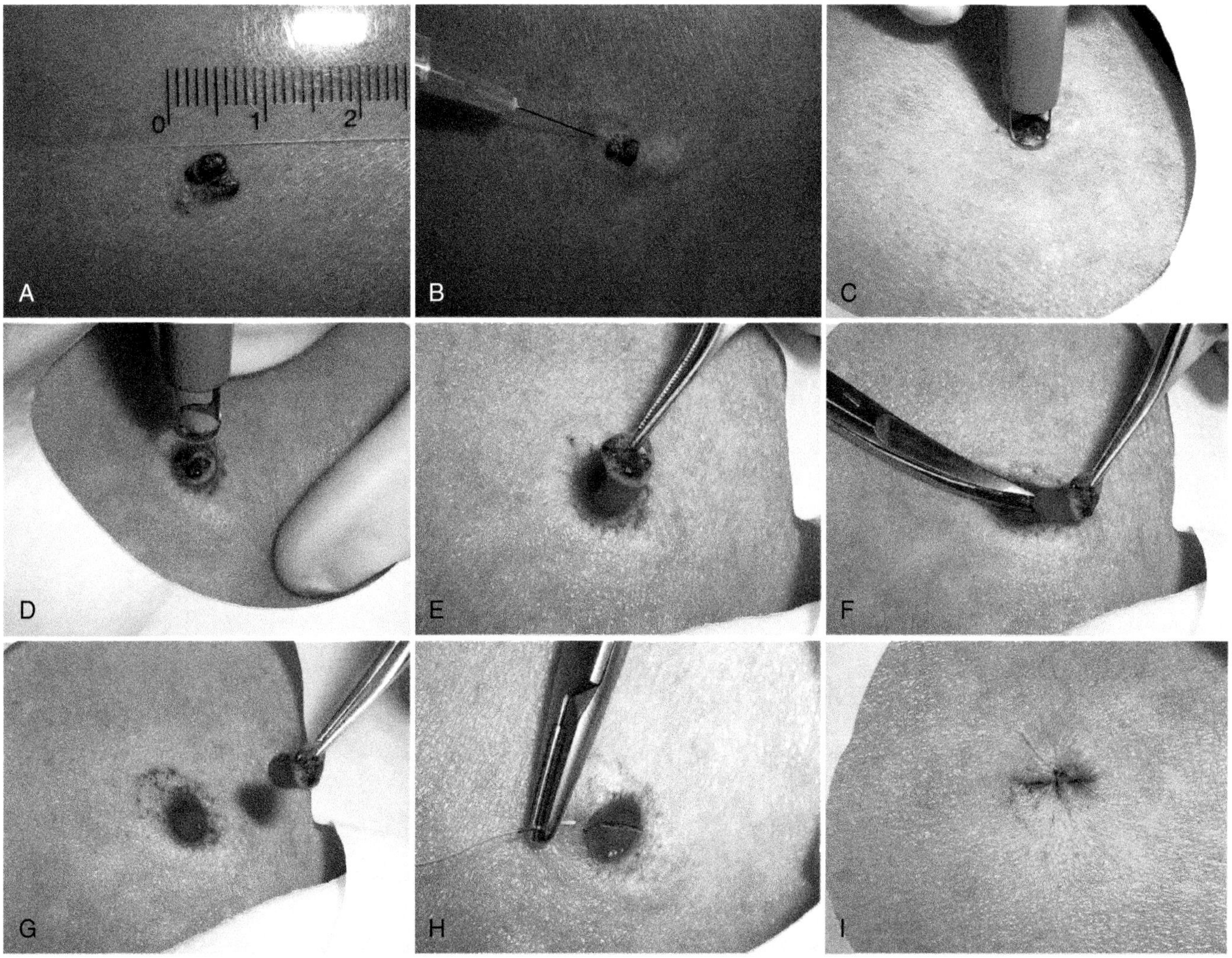

FIGURE 10-19 Punch Sequence (A) A 62-year-old woman presented with a dark spot on her back for 6 months. (B) Local anesthesia with 1% lidocaine and epinephrine was injected using a 30-gauge needle. The anesthesia is injected more deeply at first and then more superficially to make sure the punch biopsy site is completely anesthetized. (C) After sterilely prepping and draping the site, a 4-mm VisiPunch is placed on top of the lesion to make sure that it will provide an adequate biopsy. The lesion can be seen within the punch. (D) The skin is stretched perpendicular to skin lines and the punch biopsy instrument is twirled clockwise and counterclockwise until the blade cuts down to the subcutaneous fat. Once the fat layer is reached, the punch is lifted. (E) The biopsy specimen is gently lifted so that it may be snipped off with a curved sharp iris scissor. Any sharp, pointed small tissue scissor would also work. (F) The specimen is pulled to the side to make room for the scissor to snip the base. (G) The punch specimen is removed. (H) The punch defect is sewed. The tip of the needle is viewed in the hole before the stitch is completed. (I) One interrupted suture is sufficient for closure of this punch biopsy. *(Copyright Richard P. Usatine, MD.)*

See video on the DVD for further learning. 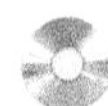

site in the direction that gravity will take the blood from the punch site.

Stretching the Skin to Prevent Standing Cones

Stretching the skin to prevent standing cones ("dog ears") is especially important when doing a punch larger than 5 mm or performing a punch on the face or other cosmetically important area. Figure 10-20 shows how stretching the skin perpendicular to skin lines will allow for a better cosmetic outcome.

Hemostasis and Repair

- If no sutures are to be placed, hemostasis can be achieved with aluminum chloride on a cotton-tipped applicator (CTA). If this does not work, electrocoagulation is another option. If the aluminum chloride solution is aqueous, there are no concerns about using electrocoagulation immediately as needed. Electrocoagulation also will cause the defect to shrink in size.
- If electrocoagulation is not working, hold pressure on the wound and consider placing a suture.

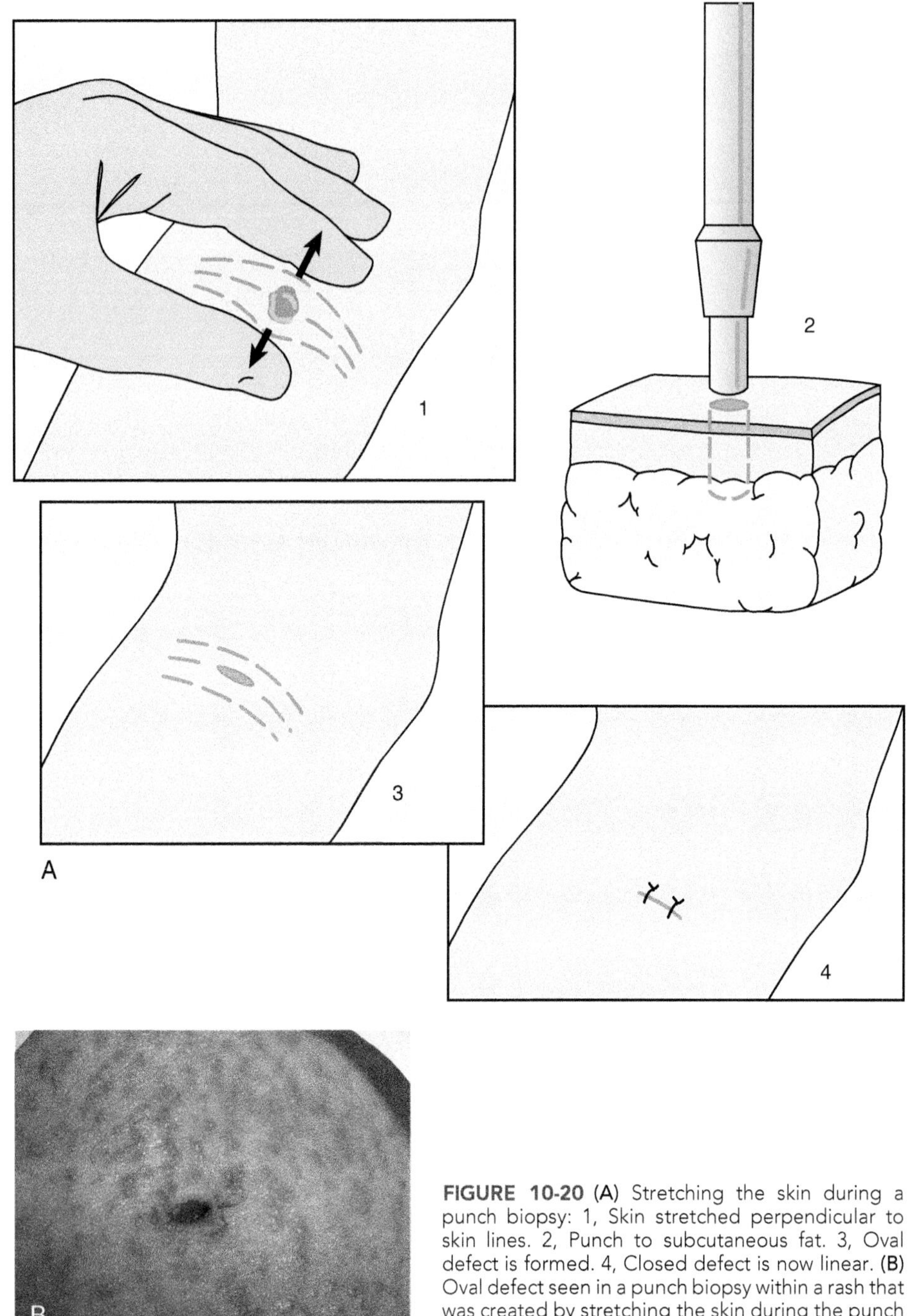

FIGURE 10-20 **(A)** Stretching the skin during a punch biopsy: 1, Skin stretched perpendicular to skin lines. 2, Punch to subcutaneous fat. 3, Oval defect is formed. 4, Closed defect is now linear. **(B)** Oval defect seen in a punch biopsy within a rash that was created by stretching the skin during the punch procedure. *(Copyright Richard P. Usatine, MD.)*

- *Preventing dog ears before suturing:* If the defect is round because the initial stretching perpendicular to skin lines was not employed and dog ears seem to be likely, try gently undermining the defect with blunt dissection using the iris scissor. This often will allow the defect to elongate along skin lines. Another option has been described using two skin hooks. The skin hooks are placed on opposite ends of the wound following skin lines and the circular defect is stretched for 1 minute. This method was found to prevent dog ears in one study.[4]
- Many choices for suturing a punch biopsy are available. Nylon suture is a good and inexpensive material to use. Usually 4-0 or 5-0 nylon is adequate. Money can be saved by purchasing sutures with a short 9-inch monofilament meant to close punch biopsies.
- Vicryl (polyglactin 910) was compared with nylon for closure of punch biopsy sites in one study.[5] Each 3-mm punch site was closed with one simple suture. The sites were evaluated at 2 weeks and 6 months for redness, infection, dehiscence, scar hypertrophy,

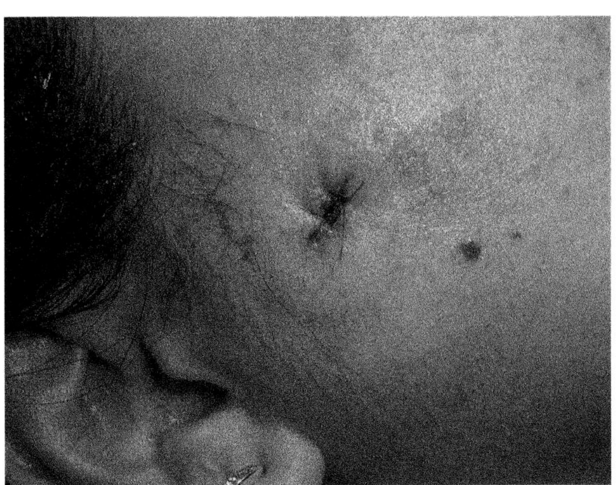

FIGURE 10-21 Punch biopsy defect closed with two interrupted 5-0 Prolene sutures after a 4-mm punch was used to excise a pyogenic granuloma on the face. *(Copyright Richard P. Usatine, MD.)*

and patient satisfaction. The authors found no statistically significant difference between the two suture materials in any of the above parameters.[5]

- Fast-absorbing gut can be used for closure if the area is not under tension and it is difficult for the patient to return for suture removal.
- One to two interrupted sutures is adequate for a 3- or 4-mm punch and two to four sutures may be needed for 5- or 6-mm punch biopsies (Figures 10-21 and 10-22).

Dressing and Aftercare

- Cover the final wound with clean petrolatum and a sterile adhesive bandage.
- If the bleeding is hard to stop or if the area is very vascular, consider applying a small pressure bandage to avoid postop bleeding.
- Explain aftercare to the patient and/or family members. We usually suggest patients keep the area dry for 24 hours then they may bath normally. See Appendix A for a patient information handout titled *Care of Your Skin after a Punch Biopsy*.
- Sutures are generally left in place for 5 to 7 days on the face and 7 to 14 days elsewhere on the body. See Chapter 35 for further details of postoperative wound care.

SUGGESTION FOR LEARNING THE PUNCH BIOPSY TECHNIQUE

When learning punch biopsy technique, it may be helpful to practice on an orange, banana, or pig's foot. The twirling motion to cut a core biopsy can be practiced on just about any fruit or meat, but the stretching of the skin against skin lines is very hard to simulate.

Less than Optimal Outcomes

Complications that may arise from a punch biopsy include the following:

- Producing a divot or indentation that persists
- Cutting a vital nerve or artery (rare)
- Erythema that may last for months and often resolves
- Slow healing for a punch on the lower leg or one that is left open
- Hypopigmentation or hyperpigmentation that can be permanent
- Infection (Figure 10-23)
- Hypertrophic or keloidal scarring may rarely occur, particularly with patients predisposed to their occurrence
- Regrowth of an incompletely excised lesion (less common than with a shave biopsy).
- Standing cones or dog ears that do not flatten

Serious complications are extremely infrequent with punch biopsy.

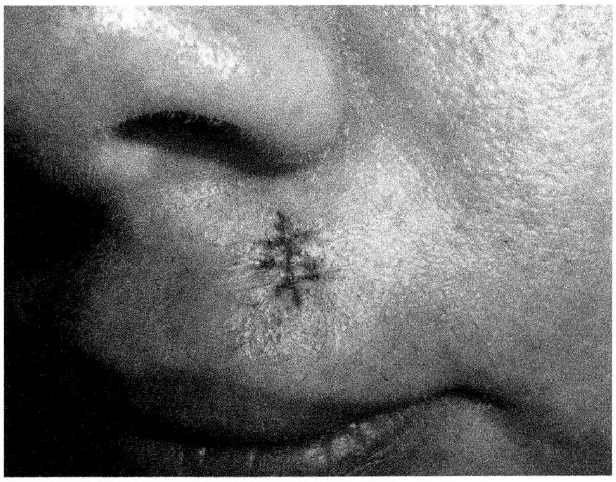

FIGURE 10-22 Punch biopsy was closed with 5-0 Prolene on the face of a young woman in which a changing pigmented lesion was excised with a 5-mm punch. To obtain a good cosmetic closure, three interrupted sutures were placed. *(Copyright Richard P. Usatine, MD.)*

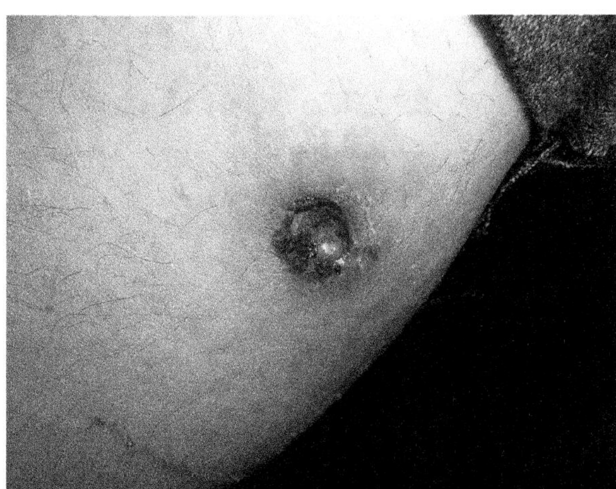

FIGURE 10-23 An infected punch biopsy 1 week after a 6-mm punch was performed with no closure. Unfortunately, silver nitrate was used for hemostasis and this large lesion was left open to heal. Most clinicians would close a punch biopsy of this size and avoid silver nitrate. *(Copyright Richard P. Usatine, MD.)*

Patients should be informed that a punch biopsy obtained on mobile areas such as the back, which is stretched each time we bend or breathe, or the arms, which are stretched each time the muscles are flexed or pumped, may well result in some stretching of the wound. The ultimate scar, while frequently flat and flesh colored, may become the size of the area that was removed via punch technique and not be a simple linear scar.

SPECIFIC EXAMPLES FOR PUNCH BIOPSIES

Erythroderma

It is important to establish the cause of erythroderma (Figure 10-24) quickly so that specific therapy can be initiated. A 4-mm punch biopsy is a good start. Call the pathologist to ask for a rush order because erythroderma can be a life-threatening condition.

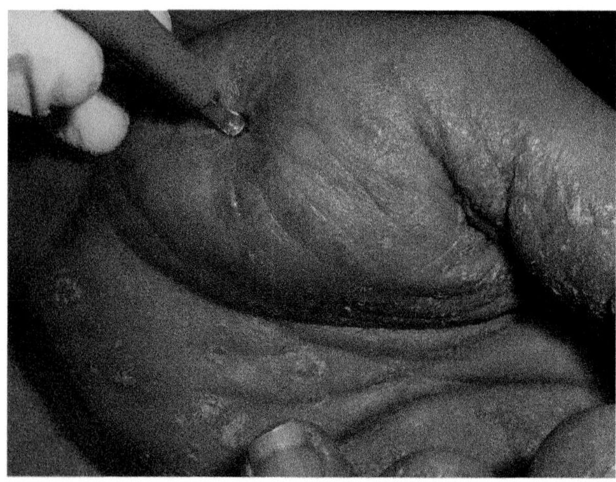

FIGURE 10-25 Hyperkeratotic plaques with scale on the hands and feet. A 3-mm punch biopsy of the hand confirms the diagnosis of palmar plantar psoriasis. *(Copyright Richard P. Usatine, MD.)*

Palmoplantar Psoriasis

The diagnosis of psoriasis can be made based on the clinical presentation in most cases by using clues such as the distribution, appearance, and chronicity of the lesions. A punch biopsy can be used to confirm the diagnosis in an atypical presentation when there is uncertainty. Sometimes it is difficult to determine whether hyperkeratosis on the palms and soles is from psoriasis or other conditions such as dyshidrotic eczema or dermatophytosis. A punch biopsy can help direct therapy (Figure 10-25). It is especially helpful to confirm a diagnosis of palmoplantar psoriasis because these patients often need potent systemic therapy with agents that are known to have serious potential risks. Perform the punch over an area of the hand that is affected but has soft tissue below it. A shave biopsy is another option.

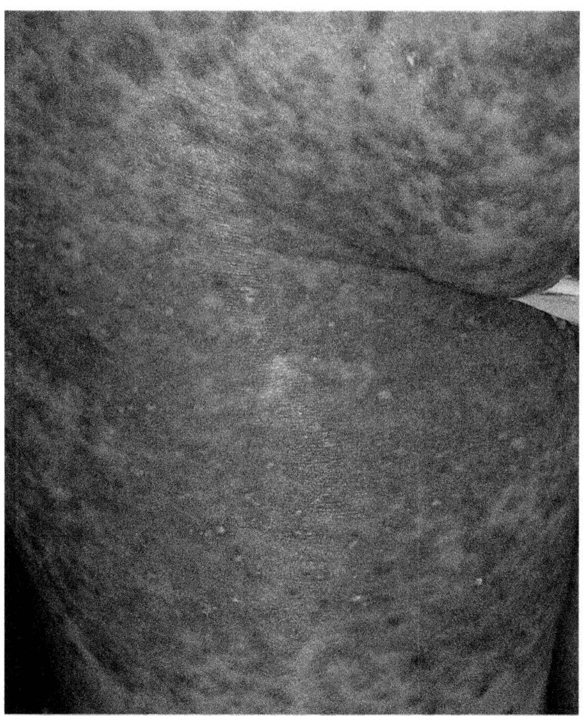

FIGURE 10-24 A patient with erythroderma and small pustules visible on the posterior thigh. While pustular psoriasis was suspected, a 4-mm punch biopsy was performed of this area and sent to pathology with a rush order. The patient was hospitalized and the following day the diagnosis of pustular psoriasis was confirmed. Intensive treatment allowed the patient to leave the hospital improved in a few days. *(Copyright Richard P. Usatine, MD.)*

Morphea

Flat atrophic shiny or wrinkled patches on the skin can be morphea (localized scleroderma) or lichen sclerosis. It is difficult to tell just by looking so a punch biopsy is very helpful. Figure 10-26A shows a 4-mm punch site from morphea on the abdomen of a young woman. In Figure 10-26B, morphea is seen on the breast of a 30-year-old woman. Diagnosis was confirmed with a 4-mm punch.

Trichotillomania versus Other Types of Alopecia

The cause of hair loss is not always obvious by history and physical exam. In Figure 10-27, a 37-year-old woman was concerned about an area of alopecia on her scalp. She admitted that her scalp was pruritic and that she was under much stress. Trichotillomania was suspected due to the story and broken hairs, but the patient did not initially admit to pulling her hairs. A 4-mm punch biopsy confirmed the suspected diagnosis. Note that the biopsy site was not closed and hemostasis was obtained with electrocoagulation. When the histology supported trichotillomania, the patient took responsibility for her behavior and was able to stop the hair pulling and excoriations.

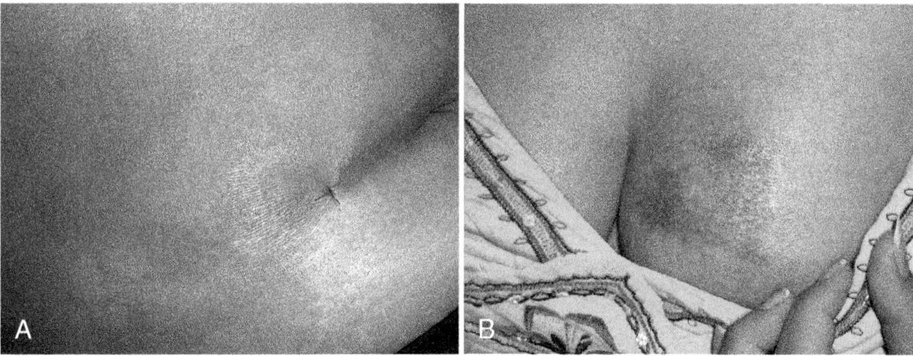

FIGURE 10-26 **(A)** Morphea or localized scleroderma on the abdomen of a young woman. Diagnosis confirmed with a 4-mm punch. **(B)** Morphea on the breast of a 30-year-old woman. *(Copyright Richard P. Usatine, MD.)*

PEMPHIGUS

A man presented with blisters on his arms. A 4-mm punch biopsy of the edge of a bulla led to the diagnosis of pemphigus vulgaris (Figure 10-28). A second 4-mm punch biopsy of perilesional skin was also sent for direct immunofluorescence in Michel's media. The result confirmed the diagnosis.

CODING AND BILLING PEARLS

The punch procedure is either used as a form of biopsy and billed under the biopsy codes or used to fully excise a lesion and then billed under excision codes. Occasionally it can be confusing sometimes to decide whether the punch procedure is a "biopsy" or "excision." Clear-cut examples of punch biopsies include sampling a possible skin cancer or removing a piece of skin to determine the cause of an unknown rash. Excision codes are used for those punch procedures that are used to remove a small benign nevus or another small benign lesion. The intent is to excise the whole lesion, and even though it is recommended to send all pigmented lesions for confirmatory pathologic diagnosis, the primary reason for the procedure was not a "biopsy" but a removal of the lesion itself. Malignant excision codes are generally not used with the punch procedure because punch instruments are small and not likely to provide for adequate margins around skin cancers for the definitive procedure.

Make sure that all documentation is consistent with the procedure that is billed. If the punch is done as a biopsy, call it a punch biopsy, but if the punch is done as an excision, call it a punch excision or just an excision.

Punch biopsy CPT codes and fees are summarized in Table 38-7 of Chapter 38, *Surviving Financially*. Note that, although these codes cover punch biopsies they also cover biopsies done by shave or curette. The codes are based on location only and not on the size of the biopsy or lesion. The codes are also independent of whether the lesion turns out to be benign or malignant, so there is no need to wait for the pathology result to submit the bill. The codes are also independent of whether or not a suture was placed to close the punch.

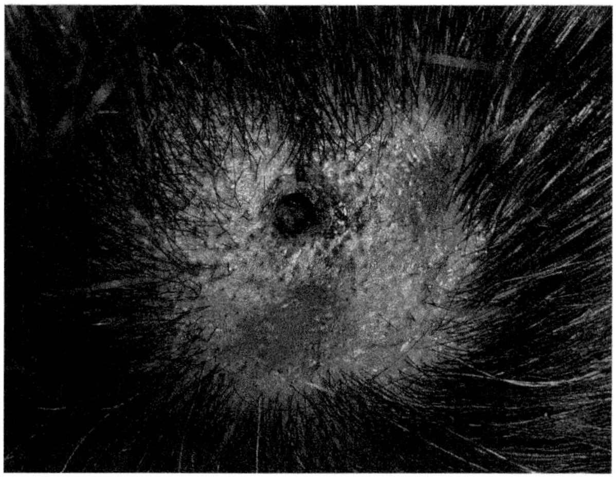

FIGURE 10-27 A 37-year-old woman with an area of alopecia on her scalp. She admitted that her scalp was pruritic and that she was under much stress. Trichotillomania was suspected due to the story and broken hairs, but the patient did not initially admit to pulling her hair. A 4-mm punch biopsy confirmed the suspected diagnosis. Note that the biopsy site was not closed and hemostasis was obtained with electrocoagulation. *(Copyright Richard P. Usatine, MD.)*

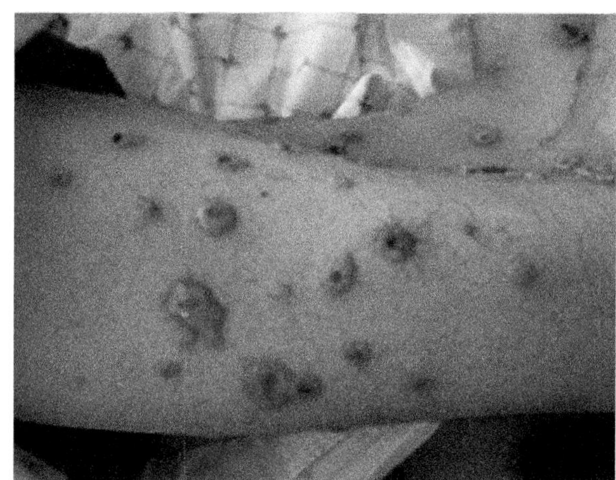

FIGURE 10-28 A man presented with blisters on his arms. A 4-mm punch biopsy of the edge of a bulla led to the diagnosis of pemphigus vulgaris. *(Courtesy of Jennifer Welsh, MD.)*

CPT codes and fees for punch excisions are the same as for small benign excisions and are provided in Table 11-2 of Chapter 11. These codes are based on size and location so it is crucial to measure the lesion before excising it. If the lesion is cutaneous and will be fully removed, then the punch size is the lesion size for billing. If the lesion is subcutaneous, such as a lipoma or deep cyst, then the lesion size is the actual measured size before surgery and not the punch size. Do not estimate the size later because estimates are usually rounded to the nearest centimeter and the reimbursement goes up 0.1 cm above each rounded number (e.g., payment is greater for an excision of a 1.1-cm lesion than a 1.0-cm lesion). The codes are also independent of whether or not a suture was placed to close the punch, but in many cases one or more sutures will be used because punch excisions tend to be larger than biopsies only.

CONCLUSION

The punch is a relatively easy and convenient procedure for getting a full-thickness biopsy. It is much easier to perform than an elliptical excision, but neither as easy nor as fast as the shave biopsy. It is preferentially used when a shave biopsy is too superficial, and a small 3- to 6-mm biopsy will provide adequate tissue sampling. Although the punch biopsy is a critical skill to master, a clinician should not be performing more punch biopsies than shave biopsies (see Chapter 9, *The Shave Biopsy*).

Resources

Delasco biopsy sutures (800-831-6273; www.delasco.com).

Huot Instruments, manufacturer of the VisiPunch (www.huotinstruments.com).

References

1. Russell EB, Carrington PR, Smoller BR. Basal cell carcinoma: a comparison of shave biopsy versus punch biopsy techniques in subtype diagnosis 4. *J Am Acad Dermatol.* 1999;41:69–71.
2. Christenson LJ, Phillips PK, Weaver AL, Otley CC. Primary closure vs second-intention treatment of skin punch biopsy sites: a randomized trial. *Arch Dermatol.* 2005;141:1093–1099.
3. Tran KT, Wright NA, Cockerell CJ. Biopsy of the pigmented lesion—when and how. *J Am Acad Dermatol.* 2008;59(5):852–871.
4. Lo SJ, Khoo C. Improving the cosmetic acceptability of punch biopsies: a simple method to reduce dog-ear formation. *Plast Reconstr Surg.* 2006;118:295–296.
5. Gabel EA, Jimenez GP, Eaglstein WH, *et al.* Performance comparison of nylon and an absorbable suture material (polyglactin 910) in the closure of punch biopsy sites. *Dermatol Surg.* 2000;26:750–752.

11 The Elliptical Excision

DANIEL L. STULBERG, MD • NIKKI KATTALANOS, PAC •
RICHARD P. USATINE, MD

An elliptical (also called fusiform) excision is a straightforward, effective way to remove lesions with lateral and deep surgical margins. The shapc of the excision lends itself well to a linear repair that can be aligned for a cosmetically pleasing result.

INDICATIONS

- Removal of suspicious lesions to obtain pathology and completely resect the lesion
- Removal of diagnosed malignant lesions for treatment
- Removal of benign lesions for cosmesis or comfort (e.g., nevi, dermatofibromas)
- Re-excision of melanoma to recommended surgical margins.

CONTRAINDICATIONS

Contraindications by lesion include the following:

- Aggressive malignant lesions with margins that are not clinically apparent should be considered for Mohs surgery (see Chapter 37, *When to Refer/Mohs Surgery*).[1] The Mohs surgeon carefully cuts and marks each specimen to be prepared for viewing under the microscope at the time of surgery. This ensures the clearest margins obtainable with the most tissue-sparing surgery.
- Recurrent basal or squamous cell cancers should be referred for Mohs surgery, because Mohs surgery has the lowest statistical rate of recurrence with excisions.[2–4]
- Other factors to consider when deciding about a referral for Mohs surgery include lesion size, histology, location, cost, patient age, immunosuppression, history of transplant, availability of a Mohs surgeon and patient preferences. (For more details, see Chapter 37.)

Contraindications by lesion include the following:

- In areas where there is not an adequate amount of tissue for closure, consider an alternate technique (flap, graft, electrodesiccation, cryosurgery, and topical treatments).
- For lesions involving the eyelids or in which the excision would put tension on the lid, refer to Mohs surgery, plastic surgery, oculoplastics, or another appropriate specialist.
- Cancers at the margin of the nose and ears and lips tend to have deeper involvement and should be considered for Mohs surgery.[1,5]
- Cancers in the H-zone on the face should also be considered for Mohs surgery (see Figure 37-12 in Chapter 37).

EQUIPMENT

The following equipment is required to perform an elliptical incision (also see Figure 11-1), although excision of small ellipses may not require all of the items on the list:

- Surgical marking pen
- 1% lidocaine with epinephrine
- Syringes, 5 to 12 mL
- Needles, 27- to 30-gauge 1¼ to 1½ inch for injection
- Sterile gloves
- Electrosurgical instrument for hemostasis (optional to have one for cutting)
- No. 15 scalpel or No. 15c and blade handle
- Adson forceps (with and without teeth)
- Iris scissors (optional to have another scissor for undermining)
- Webster needle holder (consider gold-handled holder with carbide inserts)
- 2 mosquito hemostats
- 2 skin hooks (single, sharp prong)
- Cotton-tipped applicators (CTAs) and gauze
- Designated suture scissors (optional)
- Small sterile metal basin (optional, used for cleaning and irrigating with sterile saline)
- Skin preparation solution (chlorhexidine or povidone-iodine)
- Sterile drapes and a single fenestrated drape
- Suture materials (see Chapter 5, *Suture Material*)
- Specimen container with formalin and label
- Dressings: 2 × 2 gauze, 4 × 4 gauze, adhesive tape (optional nonadherent strips, wound closure strips, dental roll for pressure dressings).

Adding clean cotton gauze and CTAs (purchased in bulk) to be autoclaved in surgical sets is an efficient way to prepare for surgery. This will save time and money over individually packaged sterile gauze and CTAs and avoid wasting the paper used in the wrapping process, hence making for a greener office.

Disposable instrument setups (Figure 11-1B) may be the only option in practices that do not do regular

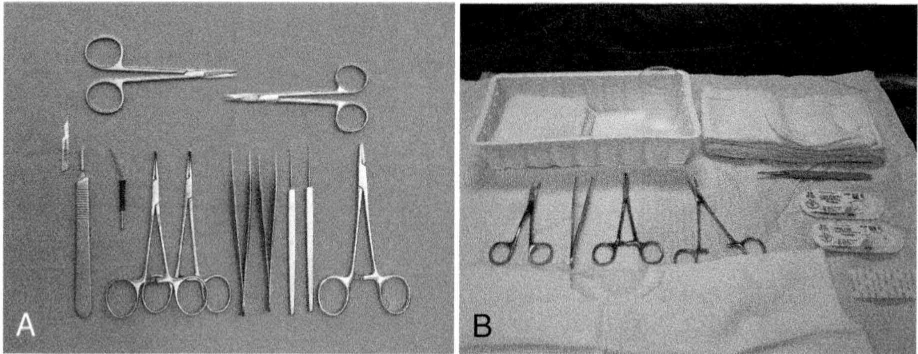

FIGURE 11-1 (**A**) Instruments for an elliptical excision from left to right: two iris scissors on top, No. 15 scalpel blade, scalpel handle, electrosurgery electrode, two mosquito hemostats, two Adson forceps, two skin hooks, needle holder. (**B**) Disposable surgical kit with sutures and adhesive strips added. *(A: Copyright Richard P. Usatine, MD; B: Copyright Daniel Stulberg, MD.)*

surgeries and don't have an autoclave. Note that disposable instruments are of lower quality than nondisposables.

THE ELLIPTICAL INCISION: STEPS AND PRINCIPLES

The major steps involved in the elliptical excision involve the following:

1. Planning and designing the excision
2. Anesthesia
3. Preparing the room, the patient, and the equipment
4. Incision
5. Hemostasis
6. Undermining
7. Wound closure (repair).

Perform a check of vital signs and be aware of coexisting medical issues such as anticoagulation before starting any surgical procedure. Obtain informed consent in writing at the time of the procedure and perform a surgical time-out before starting (see Chapter 1, *Preoperative Preparation*).

Planning and Designing the Excision

Important factors to consider when planning an excision are listed in Box 11-1.

BOX 11-1 *Factors to Consider When Planning an Excision*

Important factors to consider when planning an excision include the following:
- Avoiding vital structures
- Placement of incision lines
- Size of the surgical margin
- Whether the closure can be accomplished with a side-to-side closure
- Whether anatomic distortion will occur.

Avoiding Vital Structures

When planning an elliptical excision, it is crucial to plan how to best avoid damaging vital structures, including sensory organs, major nerves, arteries, bones, tendons, ligaments, cartilage, and internal organs. That is not to say that such damage can always be avoided because there are areas in which the risks are higher and the surgery still needs to be performed. Complications can include but are not limited to bleeding, paresthesias, paralysis, scarring, and loss of movement or expression. For example, a deep elliptical excision over the medial antecubital fossa may result in cutting the brachial artery. When possible, a shave technique can be used to perform a biopsy without the risk of cutting deep structures. Abnormal sensation at the immediate surgical site is expected and unavoidable due to damage to tiny sensory nerves. Damage to sensory nerves passing to other areas can cause more broad loss of sensation and paresthesias.

In planning the surgical excision, it is important to avoid cutting motor nerves. The temporal branch of the facial nerve is one example of a nerve at risk during facial surgery. For a superficial skin cancer in the temporal region, the clinician may choose to treat with a chemical agent or scoop shave rather than an ellipse. Referring for Mohs surgery is a good option because the temple is part of the H-zone and Mohs surgeons are very skilled surgeons.

Danger Zones

The three following areas are not the only areas at risk, but are worthy of special mention here because the motor nerves are superficial in these areas and damage to them can cause significant problems with form and function:

- *Lateral forehead.* The temporal branch of the facial nerve can be damaged by any surgery of the temple area. The nerve lies superficially within the fat layer; it can be difficult to see, and there is enough anatomic variation that its location can be unpredictable. The temporal branch emerges from the parotid gland, superiorly traveling in the subcutaneous fat to the frontalis muscle (Figure 11-2A). If the temporal

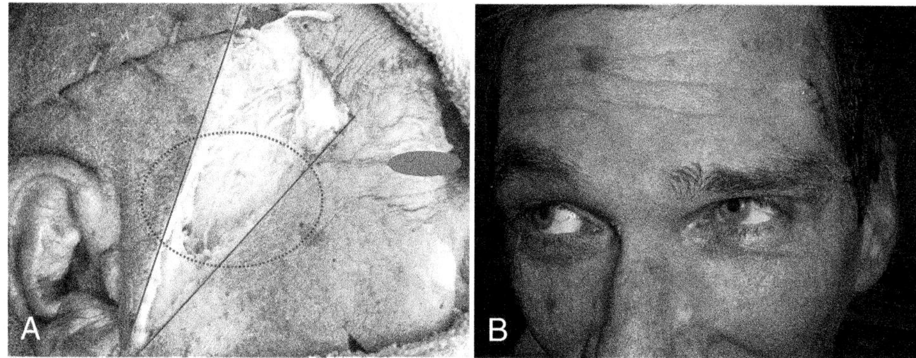

FIGURE 11-2 (A) The temporal branch of the facial nerve is superficial in the triangle formed by connecting the tragus to the lateral aspect of the eyebrow and the tragus to the most superior forehead crease. The temporal branch of the facial nerve is vulnerable to injury as it courses over the zygomatic arch within the zone. (B) This man is unable to raise his left eyebrow after receiving local anesthesia over the temporal branch of the facial nerve for the removal of a basal cell carcinoma. The effect on the nerve was temporary because the nerve was not cut. *(A: From Vidimos A, Ammirati C, Poblete-Lopez C.* Dermatologic Surgery. *London: Saunders; 2008; B: Copyright Richard P. Usatine, MD.)*

branch of the facial nerve is cut, the patient will have permanent drooping of the eyebrow and not be able to wrinkle the forehead on that side (Figure 11-2B). If any surgery is to be performed in this area, it is important for this risk to be discussed with the patient.[6] It also helps to check nerve function before administering anesthesia in this area because the anesthesia may cause a temporary facial nerve palsy.

- *Lateral midface.* The zygomatic branch of the facial nerve, the buccal branches, and the marginal mandibular branches emerge along the anterior portion of the parotid gland. The cervical branch emerges at the inferior aspect of the parotid gland (Figure 11-3).[6] Any of these nerves can be damaged with resultant areas of facial paralysis, so care should be used if entering the subcutaneous tissues anterior, superior or inferior to the parotid gland and posterior to a line dropped inferiorly from the lateral canthus of the eye.
- *Lateral neck.* The spinal accessory nerve traverses under the sternocleidomastoid muscle on its way to the trapezius muscle (Figure 11-4). Within the posterior triangle between those muscles, at the level of the thyroid cartilage, it can be superficial. If this

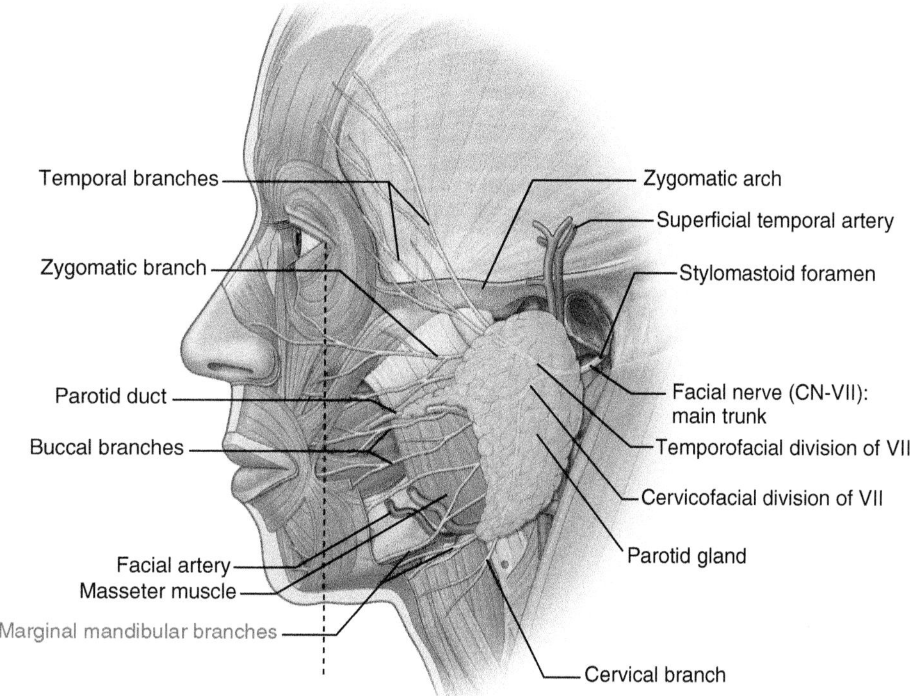

FIGURE 11-3 Five branches of the facial nerve exit the parotid gland (temporal, zygomatic, buccal, marginal mandibular, and cervical) and are less protected posterior to the line dropped from the lateral canthus. The marginal mandibular branch is vulnerable to surgical injury as it crosses the inferior edge of the mandible. *(Adapted from Vidimos A, Ammirati C, Poblete-Lopez C.* Dermatologic Surgery. *London: Saunders; 2008.)*

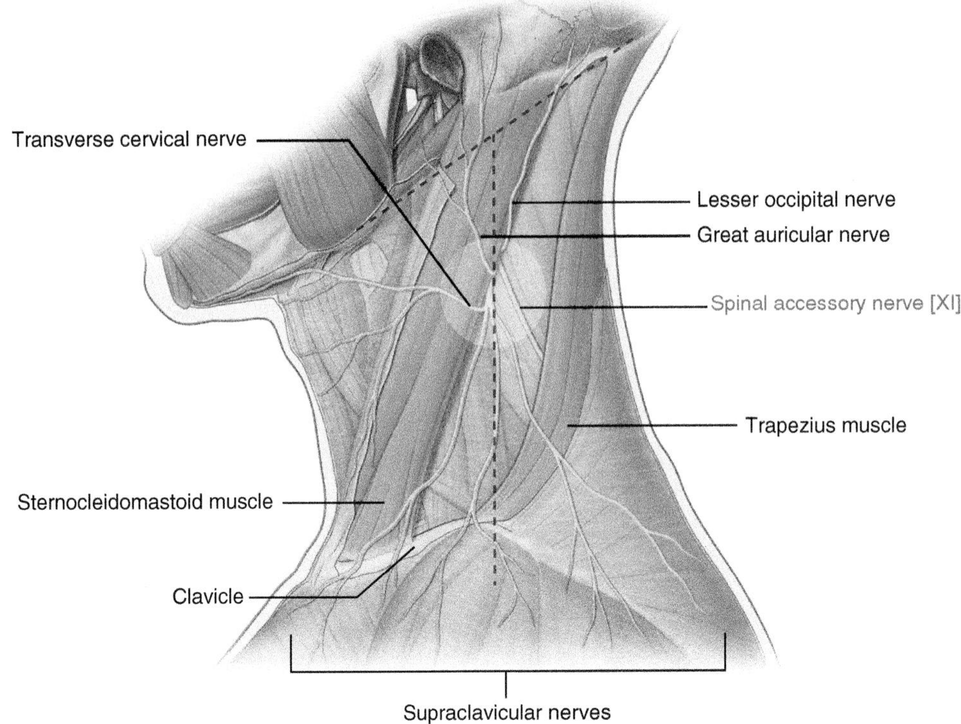

FIGURE 11-4 The spinal accessory nerve is vulnerable between the sternocleidomastoid and the trapezius at the level of the thyroid cartilage. *(From Vidimos A, Ammirati C, Poblete-Lopez C.* Dermatologic Surgery. *London: Saunders; 2008.)*

nerve is cut, the patient cannot raise the trapezius muscle. Fine hand–arm coordination can also be impaired.[6]

Placement of the Incision Line

Major factors to be considered when determining the placement of the incision line are wrinkle lines and relaxed skin tension lines (RSTLs). The design of an ellipse on the face is usually done within wrinkle lines. If wrinkles are not apparent, asking the patient to smile, lift the eyebrows or tightly close the eyes can bring out lines of facial expression (Figure 11-5A). That is because these lines run perpendicular to the muscles of facial expression (Figure 11-5B).

The RSTLs are the parallel skin lines that are seen when the skin is pinched together while the muscles are relaxed (Figure 11-5C). For example, when the skin is pinched together on the wrist, the RSTLs run horizontally from the lateral wrist to the medial wrist (Figure 11-6A). The RSTLs are used to plan the ellipse on the trunk, extremities, and on facial areas where wrinkle lines are not apparent (Figures 11-5 and 11-6).

If neither the wrinkle lines nor the RSTLs are obvious, use the circular excision method of line placement. In this method, the lesion is excised in a circular fashion, and the surgical defect is undermined in all directions. The line of closure is chosen by looking at the direction in which the circle becomes elongated. The sides that are closer together or that can be pushed together are most easily sutured. Alternatively, the sides can be pulled together with skin hooks to determine the best direction of closure. Then remove triangles from two opposite ends to orient the ellipse along the appropriate closure line.

Surgical Margin

The ellipse is designed so that the lesion is cleared with a margin. When possible, knowing the type of lesion in advance can guide the amount of tissue to be removed. The surgical margin may be 3 to 5 mm for basal cell carcinomas, 3 to 6 mm for squamous cell carcinomas, and 1 to 2 cm for diagnosed melanomas (Table 11-1).[1,2] When the suspicion for malignancy is low, a shave biopsy or an excision with smaller margins of 1 to 2 mm is usually adequate. For the initial excision of a suspected melanoma the margin should be 1 to 2 mm so as not to affect subsequent lymph node testing,[7] and additional tissue will be excised later based on depth of invasion seen on pathology. One option for some suspected melanomas is to do a scoop shave excision with 2-mm margins since a full excision may be premature before histology is obtained (see Chapter 8, *Choosing the Biopsy Type*). It is important to balance taking enough tissue to reduce the need for repeat procedures due to positive margins while minimizing impact to form and function.[8] In some cases it may be necessary to utilize Mohs surgery or take a smaller margin if the lesion is too close to vital structures.

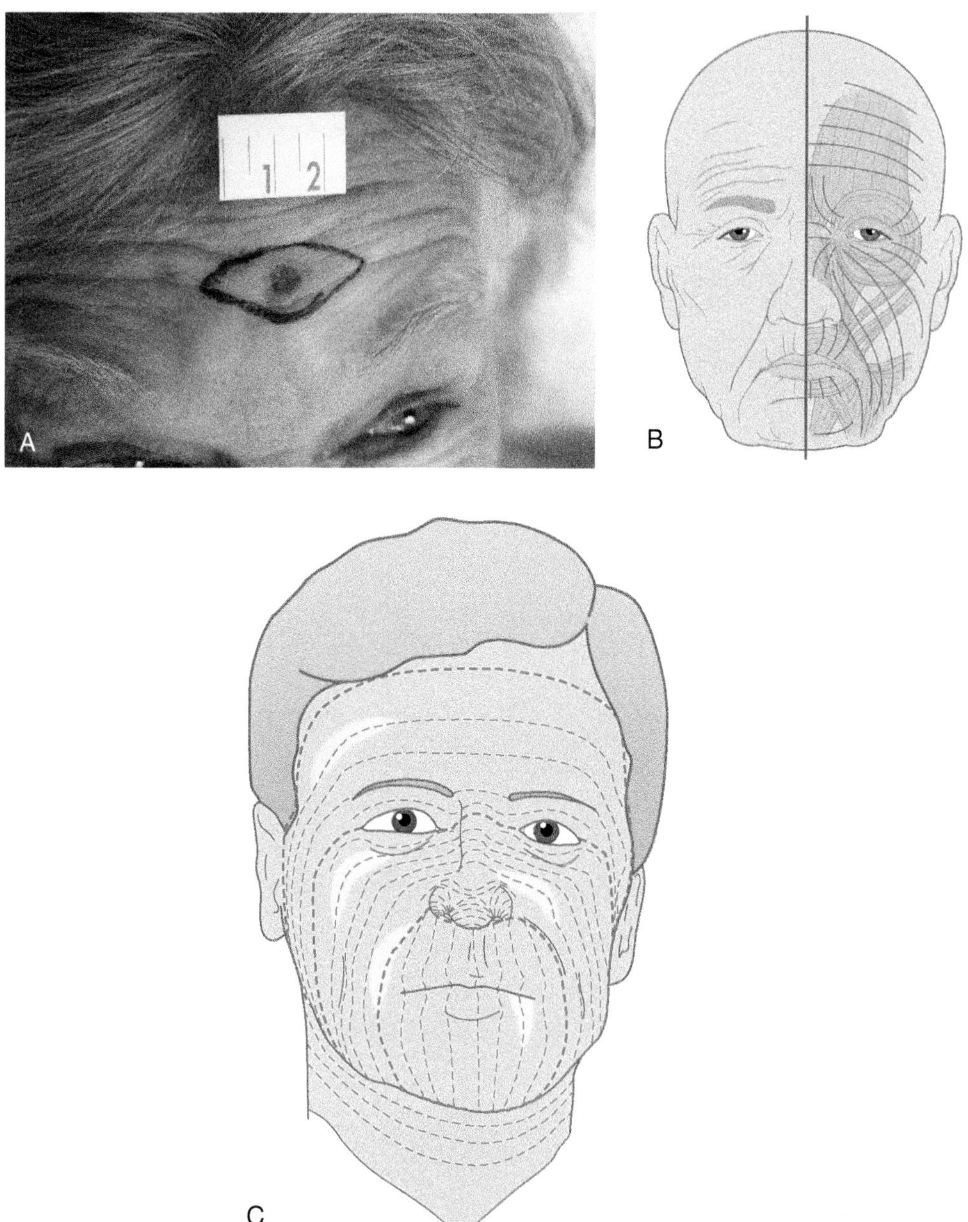

FIGURE 11-5 (A) By raising the eyebrows and wrinkling the forehead, the skin tension lines are accentuated. These lines were used to draw the ellipse around a biopsy-proven basal cell carcinoma. (B) Wrinkles, termed skin tension lines (STLs), run perpendicular to the underlying muscle fibers. For example, the STLs of the forehead are horizontal because the frontalis muscle contracts vertically. (C) The drawing shows relaxed STLs of the face. Examples of drawn optimal fusiform excisions (blue) run parallel to relaxed STLs. *(A: Courtesy of Daniel L. Stulberg, MD; B: From Vidimos A, Ammirati C, Poblete-Lopez C.* Dermatologic Surgery. *London: Saunders; 2008; C: Redrawn from Hom DB, Odland RM. Prognosis for facial scarring. In Harahap M, ed.* Surgical Techniques for Cutaneous Scar Revision. *New York: Marcel Dekker; 2000:25–37.)*

Ellipse Geometry

The ends of the ellipse should be approximately 30-degree angles so that potential dog ears (standing cones) are minimized (Figure 11-7). Standing cones consist of bulging skin at the ends of a sutured wound. Looser skin areas sometimes allow slightly larger angles at the end of the ellipse because the standing cones flatten slightly. Undermining the end of the ellipse also helps minimize these potential standing cones. A clinician should explain to patients before the surgery that the length of the incision needs to be about three times the diameter of the lesion. It is helpful to draw this for patients so they can see how large their incision will be.

It is very helpful to mark the biopsy margins with a surgical marking pen (Figure 11-8). To orient the ellipse properly, determine the wrinkle line or relaxed skin tension line that will define the axis of the ellipse. The area to be cut may be prepped with alcohol first. A clean and nonsterile surgical marking pen is acceptable if you prep the skin again after marking the lesion. The usual ellipse is drawn so that the length of the ellipse is at least three times the width of the ellipse (Figures 11-7 and 11-8). Conditions in which a greater than 3:1 ratio

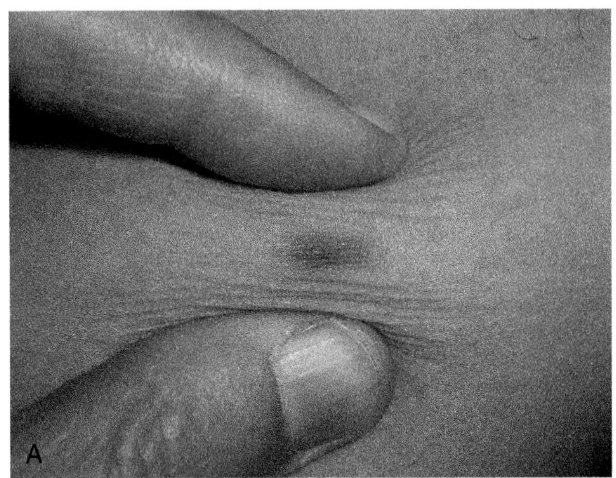

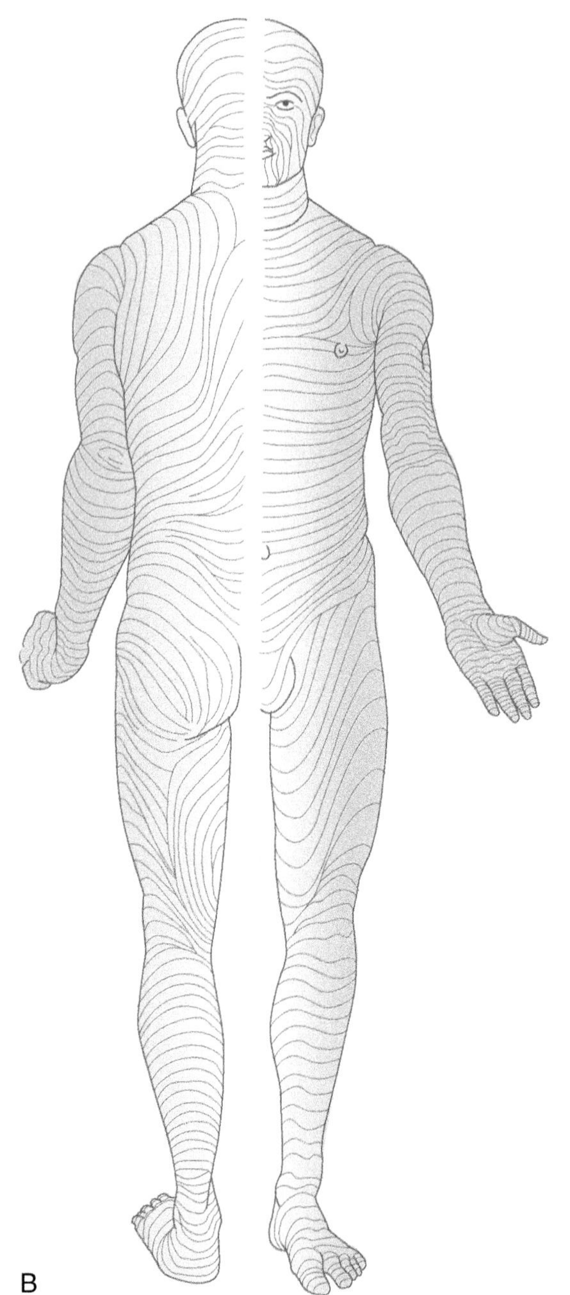

FIGURE 11-6 **(A)** Pinching the skin to determine the direction of RSTLs. **(B)** RSTLs on the body. *(B: Redrawn from Fawkes JL, Cheney ML, Pollack SV.* Illustrated Atlas of Cutaneous Surgery. *Philadelphia: Lippincott-Gower; 1992.)*

TABLE 11-1 Surgical Margins by Lesion Type[1,2,4,5,11–14]

Lesion Type	**Surgical Margin**
Uncertain	Consider shave or punch biopsy to delineate prior to elliptical excision or start with 1- to 2-mm margins to avoid unnecessary tissue removal.
Benign	Visible lesion removed.
BCC	3–5 mm
SCC	3–6 mm
Initial excision of possible melanoma	1–3 mm
Melanoma *in situ*	5 mm
Melanoma < 1 mm	10 mm (may need referral for lymph nodes 0.75 to 1 mm depending on ulceration, regression, or mitotic figures)
Melanoma > 1 mm	20 mm and lymph node evaluation

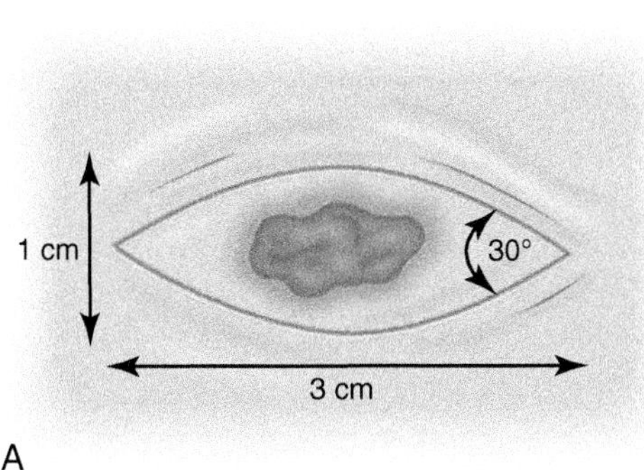

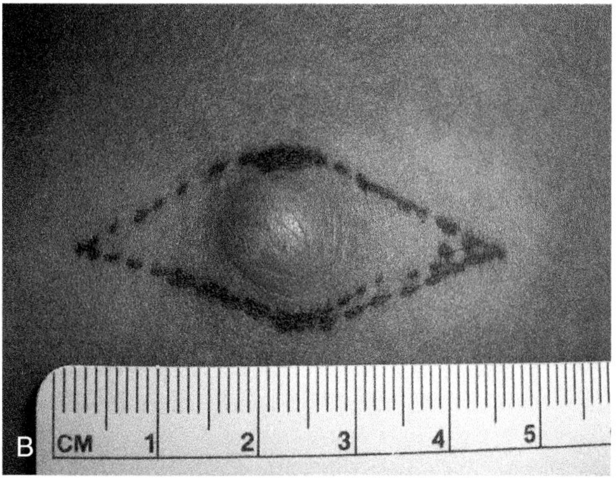

FIGURE 11-7 (A) Most ellipses should be three times longer than they are wide with approximately a 3:1 ratio. (B) Ellipse drawn around a benign pilomatricoma on the upper arm using appropriate geometry. *(A: From Vidimos A, Ammirati C, Poblete-Lopez C.* Dermatologic Surgery. *London: Saunders; 2008.)*

may be desirable include tighter skin, skin over the joints, and curved surfaces.

Once the ellipse has been drawn with a surgical marking pen, it is advisable to pinch the skin again to make sure that the ellipse can be closed and that there will be minimal anatomic distortion. Use alcohol only sparingly on the site after the marking has been performed because alcohol will remove the marking. Prepare the skin with chlorhexidine or povidone-iodine after injecting the anesthesia and before starting the procedure.

Show patients the planned excision before you begin the surgery. You can show the patient and any family in attendance your surgical markings before you start. Keep a handheld mirror nearby for excisions on the face so that your patient knows what you plan to do. This is a helpful method to make sure you truly have informed consent.

Is Side-to-Side Closure Possible?

To decide whether side-to-side closure can be accomplished, pinch the skin to determine whether the skin within the area is loose enough. The clinician has to predict from pinching the skin whether the two sides of the ellipse can be brought together. Areas such as the cheek, trunk, and arms are areas where an elliptical excision can be easily accomplished. Areas that are most difficult are over the sternum and tibia.

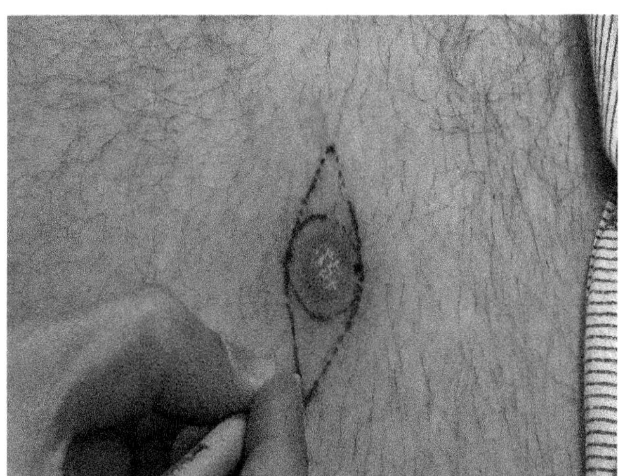

FIGURE 11-8 Ellipse being drawn around a SCC. First the margins are drawn with a circle and then the ellipse is added. *(Copyright Richard P. Usatine, MD.)*

Avoiding Distortion of Tissue

Elliptical excisions on the forehead, upper lip, and around the eye require careful planning because they can distort the eyebrow, lip, or eyelid. When possible it is better to orient an ellipse perpendicular to the eyelid or lip margin (Figure 11-5). For facial excisions, it is important to understand cosmetic units that relate to the organs of the face. Ask the patient to perform the following maneuvers: smile, show the teeth, raise the eyebrows, and purse the lips. It is best to keep the excision within one cosmetic unit rather than crossing between two units. When planning an excision, try to avoid creating functional problems with the eyes and mouth. Avoid pulling down eyelids and causing ectropion, pulling up eyebrows, cutting significant facial nerves, or distorting the look of the lip or nasal alae.

If there is doubt about whether the ellipse can be closed or if the potential exists for anatomic distortion, creation of a flap may be necessary (see Chapter 13, *Flaps*). In some instances the closure can be very tight. Wider undermining or thicker sutures may be required to accomplish the closure.

Anesthesia

See video on the DVD for further learning. 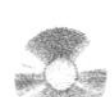

The goal is to produce adequate anesthesia with minimal pain and anxiety for the patient. Local anesthesia is obtained using 1% lidocaine with epinephrine after the ellipse has been drawn. The area of anesthesia must cover the whole ellipse including the skin that will be undermined. Use of 1% lidocaine is preferable to 2% because a larger volume can be used more safely with

1% and this volume produces greater hemostasis by distention.

Epinephrine is valuable for all elliptical excisions and is used for virtually all patients in all surgical locations. For patients with normal circulation, it is safe to use epinephrine for local anesthesia in areas such as the tip of the nose, the fingers and toes, the ears, or the penis despite old dogma. In one study there was no evidence that buffered 0.5% lidocaine with epinephrine 1:200,000 causes ischemia or necrosis when injected into digits at the surgical site (not digital blocks).[3] That was true despite a history of circulatory disorders, thrombosis, diabetes, smoking, anticoagulation, or significant preoperative hypertension.[3] However, in patients with severe peripheral vascular disease or Raynaud's phenomenon, one might discuss the risks and benefits with the patient.

Wait at least 10 minutes before making the incision so that the epinephrine can take effect, thus minimizing the bleeding. Maximal doses of 1% lidocaine (10 mg/mL) with epinephrine are calculated based on the formula of 7 mg/kg of body weight. For example, a 60-kg (132-pound) person could safely receive up to 42 mL at one time.

The amount of anesthesia needed depends on the location of the surgery and the thickness of subcutaneous tissue in the area. For example, the forehead and scalp have very little subcutaneous tissue because of the skull bones below, so a small amount of anesthesia will go far to distend tissue for hemostasis and numbness (Figure 11-9). However, excising an ellipse on the thigh or abdomen will require more anesthetic volume because the thicker subcutaneous tissues will soak up the volume faster. For an ellipse in the range of 1 × 3 cm to 2 × 6 cm, it is not unusual to need at least 20 to 30 mL of anesthesia. This should be safe for even the smallest adult. Plan ahead by drawing up at least one to two 10- to 12-mL syringes with anesthesia.

Add 8.4% bicarbonate in a 1:9 dilution to minimize pain and burning upon injection (see Chapter 3, *Anesthesia*). Pinch the skin at the area to be injected while

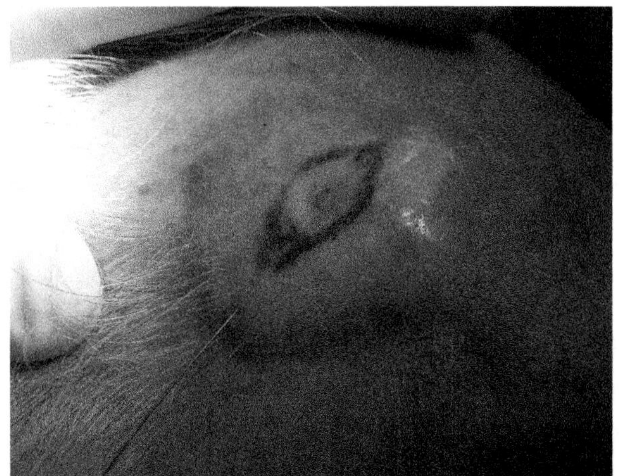

FIGURE 11-9 Injecting anesthesia before excising a BCC on the forehead. Note how the full ellipse with sufficient area to undermine can be anesthetized with a single injection using a 27-gauge, 1½-inch needle on the forehead. *(Copyright Richard P. Usatine, MD.)*

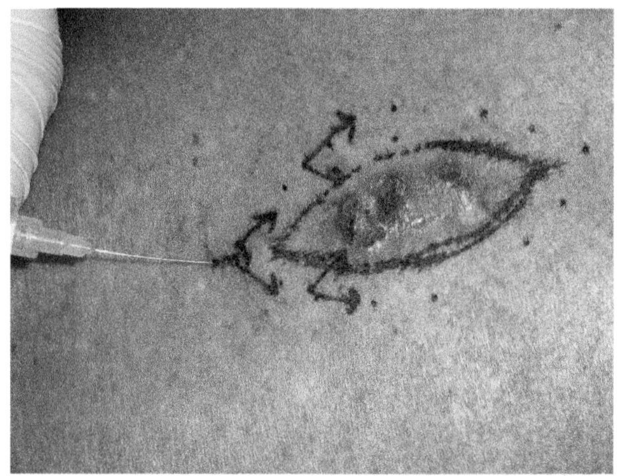

FIGURE 11-10 For a large ellipse, inject in a progressive fanlike manner from areas already anesthetized. Make sure the area to be undermined is numb. *(Copyright Richard P. Usatine, MD.)*

injecting (based on the gate theory of pain). Start with a 30-gauge needle for the most sensitive areas and use a 27-gauge needle for less sensitive areas or when the initial anesthesia begins to work. Inject slowly because tissue distention hurts.

There are many ways to cover the needed area with anesthesia. Small ellipses can be anesthetized by a single injection distal to one end of the ellipse (Figure 11-9). For large excisions, one method that will minimize the number of painful injection sites begins with a single injection at one end of the ellipse that is far enough out to get the area to be undermined. The anesthesia is then delivered in a fanlike fashion until adequate volume is given (Figure 11-10). The next injection can be placed within the area of anesthesia and the anesthetic fanned out toward the other end of the ellipse. A third or fourth injection may be needed if the ellipse is large, but each of these injections may be placed within areas already numb. Injecting in the subcutaneous layer is less painful than injecting in the dermis and gives good anesthesia and reduction of blood flow via the epinephrine effect. This is a very humane method of anesthetizing a large area for surgery.

While waiting 10 minutes for the epinephrine to take effect, make sure that all of the instruments and supplies are ready. Choose your suture and place it on the sterile tray. Consider working on charts and pathology forms while waiting. If the procedure will be time consuming, check your schedule and how many patients will be waiting while you do the surgery. To avoid feeling rushed, it often helps to do larger ellipses during designated "surgery time" and not in the middle of a busy ambulatory clinic.

Preparing the Room, the Patient, and the Equipment

If the patient is wearing clothing near the surgical site, suggest that the patient change into a gown to avoid getting bloodstains on the clothing. If hair is in the way of the surgical site, find a method to clear the field of the hair if possible using headbands, bobby pins, or hair ties. If the hair needs cutting, it is best to do this with a clean or sterile scissor and not a razor. The risk of postoperative infections increases when a razor blade is used to trim the hair at the surgical site.

Make sure the surgical table is at the right height for your work whether you choose to do the surgery sitting or standing. For those with back or feet problems, it often helps to do the surgery sitting. Once the table is in place, turn on the surgical light and point it in the right direction.

Chlorhexidine (Hibiclens) is a very good solution for a surgical prep because it does not stain the skin, very few people are allergic to it, and it does not have to dry to be effective. Povidone-iodine (Betadine) is a good alternative that has the advantage of coloring the skin so it is easy to see the area that was prepped. The disadvantages are that it does stain the skin, some people are allergic to iodine, and one must wait for it to dry before the field is sterile. It also needs to be removed from the skin after the surgery is complete to avoid causing skin irritation.

While your assistant is prepping the area, it is a good time to do a surgical scrub on your hands and forearms. Although skin surgery is not open-heart surgery, it is important to have clean hands before donning sterile surgical gloves. Do not wear a lab coat or tie that will contaminate the surgical site. It is a good idea to take off jewelry or watches and roll up your sleeves before starting the scrub. If you use a surgical loupe for magnification, eye goggles, or splash shields, put these on before you start scrubbing. Surgical masks, surgical gowns, and surgical hair coverings are optional but may protect you from blood or fluid. These might reduce the risk of postoperative infections but this has never been proven for skin surgery. Eye protection is a must to protect the surgeon, and some use a surgical mask for self-protection as well.

Once your sterile gloves are on, turn your attention to creating your sterile surgical field. Fenestrated paper fields that come in a sterilized packet are very convenient. Sterile towels may be used as an alternative. When placed on the face, patients should be able to breathe comfortably. Because these paper drapes have a tendency to move easily during surgery, it helps to place one or two sterile cloth drapes on top of the paper away from the hole, to increase the size of the sterile field and keep the paper in place (Figure 11-11).

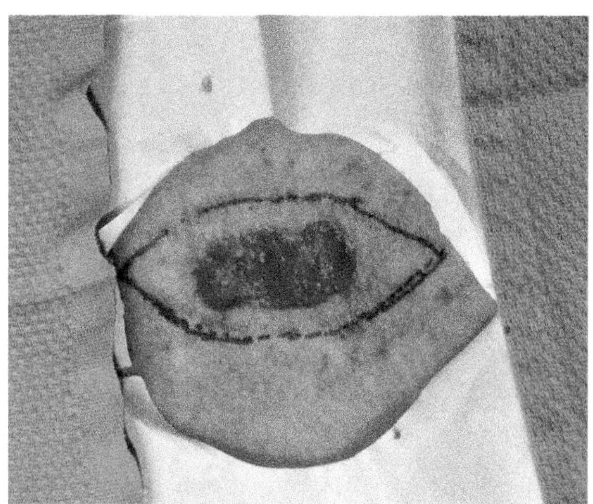

FIGURE 11-11 Fenestrated paper drape with surgical towels to extend sterile field and stabilize the drape. Note that the BCC was curetted to make sure that the margins were drawn adequately to achieve full clearance. *(Copyright Richard P. Usatine, MD.)*

Now look at your equipment and make sure that you have the following:

- Scalpel blade for cutting. Attach the scalpel to the blade holder. The individual scalpel blades tend to be sharper than the scalpel blades attached to a disposable blade holder.
- Suture material including absorbable and nonabsorbable sutures on the tray (see Chapter 5, *Suture Material*).
- Electrosurgical instrument turned on and ready for use. If the finger switch needs to be put through a sterile sheath, this is a good time to do that. Also attach the sterile electrode. If a neutral ground plate is needed and is not already in place, ask your assistant to do that.
- Instruments you expect to use. Put them in an order that makes it easy for you to reach.

For large ellipses it is very helpful to have a surgical assistant who will scrub in. If you are fortunate to have an assistant, make sure that person knows where to be and has sterile gauze in hand to help with hemostasis. Of course, it also helps to have an assistant in the room that is not scrubbed in if any additional supplies are needed.

Incision

See video on the DVD for further learning. 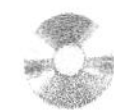

Check that the patient is numb and start your incision. The scalpel should be held like a pencil, with the hand holding the scalpel resting comfortably on the patient. The corner of the ellipse is incised with the tip of the blade. The sharper belly of the blade is used to cut the majority of the ellipse. Care should be taken to make the incision perpendicular to the skin surface (Figure 11-12). It may be helpful to stabilize the skin with your nondominant hand (Figures 11-12 and 11-13) to keep the ellipse from "stretching." Note how the scalpel is not as perpendicular as it should be in Figure 11-13. If the incision is made so that the skin is beveled inward or outward, it may be more difficult to obtain a fine-line closure. (If this error is made, it is still possible to use your scissors to straighten the skin edge before beginning the repair.)

One option is to use an electrosurgical cutting device instead of a scalpel. Although this can decrease bleeding, it does cause thermal damage to the tissue sent for pathology and to the remaining tissue of the patient.

The incision should be made straight through the dermis into the subcutaneous fat, keeping the scalpel perpendicular to the cutting axis. While making the

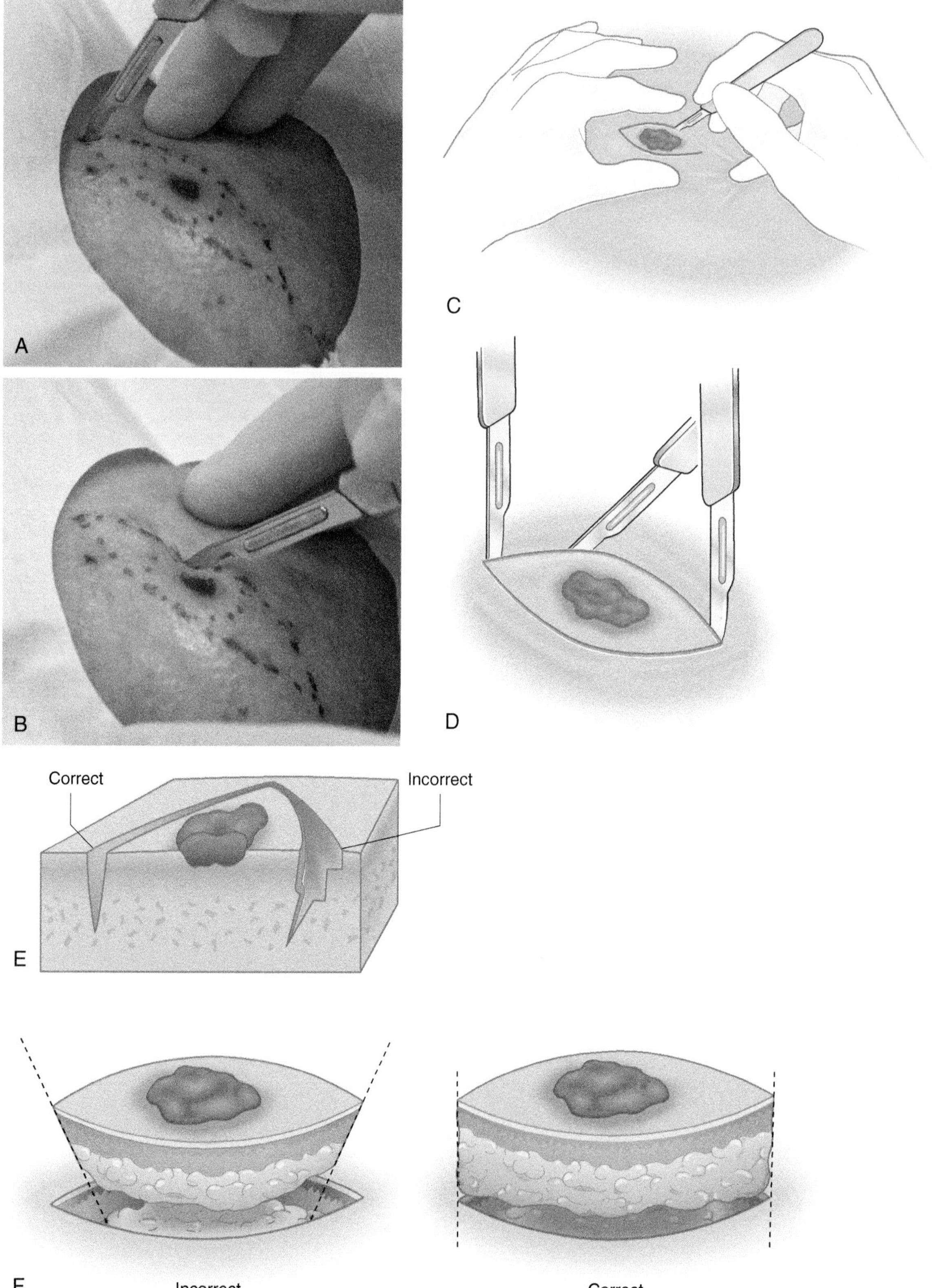

FIGURE 11-12 Cutting the ellipse holding the scalpel like a pencil and the blade perpendicular to the plane of the skin. Start with the blade close to 90 degrees at the tip of the ellipse **(A)** and then decrease the angle while cutting to use more of the belly of the blade **(B)**. **(C)** The left hand is stabilizing the surrounding skin while cutting the ellipse. **(D)** Correct blade angles for cutting the ellipse. **(E)** The ellipse should be cut using one continuous cut than multiple cuts in a "staircasing" pattern. **(F)** The ellipse should not look like a boat but should have parallel perpendicular walls.

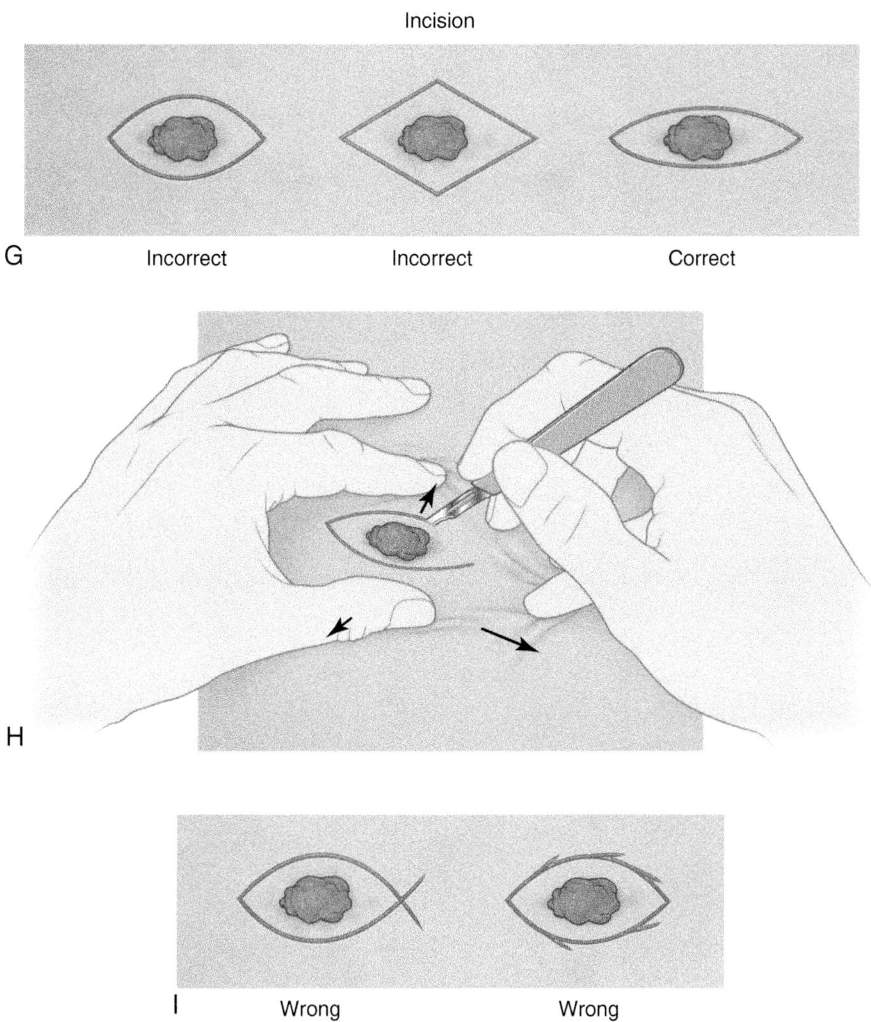

FIGURE 11-12, cont'd (G) When drawing the ellipse use a smooth curved line rather than two pointed triangles together. (H) Finger pressure outward can help cut the ellipse. (I) Do not make a fish tail at the end or allow the blade to cut outside the ellipse. *(A and B, Copyright Richard P. Usatine, MD; C–F, Adapted from Vidimos A, Ammirati C, Poblete-Lopez C.* Dermatologic Surgery. *London: Saunders; 2008; I–H, Modified from Leffell DJ, Brown M.* Manual of Skin Surgery. *New York: Wiley-Liss; 1997:156. Copyright: John Wiley & Sons.)*

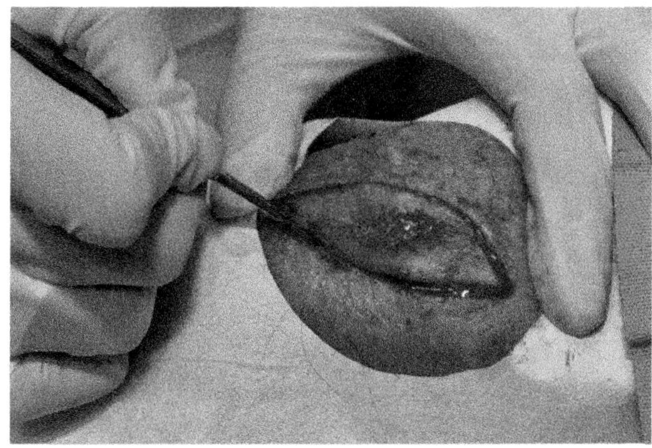

FIGURE 11-13 Stabilizing the surrounding skin while cutting the ellipse. While it is best to keep the scalpel perpendicular to the skin, this operator has allowed the scalpel to lean outward away from the lesion. A subsequent lack of a parallel margin can be corrected with a scissor prior to closure. *(Copyright Richard P. Usatine, MD.)*

incision, the skin can be spread open to ensure that the cut is perpendicular and the edges are vertical. When making a curved incision, there is a natural tendency to lean the scalpel to the outside of a curve. This is not good technique.

The incision should be carried down to subcutaneous fat. With experience and confidence this can often be performed in one or two passes of the blade. If more passes are needed, it helps to have a surgical assistant stretch the skin perpendicular to the axis of the incision so that the incised skin will separate easily. Although the patient may experience bleeding at this point, it is best to use pressure with gauze only and not stop to electrocoagulate every bleeder.

Use caution to not cut beyond the point of the ellipse causing an overcut or fish-tail pattern at the end (Figure 11-12I). It can be helpful to reverse the scalpel so that the point of the scalpel is at the second end of the ellipse to prevent cutting beyond the point of the ellipse.

Grasp one point of the ellipse with a toothed forceps and using the scalpel, scissor, or electrosurgical device

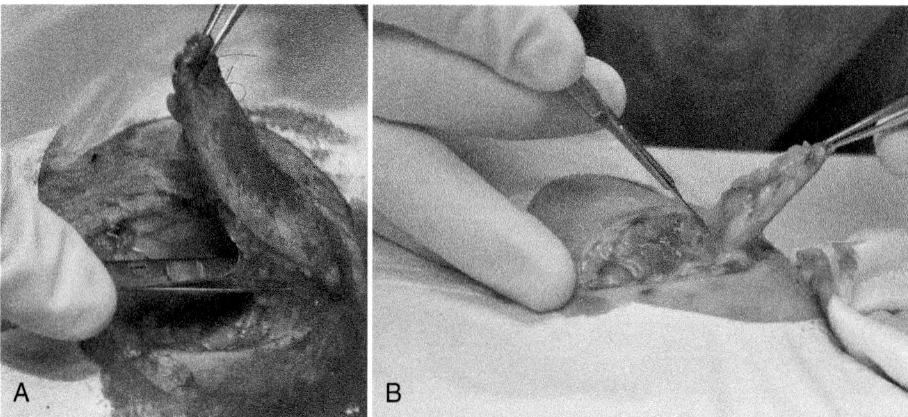

FIGURE 11-14 (A) Cutting horizontally under the ellipse using a sharp iris scissor. (B) Cutting using a scalpel. *(Copyright Richard P. Usatine, MD.)*

cut horizontally under the ellipse from that point to the other end of the ellipse (Figure 11-14). Use caution to stay at the same level in the subcutaneous fat to facilitate a good repair (Figure 11-15).

If the lesion is being sent for pathology to evaluate for clear margins, tag the excised lesion by putting a suture through one end of the sample and recording the location (medial, lateral, etc.) on the pathology slip and medical record (Figure 11-16). If your assistant can attend to the patient by putting pressure on the cut area with gauze, you can use this time to mark the excised lesion. If you are operating alone, you may put the specimen on the sterile tray in an orientation that is similar to the anatomic position within the patient. Then you may finish repairing the defect and place the marking suture at the end of the procedure. If the procedure is taking a long time so that the specimen may dry out, you can choose to place the suture and put the specimen in the formalin at a time when bleeding is controlled. Although a surgical marker may be adequate for marking the corner of an ellipse, there is a risk that the formalin will dissolve the marking and the proper direction will be lost. Using a suture to orient the pathologist provides for greater certainty if the margin is not clear.

Hemostasis

See video on the DVD for further learning. 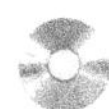

After the ellipse is out, it is time to achieve good hemostasis through electrocoagulation. The use of firm pressure by the surgical assistant and rolling cotton-tipped applicators across the surgical field will help locate the bleeding points. Firm pressure with gauze alone is very helpful to stop bleeding sites before starting to use electrocoagulation.

The major techniques to produce electrocoagulation are as follows:

1. The electrode directly contacts the bleeding site or vessel (Figure 11-17).
2. The electrode is touched to a hemostat or forceps that is grasping the bleeding tissue or vessel and then activated. When a standard electrode is not working because the field has too much blood, it may help to grasp the bleeding tissue with a hemostat or forceps and direct the current through the instrument to stop the bleeding.
3. Special bipolar forceps grasp the tissue and are activated with a foot peddle (see Figure 4-7 in Chapter

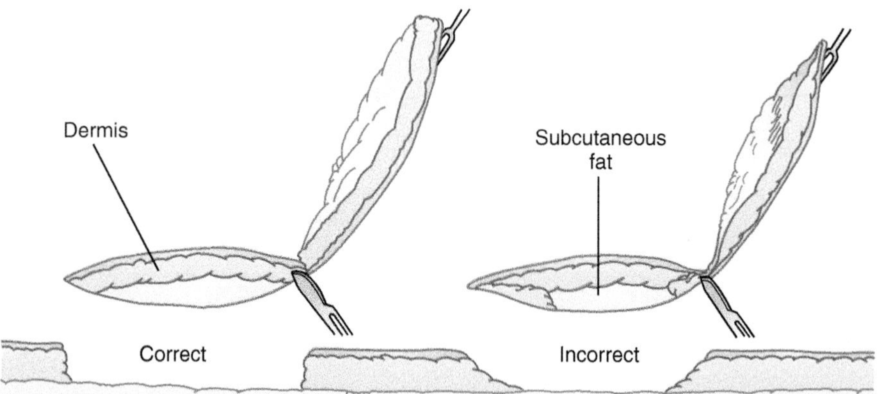

FIGURE 11-15 Incision carried down to the subcutaneous fat. Correction involves parallel walls and not leaving dermis at the tips of the ellipse. *(Redrawn from Fawkes JL, Cheney ML, Pollack SV. Illustrated Atlas of Cutaneous Surgery. Philadelphia: Lippincott-Gower; 1992.)*

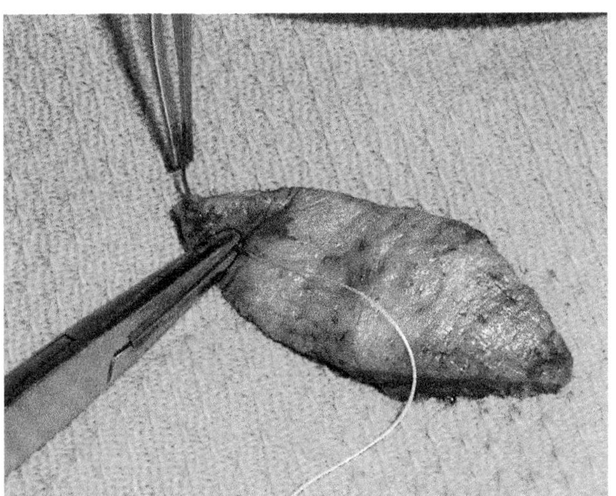

FIGURE 11-16 Tagging the specimen on one corner using a single interrupted suture. Make sure you record the corner marked in the chart and on the pathology requisition form. *(Copyright Richard P. Usatine, MD.)*

4, *Hemostasis*). Bipolar forceps have the advantage of working in a bloody field that is not entirely dry. It is still best to dry the field as much as possible, but the current can still pass through the bleeding tissue despite the presence of blood. The bipolar forceps is the safest method in a patient with a pacemaker or implantable defibrillator.

4. The ball electrode on the Surgitron can also work in a semibloody field.

Creating a dry surgical field is essential for good viewing of the tissues at the time of the final repair. Suturing with a dry field helps prevent hematoma formation, wound infection, and dehiscence.

The electrosurgical unit should be used just enough to stop significant bleeding so that tissue injury is minimized. Slight oozing at the wound edges can be left alone or stopped with pressure only because the suturing should stop this later. Avoid creating large areas of char and tissue necrosis because this can increase the risk of wound infection. When a vessel is not responding to electrocoagulation, use a suture. One method is to use absorbable suture with a small figure-of-eight around the vessel (see Figure 4-5 in Chapter 4). For example, if you are already using Vicryl for your deep sutures, just use this for the hemostatic stitch. The U-suture (square suture) is another method of obtaining hemostasis with a deep absorbable suture (see Figure 4-6 in Chapter 4).

Once hemostasis has been achieved, make sure that the whole tumor is excised. Look at and feel the base and edges of the elliptical defect and the specimen removed. If it appears that some of the tumor or cancer remains (see Figure 34-11 in Chapter 34), cut it out and explain the site and orientation of this second piece to the pathologist. It is better to do this now than to wait and discover the margins were not clear.

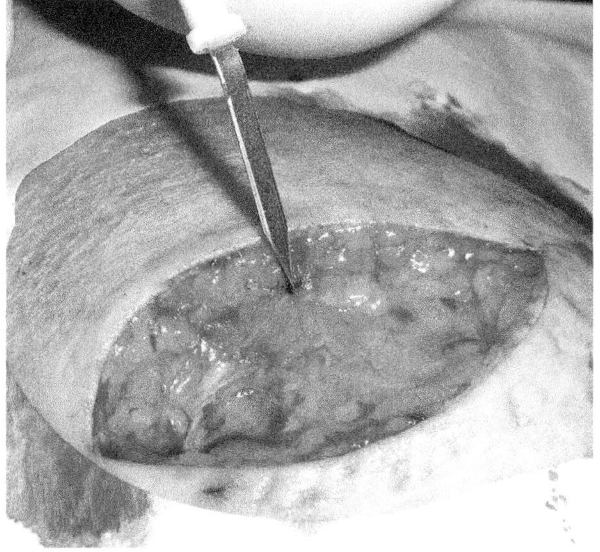

FIGURE 11-17 Electrosurgery is used for hemostasis. *(Copyright Richard P. Usatine, MD.)*

Undermining

See video on the DVD for further learning. 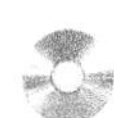

Undermining allows the clinician to mobilize the tissue so that it can be advanced to close a defect. Most small wounds will not need undermining. Determine if and how much undermining will be needed by testing to see how mobile the skin edges are using one skin hook on either side of the wound (Figure 11-18A). When skin hooks are not available, fingers and forceps can be used, but this is a less desirable method (Figure 11-18B). More tension will require more undermining. Repeat this after the undermining is done to determine if there was sufficient undermining. If not, keep going until the skin is able to close in a side-to-side fashion. Minimize undermining with patients on anticoagulation, because they are at higher risk for a hematoma.

Undermining may be performed by spreading the iris scissors (or other tissue scissor) under the edges of the incision (Figure 11-19). The skin hook is a very atraumatic way to hold up the skin edge for undermining. It is especially helpful if your assistant can hold the skin up with two skin hooks giving maximal visualization for undermining. Using blunt dissection the undermining plane is achieved with less bleeding. However, there will be some strands of connective tissue that are better and more quickly snipped than broken with blunt dissection. Therefore, the most efficient and atraumatic method of undermining involves a combination of blunt dissection and snipping (Figure 11-19).

Alternatives include using a scalpel, which will generally provoke more bleeding, or using an electrosurgical cutting device, which can minimize bleeding

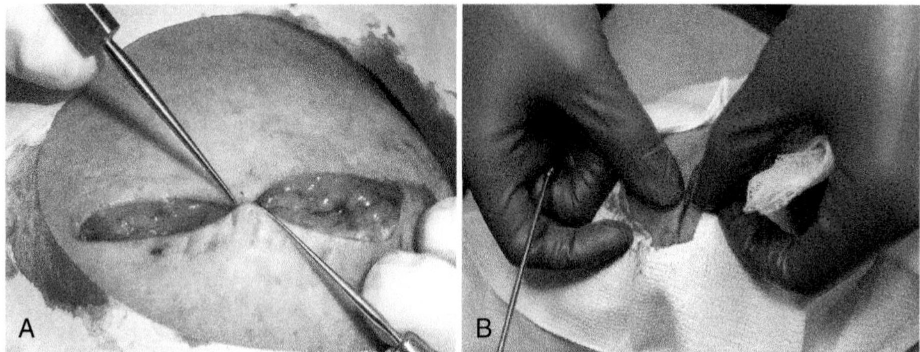

FIGURE 11-18 (A) Checking to see if the ellipse will close without too much tension using skin hooks. (B) Checking for closure with fingers. *(A: Copyright Richard P. Usatine, MD; B: Copyright Daniel L. Stulberg, MD.)*

(Figure 11-20). Because it is easier to undermine the edge furthest away from you, it might help to have an assistant standing on the other side of the table retracting the skin with two skin hooks. The roles are then reversed and the assistant undermines the side nearest you while you hold the skin hooks. Do not forget to undermine at the points of the ellipse to diminish the formation of standing cones (wrinkling or bunching of the skin) at the ends of the repair (Figure 11-19C). With the edges held up with skin hooks, electrocoagulation of bleeders can easily be achieved. Cotton-tipped applicators are helpful to look for bleeders under the undermined skin.

Most areas of the body are undermined within the subcutaneous fat. Some areas of the body, such as the scalp, are better undermined in a deeper plane. The scalp should be undermined in a subgaleal plane (below the galea and above the periosteum) because it is a bloodless, easy plane in which to widely separate the tissue. Although this may seem anxiety provoking at first, there is much less bleeding in this plane than in the subcutaneous fat and you will not damage the skull or underlying central nervous system. See Figure 11-21 for a view of the galea.

Appropriate levels of undermining include the following (Figure 11-22):

- *Scalp:* deep to the galea aponeurotica, above the periosteum (Figure 11-22B)
- *Face:* high fat to avoid facial nerves
- *Trunk and extremities:* deep subcutaneous fat above the muscle
- *Nose:* deeper fascia or connective tissue plane.

The width of undermining is determined by the size and location of the defect. Undermining is useful to loosen the surrounding skin, but should not be excessive. Undermining should allow the skin edges to come together without too much tension and allow eversion of the wound edges with suturing.

Wound Closure (Repair)

See video on the DVD for further learning. 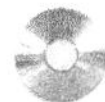

The surgical site should be dry before initiating wound closure. If the ellipse is small and narrow and not under much tension, buried sutures may not be needed. In this case, close the wound with interrupted nonabsorbable sutures such as nylon or polypropylene (Prolene). Closure by the rule of halves is a good method in these cases (Figure 11-23).

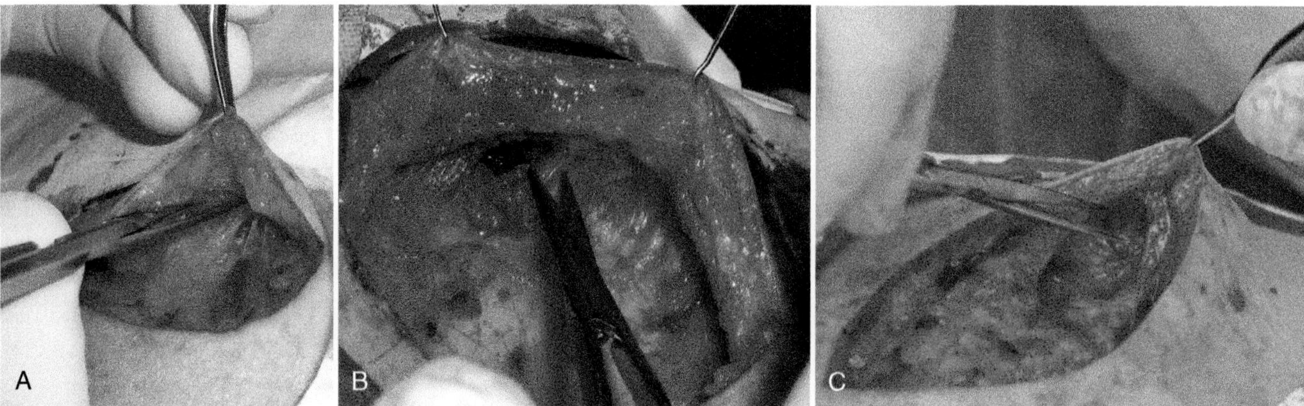

FIGURE 11-19 Undermining with scissors using skin hooks to elevate the skin: (A) Using blunt dissection; (B) snipping fibrous fascia; (C) undermining the tip of the ellipse. *(Copyright Richard P. Usatine, MD.)*

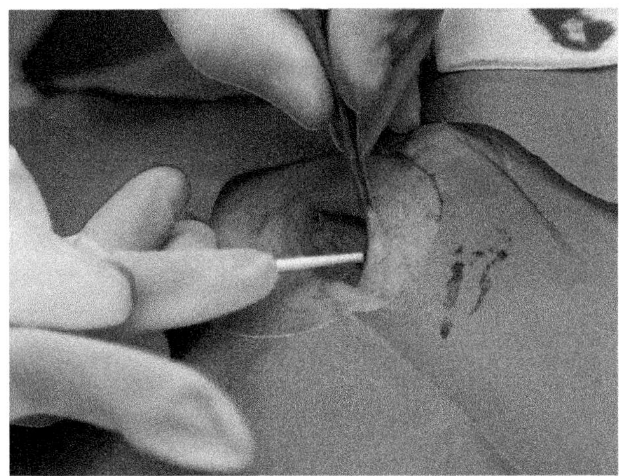

FIGURE 11-20 Undermining with electrosurgery can be less bloodless, but one must be careful to get the level correct because the electrode cuts easily at all levels. *(Copyright Daniel L. Stulberg, MD.)*

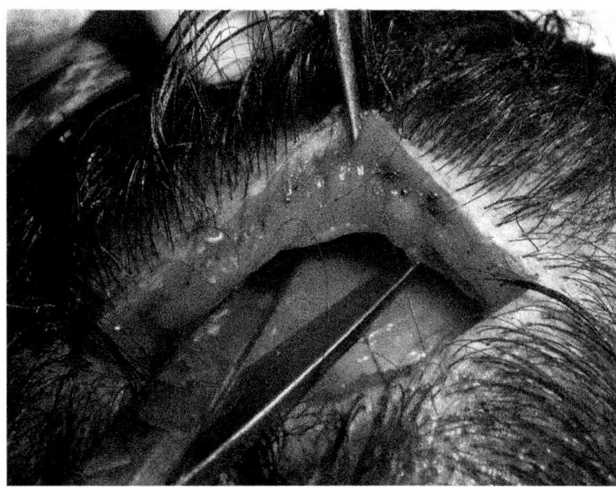

FIGURE 11-21 Undermining with blunt dissection is being performed below the galea to close this elliptical excision. Note the light-colored galea aponeurosis at the bottom of the cut scalp. The subgaleal plane has loose alveolar tissue like tissue paper. This avascular level is perfect for undermining. *(Copyright Richard P. Usatine, MD.)*

Most ellipses will benefit from using buried absorbable sutures to bring the skin edges together. The goal is to have the wound edges closely approximated using only buried sutures (buried vertical mattress sutures, deep sutures; see Chapter 6, *Suturing Techniques*).

The buried sutures take advantage of the undermined area. Use absorbable suture such as 4-0 polyglactin (Vicryl) on a 13- or 16-mm-long plastic needle (see Chapter 5, *Suture Material*). It is easiest to start the buried sutures at one end of the ellipse rather than the middle. The greatest tension is in the middle of an ellipse, and the skin edges tend to pull apart while you are trying to tie the deep suture. By starting at the apex furthest from you, you can begin to take tension off the wound in an area in which there is less tension to begin with. As you move the deep sutures from the apex toward the middle of the ellipse, the wound will narrow and the sutures will be easier to tie. If a deep suture is not placed well, do not hesitate to take it out and redo it.

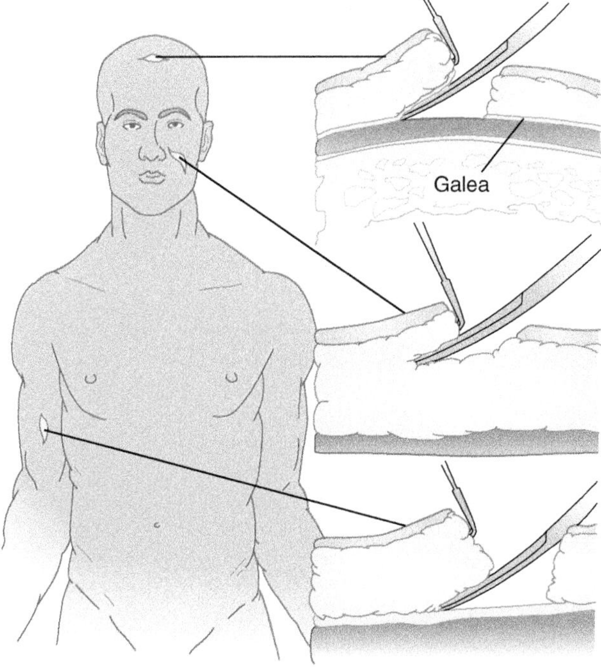

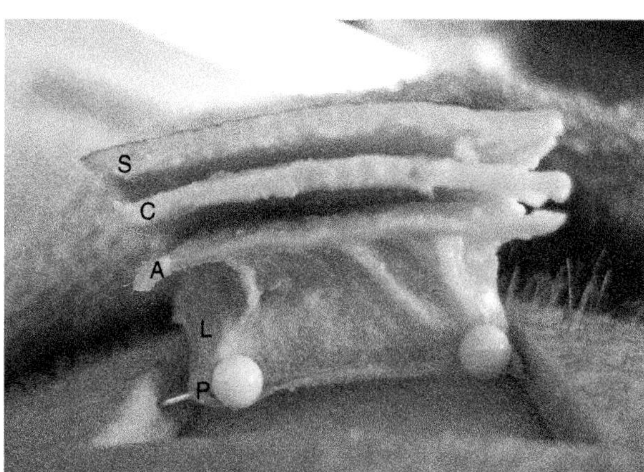

FIGURE 11-22 (A) Correct levels of undermining. (B) Levels of the scalp named using the SCALP mnemonic: S = skin, C = connective tissue, A = aponeurosis (galea), L= loose alveolar tissue (the best level for undermining as it is least vascular), P = pericranium. *(A: Redrawn from Fawkes JL, Cheney ML, Pollack SV.* Illustrated Atlas of Cutaneous Surgery. *Philadelphia: Lippincott-Gower; 1992; B: From Vidimos A, Ammirati C, Poblete-Lopez C.* Dermatologic Surgery. *London: Saunders; 2008.)*

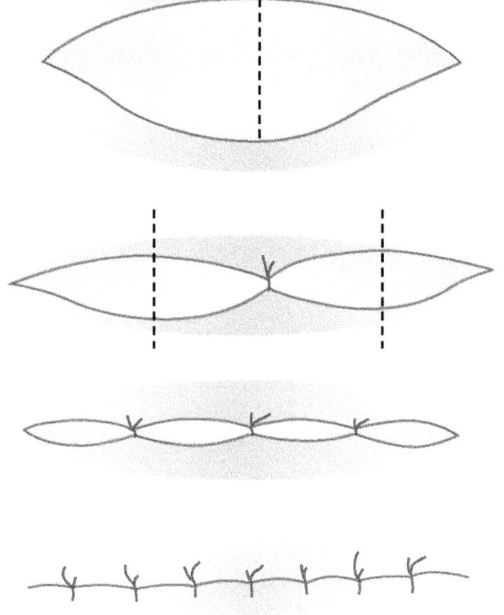

FIGURE 11-23 Using the rule of halves to close an ellipse not under tension. *(Copyright Richard P. Usatine, MD.)*

The buried suture is performed in the following manner (Figure 11-24):

- Hold up the skin edge with a skin hook or fine-toothed forceps and place the needle from the undermined area up to the upper dermis (not through the epidermis) and out or just below the dermal epidermal junction.
- Hold the needle with the forceps and reload your needle holder with the needle facing the opposite direction. Then introduce the needle at the same height with regard to the dermal-epidermal junction and bring it slightly upward and outward away from the wound.
- Using the curvature of the needle enter the undermined area and bring it out with the suture coming toward you. In this way both suture ends should be on the same side and easier to tie.
- Perform an instrument tie initially using two throws. Pull the two ends perpendicular to the wound and then change direction and pull the ends parallel to the wound. Cinch the knot down so that the skin is well approximated. Put in three more knots each with a single throw. If the skin is opening between your first and second throw, ask your assistant to hold the skin edges together with their fingers on both sides away from the edge to avoid being stuck by the needle.
- The strands of suture should be cut short but not so short as to compromise the knot below. Place the scissor above the knot, turn it 45 degrees, then cut.
- Keep repeating this process until there is no more gaping wound and the two sides have come together to form a thin line.

If the wound is well approximated, start a running suture with 4-0 to 6-0 polypropylene (Prolene) or nylon to hold the epidermal edges together for optimal healing. A single interrupted suture is placed at one end of the wound and only the short end is cut. The remainder of the suture is looped around the skin edges one throw at a time (Figure 11-25). This is taken to the end and then the knot is tied to the final loop (see Chapter 6, *Suturing Techniques*). While the running suture is quick, if it does open or needs to be opened with a wound infection, it will no longer retain its strength.

If the skin is not well approximated with the deep sutures or there continues to be much tension on the wound, use interrupted sutures rather than a running suture. Simple interrupted sutures can be very useful and can be combined with a running suture. If greater wound eversion is needed and skin tension remains high, vertical mattress sutures can be beneficial (Figure 11-25). In areas where there is natural inversion such as in the creases of the forehead, vertical mattress sutures can be used for wound eversion (see Chapter 6).

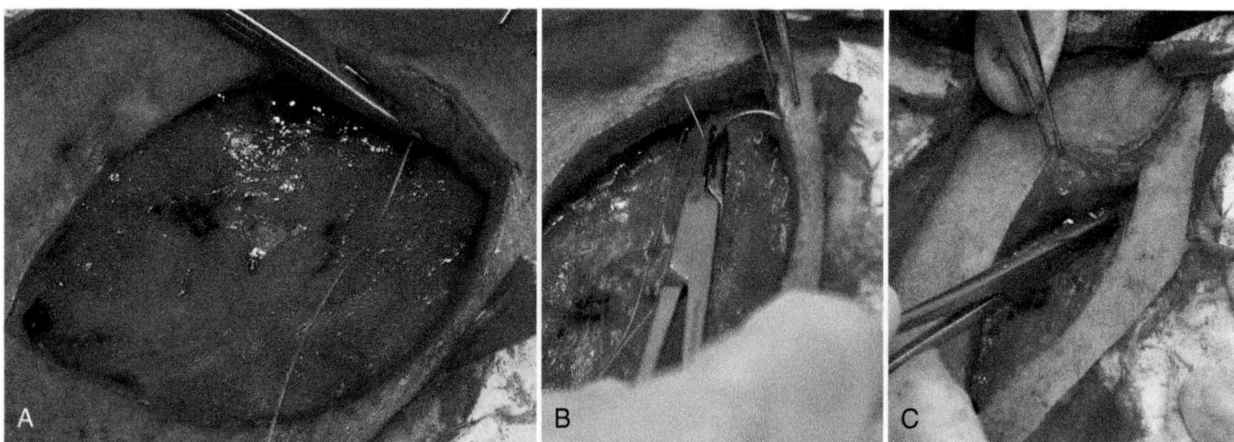

FIGURE 11-24 Closing the ellipse with deep vertical mattress sutures. **(A)** Start the first deep stitch at one end of the ellipse. The needle is inserted in the undermined area and is brought up to 1 to 2 mm below the dermal-epidermal junction. **(B)** Place the second half of the deep stitch starting from the same level and using the curvature of the needle to come out in the undermined area. **(C)** Continue to place deep sutures moving from one side of the ellipse toward the other. *(Copyright Richard P. Usatine, MD.)*

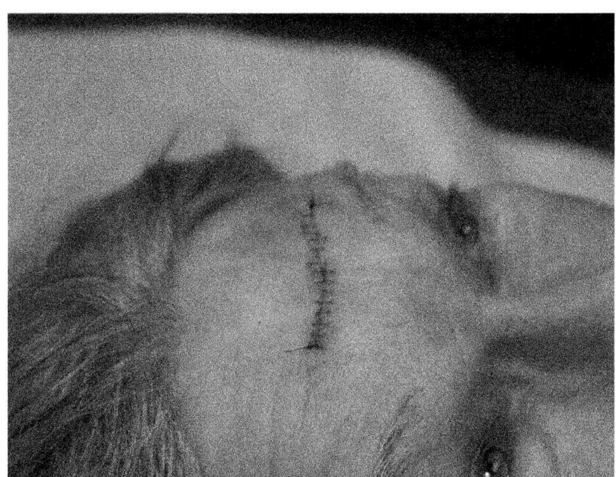

FIGURE 11-25 Running suture placed along natural wrinkle lines. *(Copyright Daniel L. Stulberg, MD.)*

Standing Cones (Dog-Ear) Repair

See video on the DVD for further learning. 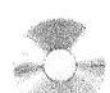

The best way to avoid standing cones is by planning and drawing your ellipse as described earlier. However, even with the best planning, a standing cone can still happen. Repair of a standing cone of tissue at either end of an elliptical excision is accomplished by extending the length of the excision (Figure 11-26). One method involves cutting a line through the center of the standing cone at a slight angle from the original incision. This results in one overhanging edge of tissue that needs to be trimmed. This trimming is done with a No. 15 blade or scissor to neatly trim the tissue to the very end of the excision. A No. 15 blade or a sharp scissor is preferred to keep the cut perpendicular with the skin. When trimming this tissue, it is important to trim only a small amount at a time so that not too much tissue is removed.

Another method involves holding the standing cone up with a skin hook or forceps and cutting the bulging portion off as you might cut off the top of a mountain. The skin is then pushed down to see if it lays flat. Regardless of which method is used, once the skin lays flat, place a single interrupted suture to complete the repair.

Some standing cones will flatten over time without repair. This works best when the skin is loose, as on an elderly person. Deciding when a standing cone should be surgically repaired is a judgment call that weighs the creation of a longer wound against the risk that the bulge will be forever unsightly.

Clean and Dress the Wound

- Make sure that there is no persistent bleeding before removing the drapes. Hold pressure on the wound with gauze and see that the bleeding has come to a stop. It is desirable to milk out any remaining blood before moving on because blood is a good medium for bacterial growth. If the bleeding has not stopped, hold pressure on the wound with gauze for 5 minutes by the clock. If bleeding persists then you will need to open some sutures and look for the bleeding site.
- Clean the wound with sterile saline before dressing it. Sterile saline can now be purchased in 1-oz plastic vials that are convenient for wound cleansing (see resources below).
- Some areas will not be amenable to dressing such as the scalp and lip. (If a scalp dressing is needed, it can be applied by wrapping gauze around the head.) For other areas it is helpful to create a pressure dressing to minimize postoperative bleeding in the first 24 hours. First apply clean petrolatum from a squeeze tube using clean or sterile cotton-tipped applicators. A sterile 2 × 2 gauze can be folded for the first layer. Alternatives include Telfa pads to decrease sticking or dental roll for good pressure application. Additional gauze is added on top and the whole dressing is tightly taped to the skin. Of course taping should not be so tight as to impair circulation but needs to be firmly adherent so that the dressing does not fall off until removed in 24 hours (see Chapter 35, *Wound Care*).
- We specifically avoid using antibiotic ointments because even bacitracin ointment is a common

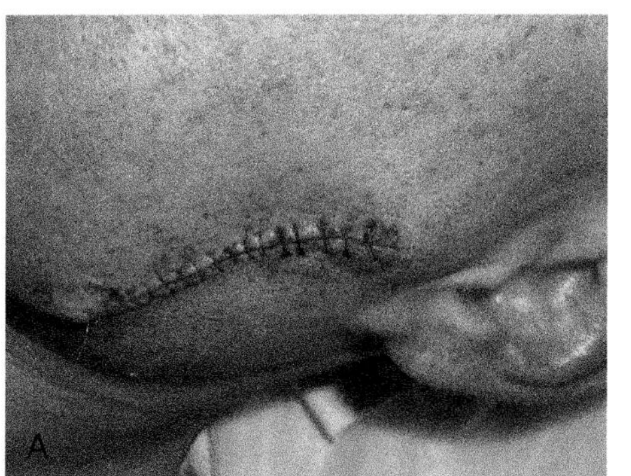

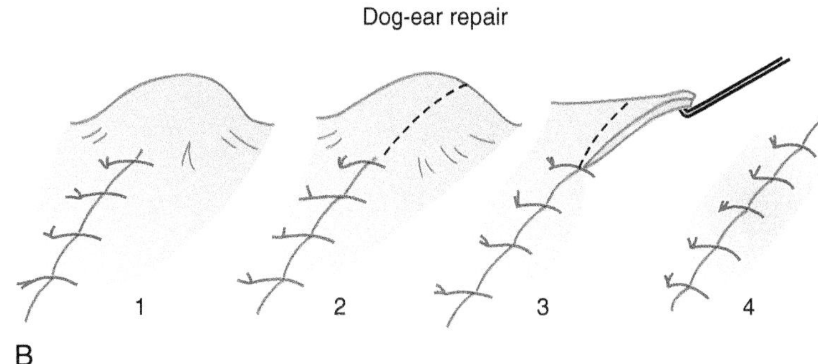

FIGURE 11-26 (A) Running suture after BCC removal produced standing cones (dog ears) on both ends of this ellipse. These flattened with time. (B) Method for standing cone removal. (1) Standing cone present. (2) Extend incision through cone along dotted line. (3) Pull over the long side and cut it off at dotted line to remove one portion of redundant skin. (4) Add one suture to flatten the cone (dog ear). *(B: Redrawn from Fawkes JL, Cheney ML, Pollack SV.* Illustrated Atlas of Cutaneous Surgery. *Philadelphia: Lippincott-Gower; 1992.)*

contact allergen. Since switching to petrolatum only we have seen no increase in postoperative wound infections.

Aftercare

- Patients may be given a handout on wound care that goes over such issues as dressing changes, pain control, bleeding complications, and wound infections (see Chapter 35). Hydrogen peroxide, alcohol, and other topical cleansers are not necessary and can be harmful to healing skin.
- The patient may shower after 24 hours, but should not soak in a bathtub or other body of water until the sutures are out. Remove sutures from the face at 5 to 7 days, trunk at 7 to 10 days, and the extremities at 10 to 14 days. Consider leaving the nonabsorbable sutures in longer if buried sutures were not used and other factors are present that might increase the risk of dehiscence. Factors that compromise wound healing such as smoking, older age, poor nutrition, and systemic steroids increase the risk of infection and wound dehiscence so decisions about the timing of suture removal may be more complex in these patients.
- Because not all patients will or can read your handouts, counsel the patient regarding the signs of wound infection and to contact the office or seek care if fever, erythema, purulence, or increasing pain develops.
- We often call our patients the following day after a large excision. This can put your mind at ease and makes the patient feel cared for and special. This is also the perfect opportunity to answer patient questions about wound care or potential wound complications. This 1- to 2-minute call has much value for the patient and your practice.

Complications and their prevention are described in detail in Chapter 36.

NOTES ON INFECTION

- Infection may occur regardless of the precautions taken to ensure sterility.
- Sterile technique is routinely used for full-thickness excisions which are sutured.[9,10] When wound infections occur the most common pathogens are *Staphylococcus aureus* and *Streptococcus pyogenes.*
- Do not overlook the possibility of MRSA infections especially if the patient has a history of previous MRSA infections.
- Culture wounds that appear infected and open sutures if needed to allow the pus to drain.
- In general, antibiotic prophylaxis is rarely indicated.
- The 2008 AAD Advisory Statement recommends antibiotic prophylaxis for subacute bacterial endocarditis in high-risk cardiac patients and high-risk patients with prosthetic joints when performing excisions that involve cutting the oral mucosa.[9] Consider antibiotic prophylaxis if significant undermining is planned (see Chapter 1, *Preoperative Preparation*).
- Consider antibiotic prophylaxis with wedge excisions of the ear or lip, excisions in the groin or leg, in the presence of extensive inflammatory disease, skin flaps of the nose, and skin grafts (see Chapter 1).

VARIATIONS

Variations in the standard ellipse include the following shapes:

1. Crescent excision
2. S-plasty
3. M-plasty
4. Partial closure.

Crescent Excision

On the cheek of the face it often looks better for the final repair to be a crescent rather than a straight line. Asking the patient to smile can show the crescentic pattern of the smile lines. See Figure 11-27 to visualize how the crescent excision is drawn and executed.

M-Plasty

In certain situations the ellipse should be shorter on one side to avoid having the ellipse cross into another cosmetic unit. See Figure 11-28 as an example of how the M-plasty is used on the face to shorten one side of the ellipse.

S-Plasty

Another variation of the ellipse that works well on convex surfaces such as the cheek is the S-plasty (Figure 11-29). Each side of the ellipse is drawn in an S configuration to avoid standing cones. Use of the rule of halves is helpful when closing this type of excision. If standing cones still form, they can be excised as described previously. Cosmetically this can give a better result than a straight line over some convex surfaces.

Partial Closure

Some large excisions on the scalp may be very difficult to close even with extensive undermining. Although the scalp may be allowed to heal by second intention, the clinician may want to obtain a partial closure to decrease the size of the area required to heal secondarily (Figure 11-30). Temporary pulley stitches are put in as step 1 to begin the closure. The wound is then closed from the apices with interrupted sutures zippering toward the center. This leaves a smaller wound to heal by second intention, thereby reducing final healing time.

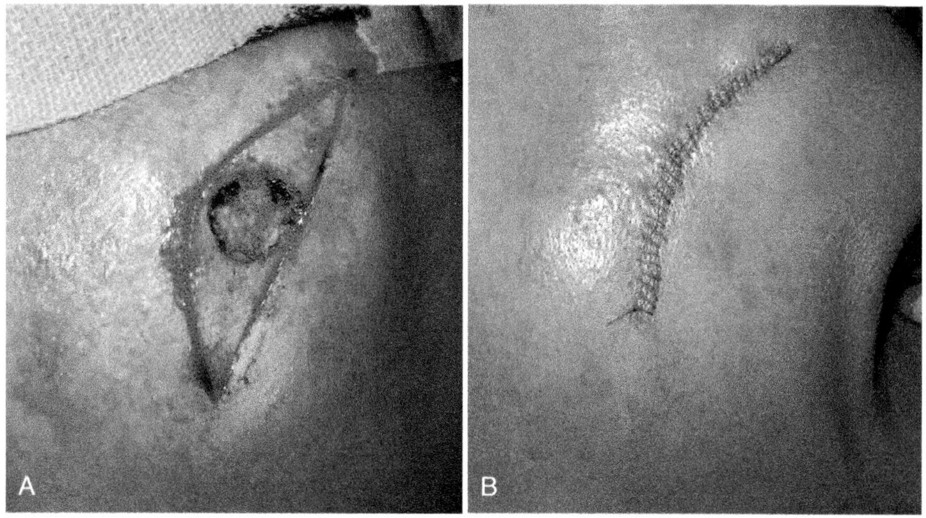

FIGURE 11-27 Crescent excision. **(A)** Circular defect on the cheek following removal of a basal cell carcinoma utilizing the Mohs method. The crescent excision is designed to result in a curvilinear line that follows the natural relaxed skin tension lines. Areas of use include the cheek over the malar eminence and the chin. **(B)** Crescentic repair follows smile lines. *(From Robinson J, Hanke W, Sengelmann R, Siegel D.* Surgery of the Skin: Procedural Dermatology, *2nd ed. Philadelphia: Mosby; 2010.)*

ALTERNATIVES TO AN ELLIPTICAL EXCISION

The alternatives to an elliptical excision include the following:

- Punch excision if the lesion is small enough
- Use of an elliptically shaped disposable cutter with a thin rotating flexible blade (Elliptipunch) (Figure 11-31)
- Use of an elliptical punch that is rocked back and forth over the area to make the cut (Elliptiscalpel) (Figure 11-32)
- Excision with flap repair (see Chapter 13, *Flaps*)
- Electrodessication and curettage for small BCCs, superficial BCCs, and SCC *in situ* (Bowen's disease) (see Chapter 14, *Electrosurgery*)
- Cryosurgical destruction with liquid nitrogen spray for superficial BCCs and SCC *in situ* (see Chapter 15, *Cryosurgery*).

SUGGESTIONS FOR LEARNING THE ELLIPTICAL EXCISION TECHNIQUE

Frozen or fresh pig's feet (not smoked) are available in many grocery stores and are good for practicing suturing and excision techniques. The skin on the pig's feet is less elastic than human skin, so practice with ellipses that are a 4:1 or 5:1 ratio.

CODING AND BILLING PEARLS

Record the location of the lesion and the width and length for coding because reimbursement varies with body location and size.

It is often best to know the diagnosis before excising a large lesion because this will determine the margins. Also larger lesions will be compensated at a higher rate and therefore may need prior approval. If an initial

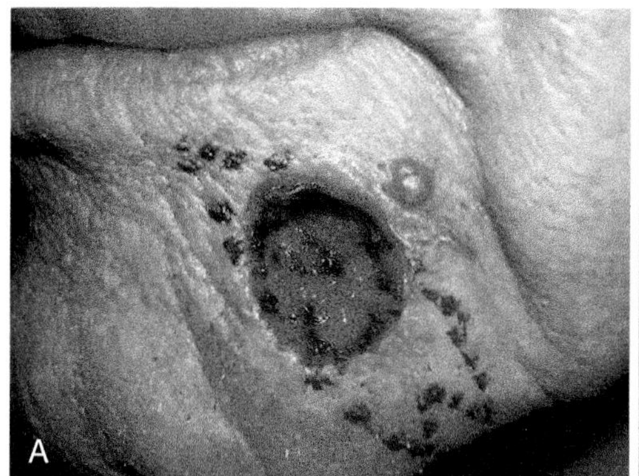

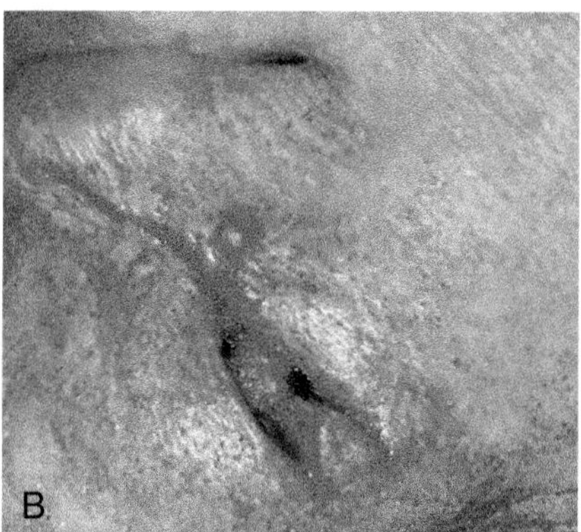

FIGURE 11-28 **(A)** M-plasty is designed to avoid crossing over into a new cosmetic unit. A tip stitch may be used to complete the M. **(B)** The final result produces a shorter scar that remains within one cosmetic unit. *(From Robinson J, Hanke W, Sengelmann R, Siegel D.* Surgery of the Skin: Procedural Dermatology, *2nd ed. Philadelphia: Mosby; 2010.)*

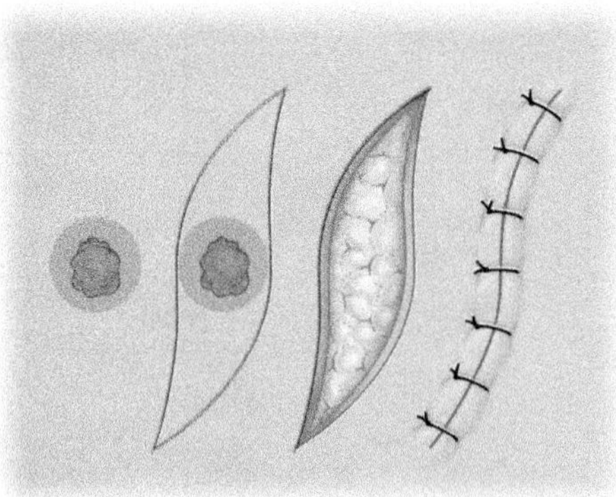

FIGURE 11-29 S-plasty with the lazy-S repair is designed by juxtaposing two S-shaped incisions around the defect. By approximating the center of each slightly offset S to the other, the final repair becomes a smooth serpentine line that contracts over convex surfaces with minimal buckling. It is useful when performing an excision along a convex surface such as the forearm or jaw. This minimizes the contraction and buckling seen along the length of the scar. Closing the wound with the rule of halves is helpful. *(From Vidimos A, Ammirati C, Poblete-Lopez C.* Dermatologic Surgery. *London: Saunders; 2008.)*

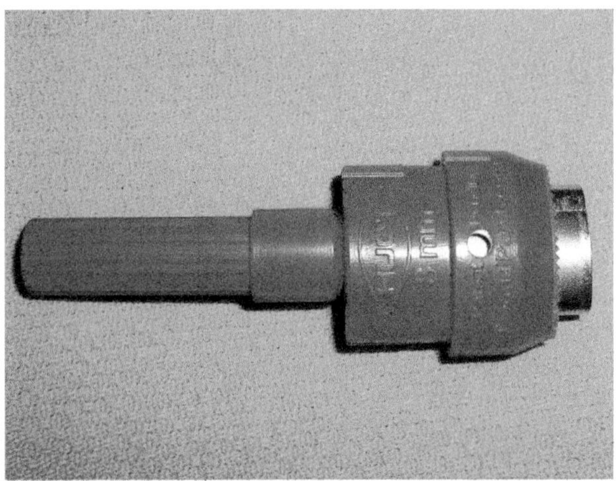

FIGURE 11-31 The Elliptipunch may be used to create an elliptical excision when the instrument fits the needed size. The blade is flexible and can be rotated to cut the skin. *(Copyright Richard P. Usatine, MD.)*

biopsy was done to determine the diagnosis, this may help to obtain prior approval for the correct procedure. If a skin cancer is suspected, the rates for reimbursement are high enough often to require prior approval for billing. Also if an intermediate repair is expected, the fee is significantly increased so prior approval is even more important. If the diagnosis is not already known, hold off on billing until the pathology returns because the codes for excision of malignant lesions receive a higher reimbursement.

Tables 11-2 and 11-3 summarize the CPT codes and Medicare fees for excisions. Note how the fee goes up 0.1 cm above each round centimeter. Do not round the measurements or make estimates; use exact numbers.

When calculating the size of the excised lesion it is important to include the necessary margins. Therefore, if you are excising a 1-cm BCC with 4-mm margins, you would bill for an excision at 1.8 cm. Do not forget to make these measurements because it is crucial to getting paid for what you do.

If the repair involves significant undermining and/or deep sutures, additional codes are supplied for these types of intermediate and complex repairs. Even the use of a single deep suture allows you to bill for an intermediate repair. The compensation for such a repair is comparable to the compensation for the rest of the excision. Therefore, using deep sutures when needed not only protects the patient from risks of dehiscence and hematoma, it also increases the compensation. When coding for intermediate repair, it helps to include the reason for the deep sutures in your operative note. The most common reasons are to "take tension off the wound" or "prevent dehiscence."

The CPT code for an intermediate repair is based on the length of the final closed wound. The codes for intermediate repairs encompass wide ranges of wound length and most of the coding will be within the 2.6- to 7.5-cm range. See Box 38-1 in Chapter 38, *Surviving Financially*, for the CPT codes and Medicare fees for intermediate repairs.

A complex repair can be billed if a lot of undermining is needed. Start by billing for intermediate repairs and make sure payments are received before attempting to bill at the complex repair level. Flaps are addressed in Chapter 13 and have their own billing codes.

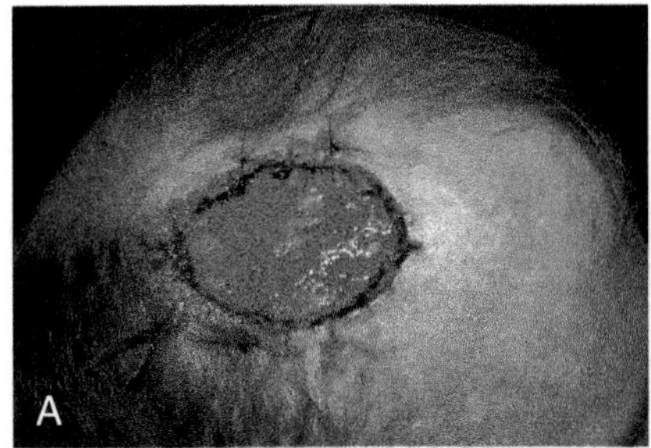

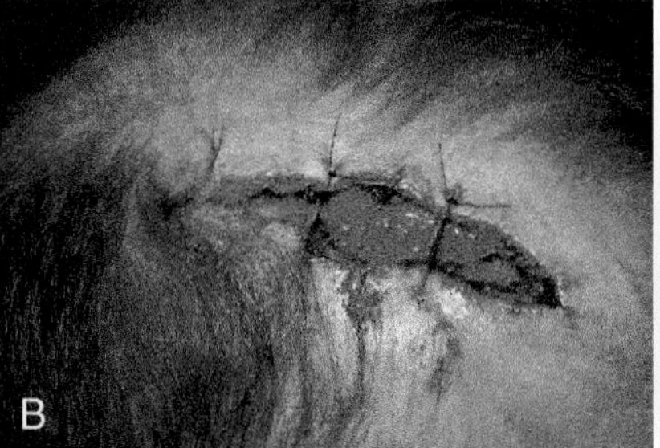

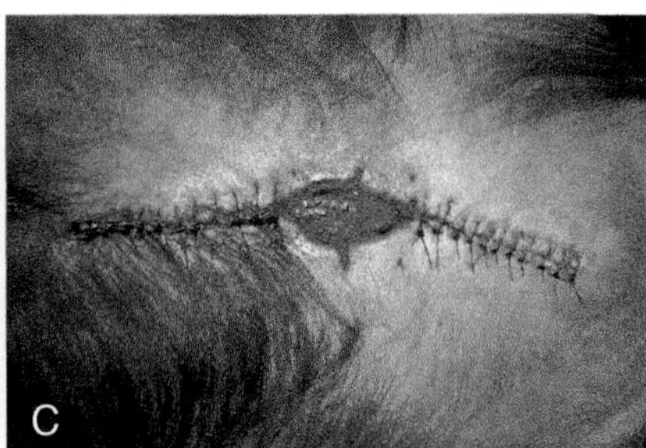

FIGURE 11-30 Partial closure: **(A)** Large basal cell carcinoma on the parietal scalp was excised with Mohs surgery. **(B)** Pulley stitches act as an intraoperative tissue expander. **(C)** Closing the wound from the apices and "zippering" toward the center leaves only a small wound to heal by second intention, thus reducing healing time. *(From Robinson J, Hanke W, Sengelmann R, Siegel D.* Surgery of the Skin: Procedural Dermatology, *2nd ed. Philadelphia: Mosby; 2010.)*

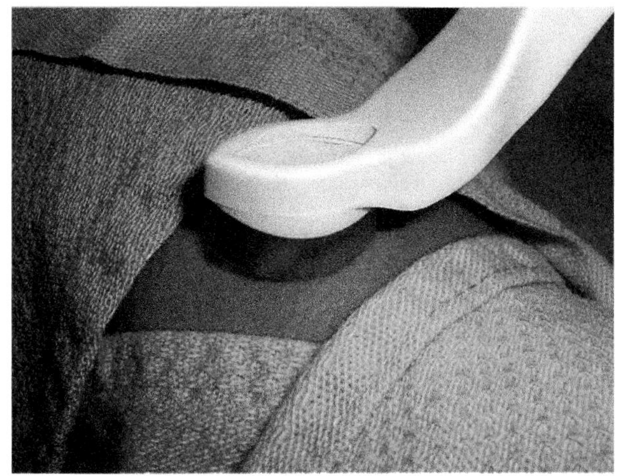

FIGURE 11-32 The Elliptiscalpel is another method of performing an ellipse by rocking the blade back and forth over the skin to be cut. *(Copyright Richard P. Usatine, MD.)*

TABLE 11-2 Excision-Benign Lesions[11–14]

CPT codes		2010 Medicare National Nonfacility Price
Trunk, Arms, or Legs		
11400	0.5 cm or less	$105
11401	0.6 to 1.0 cm	$130
11402	1.1 to 2.0 cm	$145
11403	2.1 to 3.0 cm	$168
11404	3.1 to 4.0 cm	$191
11406	Over 4.0 cm	$276
Scalp, Neck, Hands, Feet, Genitalia		
11420	0.5 cm or less	$106
11421	0.6 to 1.0 cm	$139
11422	1.1 to 2.0 cm	$155
11423	2.1 to 3.0 cm	$181
11424	3.1 to 4.0 cm	$209
11426	Over 4.0 cm	$302
Face, Ears, Eyelids, Nose, Lips, Mucous Membranes		
11440	0.5 cm or less	$117
11441	0.6 to 1.0 cm	$149
11442	1.1 to 2.0 cm	$167
11443	2.1 to 3.0 cm	$202
11444	3.1 to 4.0 cm	$255
11446	Over 4.0 cm	$352

TABLE 11-3 Excision of Malignant Lesions

CPT codes		2010 Medicare National Nonfacility Price
Trunk, Arms or Legs		
11600	0.5 cm or less	$165
11601	0.6 to 1.0 cm	$203
11602	1.1 to 2.0 cm	$222
11603	2.1 to 3.0 cm	$253
11604	3.1 to 4.0 cm	$281
11606	Over 4.0 cm	$401
Scalp, Neck, Hands, Feet, Genitalia		
11620	0.5 cm or less	$168
11621	0.6 to 1.0 cm	$204
11622	1.1 to 2.0 cm	$231
11623	2.1 to 3.0 cm	$271
11624	3.1 to 4.0 cm	$306
11626	Over 4.0 cm	$371
Face, Ears, Eyelids, Nose, Lips, Mucous Membranes		
11640	0.5 cm or less	$175
11641	0.6 to 1.0 cm	$214
11642	1.1 to 2.0 cm	$246
11643	2.1 to 3.0 cm	$292
11644	3.1 to 4.0 cm	$360
11646	Over 4.0 cm	$476

CONCLUSION

The elliptical excision is one of the most basic and useful techniques for the excision of skin lesions. It can be aligned with skin tension lines, wrinkle lines, and other structures to give a good cosmetic result. The best results are obtained when the clinician pays close attention to the fine points of planning, designing, and executing the excision as described in this chapter.

Resources

Delasco; sterile saline can now be purchased in 1 ounce plastic vials that are convenient for wound cleansing (800-831-6273; www.delasco.com/pcat/1/Wound_Care/SalJet/SalJet).

Huot Instruments, manufacturer of the Elliptipunch (8- × 20-, 10- × 25-, and 12- × 30-mm sizes and Visi-Punch biopsy units (www.huotinstruments.com).

MooreBrand® Minor Laceration Pack; contains 5-inch needle holder, 4½-inch sharp/sharp scissors, 5-inch metal tissue forceps along with drapes and gauze; these instruments are of sufficient quality to perform large elliptical excisions and are all disposable; priced at under $6 (www2.mooremedical.com).

References

1. Minton TJ. Contemporary Mohs surgery applications. *Curr Opin Otolaryngol Head Neck Surg.* 2008;16(4):376–380.
2. Thissen MR, Neumann MH, Schouten LJ. A systematic review of treatment modalities for primary basal cell carcinomas. *Arch Dermatol.* 1999;135:1177–1183.
3. Smeets NW, Krekels GA, Ostertag JU, *et al.* Surgical excision vs Mohs' micrographic surgery for basal-cell carcinoma of the face: randomised controlled trial. *Lancet.* 2004;364(9447):1766–1772.
4. Leibovitch I, Huilgol SC, Selva D, *et al.* Cutaneous squamous cell carcinoma treated with Mohs micrographic surgery in Australia I. Experience over 10 years. *J Am Acad Dermatol.* 2005;53(2):253–260.
5. Silapunt S, Peterson SR, Goldberg LH. Squamous cell carcinoma of the auricle and Mohs micrographic surgery. *Dermatol Surg.* 2005;31(11, Pt 1):1423–1427.
6. Robinson JK, Hanke CW, Sengelmann RD, *et al. Surgery of the Skin—Procedural Dermatology.* St Louis, MO: Elsevier/Mosby; 2010.
7. Tran KT, Wright, NA, Cockerell CJ. Biopsy of the pigmented lesion—when and how. *J Am Acad Dermatol.* 2008;59:852–871.
8. Kimyai-Asadi A, Alam M, Goldberg LH, *et al.* Efficacy of narrow-margin excision of well-demarcated primary facial basal cell carcinomas. *J Am Acad Dermatol.* 2005;53(3):464–468.
9. Wright TI, Baddour LM, Berbari EF, *et al.* Antibiotic prophylaxis in dermatologic surgery: advisory statement 2008. *J Am Acad Dermatol.* 2008;59(3):464–473.
10. Bennett R. Surgical complications (Chap 248). In: Wolff K, Goldsmith LA, Katz SI, *et al*, eds. *Fitzpatrick's Dermatology in General Medicine.* 7th ed. New York: McGraw-Hill; 2007.
11. Dengel L, Turza K, Noland MM, *et al.* Skin mapping with punch biopsies for defining margins in melanoma: when you don't know how far to go. *Ann Surg Oncol.* 2008;15(11):3028–3035.
12. Kimyai-Asadi A, Katz T, Goldberg LH, *et al.* Margin involvement after the excision of melanoma in situ: the need for complete en face examination of the surgical margins. *Dermatol Surg.* 2007;33(12):1434–1439; discussion: 1439–1441.
13. Thomas DJ, King AR, Peat BG. Excision margins for nonmelanotic skin cancer. *Plast Reconstr Surg.* 2003;112(1):57–63.
14. Bisson MA, Dunkin CS, Suvarna SK, Griffiths RW. Do plastic surgeons resect basal cell carcinomas too widely? A prospective study comparing surgical and histological margins. *Br J Plast Surg.* 2002;55(4):293–297.

Additional Reading

Arora A, Attwood J. Common skin cancers and their precursors. *Surg Clin North Am.* 2009;89:703–712.

Firoz B, Davis N, Goldberg LH. Local anesthesia using buffered 0.5% lidocaine with 1:200,000 epinephrine for tumors of the digits treated with Mohs micrographic surgery. *J Am Acad Dermatol.* 2009;61:639–643.

Garbe C, Hauschild A, Volkenandt M, *et al.* Evidence and interdisciplinary consensus-based German guidelines: surgical treatment and radiotherapy of melanoma. *Melanoma Res.* 2008;18:61–67.

Garbe C, Peris K, Hauschild A, *et al.* Diagnosis and treatment of melanoma: European consensus-based interdisciplinary guideline. *Eur J Cancer.* 2010;46:270–283.

Lane JE, Kent DE. Surgical margins in the treatment of nonmelanoma skin cancer and Mohs micrographic surgery. *Curr Surg.* 2005;62:518–526.

Ricotti C, Bouzari N, Agadi A, Cockerell CJ. Malignant skin neoplasms. *Med Clin North Am.* 2009;93:1241–1264.

12 Cysts and Lipomas

JONATHAN KARNES, MD • JOHN L. PFENNINGER, MD •
RICHARD P. USATINE, MD

Removing "lumps and bumps" is common in an outpatient setting. The clinician often encounters a multitude of benign cystic lesions and lipomas on physical exam. The most common reasons to remove them include pain and discomfort, growth, discharge, infection or inflammation, and cosmetic concerns. These lesions present as masses and it can sometimes be hard to differentiate them from solid tumors or lymph nodes. Subsequently they may also need to be removed to verify a diagnosis. Epidermal inclusion cysts will frequently have a central punctum (pore) over them and be smooth. There is often a history of foul-smelling drainage. Lipomas are generally softer and more irregular. This chapter discusses treatment options for epidermal inclusion cysts, lipomas, and digital mucinous cysts. These comprise a large portion of the lumps and bumps encountered. An understanding of the basic approaches to each lesion should make treating them more efficient and effective.

EPIDERMAL INCLUSION CYSTS AND VARIANTS

Epidermal inclusion cysts arise from a plugged follicular opening, resulting in a nodular cyst filled with cheesy malodorous keratin material. These are also commonly and incorrectly called *sebaceous cysts* but do not in fact contain any sebum. Unfortunately, the ICD code for these cysts is named "sebaceous cyst" so you must know this misnomer for billing purposes. Other names include *infundibular cysts, keratinous cysts,* and *epidermoid cysts.* Generally, these present as a compressible but nonfluctuant nodule, which can be diagnosed clinically due to a comedo-like central punctum that can be distinguished at the apex (Figure 12-1). Because the keratin material inside the cyst wall is highly inflammatory, any cyst that has ruptured can spark a vigorous inflammatory response that can be mistaken for cellulitis (Figure 12-2). Even if these do become superinfected, the treatment of choice is incision and drainage to remove the inflammatory and/or infected contents.

Pilar cysts (also known as *trichilemmal cysts* and commonly called *wens*) are very similar to epidermal inclusion cysts with the exception that the capsule is much thicker and the location generally on the scalp (Figures 12-3 and 12-4). Pilar cysts rarely have a punctum but the thickness of the capsule makes removal somewhat easier. These can also become very large but in most cases they are 5 to 20 mm in size. It is not unusual for the hair to become thinned or actually stop growing over the cyst (Figures 12-3 and 12-4).

One variant of the epidermal cyst is the milium cyst. *Milia* are histologically identical to classic epidermal cysts but only grow to 1 to 2 mm. They are generally located around the eyes and central portion of the face (See Figure 33-20 in Chapter 33, *Procedures to Treat Benign Conditions*).

Cysts can be located almost anywhere but are common on the trunk, neck, face, and behind the ears. They range in size from millimeters to centimeters. Epidermal inclusion cysts are benign; however, there are rare proliferating epidermal inclusion cysts that can become carcinogenic. Any cyst that does not look 100% typical on excision should be sent to the pathologist. A full differential diagnosis is given in Box 12-1.

Dermoid cysts are far less common. They occur along congenital lines of cleavage (lingually, lateral eyes, behind the ears, and base of the nose) due to sequestration of embryonic cells. Unlike the common cyst, they are usually found in children and teenagers. So, young age is a warning sign for "something different." Facial cysts in young children need to be approached with caution and may need an imaging study before performing an excision.

The occurrence of multiple true sebaceous cysts at a younger age is termed *steatocystoma multiplex,* which is a genetically inherited problem. These capsules are extremely thin. Small fluid-filled very thin-walled cysts around the eyes are called *hidrocystomas* (Figure 12-8).

Several techniques for removing epidermal inclusion cysts and pilar cysts are described below. The best approach depends on size, location, and cyst condition. The minimal excision technique is simplest. Other methods include elliptical excision and incision and drainage with iodine crystals. Each offers advantages in select cases. Familiarity with various techniques balances preventing recurrence with maximizing efficiency and cosmetic outcome.

Indications for Cyst Removal

- Rapid growth
- Slowly increasing size
- Pain or discomfort
- Drainage
- Infection or inflammation
- Uncertain etiology
- Unsightly
- Recurrence from previous removal attempt.

Contraindications for Cyst Removal

- Avoid trying to remove cysts that are *actively inflamed* (Figure 12-2). Although it can be done successfully,

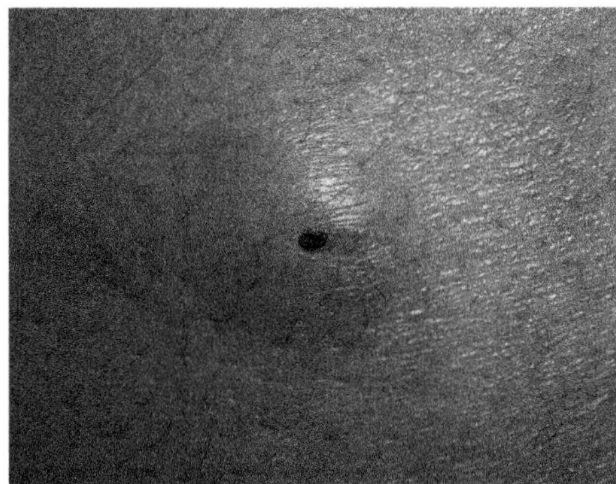

FIGURE 12-1 An epidermal inclusion cyst with a central punctum that looks like an open comedone. *(Copyright Richard P. Usatine, MD.)*

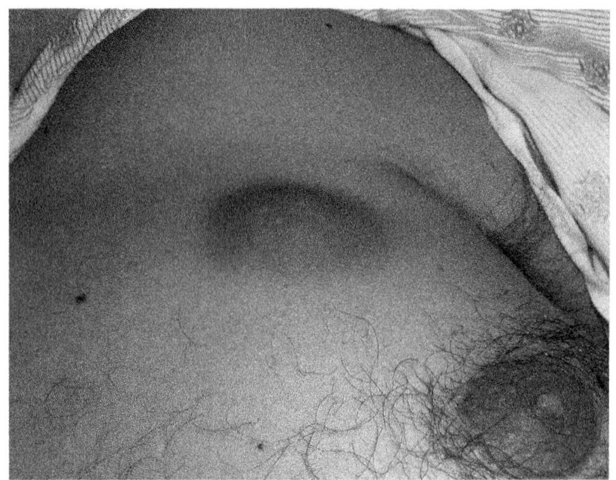

FIGURE 12-2 Local inflammation around an epidermal inclusion cyst can mimic cellulitis or an abscess. The best treatment is incision and drainage. *(Copyright Richard P. Usatine, MD.)*

BOX 12-1 ***Differential Diagnosis of Epidermal Inclusion Cysts***

Bartholin's cyst (Figure 12-5)
Branchial cleft cyst (Figure 12-6)
Comedones
Dermoid cyst
Hidradenoma (Figure 12-7)
Hidrocystoma (Figure 12-8)
Keratoacanthoma (see Figure 34-17, Chapter 34)
Lipoma
Liposarcoma
Lymphadenopathy
Milia (see Figure 33-20, Chapter 33)
Mucinous cystadenoma (Figure 12-9)
Mucoceles (See Figure 33-22, Chapter 33)
Mucoid/myxoid/ganglion cyst (Figure 12-10)
Neurofibromas (See Figure 33-30, Chapter 33)
Parotid tumor
Pilonidal cyst (Figure 12-11)
Proliferating trichilemmal cyst/malignant trichilemmal cyst
Steatocystoma
Thyroglossal duct cyst (Figure 12-12)

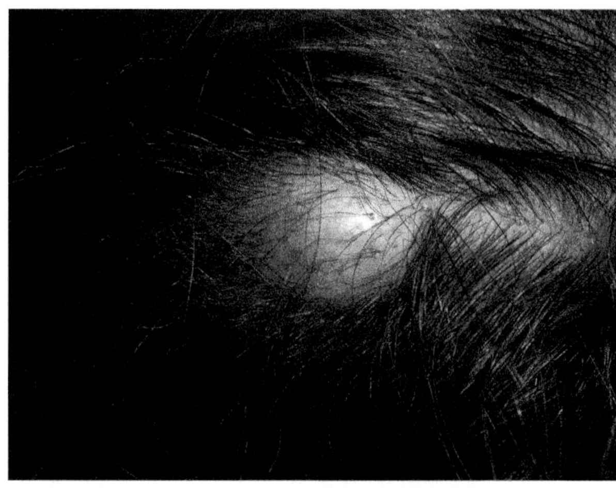

FIGURE 12-3 A typical presentation of a pilar cyst (trichilemmal cyst or wen) on the scalp. *(Copyright Richard P. Usatine, MD.)*

wound healing may be impaired. The keratinaceous material in epidermal inclusion cysts is highly immunogenic and an inflamed cyst should be treated with incision and drainage and allowed to heal before attempting to remove the cyst wall. Antibiotics are rarely helpful. Small lesions can be excised going around the entire area of inflammation.[1]

- Make note of the surrounding anatomy and the size/depth of tissue that contains the cyst. Consider deferring or referring lesions that overlie areas such as large vascular networks, special sensory organs, or cosmetically sensitive areas. With experience, these areas may be managed in the office, but this depends on comfort, experience, and support services. Be aware of the spinal accessory nerve when neck lesions are involved because the nerve lies immediately under the skin and can be easily severed, leading to difficulty in abducting the arm (See Figure 11-4 in Chapter 11). Also be careful to not cut the temporal branch of the facial nerve with cysts

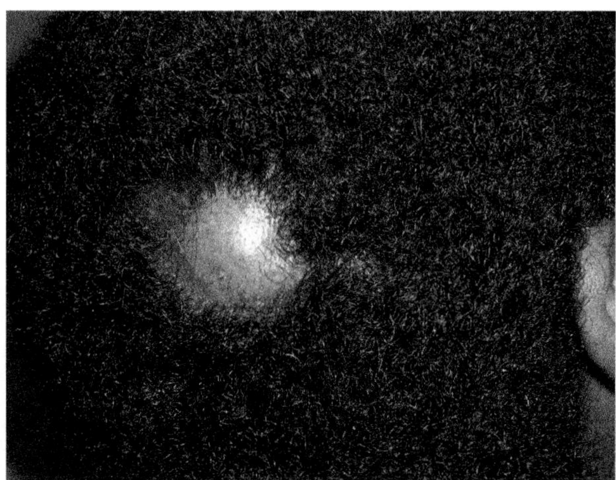

FIGURE 12-4 A fairly large pilar cyst with hair loss over the cyst. A simple ellipse over the cyst will remove redundant tissue. *(Copyright Richard P. Usatine, MD.)*

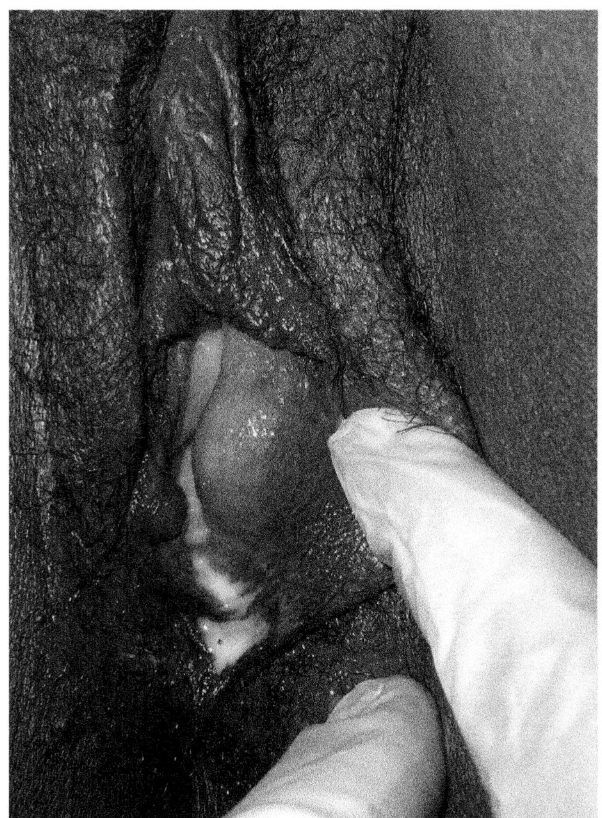

FIGURE 12-5 A Bartholin's duct cyst. *(Copyright Richard P. Usatine, MD.)*

over the temple (See Figures 11-2 and 11-3 in Chapter 11).

- Diagnosis is usually made on clinical grounds before proceeding with removal. Keep the differential in mind even though the diagnosis may seem certain (Box 12-1). For example, a dermoid cyst on the face can communicate with the cerebrospinal fluid in some circumstances. Consider imaging for a possible dermoid cyst if the cyst has been present on the face since early childhood and is midline (Figure 12-13).

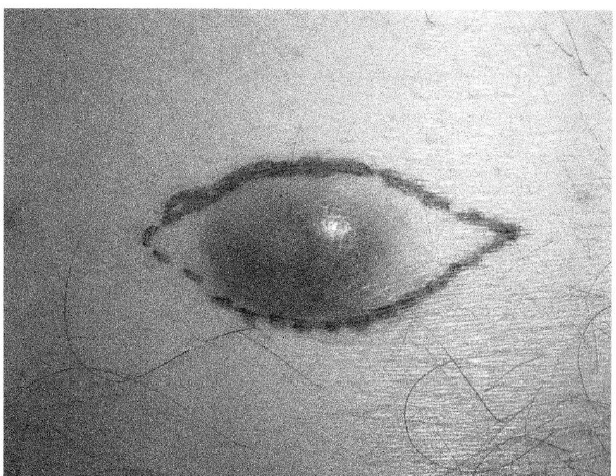

FIGURE 12-7 A solid cystic hidradenoma. *(Copyright Richard P. Usatine, MD.)*

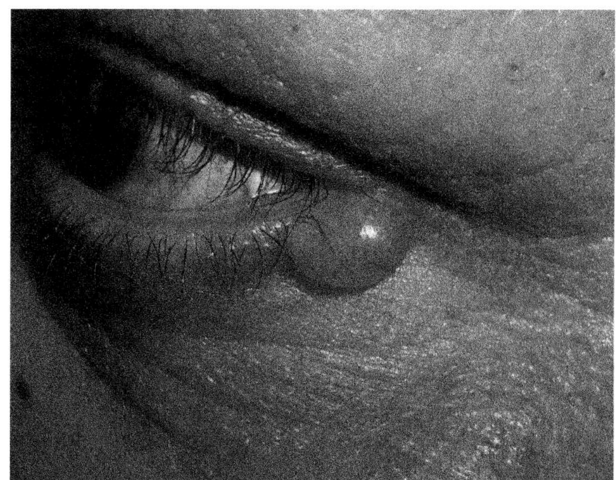

FIGURE 12-8 Hidrocystomas around the eye. It is benign and has a very thin wall that is easy to cut. *(Copyright Richard P. Usatine, MD.)*

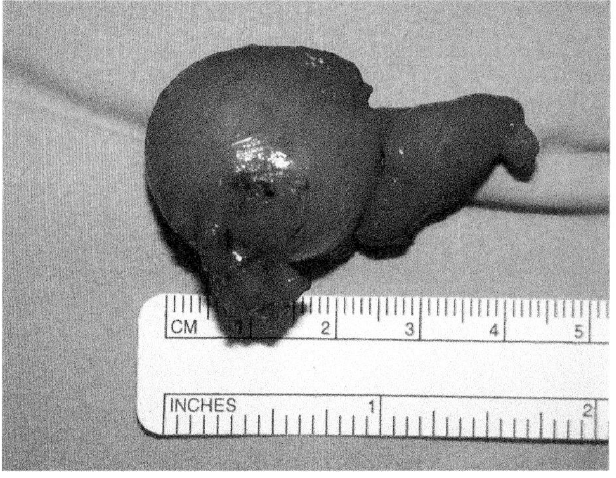

FIGURE 12-6 A branchial cleft cyst after removal. *(Courtesy of Frank Miller, MD.)*

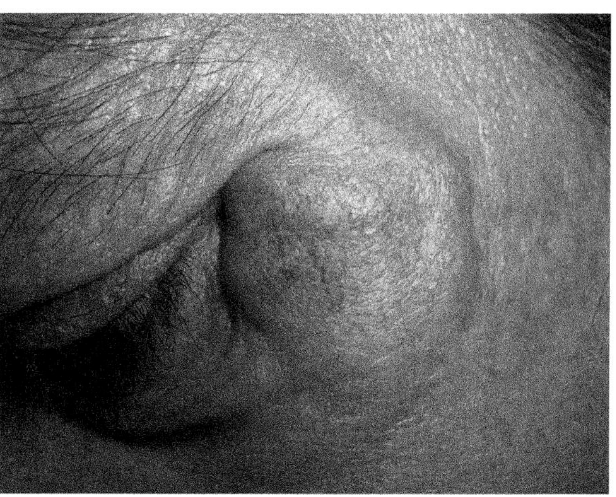

FIGURE 12-9 A mucinous cystadenoma near the eye. *(Copyright Richard P. Usatine, MD.)*

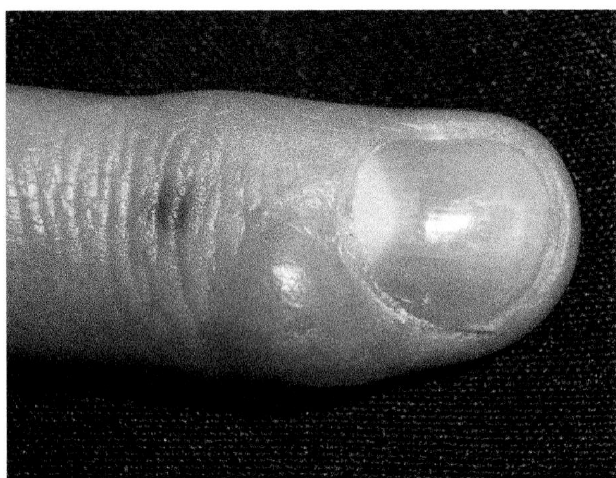

FIGURE 12-10 Digital mucous (myxoid) cyst on the finger. They are most commonly found distal to the DIP joint. *(Copyright Richard P. Usatine, MD.)*

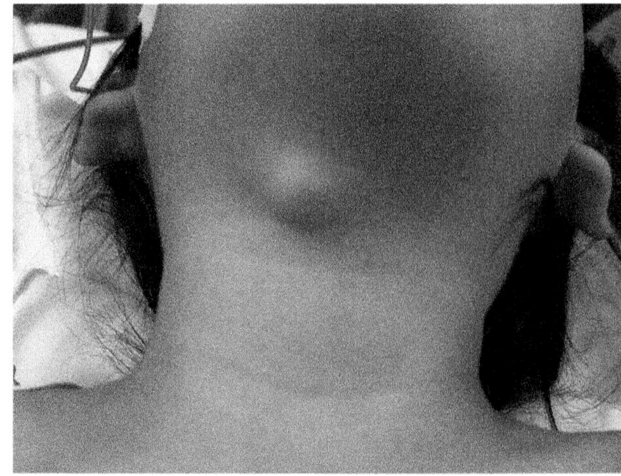

FIGURE 12-12 A thyroglossal duct cyst in a young girl. Note how it is midline. These will move up with swallowing. *(Courtesy of Frank Miller, MD.)*

When encountering something atypical, send samples to pathology, or confer with a colleague before proceeding.

MINIMAL EXCISION TECHNIQUE

See video on the DVD for further learning. 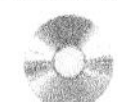

The minimal incision technique for removing cysts involves purposefully incising the cyst wall and expressing its contents allowing cyst removal through a smaller incision (linear opening or small punch rather than a larger ellipse that surrounds the cyst).

Advantages

Use of the minimal excision technique is becoming increasingly common for epidermal cyst removal. Its advantages can be subdivided into those for the physician and those for the patient.

Advantages of the minimal excision technique for the clinician include the following:

- Requires only a few routine instruments.
- Special prepping and draping are not needed.
- Utilizes a very small incision.
- May not require suture material.
- The procedure is quick.
- Easy to learn.

Advantages for the patient include the following:

- Results in excellent cosmetic outcomes.
- No need for second appointment and often no need to return for suture removal.
- Wound healing is faster.
- Generally it is a same-day treatment.

Disadvantages

Disadvantages of the minimal excision technique for the clinician include:

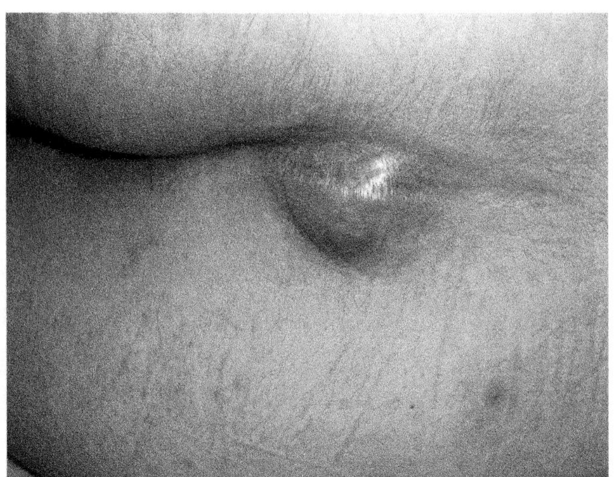

FIGURE 12-11 Pilonidal cyst. *(Copyright Richard P. Usatine, MD.)*

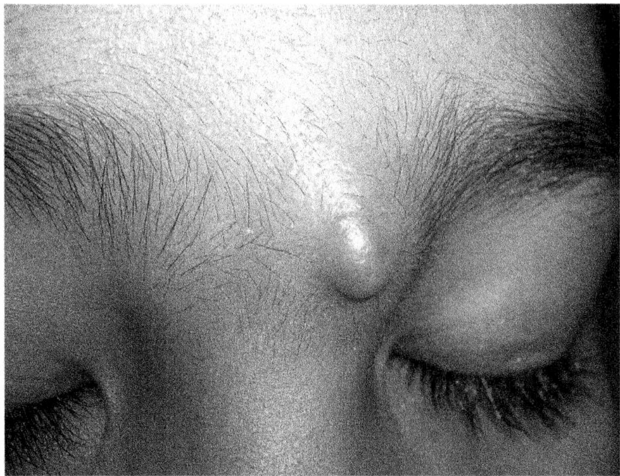

FIGURE 12-13 A midline dermoid cyst on the face of a young girl. *(Copyright Richard P. Usatine, MD.)*

- It is more challenging to remove the entire cyst wall.
- Part of the procedure involves the expression of pungent cyst contents.

Disadvantages for the patient include:

- The chance of recurrence is slightly increased.
- Not all lesions can be successfully treated with this technique.

Do not use this method if:

- The lesion is inflamed (sack is very tenuous, like wet tissue paper).
- It is a recurrent lesion.
- The lesion is large (more than 4 cm).
- The patient has manipulated the lesion significantly and there is likelihood of adhesions/scarring.

Be aware that this procedure is more difficult where the skin is very thick such as on the back.

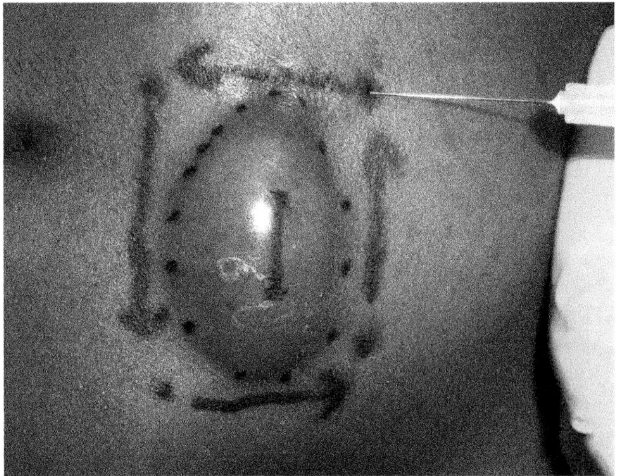

FIGURE 12-14 Epidermal cyst on the face is outlined before injecting anesthesia. The solid line is drawn to match skin lines and to be about 40% of the diameter of the cyst. A ring block is marked with four arrows and each injection starts at the end of the previous arrow. *(Copyright Richard P. Usatine, MD.)*

Equipment

For the minimal excision technique, you will need the following:

- Either a No. 11 scalpel or a 4-mm disposable punch biopsy
- Marking pen
- 3- to 5-mL syringe with a 27- to 30-gauge needle for anesthesia
- Sterile gauze
- Tissue scissors
- Forceps
- Suture or skin tape (optional).

It is helpful to use a face shield and a gown to cover your clothing while injecting the anesthesia and performing the surgery. Cysts can squirt their contents into your face and onto your clothes.

Minimal Excision Technique: Steps and Principles

See video on the DVD for further learning. 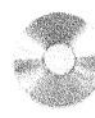

Preoperative Measures

- After determining that the minimal excision technique is the best method for the patient, obtain informed consent. (See Appendix A for an informed consent form titled *Disclosure and Consent: Medical and Surgical Procedures.*)
- Determine the apex of the lesion. This is sometimes around a punctum (Figure 12-1).
- Prep the area with an antiseptic such as chlorhexidine or alcohol. Mark the apex with a line (Figure 12-14), a small ellipse, or a small circle to orient a punch depending on which technique is chosen to enter the cyst wall. It is also worthwhile to draw a circle around the widest margins of the cyst (Figure 12-14). You may use a fenestrated drape if you plan to place a suture.
- Inject anesthetic around the cyst with a 27- to 30-gauge needle. Avoid injecting anesthesia directly into the cyst because it may squirt cyst contents out of the punctum, producing an unpleasant smell (Figure 12-14). If the anesthesia enters the cyst and does not squirt out it may cause increased pain for the patient as the pressure builds inside the cyst. It is best to plan to inject around the cyst performing a ring block. In Figure 12-14 the arrows show how you can start at one corner of a square and inject at the arrow ahead each time so that the new injection will be less painful from the effect of the preceding injection. A fifth injection may be added to the skin above the cyst at the site for the planned incision to ensure a painless surgery (Figure 12-15). In Figure 12-16 the pressure of the anesthesia has caused some keratin to be extruded from the punctum without any harm.

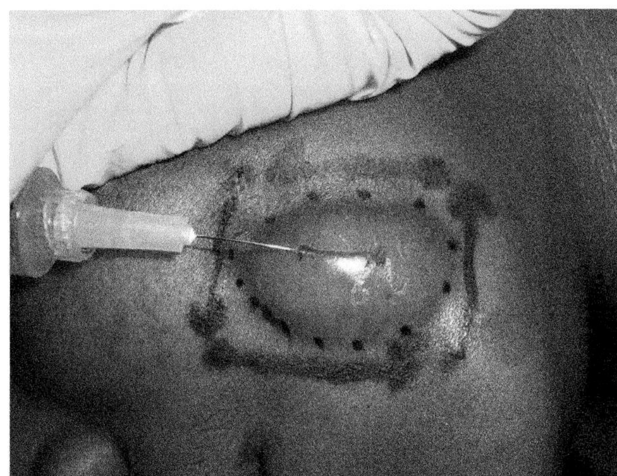

FIGURE 12-15 The ring block has been performed without injecting into the cyst. The final injection is given over the cyst to make sure that the incision line is fully anesthetized. *(Copyright Richard P. Usatine, MD.)*

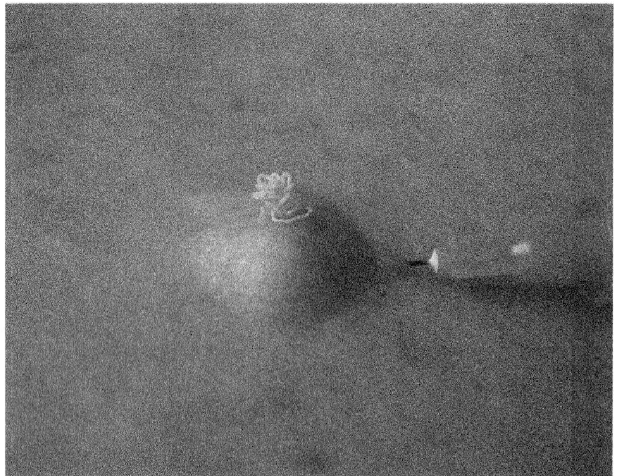

FIGURE 12-16 An otherwise invisible punctum is discovered when lidocaine creates pressure inside the cyst extruding keratin from the punctum. *(Copyright Richard P. Usatine, MD.)*

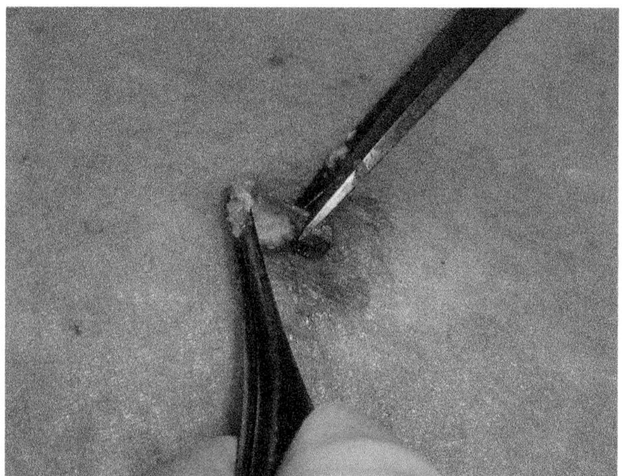

FIGURE 12-18 A small emptied cyst is pulled through a small punch opening and freed from underlying tissue using an iris scissor. *(Copyright Richard P. Usatine, MD.)*

Performing the Procedure

- Stretch the skin to anchor the lesion. Incise a linear or punch opening (Figure 12-17A and B) over the cyst apex and into the cyst itself. Alternatively, cut a small ellipse instead of a linear or circular opening.
- Express all cyst contents with firm digital pressure on the cyst and surrounding tissue (Figure 12-17C). Keep plenty of 4 × 4 gauze on the field to mop up the contents of the cyst.
- Identify the cyst wall and dissect it from surrounding tissues using blunt dissection with an iris scissor or curved hemostat. Curved iris scissors or any curved tissue scissors work very well. Once a small area has been dissected, you may grasp the cyst wall with forceps or hemostat (Figure 12-17D). Continue blunt dissection until the cyst wall is able to be pulled through your incision.
- Sometimes the skin incision needs to be extended or deepened to extract the entire cyst contents.
- If the cyst is attached to the fascia below, just snip this fibrous tissue with a scissor (Figure 12-18).
- Inspect the material removed. You should have extracted a nearly complete cyst wall (Figures 12-19 and 12-20). Pilar cysts have a thicker wall and are

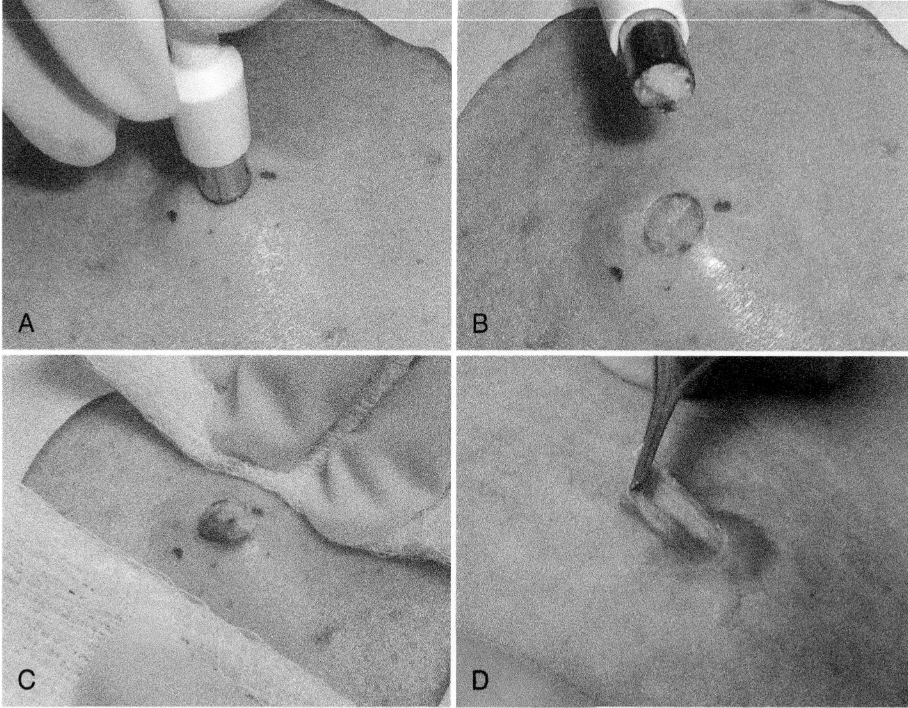

FIGURE 12-17 **(A)** A 4-mm punch creates an opening into the underlying epidermal inclusion cyst. **(B)** The punch is removed and the keratinaceous material is seen inside the punch and in the cyst. **(C)** The cyst contents are expressed with pressure from both sides. **(D)** The cyst wall is shiny and seen being pulled through the punch incision. *(Copyright Richard P. Usatine, MD.)*

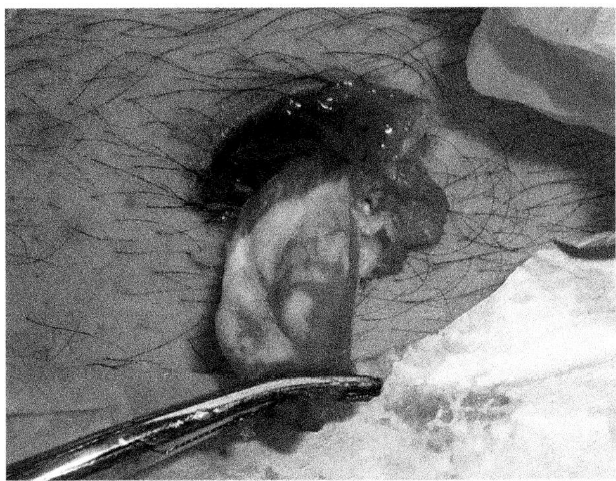

FIGURE 12-19 Pulling a large emptied cyst wall through the opening created by an ellipse in the abdominal wall. *(Copyright Richard P. Usatine, MD.)*

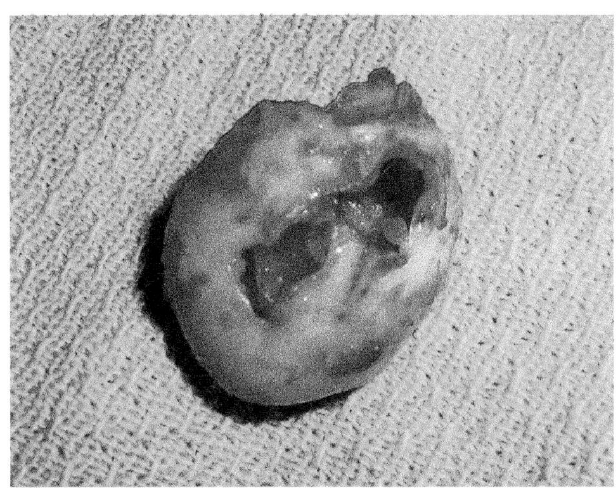

FIGURE 12-21 Pilar cyst has a thick wall and keeps its spherical anatomy in most cases even if it was cut and emptied. *(Copyright Richard P. Usatine, MD.)*

easier to extract intact than an epidermal cyst (Figure 12-21). You may be able to piece sections together like a jigsaw puzzle to make sure that the entire cyst is out.

- Inspect the cavity and be sure all of the (white) cyst wall has been removed.
- Sterile cotton-tipped applicators are useful for probing the cavity and cleaning out remaining cyst contents.
- Consider irrigating the cavity and surrounding skin with sterile saline or water especially if any cyst contents spilled into the incision.
- Repair the defect. With the minimal excision technique, often no closure is needed. If desired, the skin may be approximated with 4-0 to 6-0 nylon or polypropylene. Skin tapes may also be used. If a large cyst was removed through an elliptical excision, consider placing a deep layer of buried absorbable sutures to close the dead space. Some clinicians choose to not close small pilar cyst excisions and get good results. Sutures have the advantage of providing hemostasis and approximating the epidermis.[2]

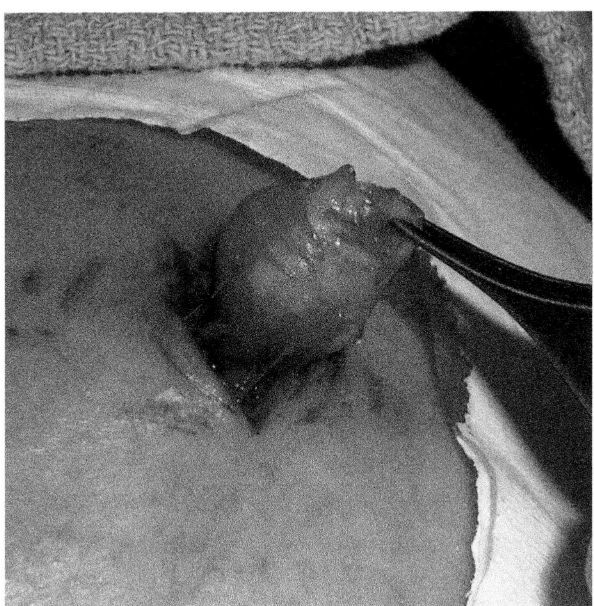

FIGURE 12-20 A relatively intact epidermal cyst near the shoulder is extracted through a linear incision. Many epidermal cysts are not so well encapsulated. *(Copyright Richard P. Usatine, MD.)*

Pathology

Benign-appearing typical cysts do not need to be sent to the pathologist. If a solid tumor is found, or if there is any irregularity about the procedure or uncertainty about the diagnosis, send the specimen. Note the possible differential diagnoses in Box 12-1.

Alternatives to the Minimal Excision Technique

A couple of alternatives to the minimal excision technique are worth discussing.

Elliptical Excision

Full elliptical excisions are covered in Chapter 11. This technique may be a good option if cysts have been heavily manipulated or have recurred. One approach is to avoid cutting into the cyst wall and attempting to remove the cyst whole. Another approach is similar to the minimal cyst removal in which the cyst is cut on purpose and the contents are evacuated to allow the cyst to be removed through a smaller ellipse. If the cyst is large and elevated, make sure the width of the ellipse is equal to the width of the cyst to avoid dog ears (standing cones).[3] This is especially true with large protuberant pilar cysts (Figure 12-22). The scalp will not lay flat unless the ellipse is as long as the cyst. The elliptical excision method is preferred with any large protuberant cysts that would leave redundant skin if the cyst is excised through a punch or a linear incision.

Incision and Drainage Plus Iodine Crystals

One alternative consists of a combination incision and drainage (I&D) of the cyst followed by placing two

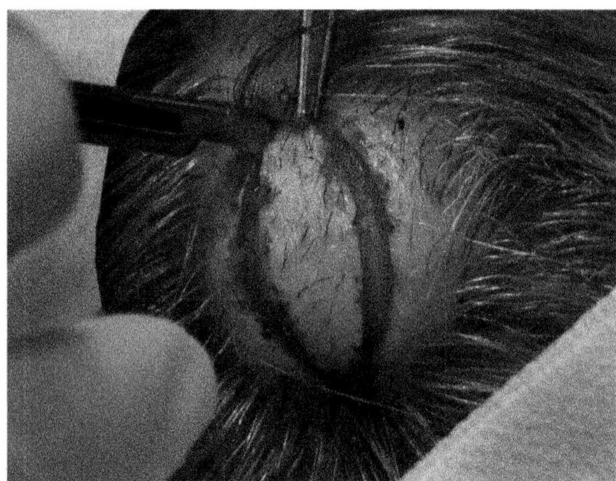

FIGURE 12-22 This large pilar cyst will be removed through an ellipse that extends across the full diameter of the cyst. This will allow the scalp to lay flat once the cyst is removed. If the ellipse is made shorter, then standing cones will result on both sides of the repaired defect. Note that the hairs were clipped with a scissor rather than shaving the scalp. Shaving increases risk of infection, but snipping with a scissor makes the surgery easier with no increased infection risks. *(Copyright Richard P. Usatine, MD.)*

iodine crystals in the center of the cyst. Over a period of several days, the cyst will harden and darken. This may then be expressed through the skin on the return visit. This is a fairly simple technique with similar cosmetic results to the minimal excision technique. It does however, require a follow-up visit and some patience as the cyst darkens and hardens. Iodine crystals USP are available from the pharmacy. The size used is dependent on the size of the cyst. It works well for cysts up to about 2 cm.[2]

Incision and Drainage of Inflamed and Infected Cysts

When patients present with an acutely inflamed or possibly infected cyst, the treatment is to incise, drain, and pack the wound. The same principles apply as those described in Chapter 17, *Incision and Drainage*. Use a ring block for anesthesia and a No. 11 blade scalpel to incise the inflamed area. Because the incision will be packed and not closed, clean technique is adequate. Antibiotics are rarely beneficial because the majority of these inflammatory changes are due to a reaction to the ruptured contents rather than a true infection. Antibiotics are not needed especially after an I&D, nor are cultures. Some clinicians may want to culture and use antibiotics in immune-suppressed patients, but even then the definitive treatment is I&D.

Hidrocystomas

Hidrocystomas (Figure 12-8) can be easily excised using pickups and cutting a small thin ellipse over the cyst with a sharp tissue scissor. The fluid will drain out easily. There should be little bleeding so pressure alone should be adequate for hemostasis.

Dermoid Cysts

Be aware of the precautions cited earlier. If a dermoid cyst (Figure 12-13) is suspected, excisional removal is indicated. If a dermoid cyst is found on the face of a young child, refer for removal under sedation or general anesthesia.

Complications

Complications of any cyst removal technique include incomplete removal of the cyst leading to recurrence, localized inflammatory reactions to retained cyst material, seroma and hematoma formation, infection, and scar formation. Careful attention to the cyst wall and to keeping the incision free of cyst contents will help with wound healing and preventing significant inflammation. Seromas and hematomas will present with swelling and pain. Usually aspiration of the underlying fluid will completely relieve these symptoms and should not affect final outcome.

LIPOMAS

Lipomas are subcutaneous benign tumors composed of adipose tissue held together with connective tissue. Although they may be encapsulated, in general they are more amorphous, lobulated masses that are either slightly lighter or darker than surrounding adipose. Often it is nearly indistinguishable from normal tissue by color, but the fat may be held together so that it is separate from the surrounding subcutaneous fat. Lesions typically arise after the fourth decade of life and present as single or multilobed soft tumors that are easily compressible and have a doughy consistency. Lipomas most commonly arise over the neck and trunk, though they can also be found on the extremities and face. Usually patients complain of lipomas when they are located on pressure-bearing areas and become painful, when they arise in cosmetically sensitive areas, or when they become very large. In these cases, and in instances of rapid growth, it is reasonable to remove them. Another indication would be if the diagnosis is in doubt.

Lipomas can usually be diagnosed clinically, although the differential diagnosis includes many of the same entities discussed for cysts (Box 12-1). Additional considerations are hematoma, panniculitis, rheumatic nodules, and metastatic cancer. Rapidly growing subcutaneous masses should be removed and sent for pathology. Several approaches are used to remove lipomas: incision and expression, elliptical excision, and liposuction.

Indications for Lipoma Removal

Indications for removal of lipomas include:

- Symptomatic lesions (causing pain, discomfort, or anxiety)
- Cosmetic concerns
- Clarifying a diagnosis

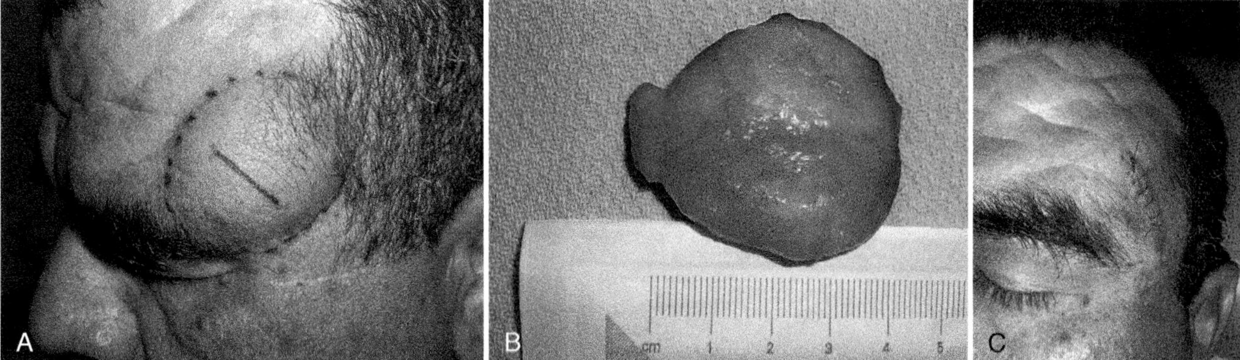

FIGURE 12-23 (A) Lipoma on the temple/forehead is marked with a dotted line around the circumference and a solid line to guide the incision along skin lines. (B) Lipoma removed without damage to the temporal branch of the facial nerve. (C) Linear incision closed with running sutures. *(Copyright Richard P. Usatine, MD.)*

- Clinical depth below the fascia
- Rapid growth.

Contraindications for Lipoma Removal

There are no contraindications other than patient preference to leave superficial lipomas alone.

General Considerations

Liposarcomas can appear similar to lipomas, but do not arise from lipomas. In the case of some worrisome lesions, first consider needle aspiration or imaging.[4,5] However, a full excision will always give the best sampling of the lesion to the pathologist.

Anatomic considerations are important as well. Lesions that present in the sacroiliac region can occasionally communicate with the spinal column. Here, consider consulting with neurosurgery or ruling out nerve involvement by obtaining an MRI. Also of note, lipomas on the forehead can track behind the fascial plane and under the frontalis muscle. Forehead lipomas are frequently removed in the office but contrary to most other lipomas, are not as discrete and thus are more difficult to remove (Figure 12-23). On exam they will generally feel larger than they actually are, causing the surgeon to question if the lesion was really removed. Despite these caveats, lipoma excisions are generally straightforward.

Preoperative

- After obtaining informed consent, prep the area with chlorhexidine. Mark the borders of the lipoma with a surgical marking pen (Figure 12-23A). Locate the best area for the linear incision or punch biopsy and mark it with the marking pen taking into account skin lines and cosmetic considerations (Figure 12-23A). The incision need not be directly in the center of the lesion.
- Inject 1% lidocaine with epinephrine directly into the lipoma and the skin above it. Make sure that the skin that will be incised is well anesthetized.

INCISION AND PRESSURE METHOD

See video on the DVD for further learning. 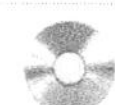

The easiest method to remove lipomas is the *incision and pressure method*. Draw out the linear incision so that it is approximately one-third to one-half the diameter of the lipoma (Figure 12-24A). Make a linear incision through the skin over the top of the lipoma. Hold the No. 11 blade perpendicular to the skin and cut through the skin into the lipoma with a sawing motion. Fortunately, lipomas are relatively avascular so little bleeding should be encountered. If there is much bleeding, reassess the diagnosis and procedure immediately.

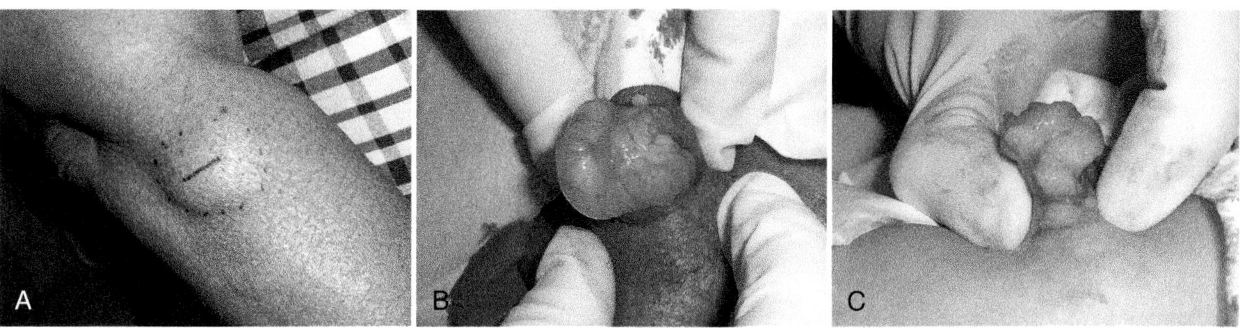

FIGURE 12-24 (A) Lipoma on the forearm marked for linear incision and removal. (B) The lipoma is extruded from the incision with the pressure from four fingers. (C) Firm pressure around and below the lipoma delivers it through the small opening with one hand. *(Copyright Richard P. Usatine, MD.)*

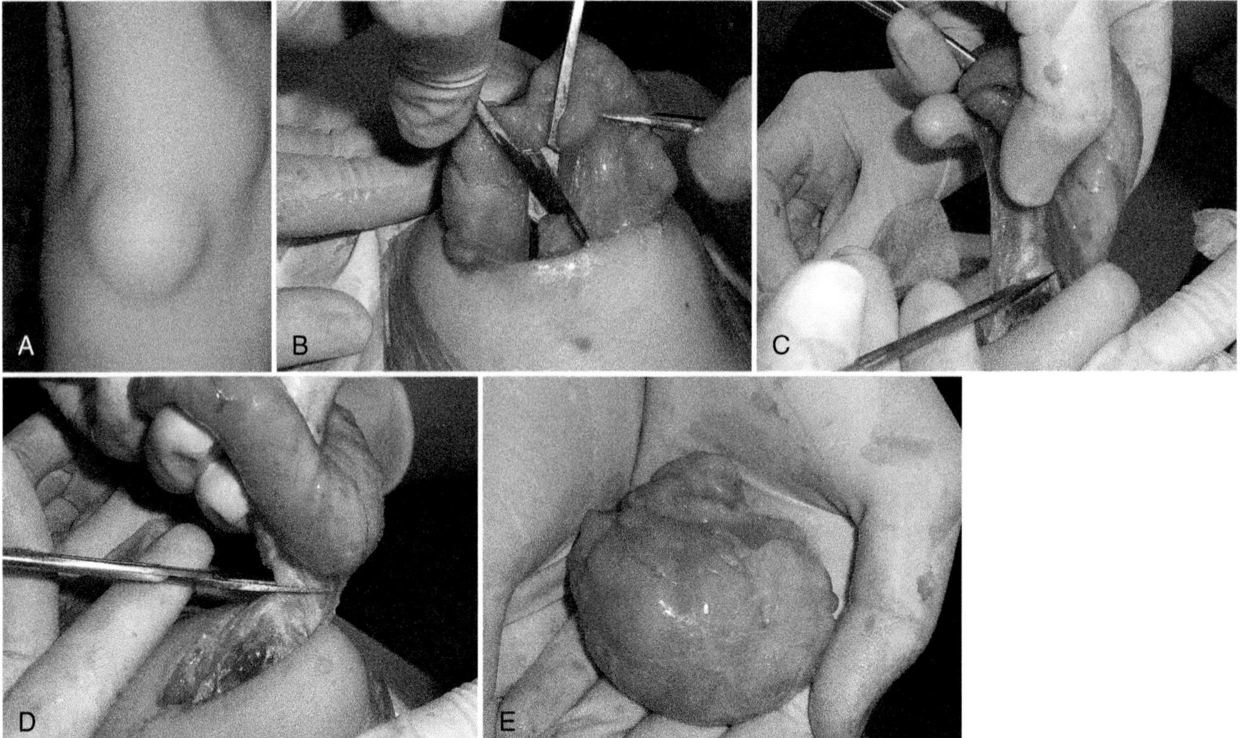

FIGURE 12-25 (A) Large lipoma overlying the left latissimus dorsi muscle of a young man. (B) Use a curved hemostat to separate the lipoma from surrounding tissues. (C) Cut the lipoma from its attachments below. (D) Final release of the lipoma shows that it was lying directly on the chest wall muscles. (E) Large partially encapsulated lipoma in the hand for examination. *(Copyright Richard P. Usatine, MD.)*

Once the incision has been made, insert and spread the curved hemostats around the edge of the lipoma to break up the fibrous bands that attach it to the surrounding tissue. Do this through 360 degrees and try to get under the lipoma as well. Then express the lipoma through the incision using digital pressure (Figure 12-24B). If this does not work, use the hemostat again to free the lipoma further. If this still does not work, consider extending the incision on both sides to give more room for the lipoma to come out. Pulling the lipoma with the hemostat clamped on it can help while an assistant is squeezing the lipoma out from below with digital pressure.

Once the lipoma is out, see if it appears whole and explore the cavity to make sure the entire lipoma has been removed. Bleeding should be nonexistent to minimal. Hold pressure on the defect to express any blood or fluid. The incision can be closed with simple interrupted sutures or subcuticular sutures. If the defect is large consider placing some deep sutures to close dead space (see Chapter 6, *Suturing Techniques*). Some clinicians use Steri-Strips with no sutures underneath a pressure dressing. With experience and efficient office staff, this procedure can be done in 10 minutes. Even a large lipoma can be removed using this method (Figure 12-25).

EXAMINATION AND PATHOLOGY

Inspect the lipoma and feel it between your fingers. It should be a contiguous yellow mass without significant vascularity or calcifications (Figure 12-25E). Any hint of abnormality or odd behavior of the tissue during the procedure should prompt you to send the specimen for pathology. Any lesions with significant vascularity, size, calcifications, or other worrisome features should be sent to pathology to confirm a benign diagnosis.

PUNCH (ENUCLEATION) TECHNIQUE

The punch technique can be used to remove lipomas. Enucleation involves entering the lipoma through a small punch through the dermis and scooping out, or enucleating, the lipoma with a small curette.

Equipment

- 4- to 6-mm punch biopsy tool
- 3-mm skin curette
- Tissue scissors
- Hemostat.

Removing the Lipoma

- Center the punch tool over the lipoma, stretching the skin perpendicular to the skin lines. With a twisting motion, punch through the dermis and into the lipoma.
- Insert the curette through the incision and using a finger as a guide and boundary on the surface, begin to free the lipoma by scraping it from the surrounding tissue.

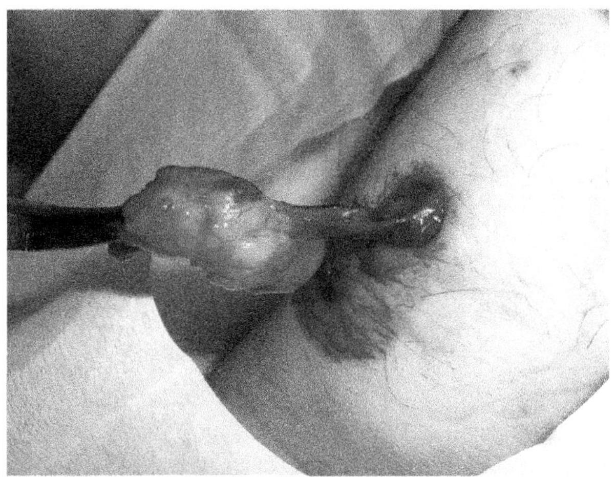

FIGURE 12-26 Small lipoma being extracted through a 6-mm punch incision. *(Copyright Richard P. Usatine, MD.)*

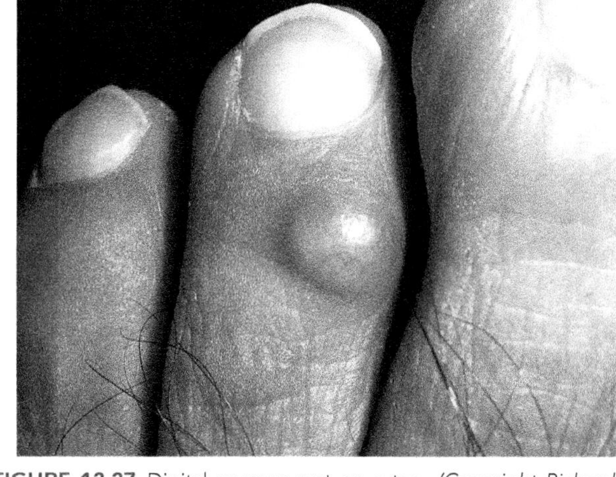

FIGURE 12-27 Digital mucous cyst on a toe. *(Copyright Richard P. Usatine, MD.)*

- Bring a section of the lipoma through the opening and grasp it with a hemostat. Continue to curette until the entire lesion is delivered out of the small opening (Figure 12-26). Firm digital pressure around the lipoma will aid in the extraction.
- For larger lipomas some advocate multiple small incisions or punches to perform segmental extraction.[6]
- A 6-mm punch may be used for larger lipomas.
- For small lipomas a punch biopsy may be used as the opening and the lipoma can be extracted manually without a curette similar to the method described for the linear incision technique.

ELLIPTICAL EXCISION OF A LIPOMA

A true *elliptical excision* for removal can be practical for larger lipomas or those under thick skin (back of the neck, posterior trunk) and with lesions that are of uncertain diagnosis or unusually firm. The elliptical excision is covered fully in Chapter 11. It may be more helpful to leave the elliptical piece of skin attached to the dermis and use the skin as a convenient handle to manipulate the lipoma with a hemostat, clamp, or forceps. The scar will be larger using this technique, but in some instances that is not a concern.

COMPLICATIONS OF LIPOMA REMOVAL

Complications to lipoma removal include scarring, formation of hematomas or seromas, infection, and recurrence. The linear incision and enucleation methods should minimize any scarring by virtue of limiting the size of the incision and having an incision that is not under pressure after the lipoma is removed. Seromas and hematomas are rare but can be treated with aspiration or expression. These are better addressed before they form by applying a pressure dressing after the surgery is completed.

DIGITAL MUCOUS (MYXOID) CYSTS

Digital mucous cysts or myxoid cysts are similar to ganglia but arise on the distal fingers and occasionally toes (Figures 12-27 and 12-28). These are the most common cysts on the hand and are benign. The exact etiology is uncertain, but the cysts likely form from the mucoid degeneration associated with arthritis. Cysts usually present after the fifth decade of life, but can present earlier when associated with arthropathy such as rheumatoid arthritis. The most common location is the distal interphalangeal joint, on the dorsal aspect. Lesions that occur in the proximal nail fold can distort the lunula, put pressure on the matrix, and cause nail deformities and pain (Figure 12-28).

When treatment is sought, options range from observation to joint surgery with osteophyte removal and flap reconstruction. In the office setting, the most common options are draining with repeat sterile needling and cryotherapy.[1,2] Alternatives include the

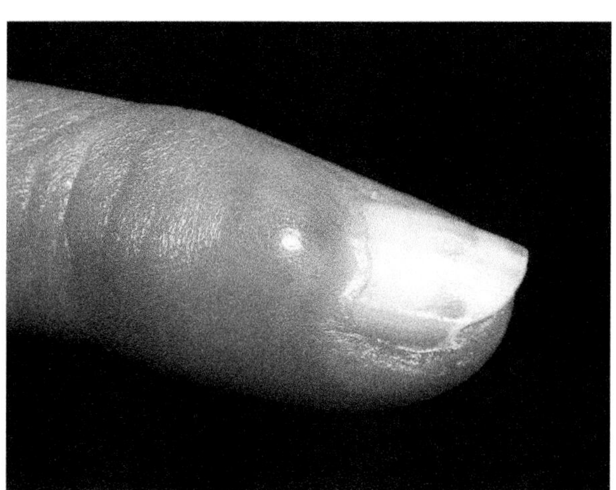

FIGURE 12-28 Digital mucous cyst causing nail deformity. The pressure of the cyst on the matrix typically causes a depressed trough. *(Copyright Richard P. Usatine, MD.)*

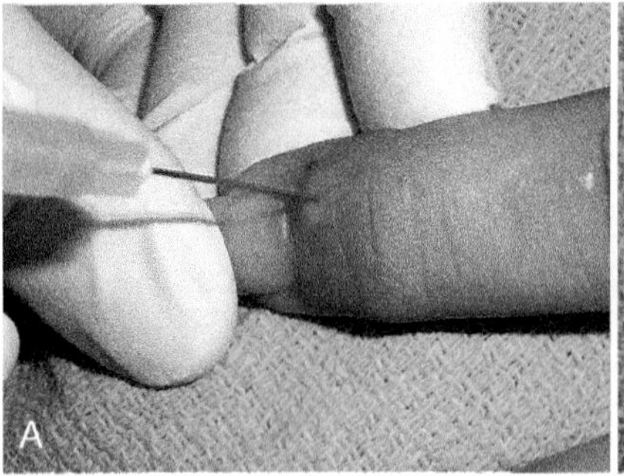

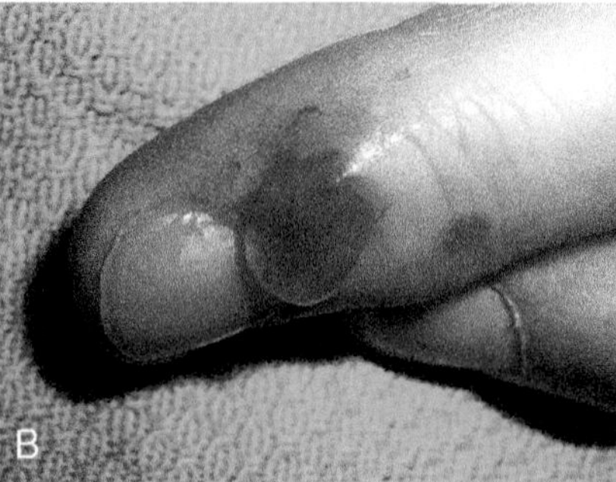

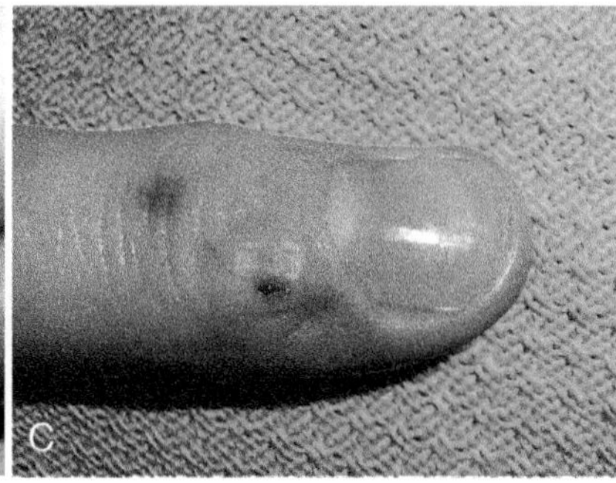

FIGURE 12-29 **(A)** Needling a digital mucous cyst. **(B)** The gelatinous material is similar to synovial fluid. **(C)** Collapsed digital mucous cyst. *(Copyright Richard P. Usatine, MD.)*

injection of sclerosing agents, steroid injections, or excision with flap repair. All options risk recurrence with radical joint surgery as the most definitive and most costly option.

Indications for Treating Digital Mucous Cysts

- Painful digital mucous cysts
- Distortion of the nail plate (Figure 12-28).

Contraindications for Treating Digital Mucous Cysts

- An infected cyst should be managed medically with antibiotics first.

Needling and Cryotherapy

- Obtain informed consent and discuss the small risk of scarring, nail deformities, infection in the joint space, and recurrence (10% to 15% with cryotherapy).[7]
- Offer to provide local anesthesia with lidocaine. This can be done with 1% to 2% lidocaine without epinephrine with a 30-gauge needle at the site of the cyst.
- Prep the area with an alcohol swab.
- Puncture the lesion with multiple needlesticks and drain out the thick clear to serous fluid inside (Figure 12-29).
- Using a cryosurgery probe or spray nozzle, create an ice ball with a diameter 2 to 3 mm beyond the extent of the cyst (Figure 12-30). Let this thaw and repeat.

Alternatives to Cryotherapy

Minami *et al.*[7] described a method of cryotherapy that involved direct contact with a probe or liquid nitrogen–soaked cotton tipped swab applied over a thin plastic film after the pseudocyst had been drained. Presumably this prevented cotton contents from adhering to the tissue. After a median of 2.64 treatments, they had an 85% to 92% cure rate.

Another very good alternative is serial needling. This can be done in the office or at home by a capable patient who is given sterile needles. The success rate is 70% with minimal expense aside from office visits.[8] Another option is excision of the cyst in the office with a small rotation flap pinned with two small sutures. This requires a digital block and a surgical tray, but the long-term cure rate may rival joint surgery.[9] A similar but simpler technique was described wherein a three-sided or fingertip-shaped pedicle is created around the cyst and undermined—creating a small flap. Then, instead of rotating or transposing the cyst containing flap, tack it back down with one or two sutures. The scarring that forms theoretically blocks a path from the joint space to the cyst.[10]

CODING AND BILLING PEARLS

Epidermal cysts (ICD-9 code 706.2) are skin lesions and as such, excisions are coded by the size of the cyst, the location, and the fact that they are benign. Simple excision and repair includes the anesthetic, the excision, the repair, and suture removal. The size is based on the size of the cyst, not the size of the incision so a minimal cyst removal is not compensated at a lower rate because the incision was shorter. Additional charges are made for an intermediate closure if deep sutures are needed to close dead space or approximate wound edges under

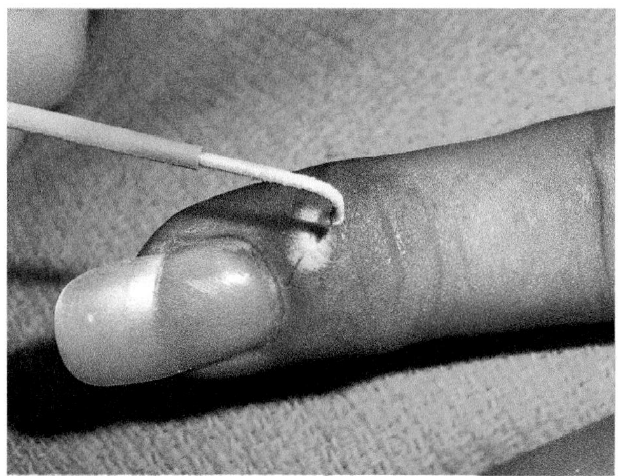

FIGURE 12-30 Cryotherapy of a digital mucous cyst after it was punctured with a needle and drained. Aim for a 2-mm margin of freeze around the lesion. *(Copyright Richard P. Usatine, MD.)*

tension. The intermediate closure charge is based on the size of the final closed wound. Make sure to document the reason for the intermediate closure to avoid a denial of the service.

If the cyst was infected or inflamed and the procedure performed was only an incision and drainage, use the code for simple I&D (10060). Use this code if the lesion was opened and drained but not packed or sutured. If multiple cysts were done, if it was complicated with the use of packing or iodine crystals, or if the sack was removed, then the correct code is 10061 for "multiple or complex removal." Note that just adding packing to the opened incision and drainage automatically qualifies the procedure as a complex I&D (10061).

Lipoma excisions may be coded as for a skin lesion or a subcutaneous tumor. If the lipoma is superficial in the subcutaneous fat below the skin, the removal may be coded the same as for an excision of an epidermal cyst (excision of a benign skin lesion). Similar to epidermal cysts, the size is based on the measurement of the lipoma and not the incision. Also, if a two-layered closure is performed, document the necessity for this and bill for an intermediate closure.

Lipomas may also be coded with the new 2010 CPT codes for excision of a subcutaneous tumor based on anatomic location. Some coders advocate using these codes only for deep lipomas including those under fascia or under muscle. Other coders state that all lipomas should be coded with these codes. See Table 38-13 in Chapter 38, *Surviving Financially*, for the specific soft tissue tumor codes based on location of the lipoma. The most commonly needed codes for lipomas are listed in Table 12-1. These soft tissue tumor codes are all inclusive. Neither the length of the incision nor the type of repair that is used matter. The large lipoma in Figure 12-25 was deep based on the visibility of the latissimus dorsi muscle at the time of excision and could easily be coded as 21931. If a decision is made to code it as a skin lesion (an acceptable alternative), then the code used would be 11446 for a benign skin lesion excised with a diameter over 4.0 cm. Both coding methods pay well and are considered legitimate for the procedure performed. The specific ICD-9 codes for lipomas are 214.0 for the face and 214.1 for other areas.

As of 2010, four new codes (21011, 21012, 21013, and 21014) are available for reporting the excisions of soft tissue tumors (including lipomas) of the face and scalp. If a lipoma is less than 2 cm in maximum dimension, report code 21011. If the lipoma is larger than 2 cm, report 21012. If the tumor is subfascial (i.e., intramuscular or subgaleal) and is less than 2 cm in maximum dimension, report code 21013. If it is larger than 2 cm, report 21014. Therefore, the excision of a 3-cm submuscular lipoma of the forehead is reported with code 21014.

Speak with staff and/or consultants who support coding and billing functions to help make decisions when the best coding strategy for a specific lipoma is not clear.

(For further tips see Chapter 38, *Surviving Financially*.)

TABLE 12-1 Subcutaneous Soft Tissue Tumor Excisions (Including Lipomas)

CPT	Description	2010 National Medicare Reimbursement
21930	Back or flank, <3 cm	430
21931	Back or flank, ≥3 cm	459
24071	Upper arm or elbow, <3 cm	395
24075	Upper arm or elbow, ≥3 cm	441
25071	Forearm and/or wrist, <3 cm	341
25075	Forearm and/or wrist, ≥3 cm	414
21011	Face or scalp, <2 cm	306
21012	Face or scalp, ≥2 cm	328

CONCLUSION

The most common "lumps and bumps" that present in an outpatient setting can be managed effectively with a combination of the techniques described in this chapter. New techniques minimize scarring and are convenient for patients and providers. Learning these few tricks should expand your capabilities and improve your efficiency and effectiveness in treating these common problems.

References

1. Diven DG, Dozier SE, Meyer DJ, Smith EB. Bacteriology of inflamed and uninflamed epidermal inclusion cysts. *Arch Dermatol.* 1998;134:49–51.
2. Zuber TJ. Minimal excision technique for epidermoid (sebaceous) cysts. *Am Fam Physician.* 2002;65:1409–1412, 1417–1418, 1420.
3. Suliman MT. Excision of epidermoid (sebaceous) cyst: description of the operative technique. *Plast Reconstr Surg.* 2005;116: 2042–2043.
4. Pandya KA, Radke F. Benign skin lesions: lipomas, epidermal inclusion cysts, muscle and nerve biopsies. *Surg Clin North Am.* 2009;89:677–687.
5. Serpell JW, Chen RY. Review of large deep lipomatous tumours. *ANZ J Surg.* 2007;77:524–529.
6. Chandawarkar RY, Rodriguez P, Roussalis J, Tantri MD. Minimal-scar segmental extraction of lipomas: study of 122 consecutive procedures. *Dermatol Surg.* 2005;31:59–63; discussion 63–64.
7. Minami S, Nakagawa N, Ito T, *et al.* A simple and effective technique for the cryotherapy of digital mucous cysts. *Dermatol Surg.* 2007;33:1280–1282.
8. Epstein E. A simple technique for managing digital mucous cysts. *Arch Dermatol.* 1979;115:1315–1316.
9. Crawford RJ, Gupta A, Risitano G, Burke FD. Mucous cyst of the distal interphalangeal joint: treatment by simple excision or excision and rotation flap. *J Hand Surg.* 1990;15:113–114.
10. Lawrence C. Skin and osteophyte removal is not required in the surgical treatment of digital mucous cysts. *Arch Dermatol.* 2005;141:1560–1564.

13 Flaps

RYAN O'QUINN, MD • RICHARD P. USATINE, MD

The proper development and implementation of the skin flap is a key skill in reconstruction of skin defects, especially facial defects, following trauma or the removal of benign skin lesions or skin cancers. Although the surgeon should always consider primary, linear closure of a skin defect, there are many circumstances in which a skin flap may be the ideal choice for reconstruction.[1,2]

Skin flaps may be chosen instead of a primary linear closure to:

- Recruit skin from areas of lower tension to areas of higher tension.
- Prevent the retraction of a free margin such as the lip or eyelid.
- Keep a reconstructive maneuver in a single cosmetic subunit.
- Realign wound closure lines in a more cosmetically acceptable manner.

In addition, flaps can also perform very well in situations that would not be ideal for skin grafts; flaps can be employed to fill deeper defects that would lead to poor contours with skin grafting or to cover anatomic structures that may prevent the use of grafts (cartilage or tendon).

It is critical to understand the advantages and disadvantages of the different types of flaps rather than apply a "cookbook" approach to flap planning. When selecting the best choice of flap for a particular defect, the relative benefits and risks of each flap should be considered beforehand. A deep understanding of both flap theory and anatomy can lead to the best results.

TERMINOLOGY

Flaps can be classified by their blood supply into *axial pattern flaps*, which have a larger, typically named artery supplying their vascular needs (such as the paramedian forehead flap, which depends on the supratrochlear arteries of the medial lower forehead), and *random pattern flaps*, which rely on the unnamed vasculature of the dermis, subcutaneous fat, and in some cases, the superficial musculature of facial structures. Because the blood supply of the skin and soft tissues of the scalp, face, and neck is so rich, the random pattern flaps enjoy very high rates of success. These local, random pattern flaps are by far the more commonly employed flaps and will be the focus of this chapter.

The random pattern flap is further classified by its movement. The three basic types of movement are (Figure 13-1):

1. Advancement
2. Transposition
3. Rotation.

The initial wound that is to be reconstructed is the *primary defect*, and here it refers to the result of the removal of a skin tumor (Figure 13-2). Once a flap has been advanced, transposed, or rotated into position to close the primary defect, the wound that remains behind at the donor site of the flap is the *secondary defect*. The *primary motion* of a flap is the movement that the flap makes when it advances, transposes, or rotates into and closes the primary defect (Figure 13-2). The *secondary motion* is the movement that the tissue adjacent to and surrounding the flap makes when the final defect is closed. Both the primary and secondary motion of a flap are important in proper flap design. The very end of the flap that fills the primary defect, furthest from the donor site is the *flap tip*. The *flap pedicle* is that portion of the flap that connects it to the surrounding skin, and is the conduit for the vascular supply of the flap. The *key suture* of a local flap is the location in which the first suture is typically placed to provide the initial correct alignment of a flap to fill the primary defect and to direct additional placement of sutures to close the secondary defect. *Standing cutaneous cones* (dog ears) are areas of local tissue redundancy that occur in wound closure, but that can be minimized, eliminated, or moved to more cosmetically advantageous locations by the correct choice of and meticulous planning for a flap.

USE OF FLAPS FOLLOWING TREATMENT OF MALIGNANT TUMORS

Although malignant tumor clearance is always very important, it is even more critical prior to employing flap reconstruction. If a flap is used, and later the surgical margins are determined to be positive histologically for persistence of tumor, the cure rate for a subsequent excision may be reduced due to the loss of the true surgical margins by the significant movement of tissue that occurs in flap mobilization. In addition, using a flap prematurely may "burn bridges" and prevent further reconstruction using adjacent tissue if a re-excision is necessary. A potentially worse scenario can arise if there is a persistence of tumor that is buried under a flap. Such tumors can grow to great size and depth before they become clinically obvious, and may lead to severe morbidity and need for extensive reconstruction at the time of re-excision. Mohs micrographic surgery can

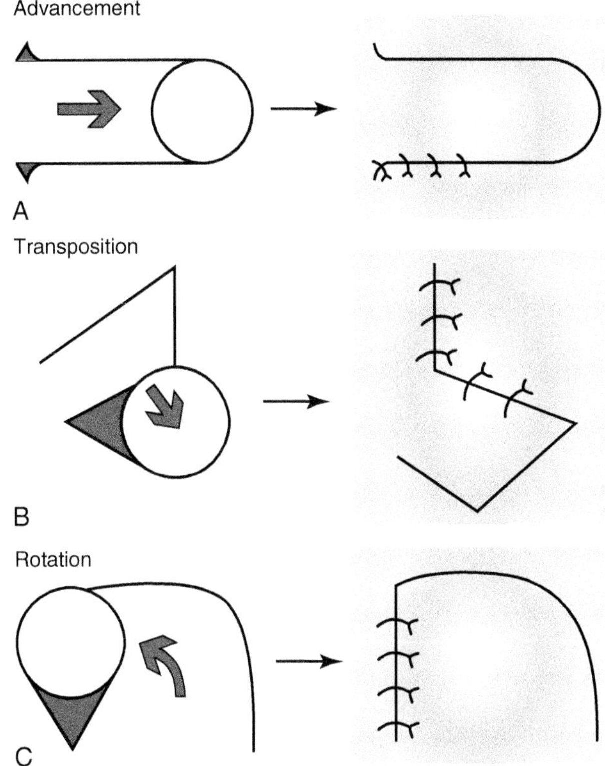

FIGURE 13-1 The three basic types of random pattern flap movement: (A) advancement; (B) transposition; (C) rotation. The circles are the primary defects. Red triangles are Burow's triangles that need excising for the flap to work.

achieve cure rates of up to 99% in primary tumors and is the gold standard for margin clearance of cutaneous malignancy. Mohs surgery should be strongly considered for more aggressive tumors or those in critical anatomic areas. Margin control of skin tumors can be achieved using standard frozen section pathology, but if this is not available, wounds can be bandaged following tumor excision with a plan for delayed repair following clearance of the tumor with permanent section pathology.

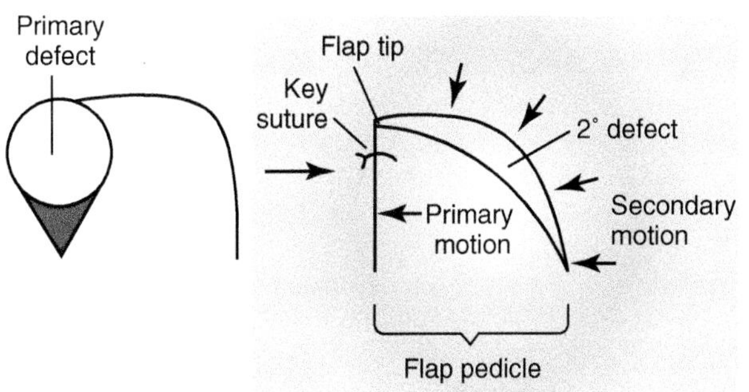

FIGURE 13-2 The initial wound to be reconstructed is the primary defect and the wound that remains behind at the donor site of the flap is the secondary defect. The primary motion of a flap is the movement that the flap makes when it advances, transposes, or rotates into and closes the primary defect. The secondary motion is the movement that the tissue adjacent to and surrounding the flap makes when the final defect is closed.

CONTRAINDICATIONS

Although there are no absolute contraindications, factors to consider when planning for the use of a flap include underlying disorders that may lead to increased rates of intraoperative or postoperative complications. These include patients who are highly anticoagulated or with bleeding diatheses who may experience troublesome intraoperative bleeding or postoperative hematoma formation. Patients who smoke excessively experience a much higher risk of flap tip necrosis and flap failure, and encouraging smoking cessation in the perioperative and postoperative course is helpful to achieve the best healing. The use of flaps must also be carefully weighed in those patients who may have underlying skin conditions that can lead to increased complications. Decreased flexibility and therefore impaired movement of skin can be seen in patients with extensive scarring from burns or other injuries, previous radiotherapy, or an underlying skin disease such as scleroderma. Decreased perfusion of skin leading to flap failure or infection can be seen in conditions such as diabetes mellitus, lung disease, or poor circulation secondary to atherosclerosis, especially in peripheral areas. Finally, the use of a flap may not be possible in patients with extremely thin skin that will not bear the stresses of flap movement. Examples includes elderly patients who have extreme photodamage or long-term users of corticosteroids.

PLANNING THE FLAP

Careful planning is essential for successful flap reconstruction. Following confirmed tumor clearance of the surgical margins, the primary defect is lightly infiltrated with local anesthetic so that it may be manipulated without patient discomfort. It is important for the surgeon not to proceed immediately with an anticipated flap procedure before carefully considering the ramifications of tissue movement for surrounding structures. At this point the defect should be evaluated for surrounding tissue laxity and any potential reservoirs of loose skin that may be recruited for repair. This may be done by pinching the skin with gloved fingers. If the fingers are inadequate in more inflexible areas, the skin hook is a very useful surgical instrument for gauging tissue movement without tissue damage even in large defects of inflexible skin. Careful flap planning will then include not only the evaluation of possible sources of skin for flap creation, but also the consideration of nearby anatomic structures that could be distorted by either the primary or secondary movement of the flap. Especially vulnerable areas are the free margins of the eyelids, lips, and the nasal tip. The vectors of flap movement should be placed perpendicular to such structures, lest tissue movement distort their anatomy.

Tissue texture, and color should be matched whenever possible; a flap from similar adjacent skin will lead to the best results. A defect on the nose should be filled with similar-appearing skin from the nose instead of skin from a flap on the cheek. Finally, anticipated tissue

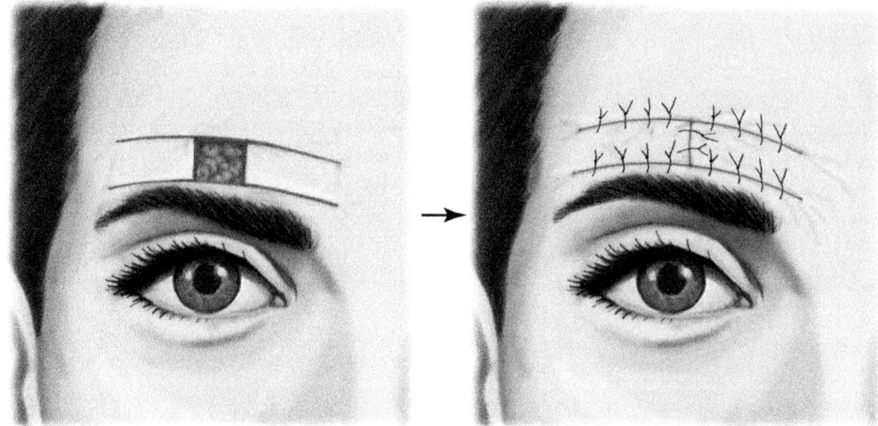

FIGURE 13-3 Double advancement flap (bidirectional) within an eyebrow to restore uninterrupted hair growth after resecting a tumor within the eyebrow.

redundancies from wound closure should be considered, with thought to how these redundancies or dog ears may be best camouflaged along anatomic borders. The proposed flap should always be drawn out prior to incision, and this may be done with a surgical marker.

ADVANCEMENT FLAP

Conceptual

The primary motion of the advancement flap is the sliding of the flap, usually in a single linear vector as it advances into the primary defect. This sliding motion may be unidirectional (single advancement flap) or bidirectional (double advancement flap).[3] Although there are several variations on this type of flap, the two main benefits of the advancement flap are as follows:

1. *Redirection of tissue movement.* It may be critical to keep the repair within a single cosmetic subunit or to selectively move certain skin into the primary defect. This can be helpful when a defect lies within an eyebrow or the mustache, and the advancing primary motion can restore uninterrupted hair growth (Figure 13-3).
2. *Reorientation of tissue redundancy.* When closing a skin defect, tissue redundancies (dog ears) are inevitable. A properly employed advancement flap can redistribute tissue redundancies to more acceptable locations that may be far from the primary defect. This is useful in moving the tissue redundancies away from a certain structure (lips or eyebrow), or aligning them along the boundary of an anatomic subunit (alar crease) to camouflage the scar (Figure 13-4).

Note that the purpose of the advancement flap is not to increase laxity to close a wound under high tension.

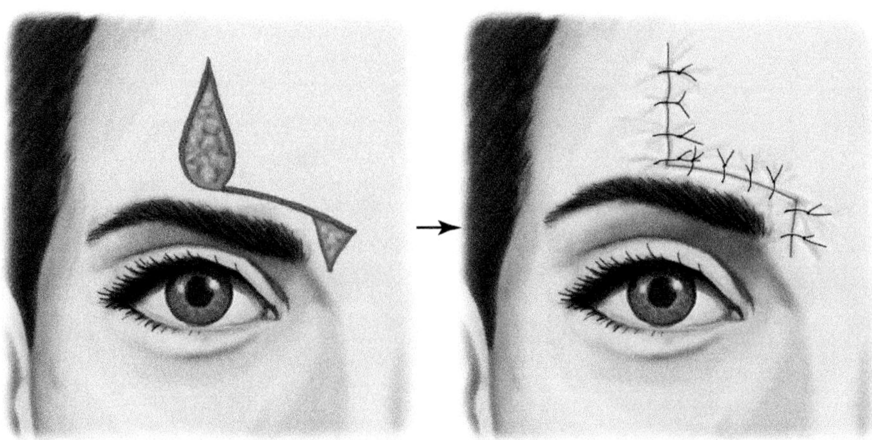

FIGURE 13-4 Reorientation of tissue redundancy to a more acceptable location away from the primary defect.

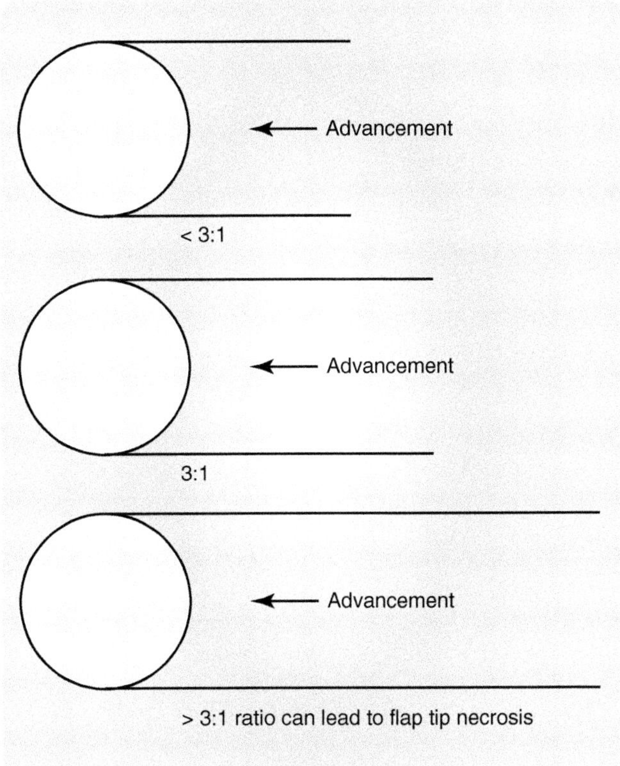

FIGURE 13-5 Advancement flaps are also limited by their blood supply so the length:width ratio should not exceed 3:1. A long, thin advancement flap in violation of this ratio runs a high risk of distal flap tip necrosis.

Although an advancement flap may appear to provide superior tissue movement over a primary linear closure, this is rarely the case. In preoperative planning, if a defect cannot be approximated primarily by pinching the skin or mobilizing the skin edges with hooks, an advancement flap will not be the best option because the amount of additional tissue movement that it provides over primary closure is often minimal.

Advancement flaps are also limited by their blood supply. The pedicle of skin and soft tissue must not be compromised. A length:width ratio should ideally not exceed 3:1. A long, thin advancement flap in violation of this ratio runs a high risk of distal flap tip necrosis (Figure 13-5).

Single-Pedicle Advancement Flap (U-Plasty)

The classic form of the advancement flap is the single-pedicle advancement flap, also known as the U-plasty (Figure 13-6). This is an older technique that has been advocated for repairs on the forehead, because it may fit in well with horizontal relaxed skin tension lines in this area. It may also be used on the sideburn or eyebrow to move hair-bearing skin together and hide the scars in the hair. A significant disadvantage to the flap is that it creates numerous surgical lines, and in an area such as the forehead, may provide an inferior surgical result compared to a primary linear closure. It has been advocated as well for use on the glabella and nasal bridge, but other flaps are nearly always preferable in these areas.

Bilateral Advancement Flap (H-Plasty)

The bilateral advancement flap is similar to the classic single-pedicle advancement flap except that another pedicled advancement flap is created on the opposite side of the defect. The two flaps need not necessarily be symmetrical or parallel, but may be curved or slightly shortened on one side as anatomic structures allow. Unfortunately, this flap creates even more incisions than the single-pedicle advancement flap and therefore its clinical usefulness is limited. This flap could be useful for the closure of a defect in the eyebrow, because the lines could be camouflaged along the brow's edges (Figure 13-7). It may also be reserved for situations in which a single pedicle is first employed and then judged inadequate to close a defect. At that point, a second pedicle is created to provide further tissue movement.

T-Plasty (O-T Flap)

The T-plasty bilateral advancement flap has great utility in facial reconstruction. It is best suited for the repair of defects at the edge of a free margin such as the lip, or at the junction of two cosmetic subunits when it is preferable to keep the repair from crossing the junction such as when closing a chin defect and preventing the closure from crossing the mental crease. The final

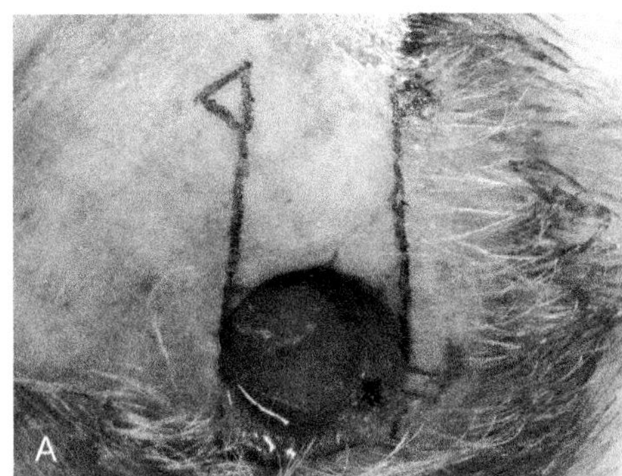

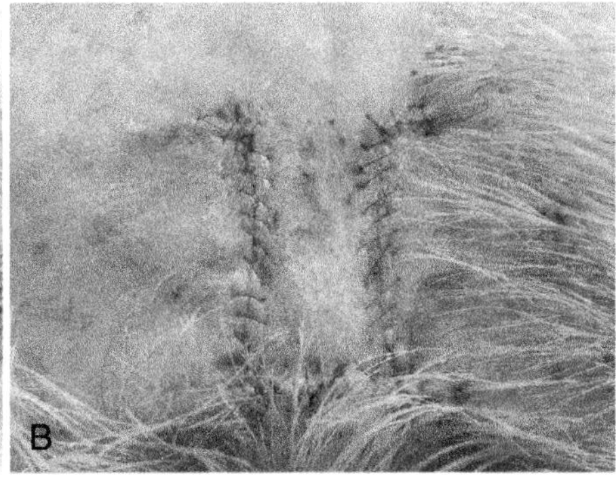

FIGURE 13-6 (A) Single-pedicle advancement flap (U-plasty) on the forehead may fit in well with horizontal relaxed skin tension lines in this area. (B) The flap is sutured in its place. *(Courtesy of Ryan O'Quinn, MD.)*

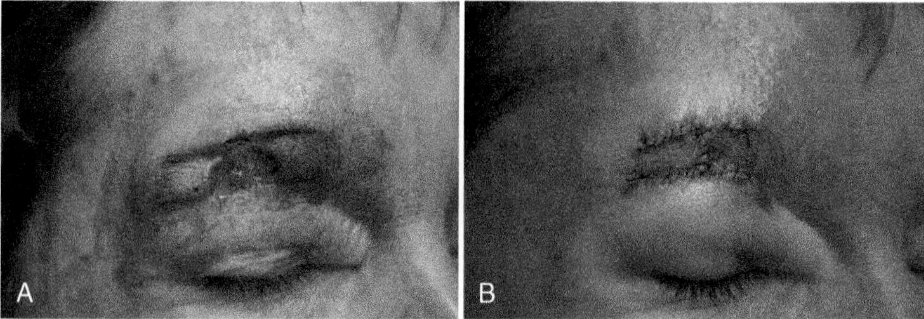

FIGURE 13-7 The bilateral advancement flap (H-plasty) could be useful for the closure of a defect in the eyebrow, because the lines could be camouflaged along the brows edges. **(A)** The "H" is cut. **(B)** The "H" is sutured in, preserving the eyebrow anatomy. *(Courtesy of Ryan O'Quinn, MD.)*

suture line in the T configuration is a result of a Burow's triangle excision on one side of the defect that is approximately the length of the defect, and two incisions (each the width of the defect) on the other side to create the bilateral flaps. These incisions need not be completely straight and can be somewhat curved and tailored to the necessary skin tension lines (Figure 13-8). The resulting redundancies along the flap edges can be sewn out by the rule of halves, or resolved with small Burow's triangle excisions.

L-Plasty

The L-plasty is a single advancement flap that is employed to redirect tissue redundancy and maintain the repair in a single cosmetic subunit. The tissue redundancy has been distributed along the edge of the advancing flap and no Burow's triangle has been excised (Figure 13-9).

Advancement Flap: Step-by-Step Instructions

1. A moderately large wound results from the removal of a BCC using the Mohs surgical technique (Figure 13-10A). The location immediately above the eyebrow presents a dilemma. Horizontal linear closure would result in unnatural elevation of the eyebrow margin. Vertical linear closure would extend the Burow's triangle through the brow into the upper eyelid.
2. A laterally based advancement flap is planned. The Burow's triangle is drawn superiorly, and the inferior edge of the flap is created running along the lateral margin of the brow (Figure 13-10B). A smaller Burow's triangle is drawn to anticipate skin redundancy.
3. The flap is incised, and both Burow's triangles removed (Figure 13-10C). The level of undermining in this area is fairly superficial with the flap containing epidermis, dermis, and several millimeters of subcutaneous fat. This is to avoid injury to the underlying superficial temporal branch of the facial nerve. All surrounding wound edges are undermined. Hemostasis was achieved with electrosurgery.
4. A skin hook illustrates the location of the buried key suture for this flap (Figure 13-10D). This initial suture advances the tissue into the defect and shows proper alignment of the final closure. At this point, the deep absorbable sutures are placed to secure the flap and hold tension. Once the flap is in place, a running polypropylene suture is placed to nicely approximate epidermal edges.
5. The final result achieves excellent closure of the primary defect without anatomic distortion (Figure 13-10E).

ISLAND PEDICLE FLAP

Conceptual

Although the primary movement is advancement of tissue into the defect, the island pedicle flap is so fundamentally different from the previously described

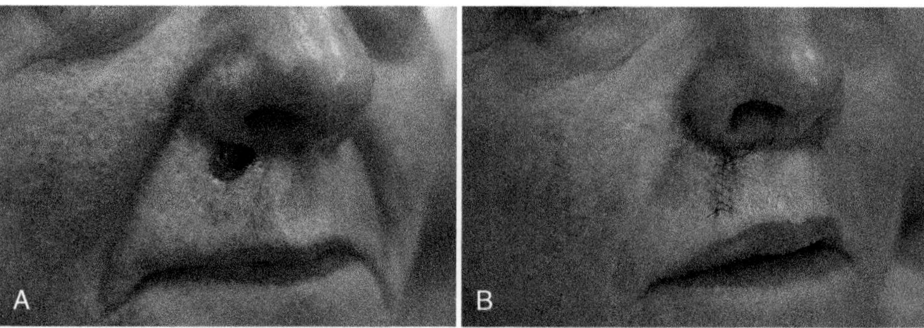

FIGURE 13-8 The T-plasty (O-T flap) is best suited for the repair of defects at the edge of a free margin such as the nasal ala or lip, or at the junction of two cosmetic subunits. **(A)** The "O"-shaped defect. **(B)** The "T"-shaped repair. *(Courtesy of Ryan O'Quinn, MD.)*

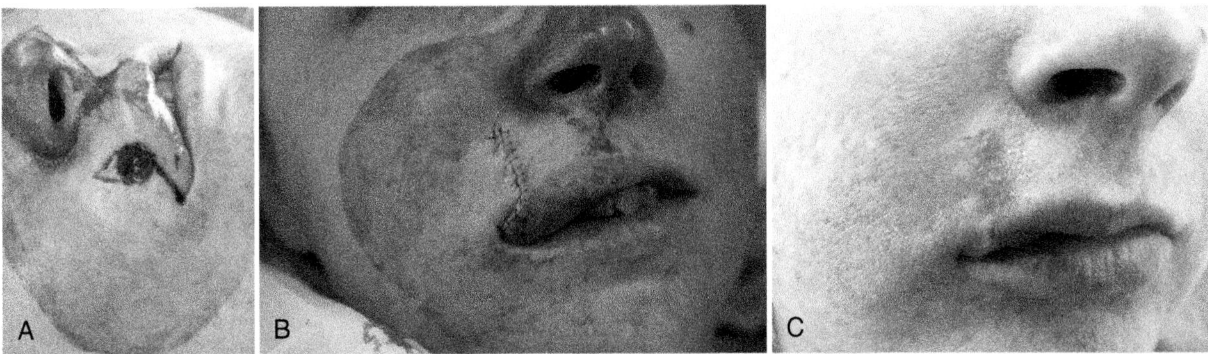

FIGURE 13-9 The L-plasty is a single advancement flap that is employed to redirect tissue redundancy and maintain the repair in a single cosmetic subunit. (A) The defect on the lip margin. (B) The "L"-shaped repair. (C) Repair healing 1 week after surgery. *(Courtesy of Ryan O'Quinn, MD.)*

advancement flaps that it occupies a class of its own. Unlike the other advancement flaps, it does provide significantly increased tissue movement over primary closure. Uniquely, the epidermis and dermis of the island pedicle flap are completely severed from the surrounding skin, and instead the pedicle is an "island" of rich, vascular subcutaneous and muscle tissue underneath the flap. Because of this, it is very rare to experience ischemic necrosis of a properly designed and executed island pedicle flap. The flap is not subject to the 3:1 rule of advancement flaps and moves a thinner flap over a greater distance. It may be an ideal choice in patients with poorly perfused skin or smokers. Another advantage of the flap is that it may limit reconstruction of a large or complex defect to a single cosmetic subunit. This is the case in the area of the lateral upper cutaneous lip, where the flap is the most useful.

Island Pedicle Flap: Step-by-Step Instructions

1. Reconstruction of a large defect of the upper cutaneous lip presents a particular challenge (Figure 13-11A). Care must be taken to avoid anatomic distortion of the upper lip and nasal ala. An island pedicle flap is drawn inferiorly and lateral to the angle of the mouth. This will allow the lax skin of the area to be moved upward into the primary defect. The lines are drawn such that the flap fits

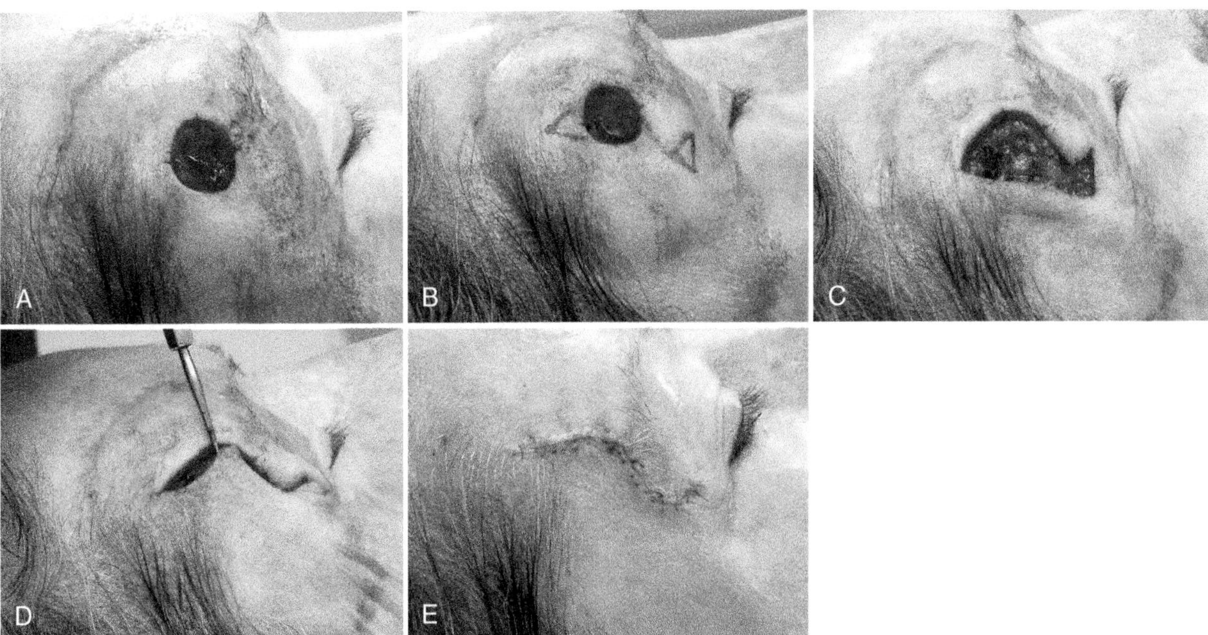

FIGURE 13-10 Advancement flap: step-by-step instructions. (A) Circular wound from the removal of a BCC using the Mohs surgical technique. (B) The Burow's triangle is drawn superiorly, and the inferior edge of the flap is created running along the lateral margin of the brow. A smaller Burow's triangle is drawn to anticipate skin redundancy. (C) The flap is incised, and both Burow's triangles removed. (D) A skin hook is used here to illustrate the location of the buried key suture for this flap. (E) The final result achieves excellent closure of the primary defect without anatomic distortion. *(Courtesy of Ryan O'Quinn, MD.)*

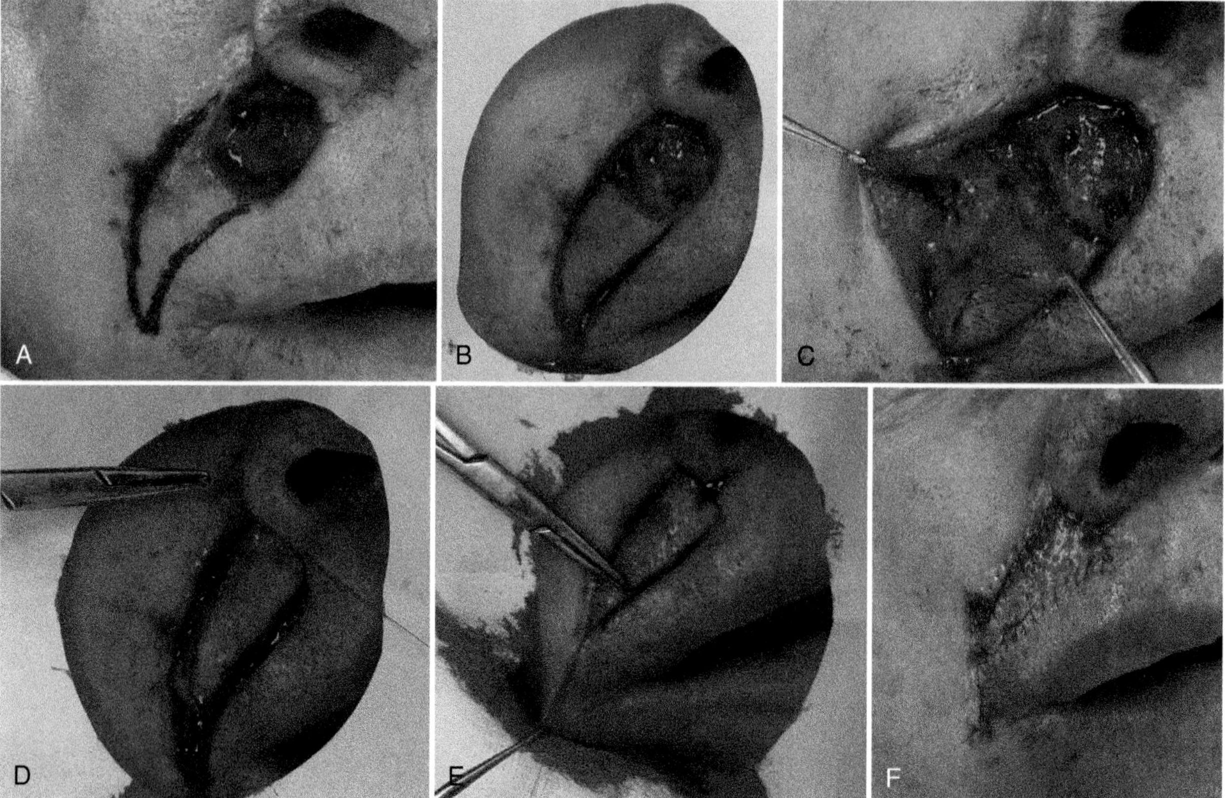

FIGURE 13-11 Island pedicle flap: step-by-step instructions. **(A)** Large defect of the upper cutaneous lip. The lines are drawn such that the flap fits nicely into the nasolabial fold laterally. The curvilinear shape of the flap ensures that the secondary defect will be closed horizontally to avoid raising the lip. **(B)** The flap is incised along planned lines. **(C)** All surrounding wound edges are undermined. The pedicle is not undermined. **(D)** The key suture is placed in the center of the advancing edge of the island pedicle flap. **(E)** The secondary defect is then closed with a buried suture at the inferior tip of the flap. The vector of tension here is horizontal, avoiding pull on the upper lip. **(F)** The final result reconstructs the upper cutaneous lip with no anatomic distortion (perioperative swelling will resolve). *(Courtesy of Ryan O'Quinn, MD.)*

nicely into the nasolabial fold laterally. The curvilinear shape of the flap ensures that the secondary defect will be closed horizontally to avoid raising the lip.

2. The flap is incised along planned lines (Figure 13-11B). The depth of incision is to the deep subcutaneous layer. The central deep portion of the flap is left undisturbed to avoid compromising vascular supply. The flap tip and primary defect edges are trimmed so that the advancing edge of the island flap fits nicely.
3. All surrounding wound edges are undermined. In Figure 13-11C the richly supplied pedicle is visible. It is not undermined to avoid vascular compromise. Hemostasis is achieved with electrosurgery.
4. The key suture is placed in the center of the advancing edge of the island pedicle flap (Figure 13-11D). As the flap is advanced, it fills the primary defect, and creates a smaller secondary defect lateral to the angle of the mouth.
5. The secondary defect is then closed with a buried suture at the inferior tip of the flap (Figure 13-11E). The vector of tension in this example is horizontal, avoiding pull on the upper lip.
6. After completion of the layered closure, the final result nicely reconstructs the upper cutaneous lip with no anatomic distortion (perioperative swelling will resolve) (Figure 13-11F).

ROTATION FLAP

Conceptual

The rotation flap consists of tissue rotating in an arc to fill the primary defect. The rotation flap differs from primary closure and the advancement flap in that the tension is directed not in a single, linear vector, but rather from several different directions. Once the flap is put into position with the first key suture, the primary defect is filled, leaving a much longer curvilinear secondary defect. Closing this secondary defect results in the redirection of wound tension, as well as the redirection of tissue redundancy. This redistribution of wound tension is the great advantage of a well-chosen rotation flap. It can recruit significant laxity from the surrounding tissue and greatly aid in closing defects under significant tension such as large, tight scalp defects, or it

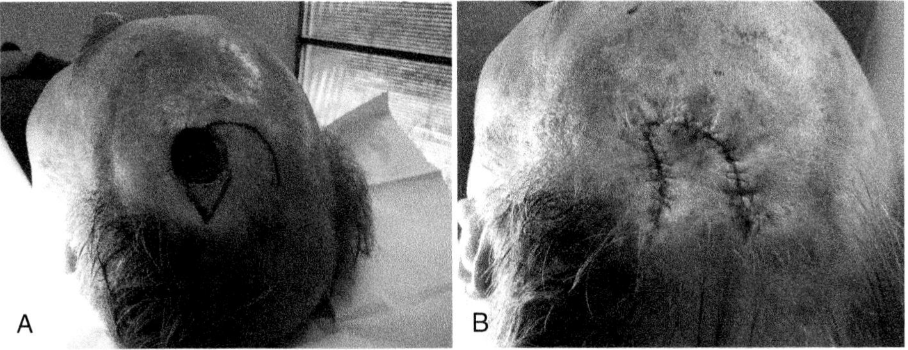

FIGURE 13-12 (A) A single rotation flap is drawn to repair this scalp defect. A single Burow's triangle is drawn to remove tissue redundancy created by primary flap movement. (B) The flap is rotated into the defect and sutured. *(Courtesy of Ryan O'Quinn, MD.)*

can result in moving the secondary motion of a flap away from a critical anatomic structure, such as when a rotation flap is used to close a wound in the infraorbital region.[4]

Single-Rotation Flap

The single-rotation flap is the rotation flap in its most basic form. A single flap is rotated into the defect. A single Burow's triangle is excised to remove tissue redundancy created by primary flap movement (Figure 13-12).

Bilateral O-Z Rotation Flap

The bilateral rotation flap is helpful with wounds under high tension. Often, a wound can be approached with a single rotation flap, and if it is inadequate to close a very tight wound, another rotation flap can be incised and rotated in to provide more movement for final wound closure. Often, no Burow's triangle need be excised (Figure 13-13).

Rotation Flap: Step-by-Step Instructions

See video on the DVD for further learning. 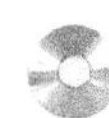

1. The rotation flap works very well in areas of inflexible skin or wounds under considerable tension where a primary closure may be impossible. In Figure 13-14A, a single rotation flap is planned, with a Burow's triangle drawn inferiorly.
2. The rotation flap is incised and the Burow's triangle removed (Figures 13-14B and C). All wound edges are widely undermined and hemostasis is achieved with electrosurgery (Figure 13-14D).
3. The flap is rotated in to fill the primary defect and the key suture is placed (Figure 13-14E). Note that a long, curved secondary defect is created.
4. The secondary defect is then closed with buried sutures by the "rule of halves" (Figure 13-14F). This effectively redistributes the tension from the initial primary defect over a much larger area.
5. Running sutures are placed to approximate the epidermis (Figure 13-14G).

TRANSPOSITION FLAP

Conceptual

Both the design and tissue movement of the transposition flap is more difficult than with the other random pattern flaps. Like the rotation flap, tissue is harvested

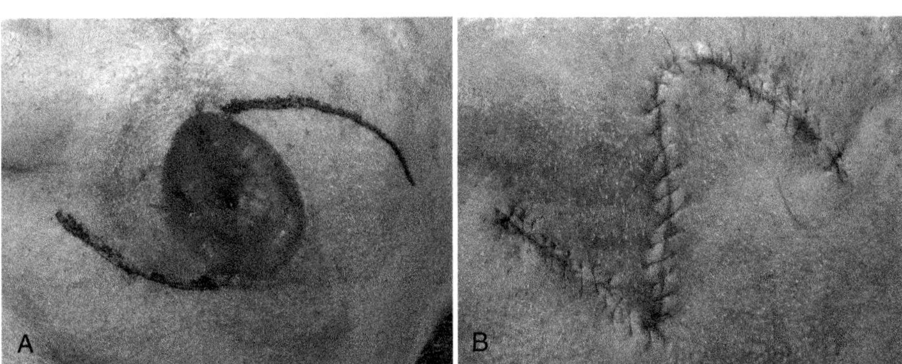

FIGURE 13-13 (A) Bilateral O-Z rotation flap on the scalp is drawn. (B) The flap is sutured and resembles a "Z." *(Courtesy of Ryan O'Quinn, MD.)*

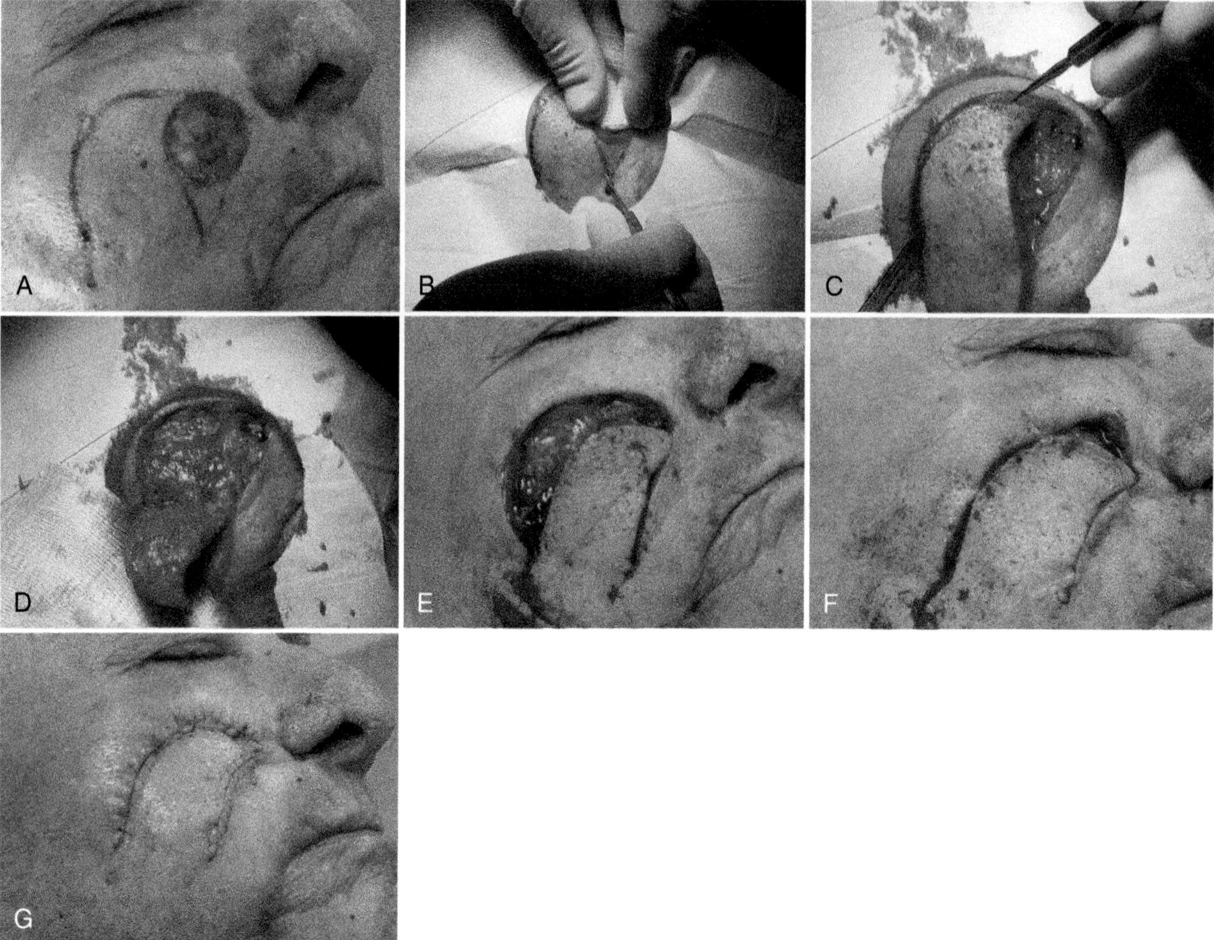

FIGURE 13-14 Rotation flap: step-by-step instructions. **(A)** The rotation flap works very well in areas of inflexible skin or wounds under considerable tension where a primary closure may be impossible. Here, a single rotation flap is planned, with a Burow's triangle drawn inferiorly. **(B)** The Burow's triangle is incised and removed. **(C)** The rotation flap is incised. **(D)** The flap and all wound edges are widely undermined and hemostasis achieved with electrosurgery. **(E)** The flap is rotated in to fill the primary defect and the key suture is placed. Note that a long, curved secondary defect is created. **(F)** The secondary defect is then closed with buried sutures by the rule of halves. This effectively redistributes the tension from the initial primary defect over a much larger area. **(G)** The final result is achieved with running sutures to approximate the epidermis. *(Courtesy of Ryan O'Quinn, MD.)*

from an area of laxity to be used to repair the primary defect, but instead of advancing or rotating into the defect, the flap is transposed over an area (Figure 13-1B) of normal skin. The great advantage of the transposition flap is its ability to redirect the wound closure tension. A wound inferior to the free margin of the lower eyelid is often at high risk for ectropion. A transposition flap can transpose skin into the defect to close the wound while reorienting the tension parallel to the eyelid margin. Similarly, a wound of the lower nose can often be difficult to close without pulling up on the nasal tip. A transposition flap can be employed to redirect the tension away from the tip, while moving more pliable skin from the upper nose to resurface the wound.

Rhombic Transposition Flap

The rhombic flap may be the most commonly used type of transposition flap. Although many variants exist, the classic rhombic flap is easily visualized as a parallelogram with the flap tip having a 60-degree angle. The primary defect may be cut to fit the flap, or the flap may be trimmed to fit the defect when it is placed. It is useful to redirect wound tension away from the primary defect. This type of flap is often deployed on the upper nose and periorbital areas (Figure 13-15).

Zitelli Bilobed Transposition Flap

The Zitelli bilobed flap is a more specialized variant of the transposition flap. Although more complex, we include it here because of its great usefulness in reconstruction of wounds of the sebaceous and inflexible skin of the lower nose. The bilobed flap is excellent for closing small to intermediate-sized wounds less than 1.5 cm in diameter. The placement of the extra lobe allows greater movement of tissue from the upper nose[5,6] (Figure 13-16).

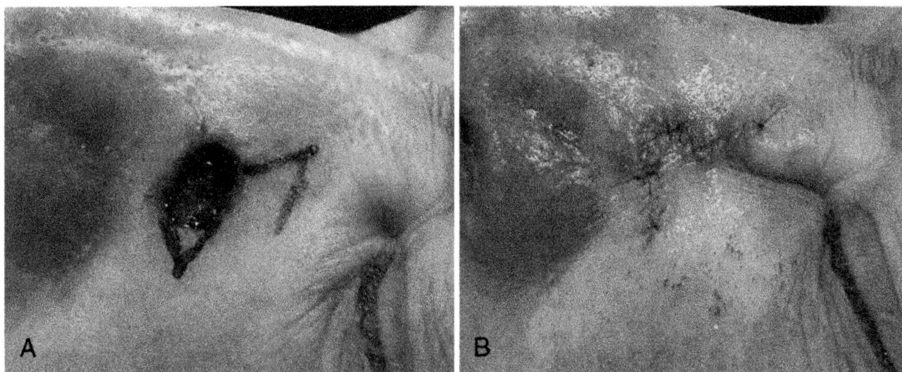

FIGURE 13-15 Rhombic transposition flap is useful to redirect wound tension away from the primary defect, and is often used on the upper nose. **(A)** Flap drawn with 60-degree angle. **(B)** Repaired flap looks like a parallelogram. *(Courtesy of Ryan O'Quinn, MD.)*

Transposition Flap: Step-by-Step Instructions

1. The primary defect is a small one of the inflexible sebaceous skin of the distal nose (Figure 13-17A). The rhombic flap taps into the more mobile skin of the proximal nose.
2. The flap is incised and the laterally placed Burow's triangle is removed (Figure 13-17B). On the mid to distal nose, the flap will be incised slightly deeper to improve flap perfusion. A small amount of nasalis musculature is included at the bottom of the flap. All wound edges are undermined and hemostasis is obtained with electrodesiccation.
3. The key suture is placed initially to close the secondary defect (Figure 13-17C). This pushes the flap into place. Usually the flap tip is trimmed to fit the primary defect.
4. The remainder of the flap is sutured in a layered fashion (Figure 13-17D).

LEARNING THE TECHNIQUES

See video on the DVD for further learning. 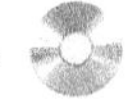

Performing cutaneous flap surgeries is an advanced skill that takes considerable experience to master. Initial experience can be gained in a workshop using pig's feet. New clinicians should start their practice on patients with the help of a mentor, such as a dermatologic, Mohs, or plastic surgeon.

CODING AND BILLING PEARLS

The adjacent tissue transfer (flaps) or rearrangement procedures (plasties) are described by the series of codes from 14000 to 14300. These codes are for the excision of the lesion and/or repair by adjacent tissue transfer or rearrangement. Routine excision of the lesion, whether it is benign or malignant, is included with codes 14000–14300 and should not be coded or billed separately.

The specific code is determined by the location and size of the defect. The term *defect* includes the primary defect resulting from the excision and the secondary defect resulting from flap design to perform the reconstruction. The areas of both defects are added together to determine the code (see Box 13-1 for the actual CPT codes).

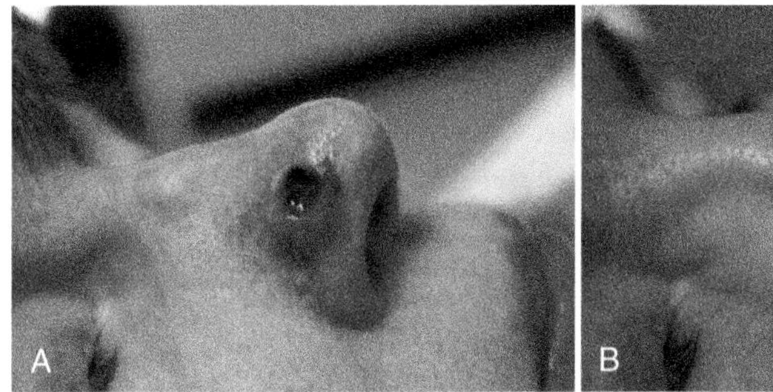

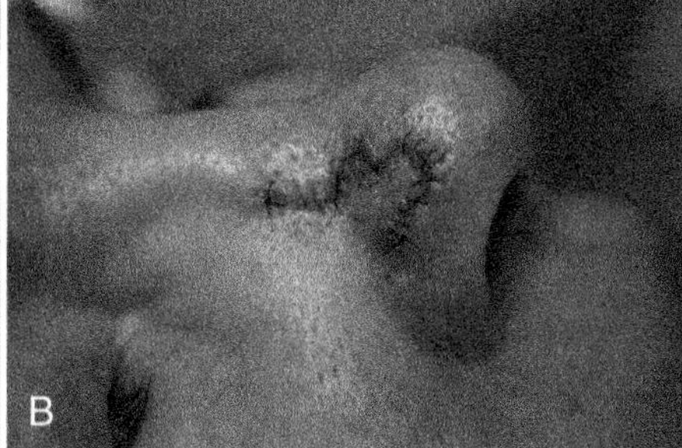

FIGURE 13-16 The bilobed transposition flap is excellent for closing small to intermediate-sized wounds less than 1.5 cm in diameter on the lower nose. The placement of the extra lobe allows greater movement of tissue from the upper nose. **(A)** Small lower nose defect after excising a BCC. **(B)** Bilobed transposition flap completed. *(Courtesy of Ryan O'Quinn, MD.)*

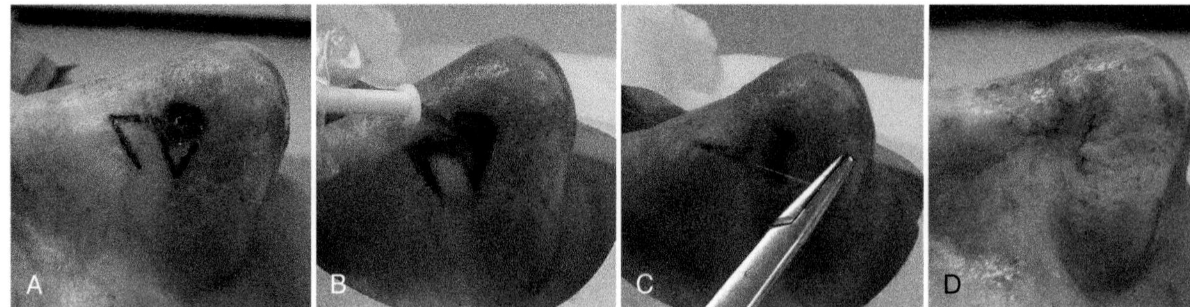

FIGURE 13-17 Transposition flap: step-by-step instructions. **(A)** The primary defect is a small one of the inflexible sebaceous skin of the lower nose. The rhombic flap is drawn to use the more mobile skin of the upper nose. **(B)** The flap is incised and the laterally placed Burow's triangle is removed. All wound edges are undermined and hemostasis is obtained with electrodesiccation. **(C)** The key suture is placed initially to close the secondary defect. This pushes the flap into place. The flap tip is trimmed to fit the primary defect. **(D)** The remainder of the flap is sutured in a layered fashion. *(Courtesy of Ryan O'Quinn, MD.)*

BOX 13-1 *CPT Codes for Adjacent Tissue Transfer (Flaps)*

14000 Trunk; defect 10 sq cm or less
14001 Trunk; defect 10.1 sq cm to 30.0 sq cm
14020 Scalp, arms, and/or legs; defect 10 sq cm or less
14021 Scalp, arms, and/or legs; defect 10.1 sq cm to 30.0 sq cm
14040 Forehead, cheeks, chin, mouth, neck, axillae, genitalia, hands, and/or feet; defect 10 sq cm or less
14041 Forehead, cheeks, chin, mouth, neck, axillae, genitalia, hands, and/or feet; defect 10.1 sq cm to 30.0 sq cm
14060 Eyelids, nose, ears, and/or lips; defect 10 sq cm or less
14061 Eyelids, nose, ears, and/or lips; defect 10.1 sq cm to 30.0 sq cm
14300 More than 30 sq cm, unusual or complicated, any area

References

1. Bowman PH, Fosko SW, Hartstein ME. Periocular reconstruction. *Semin Cutan Med Surg*. 2003;22:263–272.
2. Chen EH, Johnson TM, Ratner D. Introduction to flap movement: reconstruction of five similar nasal defects using different flaps. *Dermatol Surg*. 2005;31:982–985.
3. Krishnan R, Garman M, Nunez-Gussman J, Orengo I. Advancement flaps: a basic theme with many variations. *Dermatol Surg*. 2005;31:986–994.
4. Seline PC, Siegle RJ. Scalp reconstruction. *Dermatol Clin*. 2005;23:13–21, v.
5. Aasi SZ, Leffell DJ. Bilobed transposition flap. *Dermatol Clin*. 2005;23:55–64, vi.
6. Collins SC, Dufresne Jr RG, Jellinek NJ. The bilobed transposition flap for single-staged repair of large surgical defects involving the nasal ala. *Dermatol Surg*. 2008;34:1379–1385.

14 Electrosurgery

RICHARD P. USATINE, MD • JOHN L. PFENNINGER, MD

Electrosurgery is used in dermatologic practice to destroy benign and malignant lesions, to control bleeding, and to cut or excise tissue. Many types of electrosurgical units are available for use in the office setting. *Modern high-frequency electrosurgery* units transfer current to the patient through "cold" electrodes. The water molecules are energized to the point that cells literally vaporize as opposed to being burned. The term *electrocautery* implies that heat is transferred directly to tissue with a *heated* electrode; electrocautery is just one type of electrosurgery. The battery-powered units that produce a red wire when activated are an example of a simple cautery unit and are useful for draining a subungual hematoma and other minor procedures such as cauterizing the lumens of resected vas deferens where residual tissue damage is not an issue.

The major electrosurgical functions include fulguration, electrodesiccation, electrocoagulation, and electrosection (cutting). In *fulguration*, the electrode is held away from the skin so that there is a sparking to the surface (such as happens with lightning). In fact, the term *fulguration* comes from the Latin term *fulgur*, which means "lightning." Fulguration produces a high-intensity but more shallow level of tissue destruction (Figure 14-1). With *electrodesiccation*, the active electrode touches or is inserted into skin to produce deeper tissue destruction (Figure 14-2). Epilation is a type of desiccation in which a fine-wire electrode is inserted into a hair follicle to literally "cook it." *Electrocoagulation* is used to stop bleeding in deep and superficial surgery (Figure 14-3). In *electrosection*, the unit is set so the electrode cuts tissue (Figure 14-4). The higher the unit's operating electrical frequency (not to be confused with power), the less tissue damage is left behind when using the cutting function.

Current can be applied either in a unipolar or bipolar fashion. The majority of electrosurgical units (ESUs) are unipolar. *Unipolar* refers to the fact that the current enters a site at the point of the electrode and passes through the body to a grounding plate to complete the circuit. With *bipolar* applications, the current travels from one point of the electrode, through the tissue, to another point of the electrode (e.g., with fine forceps, from point to point). No grounding plate is needed for this type of use. This reduces possible complications from burns at unwanted sites where the current can exit. It also reduces complications with pacemakers. The bipolar units are ideal to control bleeding since forceps can pinpoint and grasp a bleeder. When the current is applied, only the tissue between the tips of the forceps is affected (Figure 14-5).

With *dual-frequency (DF) ESUs*, 1.7 MHz (1.7 million cps) is used in the bipolar function, which is better for coagulation because of the lower frequency, whereas unipolar functions (cut, blend) are at 4.0 MHz to decrease tissue damage in the cutting functions.

ADVANTAGES OF ELECTROSURGERY

- Simple to use.
- Easy to master.
- Rapid technique.
- Controls bleeding while cutting or destroying tissue.
- Equipment is compact and affordable for basic units. DF units are more expensive, however.
- When used for tissue destruction, sterile conditions or sutures are not needed.
- With high-frequency units, tissue destruction is minimized when used in the pure cutting mode.
- Infection rarely develops in wounds that are left open.
- Useful to treat a wide variety of skin lesions, especially for:
  - Superficial lesions
  - Tiny lesions (may not need anesthesia)
  - Vascular lesions
  - Premalignant lesions
  - Nonmelanoma skin cancers.

DISADVANTAGES OF ELECTROSURGERY

- Safety risk (electrical shocks, burns, fires, or interference with pacemakers).
- Hypertrophic scars, especially with poor technique.
- Smoke may carry viral particles, which have the potential to transmit infections (e.g., HPV, HIV).
- Odor of smoke plume.
- Delayed hemorrhage.
- Unsightly wound.
- Slow healing, especially if a large area is treated (healing can be slower than scalpel shave excision).
- Small lesions are obliterated, resulting in no specimen being available for histology unless a biopsy was performed first.
- Electrosurgical artifacts can occur at margins if used for excisional biopsy or removal (e.g., LEEP).

ELECTROSURGERY VERSUS CRYOSURGERY

Cryosurgery is often the treatment of choice for seborrheic and actinic keratoses as well as simple warts. It is faster and easier to perform than electrosurgery for these indications because it does not require anesthesia.

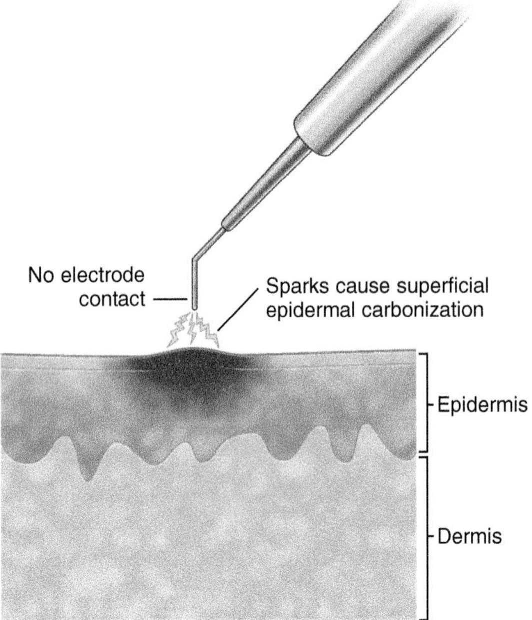

FIGURE 14-1 In *fulguration*, the electrode is held away from the skin so that there is a sparking to the surface (such as happens with *fulgur*, "lightning"). Fulguration produces a high intensity but more shallow level of tissue destruction that may reach the upper dermis. *(Adapted from Sebben JE. Electrosurgery. In Ratz JL, ed.,* Textbook of Dermatologic Surgery. *Philadelphia: Lippincott-Raven; 1998.)*

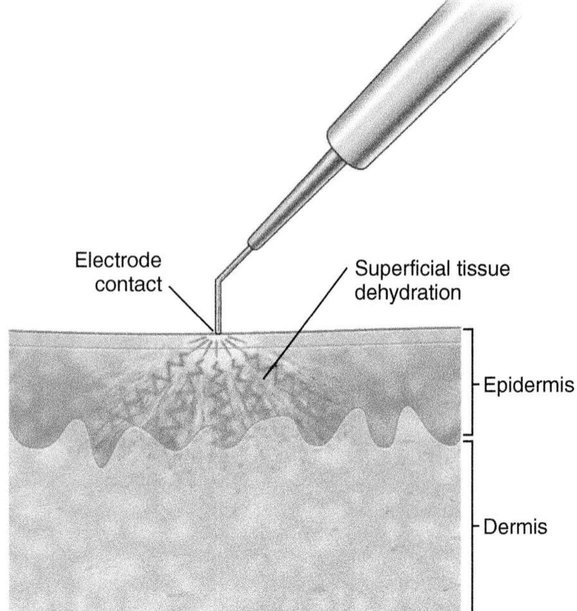

FIGURE 14-2 With *electrodesiccation*, the active electrode touches or is inserted into the skin to produce tissue destruction deeper into the dermis. *(Adapted from Sebben JE. Electrosurgery. In Ratz JL, ed.,* Textbook of Dermatologic Surgery. *Philadelphia: Lippincott-Raven; 1998.)*

Cryosurgery also tends to cause less scarring than electrosurgery especially if the lesions are very superficial. However, cryosurgery may be more likely to cause hypopigmentation because the cold destroys melanocytes. This is especially important in a more darkly pigmented person. Electrosurgery can be more effective than cryosurgery for extensive condyloma, especially if a cutting current can be used.

There may be a risk of developing human papilloma virus (HPV) in the respiratory tract from inhaling the plume (smoke) from an HPV lesion as it is being treated.[1–3] Intact HPV DNA has been isolated from the

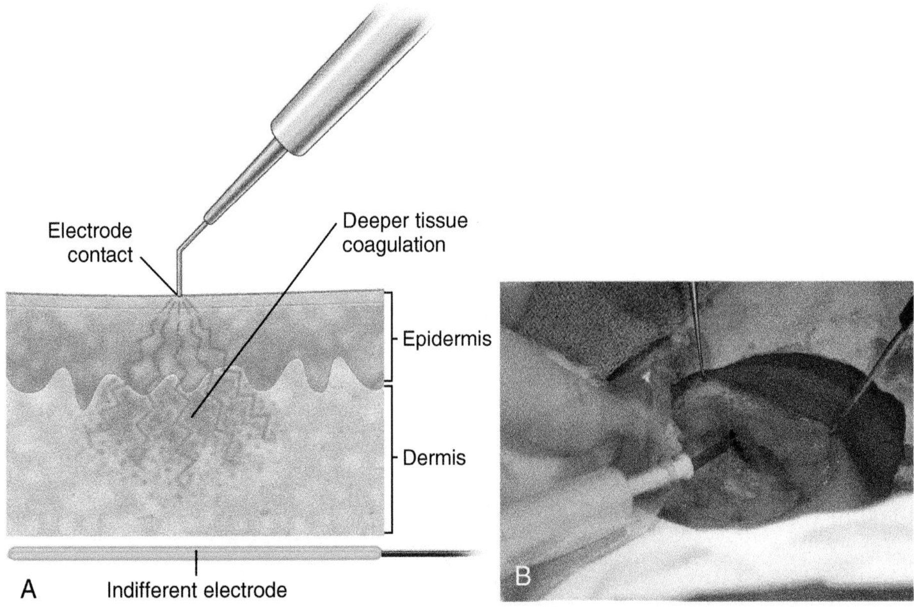

FIGURE 14-3 **(A)** *Electrocoagulation* is used to stop bleeding in deep and superficial surgery. In this image an indifferent electrode is being used to produce deeper tissue coagulation. Electrocoagulation can also be performed without an indifferent electrode. **(B)** Electrocoagulation is being performed in the undermined area of an ellipse using a Hyfrecator while the surgical assistant holds up the tissue with skin hooks. *(A: Adapted from Sebben JE. Electrosurgery. In Ratz JL, ed.,* Textbook of Dermatologic Surgery. *Philadelphia: Lippincott-Raven; 1998.)*

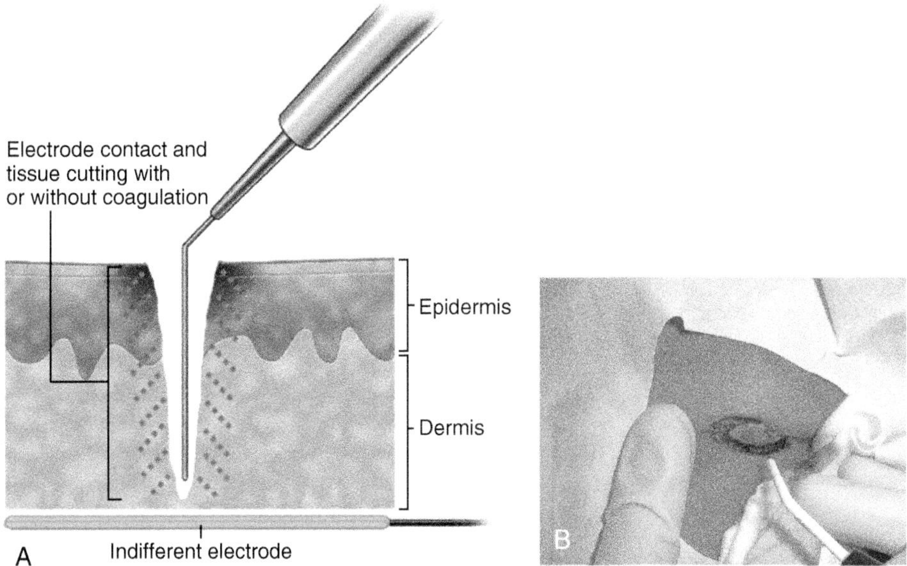

FIGURE 14-4 **(A)** In *electrosection*, the unit is set so the electrode cuts tissue. This mode requires an indifferent electrode. **(B)** Electrosection is being performed with a very tip electrode attached to a Surgitron. An indifferent electrode is placed under the patient near the surgical site. *(A: From Vidimos A, Ammirati C, Poblete-Lopez C.* Dermatologic Surgery*. London: Saunders; 2008.)*

plume of verrucae that were treated with electrosurgery and lasers. Therefore, it is prudent for all physicians to use a smoke evacuator while performing laser and electrosurgical treatment of verrucae and other viral lesions. (See *Safety Measures with Electrosurgery*, p. 167.) Unfortunately, evidence is insufficient to measure the magnitude of these risks. These personal risks, however, may be one factor used to determine the physician's choice of therapy for viral lesions.

One disadvantage of cryotherapy over electrosurgery is that with cryosurgery the final result cannot be seen immediately, and there is more subjective judgment involved in performing the treatment. However, the degree of damage can be estimated accurately with more experience and by following certain guidelines (see Chapter 15). Cryosurgery also causes more postoperative swelling, which may be uncomfortable for the patient but is only a transient phenomenon.

ELECTROSURGERY VERSUS SCALPEL

The traditional instruments for performing excisions and shave biopsies are the scalpel and razor blade. These are inexpensive, the blades are disposable, and the cuts are clean. The cold steel blades cause no heat-induced tissue damage that could obscure the pathology specimen. Using electrosurgery in place of a blade has the advantage of facilitating hemostasis while cutting. However, the lateral heat produced by the electrosurgical instrument can cause residual tissue damage that might result in slow healing as well as artifact on the edges of the biopsy specimen. The higher the frequency, the less residual damage on both the specimen removed and on the viable tissue remaining. Also, the cutting is very quick and it may go more deeply than desired, excising excessive amounts of tissue or damaging deeper nerves and vessels.

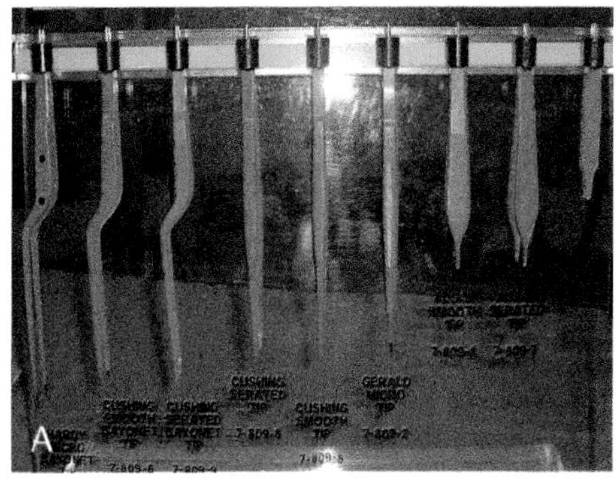

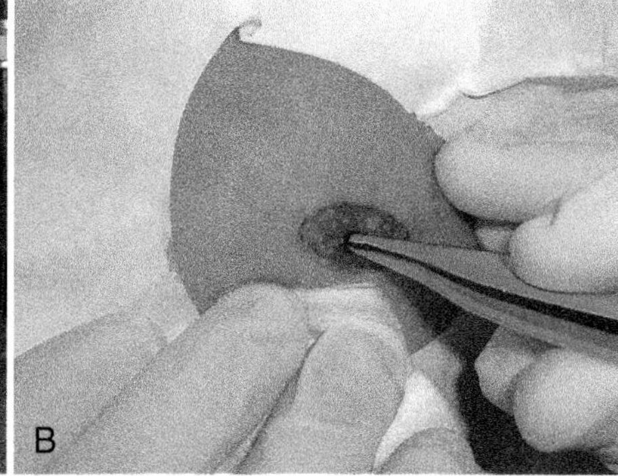

FIGURE 14-5 **(A)** Selection of bipolar forceps that could be used on a number of electrosurgical units. **(B)** Bipolar forceps in action for electrocoagulation while doing an elliptical biopsy. Note that a small gap is preserved between the ends of the bipolar forceps around the bleeding site. Clamping the forceps close together is not an effective method of electrocoagulation.

High-frequency electrosurgery on the pure cutting current will approach but not match the scalpel for producing an entirely burn artifact–free pathologic specimen. Therefore, if a malignancy (especially melanoma) is suspected, unless wide margins are being obtained, it may be best to obtain a biopsy with the scalpel (cold steel).

For excising benign lesions, the small amount of lateral heat may not interfere with wound healing when used carefully on a low-power cutting setting. A shave excision using a blade followed by electrosurgery with a loop electrode can lead to a nearly scar-free result and combines the best of both techniques to optimize the results. The mode can be set for either cutting/coagulation (blend) or preferably pure cutting only. Ideally then, the lesion (commonly a nevus or seborrheic keratosis) is shaved off with a blade and then the loop of the radio-frequency (RF) unit removes the residual tissue and controls any bleeding. If the loop will be used to perform the shave, the less the coagulation function will be used and, hence, the less damage that will result to the remaining tissue and to the biopsy specimen. Pure cutting will work just fine to make a smooth cut and control bleeding.

The Ellman Surgitron models are a high-frequency units (often termed a *radio-frequency* unit because it operates at 4.0 MHz, which is in the range of a radio). They employ a Vari-Tip fine-wire electrode that is adjustable in length for cutting through the skin for elliptical and other full-thickness excisions. On the pure cutting setting, the Vari-Tip electrode can cut with less lateral heat and can allow the physician to do quick and bloodless excision of benign lesions. A combined cold steel (blade) and electrosurgical procedure can also be used here. While the scalpel cuts through the skin to provide better depth control, deeper dissection/undermining and excision with cutting or blended cutting and coagulation can control bleeding.

In summary, no instrument can beat the scalpel (or razor blade) for cost and minimization of tissue damage. The high-frequency electrosurgery unit is more expensive to purchase and operate. A radiosurgery unit can be used to perform several kinds of surgery that have been traditionally performed with a scalpel. This may be beneficial if the lesion is benign and very vascular. However, with small biopsies it cannot match the scalpel for quality of pathologic specimen. Superior cosmetic results can be obtained when using the scalpel for a shave excision followed by light "brushing" of the RF loop over the base of the lesion on a pure cutting setting to smooth out any irregularities while at the same time controlling bleeding. This also tends to treat any sparse residual cells of the lesion that may persist.

ELECTROSURGERY VERSUS LASER

Laser is an acronym for *light amplified by stimulated emission of radiation*. Laser technology uses focused light energy to affect cells. Many types of lasers are available to perform different functions (see Chapters 26 through 30). Electrosurgery is less expensive than laser surgery but is more limited in utility. The standard electrosurgical units are a fraction of the cost of a laser (as low as $1000 to 4000 compared to laser units costing $30,000 to $200,000). Most physicians face the choice of referring a patient for laser surgery versus doing electrosurgery in their own office. As with electrosurgery, the CO_2 laser may be used to cut, coagulate, and ablate (destroy) tissue. It is most often used in the office for resurfacing procedures, such as in the treatment of rhytids (wrinkles) and skin surface irregularities; pigmentation; and small vessels. The pulsed dye laser or a similar yellow-light laser is unequivocally better than electrosurgery for treating large hemangiomas and maximizing the cosmetic result. These lasers are used very effectively to treat port-wine hemangiomas. Visible-light lasers obtain better cosmetic results when treating most other vascular lesions, such as angiomas and telangiectasias. They offer much less chance of scarring.

If high-frequency ESUs are used, the radio waves vaporize cells with much the same effect as light energy from lasers. In both cases, minimal tissue damage occurs since vaporization is accomplished using either light or radiowave energy. If cell destruction is desired (such as with the treatment of a basal cell carcinoma or verrucae) then there really is no benefit to either laser or radio-frequency compared to simpler units.

In some cases, it may be appropriate to allow the patient to choose between being treated with electrosurgery or laser treatment. It is helpful to inform the patient of the risks and benefits of the two. Ultimately, the patient needs to make the final decision (especially if the goal of therapy is purely cosmetic). Although different lasers offer more options for treatment, for the majority of conditions seen in the office, electrosurgery will be more than adequate.

EQUIPMENT

Thermal Pencil/Battery Cautery

An inexpensive thermal "pencil" cautery (Figure 14-6) is a useful device to have for small skin lesions. They

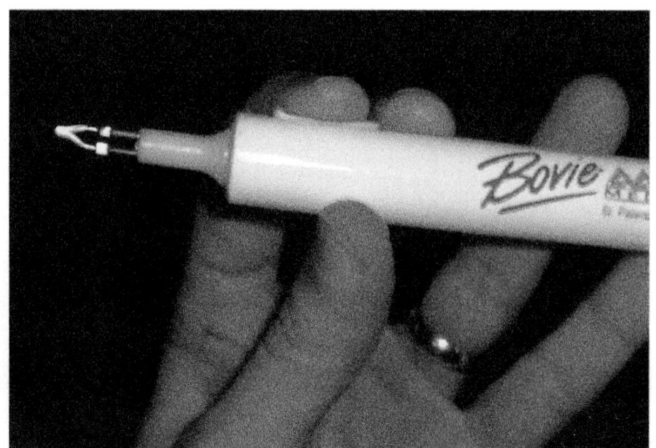

FIGURE 14-6 Note the red-hot tip of this handheld disposable electrocautery unit. This unit performs true hot electrocautery.

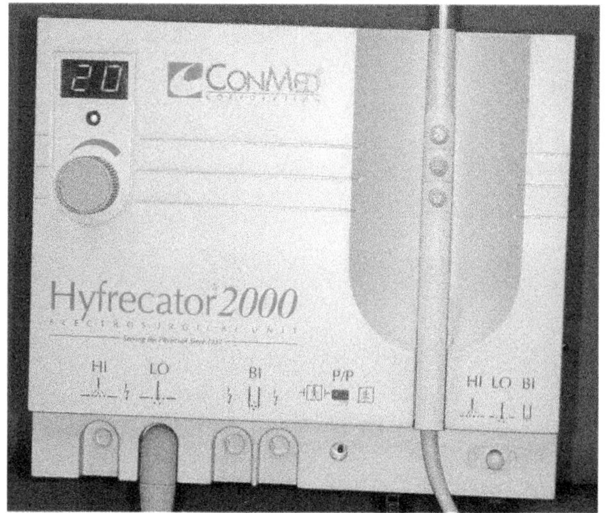

FIGURE 14-7 The Hyfrecator 2000 from the ConMed Corporation is a commonly used electrosurgical unit in the office.

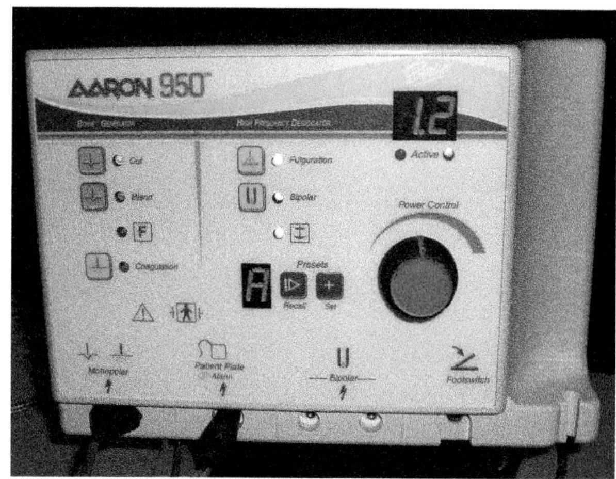

FIGURE 14-8 The Aaron 950 by Bovie is an electrosurgical unit that can be used for cutting, bipolar, and the other typical electrosurgical applications.

are also used to occlude the cut ends of the vasa when doing a vasectomy. This disposable device consists of two penlight batteries in a housing connected to a wire filament that heats up when activated. Reusable models are also available with disposable tips. These battery cautery units can be a useful tool for treatment around the eyes and on patients with pacemakers. The devices come in high- and low-temperature varieties; low-temperature devices are preferred in skin surgery.

Thermal pencil cautery units are also excellent for opening a subungual hematoma. When the hot electrode perforates the nail, the heated tip is cooled by the blood from the hematoma, preventing damage to the nail bed.

Electrosurgical Units

Basic Electrosurgical Units (Noncutting, Lower Frequency)

- Aaron 940 (Bovie)
- Electricator (Delasco)
- Hyfrecator 2000 (ConMed) (Figure 14-7)
- SurgiStat II (Valleylab).

High-Frequency Units (up to 4 MHz)

- Aaron 950 (Aaron) (Figure 14-8)
- Cameron-Miller (various models)
- Finesse (Utah Medical)
- Force FX (Valleylab)
- LEEP (CooperSurgical)
- Quantum 2000 (Wallach Surgical)
- Surgitron FFPF EMC (Ellman)—unipolar only
- System 2450 (ConMed).

Dual-Frequency Units (Unipolar 4 MHz and Bipolar 1.7 MHz)

- Surgitron AcuSect (Ellman)—unipolar and bipolar (Figure 14-9A)
- Surgitron Dual RF (Ellman) (Figure 14-9B)
- Surgitron Dual RF S5 (Ellman) with built-in cooling system and more robust transistors and transformers for procedures that take longer such as skin tightening [Pellevé]).

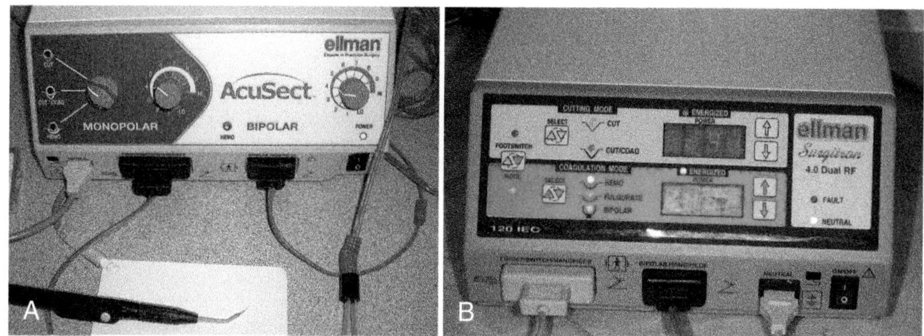

FIGURE 14-9 (A) The Ellman AcuSect is a new combined monopolar and bipolar unit that performs cutting with a reusable neutral electrode. (B) The Ellman Surgitron dual radio-frequency unit is powerful enough to use in the operating room but may also serve as an in-office all-purpose electrosurgical unit. It can perform all modes of electrosurgery discussed in this chapter.

Some RF units were primarily developed for dermatologic applications, whereas others were introduced when the large loop electrical excision procedure (LEEP) became available for cervical conizations. All units can be used for either purpose if the proper electrodes are available. Be mindful, however, that the goal for most skin procedures is to limit scarring. The higher the operating frequency of the unit, the less tissue damage that will result. For destructive procedures, frequency is of less concern.

Because the Hyfrecator and Surgitron are commonly used in the office setting, information provided here will be specific to these two instruments but it can be readily adapted to others. This is not meant as an endorsement of these units. However, their features will be used to provide practical advice for performing electrosurgery,

With many units, accessories are disposable, including grounding pads and standard handpieces. This adds a cost of $10 to $20 per procedure just for tips in addition to increasing waste. If a new grounding pad and handpiece must be used with each patient, the costs can approach $80 to $90 per procedure (e.g., when doing the LEEP procedure). When purchasing an ESU, consider whether reusable equipment is available.

Basic units will only be able to coagulate and fulgurate. To perform modern electrosurgery, units should be capable of pure cutting current, pure coagulation, or a mix of these two ("blend," "cut and coag") in addition to fulguration. "Pure cutting" will still have some coagulation function (e.g., Surgitron is 90% cutting with 10% coagulation). The more coagulation, the more tissue destruction. Higher end units are more versatile and digital settings allow the user to customize the cutting and coagulation percentages in the blend setting.

Comparison of Types of Electrosurgical Units

Radiosurgery is electrosurgery using an RF current in the electromagnetic spectrum of the AM radio. Radiosurgery is performed at a much higher frequency than that used by the other basic electrosurgery units (including the Hyfrecator). Radiosurgical units are more than three times the cost of basic ESUs, but are more versatile (especially for cutting).

True radiosurgery uses an "antenna" as the neutral or indifferent electrode. This replaces the grounding plate. This antenna does not have to make contact with the skin. When using a basic ESU, a neutral electrode is not needed. Some units incorporate safety features that will not allow the unit to operate if the patient is not grounded.

The major significant difference between radiosurgery units and a basic ESU is that the radiosurgery units allow for a cutting mode. If radiosurgery is used only for hemostasis and tissue destruction of benign and malignant lesions, there may be no real difference in outcomes between them.

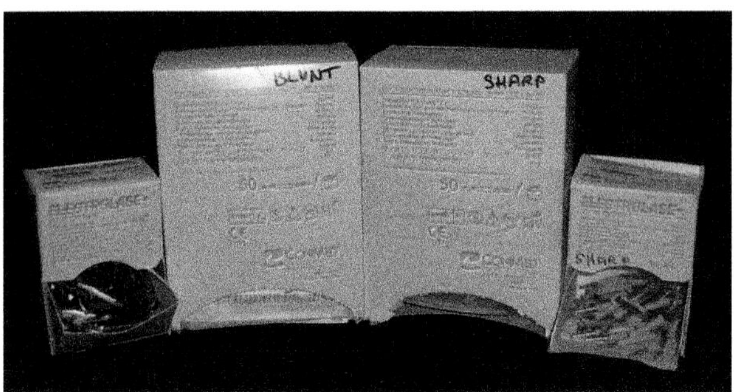

FIGURE 14-10 Commonly used disposable electrodes for the Hyfrecator 2000. These are available in blunt or sharp versions and may be purchased sterilely packaged or as nonsterile clean electrodes.

ACCESSORIES

Hyfrecator

- Electrolase blunt and sharp tips (Figure 14-10)
- Epilation needles
- Nondisposable bipolar forceps (Figure 14-5) and foot switch
- Sterile sleeves for handle (a sterile glove will work if a sterile sleeve is not available) (Figure 14-11).

Ellman Surgitron Units

- Nondisposable (autoclavable) and disposable electrodes (loops, ball, Vari-Tip) (Figure 14-12)
- LEEP electrodes (Figure 14-13)
- Nondisposable bipolar forceps (Figure 14-5)

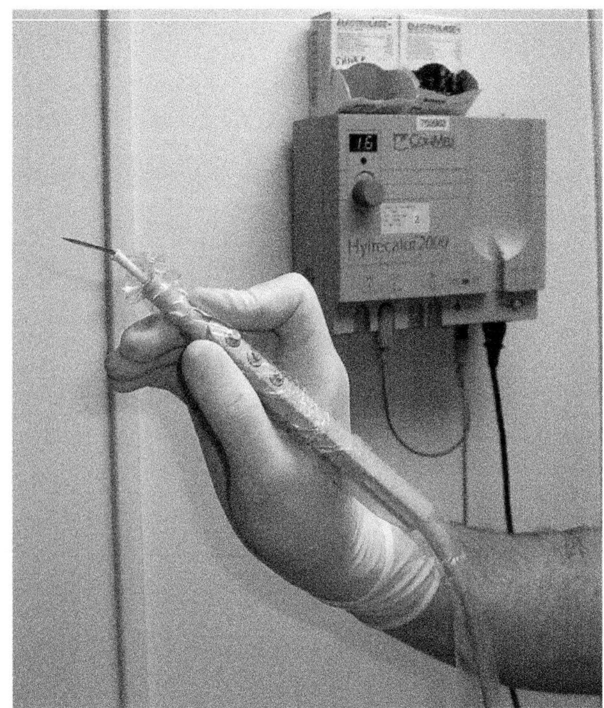

FIGURE 14-11 A sterile sheath has been applied over the Hyfrecator handle so that it can be used in a sterile surgical procedure.

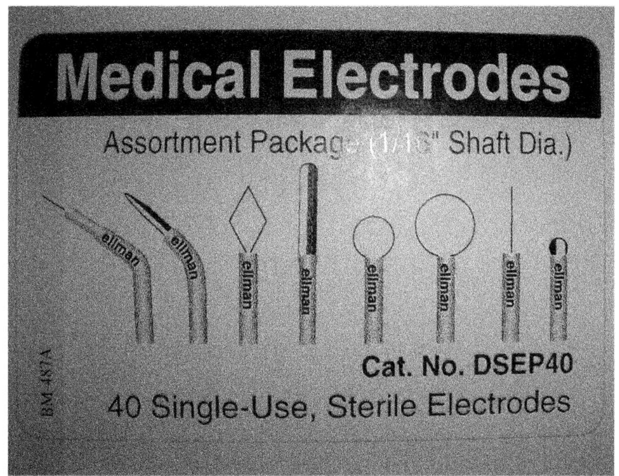

FIGURE 14-12 An assortment of medical electrodes for single use may be purchased from Ellman for use with the Surgitron.

- Control handpiece—sterile and those made to be autoclaved (Figure 14-14)
- Neutral plate (Figure 14-15).

Note that the bipolar forceps are essentially the same for both instruments. These are especially useful for coagulation of small bleeding vessels because grasping the vessel and coagulation are done in one movement. Bipolar electrosurgery can be used in a bloody field and is safer than unipolar electrosurgery for patients with pacemakers.

Units can be activated using either a hand switch or foot controls. It is a matter of preference, but the clinician may have slightly better control of the handpiece for delicate procedures when foot switches are used for activation.

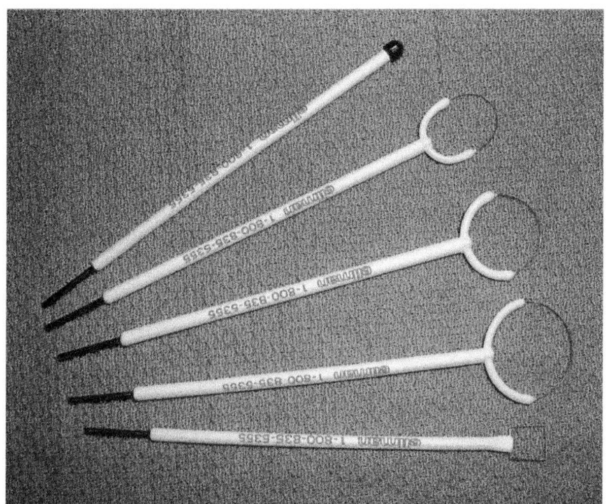

FIGURE 14-13 Reusable LEEP electrodes for the Ellman Surgitron or other cutting units. The handles on these are long and sturdy for intravaginal use. However, these electrodes can also be used for the treatment of rhinophyma.

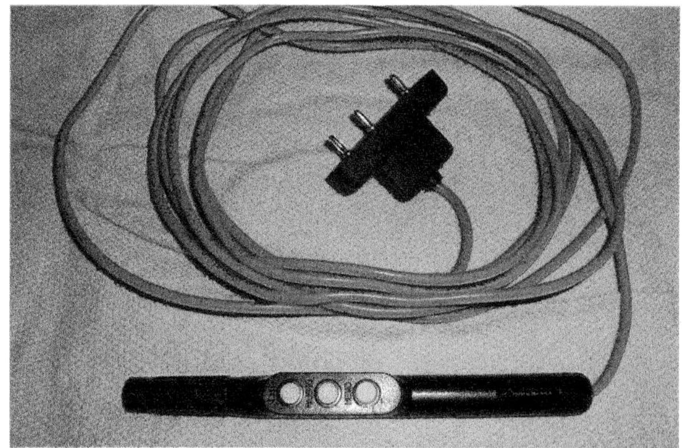

FIGURE 14-14 Reusable sterilizable hand switch for the Surgitron. Note the three buttons for cutting, cutting and coagulation blend, and hemo for pure coagulation.

Smoke Evacuators

Electrosurgery creates a plume (smoke) with a putrid smell. The smoke itself has been shown to include HPV and HIV particles although it is not known if they are infectious. It is best to use some type of smoke evacuator to remove the plume created by the surgery, especially if extensive removal/destruction is being performed. When constructing or remodeling an office, consider installing an exhaust fan (a typical bathroom fan works) to help remove the smell. Types of smoke evacuators include:

- Acu-Evac II 220 (Acuderm)
- Aaron Medical Smoke Shark (Bovie)
- Buffalo Filter
- AER Defense (ConMed) (Figure 14-16)
- OptiMumm (for use with Valleylab units)
- SaftEvac—60 to 65 dB at 1 meter (Delasco)
- Surg-e-Vac (Ellman).

INDICATIONS FOR USE OF ELECTROSURGERY

- Excising tissue
- Vaporization of tissue fragments

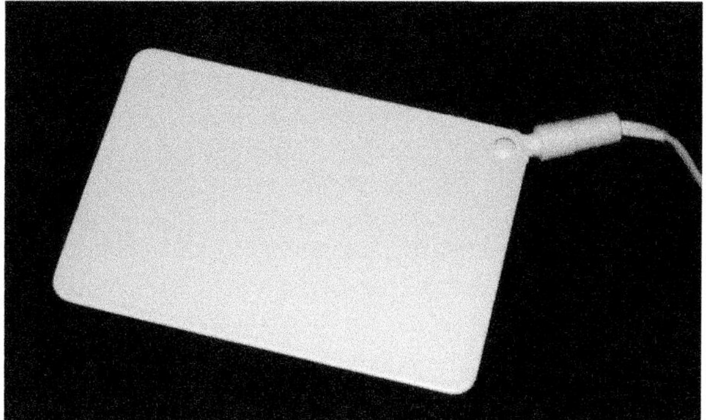

FIGURE 14-15 The reusable indifferent or neutral electrode for the Surgitron. This does not need to touch the skin of the patient as it works to receive radio-frequency waves.

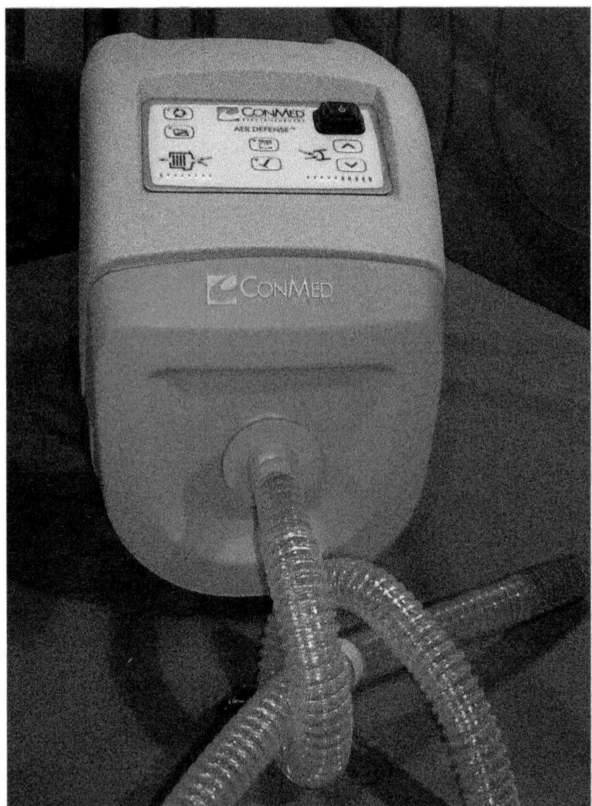

FIGURE 14-16 An example of a smoke evacuator. This one is an AER Defense by ConMed.

- Controlling bleeding (coagulation)
- Destruction of tissue
- Cosmetic functions (skin tightening)
- Nail matrixectomy
- Epilation.

One of the most common uses of high-frequency electrosurgery is the cutting current that is used to smooth out the skin at the site of a shave removal that has been performed with a blade. After removing a nevus, bleeding often occurs and an irregular surface remains. The blood makes it difficult to see the tissue. Using a large skin loop at pure cutting (level 2 or 15 to 20 W) and using a light "brushing" technique, the residual base of tissue is not only smoothed out but bleeding is controlled. Any small residual lesion can be vaporized. This all affords an excellent cosmetic result. Although the removal can be performed using the loop itself (i.e., no blade is used first), two potential problems can arise: (1) it cuts so quickly it easily goes too deep and (2) the tissue sent to the pathologist will have very minimal but definite "burn artifact," which can make interpretation difficult. If the power is set too high, the tissue can also be totally destroyed precluding any pathologic examination. For pure destruction of lesions, there is again no advantage to the high-frequency units.

CONTRAINDICATIONS

There are really no absolute contraindications to using electrosurgery but there are some precautions relative to contraindications:

- Pacemakers (see *Pacemaker Problems*, p. 168).
- Electrosurgery/cautery is not indicated as a treatment modality or for obtaining a biopsy of pigmented lesions suspicious for dysplasia or melanoma.
- Electrodesiccation and curettage (ED&C) should generally be avoided in the following circumstances:
    - Aggressive (morpheaform, sclerotic), large (greater than 1 cm), or recurrent basal cell carcinoma (BCC).
    - BCC larger than 2 cm will have a higher recurrence rate with ED&C (see Chapter 34, *Diagnosis and Treatment of Malignant and Premalignant Lesions*).
    - Squamous cell carcinoma (SCC) greater than 7 to 8 mm. Excise to be sure of complete removal because SCCs are more aggressive than BCCs by their very nature.
    - Immune-suppressed patients, especially those who have had organ transplants, may be best served by excising the lesions to ensure complete removal in all but the smaller lesions (less than 7 to 8 mm).
    - Patients with slow healing (diabetes, peripheral vascular disease) may do better with excisional rather than destructive methods.

Location is also an important consideration when using destructive techniques for nonmelanoma skin cancers (NMSCs). Higher recurrence rates are associated with NMSC in the following areas:

- Alar groove, preauricular and periocular.
- H-zone on the face. Associated with higher recurrence rates for recurrent BCC treated with surgery rather than Mohs surgery (see Chapter 37). This was not true for primary BCC in these regions treated with surgical excision. ED&C may be performed in the H-zone as long as the patient understands that there may be a higher recurrence rate than with surgery.[4]
- SCC on non–sun-exposed skin and mucous membranes such as the lip and eyelid margins (may also be more aggressive biologically).

ELECTROSURGICAL TECHNIQUES: GENERAL PRINCIPLES

Power Setting

Every electrosurgical unit is different, and the desired setting will vary for each model, procedure, lesion, or patient. Even two supposedly identical electrosurgical models may require different settings. Therefore, the setting levels provided are only starting points (Tables 14-1 to 14-3 and Box 14-1). The basic principle for setting the correct power output is to start low and

TABLE 14-1 Range of Power Settings with the Hyfrecator 2000

Lesions	Power Setting (watts on low)	Type of Electrode
Benign		
Angiomas (cherry)	2–2.5	Sharp or dull
Angiomas (spider)	2–2.5	Sharp or needle
Condyloma acuminata	12–18	Dull
Dermatosis papulosa nigra	2–2.5	Dull or sharp
Pyogenic granulomas	16–20 or switch to high	Dull
Sebaceous hyperplasia	2–2.5	Dull
Seborrheic keratosis	10–14	Dull
Skin tags (acrochordons)	2–2.5	Sharp
Syringomas	2–2.5	Sharp
Telangiectasias	2–2.5	Sharp or needle
Verrucae vulgaris	12–18	Dull
Verrucae plana	12–18	Sharp or dull
Malignant		
Basal cell carcinoma	16–20	Dull
Squamous cell carcinoma	16–20	Dull

Disclaimer: Every patient and every electrosurgical unit is different. These numbers are just suggestions and each clinician must find the best settings based on experience with their patients and unit.

increase the power until the desired outcome (destruction, coagulation, or cutting) is achieved. For ablation/destruction, the tissue should bubble or turn gray. Keep in mind that destruction of tissue below the visible area of treatment can occur. The power setting for coagulation is generally higher than the setting needed for tissue destruction. A rule of thumb is to use the lowest power setting that accomplishes a given result so as to achieve cosmetically acceptable outcomes. It helps to moisten the tissue to provide better contact and allow a lower power setting.

The usual radiofrequency modes are:

- Pure cutting current (that still has 10% coagulation)
- Blended cutting and coagulation (approximately 50% of each)
- Coagulation (hemo)
- Fulguration (similar to the Hyfrecator)
- Bipolar coagulation.

Anesthesia

Local anesthesia will be needed for virtually all electrosurgery with the exception of the treatment for telangiectasias, small skin tags, and fine angiomas where either no or topical anesthesia is adequate. Injecting 1% to 2% lidocaine with epinephrine before the procedure will provide painless electrosurgery. However, short bursts of low current can be less uncomfortable than needle anesthesia in some individuals. Topical anesthesia with ethyl chloride is contraindicated because ethyl chloride is flammable. Anesthetic creams (see Chapter 3, *Anesthesia*) can be used for anesthesia before treatment of facial telangiectasias and eliminates the effects of distortion from injectable anesthesia.

Practical Pearls Specific to Radiosurgery

1. Activate the electrode with the foot or hand switch before touching the skin/lesion with the electrode. Touching the lesion first inhibits current flow.
2. It helps to stabilize the physician's operating hand against the patient's body part so that if the patient

BOX 14-1 ***Electrosurgical Settings***

Suggested Settings for Hyfrecator 2000 or Bovie 900

Cosmetic destruction of angiomas, telangiectasias, sebaceous hyperplasia and skin tags without anesthesia: 2–2.5 W on low
ED&C: 14–18 on low
Coagulation after shave: 12–14 on low
Coagulation after removing a pyogenic granuloma: 16–20 on low
Coagulation during full-depth excision (punch, ellipse, or flap): 12–20 on low
Consider switching to high if coagulation on low at 20 is not working. However, it may be best to find and tie off a bleeding vessel or wait while applying pressure with gauze.

Suggested Starter Settings for Ellman Surgitron DF

Vari-Tip settings for cutting
3–6 on cut
6–9 on cut/coag (6 on the face and 9 on the back)
Loop settings for cutting
3–4 on cut (may use 2–3 for smaller loop)
4 on cut/coag
Large LEEP loops for cervix or treating rhinophyma
5–15 on cut
10–20 W on cut/coag
Ball electrode for coagulation: 20–35 on hemo
Fulguration for tissue destruction: 30. This is lower frequency at 1.7 MHz (like the Hyfrecator)
Bipolar: 35 on hemo
Toenail matrix ablation: 16–20 on hemo
Elliptical excision: start on cut at 3 for ellipse. Cut off specimen and do undermining on 4 with cut/coag
Disclaimer: Every patient and every electrosurgical unit is different. These numbers are just suggestions and each clinician must find the best settings based on experience with their patients and unit.

TABLE 14-2 Approximate Range of Power settings with Radio-Frequency Surgery (Using Dual-Frequency Ellman Surgitron)

Lesions	Power Setting (watts)	Electrosurgical Modality (Waveform)	Type of Electrode
Benign			
Angiomas (cherry)	2-3 (no anesthesia) 5-8 (with lidocaine)	Coag (Hemo)	Ball
Angiomas (spider)	2-3 (topical or no anesthesia)	Coag (Hemo)	Needle*
Bleeders (excisions)	25-30 (with lidocaine)	Coag (Hemo)	Ball
Condyloma acuminata	15-25 (with lidocaine)	Cut	Loop
Dermatosis papulosa nigra	2-4 (topical anesthesia) 15-20 (with lidocaine)	Coag (Hemo) Cut	Ball Loop
Epilation	2-3 (topical or no anesthesia)	Coag (Hemo)	Needle*
Incising/excising	10-20 (with lidocaine)	Cut	Vari-tip wire
Nevi (following shave with blade)	5-20 (with lidocaine)	Cut	Loop
Pyogenic granulomas	10-20 (with lidocaine) 20-25 (with lidocaine)	Cut off with loop first Coag (Hemo) with ball to stop bleeding	Loop Ball
Sebaceous hyperplasia	2-3 (topical or no anesthesia)	Coag (Hemo)	Ball
Seborrheic keratosis	10-20 (with lidocaine)	Cut	Loop
Skin tags–small (acrochordons)	2-3 (topical or no anesthesia) 5-8 (with lidocaine) 5-20 (with lidocaine)	Coag (Hemo) Cut	Ball Loop
Syringomas	2-4 (topical anesthesia)	Coag (Hemo)	Ball
Telangiectasias	2-3 (topical or no anesthesia)	Coag (Hemo)	Needle*
Verrucae vulgaris	15-20 (with lidocaine)	Cut and coag	Loop
Malignant			
Basal cell carcinoma	20-30 (with lidocaine)	Curette and coag × 3 cycles	Ball
Squamous cell carcinoma	20-30 (with lidocaine)	Curette and coag × 3 cycles	Ball

*This includes epilation needles, microinsulated needles and 33 gauge needles.

Disclaimer: Every patient and every electrosurgical unit is different. These numbers are just suggestions and each clinician must find the best settings based on experience with their patients and unit. Start with the lower settings and it can always be turned up a little more if the desired effect hasn't been obtained.

moves, the hand with the electrode moves with the patient avoiding a laceration.

3. While cutting, move the electrode using a smooth uninterrupted movement. The intensity should be adjusted until the electrode moves through the tissue like a hot knife through butter.
4. Always use a neutral plate ("antenna") or grounding plate as specified by the manufacturer. The neutral plate should be under the patient and not far from the operative site. The neutral plate does not have to touch the skin and will allow the use of lower power settings if closer to the operative site. A true grounding plate must be in direct contact with the skin and proximity to the operative site is of less importance.
5. To avoid excessive tissue damage when cutting, *minimize lateral heat.*
   Lateral heat = The **product** of *Time* that electrode contacts tissue × *Intensity* of power × *Electrode size* × Nature of the *waveform* × the *Resistance of the tissue* (increases with the lack of moisture) **divided by** the *frequency* of the current.
   - *Electrode contact time.* Keep this to a minimum.
   - *Intensity of power.* If the intensity of the power is too high, it will cause sparking and increased tissue destruction. If too low, it will cause tissue drag, which can increase lateral heat and increase the risk of bleeding as well as a less desirable cosmetic outcome.
   - *Electrode size.* Smaller electrodes with finer wire cause less lateral heat and require less power to operate than larger ones.

   The Ellman Surgitron units operate at 4.0 MHz. The Hyfrecator operates at approximately 0.5 MHz and produces more lateral heat. However, because fulguration and desiccation are used to destroy tissue, the lateral heat is not a problem. It is during cutting that tissue destruction is to be avoided.
6. Tissue must be moist to obtain the desired effect. The moisture allows for the water molecules to vaporize

TABLE 14-3 Approximate Range of Power Settings with Radio-Frequency Surgery (Using Ellman Surgitron FFPF EMC)

Lesions	Power Setting (dial)	Power Setting (watts)	Electrosurgical Modality (Waveform)	Type of Electrode
Benign				
Angiomas (cherry)	1-2	10-20 (with lidocaine)	Coag (Hemo)	Ball
Angiomas (spider)	1-1.5	10-15 (topical anesthesia)	Coag (Hemo)	Needle*
Bleeders (excisions)	2.5-3	25-30 (with lidocaine)	Coag (Hemo)	Ball
Condyloma acuminata	2-2.5	20-25 (with lidocaine)	Cut	Loop
Dermatosis papulosa nigra	1-1.5 1.5-2	10-15 (topical anesthesia) 15-20 (with lidocaine)	Coag (Hemo) Cut	Ball Loop
Epilation	1	10 (topical or no anesthesia)	Coag (Hemo)	Needle*
Incising/excising	2	20 (with lidocaine)	Cut	Vari-tip wire
Nevi (following shave with blade)	2-2.5	20-25 (with lidocaine)	Cut	Loop
Pyogenic granulomas	2-2.5	20-25 (with lidocaine)	Cut off with loop first Coag (Hemo) with ball to stop bleeding	Loop Ball
Sebaceous hyperplasia	1-2	10-20 (topical or no anesthesia)	Coag (Hemo)	Ball
Seborrheic keratosis	2.5-3	25-30 (with lidocaine)	Cut	Loop
Skin tags–small (acrochordons)	1-1.5 2	10-15 (topical or no anesthesia) 20 (with lidocaine)	Coag (Hemo) Cut	Ball Loop
Syringomas	1.5-2	15-20 (topical anesthesia)	Coag (Hemo)	Ball
Telangiectasias	1-2	10-20 (topical or no anesthesia)	Coag (Hemo)	Needle*
Verrucae vulgaris	2-3	20-25 (with lidocaine)	Cut	Loop
Malignant				
Basal cell carcinoma	2-3	20-30 (with lidocaine)	Curette and coag × 3 cycles	Ball
Squamous cell carcinoma	2-3	20-30 (with lidocaine)	Curette and coag × 3 cycles	Ball

*This includes epilation needles, microinsulated needles and 33 gauge needles.

Disclaimer: Every patient and every electrosurgical unit is different. These numbers are just suggestions and each clinician must find the best settings based on experience with their patients and unit. Start with the lower settings and it can always be turned up a little more if the desired effect hasn't been obtained.

and cause the desired effect. It will be almost impossible to obtain any effect whatsoever on highly keratinized (dry) tissue. Just wipe over most lesions with a moist 4 × 4 to provide the moisture needed.

7. Reusable electrodes must be clean and free of carbon to work well. Use fine sand paper to keep them "shiny"!

SAFETY MEASURES WITH ELECTROSURGERY

Potential Hazards of Electrosurgery (To Patient and Physician)

- Fire and burns
- Electric shock
- Transmission of infection through electrode, smoke plume, or spattering blood
- Pacemaker interference.

Safety Precautions to Avoid Potential Hazards

Fire and Burns

- Be sure the alcohol has dried if used to prepare the skin. Do not leave alcohol swabs anywhere near active electrodes.
- Do not use ethyl chloride as the local anesthetic.
- Keep oxygen and other flammable material away from electrosurgical equipment.
- Make sure a fire extinguisher is available.
- Be careful of bowel gas, which contains methane in perirectal procedures. This is more of a problem with patients under general anesthesia who lack control. The gas can explode.

Electric Shock

- Keep electrosurgical equipment functioning properly; if there are signs of malfunction, have the equipment fixed before use.

- Use a three-pronged plug connected to an outlet that is not overloaded.
- Do not use the outlet in the treatment table.
- Make sure the patient is not grasping or touching metal portions of the treatment table.

Transmission of Infection through Electrode

- Always wear disposable gloves.
- When using reusable electrodes, clean them after each use by removing the char followed by sterilizing them in an autoclave or liquid solution. The char can be removed using fine sand paper, an ultrasonic cleaner, or by activating the electrode in a moist 4 × 4 gauze folded over the tip.
- Disposable electrodes are an option.

During sterile procedures options include the following:

- Use a sterilized handle and cord (reusable is preferred as a greener option).
- Place a nonsterile handle into a sterile sheath so that it covers the hand switch and a good portion of the cord. Another option is to use a sterile glove held open while an assistant places the nonsterile handpiece into a finger of the glove by holding the attached wire and lowering it. The electrode tip can then be used to pierce a finger of the glove so it can be secured in place. The physician can then hold the handpiece, which is now within a sterile glove.
- For short procedures in which minimal electrocoagulation is needed, an assistant who is not part of the sterile field can apply the electrosurgery tip to a hemostat or to pickups that are grasping a bleeder as needed.

Transmission of Infection through Smoke Plume or Spattering Blood

Transmission of infection through a smoke plume or spattering blood is a potential risk when treating lesions of viral origin. This is especially true when treating HPV infection in all types of warts. Intact HPV DNA has been recovered in the smoke plume of verrucae treated with electrosurgery and the carbon dioxide laser.[1–3] One case report suggests that a physician acquired an HPV infection of the larynx (laryngeal papillomatosis) while performing laser therapy on HPV-infected lesions.[1]

A publication of the National Institute for Occupational Safety and Health (NIOSH) states that research studies have confirmed that smoke plume can contain toxic gases and vapors such as benzene, hydrogen cyanide, and formaldehyde, bioaerosols, dead and live cellular material (including blood fragments), and viruses.[5] At high concentrations the smoke causes ocular and upper respiratory tract irritation in health care personnel. Smoke evacuators should be used and the various filters and absorbers used in smoke evacuators should be replaced on a regular basis. These materials should be disposed of with other biohazardous waste.[5]

Although there may also be a potential risk of transmission of hepatitis, herpes, or HIV through blood splatter or smoke plume, there is even less scientific evidence showing such transmission. Nevertheless, it is best to follow certain safety measures (especially if the lesion is of viral origin or the patient is known to be infected with HIV or hepatitis).

1. Use a smoke evacuator with the intake nozzle held within 2 inches of the operative area. It is essential to use the evacuator when treating any viral lesion.
2. The physician and treatment team should wear surgical masks and eye protection. Special N95 surgical masks that filter down to 0.5 micron are available and should be used for extensive cases.
3. Consider using a different treatment modality based on evaluation of the risks and benefits of treatment.

Pacemaker Problems

Electrosurgery should be limited in patients with pacemakers, implanted defibrillators, or cardiac monitoring equipment. Electrical current (especially in the cutting mode) may activate or inactivate these devices. Although all such devices are supposedly "shielded" from these effects, if an alternative method of treatment is acceptable, it should be considered. Battery cautery can be used safely but is not as versatile as the electrosurgical units. If electrosurgery remains the best option, use the lowest power setting possible, place the antenna/ground plate next to the lesion and as far away from the pacer as possible, use only short bursts of power, and try to avoid the cutting setting. Do not perform electrosurgery in proximity to the heart.

The use of bipolar forceps or true electrocautery (with heated wire) are the preferred options of experienced cutaneous surgeons when electrosurgery is required in a patient with a pacemaker or an implantable cardioverter-defibrillator (ICD).[6] Routine precautions included utilizing short bursts of less than 5 seconds (71%), use of minimal power (61%), and avoiding use around the pacemaker or ICD (57%).[6] One hundred sixty cutaneous surgeons reported the following complications: reprogramming of a pacemaker (six patients), firing of an ICD (four patients), asystole (three patients), bradycardia (two patients), depleted battery life of a pacemaker (one patient), and an unspecified tachyarrhythmia (one patient). Overall this was a low rate of complications (0.8 case/100 years of surgical practice), with no reported significant morbidity or mortality.[6] Bipolar forceps were utilized by 19% of respondents and were not associated with any incidences of interference.[6]

TREATING SPECIFIC LESIONS

General Approach

Once the decision has been made to use electrosurgery, *turn on the unit and choose the appropriate settings including mode and power.* Some ESUs require a few moments to "warm up." Be sure the antenna or grounding plate is in the proper position. If using a foot pedal, place it within ready reach. Choose the tip to be used for the particular application and place it in the handpiece. Check to see that when the foot pedal or the finger control is pressed, the unit activates.

When used in the cutting mode, the electrode will cut continuously. When set properly, it will move through tissue smoothly without catching or "stalling." If the cutting is not smooth, try the following: make sure the mode selected is pure cutting; moisten the tissue; move slower; check to be sure the electrode tip is shiny and clean; confirm that the grounding pad/antenna is plugged in and placed properly; turn up the power. Excessive sparking and smoke means the power (wattage) is set too high and the tissue will often appear black. When adjusted properly, the newly cut tissue will appear almost normal but will not be bleeding.

When used in the fulguration or coagulation mode, be sure to leave space between the electrode tip and the tissue to produce a "spark gap." Gently tap the lesion to obtain the desired effect. If the tip is applied to the tissue in a continuous fashion, the char will often prevent further tissue effects unless the power is turned up. However, this can cause more scarring. Ideally, the power will be set just high enough to cause graying or light charring of the tissue, which is then wiped away before the electrode is applied again (if needed). For optimal effects at the lowest setting, continue to wipe over dry areas with a moist 4 × 4 gauze. When treating areas that are bleeding, such as the base of a BCC that has been coagulated, slight amounts of blood will provide excellent conduction to desiccate/destroy the tissue. Too much blood, however, can disperse the energy and prevent tissue effects. Apply pressure to the base of the lesion with gauze or a cotton-tipped applicator to reduce bleeding and remove blood before proceeding.

Benign Lesions

See video on the DVD for further learning. 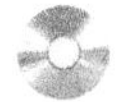

Angiomas (Cherry)

Cherry (also called capillary or senile) angiomas are usually asymptomatic and have no malignant potential. Reasons to remove them include cosmetic concerns, growth, recurrent trauma (e.g., cutting them while shaving), or bleeding. Electrosurgery is probably the most effective inexpensive treatment.

Topical or local anesthesia with epinephrine is often used if the lesions are greater than 4 mm. Larger cherry angiomas should be anesthetized and shaved off first before lightly electrodesiccating the base. Smaller cherry angiomas do not require anesthesia and can be lightly touched with the ball electrode on a low setting. The Hyfrecator is used on low at 2 to 2.5 W (Figure 14-17A). The Surgitron is used on 2 W of coagulation with the ball electrode (Figure 14-17B). The char can be wiped off with gauze or a curette. If red tissue remains, gently and briefly tap the electrode tip on the area again.

Angiomas (Spider)

Spider angiomas can be treated with the same power settings as cherry angiomas. As opposed to telangiectasias, they have a more papular or central feeding vessel with small fine vessels extending from the central area. Spider angiomas can be effectively treated with laser therapy, intense pulsed light (IPL), or electrocoagulation. Injecting lidocaine with epinephrine may obscure the lesion due to vasoconstriction. Thus, it is more common to use topical anesthetic or to treat without any anesthesia.

Electrodesiccation of the central feeding vessel should eradicate the entire angioma. This can be done with an epilation needle, a metal-hubbed 33G needle with an adapter, or a sharp electrode. When a needle is inserted into the vessel, it often bleeds preventing a good coagulation effect. A blunt/ball electrode can then be used to coagulate the central vessel. If bleeding is still a problem, apply pressure to the base of the lesion to decrease blood flow. Use caution to avoid overcoagulation leading to excessive scarring. No curettage is needed afterward. The very lowest setting that causes blanching of the vessel should be used. Using excessive energy that can cause permanent indentations should be avoided. It is normal to see skin flushing around the treatment site in the office. No special aftercare is needed. However, the patient should not scrub the treatment site vigorously while in the healing stage. Should the lesion recur, a more aggressive approach or laser can be tried.

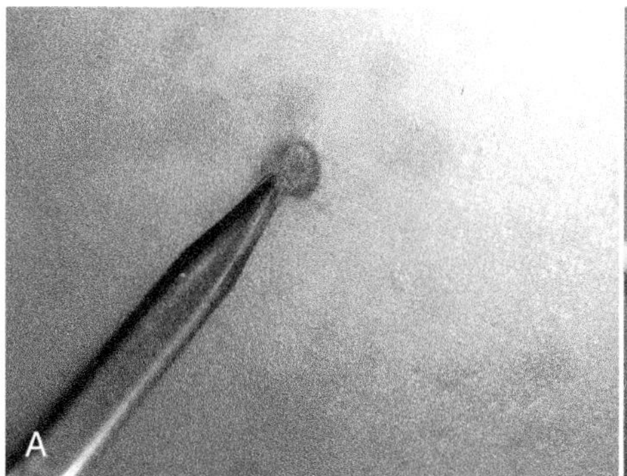

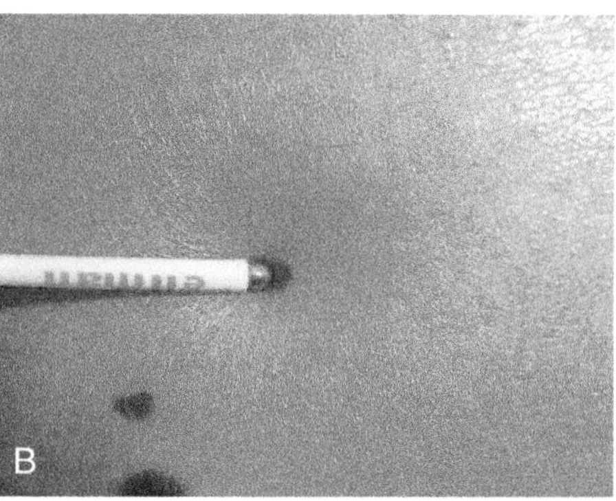

FIGURE 14-17 **(A)** A blunt Hyfrecator electrode is being used for electrodesiccation of this small cherry angioma. **(B)** The Ellman ball electrode performs electrocoagulation on this flat angioma.

Although scarring is minimal, it is not uncommon to have a very small residual hypopigmented area at the previous site of the lesion.

Condyloma Acuminata

When examining a patient for condyloma, some clinicians choose to stain the area with 3% to 5% acetic acid (vinegar). Lesions generally turn white, which makes identification easier. If electrosurgery will be performed, moist lesions will also conduct current more readily.

If there are multiple, small condylomata, it may be prudent to initiate cryosurgery or topical treatments. In the office, this may include trichloroacetic acid, which is inexpensive, quick, and effective. The patient may also be sent home with a prescription for podofilox, a purified podophyllin preparation (Condylox), or imiquimod (Aldara), but these treatments are expensive and require patient compliance. Cryosurgery is an alternative (see Chapter 15, *Cryosurgery*). For small flatter lesions, curettement using a sharp 3-mm disposable curette works well. Condyloma acuminata can be successfully and easily treated with electrosurgery using either a cutting or a desiccation method. The cutting mode and large loop are especially beneficial for extensive and/or large lesions. Laser ablation is another option albeit the equipment is expensive.

A local anesthetic should always be used before electrosurgery in the genital area. Electrosurgery can resolve condyloma with a single treatment with the sites healing in 7 to 14 days usually with minimal scarring. This may be particularly appealing to the patient who has failed multiple treatments with various chemicals and/or cryosurgery.

There are two electrosurgery options. One is to use light electrofulguration or electrodesiccation with a ball/dull electrode (coagulation or fulguration settings). This is ideal for multiple small lesions. The other is to perform radiosurgery with a loop electrode (usually not as large as the LEEP electrodes) using a pure cutting current. Using "pure cutting" generally provides enough hemostasis while also reducing the likelihood of scarring. The goal is to destroy the lesion with minimal effect to the surrounding normal skin. Note that with cryotherapy a 2-mm halo of frozen normal tissue around the lesion is needed, but with electrosurgery, only the abnormal tissue is removed.

If there are only a few small lesions, therapy can be accomplished without magnification. However, when lesions are large or extensive, removing them under magnification (magnification loupes or the colposcope) ensures complete removal, limits excessive tissue removal, and identifies lesions that are too small to be seen with the naked eye.

The unit should be set for pure cutting with the power set based on the ESU and the loop size (see Tables 14-1 to 14-3). The condyloma should be "debulked" on the first pass and then the edges should be lightly "feathered" to ensure there is no remaining tissue and to blend the treated skin into the surrounding normal tissue. *A common error is to go too deeply with the loop.* **Use caution**. The penile skin is extremely thin and the RF loops cut very fast. Going too deeply will not only increase bleeding but also the secondary scarring. The same can happen with the vulvar and perianal tissues. If one attempts to perform a flat shave with a surgical blade, one often finds it difficult to cut on the mobile skin and bleeding readily obscures the operating field. That is the beauty of high-frequency electrosurgical removal: limited if any bleeding, controllable depth, minimal tissue destruction, and little scarring even with larger lesions. Using magnification during removal enhances all of these benefits even more.

The sequence for removal of a condyloma using high-frequency electrosurgery is as follows:

1. Soak the area with acetic acid (moistened 4 × 4s or spray bottle).
2. Examine under magnification (preferred).
3. Anesthetize as needed with 1% lidocaine (with or without epinephrine). Use a 30–gauge needle. Consider a penile block in males.
4. Turn on the unit and select pure cutting mode at the appropriate level. Test the setting on the top portion of the largest condyloma until it is just right (staying away from the base of the lesion until the setting is correct).
5. With magnification assistance, remove the lesion using a loop electrode in a superficial sweep, gradually going deeper until all visible abnormal tissue has been removed (Figure 14-18).
6. Wipe treated area with a 4 × 4 gauze moistened with acetic acid and reinspect area.
7. Apply aluminum chloride to any sites that may still be bleeding (ferric subsulfate has a tendency to leave an iron deposit stain especially in the genital area).
8. When all lesions have been removed, apply ointment of choice (an antibiotic or petrolatum) to hasten healing and to prevent treated tissue from adhering to undergarments. Lidocaine ointment 5% can also be used alone or with either of the other ointments to provide an anesthetic effect.

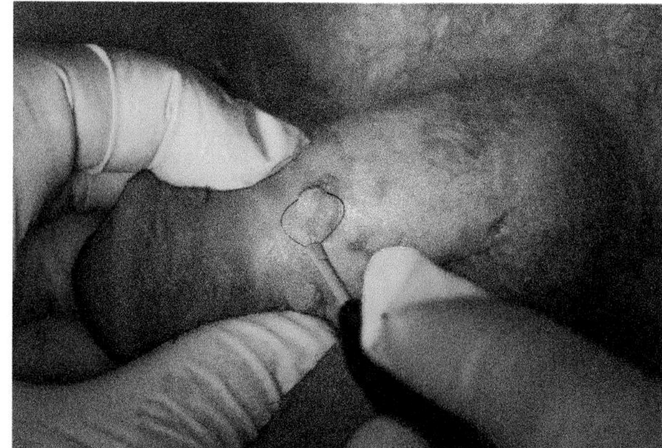

FIGURE 14-18 Removal of condyloma using radiofrequency shaving. A large dermatologic loop using a pure cutting mode is employed. Caution is needed lest the loop cut too deeply. *(Copyright John L. Pfenninger, MD.)*

9. All tissue removed should be sent to pathology since it is difficult to discern bowenoid dysplasias from classic condylomas with the naked eye.
10. Because persistence of some virus and growth of small, grossly undetectable lesions is common, a follow-up exam is generally done in 4 to 6 weeks to check for recurrences.
11. With the association of HPV and cervical cancer, be sure you have addressed all issues regarding pap smear screening, immunizations, and safe sex practices.

Neurofibromas

Neurofibromas are soft, benign tumors that are elevated above the skin surface (see Figure 33-30 in Chapter 30, *Procedures to Treat Benign Conditions*). Smaller lesions can appear to be nonpigmented nevi. However, if shaved off, a gelatinous material appears at the base, which is classic for neurofibromas and indicates the need for further treatment. Patients may request removal for cosmetic purposes, because they exist in areas of friction or trauma or because of fear that the lesion is not benign. Two possible electrosurgical methods for removal include (1) a shave with a scalpel and then electrocoagulation of the gelatinous residual or (2) a shave with a wire loop electrode using cutting and coagulation (blended) current going progressively deeper until the lesion is removed. In both instances, it is often easier to curette out the base, which often goes surprisingly deep, followed by the electrosurgery. For lesions over a centimeter in diameter, excision with suture closure provides faster healing with less scarring.

Before treating neurofibromas, advise patients that these lesions can regrow and that the area of the excision can become indented and/or hypopigmented.

Nevi (Moles) Benign

See video on the DVD for further learning. 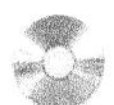

One excellent method for removal of benign nevi is to use high-frequency (radio-frequency) electrosurgery. It is this exact procedure for which RF really provides value over the other methods of simple shave excision. However, a brief discussion with some caveats is indicated regarding this approach to nevi.

If there is any suspicion that a presumed nevus is malignant, a full-thickness biopsy should be performed to rule out melanoma. It is not acceptable to do the primary removal/biopsy with electrosurgery using a loop (even the pure cutting mode) because the associated heat-induced tissue alteration, although minimal, can still interfere with the pathologic diagnosis and the determination of the depth of invasion in the case of a melanoma. If the power setting is too high or if any coagulation current is used, the "burn artifact" is even more pronounced and unacceptable.

All excised pigmented lesions regardless of method used for removal should be sent to the pathologist. Many nevi are removed because of cosmetic concerns or because of repeated trauma to them (e.g., under a bra strap, where routine shaving cuts them on the face or legs). When a lesion is almost certainly not a melanoma, a shave removal can be performed safely (see below for recommended technique). *With atypical-appearing nevi,* one has to ask the question, "Could this be a melanoma?" If the response is "Yes, it certainly could be," then biopsy for depth. If the response is that a melanoma is quite unlikely, then removal using a shave technique is preferred. Shave removal is quicker, less costly, provides an adequate diagnosis in the majority of instances, and results in less scarring providing an excellent cosmetic result, especially with the RF technique described here (see Chapter 8, *Choosing the Biopsy Type*).

Much fear has been instilled into providers that they may shave a melanoma thus preventing adequate determination of the depth of the lesion. Depth is used both for prognosis and for delineating the type of treatment required. However, there is not enough time or expertise available for every atypical nevus to be excised with suture closure. It is far better to sample atypical nevi using the method described here than to put off doing so for fear of "doing it wrong" or not having the expertise to excise and do the closure, thus missing a deadly melanoma. Another consideration is that if the patient is left with large scars after a biopsy for minor lesions, they will be less apt to return for further biopsies, which increases the risk that they will experience a more advanced melanoma later. Shave or punch biopsies that do not remove the whole melanoma at once do not negatively influence survival.

Luckily, it is rare that it makes that much clinical difference if a melanoma is transected. (Everyone practicing clinical dermatology has sooner or later transected an unsuspected melanoma.)

The following electrosurgical technique is excellent for the removal of presumed benign nevi with RF (Figure 14-19):

1. Anesthetize with 1 or 2% lidocaine with epinephrine. Be careful not to distort the lesion any more than necessary
2. Use a No. 15 scalpel blade or razor blade to shave off the lesion. If the lesion has no worrisome features, shave flat to avoid any depression of the scar. However, if there are some atypical features, shave in a saucer-like pattern with the central portion a little deeper than the margins to ensure complete removal of the entire lesion.
3. Using a high-frequency ESU and a wire loop electrode, "smooth out" the lesion to eliminate any residual tissue as well as to stop the bleeding using a light "feathering," sweeping motion. Blend in the edges of the shave with the surrounding skin. Keep the tissue moist with a dampened 4 × 4 gauze to make this step easier.
4. Send the tissue to pathology.

Although radiosurgery is used to *finish the shave*, using the loop to remove the lesion primarily, instead of using a blade, is discouraged (due to burn artifact and the chances of the excision going too deeply). A well-done shave biopsy with a blade can also be completed with nothing more than aluminum chloride for hemostasis.

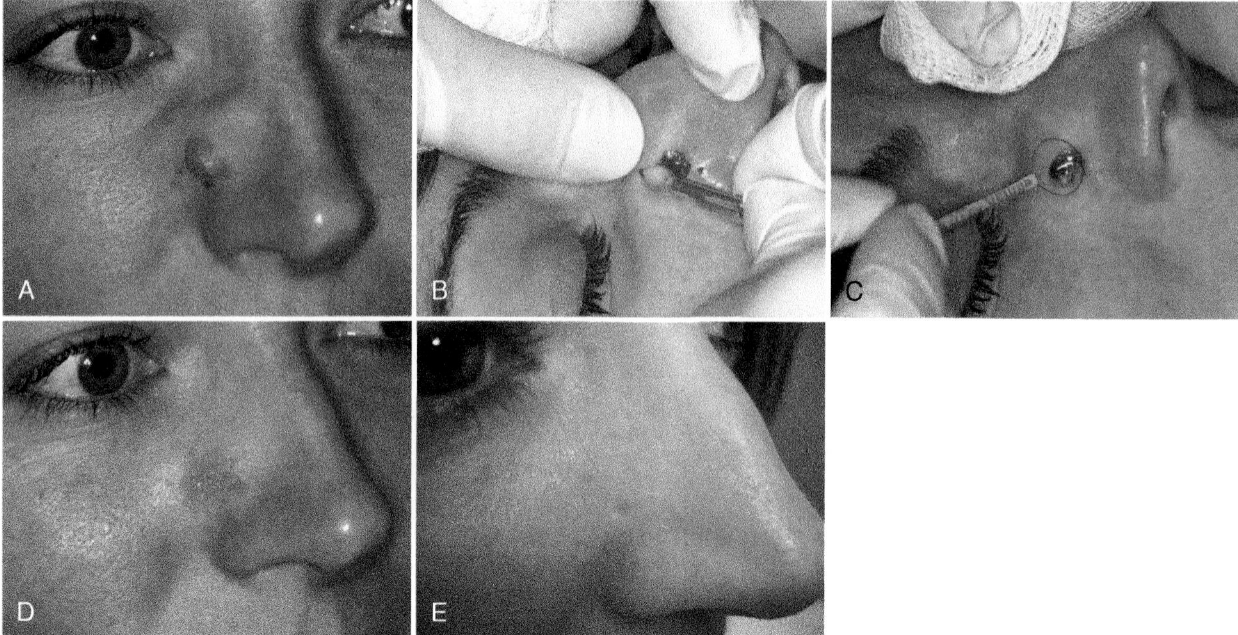

FIGURE 14-19 (**A**) A benign intradermal nevus on the face has been anesthetized prior to shave excision. (**B**) The nevus is excised with a No. 15 scalpel blade. (**C**) The remaining tissue is feathered with RF surgery using a loop electrode. (**D**) Immediate result. (**E**) Cosmetic result 1 year later. *(Copyright John L. Pfenninger, MD.)*

Pyogenic Granuloma

Pyogenic granulomas are very vascular benign tumors (Figure 14-20). They occur most commonly on the fingers, face, lips, and gingiva. Pyogenic granulomas often occur at the site of minor trauma and are more common in pregnancy. These vascular lesions are ideal for electrosurgical treatment.

In a randomized controlled study (RCT) comparing cryotherapy with liquid nitrogen versus curettage and electrodesiccation of patients with pyogenic granuloma, the curettage and electrodesiccation had the advantage of requiring fewer treatment sessions to achieve resolution and better cosmetic results.[7]

Before treatment, inject 1% lidocaine with epinephrine to cause blanching of the skin at the base of the lesion. Epinephrine is needed because of the extreme vascularity of these lesions. If the pyogenic granuloma is on a finger, start with a digital block with lidocaine

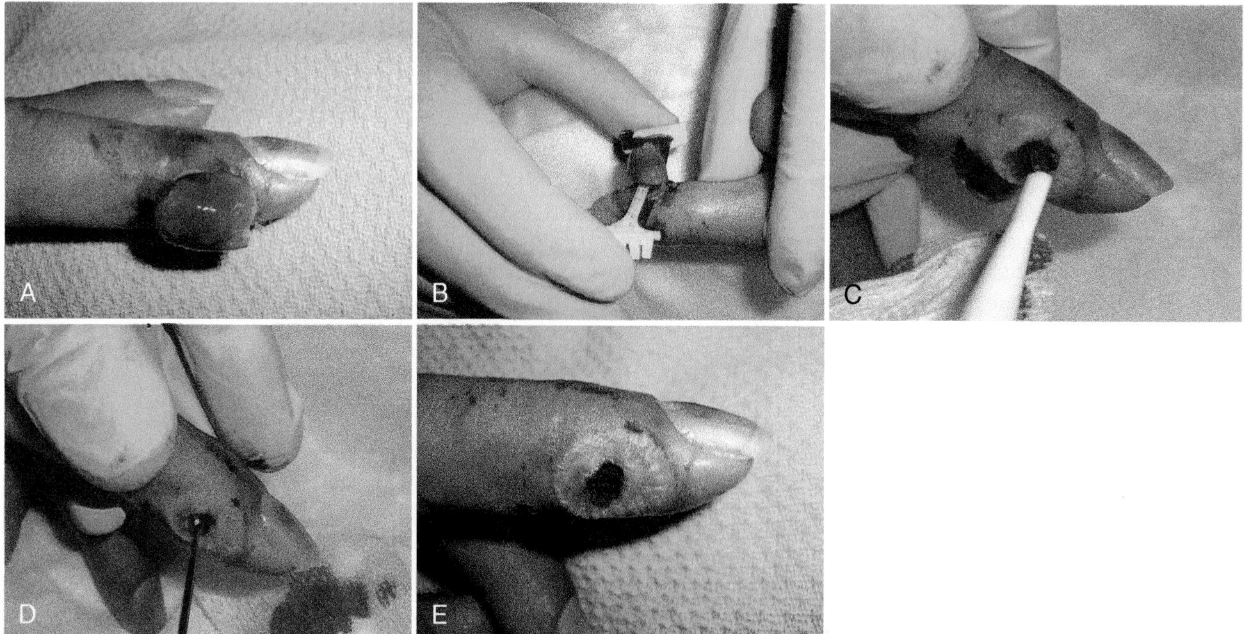

FIGURE 14-20 (**A**) Pyogenic granuloma that started during pregnancy. (**B**) Shave excision after pregnancy. (**C**) Curettage. (**D**) Electrofulguration with visible spark to the remaining vascular tissue. (**E**) Final result. More than one cycle of curettage and electrodestruction may be needed to stop the bleeding and prevent recurrence. *(Copyright Richard P. Usatine, MD.)*

and no epinephrine. Some physicians place a temporary tourniquet around the base of the finger to control bleeding during the procedure. If choosing this approach, the tourniquet may be left on for at least 30 minutes safely. (See page 217 for discussion of tourniquets.)

Wait at least a few minutes after the injection to gain the benefit of the epinephrine. Lab slips and forms can be filled out during this time. The elevated portion of the lesion is then shaved off with a scalpel blade. (Alternatively, a loop electrode using a cutting/coagulation current could have been used with the caution that it can easily penetrate too deeply, very quickly.) Send the specimen for histology to rule out the remote possibility that the lesion is an amelanotic melanoma. The base of the wound is curetted with a 3-0 to 5-0 dermal curette to remove the remaining tissue. Before electrocoagulating the base, compress the tissue with gauze to control bleeding. Pooled blood or active bleeding will diminish the efficacy of electrosurgery. In Figure 14-20, after blotting the blood away, the base is treated with electrodesiccation. (It may be necessary to use the higher power of electrocoagulation for these vascular lesions.) Further curettage and desiccation may be required a number of times to destroy the whole pyogenic granuloma and to stop the bleeding. If some tissue remains, the pyogenic granuloma will regrow.

Rhinophyma

Rhinophyma is a form of rosacea that can grossly disfigure the nose (Figure 14-21). In this case the bulbous tissue was also blocking the nostrils and impairing breathing. Patients are stared at in public places and may limit their activities to avoid public ridicule. The electrosurgical cutting devices provide an excellent treatment option for rhinophyma. Although the surgery is performed for more than cosmetic reasons, it is important to obtain prior authorization from the insurance company before proceeding with this procedure. It can be a difficult and time-consuming procedure so it is best to allocate 1 to 2 hours on the schedule. Payment is commensurate with the time invested. This is an advanced procedure and should be performed only when the clinician has significant experience with facial surgery and electrosection.

To do this procedure in the office, the patient should be in relatively good health with no unstable cardiopulmonary disease. This is a potentially bloody surgery so it does help to make sure all nonessential anticoagulants are stopped. The patient should understand that the nose will be red and raw for 1 to 2 weeks after the surgery. Make sure the patient changes into a gown and removes all upper clothing before beginning.

When first performing this procedure, consider treating only a portion of the nose and doing the surgery in two stages. This gives the patient a chance to see what the surgery and recovery periods are like without committing to having the entire nose treated in one sitting.

Appropriate-sized cutting loops are essential. The loops used for cervical LEEP procedures (Figure 14-13) are excellent for this purpose. Other large electrosurgical loops can also be used. Place the neutral plate below the patient's head. A smoke evacuator is definitely needed and it helps to have two assistants. One will be needed to hold the smoke evacuator tubing and to make adjustments in the electrosurgical settings. The other assistant can help remove the strips of skin and apply pressure for hemostasis when needed.

Perform infraorbital blocks bilaterally before starting with the local anesthetic. See Chapter 3 for a guide to regional blocks. Then inject 1% lidocaine and epinephrine into the affected area (Figure 14-21B). Although this is the nose, it is crucial to have epinephrine to keep the bleeding to a minimum.

Start by shaving down the nose with the loop. The pure cutting setting with levels as high as 30 W may be needed. Move the loop across the nose in one long continuous motion (Figure 14-21C). The assistant can hold the strip of skin up while you finish the pass (Figure 14-21D). Large white areas of sebaceous hyperplasia will be encountered (Figures 14-21E and F). Shape the nose and compare the sides for symmetry. Leave some definition of the nasal alae as they come off from the central nose. This procedure literally sculpts a new nose. The abnormal tissue will be soft and cut easily. Do not remove too much tissue. A second procedure to remove more tissue can be done if needed.

Hemostasis can be obtained along the way with pressure from gauze and electrocoagulation. A bipolar forceps attached to the same electrosurgical unit may be ideal. Alternatively, change the loop electrode over to the ball electrode as needed for hemostasis (Figure 14-21G). If a second electrosurgical unit is in the room, that unit could be dedicated to hemostasis while keeping the RF cutting unit for the loop only.

At the end of the procedure (Figure 14-21H) cover the nose with petrolatum and gauze. One way to keep the gauze in place is to wrap a long gauze around the back of the head. Send the patient home with a prescription for a pain medication such as hydrocodone and acetaminophen. Have the patient return in 2 days for a wound check to make sure there are no signs of infection and that bleeding is not a problem. Moist healing postoperative care is essential.

These patients are very appreciative because this procedure often provides a new life free from the fear of going out in public (Figure 14-21I).

Sebaceous Hyperplasia

Sebaceous gland hyperplasia of the face is a common condition as people age. It is asymptomatic and not dangerous, but patients often ask for treatment for cosmetic reasons. Occasionally it may be unclear whether what appears to be sebaceous hyperplasia may actually be a BCC. If the diagnosis is uncertain, a biopsy is indicated. It is easiest to do a shave biopsy with a scalpel or sharp curette and send the specimen for pathologic diagnosis. The base can then be cauterized lightly.

If the diagnosis is certain because the sebaceous hyperplasia is typical, the condition can be treated with tissue destruction using cryosurgery or electrodesiccation. Either of these approaches will not yield a

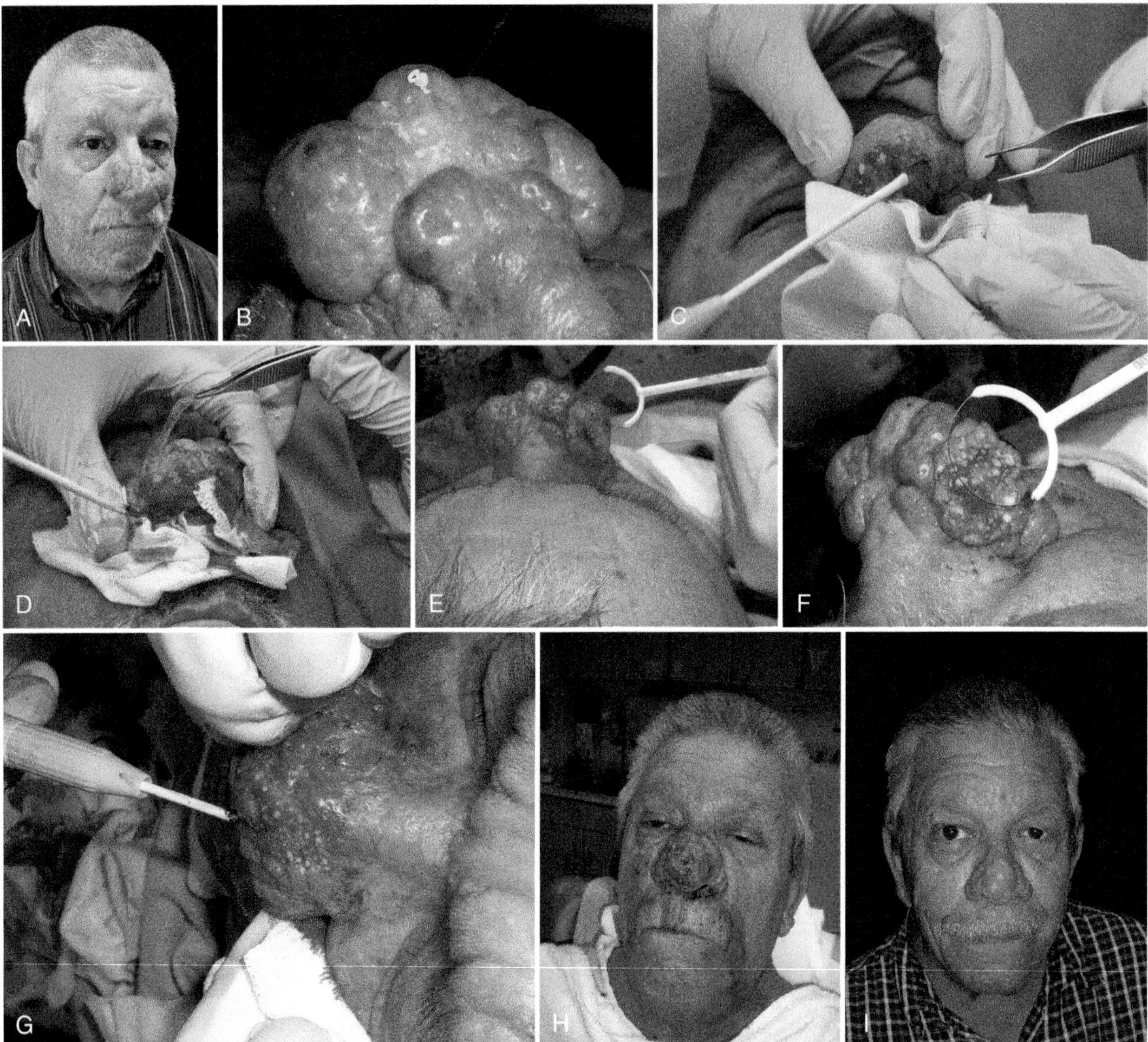

FIGURE 14-21 (A) Large disfiguring rhinophyma on a man who is not a heavy drinker. (B) A 30 gauge needle is inserted into the nose delivering lidocaine with epinephrine prior to surgery. The pressure of the anesthetic often causes sebum to exude from the dilated sebaceous glands. (C) Electrosection with a square LEEP electrode. (D) A strip of tissue is removed as the electrode cuts through the rhinophyma. (E) A semicircular LEEP electrode is being applied to the hypertrophy tissue of the nasal ala. (F) As the electrode cuts through the tissue, large white hyperplastic sebaceous glands are seen. (G) The ball electrode is used for hemostasis. (H) Much of the rhinophyma was excised, allowing the patient to breathe through unobstructed nostrils. All bleeding was stopped. (I) A happy patient after re-epithelialization from the rhinophyma electrosurgery. *(Copyright Richard P. Usatine, MD.)*

specimen for pathology. When using electrodesiccation, a low-power setting should be used to avoid scarring (Figure 14-22).

Seborrheic Keratosis

If there is any question about whether a presumed seborrheic keratosis is malignant, perform a biopsy with a scalpel or razor blade to obtain a good specimen for pathology. If the lesion is shaved or excised with electrosurgery, the heat-induced tissue destruction may interfere with the pathologic diagnosis. When removing a seborrheic keratosis with shave biopsy using a scalpel, hemostasis can be easily achieved with aluminum chloride or Monsel's solution, and electrosurgery is not needed.

When dealing with a classic, thin seborrheic keratosis, another technique is to lightly fulgurate the lesion and then wipe it off with a gauze or curette. Because this does not provide tissue for pathology, this approach should not be used if the lesion has suspicious features (i.e., may be a melanoma). The advantage to this technique is that the desiccated seborrheic keratosis is easily removed from the skin below, without going deeper than necessary (Figure 14-23). This allows for good control of the depth of removal and can minimize scarring. However, these lesions are very hyperkeratotic and thus quite dry often making any electrosurgical attempts at removal more difficult unless they are hydrated first using water-moistened 4 × 4 gauze.

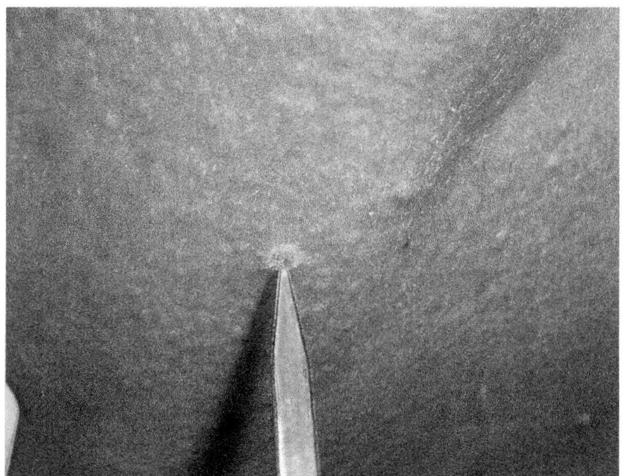

FIGURE 14-22 The blunt electrode is being used to treat sebaceous hyperplasia of the face without and no local anesthesia. The Hyfrecator is set at approximately 2 W. *(Copyright Richard P. Usatine, MD.)*

When using radiosurgery to shave these lesions, it may help to outline the lesion with a surgical pen. A large round loop electrode can be used to shave off the lesion with a single initial pass using a pure cutting setting. See Tables 14-1 to 14-3 for power settings. The skin can be smoothed, using the loop like an artist painting with a brush, while keeping the electrode at a 90-degree angle to the skin surface. Gentle strokes are used to feather the edges of the lesion into the normal skin. A moist 4 × 4 gauze is used between passes of the electrode to remove tissue and moisten the skin. Because the electrical current kills potential infectious organisms, there is no need to use sterile water or saline to moisten the gauze; tap water is fine. Remember that radiosurgery, if set at too high of a power or with any coagulation setting, may still cause more tissue destruction than just a surgical blade, so that the chance of hypopigmentation or scarring may be greater. However, using a combined technique like that described for a nevus above optimizes ease of removal while limiting complications.

Skin Tags (Acrochordons)

There is no absolute cutoff for differentiating between large, medium, and small skin tags. We define the *smallest* skin tags as those lesions that are too small to be grasped easily with a forceps and therefore are difficult to shave or snip off. The *largest* wide-based lesions are those that would be difficult to remove with a single snip of a sharp iris scissor. These are best shaved off with a scalpel.

To treat a small or medium skin tag with electrosurgery, light electrodesiccation (ball electrode) or fulguration (ball or pointed tip) should be used. After the lesion is charred, the char can be removed with a gauze or it can be allowed to fall off on its own.

The eyelid is a location where it is important to be very careful when using chemicals for hemostasis. When used carefully, light electrodesiccation allows for hemostasis without endangering the eye. For radiosurgery of a skin tag, a loop electrode with a cut and coagulation setting of 4 to 6 W should be used after lidocaine and epinephrine are injected first. The skin tag should be shaved off with the loop alone or grasped with the forceps in the loop first (Figure 14-24).

Telangiectasias

Telangiectasias (Figure 14-25) are fine veins ("spider angiomas," "spider veins") that occur commonly on the face and legs. Laser treatment can be effective but is more costly and is not as readily available as sclerotherapy or electrosurgery. Very fine veins of the lower extremities may do well with laser but generally, sclerotherapy is the treatment of choice for lesions 1 to 5 mm that are extensive. Unless the veins are very focal *on the legs*, RF/electrosurgery does not perform well. *Facial veins* are usually more limited and, without the

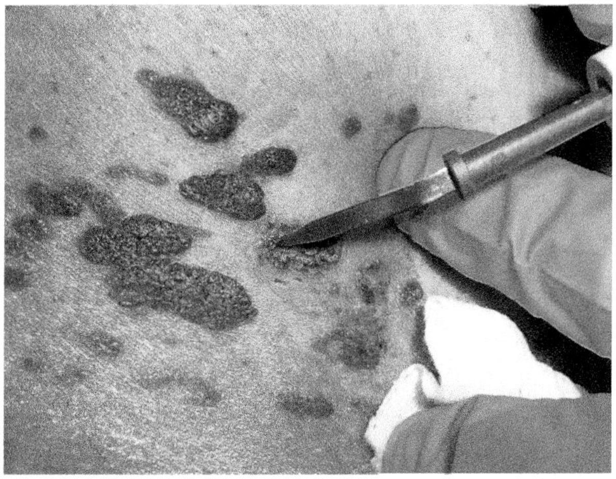

FIGURE 14-23 Electrosurgery can be used in conjunction with a curette to superficially remove seborrheic keratoses. *(Copyright Richard P. Usatine, MD.)*

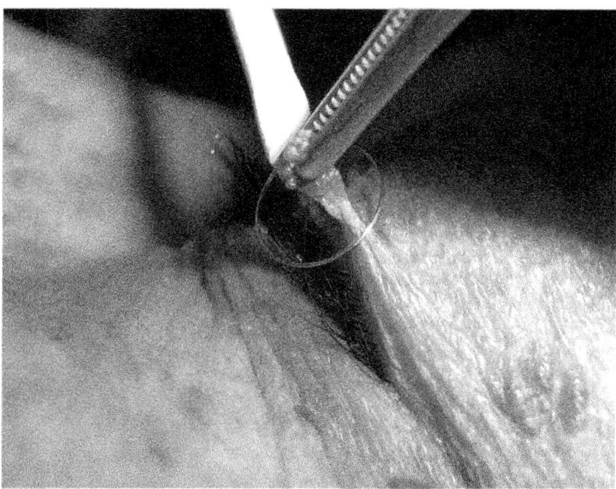

FIGURE 14-24 An electrosurgical loop on a cutting instrument is about to transect an eyelid skin tag. Local anesthetic was injected prior to cutting with RF current. This method allows for cutting and coagulation simultaneously, thereby avoiding getting blood or hemostatic chemicals into the eye. *(Copyright Richard P. Usatine, MD.)*

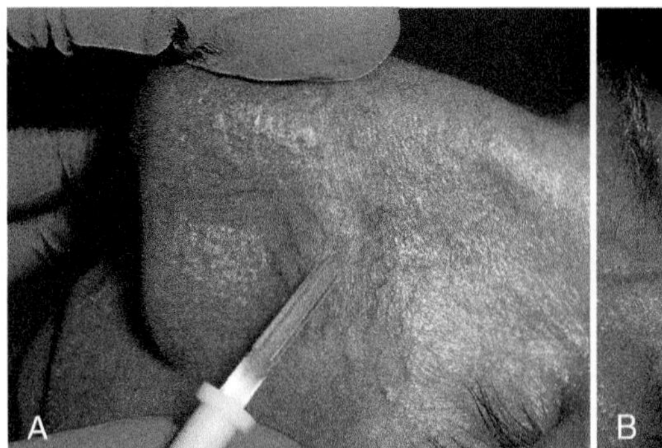

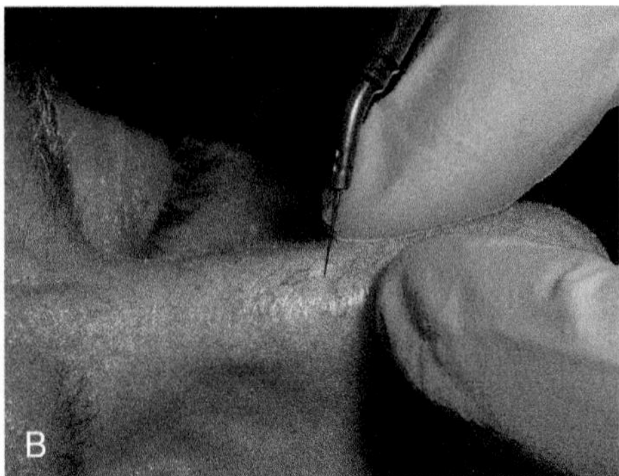

FIGURE 14-25 (A) Electrosurgical treatment of facial telangiectasias using a sharp disposable electrode with approximately 2 W of energy and no local anesthetic. (B) Electrocoagulation of nasal telangiectasias using a specialized epilation needle. The tip of the needle is inserted into the telangiectasias and the current is actuated for approximately 1 second. *(Copyright Richard P. Usatine, MD.)*

hydrostatic pressure that is present in the legs, treatment with electrosurgery can provide excellent results. Fine telangiectasias on the face are the best candidates since anything over a diameter of 1 mm is likely to bleed and persist. As with all procedures, discuss the risks and benefits of electrosurgical treatment and obtain informed consent before proceeding. Treatment of these lesions is generally for cosmetic reasons so it is even more important to review the various options and the possible complications.

Before treating telangiectasias discuss with the patient the pros and cons of using topical anesthesia.

1. It is possible to treat without anesthesia in many cases. Areas around the nose, however, are especially sensitive. If a topical anesthetic is used, allow it to remain in place at least 15 minutes. Injecting the area with a local anesthetic can obscure the lesion.
2. Choose a fine-needle (33-gauge) electrode or sharp tip of the Hyfrecator electrode. The Ellman company provides fine-needle electrodes for the Surgitron that are specially coated with Teflon for treating telangiectasias. This limits burning of the overlying skin. Only the very tip is active while the rest of the needle is shielded. ConMed also provides fine-needle electrodes for use with the Hyfrecator.
3. Magnification loops are very helpful since the smaller telangiectasias respond best and will be more easily identified.
4. Use a low-power coagulation/hemostasis setting. For the Ellman, 2 W work well. Use 2 to 2.5 W for the Hyfrecator.
5. Wipe off the topical anesthetic if used. With the patient in a supine position to limit movement, insert the fine needle into the vein superficially, enough to penetrate into the lumen. The needle may even pass through the small diameter vessel but remain as close to the surface as possible to limit tissue damage. Do not cannulate the vein; instead, place the needle in a perpendicular position to it. Generally, it is not helpful to find the "feeding trunk" since the entire vein will need to be treated anyway or they will recur. If the "feeder" is treated first, the vessel may go into spasm, making the remainder of the vein hard to find. With this in mind, start distally with the smallest part of the vein and march toward the central (larger portion) of the vessel. Keep the electrode activated and just "tap" into the vein every 3 mm along the entire path. The hand holding the handpiece should rest on the patient so that it moves with the patient should the patient suddenly jerk or pull away.
6. Bleeding is not uncommon, especially as the vessels become larger. Cautiously turn up the power slightly. If this does not help, apply pressure. If the vessel continues to bleed, it is likely that it is not occluded and chances for recurrence are higher.

Complications include the discomfort while doing the procedure, bleeding (controlled with pressure), recurrence, and persistent red or brown marks. The discoloration generally clears but takes time and is more common if the power is set too high or if sensitive skin is treated. If the vessels are extensive and very fine or, very "large" such as those seen with rhinophyma and rosacea, it is best to go with a laser treatment. Limited sclerotherapy is also an option that provides excellent results if the vessels are large enough to cannulate.

Warts (Verruca Vulgaris)

Patients seek treatment for warts (lesions caused by the human papilloma virus/HPV) because warts can cause pain, can be unsightly, and can spread to other parts of the body or to other individuals. HPV can infect many parts of the body. In this section, we will only address those HPV infections of the skin: verruca vulgaris, plantar warts, and planar (flat) warts.

In general, most warts can be treated effectively and easily with cryotherapy as described in Chapter 15 or with intralesional injection as discussed in Chapter 16. Patients may even use topical agents effectively at home. However, some warts are refractory to all treatments. Also, if the warts are small (a few millimeters) and there are only a few lesions, electrosurgery has the advantage of allowing the physician to obtain good cure rates with a single in-office treatment. Electrosurgery offers the advantage that the complete removal of the wart can be seen at the time of treatment. With cryotherapy, one must base treatment on the size of the ice ball halo, the freezing time, and most importantly the thaw time. Cryotherapy and intralesional injection methods are more likely to require multiple visits for treatment. Cryotherapy may be more painful in the days that follow the treatment and it frequently leads to an open wound (as does electrosurgery) or a blister.

Electrosurgery of warts always requires local anesthesia. If treating the digits (Figure 14-26), local infiltration with epinephrine-free anesthetic or a digital block should be used. In some cases, local infiltration with lidocaine and epinephrine can be used if the digital artery is avoided. For other locations, the use of epinephrine in the local can aid in obtaining a blood-free field. Fulguration or electrodesiccation/coagulation/hemostasis settings are used to destroy the wart (Figure 14-26B). Refer to Tables 14-1 to 14-3 for power settings. The ball or pointed tip electrode is generally used. With smaller lesions, desiccated tissue is then wiped away with a moist gauze or a curette (Figure 14-26C). If any wart tissue remains, the remaining tissue should receive additional electrosurgery and be wiped away until the final deep layer shows a uniform clear dermis (Figures 14-26D and E). The base of the lesion, however, is often charred by the treatment obscuring the underlying tissue so this needs to be wiped off to inspect the base. Warts are an epidermal lesion so care should be used not to penetrate through the dermis.

If the wart is large and protuberant, the tissue can be shaved off first ("debulked") with a scalpel, curette, or a loop electrode using a cutting or cut/coag setting. Caution is in order to ensure that the excision does not go too deep. Also, warts are very hyperkeratotic and thus very dry, so the electrosurgical application may not work. Soaking with a moistened 4x4 gauze or with K-Y jelly beforehand will help. An alternative way to remove the bulk of the tissue is to use a sharp curette. After "debulking," the residual base can then be coagulated and wiped away. Care should be taken not to burn surrounding tissue excessively, which can cause painful permanent scarring. In the fingers, use care to avoid the digital nerves and arteries on the sides of the digits.

There is no special benefit to using RF methods in the destruction of warts unless the debulking process will include loop debulking.

Possible general *complications* include significant pain, recurrence, and hypopigmentation and scarring. Caution must be used on the plantar surfaces because scarring can cause long-term problems of pain with ambulation. Treatment around the nails may lead to deformities of the nail if the matrix is injured. In some instances, before resolving, treatment can induce a paradoxical reaction where the wart may grow or multiply.

Malignant Lesions

If the nature of a lesion is in doubt, it is always best to biopsy it before definitive treatment. As one gains experience, some lesions may be able to be treated on the day of the first evaluation when they have a "classic" clinical history, appearance, and "feel." All tissue specimens are best sent for histologic confirmation whether they were biopsied previously or not. Shave or curettement biopsies are generally adequate for NMSCs. If the lesion is potentially a melanoma, a full-thickness biopsy should be performed with no further electrosurgical treatment. Performing wide excisions on a "presumed" diagnosis is costly, creates more potential for complications, and often will over- or undertreat a lesion (see Chapter 8, *Choosing the Biopsy Type*).

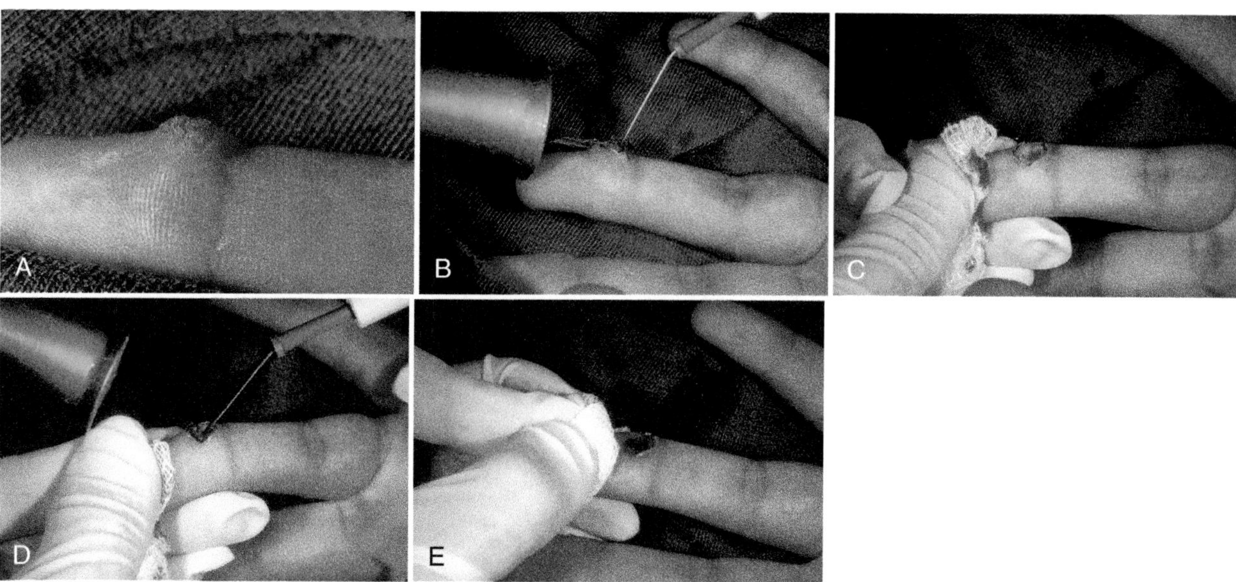

FIGURE 14-26 **(A)** Common wart not responding to cryosurgery. **(B)** Electrodesiccation with the Hyfrecator and smoke evacuator. **(C)** Charred tissue removed with gauze. **(D)** Repeat electrodesiccation. **(E)** Immediate result. *(Copyright Richard P. Usatine, MD.)*

ELECTRODESICCATION AND CURETTAGE

See video on the DVD for further learning. 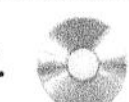

Electrodesiccation and curettage (ED&C) is a useful method of treating NMSCs. It should never be used with melanomas. With curettement, one can feel where the soft tissue ends.

There are *contraindications* for using electrosurgery to treat BCC or SCC based on the histology and location. Sclerosing (morpheaform), micronodular, "aggressive" BCCs as well as SCCs in non–sun-exposed areas over 7 to 8 mm can be more aggressive and are best treated with excision. The superficial type of BCC or SCC *in situ* may be successfully treated with ED&C.

One study compared recurrence rates of 268 consecutive primary nonmelanoma tumors (BCCs and SCCs) treated by surgical excision or ED&C. The recurrence rates between the two types of treatment were not found to be significantly different.[8] A meta-analysis of all studies reporting recurrence rates of BCC between 1947 and 1987 reported a 5-year recurrence rate of approximately 8% for ED&C.[9]

An analysis of recurrence rates of 2314 previously untreated BCCs removed by ED&C showed that increasing lesion diameter, high-risk, and middle-risk anatomic sites were independent risk factors for high recurrence rates.[10] From 1973 to 1982 the following recurrence rates were found (Figure 14-27):

- *Low-risk sites (neck, trunk, and four extremities).* BCCs of all diameters responded well to curettage-electrodesiccation with an overall 5-year recurrence rate of 3.3%.
- *Middle-risk sites (scalp, forehead, preauricular and postauricular, and malar areas).* BCCs less than 10 mm in diameter had a recurrence rate of 5.3%.
- *High-risk sites (nose, paranasal, nasal-labial groove, ear, chin, mandibular, perioral and periocular areas).* Lesions less than 6 mm in diameter had a recurrence rate of 4.5%.[10]

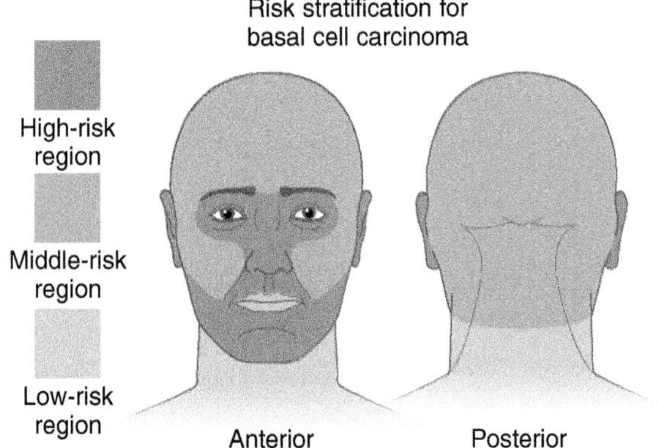

FIGURE 14-27 Risk stratification for basal cell carcinoma on the face and head. *(From Robinson J, Hanke W, Sengelmann R, Siegel D. Surgery of the Skin: Procedural Dermatology, 2nd ed. Philadelphia: Mosby; 2010.)*

The authors concluded that BCCs less than 6 mm in diameter, regardless of anatomic site, as well as selected larger BCCs depending on their anatomic site, are effectively treated by ED&C.[10]

Recurrence rates of primary NMSCs treated by excision versus ED&C ×3 were studied in a private dermatology practice. Tumors up to 2 cm in size were included. One percent of excised tumors recurred, whereas 3% treated with ED&C did. This study found the recurrence rates to be essentially the same in spite of the fact that they used electrosurgery to treat tumors larger than generally recommended. ED&C was quicker, less costly, has fewer complications, and the scars were often less.[8]

Organ transplant recipients frequently develop multiple SCCs. In one study, appropriately selected low-risk SCCs in 48 organ transplant recipients were treated by ED&C. Only histologically confirmed SCCs were considered in this study.[11] The mean follow-up time was 50 months, and 13 residual or recurrent SCCs were observed in 10 patients. The overall rate of residual or recurrent SCCs was 6%, with 7% for SCCs on the dorsum of the hands or fingers, 11% for SCCs on the head and neck, 0% for the forearms, and 5% for the remaining non–sun-exposed areas (shoulder, legs). In organ transplant recipients with many SCCs, ED&C can be a safe therapy for appropriately selected low-risk SCCs, with an acceptable cure rate.[11]

Using ED&C with BCC or SCC: Step-by-Step Instructions

See video on the DVD for further learning. 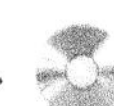

1. Inject the skin surrounding the lesion with 1% to 2% lidocaine with epinephrine.
2. Curette the softer tissue of a BCC first before using electrosurgery (Figure 14-28A). A sharp dermal curette, usually 3 to 5 mm depending on lesion size is used for this. Reusable curettes are adequate but must be sharpened periodically. Disposable curettes are always sharp but clinicians need to be careful to not remove normal tissue since they can cut through normal tissue if too much pressure is applied. Curettement is effective because the BCC is softer than the surrounding normal skin and it also has a characteristic almost gelatinous appearance. (Ice cream provides a good analogy. Think of normal tissue as being hard, frozen ice cream. It is difficult to scoop it out compared to somewhat thawed ice cream, which is very easy to scoop out. Neoplastic tissue is softer like the thawed ice cream because of abnormal connections between cells. Exceptions include morpheaform BCCs and keratoacanthomas.) The abnormal tissue is removed by scraping with the curette in all directions.
3. Then fulguration is performed at the base of the lesion including 2 mm of the surrounding normal tissue (Figure 14-28B). The general rule for a BCC is that a margin of 3 mm of normal tissue should be removed with an excision. ED&C provides this margin. Many will curette with a larger curette first

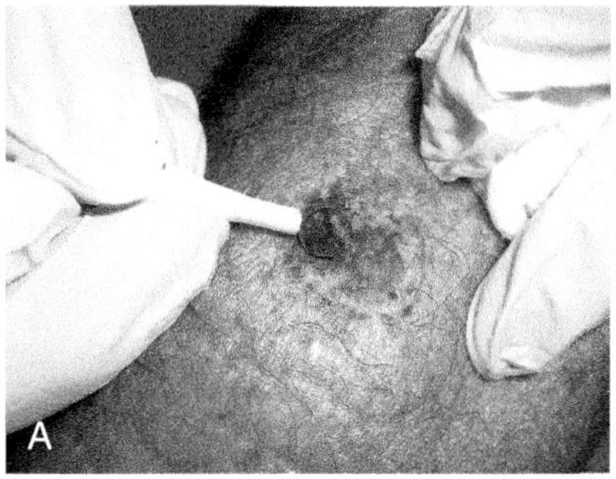

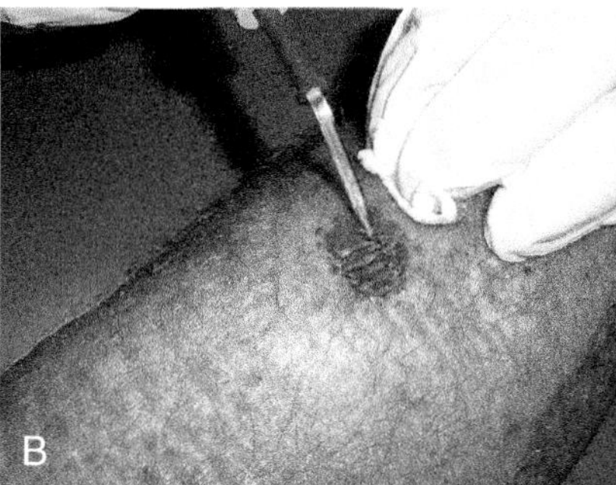

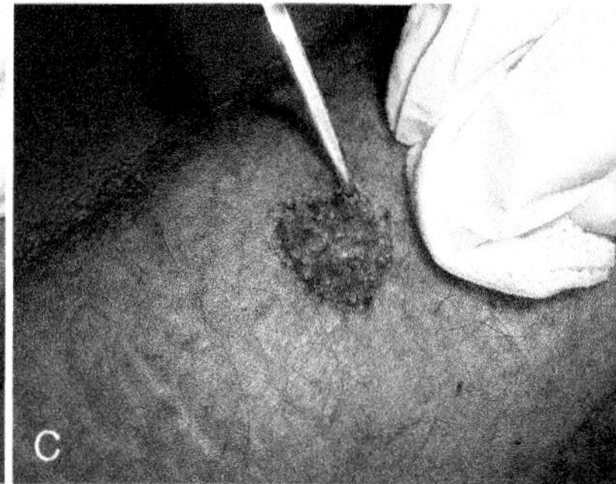

FIGURE 14-28 (A) Curettage of a nodular basal cell carcinoma on the arm. (B) Electrodesiccation after curettage of the BCC. (C) Final electrodesiccation after the third cycle of curettage. The blunt electrode is moved back and forth across the treated area and a small margin of normal tissue is treated using a circular motion around the periphery. *(Copyright Richard P. Usatine, MD.)*

(5 to 7 mm), then follow with a smaller curette (3 mm) purportedly to remove any small pockets of tissue. Although this is an interesting idea, it has not been clinically proven.
4. Two additional cycles are performed for a total of three cycles (Figure 14-28C). Treatment time is 5 minutes or less.

One caveat is that should the curettement penetrate into the subcutaneous fat, it indicates either that the tumor has invaded deeply or that the curettement was overzealous. It is best to perform a full excision at that point.

Realize that an initial shave excision or the curetted pieces are likely to be read as "margins positive" by the pathologist. Indicate in the EMR and/or on the requisition and the final report that "Margins will be positive due to nature of the procedure." This will at least document that the report was reviewed and considered.

The wound may take 3 to 4 weeks to heal, usually with some hypopigmentation. It is essential that the patient understand the principles of moist healing and adhere to them.

LEARNING THE TECHNIQUES

Regardless of the unit used, it is possible to practice the electrosurgery techniques with a piece of uncooked beef steak. The steak should be a fresh, inexpensive cut of steak that is not too fatty and without many tendinous attachments. Pig's feet can even be used (e.g., after a suturing workshop). It is not necessary to use a smoke evacuator while practicing on meat, but there will be the smell of a foul barbecue!

Practicing with the Hyfrecator

To practice with the Hyfrecator, the meat should be touched broadly with the nonoperating hand to create a ground. Begin with the handpiece plugged into the low setting. Practice activating the handpiece and coming close to the steak until the sparks of fulguration appear. Turn up the current to see how the sparking and tissue destruction (cooking of the steak) increase. Try the same exercise with the electrode touching the beef to produce electrodesiccation. Then plug the handpiece into the high setting. Observe the increased destruction of tissue.

Practicing Radiosurgery

Follow these guidelines for practicing with the Ellman Surgitron and other high-frequency units:

1. To practice cutting with the Surgitron, the meat should be placed on a paper towel sitting on top of the "antenna" plate. Begin with a round wire electrode (either small or large, with the latter requiring slightly more power but providing a flatter excision) in the handpiece, and set the unit to "cut" on a midrange setting. Be sure the meat is moist and not dried out on top. Cut through the meat, keeping the loop at a right angle to the tissue. Perform the usual sequence and activate the electrode *before* touching the meat to provide a smooth cut with minimal tissue damage. Compare how this looks and feels to activating the electrode *after* touching the meat. Note that when doing it this way, the electrode will often not cut at all.
2. Repeat this exercise after turning the power up to a much higher setting and observe more spark and smoke. The tissue will also have more char (damage). The ideal setting will provide enough power to cut smoothly through the meat without catching ("stalling"), and yet leave little tissue damage behind.
3. Now turn the power to a low setting. Note how the electrode drags. Determine which setting will allow the electrode to move through the meat without either sparking or a drag. Try this with a forceps holding the meat before activating the loop. Be sure to grasp the tissue with the forceps through the loop before starting the cutting.
4. Practice making true vertical incisions in the meat using the Vari-Tip electrode, again on the "pure cut" setting. Change the length of the electrode to see how the depth of the cut can be varied. Increase and decrease the power as above.

5. Remove the antenna plate (neutral electrode) from under the meat and try cutting with a loop on a setting that was optimal. Note that it is almost impossible to cut at all. Increasing the power may allow cutting, but there will be more tissue burn artifact. This demonstrates the value of having the neutral electrode close to the lesion.
6. The *cut and coagulation setting* should also be tried to feel how the electrode moves slightly more slowly through tissue with comparable power settings. The power most likely will have to be increased for a "smoother" cut.
7. Try the above exercises in the *coagulation* setting with the wire loop. Unless the power is set very high, the loop will not cut. Coagulation can be accomplished with any electrode (ball, pointed tip, fine needle/Vari-Tip) but most commonly will be used with the ball electrode. Use a light touch, barely touching the tissue while moving the electrode gently over the area to be coagulated. The electrode must be activated *before* touching the meat and works best when used in a gentle tapping fashion. If excessive char builds up, it must be wiped away or moistened for the tip to be effective. Bleeding can be controlled in a surgical field by grasping the bleeder with forceps or hemostats and touching any active electrode to the instrument.

One method that can be used to test ESU cutting settings on the patient without consequences to healing is to remove the tissue of concern with a circle before finishing the ellipse with two additional triangles. This circle will not be the area that needs to heal for the patient and therefore will allow for evaluation of the settings before the final cuts are made (Figure 14-29).

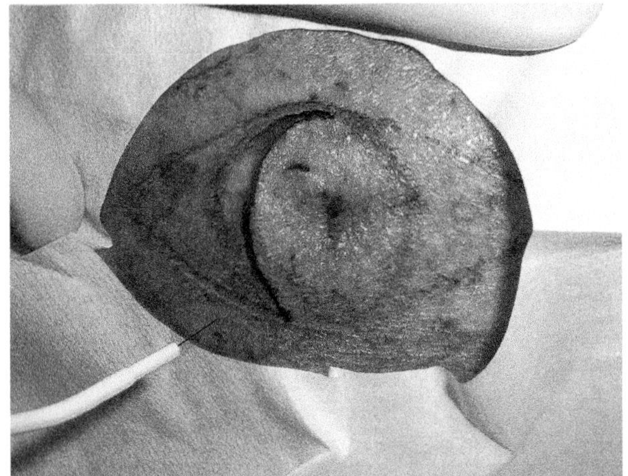

FIGURE 14-29 Testing the electrosurgical cutting settings on a patient without consequences to healing. The melanoma *in situ* is being cut out with a circle before finishing the ellipse with two additional triangles. This circle will not be the area that needs to heal for the patient and therefore will allow for evaluation of the settings before the final cuts are made to complete the ellipse. The setting is excellent as there is no bleeding and no excessive char. The Vari-Tip electrode moved smoothly through the tissue without dragging or sparking. *(Copyright Richard P. Usatine, MD.)*

BOX 14-2 *CPT General Destruction Codes*

11200	Removal of skin tags by electrosurgery or any other technique, any area, up to and including 15 (billed once only)
11201	Removal for each additional 10 lesions or portion thereof (may be billed more than once)
17110	Electrosurgery (destruction any means) warts/benign lesions other than skin tags up to 14 lesions (this is a single code used once only regardless if 1 or 14 lesions are treated)
17111	15 or more lesions (stand alone code, not per lesion)
17000	Electrosurgery (destruction any means), all premalignant lesions (AKs), first lesion
17003	Second through 14th lesion (this code is billed for each lesion from 2 to 14) (charge each lesion)
17004	15 or more lesions (stand-alone code, not per lesion)

CODING AND BILLING PEARLS

Electrosurgery is one modality used throughout dermatology for diverse procedures. When electrosurgery is used for tissue destruction, coding is based on the skin destruction codes found in Tables 38-5, 38-6, and 38-11 of Chapter 38, *Surviving Financially*. Benign and premalignant tissue destruction has essentially been divided into three types of CPT codes based on these diagnoses:

- Skin tags: 11200, 11201
- Benign other than skin tags or cutaneous vascular lesions (includes warts and seborrheic keratoses): 17110, 17111
- Premalignant (actinic keratoses): 17000, 17003, 17004.

(Note that laser destruction of cutaneous vascular lesions has separate codes.)

The general destruction codes shown in Box 14-2 are usually independent of the method of destruction and the location of the lesions. However, for destructions of benign lesions, certain specific parts of the body are reimbursed at a higher rate including the anus, penis, vulva, vagina, and eyelid. The CPT codes and typical fees charged for these are detailed in Table 38-6 of Chapter 38. Do not forget to use these codes because they do pay better than 17110 and 17111. These specific location codes are not based on the exact number of lesions and a single lesion may be reimbursed the same as many lesions.

Insurance companies will not pay for removal of skin tags unless there are documented medical reasons (strangulation, pain, or bleeding). Even with documentation many skin tag removals will be denied payment. When patients just do not like the looks of them, the procedure is considered a cosmetic removal. In this instance, patients should be advised in advance that they will be responsible for payment and an estimate should be given. Interestingly, an office visit E/M code can be charged to insurance but the removal fee is the patient's responsibility.

Note that malignant skin destruction codes (Table 38-11 in Chapter 38) are based on size and location of the cancer and not on the type of skin cancer. Electrodesiccation and curettage of BCCs and SCCs are reimbursed based on these codes.

When electrosurgery is used for cutting or coagulating during a biopsy or excision, there are no additional codes for this. The electrocoagulation is part of the procedure just as giving the local anesthetic is.

A specific code is used for rhinophyma correction. CPT code 30120 is used for excision or surgical planing of skin of nose for rhinophyma. The national Medicare reimbursement rate is $492.

CONCLUSION

Electrosurgery is a powerful and versatile tool for skin surgery. It is an important skill for the clinician to master and each unit requires specific familiarity. Caution is especially indicated in cosmetically sensitive areas (e.g., face, hands, and breasts) since the cutting modes can penetrate very quickly. Through the application of the principles and guidelines discussed in this chapter, the clinician should be able to safely master the power and benefits of electrosurgery in the office to provide needed services to patients and reduce health care costs when compared to more traditional excisional methods.

References

1. Calero L, Brusis T. [Laryngeal papillomatosis—first recognition in Germany as an occupational disease in an operating room nurse]. *Laryngorhinootologie*. 2003;82:790–793.
2. Sawchuk WS, Weber PJ, Lowy DR, Dzubow LM. Infectious papillomavirus in the vapor of warts treated with carbon dioxide laser or electrocoagulation: detection and protection. *J Am Acad Dermatol*. 1989;21:41–49.
3. Bigony L. Risks associated with exposure to surgical smoke plume: a review of the literature. *AORN J*. 2007;86:1013–1020.
4. Mosterd K, Krekels GA, Nieman FH, *et al*. Surgical excision versus Mohs' micrographic surgery for primary and recurrent basal-cell carcinoma of the face: a prospective randomised controlled trial with 5-years' follow-up. *Lancet Oncol*. 2008;9:1149–1156.
5. Control of smoke from laser/electric surgical procedures. National Institute for Occupational Safety and Health. *Appl Occup Environ Hyg*. 1999;14:71.
6. El-Gamal HM, Dufresne RG, Saddler K. Electrosurgery, pacemakers and ICDs: a survey of precautions and complications experienced by cutaneous surgeons. *Dermatol Surg*. 2001;27:385–390.
7. Ghodsi SZ, Raziei M, Taheri A, *et al*. Comparison of cryotherapy and curettage for the treatment of pyogenic granuloma: a randomized trial. *Br J Dermatol*. 2006;154:671–675.
8. Werlinger KD, Upton G, Moore AY. Recurrence rates of primary nonmelanoma skin cancers treated by surgical excision compared to electrodesiccation-curettage in a private dermatologic practice. *Dermatol Surg*. 2002;28:1138–1142.
9. Rowe DE, Carroll RJ, Day CL Jr. Long-term recurrence rates in previously untreated (primary) basal cell carcinoma: implications for patient follow-up. *J Dermatol Surg Oncol*. 1989;15:315–328.
10. Silverman MK, Kopf AW, Grin CM, *et al*. Recurrence rates of treated basal cell carcinomas. Part 2: curettage-electrodesiccation. *J Dermatol Surg Oncol*. 1991;17:720–726.
11. de Graaf YG, Basdew VR, van Zwan-Kralt N, *et al*. The occurrence of residual or recurrent squamous cell carcinomas in organ transplant recipients after curettage and electrodesiccation. *Br J Dermatol*. 2006;154:493–497.

Additional Reading

Pfenninger JL. Radiofrequency surgery (modern electrosurgery) (Chap 30). *In*: Pfenninger JL, Fowler GC, eds. *Pfenninger and Fowler's Procedures for Primary Care*. 3rd ed. Philadelphia: Mosby/Elsevier; 2011.

Soon SL, Washington CV. Curettage and electrodesiccation. *In*: Robinson JK, Hanke CW, Sengelmann RD, Siegel DM, eds. *Surgery of the Skin*. 2nd ed. New York: Elsevier; 2010.

15 Cryosurgery

RICHARD P. USATINE, MD • DANIEL L. STULBERG, MD

Cryosurgery is the most commonly performed dermatologic procedure in the United States. There are many different ways to achieve cold temperatures, but clinically, the end result is to freeze the fluid in cells, which causes crystals that damage the cells, resulting in tissue destruction. Different cell types are destroyed at different temperatures (see Table 15-1). Melanocytes are relatively fragile causing the tendency for hypopigmentation with their death. Cartilage and bone are most resistant to freezing and other cells are in between.

Cryosurgery is an easily mastered technique that is extremely useful for treating benign and premalignant lesions. In experienced hands cryosurgery is also a valuable technique for treating small, nonaggressive nonmelanoma skin cancers (NMSCs).

INDICATIONS

Cryosurgery is most often used to treat actinic keratoses and benign conditions. Table 15-2 provides recommended freeze times and margins of freeze for benign conditions (using liquid nitrogen with an open spray technique). Table 15-3 gives recommended freeze times and margins of freeze for vascular conditions (using liquid nitrogen with a closed probe or an open spray technique). Table 15-4 lists recommendations for treating premalignant and malignant conditions (using liquid nitrogen with an open spray technique). Details on how to perform these procedures follow.

CONTRAINDICATIONS

- Cryosurgery is never an appropriate treatment for melanoma.
- Nevi should not be treated with cryosurgery because if a nevus were to grow back, it might appear malignant and a biopsy could be suspicious for melanoma (pseudomelanoma).
- Cryosurgery should not be used for NMSCs that are aggressive. This includes recurrent basal cell carcinoma (BCC) or squamous cell carcinoma (SCC), any large BCC or SCC, sclerosing BCC, micronodular BCC, poorly differentiated SCC, and any skin cancer with perineural spread. Avoid cryosurgery for cancers on the ala of the nose, the lip, and the ear. If Mohs surgery is indicated, cryosurgery is not.

Contraindications for cryosurgery are listed in Table 15-5.

ADVANTAGES OF CRYOSURGERY

The advantages of cryosurgery can be categorized into those for the clinician and those for the patient. Advantages for the clinician include the following:

- Ease of procedure.
- Speed of procedure.
- Multiple lesions may be treated at the same visit
- No need for injection of anesthetic (unless treating skin cancers for which the freeze times are longer).
- Clean procedure with no contamination and preparation.
- Relatively low supply cost after initial investment.
- Has an 83% to 88% cure rate for actinic keratoses.[1–3]

Advantages for the patient include:

- Ease of procedure.
- Speed of procedure.
- No injections (in noncancerous lesions).
- Pain is tolerable (for adults and many children over age 8).
- No sutures.

DISADVANTAGES OF CRYOSURGERY

As with the advantages of cryosurgery, the disadvantages can also be categorized into those for the clinician and those for the patient. Disadvantages for the clinician include the following:

- Liquid nitrogen needs to be delivered and stored. A liquid nitrogen generator may be purchased. If that is not done, nitrous oxide tanks or other supplies will need to be replenished as needed.
- The clinician must be certain of the diagnosis because no tissue will be sent for pathology.
- Cryosurgery is not as accurate as a scalpel or laser in cosmetic work.

Disadvantages for the patient include:

- Erythema and swelling are the norm. Blistering is common.
- Pain, especially throbbing pain around the nail folds.
- Pain with walking if plantar warts are treated.
- May require multiple visits.
- Hypopigmentation (see the *Complications* section later in this chapter for more risks).

TABLE 15-1 Key Events during Freezing Including Cell Death

Temperature (°C)	Event
+11 to +3	65% of capillaries and 35% to 40% of arterioles and venules develop thrombosis.
–0.6	Freezing begins to occur in tissue.
–4 to –7	Melanocytes die.
–15 to –20	100% of blood vessels develop thrombosis.
–20	Cells in sebaceous glands and hair follicles die.
–21.8	Ice crystals theoretically form in the tissue (the eutectic temperature of sodium chloride solution).
–20 to –30	Keratinocytes and malignant cells die.
–30 to –35	Fibroblasts die.
–50 to –60	All cells die including cartilage cells.

Source: Adapted from Vidimos A, Ammirati C, Poblete-Lopez C. *Dermatologic Surgery.* London: Saunders; 2008; Table 8-3.

TABLE 15-2 Recommended Freeze Times and Margin of Freeze for Benign Conditions Using Liquid Nitrogen with an Open Spray Technique

Benign Conditions	Freeze Time Average (s)[a]	Freeze Time Range (s)[b]	Halo Diameter (mm) Margin of Freeze
Chondrodermatitis nodularis helicis	20	20–30	1
Condyloma	10	5–20	1–2
Dermatofibromas[c]	20	20–30	1
Digital mucous cyst	15	10–20	1
Granuloma annulare	15	10–20	0–1
Hypertrophic scar	10	10–20	0–1
Keloids	20	20–30	1
Lichen planus, hypertrophic	20	20–30	0–1
Molluscum contagiosum	5	5–10	0–1
Mucocele[c]	10	10–20	1
Pearly penile papules	10	5–10	0
Prurigo nodularis	15	10–30	1
Sebaceous hyperplasia	10	10–20	0
Seborrheic keratoses	15	10–20	1
Skin tags	5 or until lesion turns white using a Cryo Tweezer	5–15	0
Solar lentigines	5	5–15	0
Stucco keratoses	10	10–15	1
Syringoma	15	15–25	1
Verruca, common	10	10–20	2
Verruca, flat	5	5–10	1
Verruca, plantar	10	10–20	2
Xanthelasma	15	20–25	1

[a]The freeze time average is a good starting time for an initial treatment. It is based on times for smaller to medium sized lesions that have not been treated before.

[b]The freeze time range includes a range of times based on the variable sizes and locations of lesions. Smaller lesions on thinner more delicate skin should receive treatments at the lower end of the range. Patients receiving treatments longer than 25 s should be offered local anesthetic first. Another option is to split freeze times over 15 s in half and complete two freeze cycles with a sum of the recommended time because some patients will not tolerate one long freeze as well as two shorter freezes.

[c]Dermatofibromas and mucoceles may respond better to a closed probe technique.

Disclaimer: All times are based on the available studies and author experience.

TABLE 15-3 Recommended Freeze Times and Margin of Freeze for Vascular Conditions Using Liquid Nitrogen with a Closed Probe or an Open Spray Technique

Vascular Conditions[a]	Freeze Time Average (s)[b]	Freeze Time Range (s)[c]	Halo Diameter (mm) Margin of Freeze
Angiokeratoma	20	15–25	0–1
Angioma	15	10–20	0–1
Pyogenic granuloma	20	15–30	0–1
Vascular malformations (port-wine stain)	25	20–30	0
Venous lake	15	10–20	0–1

[a]Many vascular conditions are best treated with electrosurgery or lasers except for a venous lake, in which cryosurgery is a preferred treatment. Cryosurgery for the other vascular conditions is an option. Regardless of the vascular lesion being treated, the closed probe technique with applied pressure is most effective.

[b]The freeze time average is a good starting time for an initial treatment. It is based on times for smaller to medium sized lesions that have not been treated before.

[c]The freeze time range includes a range of times based on the variable sizes and locations of lesions. Smaller lesions on thinner, more delicate skin should receive treatments at the lower end of the range. Patients receiving treatments longer than 25 s should be offered local anesthetic first. All times are based on the available studies and author experience.

EQUIPMENT FOR LIQUID NITROGEN

- Dewar (holding container) and dispensing device (Figure 15-1)
- Spray guns (Figure 15-2)
- Cryo Tweezers (for skin tags) (Figure 15-3)
- Various tips and probes (Figure 15-4)
- Styrofoam cups for use with Cryo Tweezers.

While we suggest liquid nitrogen as the gold standard, other methods involve the following equipment:

- Compressed gas in tanks or cartridges with appropriate gun or spray tips (nitrous oxide or carbon dioxide)
- Refrigeration—mechanically cooled probe
- Refrigerant liquids that evaporate with associated cones and swabs.

CRYOSURGERY: PRINCIPLES AND GETTING STARTED

- Factors that affect the freezing of tissue are listed and explained in Table 15-6.
- If you do not know the diagnosis, do not use cryosurgery. Lesions well suited to treatment with cryosurgery are listed in Tables 15-2 to 15-4.
- Advise the patient regarding treatment options and expected results.

TABLE 15-4 Recommendations for Treating Premalignant and Malignant Conditions Using Liquid Nitrogen with an Open Spray Technique

Premalignant and Malignant[a]	Freeze Time Average (s)[b]	Freeze Time Range (s)[c]	Halo Diameter (mm) Margin of Freeze	Approximate Thaw Time (s)	Tissue Temperature (°C)	Number of Freeze/Thaw Cycles
Actinic cheilitis	15	10–20	0	10–20	−10 to −20	1
Actinic keratosis	7	5–25	1	4–20	−10 to −20	1
BCC (especially superficial or very small nodular)	2 × 30	2 × (30–40)	5	>60–90	−30 to −60	2
Keratoacanthoma	2 × 30	2 × (30–40)	5	>60–90	−30 to −60	2
SCC *in situ* (Bowen's disease)	2 × 30	2 × (30–40)	5	>60–90	−30 to −60	2
SCC (small and early)	2 × 30	2 × (30–40)	5	>60–90	−30 to −60	2

[a]Cryosurgery is one preferred treatment based on good evidence for actinic keratoses. It is also preferred for actinic cheilitis. Treatments for actinic keratoses and actinic cheilitis may be followed by topical treatments for better field treatment. Cryosurgery for the *in situ* and malignant conditions is one option among many choices including surgery, electrodesiccation and curettage, and Mohs surgery based on the lesion, location, and patient preference. Cryosurgery should not be used for sclerosing BCC and any cancer with perineural invasion.

[b]The freeze time average is a good starting time for an initial treatment. It is based on times for smaller to medium sized lesions that have not been treated before.

[c]The freeze time range includes a range of times based on the variable sizes and locations of lesions. Smaller lesions on thinner, more delicate skin should receive treatments at the lower end of the range. Patients receiving treatments longer than 25 s should be offered local anesthetic first. All times are based on the available studies and author experience.

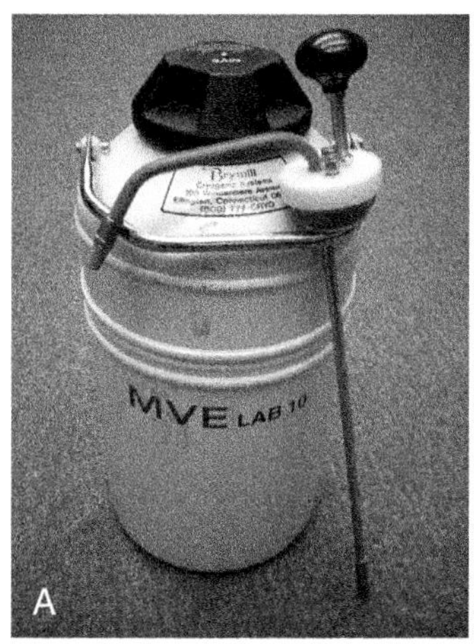
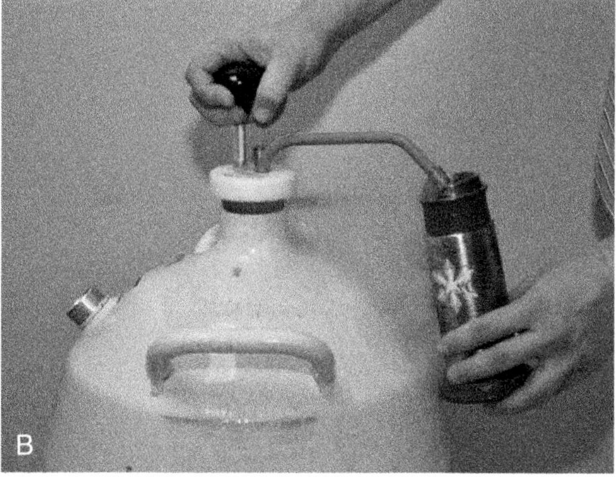

FIGURE 15-1 (A) Dewar tank and liquid nitrogen dispenser. (B) When the dispenser is placed within the tank and a seal is obtained, the liquid nitrogen rises through the metal tube and comes out through the filter at the end of the blue tube to fill the cryosurgical spray gun. *(A, Copyright Daniel Stulberg, MD; B, Copyright Richard P. Usatine, MD.)*

- Obtain informed consent at the time of the procedure based on the risks and benefits as laid out in this chapter. Most of the time, verbal consent should be adequate. If the procedure could result in hypopigmentation on the face, written consent should be obtained.

TABLE 15-5 Contraindications for Cryosurgery

Contraindications	Category
By Lesion	
Melanoma	A
Recurrent basal cell carcinoma	A
Sclerosing basal cell carcinoma (BCC)	A
Micronodular BCC	R
Nevus	A
Any undiagnosed lesion suspicious for non-melanoma malignancy (tissue should be sent for pathology first)	R
Morphea	A
By Area	
Skin cancer on ala nasi and nasolabial fold	R
Neoplasm of upper lip near vermillion border	R
Neoplasm over the shins	R
By Patient	
Previous adverse reaction to cryotherapy (e.g., cold anaphylaxis)	A
Cryoglobulinemia	R
Myeloma, lymphoma	R
Autoimmune disorders (including pyoderma gangrenosum)	R
Raynaud's disease, especially when lesion is on fingers, toes, nose, ears, penis	R

A, Absolute; R, relative.

CRYOSURGERY METHODS

Many different techniques are used to perform cryosurgery. The most common ones are listed in Table 15-7, which explains how the cryogen is applied and its temperature.

Liquid Nitrogen

Most dermatologists and many primary care providers have access to liquid nitrogen. It is the gold standard for cryosurgery. Various cryoguns are marketed that efficiently and effectively deliver the liquid nitrogen to the skin at the coldest temperatures.

Liquid nitrogen is stored in dewar containers ranging in size from 5 to 50 L. The nitrogen may be withdrawn using a ladle, a valve system, or a withdrawal tube (Figure 15-1). The withdrawal tube is the most simple and efficient way to extract liquid nitrogen from your storage container.

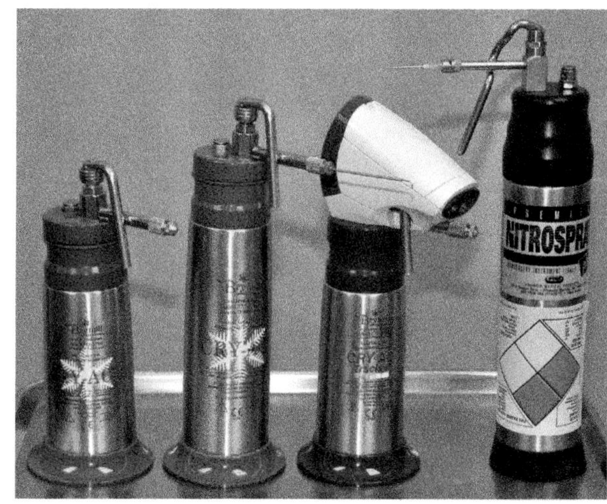

FIGURE 15-2 Two types of cryosurgical spray guns from Brymill (left) and one from Wallach (right). *(Copyright Richard P. Usatine, MD.)*

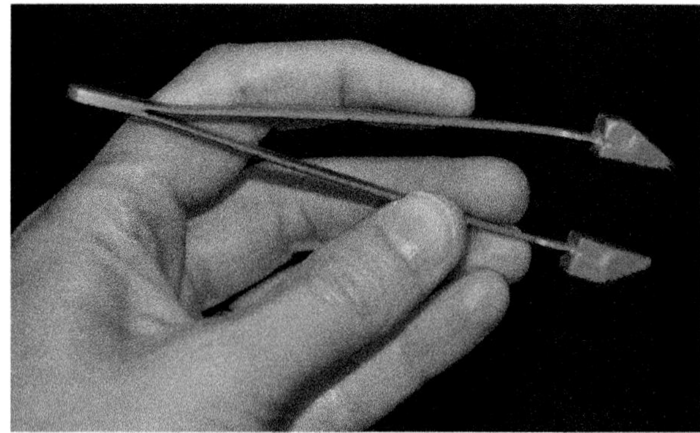

FIGURE 15-3 The Cryo Tweezer at room temperature. *(Copyright Richard P. Usatine, MD.)*

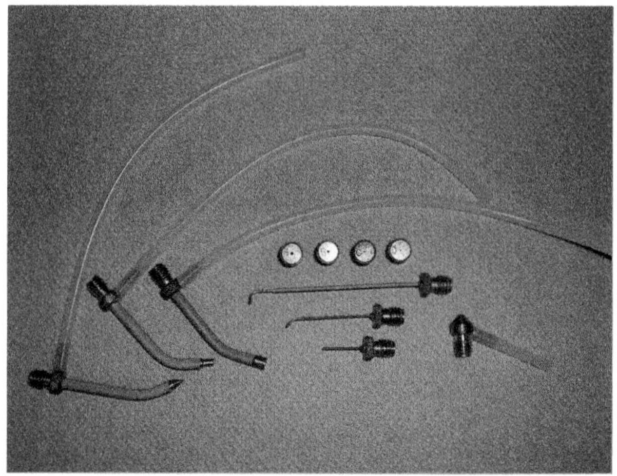

FIGURE 15-4 A large assortment of cryosurgical probes, apertures, and spray tips. *(Copyright Richard P. Usatine, MD.)*

For those clinicians who are still working with cotton-tipped applicators (CTAs) and liquid nitrogen in a cup, it is possible to do cryosurgery on benign and premalignant conditions. This method does not get cold enough for treating cancer or most vascular lesions. Dip the CTA into the liquid nitrogen and then touch the CTA to the lesion to be treated. The CTA can be unwound a bit and rewound to make a smaller point, or loose cotton from a cotton ball can be wrapped around the CTA for larger lesions to maintain the freezing temperature longer.

A more time-effective and more efficacious approach is to use a *cryogun* (Figure 15-2). Once filled, the unit can be used to treat many patients rapidly. The spray method allows the clinician to reach tissue temperatures of up to −196°C while the CTA is not likely to get below −20°C. Although there is a cost involved in the purchase of a cryogun, these units can last a clinician's full career and pay for themselves very quickly. The reimbursement for cryosurgery is excellent for only a few minutes of your time.

Michael D. Bryne developed the first handheld spray device using liquid nitrogen for medical use in 1968. His family continues to run the Brymill Corporation, which sells the most widely used cryoguns. The variety of cryoguns available from Brymill include (Figure 15-2):

- Cry-Ac®, standard 500-mL capacity—the main workhorse unit
- Cry-Ac-3, smaller capacity of 300 mL—easy handling with shorter holding time
- Cry-Ac Tracker, new device that measures the temperature of the skin when spraying liquid nitrogen using infrared sensor technology.

TABLE 15-6 Factors That Affect the Freezing of Tissue

Factor	Key Principles
Rate of tissue freezing	Rapid freezing causes more cell death. In the open spray technique, this is influenced by the rate of liquid nitrogen spray to the skin (aperture and configuration of the spray conduit).
Rate of intermittent spraying	A faster rate for an intermittent spray results in a deeper, but narrower depth of freeze. A slower rate for an intermittent spray results in a more superficial, but wider depth of freeze.
Halo diameter	The wider the halo, the deeper the freeze at the periphery of the lesion.
Distance of spray tip to tissue	The closer the tip is to the tissue, the colder the tissue may become because air is not as good a conductor as tissue.
Tissue temperature	Final tissue temperature of less than −30°C will kill malignant cells.
Duration of freezing	Having the tissue remain adequately frozen for a longer period of time causes more tissue injury. Maximum cell death rate occurs at 100 seconds.
Rate of thawing	Slow thawing causes more cell death.
Repetition of freeze/thaw cycles	More freeze/thaw cycles cause more cell death. Malignant tumors require multiple freeze/thaw cycles. All cellular structures show damage by electron microscopy after two cycles below −30°C.

Source: Adapted from Vidimos A, Ammirati C. Poblete-Lopez C. *Dermatologic Surgery.* London: Saunders; 2008; Table 8-2.

TABLE 15-7 Forms of Various Cryogens and Temperatures

Cryogens	Form	Temperatures (°C)
Liquid nitrogen	Open spray, closed probes and CTA Tissue temperature is less cold if delivered with CTA	−196
Nitrous oxide in tank	Closed probes on special gun	−89
Solidified CO_2 in tank	Closed probes on special gun	−79
CryoPen	Refrigerated closed probes	−75
Verruca-Freeze (chlorodifluoromethane and propane)	Chemical spray into cones or disposable buds with evaporation producing the cold	−70
Wartner (dimethyl ether and propane)	OTC foam applicator for warts only	−57
Histofreezer (dimethyl ether and propane)	Application is via disposable 2- and 5-mm buds	−55

Wallach makes the UltraFreeze Liquid Nitrogen Sprayer, which comes in 500- and 300-mL sizes. Whatever cryogun you use, it helps to have an assortment of apertures and tips. The tips that are available for the Brymill cryoguns include:

- Four spray tips with round apertures from 0.04 to 0.016 inch, with A being the largest and D the smallest (Figure 15-5). The C tip is a good all-purpose tip.
- Long 20-gauge bent spray with blue cover. This longer tube (3 inches) with an 80-degree angle attenuates the flow of the liquid N_2 (LN2) so that the spray is less shocking to the patient (Figure 15-5). This is good for children and adults who fear this therapy. It also allows for pinpoint accuracy on smaller lesions. It can be helpful for treating anogenital condylomas because it allows the clinician to be further from the lesions being treated.
- Shorter (1.5 inches) 20-gauge bent spray (metallic color). These have similar benefits to the long blue tube but with less attenuation of flow (Figure 15-5). They have a 45-degree angle at the end. This type of tip has one advantage over the long blue tube: it is less likely to become temporarily blocked up with repeated use. Both bent sprays can be rotated 360 degrees for greater precision when treating hard-to-reach lesions.
- Straight spray extensions range from 1.5 to 3 inches long. Straight spray needles have 16-, 18-, and 20-gauge extensions (Figure 15-5). These can be used anywhere or for lesions in body orifices.
- The Advanced Acne Aperture gives a soft, vaporized spray for superficial desquamation of cheeks, forehead, and back area in the treatment of acne (Figure 15-6).
- Closed probes are useful on vascular lesions to compress the lesion and freeze it simultaneously (Figure 15-7). Closed probes come in many sizes and shapes, ranging from 1 to 6 mm and 1 to 2.5 cm in diameter. The probes are available in round flat shapes, conical and spherical shapes, and shapes for use on the cervix. The liquid nitrogen is vented out a plastic tube so that no spray touches the patient. The spray freezes the probe tip for direct application to a lesion. One method to avoid the probe sticking to the skin is to freeze the probe before applying it to the patient. The closed probes have a "low" infection risk since there is no breach of the patient's skin. Cleaning of the closed probes can be done with an alcohol wipe prior to use.

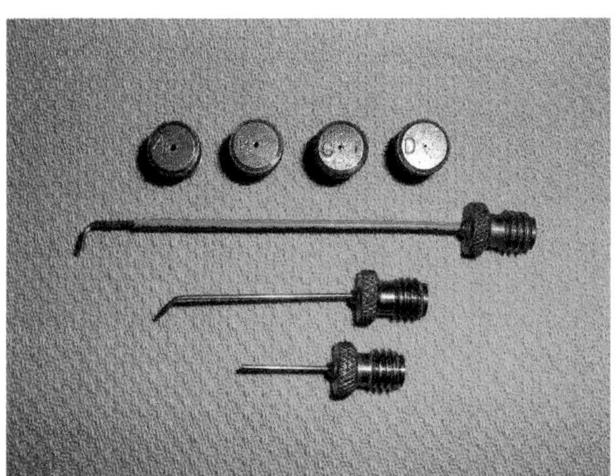

FIGURE 15-5 Spray tips A through D are arranged in order of largest aperture to the smallest aperture. Two bent spray tips and one straight spray needle (20 gauge). *(Copyright Richard P. Usatine, MD.)*

A *cryoplate* is a transparent plate with four conical openings of various diameters (3, 5, 8, and 10 mm) (Figure 15-8). Used with A - D apertures, the cryoplate

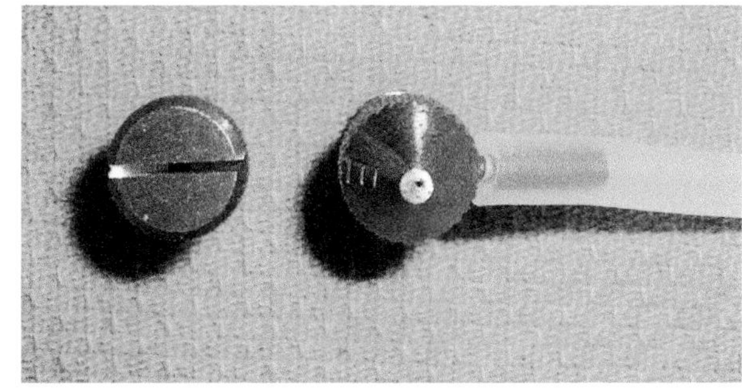

FIGURE 15-6 Acne spray tip next to a tiny E aperture tip. *(Copyright Richard P. Usatine, MD.)*

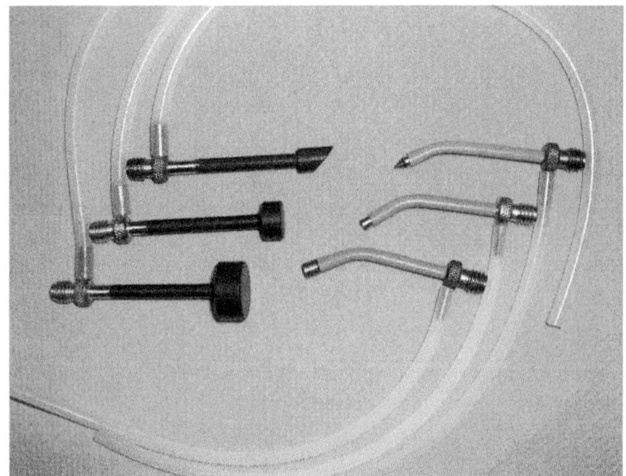

FIGURE 15-7 Closed cryoprobes with different shapes and sizes apply simultaneous pressure and freezing. These are especially helpful when treating vascular lesions. The liquid nitrogen is vented out the white plastic tube. *(Copyright Richard P. Usatine, MD.)*

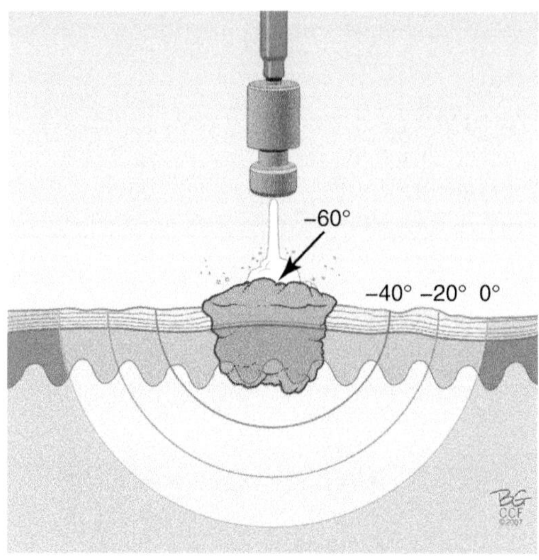

FIGURE 15-9 The liquid nitrogen sprays from the tip at –195.6°C and the cold dissipates in the tissues further from the direct spray. Even the skin at the point of initial contact does not reach the temperature of liquid nitrogen but may get as cold as –60°C. *(Modified from Vidimos A, Ammirati C, Poblete-Lopez C. Dermatologic Surgery. London: Saunders; 2008.)*

provides localization of freezing and protection of sensitive areas such as the eyes. It is good for the novice but is limited by the fact that each opening is round and includes a preset diameter.

Cryocones come as a set of six Neoprene cones of various sizes used to concentrate spray within a limited area. These can be used for irregularly shaped lesions because they can be shaped to the lesion. Sizes are 6, 11, 16, 25, 30, and 38 mm. Some people use plastic ear specula to control their freeze diameters.

Freezing Times, Thaw Times, and Halo Diameters

The amount of tissue destruction can be estimated by the duration of freezing (freeze time), the amount of thaw time (time until the ice ball is defrosted and is no longer white), and the margin of frozen tissue around the lesion (halo diameter). Factors that affect the freezing of tissue are summarized in Table 15-6.

Figure 15-9 shows how the temperature of the freeze is lowest in the middle of a continuous stationary freeze and why a halo diameter is helpful. Figure 15-10 shows the typical geometry of the hemispherical freeze that occurs in the tissues. Figures 15-11 and 15-12 demonstrate the relationship between depth and temperature of freeze to spraying factors. Intermittent spraying close to the skin can increase the depth and temperature of freeze when it is desirable to treat a deep tumor.

Cryosurgery with Liquid Nitrogen Spray: Steps and Principles

See video on the DVD for further learning. 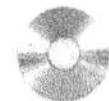

1. Hold the cryogun relatively upright to avoid having the LN2 come out of the valve and scare everyone in the room.

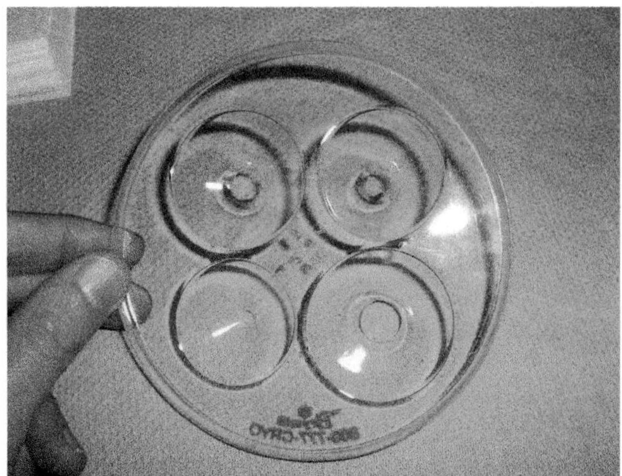

FIGURE 15-8 A cryoplate with four different size apertures for controlled freezing diameters. *(Copyright Richard P. Usatine, MD.)*

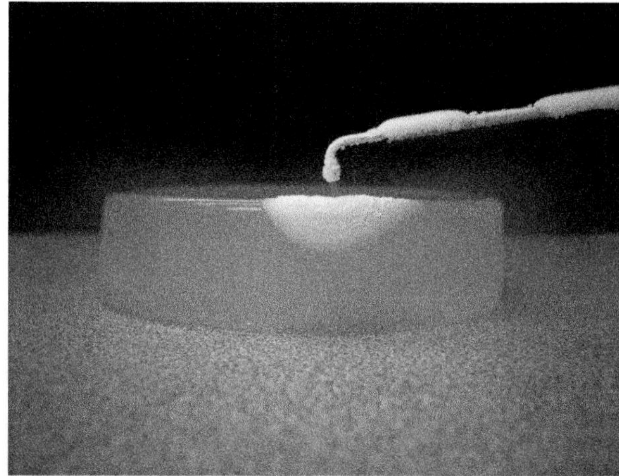

FIGURE 15-10 A real-life demonstration of the shape of the ice ball produced when liquid nitrogen is sprayed at a single-point of agar. The ice ball spreads out in a hemispherical pattern. The coldest point of the ice ball is the center. *(Copyright Daniel L. Stulberg, MD.)*

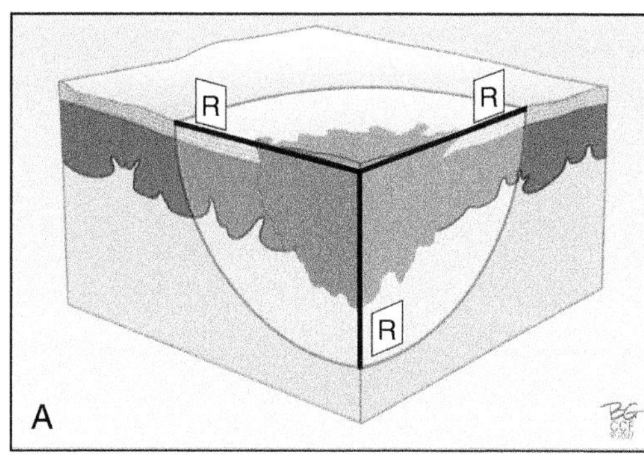

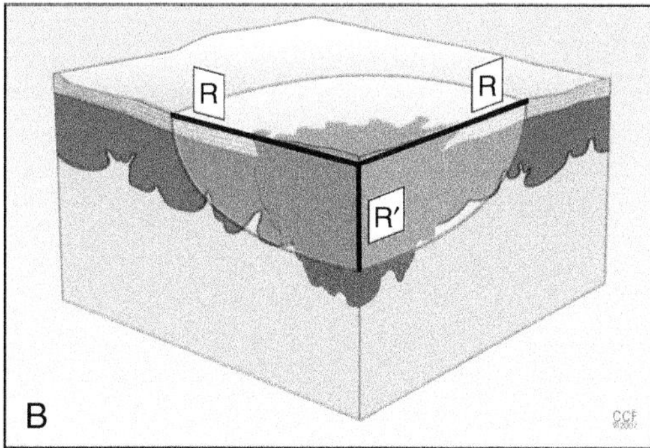

FIGURE 15-11 Relationship between depth of freeze to spraying factors. **(A)** The depth of the ice ball is equal to the surface radius of the ice ball. This tends to occur when the spray is intermittent and when the spray tip is close to the skin. **(B)** The depth of the ice ball is less than the surface radius of the ice ball (R′ < R). This tends to occur when the spray is continuous and when the spray tip is further from the skin. It can also occur when the liquid nitrogen is "painted on" and/or the rate of intermittent spray is too slow. Note that if the depth of the ice ball is too shallow, then the entire tumor may not be destroyed even though the frozen surface margins appear to be adequate. However, this type of freezing is helpful for superficial lesions. *(From Vidimos A, Ammirati C, Poblete-Lopez C.* Dermatologic Surgery. *London: Saunders; 2008.)*

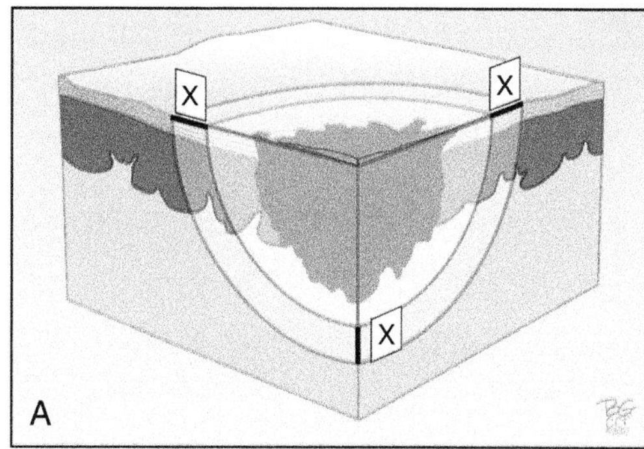

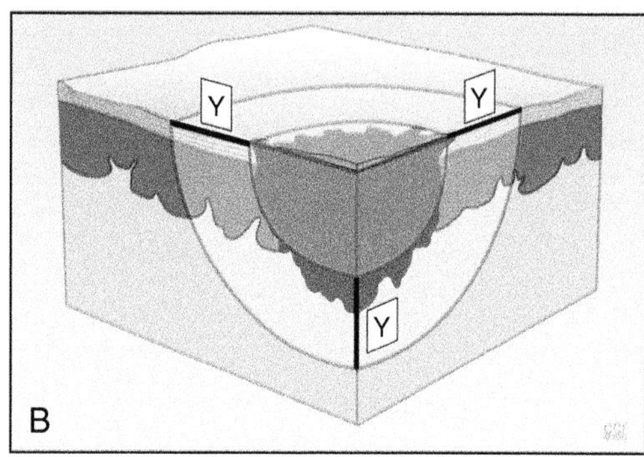

FIGURE 15-12 Relationship between the therapeutically lethal isotherm (TLI) (−30°C) and the edge of the ice ball (0°C isotherm). In both **(A)** and **(B)**, the sizes and shapes of the ice balls (0°C isotherm) are the same. **(A)** The TLI is close to the edge of the ice ball. This tends to occur when the spray is intermittent and when the spray tip is close to the skin. **(B)** The TLI is farther from the edge of the ice ball (Y > X). Note that if the location of the TLI is too far from the edge of the ice ball, the entire tumor may not be destroyed even though the frozen surface margins appear to be adequate. *(From Vidimos A, Ammirati C, Poblete-Lopez C.* Dermatologic Surgery. *London: Saunders; 2008.)*

2. Make sure that the patient is in a stable position and not a moving target. If the lesion is on the hand, see that the hand is resting on the patient or furniture so as not to move.
3. Hold the tip 1 to 2 cm from the lesion, making sure that the spray is perpendicular to the skin. If using a bent spray probe, adjust the position of the cryogun and tip to achieve a 90-degree angle (Figure 15-13). Stabilize your hands and body so that your aim will be accurate and consistent.
4. Compress the trigger to start the spray. The pattern of spray should be determined by the size, elevation, and depth of the lesion. The following techniques are options:
   - Steady continuous spray will produce a wider and more shallow freeze zone. This may be sufficient for actinic keratoses and benign lesions.
   - Pulsing the spray intermittently in one spot will cause the freeze to stay localized (less lateral spread) and deepen with the duration of spray. This is good for thicker lesions such as common warts, molluscum, dermatofibromas, and keloids.
   - Using a paintbrush technique of moving the spray in a spiral or back-and-forth motion will give a more superficial freeze for superficial lesions including actinic keratoses and lentigines. Moving the spray back and forth across the lip may be sufficient for actinic cheilitis (Figure 15-14).
   - If you are using the Cry-Ac Tracker, pay attention to the tissue temperature and use this as one extra data point to guide your treatments (Figure 15-15).

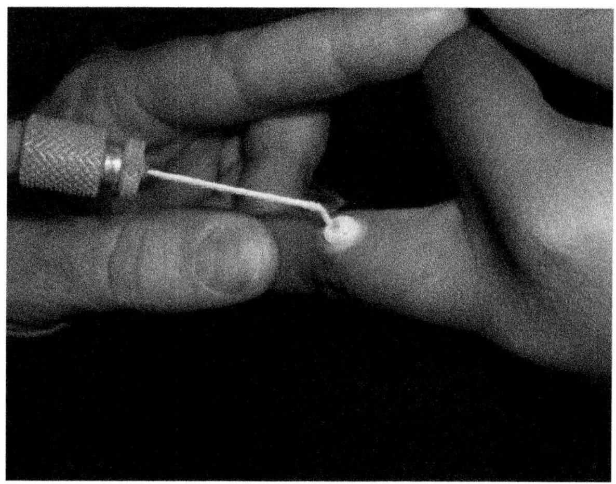

FIGURE 15-13 A common wart is treated with cryosurgery using the open spray technique and liquid nitrogen. A 2-mm margin of freeze (halo diameter) is achieved to ensure that the periphery of the wart is frozen. *(Copyright Richard P. Usatine, MD.)*

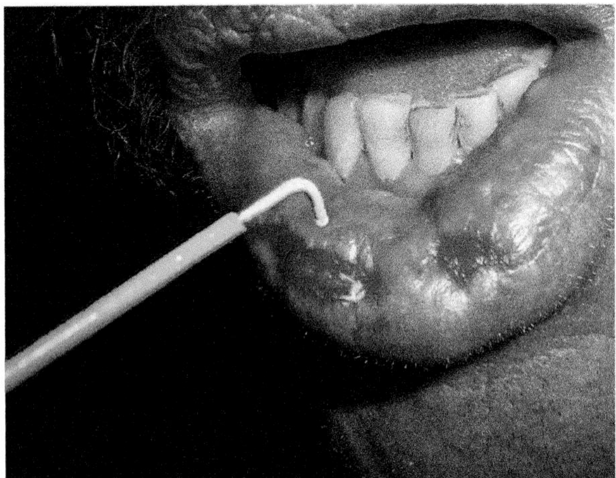

FIGURE 15-14 Biopsy-proven actinic cheilitis is being frozen using a bent spray tip and a paintbrush type motion to keep the freeze from going too deep. *(Copyright Richard P. Usatine, MD.)*

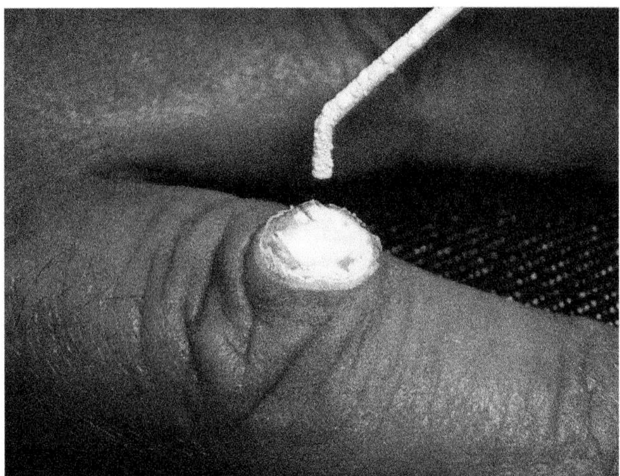

FIGURE 15-16 A wart is being frozen after excessive keratin was pared down with a sharp sterile razor. *(Copyright Richard P. Usatine, MD.)*

See Table 15-4 for guidelines on tissue temperature for treating premalignant and malignant conditions.

5. Make sure that the freeze reaches all edges of the lesion with the desired halo diameter (see Tables 15-2 to 15-4). The halo should be symmetrical around the lesion. It may be necessary to move the spray slightly back and forth to achieve an oval or linear pattern instead of a circle.
6. Freeze to the time suggested in Tables 15-2 to 15-4. Smaller lesions on thinner more delicate skin should receive treatments at the lower end of the time range.
7. Watch the thawing. If the area thaws asymmetrically, one area might not have received sufficient freeze time. You can add some freezing to that area. If the whole area thaws faster than expected, consider a second freeze/thaw cycle.
8. If the lesion is hypertrophic (especially with warts) consider paring it down with a scalpel or razor blade so that the base can be more effectively treated (Figure 15-16).
9. If you will be treating a lesion for more than 25 seconds, give the patient a choice to have a local anesthetic first. In particular, if you are treating a malignancy with two 30-second freezes, lidocaine can be very helpful. Two percent lidocaine without epinephrine is a good choice because there is no need for hemostasis or tissue distention.

Cryosurgery with Liquid Nitrogen Probes: Steps and Principles

See video on the DVD for further learning. 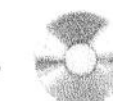

1. If you do not have a probe equal to the size of the lesion, you should choose a smaller probe and freeze the area longer than you would with a larger probe, which would unnecessarily destroy normal surrounding tissue.
2. Make sure the spray hose vent is facing away from the patient to avoid unwanted freezing.
3. Freeze the end of the probe before applying it to the patient to prevent the probe from sticking to the patient.
4. If the probe sticks to the patient, do not pull it off because significant tissue damage may occur. If the probe is taking longer than expected to detach from the patient, use your fingers or warm water to rewarm the adherent probe.

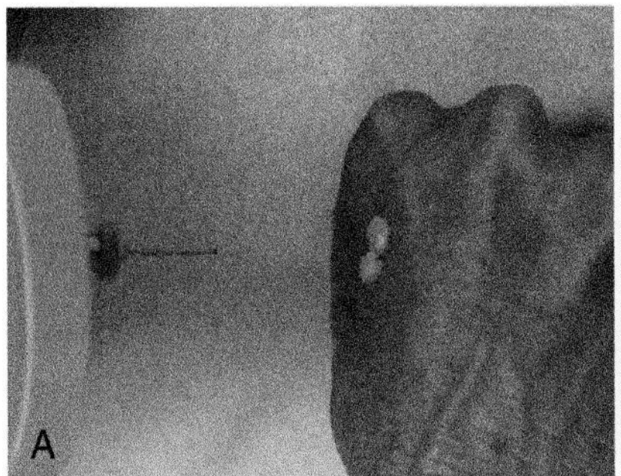

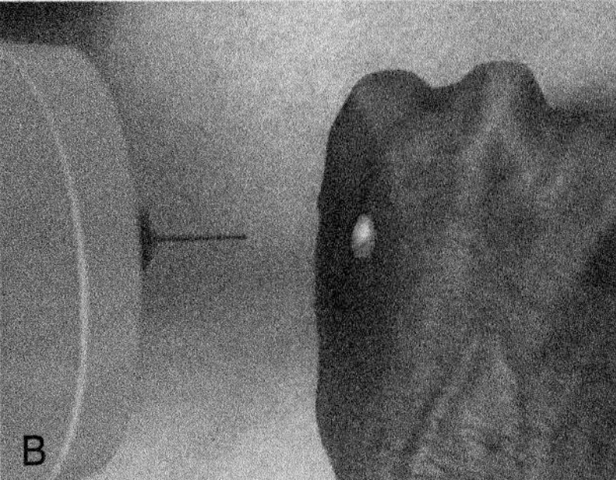

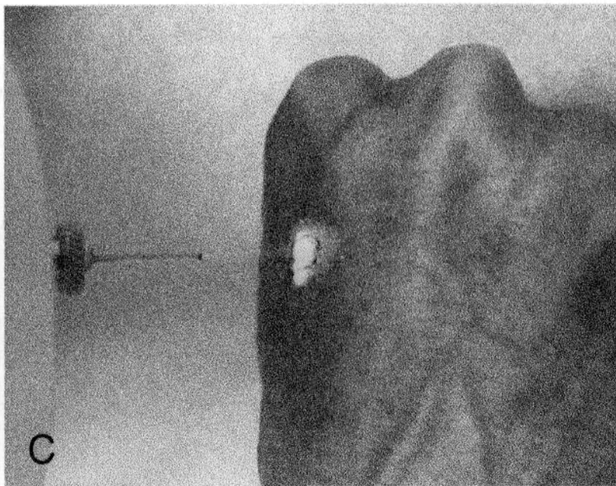

FIGURE 15-15 The Brymill Cry-Ac Tracker produces two purple lights that will converge to one light when the tracker is at the correct distance for the infrared temperature monitor to work: **(A)** too far from the skin; **(B)** correct distance. **(C)** As the spray freezes the skin, the light turns green when the temperature is below 0°C. The light will turn red when the temperature is below the variable temperature that may be set on the LCD control panel of the tracker. *(Copyright Daniel L. Stulberg, MD.)*

Liquid Nitrogen: Cryo Tweezers

See video on the DVD for further learning. 

Cryo Tweezers are designed to freeze skin tags without the overspray and inaccuracy inherent in spraying these small raised lesions. The Cryo Tweezers have a Teflon-coated brass tweezer end that holds the cold temperature after dipping them in liquid nitrogen. They have a thin "necked" portion between the heavy tweezer ends and the handle to minimize the cold spread up the handle. The tweezers should be dipped into a Styrofoam cup with LN2 so that the tips are covered, but not the handles. The initial dip should be long enough that the LN2 has stopped boiling away from the originally warm tweezer tips (about 20 seconds). The handles will get very cold, so it helps to wrap them in a 4 × 4 gauze as they are pulled out of the liquid nitrogen. Alternatively, a thick insulated glove can be used to handle the Cryo Tweezers. The skin tags are then grasped and held with the Cryo Tweezers until the freeze margin reaches normal tissue at the skin surface (Figure 15-17). The tweezers can be used to treat many skin tags before they warm up. When treating more than 10 skin tags you may need to redip the tweezers when you note that the freeze time is lengthening.

The Cryo Tweezers are particularly good for skin tags or warts on the eyelids. After grasping the elevated papule, pull the whole lid away from the eye to protect the globe from cryodamage (Figure 15-18). Then continue the freeze until the whole tag or wart is white to the base. This avoids any spray that may enter the eye. Cryo Tweezers can be cleaned between patients by dipping them into the liquid nitrogen again or using an alcohol wipe.

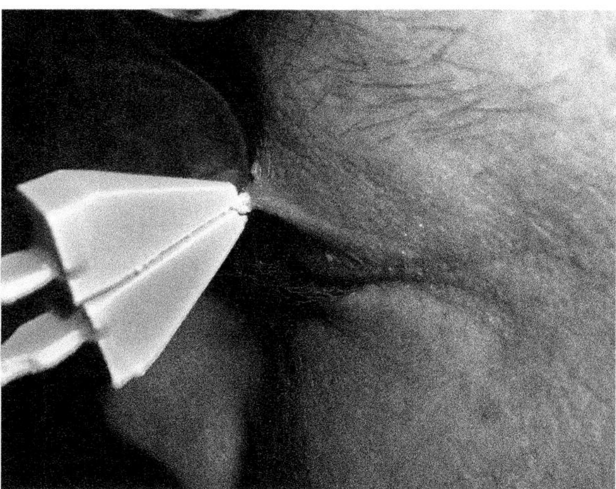

FIGURE 15-18 The Cryo Tweezer can safely treat skin tags or warts on the eyelids. The lesion is grasped carefully and pulled away from the eye; the cold will not be transmitted to the eye itself. *(Copyright Richard P. Usatine, MD.)*

Alternatives to Liquid Nitrogen

Evaporative Liquids

Volatile liquids produce cold temperatures when they evaporate. They are commercially available compressed in various spray cans. These can be directly applied to a lesion by spraying into a cone placed firmly against the patient's skin to prevent the liquid from running out. After the evaporation, the lesion and a surrounding margin, based on the cone size, will be frozen. These liquids can also be sprayed on or through (depending on the brand) a foam-tipped applicator that comes with the product and then applied to the lesion as with a CTA and liquid nitrogen (see earlier discussion). This technique has a lower initial cost for equipment, but is not as fast and versatile in its use. Also the temperatures are not as cold (see Table 15-6).

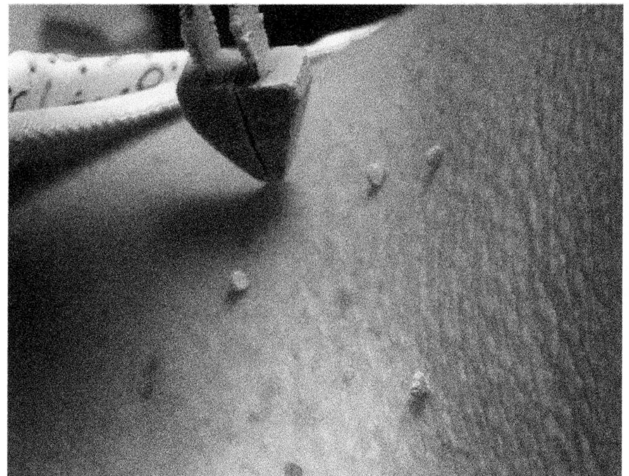

FIGURE 15-17 The Cryo Tweezer is an ideal instrument for quickly freezing small to medium skin tags with minimal pain and no bleeding. *(Copyright Daniel L. Stulberg, MD.)*

Closed Probes (Nitrous Oxide, Carbon Dioxide, or Electrical Refrigeration)

Closed probes can be chilled by guns that release compressed nitrous oxide or carbon dioxide or by an electrical refrigerating device (CryoPen). The CryoPen can be touched to the lesion, with varying size tips, similar to applying liquid nitrogen with a CTA. Other closed probes are placed against the lesion with water-soluble gel as a conductor that can also fill in gaps in the tissues. Dip the tip into a dab of water-soluble gel on a paper towel, and then touch the tip to the lesion. For efficiency touch the tip with the gel onto a number of lesions before starting the cryosurgery. After the tip is in contact with the lesion, activate the cryogun and hold in place until the desired freeze is obtained. Lifting the device and the skin after the skin has adhered due to the contact freeze may spare deeper tissues from freezing.

COMPLICATIONS

Complications of cryosurgery are listed in Box 15-1. Careful and thoughtful application of the principles in this chapter will prevent most complications.

TREATING SPECIFIC LESIONS

Condyloma

Condyloma acuminata are generally very responsive to cryosurgery. Many lesions can be treated rapidly without local anesthetic. Consider offering topical or local anesthetic to patients who have larger lesions. The bent spray tips are particularly useful for genital and perianal condyloma because the spray volume and speed are somewhat attenuated (Figure 15-20). While this may require slightly longer freeze times, it improves patient comfort during the procedure. The end of the spray tip should be held within 1 to 2 cm of the lesion to get good focused freezing. The patient may be given a prescription for a topical medication such as podofilox or imiquimod to start 2 weeks after cryosurgery. If the patient cannot afford one of these topical medications, cryosurgery may be repeated every 2 weeks until the lesions are gone.

If the perianal lesions are on the anal mucosa or are particularly large, some form of endoscopy should be performed to rule out internal HPV infection in the rectum (Figure 15-21). For perianal lesions in HIV-positive patients, consider a biopsy to rule out squamous cell carcinoma before initiating therapy.

Make sure you use site-specific billing codes for cryosurgery of the penis, vulva, or perianal area. These do pay at a higher rate (see Table 38-6 in Chapter 38).

BOX 15-1 *Pitfalls in Cryosurgery*

Expected (More Often with Longer, Deeper Freezes)

- Pain during freezing, thawing, and healing
- Blister formation—sometimes hemorrhagic (Figure 15-19)
- Intradermal hemorrhage
- Edema around treatment site
- Weeping of fluid (especially after treating cancer)

Immediate and Less Common

- Headache affecting forehead, temples, and scalp
- Syncope

Delayed and Rare

- Infection of the wound site
- Hemorrhage from the wound site
- Pyogenic granuloma

Prolonged and Rare

- Milia
- Hypertrophic scars
- Neuropathic pain at cryosurgery site

Occasional Permanent Unintended Consequences

- Hypopigmentation (most common and most visible in persons of color)
- Nail dystrophy (when treating periungual warts)
- Ectropion and notching of eyelids
- Tenting or notching of the vermilion border of the lip, ear or ala of nose
- Atrophic or depressed scar
- Alopecia

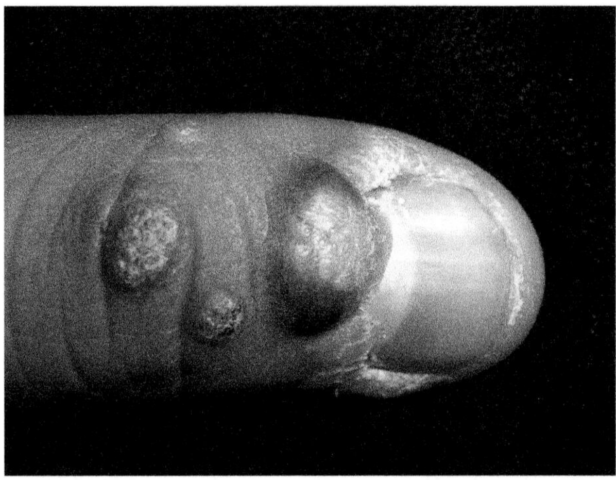

FIGURE 15-19 Hemorrhagic blisters formed after a vigorous freeze of periungual warts. This is not an uncommon reaction to cryosurgery and will resolve with no treatment and no harm. *(Copyright Richard P. Usatine, MD.)*

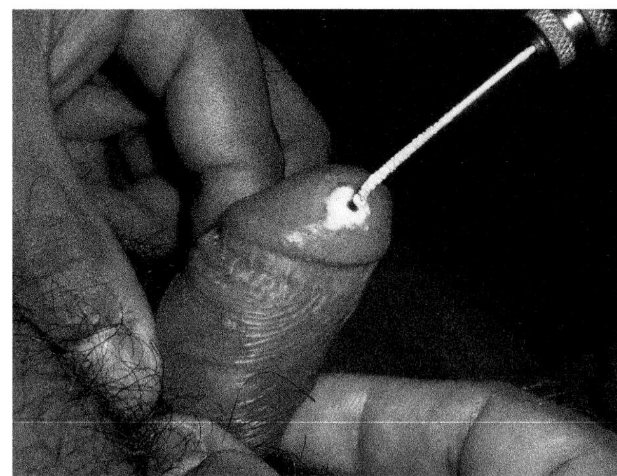

FIGURE 15-20 An open spray technique is being used to treat condyloma on the glans of a patient's penis. The spray tip is held close to the mucosa so that the freeze can be carefully controlled. *(Copyright Richard P. Usatine, MD.)*

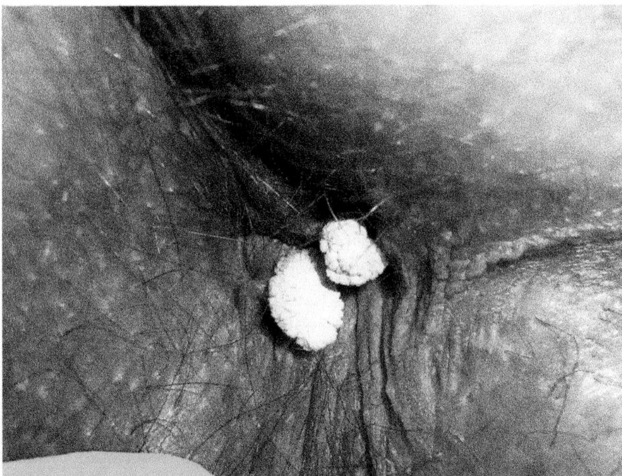

FIGURE 15-21 Condyloma acuminata in the perianal region after liquid nitrogen cryosurgery with a bent tip open spray technique. *(Copyright Richard P. Usatine, MD.)*

Dermatosis Papulosis Nigra

The many small seborrheic keratoses that make up dermatosis papulosis nigra (DPN) can be treated with cryosurgery. Because DPN is more frequently found on the face of women of color, it is important to avoid causing permanent hypopigmentation. This risk should be clearly spelled out and accepted by the patient before starting therapy. This is one time when we suggest getting a written consent signed. It also is prudent to test the cryosurgery out on a few lesions away from the midface to see how the patient will respond before treating many central lesions. The patient in Figure 15-22 was very pleased with her results. She was willing to except some temporary or permanent hypopigmentation just to make sure that her seborrheic keratoses were flattened so they would not show under makeup.

Keloids and Hypertrophic Scars

See video on the DVD for further learning. 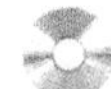

Keloids and hypertrophic scars can be a frustrating and cosmetically disfiguring complication of injury or irritation to the skin. Treatments have included applying silicone sheeting, excising and injecting the margins with steroids, injection alone, and cryotherapy alone or in conjunction with steroid injection. The data on the use of cryotherapy is nicely summarized in Table 15-8.

Molluscum Contagiosum

Cryosurgery is an excellent treatment method for molluscum. The greatest limiting factor is the age and maturity of the patient. This technique should not be used with young and fearful children. For older children and adults, molluscum can be treated using the open spray technique or a small closed probe. Because molluscum can be so small, choose a tip with a small aperture or a probe with a small diameter. The bent spray tips are particularly nice for molluscum. Usually a 5-second freeze time to the edge of the lesion is adequate.

Seborrheic Keratosis

See video on the DVD for further learning. 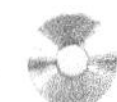

Seborrheic keratoses are frequently treated with cryosurgery. Very good cosmetic results can be obtained with cryosurgery of seborrheic keratoses from the scalp down to the legs. The open spray technique is a very fast and easy method of treating one or many seborrheic keratoses. The freeze time should be determined by the thickness and location of the seborrheic keratosis. It is better to underfreeze and have to do a second freeze than to overfreeze and cause permanent hypopigmentation, scarring, or atrophy. Some clinicians combine curettage with cryosurgery just as curettage is combined with electrodesiccation in the treatment of seborrheic keratoses. Large seborrheic keratoses can be treated in multiple sessions if needed.

Solar Lentigines

Solar lentigines may be quite responsive to depigmentation with cryosurgery. However, there is a risk of hypopigmentation or postinflammatory hyperpigmentation. It may be best to try this treatment on the dorsum of the hand before performing it on the face. For facial lesions you should obtain written consent and make sure the patient understands the potential risks. Make sure you are certain of the diagnosis before

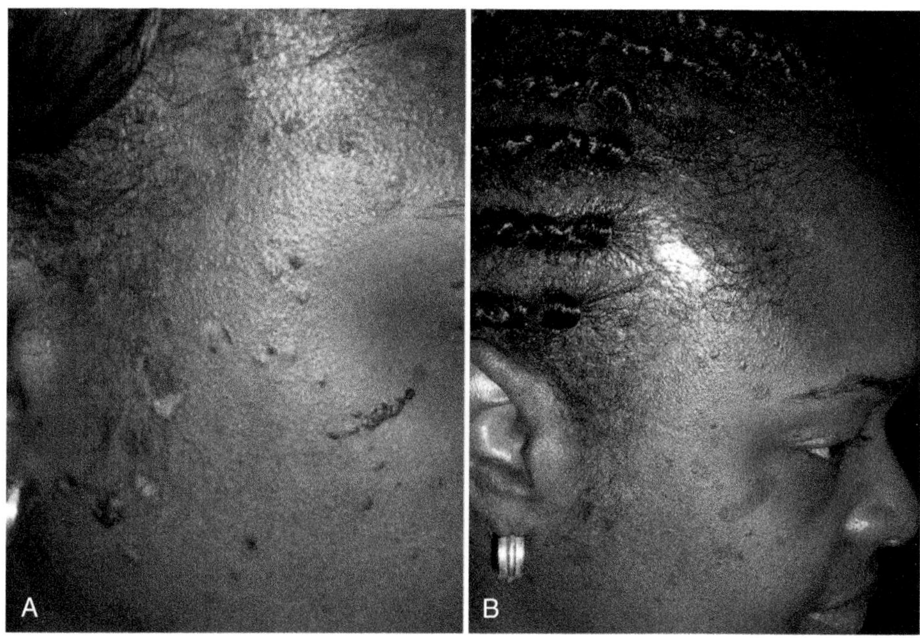

FIGURE 15-22 Dermatosis papulosis nigra that was treated with liquid nitrogen using an open spray technique. **(A)** Hypopigmentation occurred around many of the treated lesions within the first month. **(B)** The hypopigmentation was temporary and the patient was delighted with the final result of treatment. *(Copyright Richard P. Usatine, MD.)*

TABLE 15-8 Cryosurgery of Keloids and Hypertrophic Scars: Clinical Results

Study	Total Number of Patients	*Significant to Complete Remission*		*Recurrences*	
		Number	**%**	**Number**	**%**
Cryosurgery as Monotherapy					
Keloids					
Mende[5]	7	5	71		
Zouboulis et al.[6]	55	28	51	–	
Rusciani et al.[7]	40	34	85	–	
Ernst & Hundeiker[8]	234	158	68	9	4
Zouridaki et al.[9]	20	16	80	–	
Total	356	241	68%	9	3%
Hypertrophic Scars					
Zouboulis et al.[6]	38	29	76	–	
Ernst & Hundeiker[8]	51	43	84	2	4
Total	89	72	81%	2	2%
Cryosurgery Combined with Intralesional Corticosteroids					
Keloids					
Hirshowitz[10]	58	41	71	9	16
Ernst & Hundeiker[8]	56	38	68	2	4
Zouridaki et al.[9]	20	19	95	–	
Banfalvi et al.[11]	25	21	84	–	
Total	159	119	75%	11	7%

Source: From Robinson J, Hanke W, Sengelmann R, Siegel D. *Surgery of the Skin: Procedural Dermatology*, 2nd ed. Philadelphia: Mosby; 2010; Table 10.3.

proceeding. Visual diagnosis may be adequate in most cases and a dermatoscope can help confirm the clinical impression. While it is possible to perform cryosurgery on a lentigo maligna, it is best to know what you were treating because a lentigo maligna is a precancer and can go on to lentigo maligna melanoma. Because solar lentigines can be large and superficial, a paintbrush method with an open spray technique is useful.

Syringomas

Syringomas are benign tumors that occur bilaterally around the eyes, usually on the lower eyelids. They can be treated with cryosurgery using a bent spray method. One simple way to protect the eye is to place a wooden tongue depressor between the syringomas being treated and the closed eye (Figure 15-23).

Warts

Warts are covered in detail in Chapter 33, *Procedures to Treat Benign Conditions*.

Vascular Lesions

Hemangiomas

Small or large hemangiomas can be compressed with an adherent cryoprobe and then frozen destroying the vascular tissue. Freeze the cryoprobe first before applying when using liquid nitrogen (Figure 15-24). By freezing the probe first, the probe will not stick to the skin and can be moved to other parts of the hemangioma if the probe is smaller than the hemangioma.

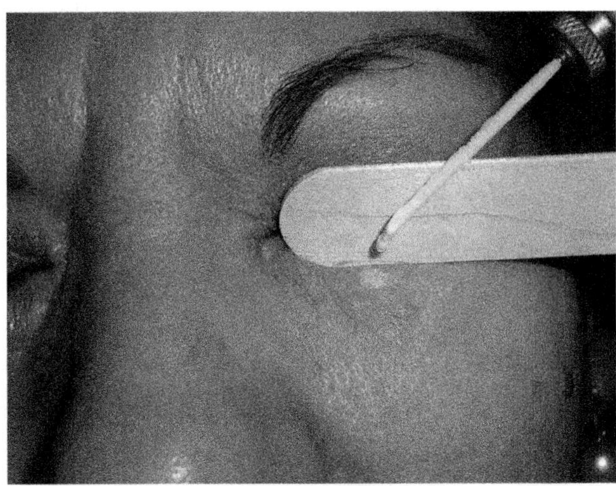

FIGURE 15-23 Syringoma are being treated with a bent tip open spray. A wooden tongue depressor is used as a barrier to protect the eye from the spray. Although patients are always directed to close their eyes, the tongue depressor provides additional security. *(Copyright Richard P. Usatine, MD.)*

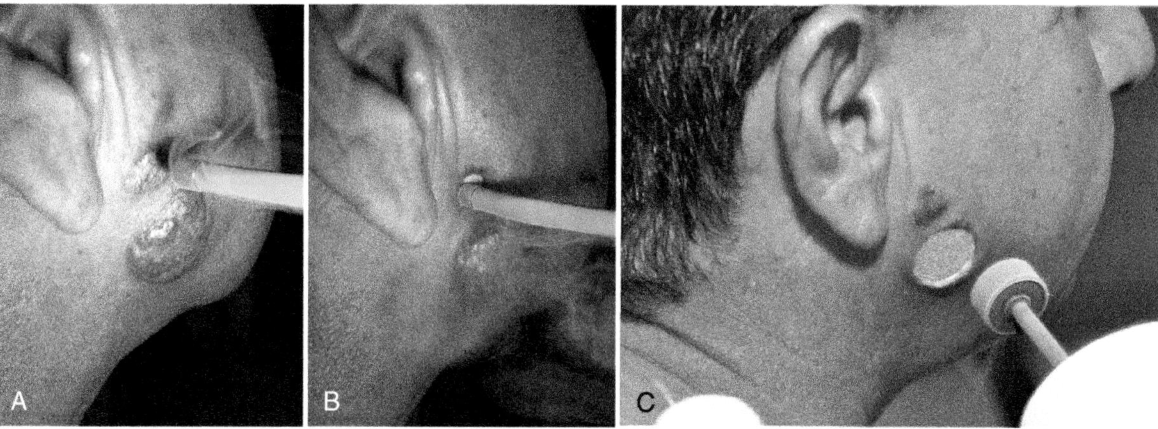

FIGURE 15-24 A 31-year-old man requested treatment of a strawberry hemangioma that he had had since infancy. Because he could not afford laser treatment, he was offered cryosurgery. The initial treatment is being performed with a closed probe and liquid nitrogen. **(A)** The closed probe is frozen first before touching the skin to avoid sticking to the skin. **(B)** The probe compresses the hemangioma while additional liquid nitrogen is used to keep the probe at a low temperature. **(C)** The larger hemangioma is treated with a larger probe using the same technique. Note the freeze ball and the compression obtained. The probe did not stick to the skin. Cryosurgery was repeated two times and the patient was happy with the final result. *(Copyright Richard P. Usatine, MD.)*

Pyogenic Granuloma

While the success rate for treating a pyogenic granuloma should be higher with a shave excision and electrosurgical destruction, some children will allow you to freeze their lesion but will not permit you to inject local anesthetic for the preferred surgical method. In these cases cryosurgery with a closed probe is preferred over the open spray technique. Because the closed probe can compress the pyogenic granuloma, the freeze can reach the base to decrease the chance of recurrence (Figure 15-25). An alternative is to compress the lesion with a Cryo Tweezer (Figure 15-26).

Venous Lakes

Venous lakes are vascular tumors that appear most commonly on the lower lip. They can be compressed with an adherent cryoprobe and then frozen, destroying the venous lake. Freeze the cryoprobe with liquid nitrogen first before applying (Figure 15-27) so that the probe does not stick to the lip when the freeze is complete.

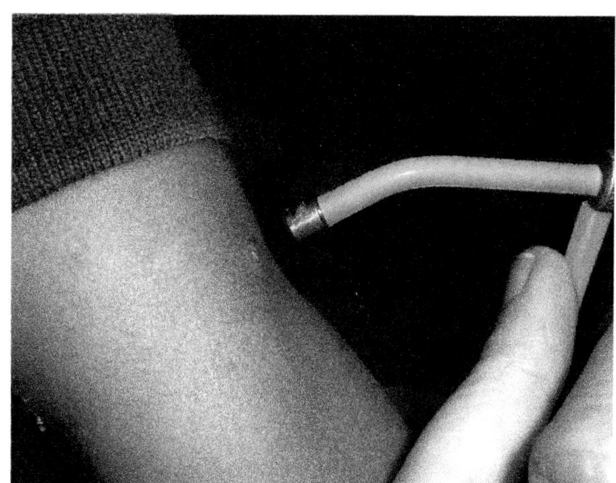

FIGURE 15-25 A closed probe is about to be applied to a pyogenic granuloma in a 7-year-old boy. While he was unwilling to allow an injection of local lidocaine for electrosurgical treatment, he was able to tolerate a cryosurgery with no anesthesia. The closed probe was chosen to compress the vascular tissue of this lobulated hemangioma. *(Copyright Richard P. Usatine, MD.)*

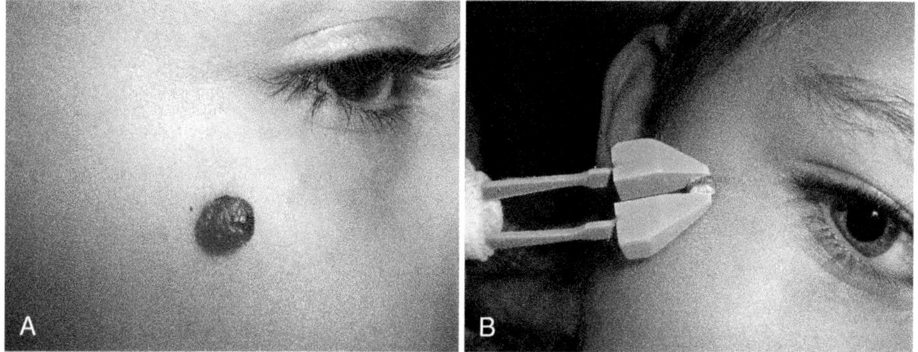

FIGURE 15-26 **(A)** Pyogenic granuloma on the face of a young girl. **(B)** The Cryo Tweezer is freezing and compressing the pyogenic granuloma laterally. Note the end of the 4 × 4 gauze wrapped around the handle of the Cryo Tweezer to prevent a freezing injury to the clinician's hand. *(Copyright Richard P. Usatine, MD.)*

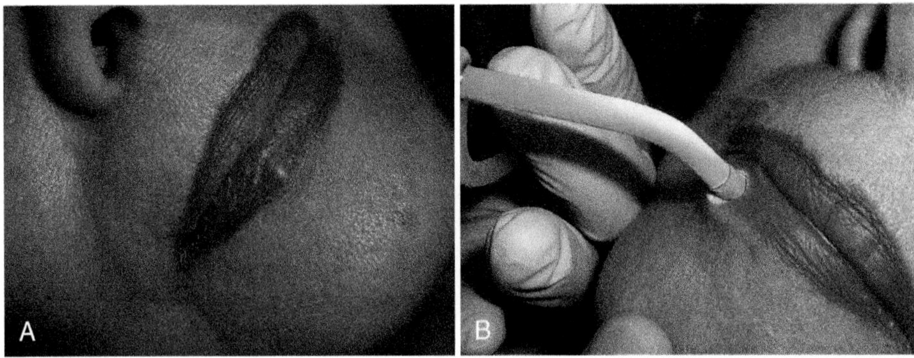

FIGURE 15-27 (A) Venous lake on the lip. (B) Venous lake being frozen with liquid nitrogen and a closed probe. *(Copyright Richard P. Usatine, MD.)*

Premalignant Lesions

Actinic Keratoses

Actinic keratoses (AKs) are very amenable to treatment with cryosurgery. Any of the open spray techniques can be used with the cryogun. The smaller lesions can be treated for 5 to 10 seconds, whereas the thicker more hypertrophic lesions should be treated for 10 to 20 seconds. A single freeze cycle should be adequate unless the thaw time appears too short. Table 15-9 shows the percentage cure of actinic keratoses with a single freeze/thaw cycle. Tissue destruction increases if longer freeze times or repeated freeze thaw cycles are performed.[3]

The most efficient method of treating many AKs is to have your cryogun with you in the exam room when examining a patient with many AKs. Once you and the patient determine that cryosurgery is to be done, freeze each AK as you find it so that you do not need to find each AK twice (once without and once with the cryogun). Also if you look closely, you will see that the borders of the AK become more visible as the freezing is occurring. Another option is to mark the location of AKs because they are often more easily palpated than seen (Figure 15-28).

Count your AKs as you go because you are paid individually for each AK until you reach 15. Then one global CPT code is used for 15 AKs and above.

Malignant Lesions

After developing proficiency with all kinds of benign lesions, it is reasonable to consider using cryosurgery for the least aggressive nonmelanoma skin cancers. Studies have shown that cryosurgery has similar effectiveness to electrodesiccation and curettage for correctly chosen BCCs. The most commonly recommended regimen is to maintain a freeze for 30 seconds, allow full thawing, and then repeat the 30-second freeze.[4] Clinical cure rates are approximately 90%, so appropriate follow-up is important.[4] If the lesion recurs after treatment, surgical excision or Mohs surgery may be indicated. These longer freeze times can be painful and difficult to tolerate, so inject with lidocaine for anesthesia prior to treatment. Efficacy and appearance are not as highly rated as surgical management, and after treatment there will likely be a prolonged period (weeks) of erythema, exudate, and healing, so judgment should be used in picking cryotherapy over surgical management.[4] It is typical to have some hypopigmentation and skin atrophy after healing.

The Cry-Ac Tracker can help the clinician develop confidence in the treatment of appropriate skin cancers with cryosurgery. The Cry-Ac Tracker allows the clinician to see and read the tissue temperatures during treatment. It also has a stopwatch timer and at the end of one burst of treatment will provide the number of seconds in which the coldest temperature was

TABLE 15-9 Actinic Keratoses of the Face and Scalp Larger Than 5 mm—Cure Rates with a Single Freeze[3]

Single Freeze Time (s)	Cure Rate (%)
<5	39
5–20	69
>20	83

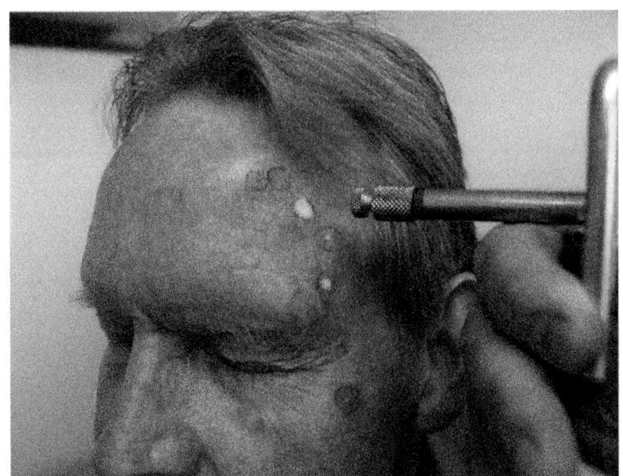

FIGURE 15-28 Multiple actinic keratoses being treated with a "C" aperture tip. The AKs were marked first prior to treatment. *(Copyright Daniel L. Stulberg, MD.)*

maintained. Previous studies recommending specific temperatures for cancer treatment were based on the use of thermocouples. The Cry-Ac Tracker measures surface temperature using infrared technology. Based on expert opinion and previous thermocouple data, it appears that skin cancers should be treated to a temperature below −30°C. The 30-second pulses are based on total freeze time and not a freeze time of less than −30°C. To reach a cold temperature faster, use a B or C tip aperture or a straight needle tip. All three of these choices work well with the Cry-Ac Tracker. Do not use a bent spray tip for treating skin cancer because the flow rate of liquid nitrogen is slower and the Cry-Ac Tracker does not work with the geometric configuration of a bent tip spray.

Use a surgical marker and circle the full skin cancer. If the margins are not clear, do not use cryosurgery for treatment. Measure 5 mm around the border and draw the desired halo diameter (Figure 15-29). Start the freeze and a stopwatch simultaneously—do not just estimate the 30-second freeze time. It helps to have a second person in the room to watch the time on a watch, smart phone, or the Cry-Ac Tracker. In most cases the spray can be held wide open, and intermittent pulsing only needs to be initiated if the freeze ball extends beyond the halo diameter.

Basal Cell Carcinoma

Superficial BCCs and small nodular BCCs can be treated with cryosurgery using liquid nitrogen spray guns because they produce the lowest temperatures in comparison with other cryosurgical techniques. See Contraindications on p.182 for the types of BCCs that should not be treated with cryosurgery.

Squamous Cell Carcinoma

Squamous cell carcinoma *in situ* responds well to cryosurgery. Small and early squamous cell carcinomas are also candidates for cryosurgery depending on the location and the patient. Decisions made on the choice of therapy for skin cancers involve many factors. See Chapter 34 for a more extensive discussion of these factors. If cryosurgery is chosen as the treatment method, the typical technique involves two 30-second freeze times separated by at least a 1-minute thaw time. As mentioned earlier, most patients will tolerate this best if lidocaine is injected prior to therapy. A keratoacanthoma is one type of well-differentiated squamous cell carcinoma and is amenable to cryotherapy using the same treatment technique. The open spray technique with liquid nitrogen is preferred for treating all of these skin cancers.

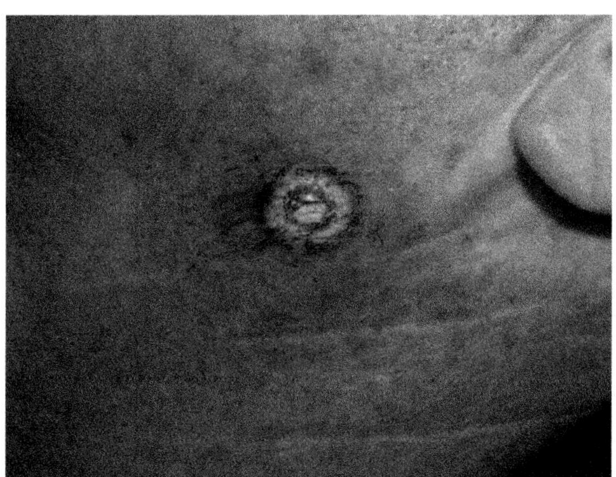

FIGURE 15-29 A small biopsy-proven squamous cell carcinoma *in situ* was found on the face. The patient chose cryosurgery as his method of treatment. The lesion was circled and a 5-mm margin was drawn around it. Some local anesthetic was injected and the patient received two 30-second freeze cycles. Each thaw cycle was over 60 seconds in length. *(Copyright Richard P. Usatine, MD.)*

Palliation

As our population ages we see more and more patients who are frail and elderly with nonmelanoma skin cancers. Some of these patients will do well with surgical excisions for the cancers. For those patients who may not be able to tolerate excisional surgery, cryosurgery may be used to shrink a skin cancer for palliation.

LEARNING THE TECHNIQUES

See video on the DVD for further learning. 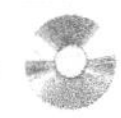

Bananas, agar plates (Figure 15-10), or uncooked chicken provide good models for practicing cryosurgery. You may observe the pattern of freeze ball that develops based on the aperture used, the rate of flow, and the intermittent spray technique used. If you use a banana or chicken, cut open the frozen area quickly to see the depth and geometry of the freeze. Try rotary or back-and-forth spray motions to cover broader areas for more superficial freezes.

AFTERCARE

Advise the patient that swelling, erythema, and blistering are the norm with cryosurgery and that the treated skin will subsequently slough off in the coming 1 to 2 weeks. Elevating an extremity postprocedure can reduce throbbing in cryosurgery of the digits. Adhesive bandages may be used to protect the area if blistering develops. If the blister pops, some clean petrolatum covered by a bandage allows for moist comfortable healing. Give the patient permission to call for a return appointment if the skin condition does not resolve.

CODING AND BILLING PEARLS

When cryosurgery is used for tissue destruction, coding is based on the skin destruction codes found in Tables 38-5, 38-6, and 38-11 of Chapter 38, *Surviving Financially*. Benign and premalignant tissue destruction has essentially been divided into three types of CPT codes based on these diagnoses:

BOX 15-2 *CPT General Destruction Codes*

11200 Removal of skin tags by cryosurgery or any other destructive technique, any area, up to and including 15 (billed once only)
11201 Removal for each additional 10 skin tags or portion thereof (may be billed more than once)
17110 Cryosurgery (destruction any means) warts/benign lesions other than skin tags up to 14 lesions (this is a single code used once only regardless if 1 or 14 lesions are treated)
17111 15 or more lesions (stand alone code, not per lesion)
17000 Cryosurgery (destruction any means), all premalignant lesions (AKs), first lesion
17003 Second through 14th lesion (this code is billed for each lesion from 2 to 14) (charge each lesion)
17004 15 or more lesions (stand-alone code, not per lesion)

- Skin tags: 11200, 11201
- Benign other than skin tags or cutaneous vascular lesions (includes warts and seborrheic keratoses): 17110, 17111
- Premalignant (actinic keratoses): 17000, 17003, 17004.

The general destruction codes shown in Box 15-2 are usually independent of the method of destruction and the location of the lesions. However, for destructions of benign lesions, certain specific parts of the body are reimbursed at a higher rate including the anus, penis, vulva, vagina, and eyelid. The CPT codes and typical fees charged for these are detailed in Table 38-6 of Chapter 38. Do not forget to use these codes because they do pay better than 17110 and 17111. These specific location codes are not based on the exact number of lesions and a single lesion may be reimbursed the same as many lesions.

Insurance companies will not pay for removal of skin tags unless there are documented medical reasons (strangulation, pain, or bleeding). Most insurance will deny payment for skin tags no matter what is documented. When patients just do not like the way the skin tags look, the procedure is considered a cosmetic removal. In this instance, patients should be advised in advance that they will be responsible for payment and an estimate should be given. Interestingly, an office visit E/M code can be charged to insurance but the removal fee is the patient's responsibility.

CONCLUSION

Cryosurgery is a quick and effective treatment for many skin lesions and should be part of the treatment options that a clinician treating skin offers.

References

1. Kaufmann R, Spelman L, Weightman W, *et al.* Multicentre intra-individual randomized trial of topical methyl aminolaevulinate-photodynamic therapy vs. cryotherapy for multiple actinic keratoses on the extremities. *Br J Dermatol.* 2008;158:994–999.
2. Morton C, Campbell S, Gupta G, *et al.* Intraindividual, right-left comparison of topical methyl aminolaevulinate-photodynamic therapy and cryotherapy in subjects with actinic keratoses: a multicentre, randomized controlled study. *Br J Dermatol.* 2006; 155:1029–1036.
3. Thai KE, Fergin P, Freeman M, *et al.* A prospective study of the use of cryosurgery for the treatment of actinic keratoses. *Int J Dermatol.* 2004;43:687–692.
4. Mallon E, Dawber R. Cryosurgery in the treatment of basal cell carcinoma. Assessment of one and two freeze-thaw cycle schedules. *Dermatol Surg.* 1996;22:854–858.
5. Mende B. [Treatment of keloids by cryotherapy]. *Z Hautkr.* 1987;62:1348, 1351–1352, 1355.
6. Zouboulis CC, Blume U, Buttner P, Orfanos CE. Outcomes of cryosurgery in keloids and hypertrophic scars. A prospective consecutive trial of case series. *Arch Dermatol.* 1993;129:1146–1151.
7. Rusciani L, Rossi G, Bono R. Use of cryotherapy in the treatment of keloids. *J Dermatol Surg Oncol.* 1993;19:529–534.
8. Ernst K, Hundeiker M. [Results of cryosurgery in 394 patients with hypertrophic scars and keloids]. *Hautarzt.* 1995;46: 462–466.
9. Zouboulis CC, Zouridaki E, Rosenberger A, Dalkowski A. Current developments and uses of cryosurgery in the treatment of keloids and hypertrophic scars. *Wound Repair Regen.* 2002;10:98–102.
10. Hirshowitz B. Treatment of scars and keloids. *Br J Plast Surg.* 1991;44:318.
11. Banfalvi T, Boer A, Remenar E, Oberna F. [Treatment of keloids (review of the literature, therapeutic suggestions)]. *Orv Hetil.* 1996;137:1861–1864.

16 Intralesional Injections

RICHARD P. USATINE, MD • JOHN L. PFENNINGER, MD

Intralesional injections of steroids are used to decrease inflammation in lesions such as cystic acne and granuloma annulare, to flatten keloids and hypertrophic scars, and to increase hair regrowth in alopecia areata. The standard injectable steroid in dermatology is triamcinolone acetonide (Kenalog). Diluting the steroid and injecting the steroid into the correct location are the most crucial aspects of this process. This chapter focuses on injectable steroids, but will also address injectable Candida antigen and bleomycin for the intralesional treatment of verrucae.

INDICATIONS

Indications for the use of intralesional steroid injections in dermatology include the following:

- Acne cysts
- Acne keloidalis nuchae
- Alopecia areata
- Discoid lupus
- Granuloma annulare
- Hidradenitis suppurativa
- Hypertrophic scars
- Keloids
- Lichen simplex chronicus
- Prurigo nodularis
- Psoriasis
- Sarcoidosis.

CONTRAINDICATIONS

Intralesional injection of steroids should be avoided in these situations:

- When lesions are too extensive.
- When there is a local infection.
- When the patient is not willing to accept the potential of skin atrophy and hypopigmentation as a side effect.

EQUIPMENT

The equipment used for intralesional injections is listed here and shown in Figure 16-1:

- Injectable steroids (triamcinolone acetonide, 10 and 40 mg/mL)
- Needles (25, 27, and 30 gauge)
- Syringes (1 or 3 mL [Luer-Lok preferable when injections are under pressure])
- As an alternative, the MadaJet can be used to administer the steroid (Figure 16-2)
- Vials of sterile saline or 1 or 2% lidocaine without epinephrine (for dilution).

The MadaJet injects 0.1 mL of solution into the dermis under pressure. Two variations are available so select the dermatologic version. (The other is for performing no-needle vasectomies.)

INFORMED CONSENT

Patients should be informed of the risks of skin atrophy, incomplete resolution of the lesion, and hypopigmentation. Have the patient sign a consent form, especially if the lesion is on the face. Special care should be taken when treating lesions on the face in darkly pigmented individuals because hypopigmentation can be a particularly unacceptable side effect. As with all informed consents, the patient should be made aware of alternative therapies. Alternative therapies for keloids are listed in Table 16-1.

STEROID STRENGTH

Once the appropriate-strength steroid for the injection has been chosen, the standard-strength preparations may need to be diluted to produce the desired strength. Recommendations for steroid strength and needle size are listed in Table 16-2. Triamcinolone acetonide suspension is available in two strengths: 10 and 40 mg/mL. It is essential to dilute the steroid, especially for injections of cystic acne of the face. Dilution may be done for each patient just before giving the injection or may be done in a sterile vial of saline and saved for the injection of multiple patients over time. Unless giving intralesional injections frequently, it is probably better to perform the dilution for each patient. Diluted vials can lose their potency and have a higher theoretical risk of contamination.

Triamcinolone is most often diluted with sterile normal saline for injection. Alternatives include sterile water or 1 or 2% lidocaine (without epinephrine). The isotonicity and neutral pH of sterile saline makes it the preferred solution for dilution.

A 1-mL Luer-Lok or tuberculin syringe is useful for making a single dilution before injection. To create a 2 mg/mL concentration, draw 0.4 mL of sterile saline into a 1-mL syringe and add 0.1 mL of 10 mg/mL triamcinolone. Other dilutions are listed in Table 16-3. Turn the syringe upside down a number of times to mix the new suspension. It is recommended that the saline be drawn up first because it is more acceptable to get a little saline into the triamcinolone than vice versa. Recommended needle sizes by lesion are listed in Table 16-2.

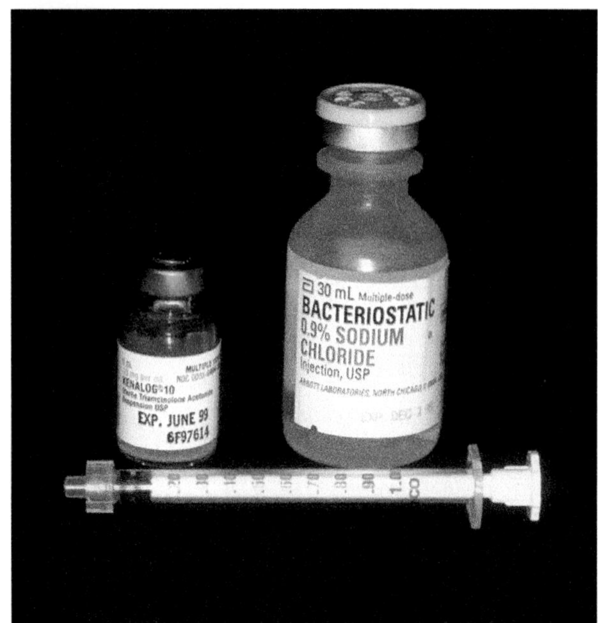

FIGURE 16-1 Injectable triamcinolone acetonide with injectable sterile saline and a Luer-Lok 1-mL syringe used for intralesional injections. *(Copyright Richard P. Usatine, MD.)*

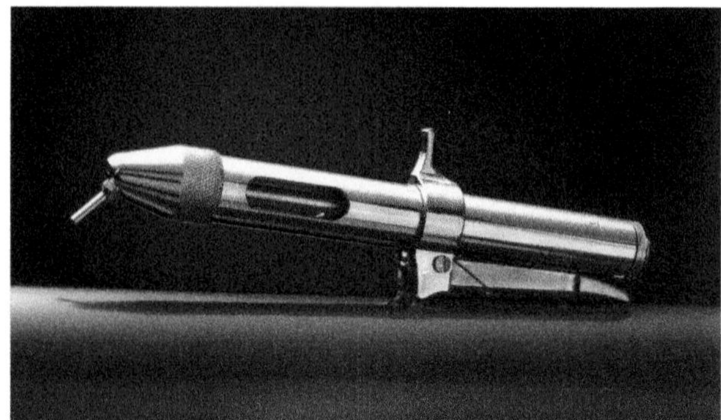

FIGURE 16-2 Needle-free jet injector. *(Courtesy of Mada Medical, Carlstadt, NJ.)*

TABLE 16-1 Therapies for Keloids

Topical	
	Corticosteroids Retinoids Imiquimod Mederma Vitamin E
Injectable	
	Corticosteroids Interferons 5-Fluorouracil Verapamil Bleomycin
Surgical	
	Surgical debulking or excision Laser debulking or excision Radio-frequency electrosurgery planing
Physical	
	Laser therapy Radiation therapy Compression therapy Silicone sheeting Cryotherapy Fractional laser ablation

Source: Adapted from Baldwin H. Keloid management (Chap 44). *In:* Robinson JK, et al., eds., *Surgery of the Skin: Procedural Dermatology.* Philadelphia: Elsevier; 2005.

TABLE 16-2 Recommended Steroid Strength and Needle Size for Intralesional Injections

Lesions	**Triamcinolone (mg/mL)**[a]	**Needle size (gauge)**
Acne cysts (face and neck)	1–2	30
Acne cysts (trunk)	2–3.3	27–30
Acne keloidalis nuchae	5–10	25–27
Alopecia areata	5 for scalp and 3.3 for face	27
Discoid lupus	2.5–5	27
Granuloma annulare	5	27
Hidradenitis suppurativa	3.3–5	27
Hypertrophic scars	10–20	25–27
Keloids	10–40	25–27
Lichen simplex chronicus	2.5–5	27
Prurigo nodularis	5	27
Psoriasis	2.5–5	27
Sarcoidosis	2.5 on face and 5 on body	27–30

[a]For lesions on the face, always start with lower concentrations.

TABLE 16-3 Common Triamcinolone Dilutions in a 1-mL Syringe

Concentration (mg/mL)	**mL of Triamcinolone 10 mg/mL**	**mL of Sterile Saline for Injection**
1	0.1	0.8
2	0.1	0.4
2.5	0.2	0.6
3.3	0.2	0.4
5	0.3	0.3

A disadvantage of using the MadaJet is that approximately 1 mL of liquid is needed to prime it. Steroid is relatively inexpensive so this is a minor problem.

TREATING SPECIFIC LESIONS

Acne Nodules and Cysts

Patients with tender large nodulocystic lesions can expect to get symptomatic relief within 24 hours of an intralesional injection. The lesion will flatten within 2 to 3 days with an effective injection.[1] Although this should not be the primary treatment of acne, it can provide short-term relief while employing more long-term treatment regimens.

One small study evaluated the effectiveness of intralesional injections of steroids in the therapy of nodulocystic acne.[1] They found that 0.63 mg/mL of triamcinolone was as effective as 2.5 mg/mL.[1] Betamethasone injections were no better than saline controls.[1] One review article states that concentrations of 3.3 and 5 mg/mL of triamcinolone are standard dilutions for intralesional acne injections.[2]

We recommend using 1 to 3.3 mg/mL of triamcinolone for nodulocystic acne depending on the location of the lesions and the experience of the clinician and patient. Triamcinolone can be injected with minimal pain using a 30-gauge needle on a 1-mL syringe at a 45- to 90-degree angle with the skin (Figure 16-3).

For acne cysts on the face, it is safer to use 1 to 2 mg/mL to make sure that atrophy does not occur. On the trunk consider using 2 to 3.3 mg/mL of triamcinolone. Enough suspension should be injected to see and feel the cyst become distended, but no more than 0.1 mL is needed for any one cyst. One injection site per acne cyst should be adequate. If the cyst is large and soft, do not inject more volume because that can lead to atrophy. If there is a lot of purulent material inside the cyst, a quick incision and drainage (with lidocaine and a No. 11 scalpel) before injecting the steroid may be helpful.

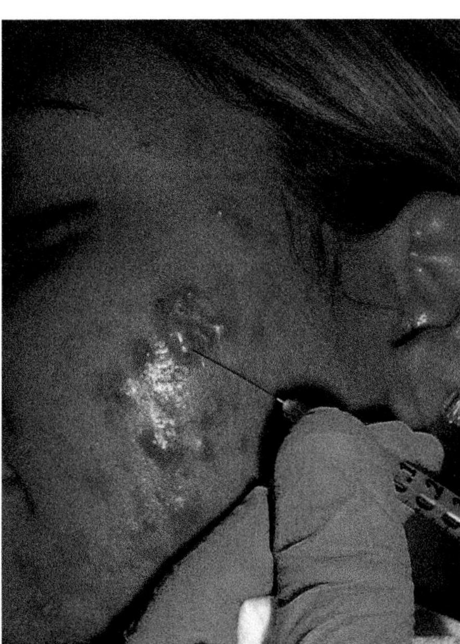

FIGURE 16-3 Nodulocystic acne being injected with dilute triamcinolone. *(Copyright Richard P. Usatine, MD.)*

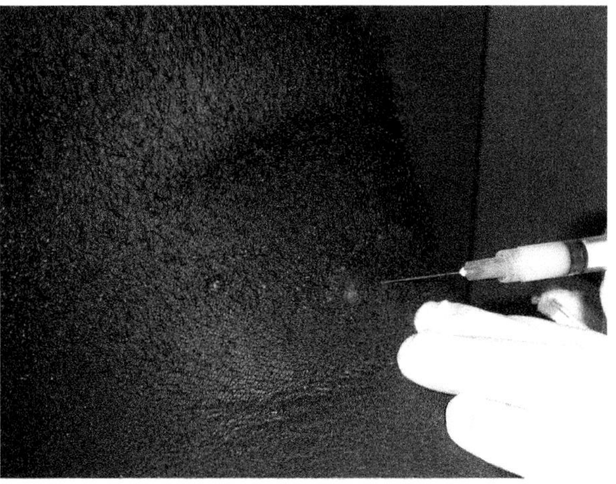

FIGURE 16-4 Acne keloidalis nuchae being treated with intralesional steroids. *(Copyright Richard P. Usatine, MD.)*

Acne Keloidalis Nuchae

Acne keloidalis (Figure 16-4) occurs on the posterior neck most commonly in men with highly pigmented skin. It is an inflammatory condition that is exacerbated by shaving the back of the neck. It has features of acne and folliculitis. Over time keloidal-type scars occur and can become very large. Treatment and prevention include not cutting the hair too short and using topical steroids and topical retinoids. Tender and painful keloidal nodules can be injected with triamcinolone for some relief. Concentrations of 5 to 10 mg/mL can be used. The heavier the fibrosis and scarring, the larger the needle needed to inject the lesion.

Alopecia Areata (Figure 16-5)

Although a recent Cochrane review on the treatment of alopecia areata (Figure 16-5) found no RCTs on the use of intralesional steroids (and many other treatments), they did acknowledge that this is a commonly used treatment for alopecia areata.[3] Considering the possibility of spontaneous remission in the early stages of the disease, it is reasonable to reassure the patient and recommend tincture of time. However, many patients are seeking an active treatment. Intralesional steroid for alopecia areata is a well-accepted standard treatment and often gives patients hope that they will regain their hair. Recommended concentrations of triamcinolone range from 5 to 10 mg/mL for the scalp, but the higher concentrations often cause scalp atrophy. Therefore we recommend using 5 mg/mL of triamcinolone for the scalp. Alopecia areata can affect the eyebrows and the beard. For those regions it is safer to stick with a lower concentration of triamcinolone such as 3.3 mg/mL. A long 27-gauge needle (1.25 to 1.5 inches) will allow for treatment of larger areas with fewer injections per site.

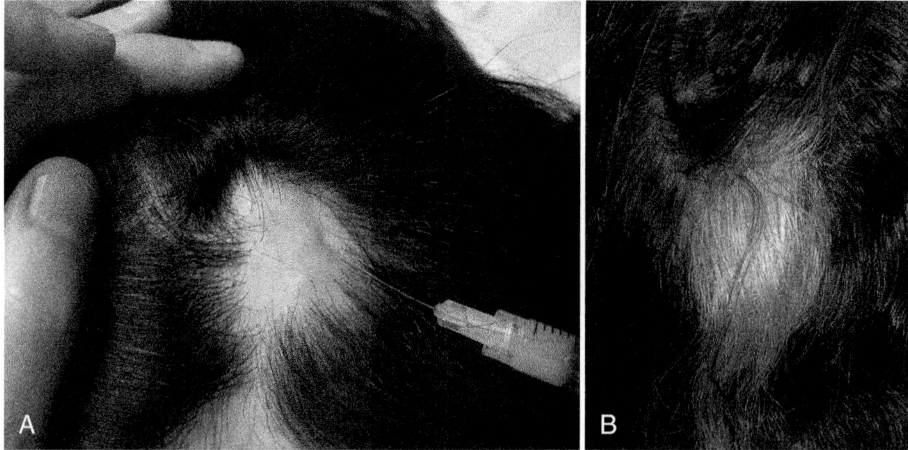

FIGURE 16-5 (A) Alopecia areata being injected with triamcinolone. (B) Regrowth of hair at a site of alopecia areata that had been previously injected with triamcinolone. Note how the new hair is white. This is not a side effect of the triamcinolone injection but a common characteristic of hair regrowth at the site of alopecia areata. *(Copyright Richard P. Usatine, MD.)*

Cutaneous Lupus

Intralesional steroids have been used for decades to treat patients with all types of localized cutaneous lupus (Figure 16-6).[4,5] Widespread cutaneous lupus is best treated with topical steroids and systemic agents when indicated. For specific local lesions that are not responding well, discuss the option of intralesional steroids with the patient. Our recommendation is to use from 2.5 to 5 mg/mL depending on the site. Special care should be taken when treating lupus on the face in a darkly pigmented individual because hypopigmentation can be a particularly unacceptable adverse effect.

Hidradenitis Suppurativa

Injecting painful acute hidradenitis suppurativa cysts (Figure 16-7) is similar to injecting acne cysts, but a higher concentration of triamcinolone (3.3 to 5 mg/mL) is acceptable because these lesions are usually in the axilla, chest, or groin and less prone to atrophy. Also a little skin atrophy is generally more acceptable in these locations than the face. It may be best to use the lower end of this range when injecting hidradenitis around the breasts because this area is of more cosmetic concern. Because the cysts are often larger than acne, a 3-mL syringe may be needed to provide more volume for injection. Large, purulent cysts can be drained with a No. 11 scalpel first before injecting the steroid.

Granuloma Annulare

Granuloma annulare (Figure 16-8) is an idiopathic granulomatous disease that typically appears in ringlike formations. Treatments for localized disease include high-potency topical steroids and injections of triamcinolone. We recommend using 5 mg/mL of triamcinolone and a 27-gauge needle. Four injection sites are usually needed to cover one annular lesion, so a syringe larger than 1 mL is often needed. We prefer not to inject more than 4 mL total. Inject into the granulomatous lesion and not below the lesion. Our experience has

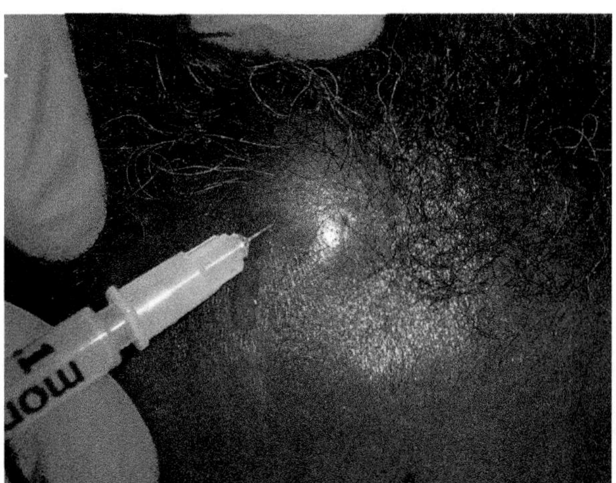

FIGURE 16-6 Discoid lupus. This patient had biopsy proven lupus paniculitis at that site and had relief of her pain after the intralesional steroid injection. *(Copyright Richard P. Usatine, MD.)*

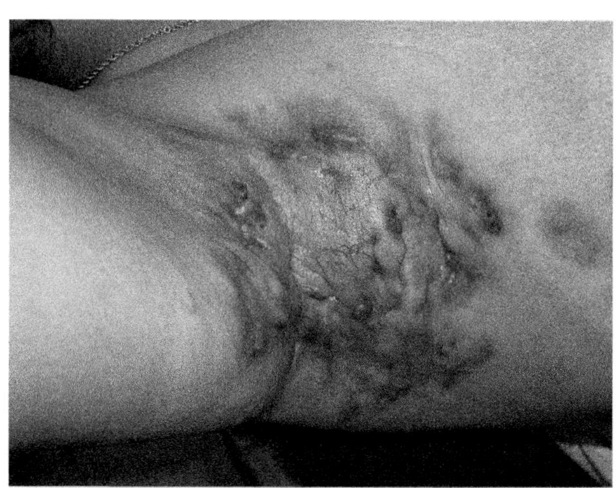

FIGURE 16-7 Chronic and acute hidradenitis suppurativa prior to steroid injections. *(Copyright Richard P. Usatine, MD.)*

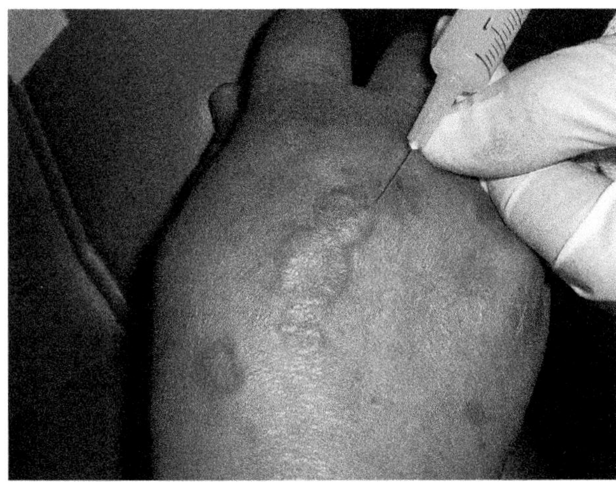

FIGURE 16-8 Granuloma annulare being injected with triamcinolone. *(Copyright Richard P. Usatine, MD.)*

shown steroid injections to be more effective than topical steroids. If the condition is disseminated, there are other treatments to consider.

Hypertrophic Scars and Keloids

See video on the DVD for further learning. 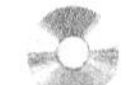

A *hypertrophic scar* (Figure 16-9) is one in which the scar tissue is raised and prominent over the area that was cut, burned, or traumatized. It may show prominent suture marks and can be redder or differently pigmented compared with the surrounding tissue. Hypertrophic scars frequently regress over a few years. A *keloid* is similar to a hypertrophic scar but it grows beyond the limits of the original surgery. Keloids tend to become quite raised and enlarged. There are histologic differences between hypertrophic scars and keloids. For the purpose of intralesional injection, however, they are treated identically.

Persons with darker skin are at higher risk than light-skinned persons of developing keloids. Keloids most commonly occur on the chest, shoulders, and other areas of increased skin tension but can occur anywhere on the skin. They tend to be more common after a traumatic lesion. Keloids frequently occur after ear piercing and acne scarring. Table 16-1 provides a list of possible treatments for keloids. Surgical excision frequently induces more scarring exacerbating the original problem. If excision is deemed necessary, scarring can be limited by including dilute steroids in the anesthetic, injecting steroids into the surgical site after surgery, using minimal tissue pressure techniques, and postoperative occlusion with silicone sheets for several months.

Initially start with 10 mg/mL of triamcinolone for the first treatment of a keloid or hypertrophic scar. The needle should be introduced into the body of the keloid at a 20- to 30-degree angle with the skin. It is important that the tip of the needle is *within* the keloid and not below it. Proper needle position should result in significant pressure while injecting and a blanching of the keloid as the suspension is injected into the area. If the solution flows in easily, the needle is most probably too deep. If the needle is too deep, reposition it and restart the injection. Inject firmly while advancing the needle and observing the keloid blanch.

If the MadaJet is being used, activate it by cocking the lever, place the tip lightly on the tissue and release the unit by pushing the button with the thumb. A whitening change will be seen. Apply the next "shot" right next to the original one and progress until the entire lesion is treated.

Large keloids may need multiple injections at one time to adequately infiltrate the lesion. Sometimes the needle can be pulled back and reoriented for the next injection from the same puncture site. The quantity injected should be just enough to blanch the entire keloid white. Hypertrophic scars are injected using the same technique. A 3-mL Luer-Lok syringe facilitates the injection into these firm structures. Without the Luer-Lok it is easy for the needle to come off and spray the clinician in the eyes. Even with a Luer-Lok syringe it is important to wear eye protection when injecting lesions under pressure.

Keloids can be treated with cryosurgery alone or in combination with intralesional steroids. In one small controlled study, ten patients with keloids were treated with intralesional steroid and cryosurgery vs. intralesional steroid or cryosurgery alone.[6] Patients were treated at least three times 4 weeks apart. In terms of keloid thickness, the keloids responded significantly

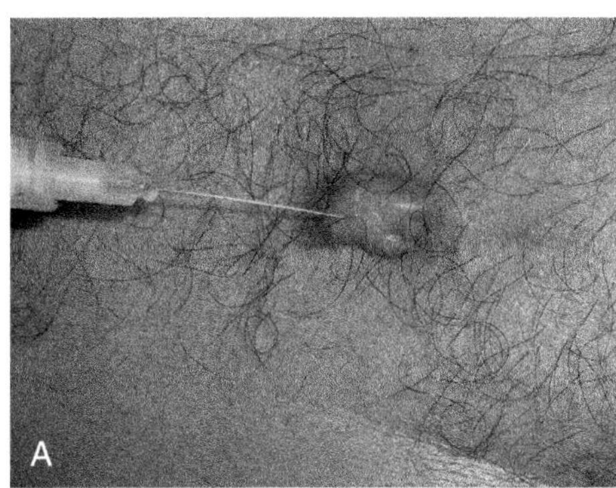

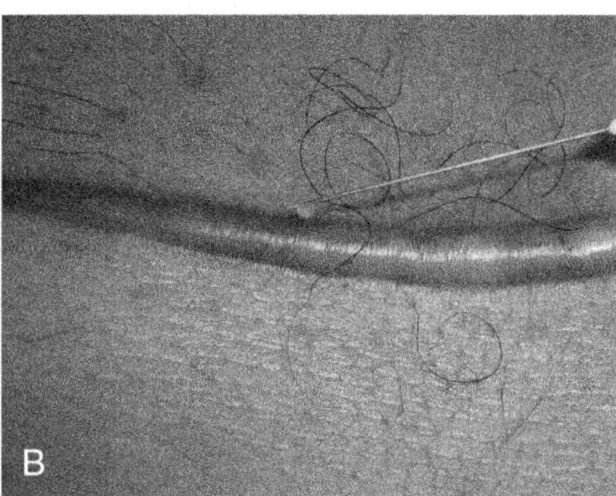

FIGURE 16-9 **(A)** Acne keloid being injected with triamcinolone. **(B)** Hypertrophic scar after a knife wound being injected with triamcinolone. *(Copyright Richard P. Usatine, MD.)*

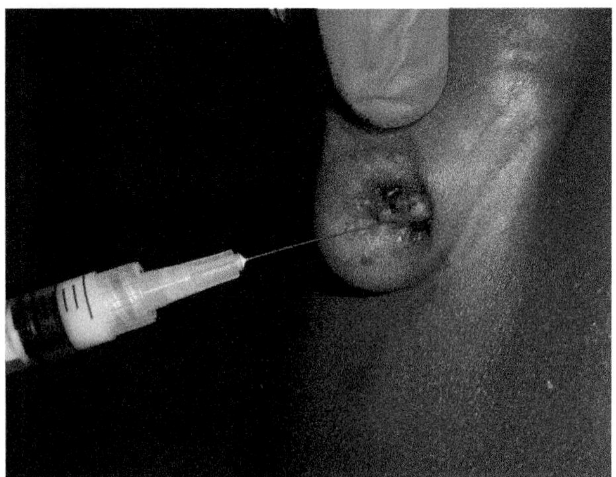

FIGURE 16-10 A keloid was shaved from the ear lobe and the bleeding stopped using electrocoagulation. The base is being injected with 40 mg/mL triamcinolone to prevent regrowth. *(Copyright Richard P. Usatine, MD.)*

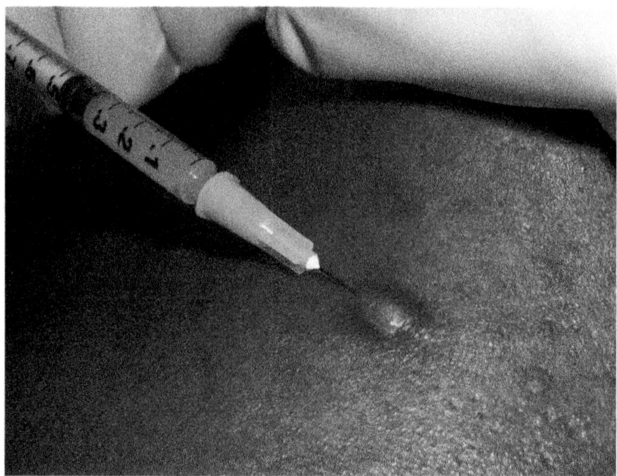

FIGURE 16-11 Prurigo nodularis is being injected with triamcinolone. *(Copyright Richard P. Usatine, MD.)*

better to combined cryosurgery and triamcinolone vs. triamcinolone alone or cryotherapy alone. Pain intensity was significantly lowered with all treatment modalities. Pruritus was lowered only with the combined treatment and intralesional corticosteroid alone.[6]

In another study 20 patients with hypertrophic and keloidal scars received two 15-second cycles (total 30 seconds) of cryosurgery treatments once monthly for 12 months with intralesional injections of 10 to 40 mg/mL triamcinolone once monthly for 3 months.[7] Topical application of silicone gel was added three times daily for 12 months. The control group included 10 patients who received treatment with silicone sheeting only. After 1 year, improvement was seen in all parameters, especially in terms of symptoms, cosmetic appearance, and associated signs compared to baseline and compared to the control group.[7]

Layton et al. reported that the intralesional injection of a steroid is helpful but cryotherapy is more effective (85% improvement in terms of flattening) for recent acne keloids located on the back.[8] Treatment with intralesional triamcinolone was beneficial, but the response to cryosurgery was significantly better in early, vascular lesions.[8]

If the keloid is older and/or firmer, it may not respond to injection therapy as well as softer and newer lesions. In such cases, it may help to pretreat the keloid with cryotherapy. It is not necessary to freeze a margin of normal tissue. After liquid nitrogen or another freezing modality is applied to the keloid, it is allowed to thaw and develop edema. This generally takes 1 to 2 minutes, which allows for easier introduction of intralesional steroids into the lesions.

In one double-blind clinical trial, 40 patients were randomized to receive intralesional triamcinolone (TAC) or a combination of TAC and 5-fluorouracil (5-FU).[9] Both groups received injections at weekly intervals for 8 weeks and lesions were assessed for erythema, pruritus, pliability, height, length, and width. Both groups showed an acceptable improvement in nearly all parameters, but these were more significant improvement in the TAC + 5-FU group ($P < 0.05$ for all except pruritus and percentage of itch reduction). Good to excellent improvement were reported by 20% of the patients receiving TAC alone and 55% of the patients in the group receiving TAC and 5-FU.[9]

Earlobe keloids may be excised with a shave excision and injection of the base with steroid (Figure 16-10). It is hard to get much volume of steroid into the base of these keloids, so 40 mg/mL triamcinolone is preferred as the concentration for injection. Another option is to use the radio-frequency electrosurgery technique with a pure cutting setting and a steroid in the anesthetic.

According to one article, simple excision of earlobe keloids can result in recurrence rates approaching 80%.[10] A randomized prospective trial comparing steroid injections versus radiation therapy found that 2 of 16 keloids (12.5%) recurred after surgery and radiation therapy, whereas 4 of 12 (33%) recurred after surgery and steroid injections. These results did not produce a statistically significant difference. No alteration of skin pigmentation, wound dehiscence, or chronic dermatitis was observed in any patient in either group.[10] While radiation therapy was considered easy to obtain in this study, it is reasonable to use steroid injections in office practice.

Localized Dermatitis (Lichen Simplex Chronicus, Prurigo Nodularis)

In a recent review paper, no studies were found on the use of intralesional steroids for psoriasis or localized dermatitis since the 1960s.[11] The authors describe their personal experience as excellent using 2.5 mg/mL triamcinolone for localized dermatitis (such as lichen simplex chronicus, prurigo nodularis, and nonspecific eczema).[11] We recommend using 2.5 to 5.0 mg/mL triamcinolone with a 27-gauge needle for the treatment of localized dermatitis. Because prurigo nodularis (Figure 16-11) can be particularly difficult to treat, the higher concentration may be needed.

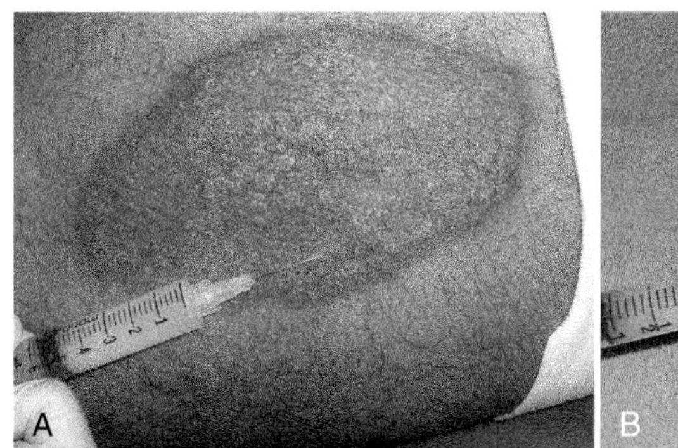

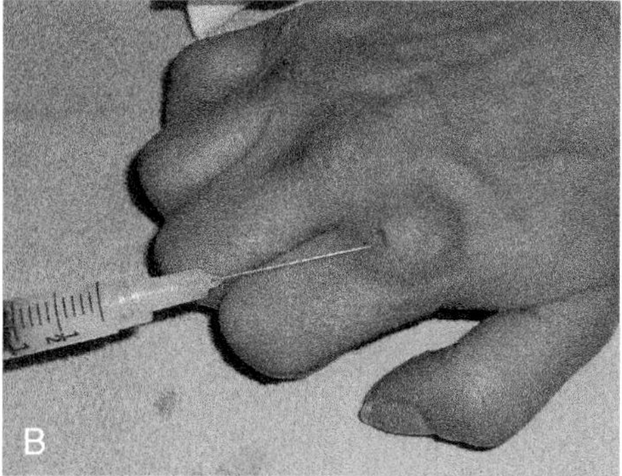

FIGURE 16-12 **(A)** Plaque psoriasis on the leg being injected with triamcinolone. **(B)** Plaque psoriasis over the MCP joints being injected with triamcinolone. *(Copyright Richard P. Usatine, MD.)*

Psoriasis

In the same review paper, no good clinical studies were found on the use of intralesional steroids for psoriasis (Figure 16-12).[11] The authors describe their personal experience as virtually 100% effective using 2.5 mg/mL triamcinolone for small plaques of psoriasis on the trunk and limbs.[11] In one small series, five patients with chronic intermittent palmoplantar pustulosis were treated with intralesional injections of 3.3 to 5.0 mg/mL of triamcinolone acetonide.[12] Prompt clearing of symptoms and lesions occurred and lasted 3 to 6 months. Despite the discomfort experienced from the injections, patients preferred this treatment modality over others available in 1984. Side effects included hypopigmentation, cutaneous atrophy, and, in one patient, exacerbation of a latent dermatophyte infection.[12] Despite the lack of evidence for the use of intralesional steroid injections for localized psoriasis, it is an accepted treatment option. We recommend using from 2.5 to 5.0 mg/mL with a 27-gauge needle for injection.

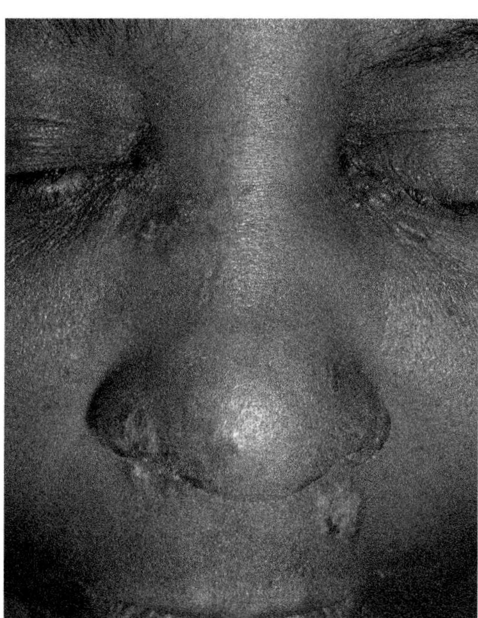

FIGURE 16-13 Sarcoidosis on the face of a black woman. One option for treatment is the use of intralesional triamcinolone. *(Copyright Richard P. Usatine, MD.)*

Sarcoidosis

Cutaneous sarcoidosis (Figure 16-13) may respond to intralesional steroids in a similar manner as other granulomatous diseases such as granuloma annulare. Cutaneous sarcoidosis is often found on the face of black women so the concentration of steroid must take the risks of atrophy and hypopigmentation into account. Concentrations of 2.5 mg/mL on the face and 5 mg/mL on the body should provide some relief from cutaneous sarcoidosis.

Tattoo Reactions

Occasionally someone will react with painful swelling and edema around the dye of a new tattoo. Most often it is the red dye (Figure 16-15). When that occurs, one treatment option is to inject the areas of inflammation with triamcinolone.

COMPLICATIONS OF STEROID INJECTIONS

Complications of steroid injections include skin atrophy and hypopigmentation (Figure 16-14). If skin atrophy

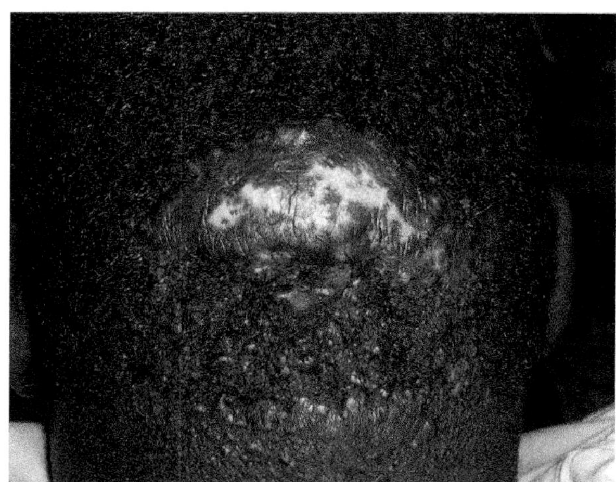

FIGURE 16-14 Hypopigmentation from cryosurgery and intralesional triamcinolone used to treat acne keloidalis nuchae. *(Copyright Richard P. Usatine, MD.)*

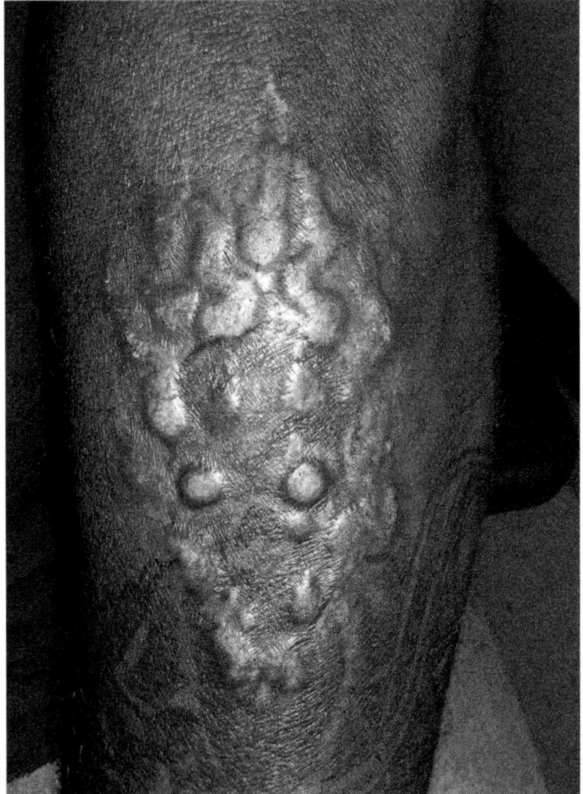

FIGURE 16-15 The red dye in the tattoo of the devil caused an allergic reaction on this man's arm. The only treatment that gave him relief was intralesional triamcinolone 5 mg/mL. *(Copyright Richard P. Usatine, MD.)*

occurs, it is worth waiting a number of months to see if the atrophy will resolve. If the atrophy is particularly bothersome after 4 months, the patient could be referred for injections of their own fat to restore the depressed area. This can be performed with liposuction and injection technique.

CANDIDA ANTIGEN AND BLEOMYCIN INTRALESIONAL INJECTIONS

Candida Antigen

Steroids are not the only injectables that can be used for dermatologic conditions. Verrucae (warts) can be treated with intralesional Candida antigen or bleomycin sulfate. Verrucae can and often do resolve spontaneously on their own. However, they can persist for years, multiply, or cause pain as well as cosmetic concerns. Treatment is often attempted with over-the-counter remedies (topical acids, occlusive techniques, and most recently with cryorefrigerants) and can be successful. When this fails, more aggressive treatments are often tried in a physician's office including cryotherapy, debridement with application of stronger acids, curettement with or without cautery, laser, and more. Each of these is generally accompanied by pain and various levels of disability as well as an open wound. Failures and recurrences even with aggressive treatment are common. Add to this the clinical scenarios where patients present with hundreds of warts, huge mosaic warts, and extensive periungual warts and one can understand the frustration patients and their caregivers often feel when treating this common problem.

Faced with the difficulty of treating warts, a new approach was taken in 1992. The idea was to somehow focus the immune system on the area where the wart existed. Candida antigen causes an immune response of erythema and occasionally pruritus in the majority of immune-competent individuals. The thought was that if the Candida were injected into the warts the immune response would eliminate the wart due to the increased immunologic activity in the area.

The first study of more than 100 patients who were treated with intralesional Candida was published in 2000. It reported that 85% of patients were completely cleared after three injections at 1-month intervals.[13] The advantages to this method of treatment are that if the patient's immune system recognizes the verrucous protein as foreign, then all lesions disappear, recurrences are rare, and there are no open wounds to deal with after treatment.

Candida antigen is an excellent method of treating most common warts, considering the results, cost, ease of administration, lack of scarring, and virtually no lasting side effects (after nearly 20 years of use).

This technique has not been tried on condyloma but can be used for virtually all other warts.

Candida antigen has been used for tuberculosis testing for 50 years or more but does not have FDA approval for the treatment of warts. Because it is approved for human use, malpractice policies will cover its administration should any unforeseen problems arise.

Contraindications

A history of sensitivity to Candida is a contraindication. Because the Candida is not live, it can be used on anyone. However, those who are immunocompromised are less likely to respond.

The Pfenninger Candida Protocol: Steps and Principles[13,14]

1. Obtain the Candida antigen (generic 1:1000 or proprietary Candin 1:500). Use caution if using allergy extracts to be sure the concentration is not too high.
2. For Candin, dilute 1:1 with 2% lidocaine without epinephrine. For generic, mix 1:4. This is counterintuitive but the generic seems to produce more of a reaction. See Table 16-4 for specific dilutions. Concentrations can be increased slowly if no

TABLE 16-4 Candida Dilutions

Creating 1.0 mL for Injection	Candida Antigen (mL)	2% Lidocaine (no Epinephrine) (mL)
Generic 1:1000	0.25	0.75
Candin 1:500	0.5	0.5

immunologic response (e.g., redness, pain) is observed after the initial treatment.

3. Apply a topical anesthetic at least 15 minutes prior or use a cryorefrigerant to ease the pain of injection. The majority of warts occur on the fingers, toes, and feet, which are all very sensitive areas.
4. Inject 0.1 mL (maximum of 0.3 mL depending on the size of the lesion) of solution *intralesionally or intradermally*. Several points need to be made:
   - The injection should take some force. If it goes in too easily, the needle is subdermal and the needed response will not occur. Inject as if you were trying to obtain a wheal although it will not happen due to the fibrous nature of the wart tissue (Figure 16-16).
   - Wear protective face shield since the solution often "squirts out" of the wart.
   - Use a Luer-Lok syringe since the needle frequently pops off with the pressure applied unless it is locked in place. A 30-gauge needle limits the pain of injection.
5. The total amount injected per visit is limited to 1 mL. Very little material is needed to incite an immune response. If there are 20 warts, try for 0.05 mL per lesion. Obviously, if there are 40 or 50 warts, it will be impossible to treat them all. However, all warts may disappear with treatment of less than the entirety due to the immune response. Some have suggested just pricking the needle into the warts if there is extensive disease. Again, this is just one of many possibilities that have not been studied.
6. Establish a return visit for 1 month. Should the warts resolve, the visit can be cancelled. If the warts persist, another treatment can be given using the same parameters. A third visit should be set up after the second if needed.
7. If after three injections at monthly intervals the warts persist, there are several options.
   - If the verrucae are smaller, continue with the Candida antigen if so desired.
   - Other traditional physical treatments can be tried. Often the warts are at least diminished in size, which now makes this a more tolerable option.
   - Bleomycin injections can be used. In the case of hundreds of lesions, bleomycin can be used on some of the lesions while Candida is used on others (see below).
8. In the absence of immunocompromised conditions (including smoking), expect 65% to 75% of lesions to resolve after the first visit. Younger patients and lesions present less than a year appear to respond best. With each succeeding treatment, approximately 50% of patients will respond.
9. Expect tenderness for a few days, erythema, peeling, and occasionally some pruritus (Figure 16-16B). Occasionally there can be a vigorous immune response with erythema and tenderness (as also occurs with too concentrated or too much volume of solution). There will be no scarring, hypo- or hyperpigmentation, or open wounds.
10. Patients may resume normal activities including bathing and group sports immediately after injection being limited by pain only. See Appendix A for a patient information handout titled *Wart Therapy*.

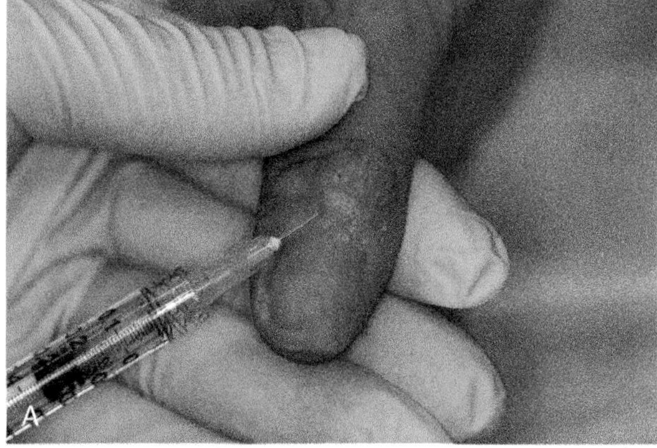

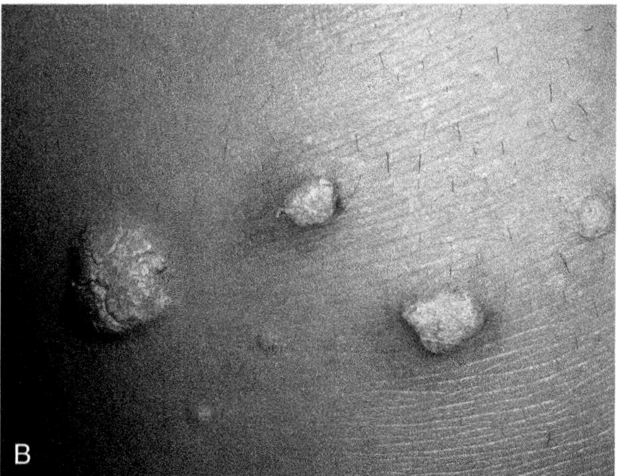

FIGURE 16-16 (A) Candida antigen injection of periungual warts. (B) It is not unusual for erythema to develop around warts injected with Candida antigen. These warts on the leg were injected the day before this photo was taken. *(A: Courtesy of John L. Pfenninger, MD; B: Copyright Richard P. Usatine, MD.)*

There is no J-code (a number assigned to each medication for billing) for Candida antigen treatment, therefore the cost of the antigen cannot be billed to insurance. It is quite expensive, especially if the proprietary type is used. Generally, it works out best if the antigen is supplied by the physician for the first visit. The patient is then given a prescription to be filled at the pharmacy to bring with them to the next visit. Make sure that patient knows that the Candida antigen must be refrigerated while storing it at home.

Your prescription should say "Candin antigen (or generic Candida antigen), 1 vial for therapeutic use to treat warts."

The remainder of the antigen in the leftover vial will build up a supply for the clinician to use for future patients for their "first visit." Reimbursement for either the lesion injection codes or lesion destruction codes alone is inadequate to cover the costs of antigen so patients should be made aware that they will need to pay for that in addition to the injection fee. Some insurance plans will pay the pharmacist (even though they will not reimburse the physician).

Bleomycin

Bleomycin sulfate is a chemotherapeutic agent. Like Candida antigen, it too has not been approved by the FDA for the treatment of verrucae but it has been well studied and used for more than 20 years.[15,16] Its efficacy is similar to that of Candida antigen but reactions are often more robust. It has not been used for the treatment of condyloma but can be used in all other areas where warts develop.

Contraindications

- Pregnancy
- Allergy to bleomycin
- Injection over the proximal fingernail, which can cause distortion to the nail
- Relative contraindications: very young children because of their thin skin.

Bleomycin Injections: Steps and Principles

1. Dilute a 15 unit vial of bleomycin (Blenoxane, Bristol Myers) with 5 mL of bacteriostatic water or 0.9% sodium chloride. This will provide 3 unit/mL of solution. Once reconstituted, it must be kept refrigerated and be used within 4 months.
2. Just prior to use, further dilute by mixing 1 mL (3 unit) with 5 mL of 1% lidocaine without epinephrine. This provides 6 mL at a concentration of 0.5 unit of bleomycin per milliliter.
3. Use a 6- to 10-mL Luer-Lok syringe with a 30-gauge needle.
4. The amount injected is based on wart size. See Table 16-5.
5. Expect more tenderness than with Candida. A darkened hemorrhagic area often appears. Peeling is common with erythema for a longer period of time especially with larger volumes.
6. Activities are limited only by pain.
7. Schedule a follow-up appointment for 1 month. It can be cancelled if the warts resolve. If they persist, a repeat injection can be given. There is no set limit to the number of 1-month visits but, generally, progress should be seen by at least the third visit although usually progress will be visible after the first injection.
8. Candida antigen can be given at the same visit while giving bleomycin (separate syringes to separate sites) if there are multiple, extensive verrucae.

TABLE 16-5 Bleomycin for Wart Treatment

Wart Size	Amount of Solution (0.5 unit/mL)
<5 mm	0.1-0.2 mL
5–10 mm	0.2-0.4 mL
>10 mm	Up to a maximum of 1 mL (rarely needed)
Multiple warts	Up to 3 mL (1.5 unit) per visit

BOX 16-1 *CPT Codes and Their Medicare Reimbursement Amounts*

11900 Intralesional Injection (up to 7) $51
11901 Intralesional Injection (more than 7) $66

Bleomycin is costly. It is easiest to provide a prescription to patients and have them bring the medication to the office for the following visit, as explained in the Candida antigen discussion above.

AFTERCARE FOR ALL INTRALESIONAL INJECTIONS

No special aftercare is needed other than follow-up for inspection of the results and consideration of additional treatments.

CODING AND BILLING PEARLS

Intralesional injections have two CPT codes for giving the injections (see Box 16-1). These should be simple to use since there is one code for up to and including seven lesions (not separate injections) and one code for eight lesions and above. If it takes three injections to inject one large plaque of psoriasis, this is still counted as one lesion.

J-codes are used to bill for the injectable material:

J3301 Injection, triamcinolone acetonide, not otherwise specified, per 10 mg
J9040 Injection, bleomycin sulfate, 15 units.

References

1. Levine RM, Rasmussen JE. Intralesional corticosteroids in the treatment of nodulocystic acne. *Arch Dermatol.* 1983;119:480–481.
2. Taub AF. Procedural treatments for acne vulgaris. *Dermatol Surg.* 2007;33:1005–1026.
3. Delamere FM, Sladden MM, Dobbins HM, Leonardi-Bee J. Interventions for alopecia areata. *Cochrane Database Syst Rev.* 2008;CD004413.
4. Verbov J. The place of intralesional steroid therapy in dermatology. *Br J Dermatol.* 1976;94(suppl 12):51–58.
5. Callen JP. Treatment of cutaneous lesions in patients with lupus erythematosus. *Dermatol Clin.* 1994;12:201–206.
6. Yosipovitch G, Widijanti SM, Goon A, *et al.* A comparison of the combined effect of cryotherapy and corticosteroid injections versus corticosteroids and cryotherapy alone on keloids: a controlled study. *J Dermatolog Treat.* 2001;12:87–90.
7. Boutli-Kasapidou F, Tsakiri A, Anagnostou E, Mourellou O. Hypertrophic and keloidal scars: an approach to polytherapy. *Int J Dermatol.* 2005;44:324–327.
8. Layton AM, Yip J, Cunliffe WJ. A comparison of intralesional triamcinolone and cryosurgery in the treatment of acne keloids. *Br J Dermatol.* 1994;130:498–501.
9. Darougheh A, Asilian A, Shariati F. Intralesional triamcinolone alone or in combination with 5-fluorouracil for the treatment of keloid and hypertrophic scars. *Clin Exp Dermatol.* 2009;34:219–223.
10. Sclafani AP, Gordon L, Chadha M, Romo T, III. Prevention of earlobe keloid recurrence with postoperative corticosteroid

injections versus radiation therapy: a randomized, prospective study and review of the literature. *Dermatol Surg*. 1996;22: 569–574.
11. Richards RN. Update on intralesional steroid: focus on dermatoses. *J Cutan Med Surg*. 2010;14:19–23.
12. Goette DK, Morgan AM, Fox BJ, Horn RT. Treatment of palmoplantar pustulosis with intralesional triamcinolone injections. *Arch Dermatol*. 1984;120:319–323.
13. Phillips RC, Ruhl TS, Pfenninger JL, Garber MR. Treatment of warts with Candida antigen injection. *Arch Dermatol*. 2000; 136:1274–1275.
14. Pfenninger JL, Fowler GC. *Pfenninger and Fowler's Procedures for Primary Care*. 3rd ed. Philadelphia: Elsevier; 2010.
15. Amer M, Diab N, Ramadan A, *et al*. Therapeutic evaluation for intralesional injection of bleomycin sulfate in 143 resistant warts. *J Am Acad Dermatol*. 1988;18:1313–1316.
16. Sollitto RJ, Pizzano DM. Bleomycin sulfate in the treatment of mosaic plantar verrucae: a follow-up study. *J Foot Ankle Surg*. 1996;35:169–172.

Additional Reading

Mones H, LaRavia D. Hypertrophic scars and keloids. *In*: Pfenninger JL, Fowler GC, eds. *Procedures for Primary Care*. Philadelphia: Elsevier; 2010.

17 Incision and Drainage

DANIEL L. STULBERG, MD • PATRICK MORAN, DO

Incision and drainage (I&D) is a simple in-office procedure that in most cases is curative for superficial abscesses and related infections including uncomplicated methicillin-resistant *Staphylococcus aureus* (MRSA) abscesses. Commonly, patients will present with the acute onset of localized pain, swelling, and erythema indicating abscess formation (Figure 17-1). These can be the result of trauma, injection drug use, insect stings or bites, a secondary infection or inflammation of an epidermoid cyst, or paronychia from nail biting or manipulation, or they may arise without a clear inciting event.

The most common pathogens are *Staphylococcus aureus* and *Streptococcus* bacteria. Systemic antibiotics should usually only be given if there is surrounding cellulitis (Figure 17-2) or other signs or symptoms of further infection. There is no clear need for antibiotics even if localized MRSA is present, and there is also no clear indication for antibiotics in a patient with diabetes or an immune-compromised patient as long as the infection is a localized one that can be drained.[1,2] Some patients may be colonized with MRSA and develop recurrent abscesses. In this situation, treatment with systemic antibiotics such as trimethoprim/sulfamethoxazole, doxycycline, or clindamycin based on local sensitivity patterns may help. Mupirocin is applied inside the nares twice daily for 5 days and topical chlorhexidine skin washing is commonly used to try to clear the carrier state, although the literature does not clearly support these practices.[3,4]

INDICATIONS

The following lesions should be treated with incision and drainage:

- Abscess
- Abscessed epidermoid cyst
- Furuncle—abscess related to the hair follicle
- Carbuncle—coalescence of furuncles
- Paronychia—abscess at the nail margin.

CONTRAINDICATIONS AND CAUTIONS

- This chapter deals with superficial abscesses seen in routine office practice. Deep abscesses and those of body compartments including the palm of the hand require more extensive surgical intervention.
- Perirectal abscesses should be approached cautiously. They may be associated with deep disease or underlying inflammatory bowel disease and care should be taken not to damage the anal sphincter, which can cause incontinence.[5]
- Incision and drainage of abscesses of the face can lead to scarring, so choose the line of incision along skin tension lines, wrinkles, or other structures to minimize the prominence of the scar. Needle aspiration and antibiotics can be tried as initial treatment with close follow-up and an informed patient understanding that incision and drainage may ultimately be necessary.
- Be cautious to avoid damage to underlying structures including nerves and blood vessels.
- Abscesses and infections in closed spaces including the hand, foot, and orbits require additional intervention and consultation.
- Crepitus or gas seen on imaging suggests a more serious infection such as necrotizing fasciitis. This is a surgical emergency requiring a STAT surgical consult.
- Breast abscesses in a nonlactating woman should prompt evaluation for possible cancer (Figure 17-2).
- Abscesses of the central face in the "danger triangle" between the bridge of the nose and the angles of the mouth may lead to further complications such as a cavernous sinus thrombosis. These are best treated with antibiotics and warm compresses early to prevent a cavernous sinus thrombosis.[6]

ADVANTAGES OF INCISION AND DRAINAGE

The advantages of I&D can be categorized into those for the clinician and those for the patient. Advantages for the clinician include the following:

- Patient results are usually excellent.
- The procedure is simple to perform.
- Most are amenable to being performed in the office setting.

Advantages for the patient include:

- Results are usually excellent.
- Reduction in pain may occur quickly.
- This is an office procedure that can save a patient the higher copays and bills that result from an emergency department or surgical center visit.
- Family member or friend can be instructed to do the repacking when needed.

DISADVANTAGES OF INCISION AND DRAINAGE

As with the advantages of I&D, the disadvantages can also be categorized into those for the clinician and those

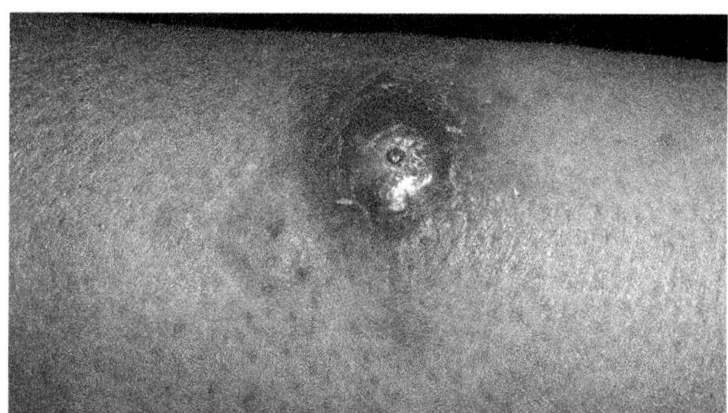

FIGURE 17-1 Abscess with raised fluctuant center on the arm. *(Copyright Richard P. Usatine, MD.)*

for the patient. Disadvantages for the clinician include the following:

- Time to collect supplies and perform the procedure
- Possibility of body fluid exposure.

Disadvantages for the patient include:

- Pain of procedure
- Scarring.

EQUIPMENT

- Alcohol, povidone-iodine, and/or chlorhexidine for skin preparation
- Lidocaine, plain or with epinephrine
- Ethyl chloride spray (This is an optional topical anesthesia that is used to drain a paronychia or prior to a lidocaine injection.)
- 3- to 10-mL syringe based on size of abscess
- 18-gauge or large needle to draw up anesthesia
- 27-gauge 1.5-inch needle for anesthesia injections
- Clean gloves
- No. 11 blade with disposable or nondisposable scalpel handle
- Hemostat (Many clinicians prefer a curved hemostat to more easily get to loculations.)
- Scissors
- 4 × 4 gauze pads
- Ribbon gauze, ¼ or ½ inch depending on lesion size
- Culture swab and transport media if desired
- Dressing 4 × 4 gauze or nonadherent dressing and tape, or large adhesive dressing.

Some clinicians also use the following:

- Sterile saline for irrigation
- Irrigation syringe and catheter, or angiocath with the needle removed.

INCISION AND DRAINAGE: STEPS AND PRINCIPLES

1. Counsel the patient regarding the diagnosis of abscess and that the recommended treatment is incision and drainage followed by packing with gauze. Obtain informed consent verbally and in writing.
2. Abscesses tend to be more difficult to anesthetize than routine lesions because the acidic environment caused by the bacteria does not respond as well to lidocaine. After prepping the skin with alcohol, inject 1% lidocaine with epinephrine to start the process. One method is to use a fan pattern lateral to one side of the abscess then lateral to the other side of the lesion and underneath the lesion (Figure 17-3). A ring block is also commonly used for an abscess (see Figure 3-11 in Chapter 3, *Anesthesia*). Avoid injecting into the abscess itself, because that will increase pressure and pain and

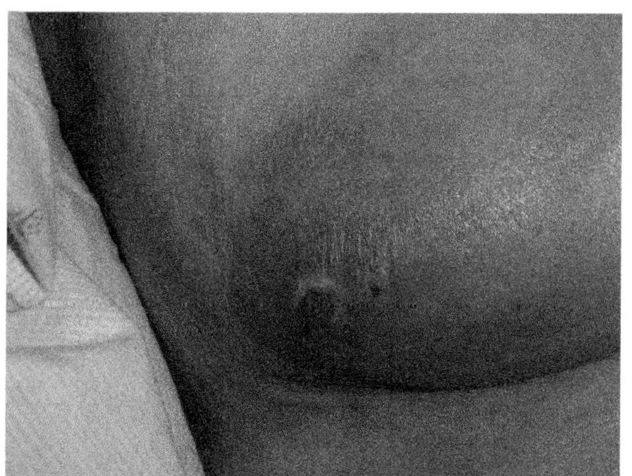

FIGURE 17-2 Abscess with cellulitis. Note the erythema around this breast abscess. This presentation prompted an investigation for underlying breast cancer. *(Copyright Richard P. Usatine, MD.)*

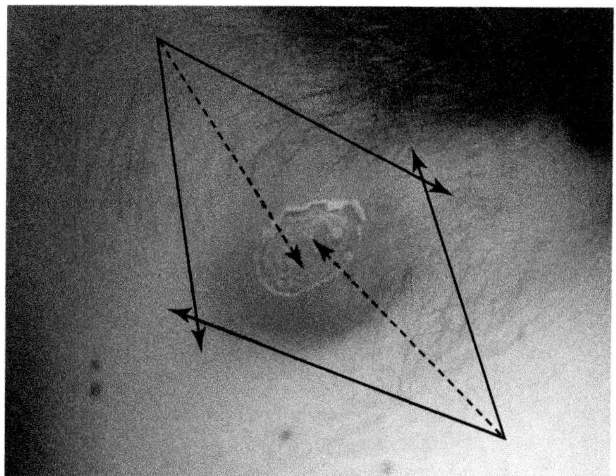

FIGURE 17-3 Injecting laterally and deep to the abscess for anesthesia. *(Copyright Richard P. Usatine, MD.)*

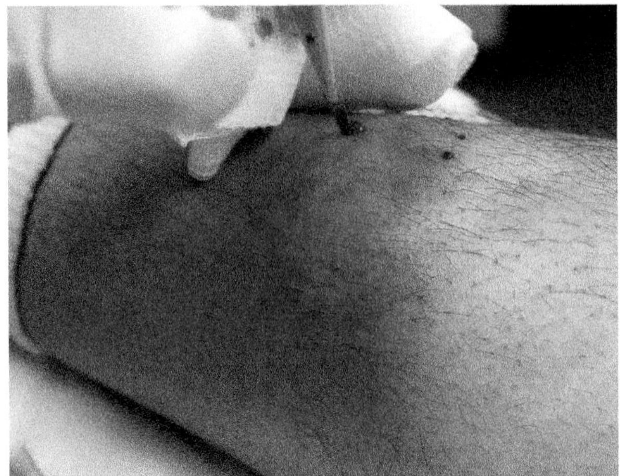

FIGURE 17-4 Incising the abscess. *(Copyright Daniel L. Stulberg, MD.)*

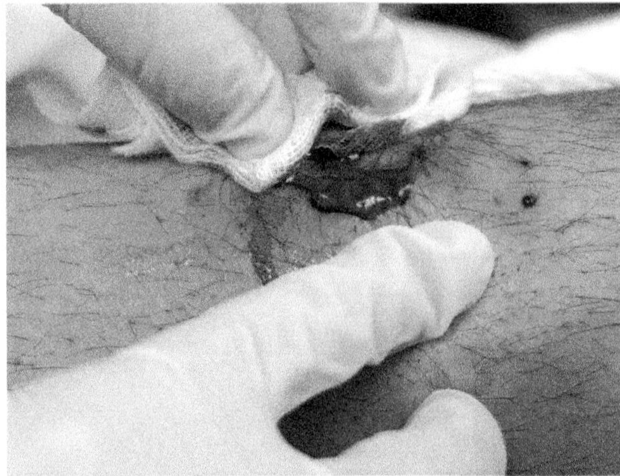

FIGURE 17-6 Expressing the purulent material. *(Copyright Daniel L. Stulberg, MD.)*

may cause the abscess to spontaneously rupture under pressure, spraying out its contents and increasing the risk of exposure to care providers. For this reason and because the lesion may already be under pressure, proper eye and barrier protection is recommended. A full face shield (e.g., the Splash Shield as seen in Figure 2-14 of Chapter 2) and a disposable gown provide good protection in this setting.

3. While the anesthetic is taking effect, set up the rest of the instruments listed above. Clean gloves and a clean technique are used. Open the bottle of strip gauze and using the forceps pick up the end and extract a length of gauze that will be more than enough to pack into the abscess cavity. Cut the strip with the scissors just above the bottle and the end will fall back cleanly into the bottle. Some clinicians use iodoform gauze to pack abscesses. This author uses plain gauze because it seems to cause less burning discomfort, and iodine even in dilute concentrations is toxic to new tissue growth.
4. In cosmetically sensitive areas, and whenever possible, align the incision along the normal skin tension lines or along structures where the scar will be less visible after healing. Using the No. 11 blade perpendicular to the skin, incise the lesion at the area of "pointing" if present where the skin has already thinned out and the purulence can be seen through the skin (Figure 17-4). Extend the incision to allow adequate exploration, drainage, and packing.
5. The pus will usually spontaneously drain (Figure 17-5) or may spray out under pressure. Express the remaining purulent material by compressing toward the abscess from both sides with gauze in hands (Figure 17-6).
6. Use the hemostats to explore the cavity and break up any loculations (Figure 17-7). If the abscess is from an inflamed or infected epidermoid cyst, use the hemostat to pull out visible portions of the cyst wall to try and prevent recurrence. Then express any remaining purulence.

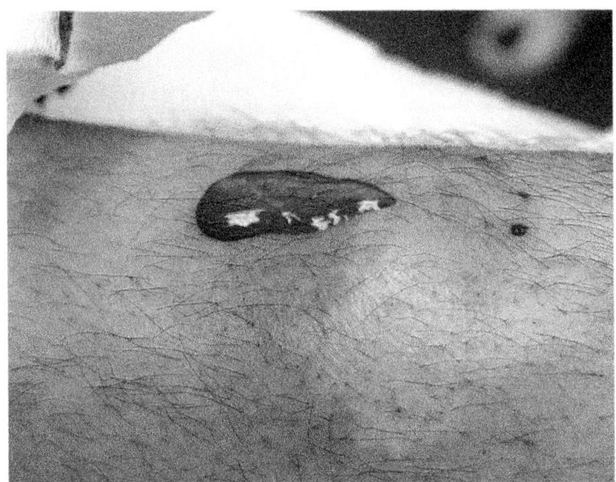

FIGURE 17-5 Release of pus. *(Copyright Daniel L. Stulberg, MD.)*

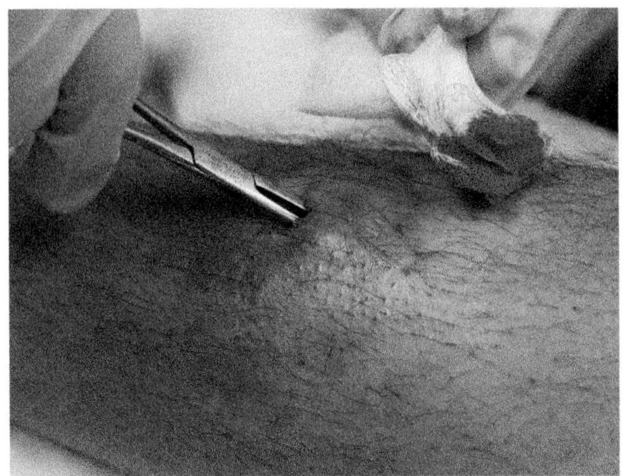

FIGURE 17-7 Breaking up loculations. *(Copyright Daniel L. Stulberg, MD.)*

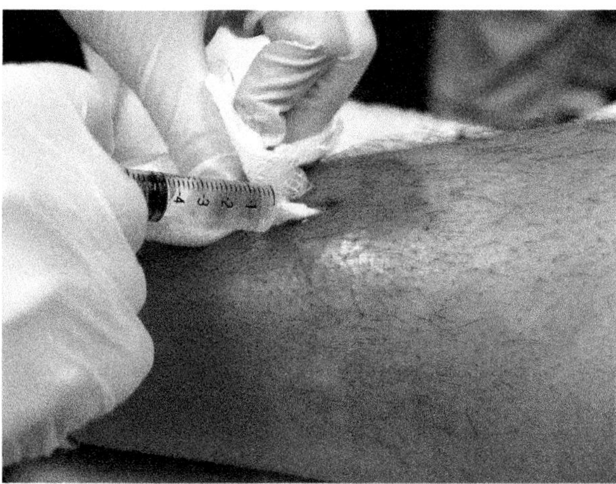

FIGURE 17-8 Irrigating the abscess cavity. *(Copyright Daniel L. Stulberg, MD.)*

7. Use cotton-tipped applicators (CTAs) to explore the cavity and clean out remaining bits of infected tissue and purulence.
8. Some clinicians will irrigate at this stage with sterile saline (Figure 17-8). This is a common practice, but a literature review found no concrete evidence to support the practice.[7]
9. Using the forceps (without teeth works better) grasp the strip gauze and start packing it into the deepest portion of the abscess cavity (Figure 17-9). Using the stick end of a CTA can help when pushing the gauze into the cavity. Continue to pack the gauze until the cavity is full and then leave a 3- to 4-cm tail outside of the wound to facilitate later removal.
10. Cover the gauze tail with gauze or a nonadherent dressing and tape. Ask the patient to keep the dressing dry for 48 hours.
11. If no further packing will be needed, show the patient how to remove the strip gauze in 2 days at home. Often this may be done in the shower. If the patient cannot reach the gauze then help will be needed.
12. If the follow-up is done in 2 days, grasp the tail of the strip gauze and in one long swift movement remove the entire strip of gauze. This is painful, but preferable to prolonging the discomfort of tugging out the gauze inch by inch.

AFTERCARE

Repacking can be done during office visits or at home if a reliable friend or family member is available to help. Repacking is uncomfortable, but usually tolerable without anesthetic.

There are no RCTs to inform us on how often and for how long a healing abscess should be packed.[8] A small abscess can often be packed only once at the time of the I&D and then the patient can be directed to remove the packing at home in 2 days. A very large abscess may need repacking every other day for 1 to 2 weeks. Consider that each time an abscess is unpacked and repacked, it causes pain to the patient. Also the packing will delay the ultimate healing but may be needed when there is a risk that premature closure will allow a new abscess to form. Therefore, the decision on how often and how long an abscess is packed is based on physician experience, patient preferences as well as size and location.

PARONYCHIA

Paronychia is a local bacterial infection of the nail fold. These infections are often caused by nail biting or manipulating the nail or nail margins (Figure 17-10). Prior to opening the abscess the paronychia can be locally anesthetized with ethyl chloride spray. It is important to be ready to make the cut in the paronychia quickly because the anesthetic effect is very brief. A No. 11 scalpel can be used to incise the abscess at the nail margin (Figure 17-11). These lesions are usually too small to allow packing. In more severe cases, a digital block or lidocaine injected locally may be needed.

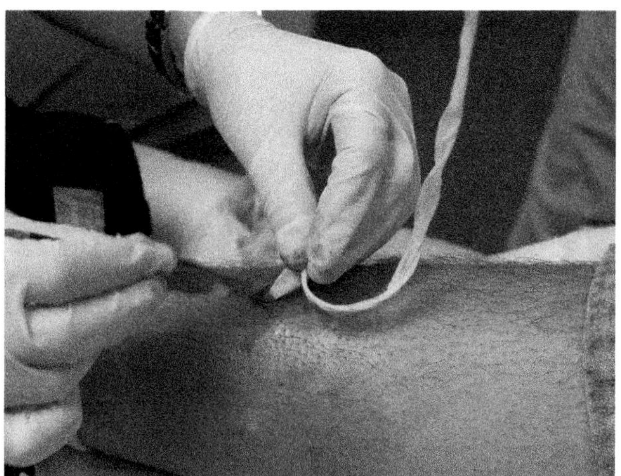

FIGURE 17-9 Packing the abscess cavity with strip gauze. *(Copyright Daniel L. Stulberg, MD.)*

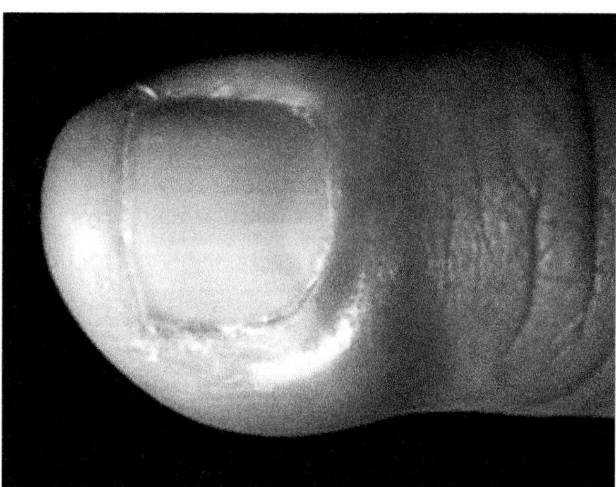

FIGURE 17-10 Paronychia. *(Copyright Richard P. Usatine, MD.)*

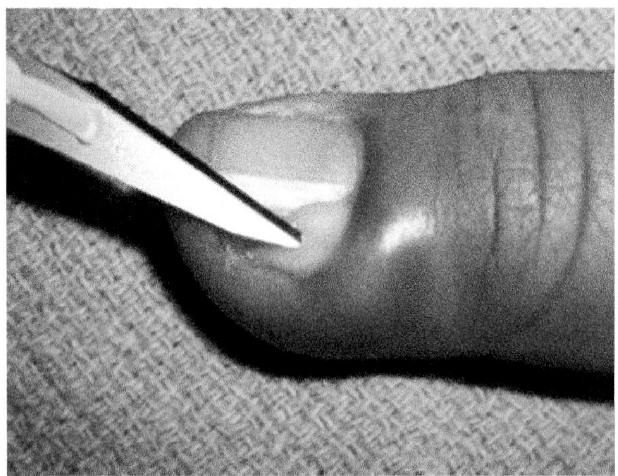

FIGURE 17-11 Incision of paronychia. *(Copyright Richard P. Usatine, MD.)*

Counsel the patient to use warm soaks three times a day and to open the abscess manually if it closes and express any purulence until it heals.

COMPLICATIONS

- Scarring will occur from an abscess rupturing and thinning the skin. A well-placed incision can lessen the scar or its prominence, but a scar will be present nonetheless.
- Reoccurrence is not unusual due to the wound closing too early or an undiagnosed loculation or due to underlying deeper infection (i.e., osteomyelitis).
- Septicemia, or an advancing deep infection, may occur in association with an abscess (e.g., necrotizing fasciitis).
- Bleeding may occur from damage to blood vessels during the course of incision and drainage or as a result of infection eroding into adjacent vessels.
- Damage to other adjacent structures may also occur as a result of infection eroding into adjacent structures or causing inflammation of nearby structures.

TREATING SPECIFIC LESIONS

- MRSA involvement has increased in recent years, but as mentioned above, evidence does not support the use of antibiotics in addition to I&D in uncomplicated abscesses.
- Because facial abscesses are in a cosmetically sensitive area for scarring, the clinician may initially manage them cautiously with needle aspiration and antibiotics and close follow-up.
- Perirectal abscesses occur in proximity to the anal sphincter and care should be taken to avoid cutting across the sphincter. As with facial abscesses they may be initially managed cautiously with needle aspiration and antibiotics and close follow-up, but have a higher risk of deeper infection and fistula tracking especially with inflammatory bowel disease.

BOX 17-1 *I&D CPT Codes*

10060	Incision and drainage of abscess (cutaneous, subcutaneous abscess, cyst, or paronychia)—simple
10061	Incision and drainage of abscess—multiple or complex (with wound packing)

Perirectal abscesses more commonly involve anaerobic and gram-negative bacteria.

SPECIAL POPULATIONS

Immune-compromised patients may be particularly susceptible to localized or systemic infections that present as abscesses or skin infections. Evaluation should take into account the patient's history, current symptoms, and physical findings. Laboratory testing, imaging studies, and systemic antibiotics may be needed and should be determined based on the overall clinical picture.[9] In contrast to routine superficial abscesses, in which culture of the abscess fluid or cavity is not usually required, cultures may be helpful in these patients to guide antibiotic therapy of atypical organisms that may be present.

CODING AND BILLING PEARLS

The CPT codes for I&D are shown in Box 17-1. Note that some specific locations have their own CPT codes. Those specific codes should be used rather than the generic ones since they often reimburse more. These areas include such cutaneous sites as the vulva, eyelid, and pinna. See Table 38-8 in Chapter 38, *Surviving Financially*, for a full listing of these sites and their reimbursement.

CONCLUSION

Patients will present with abscesses as a result of routine situations and sometimes will develop abscesses or wound infections subsequent to procedures performed by the provider. It is important for clinicians treating skin disorders to stock the appropriate items and have the appropriate skills to be able to treat skin abscesses and infections; otherwise, they will have to refer patients in these situations to another provider or facility. Having the skills and equipment to manage these patients adds to the breadth of a provider's practice.

References

1. Lee MC, Rios AM, Aten MF, *et al*. Management and outcome of children with skin and soft tissue abscesses caused by community-acquired methicillin-resistant *Staphylococcus aureus*. *Pediatr Infect Dis J*. 2004;23(2):123–127.
2. Rajendran PM, Young D, Maurer T, *et al*. Randomized, double-blind, placebo-controlled trial of cephalexin for treatment of uncomplicated skin abscesses in a population at risk for

community-acquired methicillin-resistant *Staphylococcus aureus* infection. *Antimicrob Agents Chemother.* 2007;51(11):4044–4048.
3. Loeb M, Main C, Walker-Dilks C, *et al.* Antimicrobial drugs for treating methicillin-resistant Staphylococcus aureus colonization. *Cochrane Database Syst Rev.* 2003(4):CD00340.
4. Wendt C, Schinke S, Wurtemberger M, *et al.* Value of whole-body washing with chlorhexidine for the eradication of methicillin-resistant *Staphylococcus aureus*: a randomized, placebo-controlled, double-blind clinical trial. *Infect Control Hosp Epidemiol.* 2007; 28(9):1036–1043.
5. Ho YH, Tan M, Chui CH, *et al.* Randomized controlled trial of primary fistulotomy with drainage alone for perianal abscesses. *Dis Colon Rectum.* 1997;40(12):1435–1438.
6. Puymirat E. A Lemierre syndrome variant caused by *Staphylococcus aureus. Am J Emerg Med.* 2008;26(3):380.e5–7.
7. Korownyk C, Allan GM. Evidence-based approach to abscess management. *Can Fam Physician.* 2007;53(10):1680–1684.
8. Fitch MT, Manthey DE, McGinnis HD, *et al.* Videos in clinical medicine. Abscess incision and drainage. *N Engl J Med.* 2007; 357(19):e20.
9. Stevens DL, Bisno AL, Chambers HF, *et al.* Practice guidelines for the diagnosis and management of skin and soft-tissue infections. *Clin Infect Dis.* 2005;41(10):1373–1406.

18 Nail Procedures

RICHARD P. USATINE, MD

Nails serve an important function to protect the ends of our fingers and toes, to increase mechanical traction, and to enhance fine touch. Nails also serve important social functions such as scratching, grooming, and to serve as aesthetic adornments (Figure 18-1).

Nails can be traumatized, infected, or become dysmorphic secondary to cutaneous or systemic disease. Skin cancers can form under or around nails. This chapter covers the various types of specialized surgical procedures and biopsies performed on the nail and the nail unit.

ANATOMY OF THE NAIL UNIT

What we call the "nail" is actually the nail plate that sits on the nail bed and is surrounded by the nail folds. The nail plate is made of keratin and is produced by the nail matrix found below the proximal nail fold. Figure 18-2 shows the detailed anatomy of a nail.

NAIL PROCEDURES

Nail procedures include the following:

- Digital and wing blocks
- Partial nail removal—ingrown nail and pincer nail
- Matrixectomy—chemical and physical
- Nail removal (nail evulsion)
- Biopsies to diagnose skin cancers—punch, shave, longitudinal excision
- Subungual hematoma evacuation.

Some common nail conditions that require nail procedures include the following:

- Ingrown nail requiring partial nail excision
- Deformed and painful nail requiring full nail plate avulsion
- Pincer nail when painful
- Longitudinal melanonychia requiring biopsy of nail matrix
- Subungual hematoma requiring drainage.

EQUIPMENT

Equipment Needed for Nail Plate Removal *(Figure 18-3)*

- 1 nail elevator (periosteal elevator, septum elevator, or Freer elevator)
- 1 nail splitter (English anvil type)
- 1 straight hemostat.

Additional Equipment Needed for Other Nail Surgeries

- 1 curved sharp iris scissor, Gradle scissor, or other fine-tipped scissor
- Needle holder
- Adson forceps (no teeth or fine teeth only)
- Skin hooks (single or double pronged).

NAIL PROCEDURES: COMMON STEPS

Local anesthesia is most effective with a digital block, wing block, or both (Figure 18-4). These blocks are explained fully in Chapter 3, *Anesthesia*. Neither of them is difficult to perform. In my experience asking patients who have had both blocks, the digital block is somewhat less painful than the wing block. The wing block has the benefit of producing local hemostasis because it distends the tissues near the area of surgery and epinephrine may be used so additional hemostasis is obtained.

A digital block may be performed with 1% or 2% lidocaine (no epinephrine). I prefer 2% lidocaine. Because there is not much room for a large volume of anesthesia, a more concentrated solution has the advantage of delivering more anesthetic in less volume. I use 3 to 4 mL to avoid too much volume and pressure. The anesthesia may be given at the base of the digit or in the web space (Figures 18-4A and B).

A wing block can be performed using epinephrine if the patient has no vascular diseases that would contraindicate its use. I mix 2% lidocaine without epinephrine with 1% lidocaine with epinephrine 1:1 to produce 1.5% lidocaine and ½ strength epinephrine. The onset of anesthesia is fast and it provides better hemostasis at the site of surgery (Figure 18-4C). As always, make sure that good anesthesia has been obtained before starting the procedure. If a tourniquet is used, the wing block can be performed with lidocaine only.

Povidone-iodine (Betadine), chlorhexidine (Hibiclens), or chlorhexidine-alcohol may be used to clean the surgical site for all procedures that follow. New data on surgical scrubs indicates that chlorhexidine-based scrubs are most effective in decreasing postop infection rates.[1]

Use of Glove for Tourniquet and Sterile Field

A tourniquet is not needed for nail plate removal surgeries (partial or complete). It is worth using a tourniquet for nail matrix biopsies to allow for better visualization during the biopsy. Even this procedure

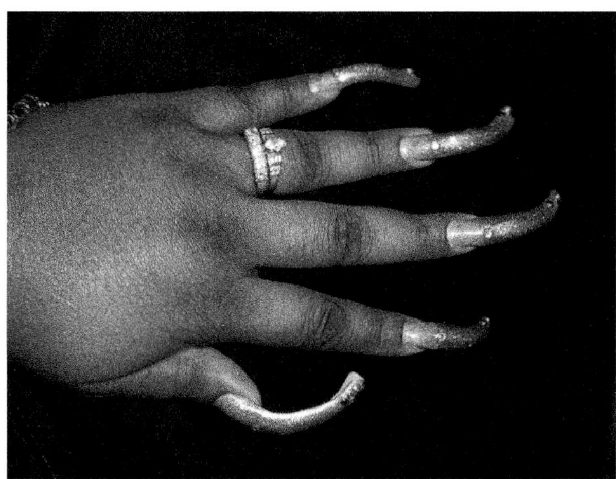

FIGURE 18-1 Nails serve important social functions including being aesthetic adornments. *(Copyright Richard P. Usatine, MD.)*

does not require a tourniquet but may be less vascular and easier to perform if a tourniquet is used.

Finger Nail Matrix Biopsies

1. Place sterile glove on patient after the patient's hand and finger have been cleaned and/or scrubbed.
2. Cut a slit in the glove finger with a sterile scissor to be able to roll back the glove over the involved finger (Figure 18-5).

Toe Nail Matrix Biopsies

1. A finger of a sterile glove can be used to make a sterile tourniquet along with a hemostat (Figure 18-6A–C). You can also use a large sterile glove on the foot to help with sterility.
2. Use a sterile hemostat to twist the glove material tighter around the digit as needed during the surgery (Figure 18-6C). Time limit recommendations for tourniquets in the literature vary from 30 minutes to over 2 hours. In a large study of tourniquet use in hand surgery, even those 60 patients whose tourniquet time exceeded 2 hours showed no postoperative complications.[2]

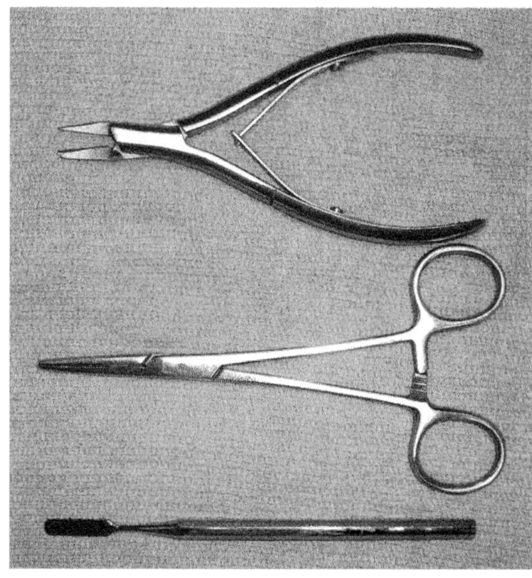

FIGURE 18-3 Instruments for nail surgery: nail splitter, straight hemostat, and nail elevator. *(Copyright Richard P. Usatine, MD.)*

PARTIAL NAIL PLATE EXCISION

See video on the DVD for further learning. 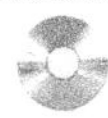

The most common indication for partial nail plate excision is an ingrown nail (especially the large toenail). An ingrown nail (onychocryptosis) occurs when the nail

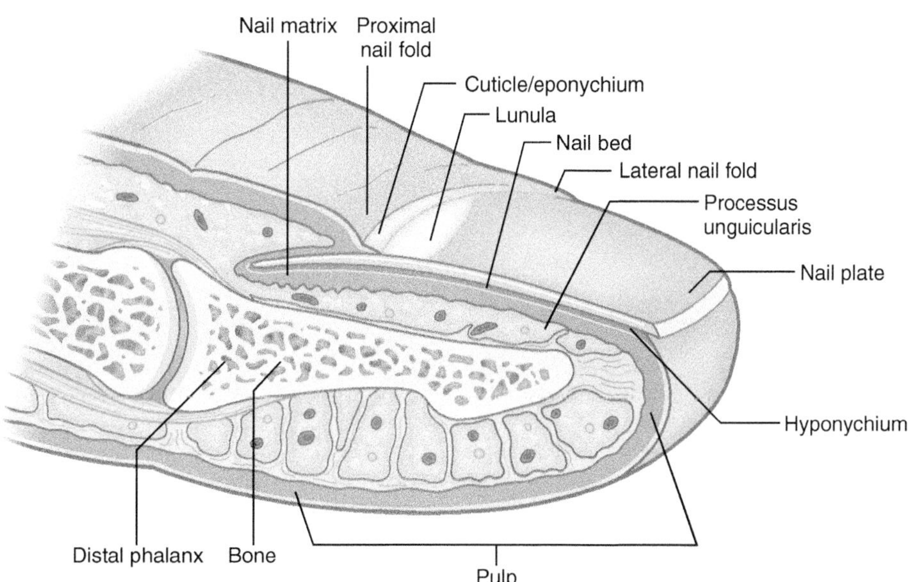

FIGURE 18-2 Detailed anatomy of the nail unit. *(Modified from Vidimos A, Ammirati C, Poblete-Lopez C. Dermatologic Surgery. London: Saunders; 2008.)*

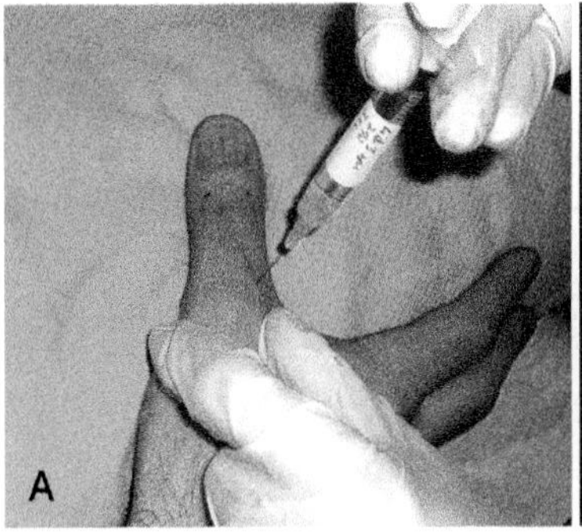

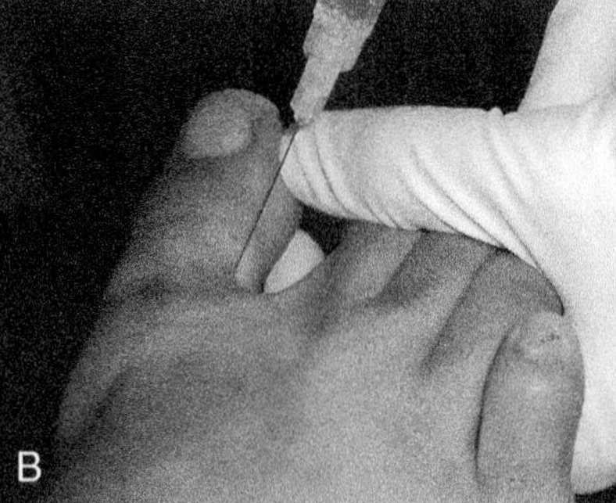

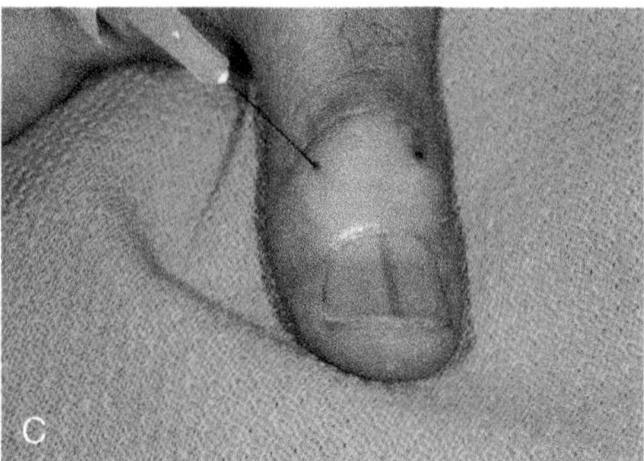

FIGURE 18-4 **(A)** Digital block of the thumb using 2% lidocaine without epinephrine. **(B)** Digital block of the large toe with needle pointed toward the web space. **(C)** Wing block using lidocaine with half-strength epinephrine. This was accomplished by mixing 2% lidocaine with 1% lidocaine including epinephrine in a one-to-one mixture. *(Copyright Richard P. Usatine, MD.)*

plate is too large for the nail bed (Figures 18-7 and 18-8). The nail plate puts pressure on the lateral nail fold and does not fit properly in the lateral nail groove. The treatment for this is to make the nail plate less wide on the involved side. The best way to prevent this from recurring is to ablate the nail matrix on the involved side using chemical or electrosurgical destruction.

Ingrown Toenail Removal Procedure Steps

See video on the DVD for further learning.

1. Anesthetize and sterilize the affected digit as described above (Figure 18-8A).
2. Use nail elevator to free the proximal nail fold from the nail plate below it (Figure 18-8B).
3. Now insert the nail elevator under the nail plate to separate the nail plate from the nail bed. Insert the elevator all the way back to the nail matrix (Figure 18-8C).
4. Use a nail splitter to cut a portion of nail to be removed (Figure 18-8D).
5. Insert a straight hemostat under the free portion of the nail and clamp down on this nail segment. Twist and turn the nail segment until the corner nail spicule is released and the portion of the nail is fully removed (Figure 18-8E).
6. Bleeding can be stopped with direct pressure, electrocoagulation, or a chemical hemostatic agent such as aluminum chloride, Monsel's solution, or silver nitrate. If a tourniquet is used there may be little to no bleeding.
7. If the matrix is to be destroyed, use phenol or electrosurgery (Figure 18-8F).
8. Granulation tissue or swelling of the lateral nail fold can be ignored, because it will resolve during the healing process (Figure 18-8G).
9. Encourage the patient to soak the foot twice daily with dilute povidone-iodine in water or another disinfectant soap solution to prevent infection and accelerate healing.[3]

FIGURE 18-5 A sterile surgical glove is used to provide a tourniquet for nail surgery and a sterile field. *(Copyright Richard P. Usatine, MD.)*

DESTRUCTION OF NAIL MATRIX

See video on the DVD for further learning. 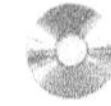

Chemical

Chemical matrixectomy is performed mainly by phenol (full-strength 88%) or 10% sodium hydroxide. In a comparison study of the use of chemical matrixectomy for the treatment of ingrown toenails, the overall success rates were 95% for both phenol and sodium hydroxide.[4] A 1-minute application of 10% sodium hydroxide was used and the details for the phenol application were not specified. The sodium hydroxide group had more pain in the first 2 days postoperatively, but all patients became pain free after that. The incidence and duration of drainage and peripheral tissue destruction was higher in the phenol group. The mean period for complete recovery was 11 days in the sodium hydroxide group and 18 days in the phenol group.[4]

In a Cochrane systematic review of surgical treatments for ingrown toenails, nail avulsion with the use

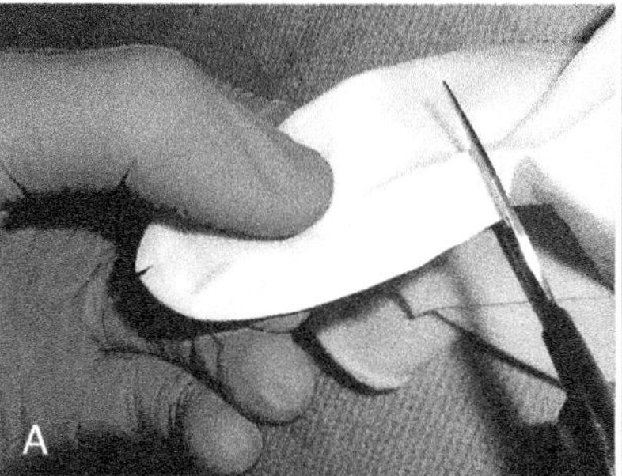

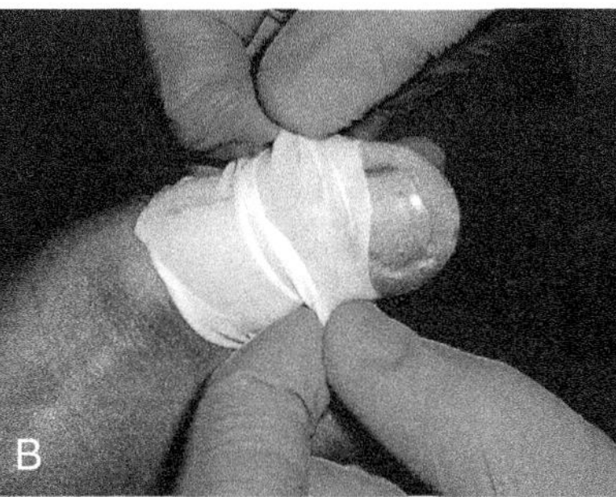

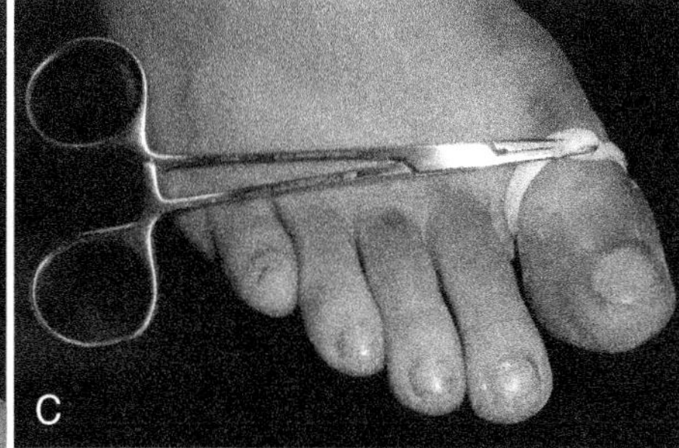

FIGURE 18-6 Creating a tourniquet from a latex glove. **(A)** Make a small snip at the end of one finger and then cut off the finger of that glove. **(B)** Roll the finger on to the digit allowing the digit to expand the small hole at the end of the "finger." This should fit snugly. **(C)** Grasp the glove material with a hemostat and turn it around to tighten the tourniquet. *(Copyright Richard P. Usatine, MD.)*

of phenol is more effective at preventing symptomatic recurrence than nail avulsion without the use of phenol.[5] Unfortunately, the use of phenol does increase the risk of postoperative infection (by 5 times) compared with simple nail avulsion.[5]

Phenol Application

Bleeding is stopped by applying a tourniquet for 3 to 4 minutes and phenol is vigorously rubbed into the matrix and grooves for 2 to 3 minutes (Figure 18-9). The matrix area must be bloodless before the phenol is applied or the phenol will not work as well. The application is best done with a cotton-tipped applicator (CTA) with a small cotton tip. During each 1-minute application the cotton tip should be rotated over the matrix. For each subsequent 1-minute application a new CTA should be chosen. Some authors suggest neutralizing the phenol after application with alcohol or saline, while others state that this is unnecessary as long as the phenol is wiped away from any normal tissue. Be very careful handling phenol because it is very caustic to normal tissues. This same method is used for the sodium hydroxide except only a single 1-minute application is needed.

One study found that partial nail avulsion with phenolization gave better results than partial avulsion with matrix excision.[6] Local antibiotics applied to the surgical site did not reduce signs of infection or recurrence. The use of phenol did not produce more signs of infection than matrix excision.[6]

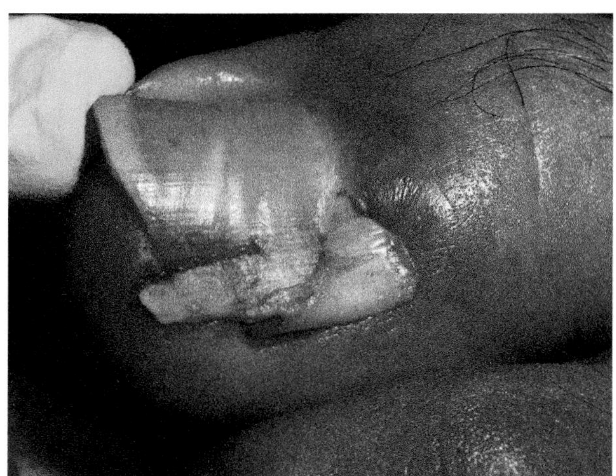

FIGURE 18-7 Partial nail plate excision to treat an ingrown toenail. *(Copyright Richard P. Usatine, MD.)*

One way to purchase phenol now is as Phenol EZ Swabs. These come in a package with phenol in a sealed ampule and dedicated swab sticks. It is more expensive per patient but does reduce the possibility of a phenol spill from an open bottle.

Physical Matrixectomy (Electrodestruction)

Another matrixectomy method involves the use of electrofulguration. This can be performed with a standard electrode or a special matrixectomy electrode that has a Teflon-coated top and a metallic bottom. The Teflon prevents damage to the upper nail fold. This matrixectomy electrode is produced by Ellman and is made to be used with their radio-frequency electrosurgical units (Figure 18-10). However, a standard electrosurgery disposable electrode can be used with a Hyfrecator or similar electrosurgical unit and the tip may be placed close to the matrix so that most of the electrical energy reaches the matrix but not the upper nail fold.

The best method for electrodestruction in this procedure is fulguration in which the electrical energy sparks to the matrix. The matrixectomy electrode should be used in the electrocoagulation setting (16 to 20 on hemo using the dual-frequency Surgitron). The electrode should be kept slightly above the matrix so that the spark of electricity can be seen and heard. Some authors recommend curetting the nail matrix before using electrosurgery (a 3-mm round skin curette can be used or a special nail curette).[3] Unfortunately, we were unable to find any published clinical studies on electrodestruction as a method of matrixectomy.

Wound Dressings

There are many ways to dress the remaining wound. Place a dab of petrolatum or antibiotic ointment on the site and cover it with gauze. A light pressure dressing may be applied, especially if there was a significant amount of bleeding (Figure 18-11).

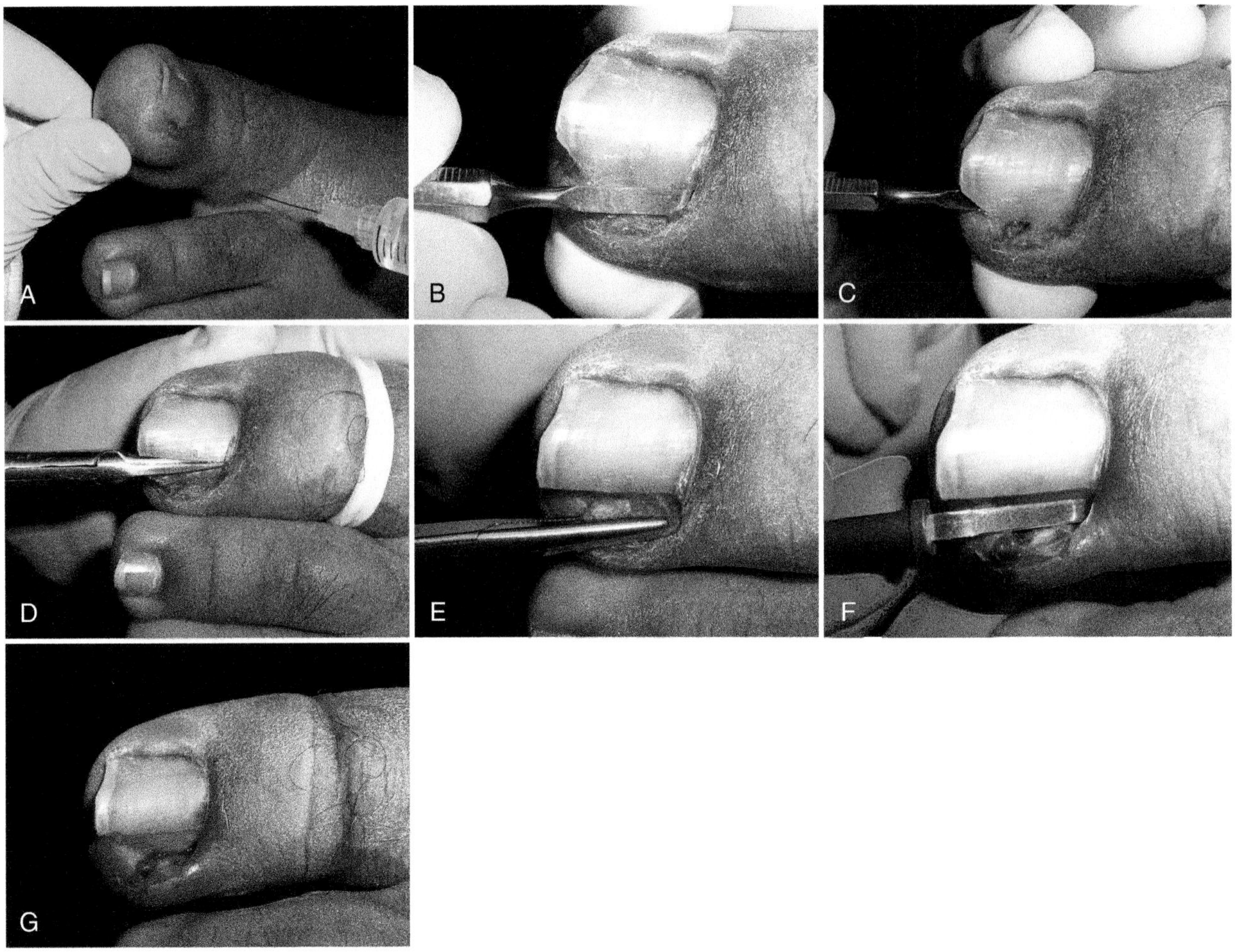

FIGURE 18-8 (A) Digital block. (B) Nail elevator used to free the nail fold from nail plate. (C) Nail elevator separating the nail plate from the nail bed. (D) Nail splitter cutting nail plate. (E) Hemostat twisting out nail segment to be removed. (F) Electrosurgery to destroy nail matrix. (G) Final result with tourniquet removed. *(Copyright Richard P. Usatine, MD.)*

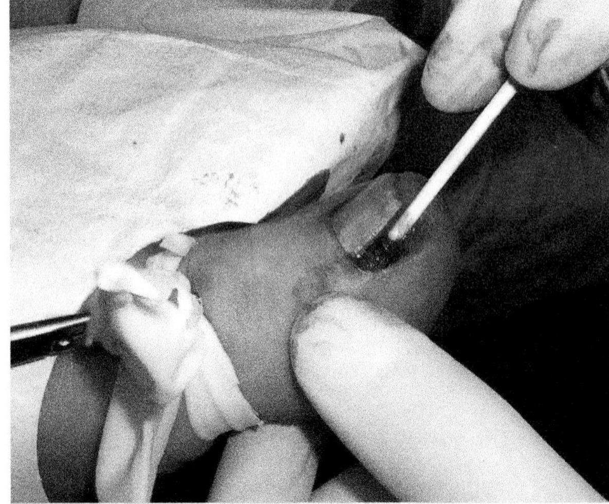

FIGURE 18-9 Applying phenol to a CTA destroys a portion of the nail matrix, which prevents a recurrent ingrown toenail. *(Copyright Richard P. Usatine, MD.)*

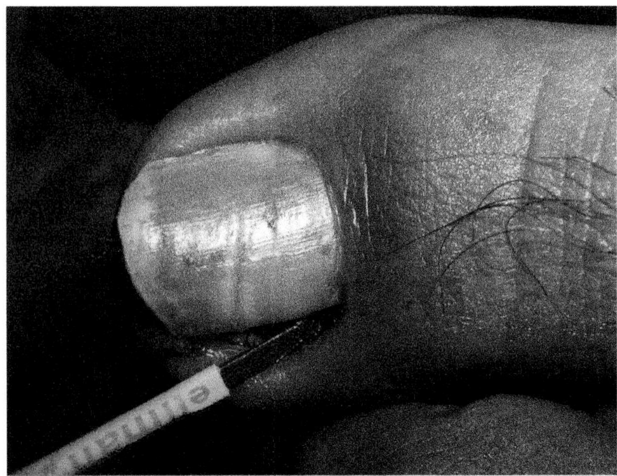

FIGURE 18-10 Performing a physical matrixectomy using a special electrode with a Teflon-coated top and a metallic bottom. The Teflon prevents damage to the upper nailfold, while the metal bottom conducts the radio-frequency to destroy the matrix in that region. *(Copyright Richard P. Usatine, MD.)*

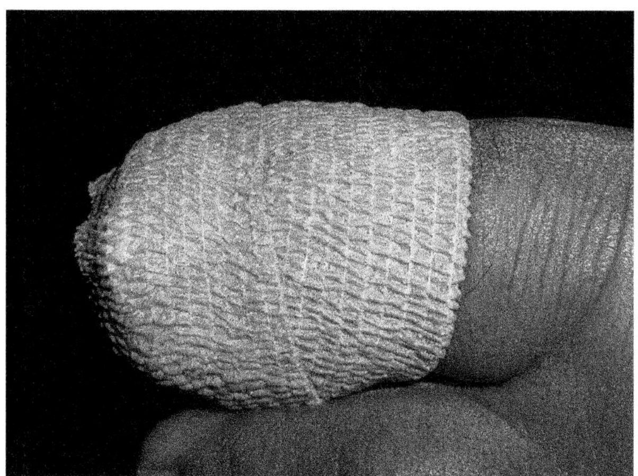

FIGURE 18-11 Light pressure dressing after partial avulsion of nail with ingrown toenail. *(Copyright Richard P. Usatine, MD.)*

FULL NAIL PLATE REMOVAL (NAIL AVULSION)

Patients with severely hyperkeratotic nails that cannot be easily clipped may request a full nail plate removal. While a warm bath or the application of 40% urea may make it easier to clip such nails, some patients will want them removed completely. The nail matrix should be permanently destroyed if the patient does not want the nail to regrow. This may be performed with phenol or electrodestruction.

Procedure Steps

Distal Nail Avulsion

1. The procedure is performed in an identical manner to the partial nail removal except that the full nail is excised (Figure 18-12).
2. Use a nail elevator to free the nail plate from the surrounding proximal nail fold.
3. Clamp a hemostat on the central portion of the nail plate and twist and pull until the nail plate dislodges from the nail unit.
4. Another option is to clamp a hemostat on the edge of the nail and curl the nail plate off the nail bed.
5. Use chemical and/or electrocoagulation to stop any significant bleeding.
6. Matrix destruction should only be formed when the goal is to prevent the nail from growing back. Phenol, sodium hydroxide, or electrodestruction are the preferred methods.

Proximal Nail Evulsion

Some experts claim that proximal nail evulsion causes less trauma to the nail bed than a distal nail avulsion.[3] The proximal nail avulsion is especially helpful when thick subungual hyperkeratosis is present or when the distal groove has disappeared.[3]

1. Separate the proximal nail fold from the nail plate using the nail elevator (Figure 18-13A).

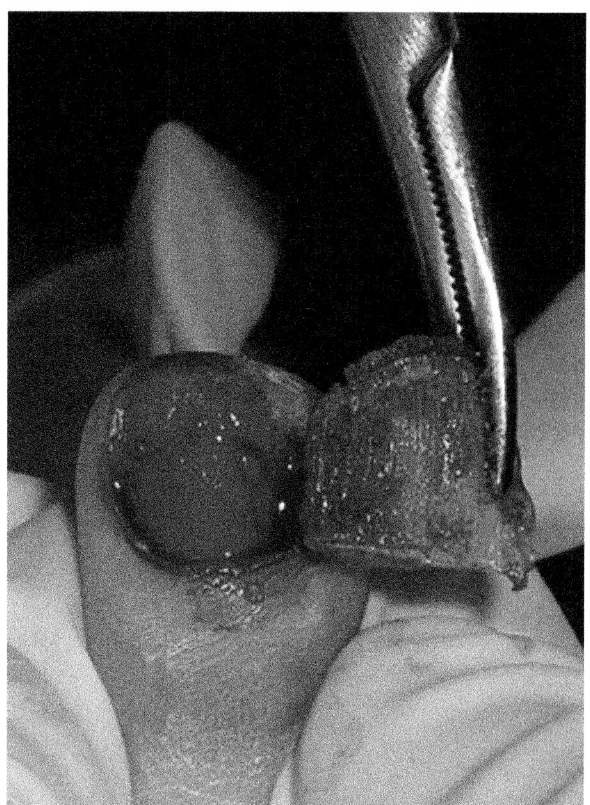

FIGURE 18-12 A painful dysmorphic nail is being avulsed using the distal approach and the lateral curl technique. Note the ridges on the underside of the nail plate that normally keep the nail plate attached to the nail bed. *(Copyright Richard P. Usatine, MD.)*

2. While leaving the tip in the end of the nail pocket, the nail elevator is turned about 160 degrees and inserted under the proximal edge of the nail plate and pushed distally to separate the nail from the matrix and nail bed with back-and-forth motions (Figure 18-13B).

BIOPSIES TO DIAGNOSE PIGMENTED NAIL CHANGES

Hyperpigmentation of the nail plate has many benign causes such as racial (ethnic) melanonychia and melanocytic hyperplasia (Figure 18-14A). However, it is crucial for clinicians not to miss a case of nail melanoma (acral lentiginous melanoma) (Figures 18-14B and C). Squamous cell carcinomas and glomus tumors are other neoplasms that may also involve the nail unit. Longitudinal melanonychia is a pigmented band that occurs in the nail plate from the proximal to the distal aspect. Racial melanonychia is the most common cause of longitudinal melanonychia. Other common benign causes are benign melanocytic hyperplasia, nevi, trauma, fungal, and medications.

We next describe four biopsy techniques to be used to diagnose nail melanoma and other malignancies that can occur in the nail unit. The easiest biopsy to perform is a 3-mm punch biopsy of the nail matrix at the origin of the pigmented band. Occasionally a shave biopsy is

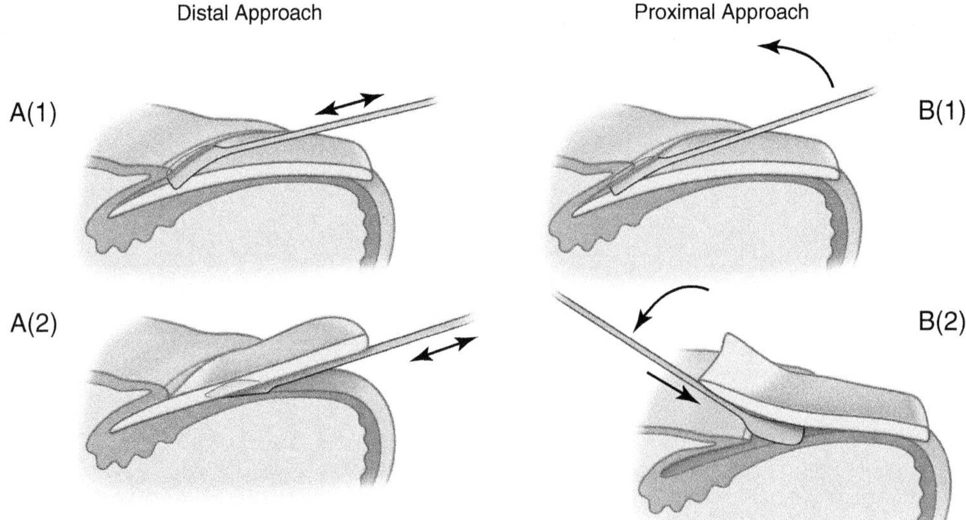

FIGURE 18-13 Comparison of the distal and proximal approaches to complete nail avulsion. **(A1)** Nail elevator used to free the proximal nail fold from nail plate. **(A2)** Nail elevator inserted distally to separate the nail plate from the nail bed. **(B1)** Nail elevator used to free the proximal nail fold from nail plate and then rotated upward. **(B2)** Nail elevator has slipped under the proximal nail plate and is lifting it from the nail bed. *(Adapted from Robinson J, Hanke CW, Siegel D, Fratila A.* Surgery of the Skin. *London: Mosby; 2010, Figure 46-4.)*

preferred if the pigmented band is wide. When the pigment is in the lateral nail and nail fold, a lateral longitudinal excision may be needed.[7]

Box 18-1 summarizes when longitudinal melanonychia should be biopsied. Hutchinson's sign is the extension of pigmentation to the skin adjacent to the nail plate involving the nail folds or the tip of the digit. This is an important indicator for nail melanoma and warrants a biopsy. In one study, dermoscopic features of nail melanoma were significantly associated with a brown coloration of the background and the presence of irregular longitudinal lines (in their color, spacing, thickness, and parallelism).[8] Box 18-2 gives the details of the ABCDEF mnemonic system for detecting nail melanoma.[9]

Before starting a biopsy it is helpful to know if the nail plate pigment is coming from the proximal or distal matrix. The proximal matrix generates pigment on top of the nail plate, whereas the distal matrix generates pigment on the bottom or ventral portion of the nail plate. Look at the edge of the nail with a good source of light and magnification before starting a biopsy. The use of a dermatoscope with clear gel applied directly to the edge of the nail is an excellent method for determining the location of the pigment and the origin of the pigment band (Figure 18-15).

Punch Biopsy of the Nail Matrix

A 3-mm punch biopsy of the nail matrix is done at the origin of the pigmented band.

Procedure Steps

1. Perform a digital block (lidocaine without epinephrine) first so that the wing block is not painful (Figure 18-4A).

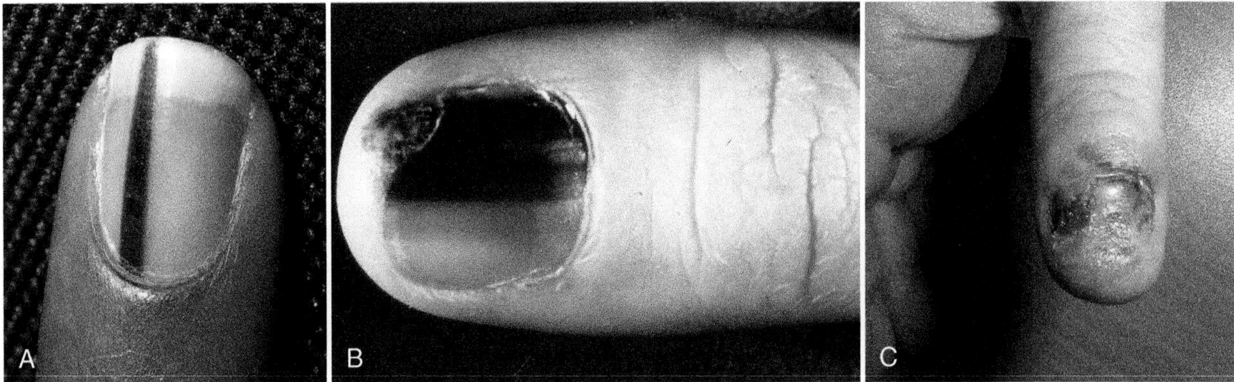

FIGURE 18-14 Nail tumors that call for biopsies. **(A)** New longitudinal melanonychia that was shown to be a benign nevus with biopsy. **(B)** A wide band of longitudinal melanonychia caused by a subungual melanoma. **(C)** Acral lentiginous melanoma showing nail destruction and a positive Hutchinson sign *(A: Copyright Richard P. Usatine, MD; B: Courtesy of the Skin Cancer Foundation, New York, NY; C: Courtesy of Dr. Dubin, www.skinatlas.com.)*

BOX 18-1 *Longitudinal Melanonychia*

Longitudinal melanonychia should be biopsied if:
- The pigment is >6 mm wide.
- It is the only nail with a dark and significant color variation.
- It is associated with nail dystrophy or deformity.
- There is a positive Hutchinson's sign.

2. Perform a wing block (lidocaine with epinephrine) to obtain good anesthesia and hemostasis (Figure 18-4C).
3. Place a tourniquet on the involved digit (Figure 18-5).
4. If there is pigment on the proximal nail fold (Hutchinson's sign), perform a shave biopsy of this area.
5. Use a nail elevator to separate the proximal nail fold from the nail plate (Figure 18-16A).
6. Use a No. 15 scalpel to cut incisions at the junction of the proximal and lateral nail folds bilaterally. Consider using the nail elevator to protect the tissues below the nail fold while cutting with the scalpel (Figure 18-16B). This can be bloody, so be prepared to hold pressure before proceeding to reflect the nail fold. The nail elevator can help further separate the proximal nail fold from the nail plate once the cuts have been made.
7. Reflect nail fold back using skin hooks to see the entire matrix (Figure 18-16C). An alternative method is to place nylon sutures on each side of the nail fold and pull the fold back using the nylon to grasp the edges.
8. Use a good light source and/or a dermatoscope (not touching surface) to look for the origin of the pigmented band.
9. Biopsy the origin of the pigmented band with a 3-mm punch through the nail plate and down to the bone (Figure 18-16D). Fewer nail deformities will result if the biopsy is in the distal matrix, but if the proximal matrix is the origin of the pigment the biopsy must be at that site.[7]
10. The friable matrix tissue may end up in the end of the biopsy instrument (Figure 18-16E). Using a VisiPunch (punch instrument with window) makes it easier to see any adherent tissue and remove the tissue without damaging it for the pathologist. If tissue remains in the punch site, use a fine-tipped scissor and snip around the specimen vertically and circumferentially for 360 degrees (Figure 18-16F).[7] Use fine-tipped scissors to gently lift the specimen and cut it off at the base if needed. If this can be performed without forceps, the tissue will have less crush artifact for the pathologist. Send the small circular nail plate specimen along with the matrix tissue for analysis because it may contain blood, melanocytic pigmentation, or even fungi.
11. Return the proximal nail fold to its original location and reapproximate the incision edges. This may be performed with 5-0 nylon or polypropylene (Prolene), Steri-Strips, or the application of a pressure dressing (Figure 18-16G).
12. *Optional:* Consider injecting 0.5 mL of Marcaine in the wing block area for extended pain relief. Either way, advise the patient on the use of pain medications as needed. Consider prescribing a pain medication for the first few days.
13. Apply petrolatum or antibiotic ointment and a pressure dressing (not too tight).
    Remove sutures in 7 to 9 days.

BOX 18-2 *ABCDEF Mnemonic System for Detecting Nail Melanoma*

The ABCDEF mnemonic system[9] was developed to detect nail melanoma. Use this system to determine the need for a nail biopsy.

A stands for age (peak incidence being between the 5th to 7th decades), and African Americans, Asians, and Native Americans in whom acral lentiginous melanoma accounts for one-third of melanoma cases.
B stands for "brown to black" and with "breadth" of 3 mm or more.
C stands for change in the nail band coloration or lack of change after adequate treatment.
D stands for the digit most commonly involved (thumb or big toe)
E stands for extension of the pigment onto the proximal and/or lateral nailfold (Hutchinson's sign)
F stands for family or personal history of dysplastic nevus or melanoma.

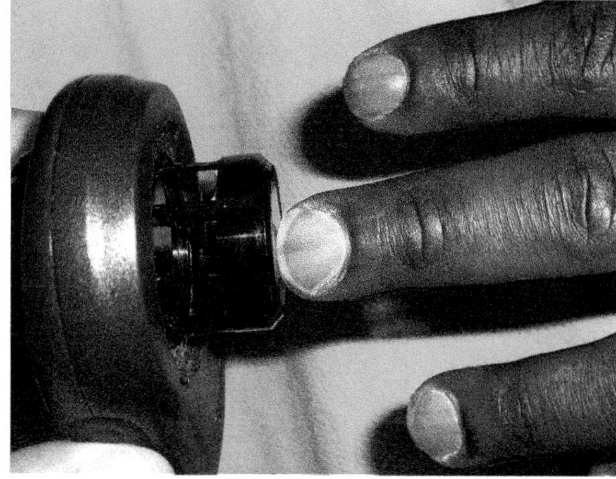

FIGURE 18-15 Dermoscopy on the edge of the nail plate with longitudinal melanonychia to determine whether the pigment is being produced in the proximal or distal nail matrix. *(Copyright Richard P. Usatine, MD.)*

Shave Biopsy of the Nail Matrix

The shave biopsy of the nail matrix[7] provides adequate samples of wider bands and is less invasive than a transversely oriented matrix excision. The reflected proximal nail plate readheres to the nail bed postoperatively and grows out with the nail unit. Despite wide matrix biopsies, long-term dystrophy is minimal.[7]

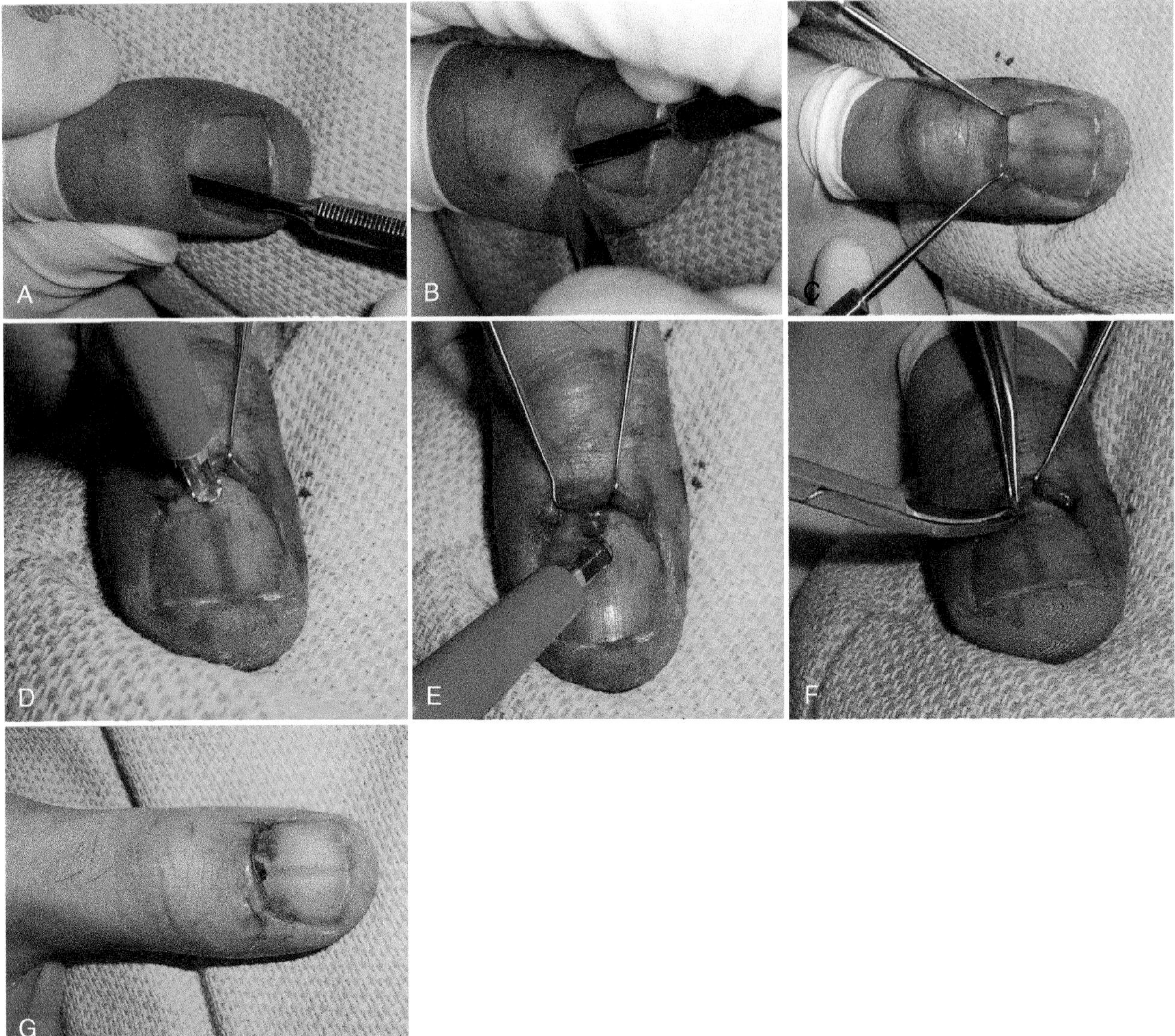

FIGURE 18-16 Punch biopsy of the nail matrix. **(A)** Nail elevator is separating the proximal nail fold from the nail plate. **(B)** No. 15 scalpel cutting incisions at the junction of the proximal and lateral nail folds bilaterally. Nail elevator used to protect the tissues below the nail fold. **(C)** Nail fold reflected back using skin hooks to see the matrix. **(D)** A 3-mm punch placed over the origin of the pigmented band. **(E)** The cut is through the nail plate and down to the bone. Friable matrix tissue is seen in the end of the biopsy instrument. The VisiPunch makes it easier to see and remove any adherent tissue. **(F)** In case any tissue remains in the punch site, fine-tipped scissors are used to gently lift the specimen and cut it off at the base. **(G)** The first incision edge has been approximated with 5-0 polypropylene. *(Copyright Richard P. Usatine, MD.)*

The shave biopsy is not recommended for tumors that grossly involve the nail unit, those associated with nail plate destruction, those with extensive pigmentation of the proximal or lateral nail folds, or those that in any way have a high preoperative likelihood of invasive melanoma.[7] A shave biopsy may not provide accurate depth for deeply invasive melanomas. In this case, a full-thickness elliptical nail matrix biopsy is most helpful.

Procedure Steps

1. Perform anesthesia using the same approach as for the punch biopsy of the matrix.
2. Follow steps 3 through 6 above to reflect the proximal nail fold.
3. Proximal nail plate evulsion is performed using a nail splitter delicately inserted transversely in one nail sulcus at the level of the proximal third of the nail plate. It is advanced under the plate transversely until the full width of the nail plate is cut. The proximal plate is then reflected laterally and secured with a hemostat. This is like opening the hood of a car in that the proximal nail plate is not actually fully removed from its anatomic position.[7]
4. The matrix is examined to identify the origin of the melanonychia using good light and a dermatoscope (not touching the tissue) if available. Ask your surgical assistant to confirm the origin of the melanonychia and document that in the chart.

5. A shave biopsy is performed of the origin with 1- to 2-mm margins. This can be performed with a razor blade or scalpel blade. If a No. 15 scalpel blade is used, score the margins first then turn the blade horizontally, parallel to the matrix surface, to shave the scored specimen (Figure 18-17). The specimen may only be 1 mm in thickness but should still provide adequate sampling of the matrix epithelium and a significant portion of dermis.[7]
6. To improve processing and sectioning, it may help to place the specimen on a piece of paper or cardboard before placing it into the formalin.[7] This will keep the specimen flat rather than allowing it to roll and curl.
7. Trim the reflected nail plate at its lateral free edge by 2 to 3 mm and return it to its original position. Trimming the lateral plate will reduce lateral embedding and pain with postoperative edema.[7]
8. The proximal nail fold is returned to its anatomic position and sutured in place using one interrupted suture on each side. Use 5-0 nylon or polypropylene (Prolene) suture.
9. Apply petrolatum or antibiotic ointment and a pressure dressing (not too tight).
10. Remove sutures in 7 to 10 days and apply adhesive wound closures (Steri-Strips) to keep the integrity of the wound for another week.

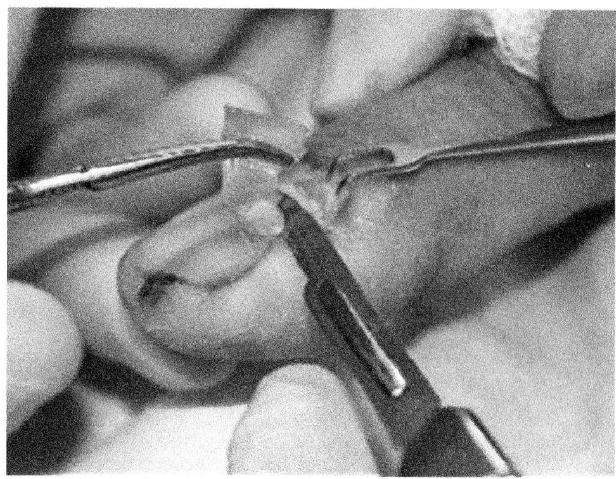

FIGURE 18-17 Shave biopsy of the nail matrix. No. 15 scalpel blade glides parallel to the epithelium after scoring 1- to 2-mm margins around origin of pigmented band. *(From Jellinek N. Nail matrix biopsy of longitudinal melanonychia: diagnostic algorithm including the matrix shave biopsy.* J Am Acad Dermatol. *2007;56:803–810.)*

Full-Thickness Nail Matrix Biopsy

A full-thickness nail matrix biopsy procedure (Figure 18-18) is performed just as the shave biopsy above except that the tissue is excised using a small elliptical

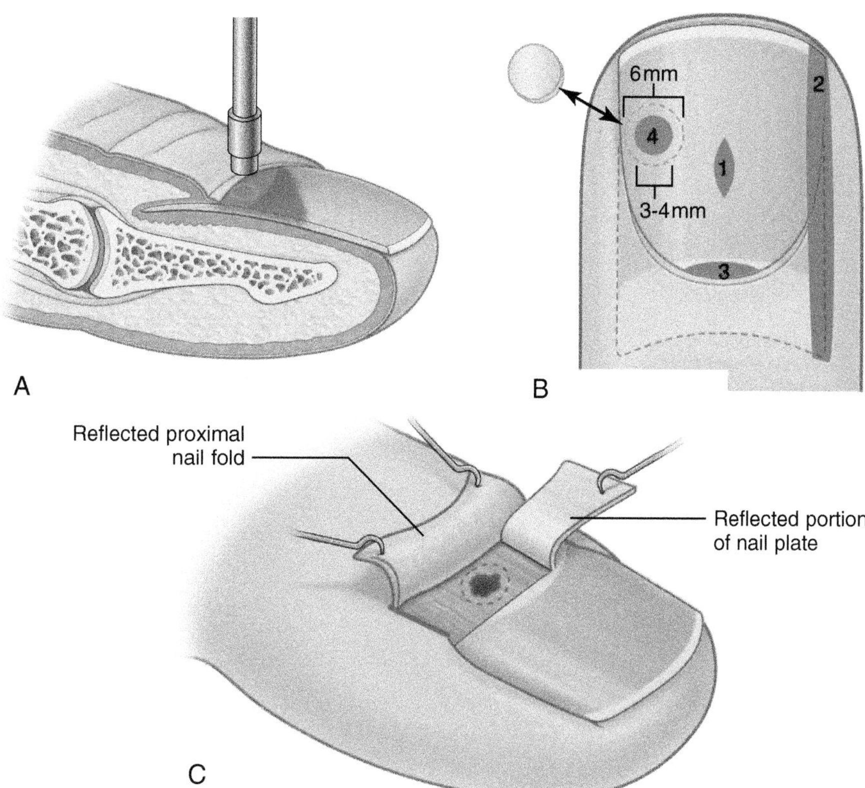

FIGURE 18-18 Types of nail biopsies. **(A)** Punch biopsy of the nail plate. **(B)** Nail bed biopsies: (1) Fusiform nail bed biopsy. (2) Lateral longitudinal biopsy of nail bed. (3) Matrix biopsy. (4) Punch biopsy of nail bed through nail plate using a 6 mm punch to remove nail plate and then a 3 to 4 mm punch for the underlying nail bed. Some surgeons choose to replace the nail disk at the end of the operation. **(C)** Matrix biopsy with the proximal nail fold reflected. *(Adapted from Robinson J, Hanke CW, Siegel D, Fratila A.* Surgery of the Skin. *London: Mosby; 2010, Figure 46-3.)*

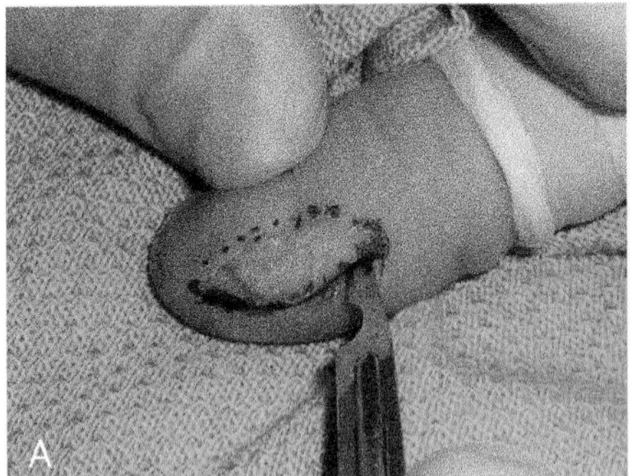

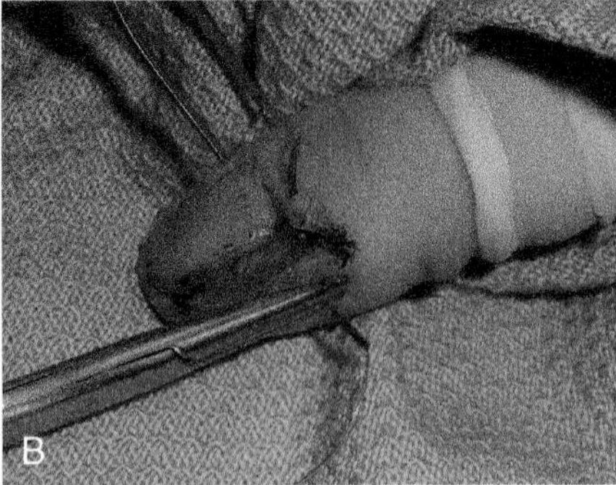

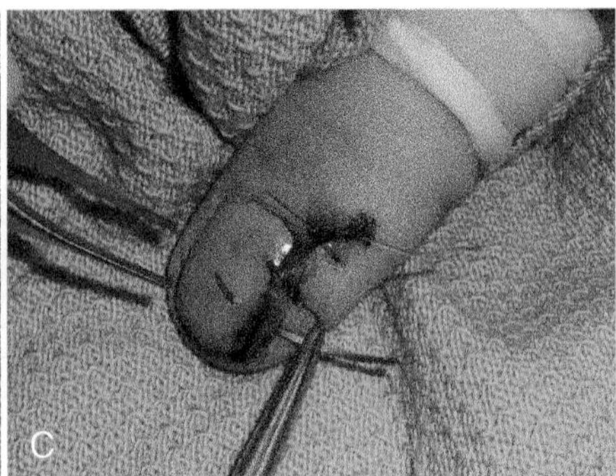

FIGURE 18-19 Lateral longitudinal excision of a nail fold tumor. **(A)** An ellipse is cut around the tumor including a portion of the nail plate. The ellipse is cut down to the bone. **(B)** Suturing is performed with 4-0 Prolene on a large plastics needle. Note the depth of the incision. **(C)** The needle can be passed through the nail as it is sharp and sturdy. *(Copyright Richard P. Usatine, MD.)*

excision. This elliptical defect is closed with 5-0 absorbable sutures and the repair is the same as described for the shave biopsy above.

Lateral Longitudinal Excision

A lateral longitudinal excision[7] (Figure 18-19) is a more technically difficult procedure and is used when there is a lateral pigment band or tumor on the edge of the nail unit. This is also a good procedure for the treatment of SCC *in situ* of the lateral nail fold.

Procedure Steps

1. Perform anesthesia using the same approach as for the punch biopsy of the matrix.
2. Soak the finger in chlorhexidine in water for 10 to 15 minutes to soften the nail plate.
3. Perform an elliptical excision with narrow margins around the tumor. Use a No. 15C scalpel and include the lateral matrix horn. Extend the incision 3 mm distally onto the digital tip. Cut down to the level of bone (Figure 18-19A).
4. Use fine-tipped scissors or the scalpel to remove the tissue to the level of the periosteum. The tissue may be stabilized with a skin hook or held gently with forceps to avoid crush injuries. Use the scissors in a "tips down" position while cutting out this wedge.
5. Excision must remove the entire lateral matrix horn because small matrix remnants can cause postoperative cysts, spicules, and/or pain.[7] A small curette may be used to remove any residual matrix fragments. This is optional because it may increase the risk of periostitis and postoperative pain while decreasing the risk of spicules or cysts.[7]
6. Repair the tissue with interrupted 4-0 nylon or polypropylene (Prolene) using a large (e.g., 19 mm) plastics needle to be able to pierce the nail (Figures 18-19B and C).
7. Apply petrolatum or antibiotic ointment and a pressure dressing (not too tight).
8. Remove sutures in 10 to 14 days.[7]
9. If this is a biopsy of melanonychia, request the pathologist cut the tissue longitudinally and not in the traditional "bread loaf" manner.[7]

Subungual Hematoma Evacuation

Subungual hematomas form when a nail is subjected to significant trauma. The pressure of the hematoma can be exquisitely painful and the patient's pain can be relieved by draining the hematoma through the intact nail. Depending on the mechanism of trauma and the physical exam, an x-ray of the distal digit may be indicated to investigate for fractures.

Procedure Steps

1. This procedure can be performed without local anesthesia or a tourniquet.
2. The nail plate can be pierced in any number of ways, including using a No. 11 scalpel, an 18-gauge needle, a 2-mm punch, a portable hot wire cautery device, or a hot paper clip.
3. The simplest and least expensive method involves heating a paper clip and melting through the nail plate. The paper clip is unbent and can be held in a hemostat. The end of the paper clip is heated with a lighter or other flame (Figure 18-20A).
4. Hold the paper clip against the nail and apply some pressure until the paper clip pierces the nail plate and blood runs out (Figures 18-20A and B). The patient should only feel pressure and not direct pain.
5. Any remaining blood can be expressed out of the nail opening to decrease the pain of the hematoma.

TREATING OTHER TYPES OF LESIONS

Pincer nails occur when the lateral nail plates dig into the soft tissue of the digits (Figure 18-21). This can eventually lead to pain and discomfort. Partial nail plate excisions bilaterally with destruction of the lateral matrix horn will often give patients relief from this condition (Figure 18-22). In more severe cases, exophytes and dorsal hyperostosis of the distal phalanx may need to be imaged and treated surgically.[10]

Onychogryphosis occurs when a nail plate becomes thickened and curved like a ram's horn (Figure 18-23). While a warm bath or the application of 40% urea

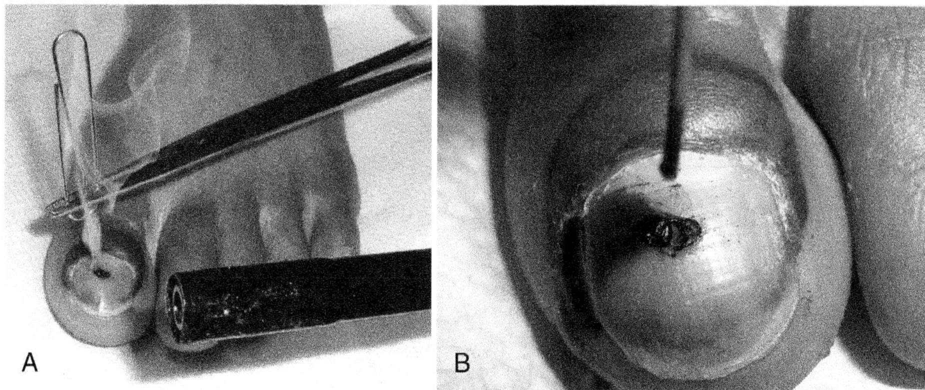

FIGURE 18-20 Subungual hematoma evacuation. **(A)** A paperclip was held in a hemostat and heated to pierce the patient's nail plate. With minimal pressure the hot point melted through the nail plate. **(B)** The hot paperclip formed a painless hole in the nail plate and the blood drained out spontaneously. This relieved the pressure and gave the patient immediate pain relief. *(Copyright Richard P. Usatine, MD.)*

cream may make it easier to clip this nail, some patients will want it removed completely. For this condition the proximal nail evulsion procedure is best, and the nail matrix should be permanently destroyed if the patient does not want the nail to regrow. This may be performed using phenol or electrodestruction.

COMPLICATIONS

The most common complications of nail surgery are pain that may be prolonged, infections and permanent nail deformities. In particular, nail matrix biopsy may result in a split nail deformity. Patients should be informed of the risk of permanent nail deformity prior to surgery. Other less common complications include pyogenic granuloma at the surgery site or persistent pain.[11]

AFTERCARE

To prevent some of the pain and throbbing that can occur after any nail surgery, explain to patients to keep their hand or foot elevated once anesthesia wears off or periodically raise the limb during the day. Oral pain medications may be needed.

If the patient is having trouble with footwear, the diabetic foot shoes with Velcro on top are a good choice while the toe is healing.

After 24 to 48 hours of keeping the digit dry, the patient should begin soaking the digit in warm, soapy water three times a day. Then have the patient apply clean petrolatum or an antibiotic ointment and a clean bandage. This should be continued for 1 to 2 weeks after surgery.

Some amount of pain, redness, and drainage is normal. However, if these signs and symptoms worsen over time, this may be an infection requiring oral antibiotics.

CODING AND BILLING PEARLS

The CPT codes shown in Box 18-3 are used when billing for nail procedures. When treating an ingrown toenail, the partial removal of the nail plate is coded using CPT

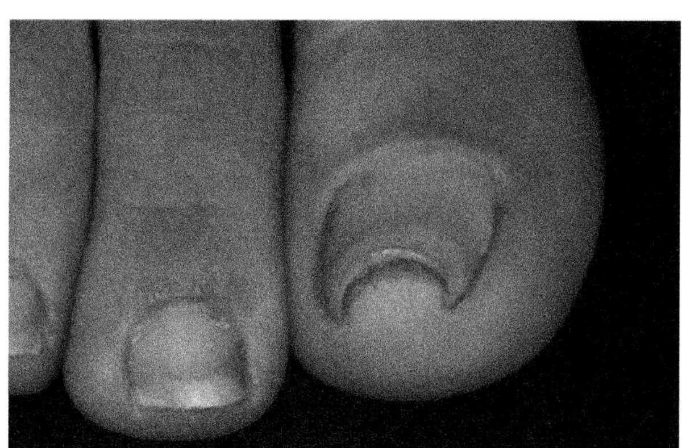

FIGURE 18-21 Pincer nail. This older man wanted surgery to decrease the pain of this condition. *(Copyright Richard P. Usatine, MD.)*

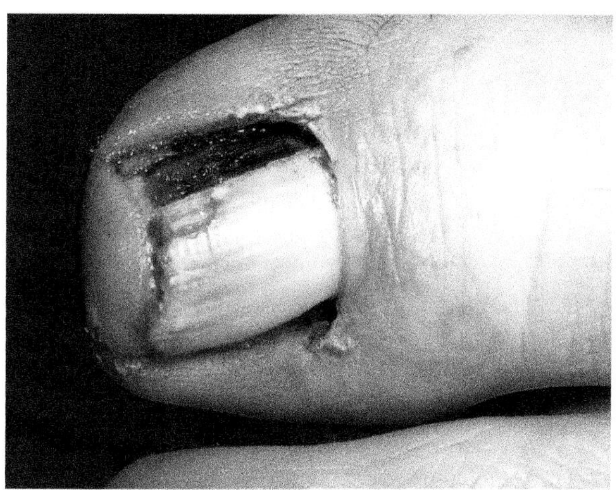

FIGURE 18-22 One simple method to treat a pincer nail involves partial nail plate removals on both sides along with matrixectomy to prevent regrowth. *(Copyright Richard P. Usatine, MD.)*

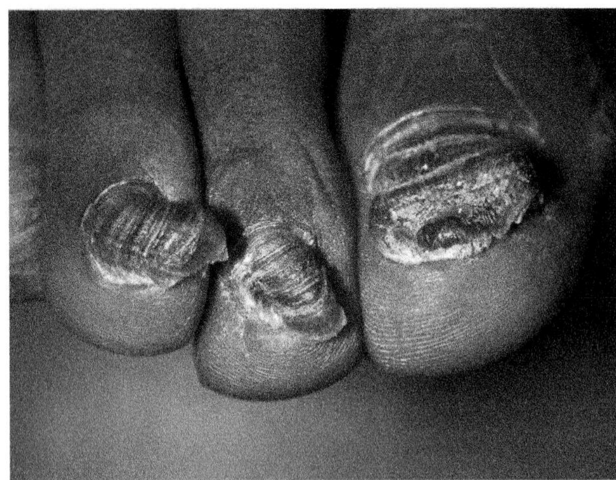

FIGURE 18-23 Ram's horn nails in an older man. Also known as onychogryphosis. Some patients choose to have a complete nail evulsion with destruction of the matrix to prevent regrowth. *(Copyright Richard P. Usatine, MD.)*

11730. If a partial matrixectomy (chemical or physical) is performed as well, a CPT code of 11750 is added. This is not only good medical practice for recurring ingrown toenails but also results in greater compensation.

Debridement of a nail is a procedure that is intended to remove excessive material (e.g., to significantly reduce nail thickness/bulk) or excessive curvature from a clinically and significantly thickened dystrophic or diseased nail. Although podiatrists may be more likely to do this procedure, the code is independent of the clinician performing the procedure.

BOX 18-3 *CPT Codes for Nail Procedures*

11719 Trimming of nondystrophic nails, any number
11720 Debridement of nail(s) by any method(s); 1 to 5 nails
11721 Debridement of nail(s) by any method(s); 6 or more nails
11730 Removal (avulsion) of one nail plate, partial or complete, simple; single nail
11732 Removal (avulsion) of additional nail plates, partial or complete, simple
11755 Biopsy of nail unit (e.g., plate, bed, matrix, hyponychium, proximal, and lateral nail folds)
11750 Removal of nail bed or nail matrix, partial or complete (e.g., ingrown or deformed nail), for permanent removal.
11760 Repair of nail bed
11765 Wedge excision of skin of nail fold (e.g., for ingrown toenail)
11740 Subungual hematoma drainage

CONCLUSION

Many types of nail problems require surgical intervention. We have covered the most common nail problems in this chapter. With good anesthetic techniques, surgery of the nail may be performed in the office setting.

Resources

Phenol can be purchased at Delasco (www.delasco.com/pcat/1/Chemicals/Phenol_(Carbolic_Acid)/dlmip022). *Note:* 1-oz bottles (up to 24) are no longer hazardous by air under the limited quantity exemption. All bottle sizes larger than 1 oz are still subject to hazardous materials regulations and fees.

Phenol EZ Swab packets can be purchased through Moore Medical (www1.mooremedical.com/index.cfm?PG=CTL&FN=ProductDetail&PID=4971).

Sodium hydroxide, 10% solution for medical use, can be purchased at eGeneralMedical (www.egeneralmedical.com/mme-43360.html).

References

1. Darouiche RO, Wall MJ Jr, Itani KM, *et al.* Chlorhexidine-alcohol versus povidone-iodine for surgical-site antisepsis. *N Engl J Med.* 2010;362:18–26.
2. Flatt AE. Tourniquet time in hand surgery. *AMA Arch Surg.* 1972;104:190–192.
3. Robinson J, Hanke C, Siegel D, Fratila A. *Surgery of the Skin—Procedural Dermatology.* 2nd ed. Philadelphia: Mosby/Elsevier; 2010.
4. Bostanci S, Kocyigit P, Gurgey E. Comparison of phenol and sodium hydroxide chemical matricectomies for the treatment of ingrowing toenails. *Dermatol Surg.* 2007;33:680–685.
5. Rounding C, Bloomfield S. Surgical treatments for ingrowing toenails. *Cochrane Database Syst Rev.* 2005; CD001541.
6. Bos AM, van Tilburg MW, van Sorge AA, Klinkenbijl JH. Randomized clinical trial of surgical technique and local antibiotics for ingrowing toenail. *Br J Surg.* 2007;94:292–296.
7. Jellinek N. Nail matrix biopsy of longitudinal melanonychia: diagnostic algorithm including the matrix shave biopsy. *J Am Acad Dermatol.* 2007;56:803–810.
8. Ronger S, Touzet S, Ligeron C, *et al.* Dermoscopic examination of nail pigmentation. *Arch Dermatol.* 2002;138:1327–1333.
9. Levit EK, Kagen MH, Scher RK, *et al.* The ABC rule for clinical detection of subungual melanoma. *J Am Acad Dermatol.* 2000; 42:269–274.
10. Baran R, Haneke E, Richert B. Pincer nails: definition and surgical treatment. *Dermatol Surg.* 2001;27:261–266.
11. Moossavi M, Scher RK. Complications of nail surgery: a review of the literature. *Dermatol Surg.* 2001;27:225–228.

Additional Reading

Haneke E, Lawry M. Nail surgery. *In:* Robinson J, Henke C, Sengelman R, Siegel D, eds. *Surgery of the Skin—Procedural Dermatology.* Philadelphia: Mosby/Elsevier; 2005.

SECTION THREE

Cosmetic Procedures

19 Aesthetic Principles and Consultation

REBECCA SMALL, MD

Minimally invasive aesthetic procedures have become the treatments of choice for rejuvenation of aging skin and facial enhancement.[1] Since approval of botulinum toxin, dermal fillers, and lasers by the Food and Drug Administration (FDA) for cosmetic use, there has been a shift away from more traditional invasive surgical procedures that may radically alter appearance toward procedures that can enhance appearance in more natural and subtle ways. According to statistics from the American Society for Aesthetic Plastic Surgery, over 10 million aesthetic procedures are performed in the United States and more than 80% are minimally invasive.[2] The most commonly performed procedures include onabotulinumtoxinA (Botox; formerly known as botulinum toxin type A) and dermal filler injections for treatment of wrinkles; lasers and intense pulsed light technologies for hair reduction, skin resurfacing, and photorejuvenation; and chemical peels and microdermabrasion for exfoliation.

These aesthetic procedures are associated with high patient and provider satisfaction because they are efficacious, have low risks of side effects, involve minimal patient discomfort with short recovery times, and can be safely performed in the office setting.[3,4] As the popularity and demand for minimally invasive aesthetic procedures continues to grow, more health care providers are choosing to incorporate these types of treatments into their practice. This introduction to the aesthetic section of the book presents basic aesthetic principles for providers who wish to get started with aesthetic medicine. The succeeding chapters demonstrate the most commonly performed aesthetic procedures that can be readily incorporated into office practice.

FACIAL AGING

Facial aging is associated with a gradual thinning of the skin and loss of elasticity over time accompanied by the diminishment of dermal collagen, hyaluronic acid, and elastin. Ultraviolet (UV) radiation from sun exposure accelerates this process at a higher rate than does chronologic aging. This UV aging process is termed *photoaging*. To appreciate the contribution of photoaging to the appearance of aged skin, one needs only compare photoprotected skin, such as skin on the inside of the upper forearm or under the chin, to the appearance and texture of skin on face and back of the hands. Photoaged skin typically exhibits the following changes (Figure 19-1 for a computer-enhanced image demonstrating these signs)[5]:

- Textural changes
  - Wrinkles (also called rhytids)
  - Dry and rough skin
- Dyschromia
  - Solar lentigines
  - Mottled pigmentation
  - Postinflammatory hyperpigmentation
- Vascular ectasias
  - Telangiectasias
  - Rosacea
  - Erythema
- Degenerative changes
  - Benign
  - Preneoplastic and neoplastic.

In a study by New York plastic surgeon Dr. D. Antell on aging in identical twins, extrinsic factors, such as prolonged sun exposure, resulted in advanced aging changes (Figure 19-2A) relative to the intrinsic aging seen in non–sun-exposed twins (Figure 19-2B).[6] Habitual facial expressions also contribute to formation of visible lines and wrinkles, particularly in the upper one-third of the face, because repetitive muscle contractions etch in frown lines between eyebrows and crow's feet radiating from the corner of the eyes. In addition to skin laxity, volume loss, and dynamic musculature, facial aging also results from biometric facial changes such as descent of malar fat pads, which contributes to deepened nasolabial folds, and resorption of maxillary and mandibular bone, which contributes to radial lip lines and mental crease formation.[7,8]

SKIN ANATOMY

The skin is divided into three layers: the epidermis, dermis, and hypodermis or subcutaneous layer (Figure 19-3). The *epidermis* is the top layer of the skin and is composed of four cell types: keratinocytes, melanocytes, Langerhans cells, and Merkel cells. The epidermis is further divided into the outermost nonliving layer, the stratum corneum, and the living cellular layers of the stratum granulosum, stratum spinosum, and stratum basale.

The stratum corneum is composed of corneocytes and lipids, which serves as a barrier against microbial pathogens and environmental irritants and also keeps the skin hydrated and protected from injury. Constant renewal is necessary for the epidermis to maintain its integrity and function effectively. In healthy young skin, it takes approximately 1 month for keratinocytes to migrate from the living basal layer of the epidermis to the stratum corneum surface and desquamate, during the process of epidermal renewal. Figure 19-4 shows the structure of the epidermis with the keratinocyte maturation highlighted. Photoaged skin demonstrates

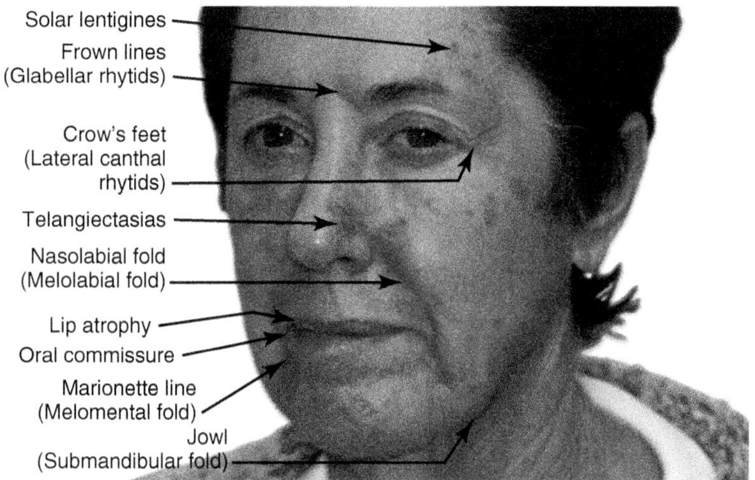

FIGURE 19-1 Photoaging changes (computer-enhanced image). *(Copyright Rebecca Small, MD.)*

slower keratinocyte maturation and abnormal retention of cells in the epidermis. This results in a rough and thickened stratum corneum with impaired barrier function, reduced hydration capabilities, and increased pigmentation from retention of melanin-laden keratinocytes in the epidermis.

The distribution of melanin within the epidermis determines skin coloration. While the number of melanocytes is similar for both light and dark skin types, melanin is concentrated in small aggregated melanosomes in light skin and is more disbursed in darker skin.[9]

The *dermis* lies beneath the epidermis and is divided into the more superficial papillary dermis and deeper reticular dermis. The main cell type in the dermis is the fibroblast, which is more abundant in the papillary dermis and sparse in the reticular dermis. Below the dermis and above the underlying muscle is the *subcutaneous layer,* also called the hypodermis, subcutis or superficial fascia. This layer has both fatty and fibrous components.

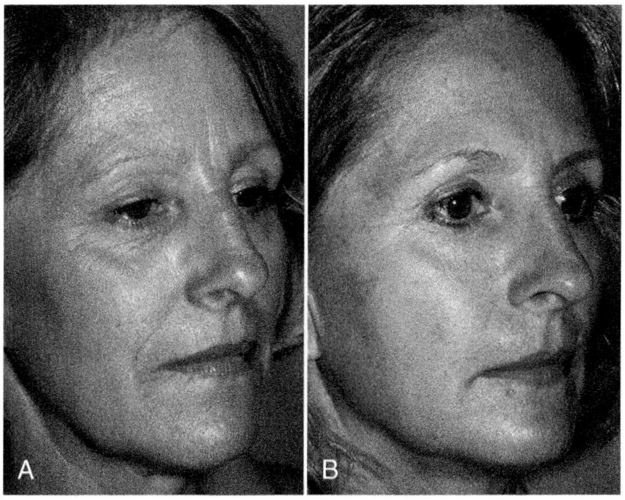

FIGURE 19-2 Facial aging differences in identical twins. Advanced photoaging changes of **(A)** skin wrinkling and laxity with prolonged sun exposure and **(B)** mild changes with minimal sun exposure. *(Courtesy of Dr. D. Antell, New York City, www.Antell-md.com.)*

AESTHETIC CONSULTATION

Aesthetic consultation is an important part of successfully performing aesthetic treatments. The patient's medical history is reviewed, including past medical history, medications, allergies, and past cosmetic history (including results from previous treatments and side effects if any, surgeries, and satisfaction with outcomes). Figure 19-5 is an example of an aesthetic intake form that clinicians may use. Repeated dissatisfaction with past aesthetic treatments can be associated with unrealistic expectations or body dysmorphic disorder and is a contraindication to treatment.

The main areas of concern should be determined and prioritized by the patient at the time of consultation. It is recommended that the patient view these areas using a handheld mirror, so that the provider and patient may simultaneously examine the desired treatment areas. Asymmetries, such as uneven eyebrow height, are pointed out to the patient, noted in the chart, and photographed.[10] Pigmented lesions in the treatment area are evaluated and lesions suspected of melanoma biopsied with results reviewed prior to proceeding with treatments.

Early on in the consultation process, providers should assess whether patients will benefit most from surgical intervention, or if minimally invasive treatments will address their concerns adequately particularly for patients presenting with severe wrinkles and excessive skin laxity. Treatment options and recommendations should be discussed along with anticipated results, risks of side effects and complications, recovery time, and costs. Based on this discussion, an individualized aesthetic rejuvenation treatment plan is created.

Baseline assessments of the patient's skin type and severity of photoaging are typically performed at the time of consultation using the Glogau classification of photoaging and Fitzpatrick skin type classification, respectively, as discussed next.

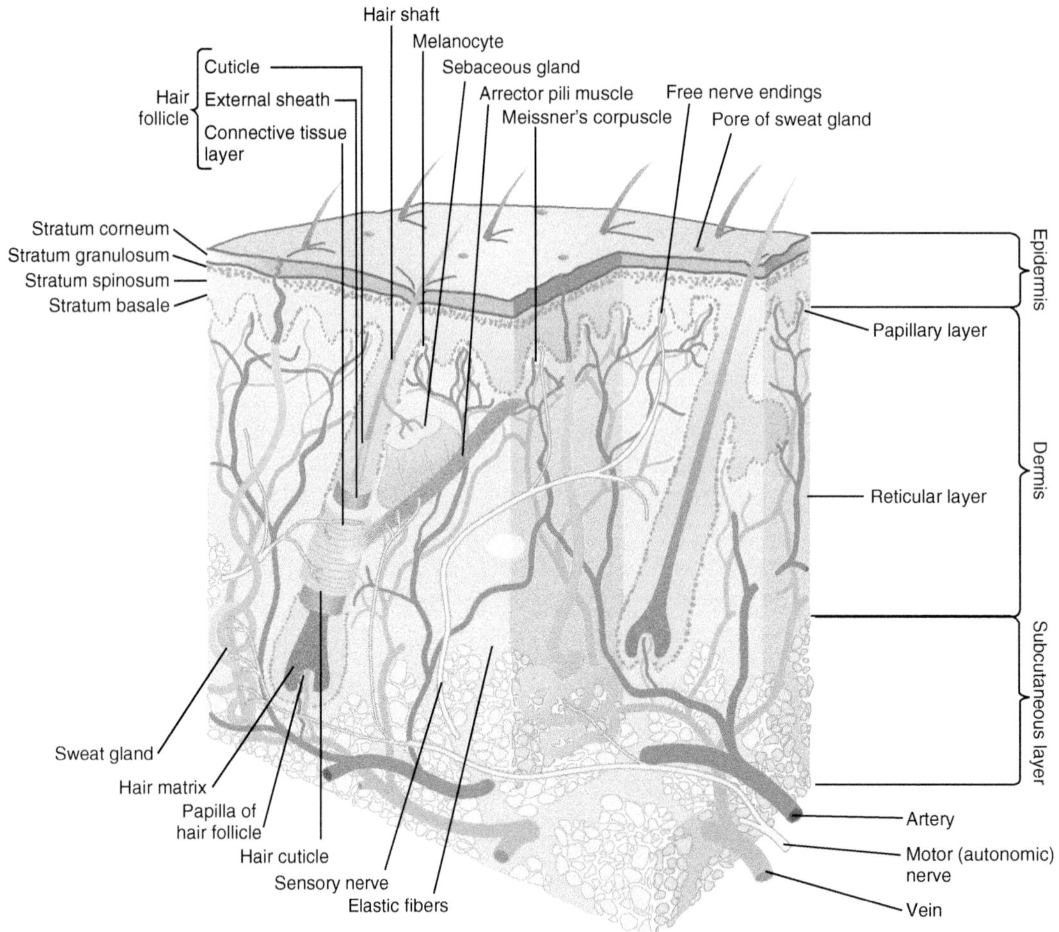

FIGURE 19-3 Skin anatomy. *(Modified from White CR, Bigby M, Sangueza OP. What is normal skin? In: Arndt KA, LeBoit PE, Robinson JK, Wintroub BU, eds.,* Cutaneous Medicine and Surgery. *Philadelphia: Saunders; 1996:3–41.)*

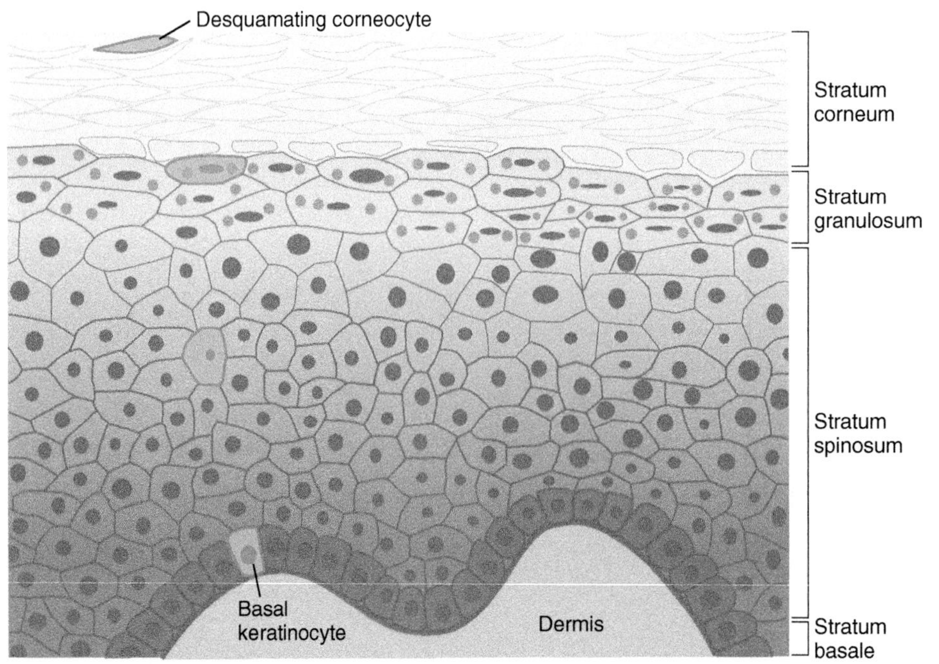

FIGURE 19-4 Epidermis structure showing keratinocyte maturation process from basal keratinocyte to desquamating corneocyte.

PATIENT INTAKE FORM Date:_______________

NAME:____ AGE:__________ * DOB:______________
Last First
ADDRESS:_______________________________________ CITY:______________ ZIP:______________

HOME PHONE:_______________________________________ ☐ OK TO CONTACT/LEAVE MESSAGE HERE

MOBILE PHONE:_____________________________________ ☐ OK TO CONTACT/LEAVE MESSAGE HERE

WORK PHONE:_______________________________________ ☐ OK TO CONTACT/LEAVE MESSAGE HERE

E-MAIL:____ ☐ OK TO CONTACT/LEAVE MESSAGE HERE

OCCUPATION:_______________________________________ REFERRED BY:__________________________

In order of importance, beginning with 1, make a wish list of what you would like to see improved in your skin in the next 30 days:
_____ Reduction of fine lines _____ Reduction of oil/acne _____ Reduction of redness _____ Reduction of brown spots/sun damage
_____ Reduction of hair _____ Acne scars diminished _____ Tattoo *For minors, please list guardian info.

Medical history	Yes	No
Are you or is it possible that you may be pregnant?		
Are you breastfeeding?		
Do you form thick or raised scars from cuts or burns?		
After injury to the skin (such as cuts/burns) do you have: (circle) Darkening of the skin in that area (hyperpigmentation) Lightening of the skin in that area (hypopigmentation)		
Hair removal by plucking, waxing, electrolysis in the last 4 weeks?		
Tanning (tanning bed) or sun exposure in the last 4 weeks? (circle)		
Tanning products or spray on tan in the last 2 weeks?		
Do you have a tan now in the area to be treated?		
Do you use sunscreen daily with spf 30 or higher?		
History of skin cancer or unusual moles?		
Have you ever had a photosensitive disorder? (E.g. lupus)		
History of seizures?		
Permanent make-up or tattoos? Where ______________		
Have you used Accutane in last 6 months?		
Are you currently taking antibiotics? Which ______________		
Are you using Retin-A or Glycolic products? (circle)		
Are you currently under the care of a physician?		
Do you currently smoke?		
Do you have an allergy or sensitivity to lidocaine, latex, sulfa medications, hydroquinone, aloe, bee stings? (circle)		
Life threatening allergy to anything?		
Do you have scars on the face?		

Explanation of items marked "Yes":
____
____

Yes	No	Please check all medical conditions past or present
☐	☐	Keloid scarring
☐	☐	Cold sores
☐	☐	Herpes (genital)
☐	☐	Easy bruising or bleeding
☐	☐	Active skin infection
☐	☐	Moles that changed, itched, or bled
☐	☐	Recent increase in amount of hair
☐	☐	Asthma
☐	☐	Seasonal allergies/allergic rhinitis
☐	☐	Eczema
☐	☐	Thyroid imbalance
☐	☐	Poor healing
☐	☐	Diabetes
☐	☐	Heart condition
☐	☐	High blood pressure
☐	☐	Pacemaker
☐	☐	Disease of nerves or muscles (e.g. ALS, myasthenia gravis, Lambert-Eaton or other)
☐	☐	Cancer
☐	☐	HIV/AIDS
☐	☐	Autoimmune disease (e.g. rheumatoid arthritis, scleroderma)
☐	☐	Hepatitis
☐	☐	Shingles
☐	☐	Migraine headaches
☐	☐	Other illness, health problems or medical conditions not listed.

Explanation of items marked "Yes":
____
____

I certify that the medical information I have given is complete and accurate. _______ Initials

For Internal Use Only Below This Line

____
____

FIGURE 19-5 Aesthetic patient intake form.

TABLE 19-1 Glogau Classification of Photoaging

Glogau Type	Photoaging	Typical Age	Skin Characteristics
I	Mild	20s to 30s	Minimal wrinkles No lentigines No keratoses
II	Moderate	30s to 40s	Wrinkles in motion Rare, faint lentigines Skin pores more prominent Keratose palpable but not visible
III	Advanced	50s to 60s	Wrinkles at rest Prominent lentigines Capillaries (telangiectasias) Visible keratose
IV	Severe	60s and Older	Wrinkles throughout Numerous lentigines Coarse pores Yellowish skin color Skin malignancies and premalignant lesions

Glogau Classification of Photoaging

The Glogau classification system was developed to assess the severity of photoaging, especially with regard to wrinkles (see Table 19-1). It is used as a baseline measure at the time of aesthetic consultation and may be used as a gross guide to therapy. In general, Glogau types I, II, and III tend to show the most noticeable improvements with less aggressive minimally invasive aesthetic treatments such as botulinum toxin and dermal filler injections, nonablative lasers, superficial and fractional ablative lasers, and superficial skin resurfacing procedures such as light chemical peels and microdermabrasion. Glogau type IV patients often require deep ablative laser treatments and/or surgery for significant results.

Fitzpatrick Skin Types

The Fitzpatrick skin type classification was developed to categorize a skin color and response to sunlight exposure. Skin types I, II, and III are white or Caucasian; types IV and V have olive skin tones, as seen in persons of Mediterranean, Asian, and Latin descent; and type VI is black, often of African American descent (see Table 19-2).[11] Fitzpatrick skin type may be used as a guide to the type and aggressiveness of aesthetic treatments, and may grossly predict skin response to

TABLE 19-2 Fitzpatrick Skin Type Classification

Fitzpatrick Skin Type	Characteristics	Response to Sun Exposure
I	White skin Red or blond hair Blue eyes Freckles	Always burns Never tans
II	White skin Red or blond hair Blue, hazel, or green eyes	Usually burns Difficulty tanning
III	White skin Any hair color Any eye color	Sometimes mild burn Gradually tans
IV	Light brown or olive skin Brown or black hair Dark eye color	Rarely burns Easily tans
V	Dark brown skin Dark brown or black hair Dark eye color	Very rarely burns Very easily tans
VI	Black skin Black hair Brown or black eyes	Never burns Very easily tans

treatments. For example, patients with Fitzpatrick skin types I, II, and III can generally tolerate aggressive treatments and have low risks of pigmentary changes. Patients with darker Fitzpatrick skin types (types IV through VI) have greater risks of pigmentary alterations, such as hyperpigmentation and hypopigmentation and require more conservative treatments to minimize the likelihood of these complications.

Photodocumentation

Photodocumentation, where photographs are used to demonstrate clinical findings, is an essential component of aesthetic treatments both for the patient's reference and for medical-legal purposes.[12] Photographs prior to treatment, midway through a series of treatments, and post-treatment are helpful and recommended. Consent for photographs is typically included in the procedure consent form and obtained prior to taking photographs. Recommended photographs include the full face and specific treatment areas which are photographed from the front, 45 and 90 degrees while the patient is positioned fully upright looking straight ahead. For injection treatments, photographs are taken with the face at rest and with active facial movement of the treatment areas. There are commercial photographic systems available that provide standardized angles and lighting to facilitate consistent photography.

Informed Consent

Patients seeking elective aesthetic treatments typically have high expectations of treatment outcomes and low tolerance for side effects. It is recommended that all aspects of the informed consent process be addressed[13]:

- Discuss the risks, potential benefits (with emphasis on realistic expectations), alternatives (including those not performed at your facility), and possible complications of the procedure.
- Provide adequate opportunity for all questions to be asked and answered.
- Educate the patient about the nature of their aesthetic issue and details of the procedure.
- Place a consent form signed by the patient in the chart.
- Document the informed consent process in the chart.

Safety Zones

The recommended regions for treatment on the face are identified as Safety Zones throughout the book and are intended as a guide for providers getting started with aesthetic procedures. Providers with more advanced procedural skill may choose to treat areas outside of the Safety Zones.

LASER TREATMENT PRINCIPLES

*Laser** devices produce monochromatic light of a single wavelength that is highly focused in a collimated beam (defined as parallel rays of light that disperse minimally). *Intense pulsed light* (IPL) devices emit a spectrum of wavelengths and employ filters to refine the energy output. Treatments with lasers and IPL devices (collectively referred to as *lasers* in this book) are based on the principle of *selective photothermolysis*. According to this principle, light of a specific wavelength is selectively absorbed by the "undesired" target in the skin such as a solar lentigo; the target is heated, damaged, and eliminated, while the surrounding skin is left unaffected. Figure 19-6 illustrates the principle of selective photothermolysis with treatment of solar lentigines and telangiectasias.[14]

When laser energy impacts skin, the beam may be absorbed, reflected, transmitted, or scattered. All four interactions occur to some degree, but absorption is the most important clinically. The degree of absorption depends on the chromophores, or light-absorbing substances, in skin. The primary chromophores in skin are melanin, oxyhemoglobin, and water, and each has a unique wavelength absorption spectrum (Figure 19-7). Treatment wavelengths are selected such that they are absorbed better by the target chromophores than by chromophores in the surrounding skin. Target chromophores for laser treatments are shown in Table 19-3.

*Refers to laser and light-based technologies.

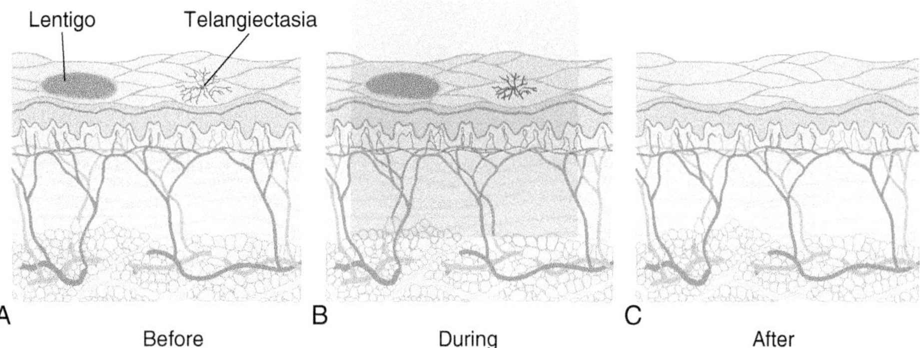

FIGURE 19-6 Selective photothermolysis. Wavelengths of light are selectively absorbed by targets in the skin, such as lentigos and telangiectasias (**A**). During laser treatments the targets are heated (**B**), damaged and eliminated while the surrounding skin is left unaffected (**C**).

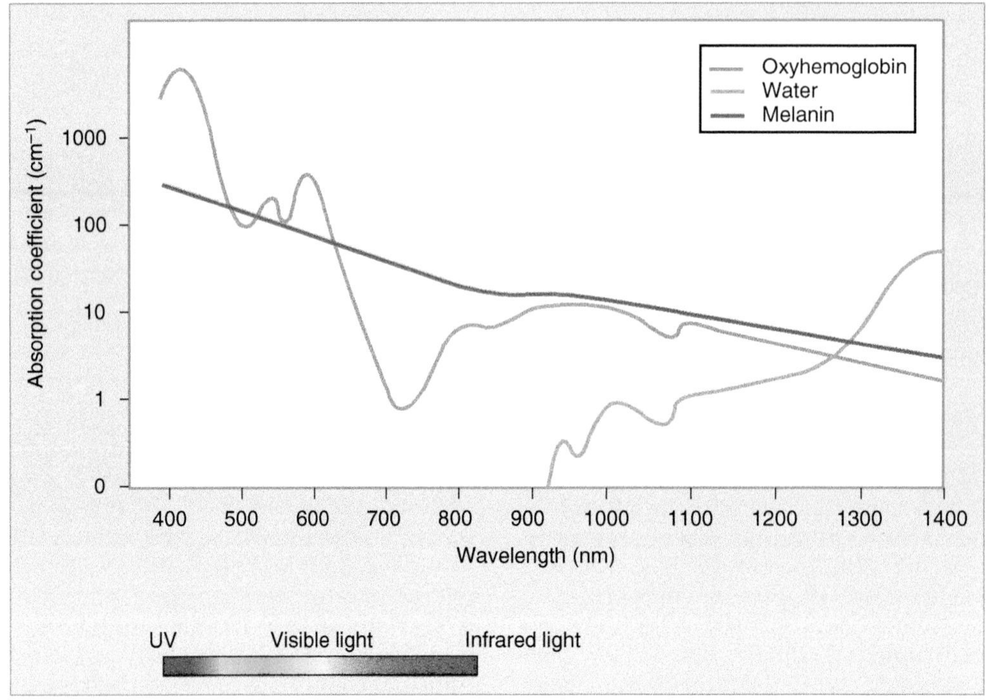

FIGURE 19-7 Absorption spectra for tissue chromophores: melanin, oxyhemoglobin, and water.

Figure 19-8 summarizes lasers commonly used for treatment of aesthetic conditions including: dyschromia, vascular ectasias, rhytids, and hair reduction.

LASER PARAMETERS

To achieve efficacious treatments with maximal safety, the provider must have an understanding of basic laser parameters, as well as the properties of the targets being treated in the skin. Laser parameter definitions and key concepts are summarized below[15]:

- *Wavelength* (measured in nanometers) determines chromophore specificity and the depth of laser penetration into the skin. As wavelength increases, so does the depth of penetration.
- *Pulse width*, or pulse duration (typically measured in milliseconds), is the amount of time that laser light is in contact with the skin. Longer pulse widths have greater depth of penetration.

TABLE 19-3 Target Chromophores for Laser Treatments

Treatment	*Chromophore*
Hair reduction	Melanin
Photorejuvenation:	
Pigmented lesions	Melanin
Red vascular lesions	Oxyhemoglobin
Tattoos	Tattoo ink
Wrinkle reduction	Water

- *Thermal relaxation time* (measured in milliseconds) is defined as the time required for an object to dissipate one-half of its heat. Energy is confined to the target when the laser pulse width is shorter than the thermal relaxation time of the target. The goal with laser treatments is to supply energy to the target faster than it is conducted to the surrounding tissue, to minimize surrounding thermal injury.
- *Spot size* (measured in millimeters) is the diameter of the laser beam on the skin surface. A larger spot size has less photon scatter in the laser beam and greater tissue penetration.
- *Fluence* is the energy output, also known as the power density (measured in joules per square centimeter). It is defined as the amount of energy delivered per unit area.
- *Multiple pulse modes* are used by some lasers. Pulsed modes of irradiation alternate power-on periods with power-off periods. During the off periods, heat is allowed to dissipate. If the off periods are longer than the thermal relaxation time of the target, there is less chance of thermal damage to the surrounding tissue by heat conduction.
- *Cooling* can also impact laser–tissue effects. The epidermis can be protected by cooling during treatment using methods such as cryogen sprays and contact cooling. However, over cooling may reduce treatment efficacy. In summary, deeper laser penetration into the skin is associated with longer wavelengths, higher fluences, larger spot sizes, longer pulsewidths and greater epidermal safety.

A typical laser is shown in Figure 19-9 with its component parts, including a computerized touch screen

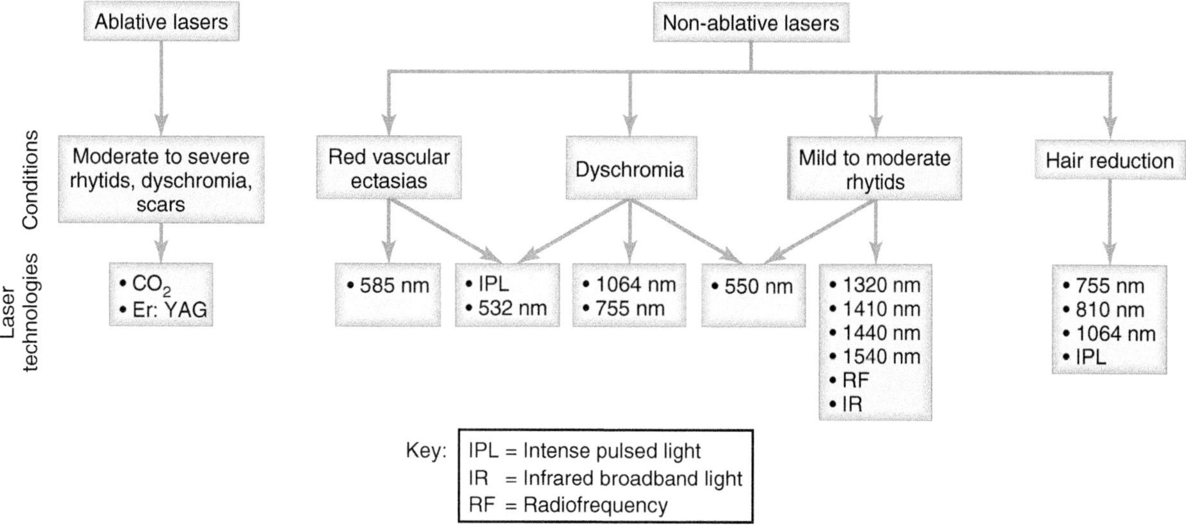

FIGURE 19-8 Lasers commonly used for aesthetic skin conditions.

commonly used to select laser parameters, a laser handpiece and distance guide.

Fractional Lasers

"Fractional" refers to a method of laser energy delivery, it does not refer to a particular wavelength. Fractional devices deliver laser energy in microscopic columns, called *microthermal zones* (Figure 19-10). The two main types of fractional laser devices are ablative (e.g., CO_2 and Er:YAG) and nonablative (e.g., 1550 and 1410 nm). Most fractional devices are used for skin resurfacing to reduce wrinkles and improve dyschromia. Only a portion of the skin is treated with this fractional method of delivery, resulting in significantly shortened recovery times particularly for ablative lasers.

Q-Switched Lasers

Q-switched lasers are lasers that have a special mechanism, a Q-switch, that allows energy to be stored and released in very short, intense pulses. The short pulse widths of Q-switched lasers (nanoseconds) make them ideal for treating pigmented lesions and for tattoo removal (e.g., 755 nm, 1064 nm, and 532 nm). As with other lasers, they operate under the basic principle of selective photothermolysis and, they also employ photoacoustic vibration, which fragments targets into smaller particles, further enhancing lesion destruction and removal.

LASER SAFETY

When using lasers, a laser safety officer should be designated, the American National Standards Institute (ANSI) laser safety requirements met,[16–18] and specific device manufacturer's guidelines for safety and maintenance follow. Wavelength-specific eyewear must be worn to protect patients and providers from ocular injury. Mirrors and windows are covered, laser warning signs posted, and a laser safety checklist reviewed prior to performing each treatment.

SKIN RESURFACING

Skin resurfacing is a common aesthetic rejuvenation practice based on the principles of wound healing. By wounding and removing superficial skin layers (also

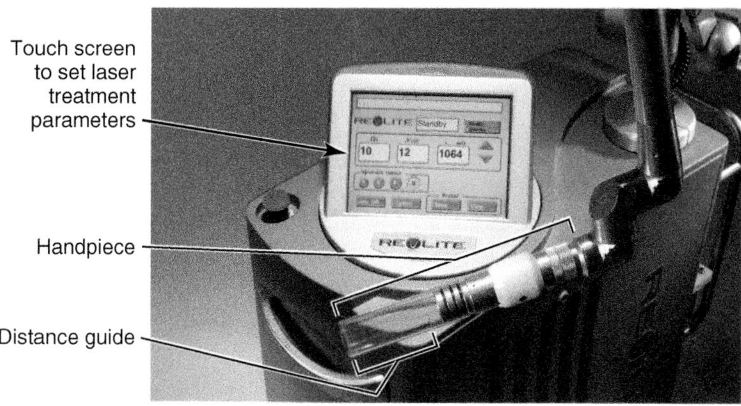

FIGURE 19-9 Laser parts. *(RevLite™ courtesy of HOYA ConBio, Fremont, CA, with modifications.)*

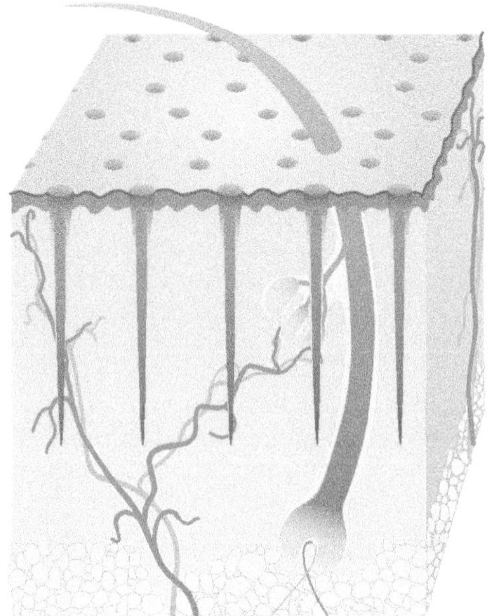

FIGURE 19-10 Fractional laser energy delivery.

called exfoliation) in a controlled manner, epidermal and dermal renewal is stimulated. Many methods of skin resurfacing are available. They can be broadly classified according to the method of skin injury:

- Mechanical, utilizing an abrasive element (e.g., microdermabrasion)
- Chemical, utilizing a topical chemical agent (e.g., chemical peels)
- Thermal, utilizing lasers to heat or vaporize tissue (e.g., resurfacing lasers).

Skin resurfacing can be performed to varying degrees of aggressiveness based on the depth of skin penetration. Figure 19-11 shows standard definitions for very superficial (stratum corneum), superficial (typically to the base of the epidermis, but may include the upper papillary dermis), medium (upper reticular dermis), and deep (midreticular dermis) skin resurfacing. Figure 19-12 illustrates the typical depths achieved with different resurfacing procedures. In general, the greater the depth of wounding, the more dramatic the results achieved. However, greater wound depths are also associated with longer recovery time, more intensive post-procedure care, and greater risks of side effects and complications. Penetration into or below the papillary dermis, which is usually associated with bleeding, has a greater risk of scarring than more superficial resurfacing of the epidermis.

AESTHETIC PROCEDURES: GETTING STARTED

Many of the aesthetic procedures discussed in this book are ideal for providers who wish to incorporate aesthetic care into practice. They are highly efficacious with rapid results that require minimal recovery time and they have relatively low risks of side effects. These core aesthetic procedures include:

- *Botulinum toxin* treatment for frown lines, crow's feet, and horizontal forehead lines
- *Dermal filler* treatment for nasolabial folds
- *Laser* treatment for hair reduction, photorejuvenation of benign vascular and pigmented lesions, and tattoo removal
- *Microdermabrasion, chemical peels* and *topical products* for skin care.

Once skill and proficiency with these core procedures has been acquired, providers may choose to undertake more advanced aesthetic procedures. Advanced

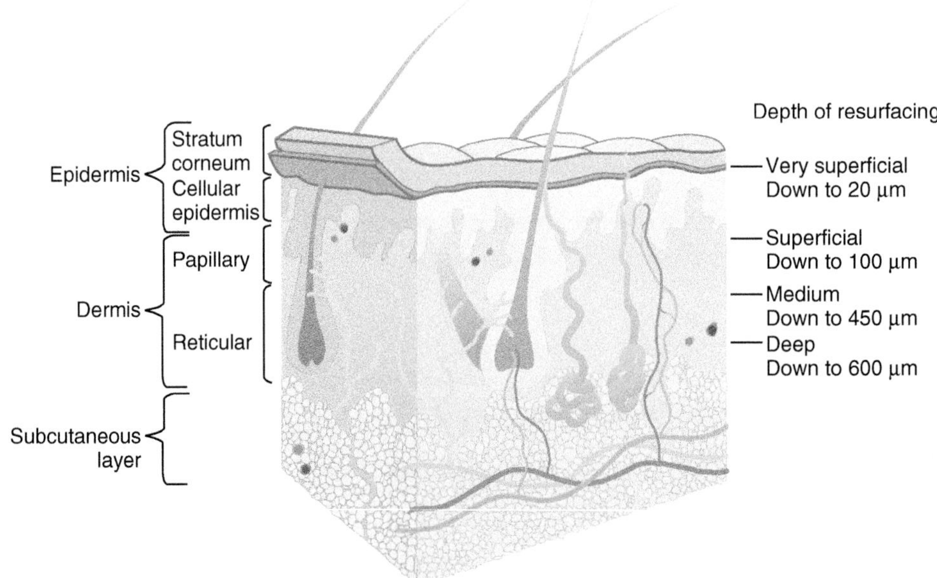

FIGURE 19-11 Skin resurfacing terminology.

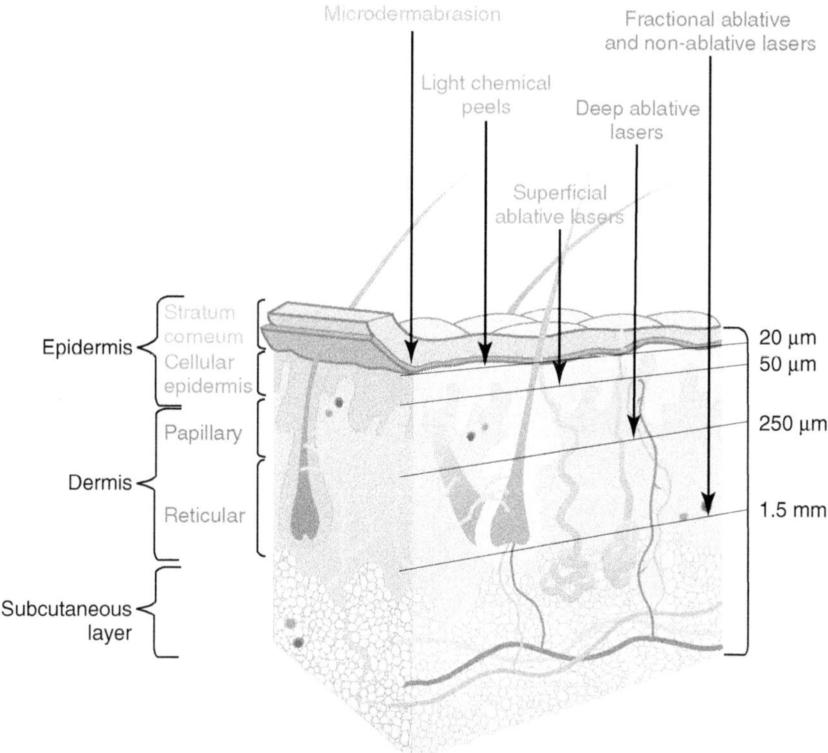

FIGURE 19-12 Depths of penetration with common skin resurfacing procedures.

procedures can be associated with longer recovery times, as with ablative lasers, or demonstrate subtle results, as with nonablative lasers for wrinkle reduction. Certain procedures require advanced procedural skill and knowledge. These include botulinum toxin injections in the lower two-thirds of the face and neck, and dermal filler injections that utilize layering techniques and semipermanent products and are used for facial contouring. In addition, procedures can be intensified and results enhanced by combining procedures over several visits or on the same day in multimodality visits.

Resources

Laser-Safe Eyewear Glendale by Honeywell
Phone: 800-500-4739
www.glendale-laser.com

Oculo-Plastik
Phone: 888-381-3292
www.oculoplastik.com

References

1. Small R. Aesthetic procedures in office practice. *Am Fam Physician.* 2009;80(11):1231–1237.
2. *Cosmetic Surgery National Data Bank 2010 statistics.* American Society for Aesthetic Plastic Surgery. 2010.
3. de Maio M. The minimal approach: an innovation in facial cosmetic procedures. *Aesthetic Plast Surg.* 2004;28:295–300.
4. Sommer B, Zschocke I, Bergfeld D, *et al.* Satisfaction of patients after treatment with botulinum toxin for dynamic facial lines. *Derm Surg.* 2003;29(5):456–460.
5. Lockman AR, Lockman DW. Skin changes in the maturing woman. *Clin Fam Pract.* 2002;4(1):113–134.
6. Antell D. How environment and lifestyle choices influence the aging process. *Ann Plast Surg.* 2009;43(6):585–588.
7. Zimbler MS, Kokoska MS, Thomas JR. Anatomy and pathophysiology of facial aging. *Facial Plast Surg Clin North Am.* 2001;9(2):179–187, vii.
8. Werschler P. Combining advanced injection techniques: Integrating new therapies into clinical practice. *Cosmetic Dermatol.* 2008;21(2 S1):3–6.
9. Szabo G, Gerald AB, Pathak MA, *et al.* Racial differences in the fate of melanosomes in human epidermis. *Nature.* 1969; 222(5198):1081–1082.
10. Small R. Aesthetic procedures introduction. *In:* Mayeaux E, ed. *The Essential Guide to Primary Care Procedures.* Philadelphia: Lippincott Williams & Wilkins; 2009:195–199.
11. Fitzpatrick TB. The validity and practicality of sun-reactive skin types I through VI. *Arch Dermatol.* 1998;124(6):869–871.
12. Kuhnel T, Wolf S. Mirror system for photodocumentation in plastic and aesthetic surgery. *Brit J Plast Surg.* 2005;58(6): 830–832.
13. Informed consent update, Claims Rx. Norcal Mutual Insurance Company. 2007.
14. Anderson RR, Parrish JA. Selective photothermolysis: precise microsurgery by selective absorption of pulsed radiation. *Science.* 1983;220(4596):524–527.
15. Levins P. Selective photothermolysis. *In:* Keller GS, Lacombe V, Lee P, Watson J, eds. *Lasers in Aesthetic Surgery.* New York: Thieme Medical Publishers; 2001:34–40.
16. American National Standards Institute. *American National Standard for the Safe Use of Lasers.* Z136.1–2007.
17. American National Standards Institute. *American National Standard for the Safe Use of Lasers in Health Care Facilities.* Z136.3–2005.
18. Recommended practices for laser safety in practice setting. *In: Perioperative Standards and Recommended Practices.* Denver, CO: Association of Perioperative Registered Nurses; 2008:447–452.

Additional Reading

Alibhai H. Introduction to aesthetic medicine. *In:* Pfenninger JL, Fowler GC, eds. *Pfenninger and Fowler's Procedures for Primary Care.* 3rd ed. Philadelphia: Mosby/Elsevier; 2010.

Small R, Hoang D. Botulinum toxin introduction and foundation concepts. *In:* Small R, Hoang D, eds. *A Practical Guide to Botulinum Toxin Procedures.* Philadelphia: Lippincott Williams & Wilkins; 2011.

Small R, Hoang D. Dermal filler introduction and foundation concepts. *In:* Small R, Hoang D, eds. *A Practical Guide to Dermal Filler Procedures.* Philadelphia: Lippincott Williams & Wilkins; 2011.

Small R, Linder J. Skin care introduction and foundation concepts. *In:* Small R, Linder J, eds. *A Practical Guide to Skin Care Procedures and Products.* Philadelphia: Lippincott Williams & Wilkins; 2011.

Small R. Laser introduction and foundation concepts. *In:* Small R, ed. *A Practical Guide to Cosmetic Lasers.* Philadelphia: Lippincott Williams & Wilkins, 2012.

20 Anesthesia for Cosmetic Procedures

REBECCA SMALL, MD

Providing adequate anesthesia is an essential part of performing cosmetic procedures and successfully incorporating them into practice. In addition to offering the patient a better procedural experience, minimizing discomfort ensures greater treatment precision and may improve outcomes.[1] Cosmetic treatments that commonly require anesthesia include laser treatments, such as ablative skin resurfacing, tattoo removal and hair reduction, dermal filler injections, and occasionally botulinum toxin injections.[2]

Four anesthesia modalities are commonly used with cosmetic procedures:

1. Injectable anesthetics (e.g., local infiltration and regional blocks)
2. Topical anesthetics
3. Contact cooling (e.g., ice)
4. Analgesic devices.

The anesthetic modality chosen is dependent on the discomfort level associated with the procedure, procedure duration, and patient tolerance for pain. Anesthesia for less painful procedures, such as botulinum toxin and laser hair reduction, can be accomplished with contact cooling using ice or a contact cooling device and topical anesthetics. More painful procedures such as dermal fillers typically require injectable anesthetics, and prolonged procedures, such as ablative laser resurfacing, often require a combination of methods such as topical anesthetic, oral analgesic, and cool air blower (see Table 20-1).

INJECTABLE ANESTHETICS

Injectable lidocaine (1% to 2%) reduces pain by blocking neural cell membrane sodium channels and inhibiting impulse propagation. Initially, small delta nerve fibers, which are responsible for pain and temperature sensations, are blocked. Larger beta nerve fibers, which are responsible for pressure and vibration, take longer to anesthetize. For this reason, injectable anesthetics have a rapid reduction of pain but a slower reduction in sensations of pressure and pulling.[3]

Lidocaine may be buffered with sodium bicarbonate in a 1:8 or 1:10 ratio to reduce the burning sensation upon injection of anesthetic. See Chapter 3, *Anesthesia*, for information on side effects and toxicity with lidocaine and alternative options for lidocaine allergic patients.

Local Infiltration

Lidocaine with epinephrine is typically used for infiltration with cosmetic procedures because a rapid onset of anesthesia is desirable, as is the associated vasoconstriction and reduced risk of bruising associated with epinephrine. Anesthetic infiltration results in tissue edema and distortion. Care should be taken to inject the smallest possible anesthetic volumes necessary when using local infiltration for cosmetic procedures. See Chapter 3, *Anesthesia* for local infiltration injection techniques.

Local infiltration is commonly used to provide anesthesia for dermal filler treatments and may be used for patients who cannot tolerate laser tattoo removal. Anesthetic infiltration significantly lengthens the time of treatment, and some providers suggest that edema caused by local infiltration may reduce the efficacy of laser tattoo treatments (see Chapter 30, *Tattoo Removal with Lasers*).

Regional Nerve Blocks

Lidocaine without epinephrine is used for nerve blocks. Facial nerve blocks are beneficial for cosmetic procedures because anesthetic is placed outside of the treatment area. Profound anesthesia can be achieved with minimal distortion of the treatment area, which is particularly useful with dermal filler treatments.[2,4] Nerve blocks are also useful for painful procedures such as ablative laser resurfacing, particularly in the sensitive perioral area.

Infraorbital and mental nerve blocks are most commonly used with facial cosmetic procedures. The locations of the infraorbital and mental nerves are shown in Figure 20-1 and can be identified by palpating the nerve foramina. The infraorbital and mental nerves lie along a vertical line extending from the supraorbital notch to the mandible. The supraorbital notch lies along the upper border of the orbit and is palpable approximately 2.5 cm lateral to the midline of the face. The infraorbital foramen is palpable approximately 1 cm inferior to the infraorbital bony margin, and the mental nerve is palpable just above the margin of the mandible.

Equipment

- 5.0-mL syringe
- Lidocaine HCl 1% to 2%
- 18-gauge, 1.5-inch needles to draw up anesthetic
- 30-gauge, 0.5-inch needles for injection.

Infraorbital Nerve Block

The infraorbital nerve innervates most of the upper lip, lower eyelid, lateral portion of the nose, and medial cheek. An infraorbital nerve block can anesthetize all of these regions (Figure 20-2).[3] The intent of the infraorbital nerve block technique described here,

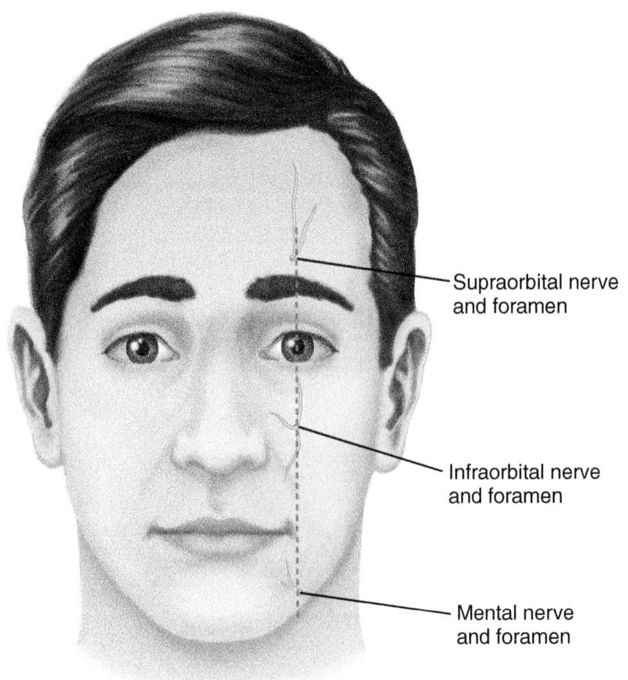

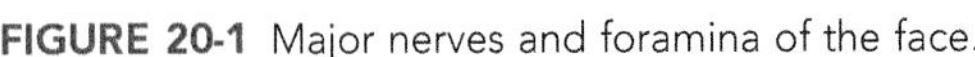

FIGURE 20-1 Major nerves and foramina of the face.

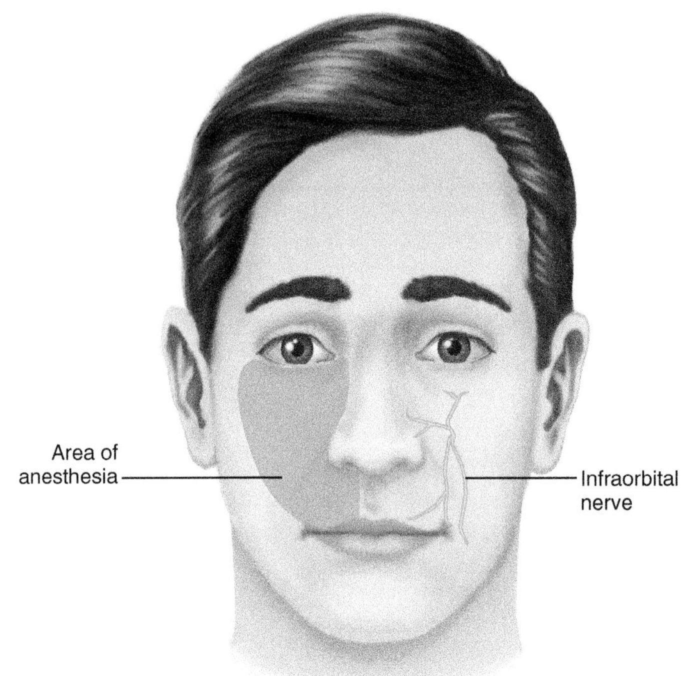

FIGURE 20-2 Infraorbital nerve and area of anesthesia with nerve block.

utilizing a short 0.5-inch needle, is to reach the distal portions of the infraorbital nerve, not the nerve foramen, which would require a longer needle (approximately 1¼ inches long). The philtrum and the corners of the mouth are typically poorly anesthetized with infraorbital blocks, and additional local infiltration is also required when treating these areas.

TABLE 20-1 Anesthetic Modalities Used for Cosmetic Procedures

Anesthetic Modalities	Cosmetic Procedures
Injectable anesthetics	
Local infiltration	Dermal fillers Laser tattoo removal
Regional block	Dermal fillers Ablative lasers
Topical anesthetics	Botulinum toxin Dermal fillers Laser hair reduction Laser tattoo removal Laser photorejuvenation for pigmented lesions Ablative lasers
Contact cooling	Botulinum toxin Dermal fillers Laser hair reduction
Analgesic devices	Laser hair reduction Ablative lasers

Procedure Steps

1. Comfortably position the patient upright at about 65 degrees with the chin tipped upward.
2. Stand on the contralateral side of the patient.
3. Lift the upper lip for good visualization of the gingivobuccal margin.
4. Insert a 30-gauge, 0.5-inch needle at the gingivobuccal margin just lateral to the maxillary canine (third tooth from the midline) and direct the needle superiorly, angling toward the pupil (Figure 20-3).
5. Advance the needle almost the full length and inject 0.5 to 1.0 mL of lidocaine. The anesthetic should flow easily.
6. After removing the needle, compress the deep palpable wheal of lidocaine superiorly toward the infraorbital foramen.
7. Repeat for the contralateral infraorbital nerve.
8. The philtral area requires additional infiltration of local anesthetic to achieve adequate anesthesia. Inject 0.1 mL of lidocaine intraorally in the mucosa just lateral to the upper lip frenulum (Figure 20-4). After the needle is removed, compress the injection site to distribute the lidocaine, and repeat for the other side of the upper lip frenulum.
9. The onset of anesthetic effect is typically 5 to 10 minutes.

Mental Nerve Block

The mental nerve innervates most of the lower lip, and a mental nerve block can anesthetize this region (Figure 20-5).[3] The corner of the mouth is typically poorly

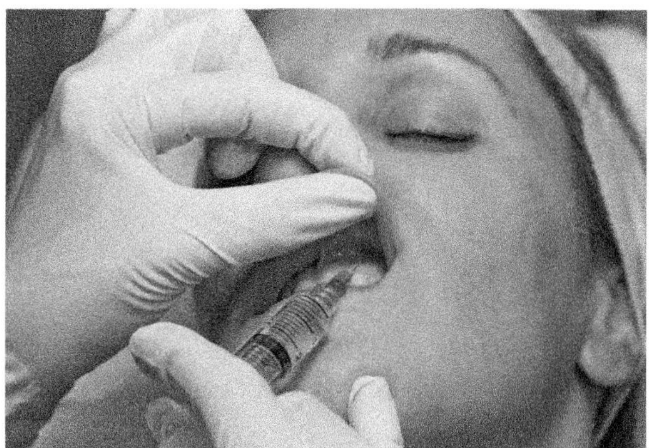

FIGURE 20-3 Technique for intraoral infraorbital nerve block. *(Copyright Rebecca Small, MD.)*

anesthetized, and additional local infiltration is also required when treating this area.

Procedure Steps

1. Comfortably position the patient upright at about 65 degrees, with the chin tipped downward.
2. Stand on the contralateral side of the patient.
3. Lift the lower lip for good visualization of the gingivobuccal margin.
4. Insert a 30-gauge, 0.5-inch needle at the gingivobuccal margin just lateral to the first mandibular bicuspid (also called the first premolar, which is the fourth tooth from the midline) (Figure 20-6) and direct the needle inferior-laterally toward the mental nerve foramen.
5. Advance the needle halfway to the hub, and inject 0.5 to 1.0 mL of lidocaine. The anesthetic should flow easily.
6. After removing the needle, compress the deep palpable wheal of lidocaine inferiorly toward the mental nerve foramen.
7. Repeat for the contralateral mental nerve.
8. The lateral corners of the mouth require additional infiltration of local anesthetic to achieve adequate anesthesia. Inject 0.1 mL of lidocaine intraorally in the mucosa at the corner of the mouth (Figure 20-7). After the needle is removed, compress the injection site to disburse the lidocaine, and repeat for the contralateral corner of the mouth.
9. The onset of anesthetic effect for nerve blocks is typically within 5 to 10 minutes.
   TIP: If adequate anesthesia is not achieved, repeat the procedure, injecting an additional 0.5 mL of lidocaine, and wait an additional 10 minutes.
   CAUTION: If the needle is angled too anteriorly, lidocaine may be placed in the dermis, which can be felt as resistance during injection, and adequate anesthesia may not be obtained.

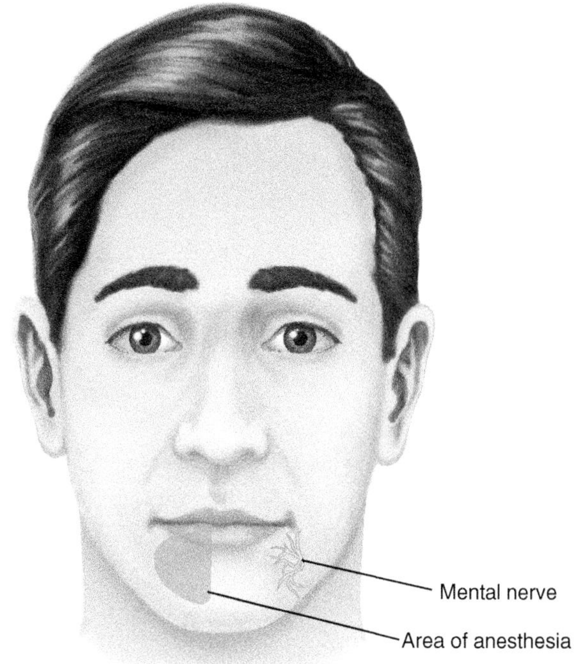

FIGURE 20-5 Mental nerve and area of anesthesia with nerve block.

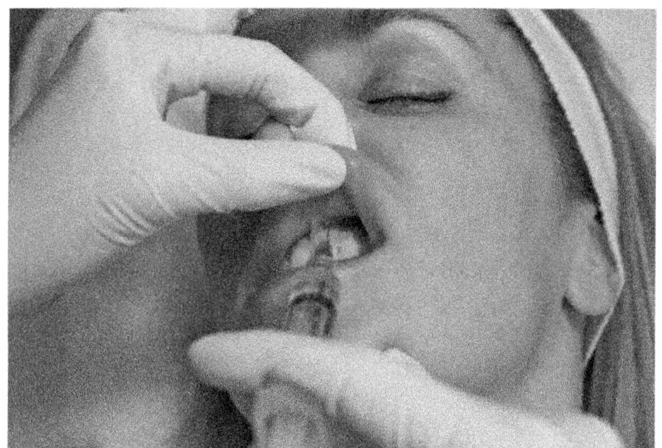

FIGURE 20-4 Technique for intraoral anesthetic infiltration of the upper lip frenulum. *(Copyright Rebecca Small, MD.)*

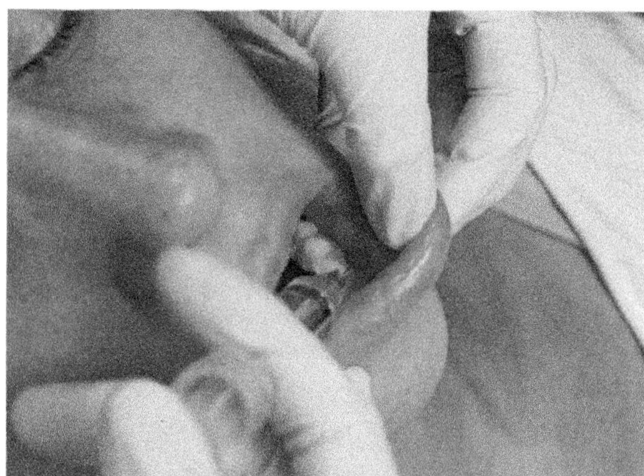

FIGURE 20-6 Technique for intraoral mental nerve block. *(Copyright Rebecca Small, MD.)*

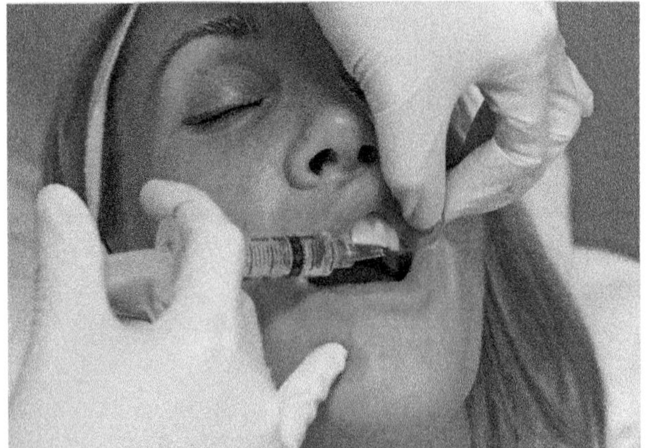

FIGURE 20-7 Technique for intraoral anesthetic infiltration in the corner of the mouth. *(Copyright Rebecca Small, MD.)*

CAUTION: Do not insert the needle to the hub to avoid the rare risk of a buried broken needle.

Patients will frequently report that their lips feel enlarged or report a sensation of drooling after infraocular and mental nerve blocks, which are good indicators of anesthetic effect. Motor nerves are also affected and patients may have slurred speech due to impaired lip function and limited pucker or smile. Patients may be reassured that these effects are temporary and once the anesthetic effect wears off they will regain sensation and motor function. See Chapter 3, *Anesthesia*, for additional information about nerve blocks.

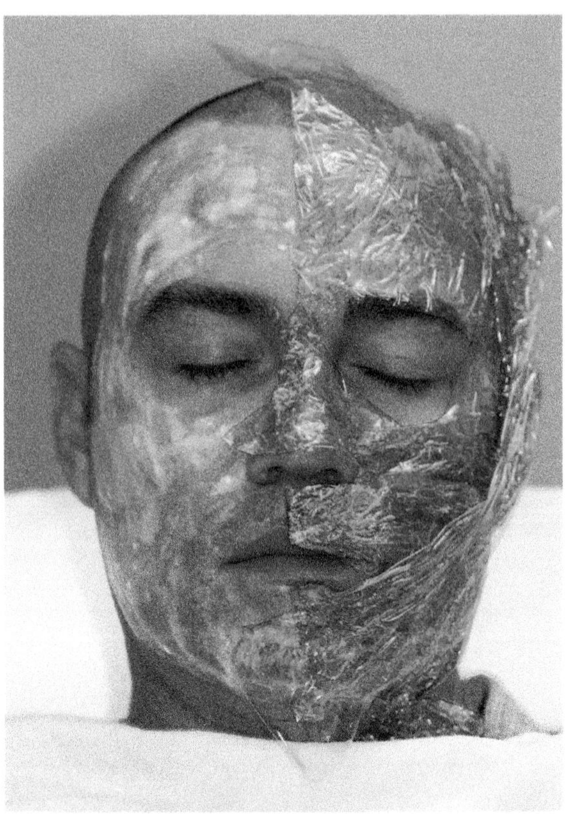

FIGURE 20-8 Topical anesthetic on the right side of the face with Pliaglis unoccluded, and left side with BLT under occlusion with plastic wrap. *(Copyright Rebecca Small, MD.)*

TOPICAL ANESTHETICS

Topical anesthetics are frequently used with cosmetic procedures due to their ease of application (see Table 20-2). They have the same mechanism of action as injectable anesthetics whereby sensory nerves are blocked by neuronal impulse inhibition.

The skin is degreased with alcohol prior to application, and for ointment- and cream-based anesthetics, the product is rubbed gently into the treatment area and then occluded with plastic wrap, taking care not to occlude the nose and mouth. Figure 20-8 shows half the face treated with BLT under occlusion with plastic wrap and the other half face with Pliaglis, a self-occluding topical anesthetic. Pliaglis, temporarily removed from the market for reformulation, is applied as a thick cream and dries on exposure to air, becoming a flexible membrane that is peeled off. The face has a relatively small surface area and there are few complications with topical anesthetics. However, caution must be used with larger areas such as the extremities or the back as systemic absorption is significant, and severe complications have been reported from topical anesthetic toxicity, including death, when applied under occlusion to large skin surface areas.

TABLE 20-2 Commonly Used Topical Anesthetic Products for Cosmetic Procedures[a]

L-M-X	Lidocaine 4% to 5%; over-the-counter product
EMLA	Lidocaine 2.5% : prilocaine 2.5%; prescription
BLT	Benzocaine 20% : lidocaine 6% : tetracaine 4%; compounded by a pharmacy

[a]See the *Resources* section at the end of the chapter for suppliers.

The degree of anesthesia achieved with a topical anesthetic is related to the strength of the product, duration, and method of application. There are many topical anesthetics of different strengths, and it is simplest to select one product for use in the office and vary the time and method of application to suit the degree of anesthesia required for a procedure. For less painful procedures, such as laser hair reduction, topical anesthetics (e.g., BLT) can be applied for shorter duration such as 15 minutes without occlusion, whereas more painful procedures, such as tattoo removal or ablative laser resurfacing, require BLT application for 45 to 60 minutes under occlusion.[5] Relative to injectable anesthetics, topical anesthetics have the disadvantage of increased visit times required for anesthesia to take effect and greater cost.

Toxicity of topical anesthetics is due to systemic absorption of the product. Several factors affect systemic absorption including the product used, surface area covered, duration of application, and the presence of an intact skin barrier. Anesthetic creams with standard formulas have better safety profiles as it is easier to predict systemic blood levels that will be obtained. For most topical anesthetic creams, systemic blood levels reached with proper use are a small fraction of the blood levels that produce toxicity. For example, 60 g of EMLA cream placed on a 400-cm^2 area (equivalent to half a back) for 4 hours produces peak blood levels of lidocaine that are 1/20th the systemic toxic level of lidocaine and 1/36th the toxic level of prilocaine. This makes its application very safe, with levels well below the concentration that would cause systemic toxicity.[6] Cases where topical anesthetic use has resulted in toxicity are mainly a result of patient self-application of large quantities to large surface areas or when procedures are used that disrupt the skin barrier, such as fractional laser resurfacing. Systemic lidocaine toxicity signs and symptoms range from mild dizziness to respiratory depression and correlate with serum levels.[7] Higher strength topical anesthetics, such as BLT and Pliaglis, should be applied in-office for safety.[8] See Chapter 3, *Anesthesia* for more information on topical anesthetics.

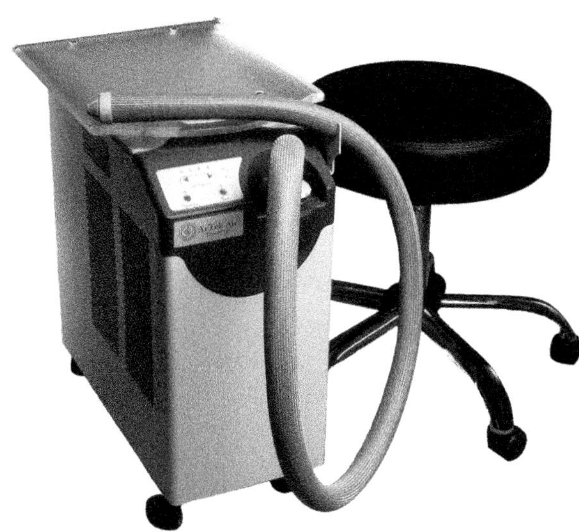

FIGURE 20-10 Air cooling device (ArTek Air by ThermoTek). *(Courtesy of ThermoTek, Flower Mound, Texas.)*

CONTACT COOLING

Ice or contact cooling devices are excellent modalities for achieving anesthesia, and they also improve safety with laser treatments by providing epidermal protection from thermal injury. Contact cooling may be used alone or adjunctively with the other modalities above, for laser hair reduction as well as botulinum toxin and dermal filler injections. Figure 20-9 shows a contact cooling device with adjustable temperature and a contoured tip that can be used for the face. Anesthesia is achieved by applying contact cooling immediately before treatment for approximately 1 to 3 minutes or until the skin is erythematous. The goal temperature for contact cooling is 5°C.[9] Overcooling, with prolonged blanching of the skin, can result in epidermal injury.

ANALGESIC DEVICES

Analgesic devices can be used with laser treatments to reduce patient discomfort and to reduce the risk of complications from thermal injury. Many lasers have built-in cooling mechanisms. Those that do not have built-in cooling mechanisms can use external analgesic devices such as cool air blowers or pneumatic skin flattening. Cool air blowers force air through a hose that is directed over the treatment area to achieve a goal skin temperature of 20°C.[10] (Figure 20-10 shows an example of a forced air cooling device, the ArTek Air by ThermoTek.) This noncontact method of cooling is particularly useful with ablative laser treatments.

Pneumatic skin flattening utilizes negative pressure to elevate and flatten skin against the device window (Figure 20-11A). The mechanism of action of these devices is based on the gate theory of pain, whereby the pressure generated by the pneumatic device inhibits pain sensation through overwhelming and blocking the pain pathways (Figure 20-11B). Some laser devices have pneumatic skin flattening incorporated into the laser and others have a separate pneumatic device that is attached to the treatment tip (Figure 20-12).[11] The disadvantages of assistive external cooling devices are the additional use of space, cost of the device, and for air blowers, an occasional requirement for an assistant and risk of overcooling if the device remains stationary in one spot on the skin.

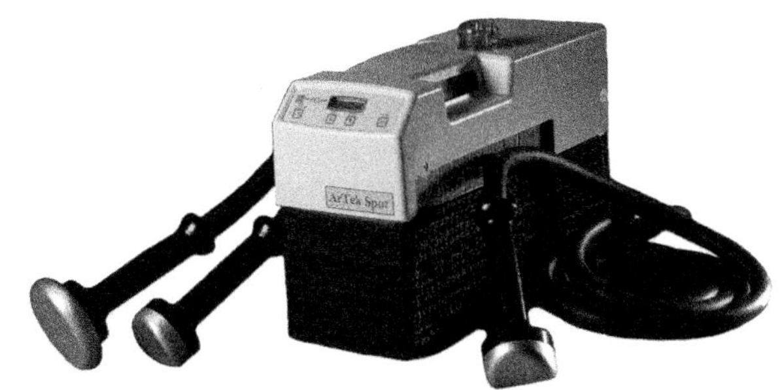

FIGURE 20-9 Contact cooling device (ArTek Spot by ThermoTek). *(Courtesy of ThermoTek, Flower Mound, Texas.)*

CONCLUSION

Certain minimally invasive aesthetic procedures, such as dermal filler injections, laser hair reduction, tattoo removal and laser skin resurfacing require anesthesia. Adequate anesthesia reduces anxiety, offers the patient a more pleasant experience, and allows for greater treatment precision and optimal technique to achieve the best possible results. Providing anesthesia is an essential part of performing cosmetic procedures and successfully incorporating them into office practice.

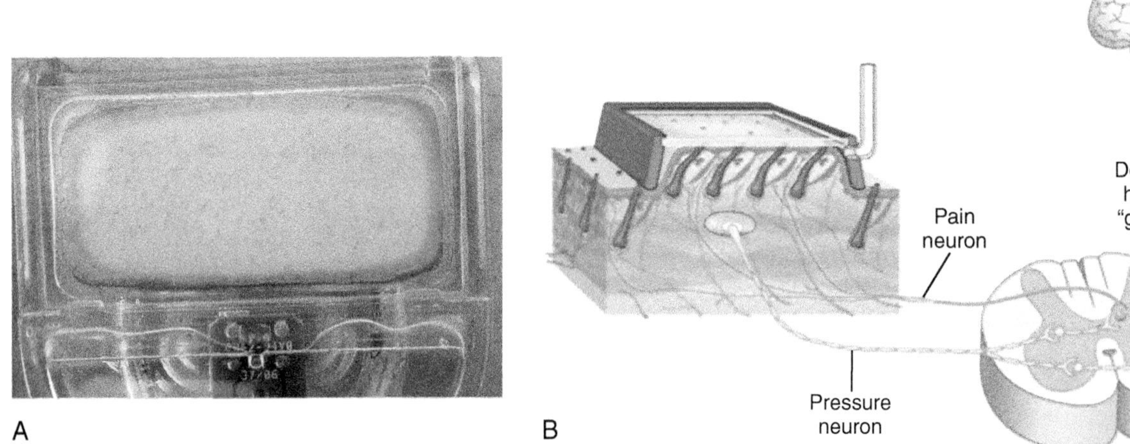

FIGURE 20-11 (A) Pneumatic skin flattening window utilizes the gate theory of pain inhibition. (B) Pressure-sensing nerves block the synaptic gate in the dorsal horn that transmits pain impulses to the brain (Serenity by Candela). *(Courtesy of Candela Corp, Wayland, MA.)*

Resources

Topical Anesthetics

American Health Solutions Pharmacy (BLT)
Phone: 310-838-7422
www.AHSRx.com

APP Pharmaceuticals (EMLA)
Phone: 847-413-2075
www.apppharma.com

PharmaDerm (L-M-X)
Phone: 973-514-4240
www.pharmaderm.com

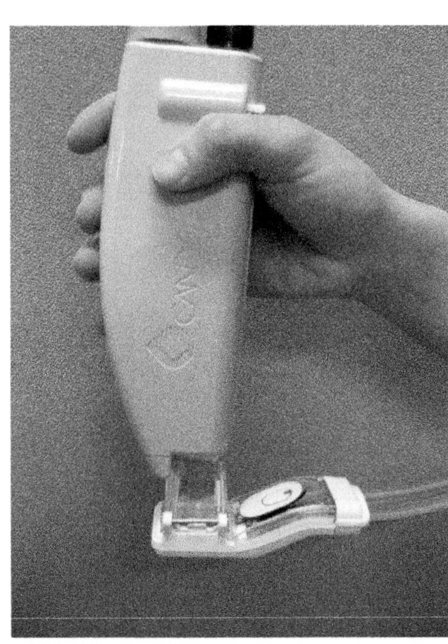

FIGURE 20-12 Pneumatic skin flattening device attached to an intense pulsed light treatment head (Serenity by Candela). *(Courtesy of Candela Corp, Wayland, MA.)*

Galderma Laboratories (Pliaglis)
Phone: 866-735-4137
www.galdermausa.com

Assistive External Devices

LaserMed (Zimmer™ cool air device)
Phone: 203-929-6354
www.zimmercoolers.com

ThermoTek (ArTek Spot™ contact cooling and ArTek Air™ cool air device)
Phone: 972-874-4949
www.thermotek.com

Candela (Serenity™ pneumatic skin flattening device)
Phone: 800-733-8550
www.candelalaser.com

References

1. Small R. Aesthetic procedures introduction. *In:* Mayeaux E, ed. *The Essential Guide to Primary Care Procedures.* Philadelphia: Lippincott Williams & Wilkins; 2009:195–199.
2. Small R. Dermal fillers for facial rejuvenation. *In:* Mayeaux E, ed. *The Essential Guide to Primary Care Procedures.* Philadelphia: Lippincott Williams & Wilkins; 2009:214–233.
3. Foley K, Pianalto D. Facial anesthesia. *Emerg Med.* 2005;30–34.
4. Salam GA. Regional anesthesia for office procedures: part I. Head and neck surgeries 4. *Am Fam Physician.* 2004;69(3):585–590.
5. Lee MS. Topical triple-anesthetic gel compared with 3 topical anesthetics. *Cosmetic Dermatol.* 2003;26(61):35–38.
6. Kaweski S. Topical anesthetic creams. *Plast Reconstr Surg.* 2008;121(6):2161–2165.
7. Marra DE, Yip D, Fincher EF, *et al.* Systemic toxicity from topically applied lidocaine in conjunction with fractional photothermolysis. *Arch Dermatol.* 2006;142(8):1024–1026.
8. Achar S. Topical anesthetic complications. In: Pfenninger JL, Fowler GC, eds. *Pfenninger and Fowler's Procedures for Primary Care.* Philadelphia: Mosby/Elsevier; 2010.
9. Altschuler GB, Zenzie HH, Erofeev AV, *et al.* Contact cooling of the skin. *Phys Med Biol.* 1999;44:1003–1023.
10. Raulin C, Greve B, Hammes S. Cold air in laser therapy. *Lasers Surg Med.* 2000;27:404–410.

11. Lask G, Friedman D, Eman M, *et al.* Pneumatic skin flattening (PSF): a novel technology for marked pain reduction in hair removal with high energy density lasers and IPLs. *J Cosmet Laser Ther.* 2006;8(2):76–81.

Additional Reading

Achar S, Chan J. Topical anesthesia. *In:* Pfenninger JL, Fowler GC, eds. *Pfenninger and Fowler's Procedures for Primary Care.* 3rd ed. Philadelphia: Mosby/Elsevier; 2010.

Amundsen GA. Local anesthesia. *In:* Pfenninger JL, Fowler GC, eds. *Pfenninger and Fowler's Procedures for Primary Care.* 3rd ed. Philadelphia: Mosby/Elsevier; 2010.

Khodaee M, Kelly BF. Peripheral nerve blocks. *In:* Pfenninger JL, Fowler GC, eds. *Pfenninger and Fowler's Procedures for Primary Care.* 3rd ed. Philadelphia: Mosby/Elsevier; 2010.

McDaniel WL, Jarris R. Local and topical anesthesia. *In:* Pfenninger JL, Fowler GC, eds. *Pfenninger and Fowler's Procedures for Primary Care.* 3rd ed. Philadelphia: Mosby/Elsevier; 2010.

Skoczlas L. Oral/facial anesthesia. *In:* Pfenninger JL, Fowler GC, eds. *Pfenninger and Fowler's Procedures for Primary Care.* 3rd ed. Philadelphia: Mosby/Elsevier; 2010.

Small R, Hoang D. Anesthesia. *In:* Small R, Hoang D, eds. *A Practical Guide to Dermal Filler Procedures.* Philadelphia: Lippincott Williams & Wilkins; 2011.

Small R, Zimmerman EM. Anesthesia. *In:* Small R, Zimmerman EM, eds. *A Practical Guide to Cosmetic Lasers.* Philadelphia: Lippincott Williams & Wilkins; 2012.

21 Botulinum Toxin

REBECCA SMALL, MD

Treatment of facial lines and wrinkles (also called rhytids) with botulinum toxin has become the most frequently performed cosmetic procedure in the United States, according to statistics from the American Society for Aesthetic Plastic Surgery.[1] It is also one of the most common entry procedures for health care professionals seeking to incorporate aesthetic procedures into their practice.[2]

As we age, the skin naturally thins, and repetitive contraction of the underlying facial musculature causes visible lines and wrinkles. Initially, these lines are seen only during facial expression with frowning, laughing, or smiling and are referred to as dynamic lines. Over time, however, dynamic lines may become etched into the skin, resulting in permanent or static lines. Botulinum toxin reduces unwanted dynamic lines, and to a lesser degree static lines, by relaxing hyperdynamic facial muscles and smoothing the overlying skin.

Botulinum toxin is a potent neurotoxin protein derived from the Clostridium botulinum bacterium. It reduces muscular contraction through inhibiting release of acetylcholine at the neuromuscular junction. Injection of small quantities of botulinum toxin into specifically targeted muscles causes localized, temporary chemical denervation with resultant muscle relaxation.[3]

Botulinum toxin has been used for more than 20 years to treat a variety of clinical conditions such as blepharospasm, strabismus, cervical dystonia, hyperhidrosis, migraines, and muscle spasticity.[4–6] Botulinum toxin is used in numerous facial aesthetic areas. However, treatment of the glabellar complex,[7] frontalis[8] and orbicularis oculi muscles,[9] which contribute to formation of frown lines, horizontal forehead lines, and crow's feet, respectively, offers the most predictable results, greatest efficacy, and fewest side effects.[10,11] Botulinum toxin treatment of hyperdynamic muscles in the upper one-third of the face are a core aesthetic procedure for providers interested in incorporating aesthetic care into office practice.[12]

COSMETIC INDICATIONS

- FDA approved for the temporary improvement of moderate to severe dynamic glabellar frown lines.
- FDA approved for adults ages 18 to 65. It is commonly used in patients older than 65, but treatments may be less effective if severe static wrinkling is present.
- Other cosmetic uses include reduction of wrinkles in upper, mid and lower face, neck, and upper chest.

ALTERNATIVE THERAPIES

Botulinum toxin is the only FDA-approved treatment for dynamic wrinkles. Static wrinkles can also be treated with chemical peels, microdermabrasion, topical products such as retinoids, nonablative lasers for soft-tissue coagulation and tightening using infrared and radio-frequency, nonablative lasers for collagen remodeling using 1320 and 1540 nm Q-switched lasers and others, and ablative and fractional ablative lasers using erbium and carbon dioxide. Limited data suggest that an acetylcholine blocker found in topical skin care products, acetyl hexapeptide-8, may reduce wrinkles.[13] However, additional studies are necessary to support this finding.

PRODUCTS CURRENTLY AVAILABLE

Clostridium botulinum produces eight serotypes of botulinum toxin proteins (A, B, Cα, Cβ, D, E, F, and G). Once activated, the botulinum toxin protein cleaves a docking protein on the internal surface of the neuronal membrane, SNAP-25, thereby inhibiting fusion and release of acetylcholine vesicles in the neuromuscular junction. Botulinum toxin serotype A is the most potent and is used for cosmetic treatments; serotype B is used for therapeutic indications. As of 2011, two botulinum toxin serotype A products had been approved by the U.S. Food and Drug Administration (FDA) for cosmetic use to treat the glabellar complex muscles that form frown lines: onabotulinumtoxinA (trade name Botox®) and abobotulinumtoxinA (trade name Dysport®). Both of these were formerly known as botulinum toxin type A. Botulinum toxin products are not interchangeable because they vary in their formulation characteristics, dosing, response, and complications. All references in this chapter to botulinum toxin refer specifically to onabotulinumtoxinA manufactured by Allergan as Botox.

CONTRAINDICATIONS

- Pregnancy or nursing
- Active infection in the treatment area (e.g., herpes simplex, pustular acne, or cellulitis)
- Hypertrophic or keloidal scarring
- Bleeding abnormality (e.g., thrombocytopenia or anticoagulant use)
- Impaired healing (e.g., due to immunosuppression)

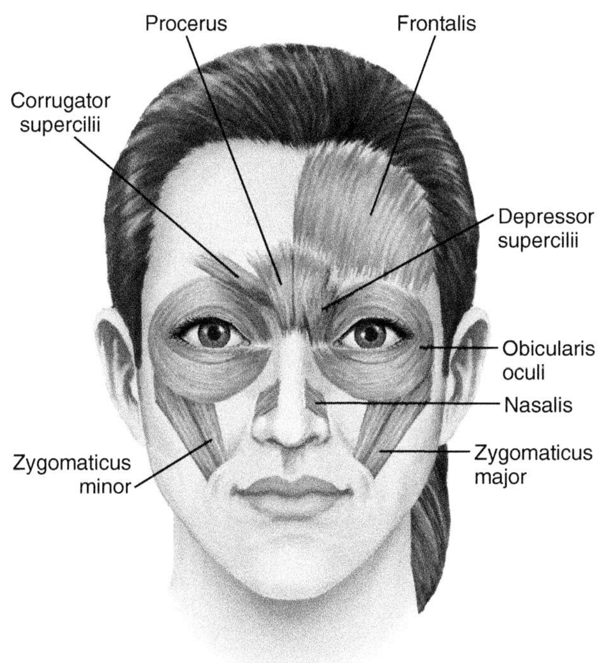

FIGURE 21-1 Musculature of the face.

- Skin atrophy (e.g., chronic oral steroid use or genetic syndromes such as Ehlers-Danlos syndrome)
- Dermatoses such as active psoriasis or eczema in the treatment area
- Uncontrolled systemic condition
- Sensitivity or allergy to constituents of Botox (i.e., botulinum toxin serotype A, human albumin, lactose, or sodium succinate)
- Gross motor weakness in the treatment area (e.g., due to a history of polio or Bell's palsy)
- Neuromuscular disorder including, but not limited to, amyotrophic lateral sclerosis, myasthenia gravis, Lambert-Eaton syndrome, and myopathies
- Inability to actively contract muscles in the treatment area prior to treatment
- Periocular/ocular surgery within the previous 6 months (e.g., laser-assisted *in situ* keratomileusis [LASIK] or blepharoplasty)
- Medications that inhibit neuromuscular signaling and may potentiate botulinum toxin effects, such as aminoglycosides, penicillamine, quinine, and calcium channel blockers
- Body dysmorphic disorder
- Unrealistic expectations
- Dependency on facial expression for livelihood (e.g., actors, singers).

ADVANTAGES OF BOTULINUM TOXIN

- Technically straightforward with short procedure time
- Safe and effective, particularly in the upper one-third of the face
- High patient satisfaction.

DISADVANTAGES OF BOTULINUM TOXIN

- Short duration of action relative to other cosmetic procedures, although effects are cumulative over time with recurring treatments.

ANATOMY

A thorough understanding of facial anatomy in the treatment areas is essential prior to performing botulinum toxin procedures (Figure 21-1). The muscles of facial expression are unique because, unlike most muscles, which have bony attachments, they have soft tissue attachments to the skin through the superficial muscular aponeurotic system. When a muscle contracts, the overlying skin moves with it and wrinkles are formed perpendicular to the direction of the muscle contraction. Figure 21-2 shows lines and wrinkles in the upper one-third of the face and the corresponding underlying musculature.

Glabellar wrinkles, or frown lines, are vertical lines that occur between the medial aspects of the eyebrows. The muscles that contribute to formation of frown lines are the glabellar complex depressor muscles, which pull the brows medially and inferiorly and include the corrugator supercilii, procerus, depressor

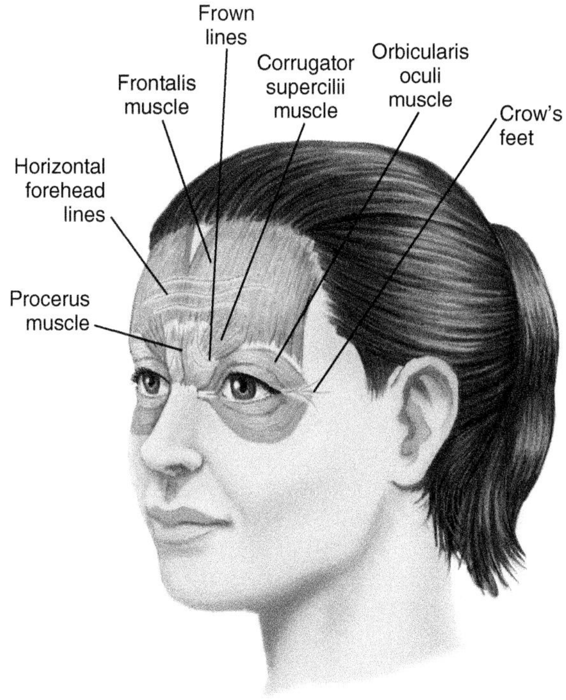

FIGURE 21-2 Musculature and wrinkles of the upper face.

Facial lines	Muscles	Actions
Frown lines	Corrugator supercilii	Eyebrows drawn medially
	Procerus and Depressor supercilii	Eyebrow depressors
Horizontal forehead lines	Frontalis	Eyebrow elevators
Crow's feet	Lateral orbicularis oculi	Eyebrow depressors

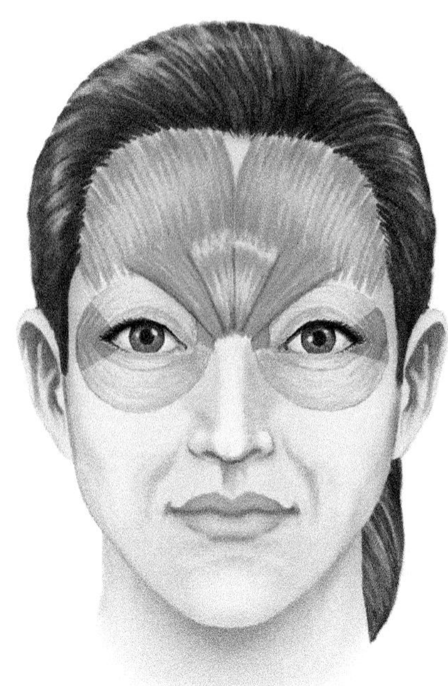

FIGURE 21-3 Functional anatomy of the upper face.

supercilii, and medial orbicularis oculi (Figures 21-1, 21-2 and 21-3).

Horizontal forehead lines result from contraction of the broad frontalis muscle, which spans the forehead between the temporal fusion lines (see Figures 21-1, 21-2 and 21-3). The muscle fibers are vertically oriented and contraction of this levator muscle raises the eyebrows. The inferior 2-cm portion has the most marked effect on eyebrow height and shape. The goal of treatment in this area is to partially inhibit activity of the frontalis muscle to reduce horizontal forehead lines while maintaining a desirable eyebrow shape and height.

Periorbital wrinkles, commonly known as crow's feet, result from contraction of the lateral portion of the orbicularis oculi, a thin, superficial muscle that encircles the eye (see Figures 21-1, 21-2 and 21-3). Contraction of the palpebral portion of the orbicularis oculi muscle results in closure of the eyelid. The goal of treatment in this area is to focally inhibit the lateral orbicularis oculi to reduce crow's feet without excessive orbicularis oculi muscle relaxation.

Many of the muscles of facial expression interdigitate with one another and, while providing treatment with botulinum toxin to one area in isolation will often provide adequate wrinkle reduction results, in some cases an adjacent muscle group may require concomitant treatment to achieve the desired results. For example, the glabellar complex muscles interdigitate to a greater or lesser degree with the frontalis muscle, and treatment of the frontalis in addition to treatment of the glabellar complex muscles may be required to smooth frown lines in some cases[14].

EQUIPMENT

Botox Reconstitution

- 5.0-mL syringe
- Botox, 100-unit vial
- 0.9% nonpreserved sterile saline, 10-mL vial
- 18-gauge 0.5-inch needle.

Botox Treatment

- Reconstituted Botox
- 1-mL BD Luer-Lok tip syringe
- 30-gauge 1-inch needle
- 30-gauge 0.5-inch needle
- 32-gauge 0.5-inch needle
- Gauze, 3 × 3 nonwoven
- Gloves, nonsterile
- Alcohol pads
- Ice pack.

RECONSTITUTION

Botox Cosmetic® is supplied as a powder which is reconstituted using saline. The manufacturer recommends using nonpreserved saline for reconstitution because it is alcohol free; however, some providers used preserved saline.

Injectors reconstitute Botox with differing amounts of saline and there is no standardized reconstitution protocol. Botox efficacy is based on the number of units injected rather than the dilution. However, diffusion and the risk of complications are related to greater dilution volumes.[15] The author's reconstitution technique is outlined below.

Reconstitute a 100-unit vial of Botox with 4.0 mL of 0.9% nonpreserved sterile saline. Using an 18-gauge needle with a 5.0-mL syringe, draw up 4.0 mL of saline. Insert the needle at a 45-degree angle into the Botox vial and inject saline slowly, maintaining upward plunger pressure so that the diluent runs down the sides of the vial. Gently swirl the reconstituted Botox vial and record the date and time of reconstitution on the vial. Note that alcohol can denature botulinum toxin and, therefore, bottle stoppers must be fully dry. Reconstitution of Botox powder using 4.0 mL of saline results in a concentration of 100 units of botulinum toxin per 4 mL (100 units/4 mL) or 2.5 units botulinum toxin per 0.1 mL increment on the 1.0-mL treatment syringe.

HANDLING AND STORAGE

Botox is shipped frozen, on dry ice. Prior to and after reconstitution it should be stored in the refrigerator at a temperature of 2 to 8°C (35.6 to 46.4°F). Prior to reconstitution it may be stored for 24 months. While the manufacturer recommends using Botox within 24 hours of reconstitution, the American Society for Plastic Surgery Botox Consensus Panel recommends using Botox within 6 weeks and notes no loss of potency during that time.[3,16]

PROCEDURE PREPARATION

1. Perform an aesthetic consultation and review the patient's medical history (see Chapter 19, *Aesthetic Principles and Consultation*).
2. Formulate a cosmetic treatment plan and record in the chart (see Chapter 19).
3. Obtain informed consent (see Chapter 19; also see Appendix A for an informed consent form and patient information handout titled *Botulinum Toxin Treatments*).
4. Take pretreatment photographs with the patient actively contracting the muscles in the intended treatment area and with the muscles at rest.
5. Document and discuss any notable asymmetries prior to treatment.
6. Minimize bruising by discontinuation of aspirin, vitamin E, St. John's wort, and other dietary supplements including ginkgo biloba, evening primrose oil, garlic, feverfew, and ginseng for 2 weeks prior to treatment. Discontinue other nonsteroidal anti-inflammatory medications and alcohol consumption 2 days prior to treatment.
7. Position the patient comfortably in a reclined position for the procedure, at about 65 degrees.
8. Cleanse the treatment areas with alcohol prior to injection and allow the alcohol to dry.
9. Anesthesia is not typically required for botulinum toxin treatments. If necessary, ice may be used prior to injections in all treatment areas except the crow's feet, because this makes identification and avoidance of veins more difficult.

BOTULINUM TOXIN: STEPS AND PRINCIPLES

General Treatment Technique

1. Injections are made into the "hill" of the contracted muscle.
2. Botulinum toxin is injected as the needle is withdrawn and should flow very easily, requiring only a light touch. If resistance is encountered, fully withdraw the needle and reinsert.
3. Avoid intravascular injection. Intravascular injection is apparent when the surrounding skin blanches during injection. If this occurs, withdraw the needle partially from the blanched site, reposition, and inject.
4. Avoid hitting the periosteum, particularly with frontalis muscle treatments, because this is painful and dulls the needle.
5. If bleeding occurs, apply firm pressure directed away from the eye and achieve hemostasis before proceeding to subsequent injection points.
6. The recommended starting doses in the following sections are intended as general guidelines and may be adjusted at the time of treatment. The botulinum toxin dose required for an effective treatment is based on the muscle mass present, which can vary between individuals. For example, men typically have greater muscle mass and, therefore, require larger doses than women for treatment of the same muscle groups.

FROWN LINES

Frown lines often convey anger, frustration, and irritation, and reduction of frown lines is a common aesthetic request. Botulinum toxin treatment of the glabellar complex muscles offers dramatic improvements in frown lines.

Botulinum toxin is placed within the Glabellar Complex Safety Zone. This region is bounded by two vertical lines at the lateral limbus that extend superiorly from the supraorbital ridge to the hair line. The lateral-most injection point for corrugator muscle injections should be 1 cm or above the supraorbital ridge at the lateral limbus line (Figure 21-4) to minimize the risk of blepharoptosis (droopy upper eyelid).

Most patients desire little to no movement of the glabellar complex muscles, however, this should be discussed with the patient prior to treatment. An overview of botulinum toxin injection points and starting doses for treatment of frown lines is shown in Figure 21-5. The starting dose for women is 20 units (0.8 mL of Botox reconstituted to 100 units/4 mL) and for men 25 units (1.0 mL of Botox reconstituted to 100 units/4 mL).

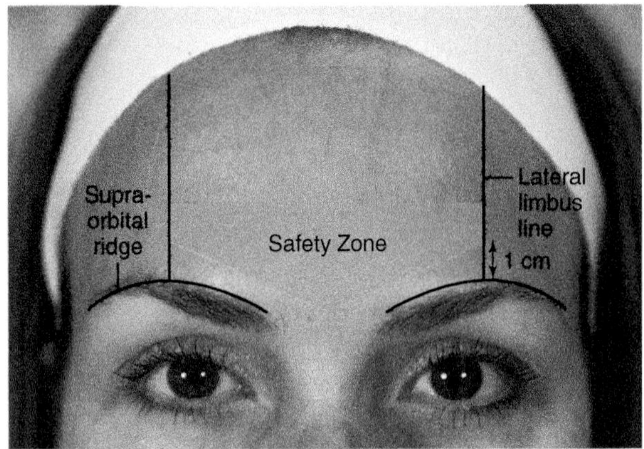

FIGURE 21-4 Glabellar Complex Safety Zone. *(Copyright Rebecca Small, MD.)*

Performing Botulinum Toxin Injections for Frown Lines

1. The glabellar muscles require deep intramuscular injection and a 30-gauge 1-inch needle is used.
2. The first injection point is at the lateral margin of the corrugator within the Glabellar Complex Safety Zone. Identify the lateral margin of the corrugator by directing the patient to actively frown. Inject 2.5 units of botulinum toxin 1 cm above the supraorbital ridge, at the visible margin of the corrugator. Insert the needle to one-half depth.

   CAUTION: Injection interior to the Safety Zone at the lateral limbus line increases the risk of blepharoptosis.

   CAUTION: Injection lateral to the Safety Zone increases the risk of eyebrow ptosis (droopy upper eyelid).
3. The second injection point is in the body of the corrugator, approximately 1 cm medial and inferior to the first injection point, closer to the eyebrow. Direct the needle toward the procerus muscle, inserting the needle to the hub, and inject 5 units of botulinum toxin. Repeat corrugator muscle injections for the contralateral side of the face.
4. The third injection point is in the procerus muscle. The procerus is approached inferiorly with the needle directed toward the forehead. While the patient frowns, insert the needle into the procerus to one-half depth and inject 2.5 to 5 units of botulinum toxin.

HORIZONTAL FOREHEAD LINES

Treatment of the frontalis muscle with botulinum toxin reduces horizontal forehead lines and can also affect eyebrow shape and height. Patients are assessed prior to treatment for the presence of eyebrow ptosis and dermatochalasis (upper eyelid laxity) with the frontalis muscle at rest. Frontalis muscle contraction is often compensatory to elevate low-set eyebrows or alleviate upper eyelid skin laxity, and treatment should be avoided in patients with these characteristics.

Botulinum toxin is placed within the Frontalis Safety Zone to minimize the risk of eyebrow ptosis and preserve eyebrow shape and height. The Frontalis Safety Zone is bounded by two vertical lines at the lateral limbus, and includes the area 2 cm above the supraorbital ridge to the hair line, as well as a small area lateral to the vertical lines approximately 2 cm inferior to the hair line (Figure 21-6).

The goal of frontalis muscle treatment is to reduce horizontal forehead lines while maintaining a desirable eyebrow shape. In women, high arched eyebrows are often desired and minimizing botulinum toxin placement in the lateral frontalis muscle will help preserve the arch. In men, a flat eyebrow shape is usually preferable, and can be achieved by placement of botulinum toxin more inferiorly in the lateral frontalis, taking care to avoid eyebrow ptosis.

An overview of botulinum toxin injection points and starting doses for treatment of horizontal forehead lines is shown in Figure 21-7. The starting dose for women is 15 to 22.5 units (0.6 to 0.9 mL of Botox reconstituted to 100 units/4 mL) and for men 20 to 25 units (0.8 to 1.0 mL of Botox reconstituted to 100 units/4 mL).

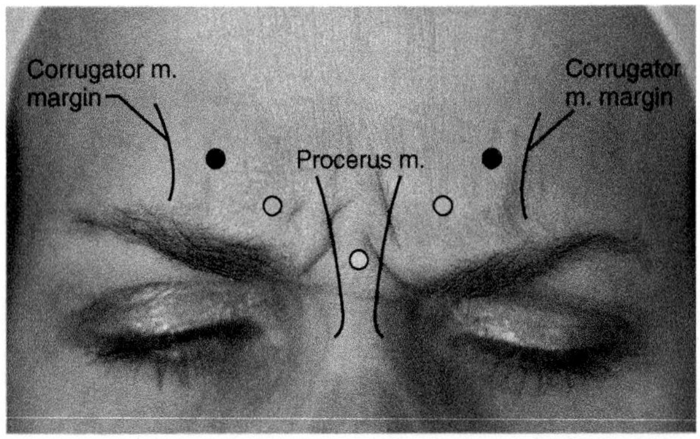

FIGURE 21-5 Glabellar complex botulinum toxin injection points and doses. *(Copyright Rebecca Small, MD.)*

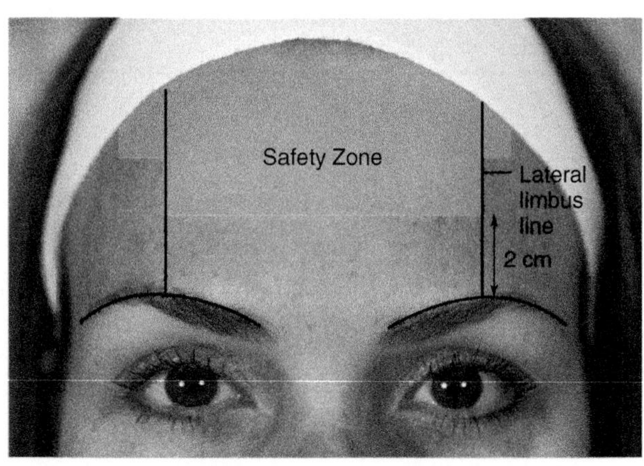

FIGURE 21-6 Frontalis Safety Zone. *(Copyright Rebecca Small, MD.)*

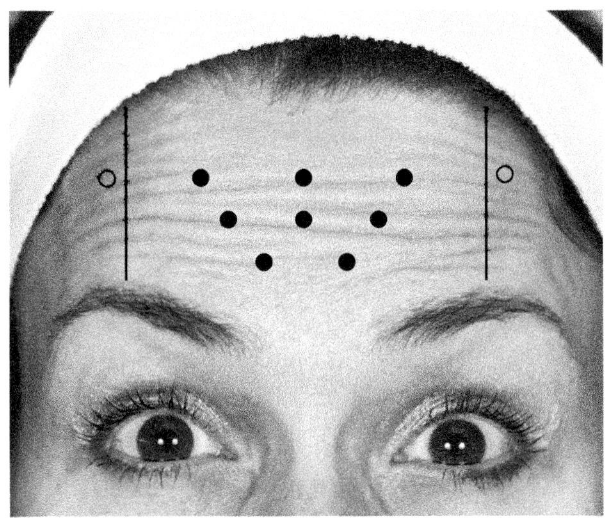

FIGURE 21-7 Frontalis muscle botulinum toxin injection points and doses. *(Copyright Rebecca Small, MD.)*

Performing Botulinum Toxin Injections for Horizontal Forehead Lines

1. Identify the horizontal ridges of the frontalis muscle by directing the patient to actively raise the eyebrows as if surprised. While standing in front of the patient, insert a 30-gauge 0.5-inch needle at a 30-degree angle to the forehead, into the "hill" of the contracted muscle. Inject 2.5 units of botulinum toxin to raise a wheal.
   CAUTION: Avoid injecting too deeply and hitting the periosteum.
2. Continue laterally along each horizontal ridge of frontalis muscle within the Frontalis Safety Zone lines, injecting 2.5 units of botulinum toxin approximately 1 cm apart. Perform botulinum toxin injections evenly across the forehead to achieve symmetry.
   TIP: Changing needles after six or more injections will maintain a sharp needle and minimize discomfort.
3. The last injection is placed at the maximal point of eyebrow elevation, typically located just lateral to the Safety Zone line, about 2 cm below the hairline, and 1.25 units of botulinum toxin are injected. Repeat for the contralateral side.
   TIP: Omission of this injection may result in a peaked eyebrow shape and subsequently require a touch-up procedure.
   TIP: As a general rule, injections are placed above the lowest forehead wrinkle to minimize effects on eyebrow height and to concentrate botulinum toxin only in the frontalis muscle.

CROW'S FEET

Botulinum toxin can dramatically reduce the appearance of periocular lines, or crow's feet by relaxing the lateral portion of the orbicularis oculi muscles. The pattern of crow's feet varies, with some extending superiorly toward the eyebrow and others extending inferiorly toward the cheek. Optimal results with botulinum toxin treatments in the crow's feet area are achieved by adapting the injection technique outlined below to the patient's pattern of crow's feet.

Botulinum toxin is placed within the Crow's Feet Safety Zone to minimize the risk of globe trauma and upper lip ptosis. The Crow's Feet Safety Zone is 1 cm outside of the orbital rim, above the level of the zygoma; it extends under the eyebrow to the lateral limbus line (Figures 21-8A and B). Botulinum toxin is concentrated within the Central Crow's Feet Safety Zone, but injections may be placed in the Extended Safety Zone according to the patient's anatomy.

The goal of treatment in the lateral orbicularis oculi muscle is to reduce crow's feet lines and elevate the lateral eyebrow. An overview of botulinum toxin injection points and doses for treatment of crow's feet is shown in Figure 21-9. The total (bilateral) starting dose for women is 15 to 20 units (0.6 to 0.8 mL of Botox reconstituted to 100 units/4 mL) and for men 20 to 25 units (0.8 to 1.0 mL of Botox reconstituted to 100 units/4 mL).

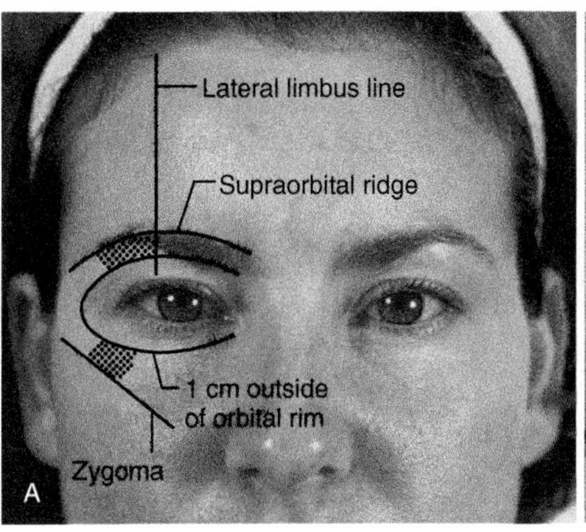

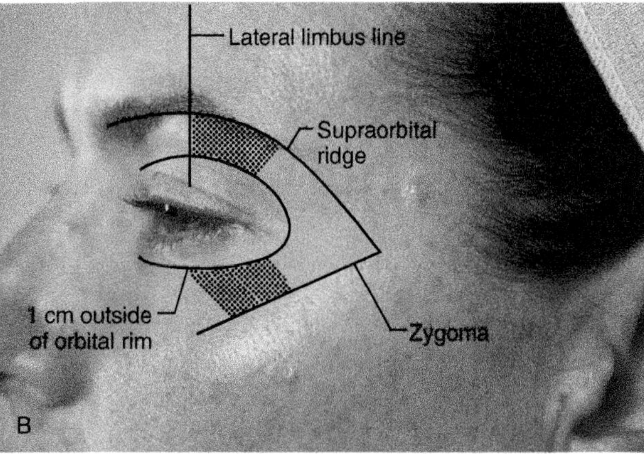

□ Central Crow's Feet Safety Zone ▦ Extended Crow's Feet Safety Zone

FIGURE 21-8 (A, B) Crow's Feet Safety Zone. *(Copyright Rebecca Small, MD.)*

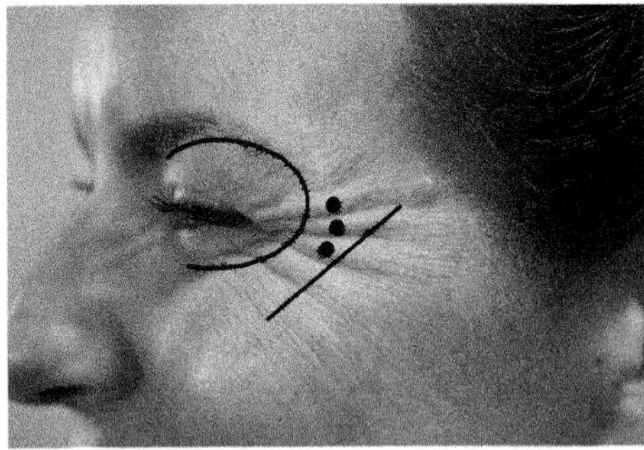

FIGURE 21-9 Orbicularis oculi muscle botulinum toxin injection points and doses. *(Copyright Rebecca Small, MD.)*

Performing Botulinum Toxin Injections for Crow's Feet

1. The orbicularis oculi muscle is a thin, superficial muscle, and botulinum toxin is placed subdermally using a 30- or 32-gauge 0.5-inch needle to raise a wheal at each injection point. After each injection, apply firm pressure away from the eye to compress the wheal.
2. The first injection point is at the lateral canthal line, 1 cm outside of the orbital rim. Direct the patient to first smile and then squint to elicit contraction of the orbicularis oculi muscle. Inject 2.5 units of botulinum toxin subdermally into the "hill" of the contracted muscle.
3. The second injection point is approximately 0.5 cm superior to the first injection point and 2.5 units of botulinum should be injected.
4. The third injection point is approximately 0.5 cm inferior to the first injection point. The needle should be angled inferiorly and threaded superficially to the hub, and 2.5 units of botulinum toxin injected as the needle is withdrawn. Repeat injections for the contralateral orbicularis oculi muscle.
   TIP: Bruising is the most common side effect of the crow's feet procedure. Look for and avoid veins, which are best seen with oblique lighting.
   CAUTION: Avoid injecting too deeply and too inferiorly below the level of the zygoma, to avoid the zygomatic muscles. Relaxation of these muscles may result in cheek and lip ptosis.

RESULTS AND FOLLOW-UP

Partial reduction in muscle function is typically seen by the third day after botulinum toxin treatment. Maximal reduction in function of the targeted muscles is visible 1 to 2 weeks after treatment. Botulinum toxin effects are most noticeable for treatment of dynamic lines. Static lines are slower to respond, usually requiring two or three consecutive botulinum toxin treatments. Deep, static lines, particularly in the glabellar complex area may not fully respond even after multiple treatments, and combination treatment with dermal fillers may be necessary to achieve reduction of these severe frown lines.

If excessive muscle activity persists in the treated area, a touch-up procedure may be performed 2 weeks after the initial treatment. The touch-up dose is based on the degree of movement remaining in the treated muscle and may range from 2.5 to 10 units. Reassess the treatment area 2 weeks after the touch-up procedure. Photographs are taken at each visit for documentation.

Return of muscle function in the treated area is gradual, typically 2½ to 4 months after treatment, based on the area treated and botulinum toxin dose. Patients should follow up for subsequent treatments when muscles in the treated areas begin to contract, prior to facial lines returning to their pretreatment appearance.[17]

Treatment of the glabellar complex muscles with botulinum toxin results in a dramatic improvement of dynamic frown lines, as well as marked elevation in medial eyebrow position post-treatment due to the lack of depressor muscle function (Figures 21-10A and B). The duration of botulinum toxin effects in the glabellar complex for frown lines is typically 3 to 4 months.

Patients receiving botulinum toxin treatments for horizontal forehead lines are usually seen in follow-up 2 weeks after treatment to evaluate eyebrow symmetry and shape at rest and with active elevation. Figure 21-11A shows a patient with dynamic horizontal forehead lines prior to treatment, and Figure 21-11B shows the patient 1 week after receiving 22.5 units of botulinum toxin in the frontalis muscle with mildly peaked eyebrows. A peaked eyebrow shape, or "quizzical brow" is treated with 1.25 to 2.5 units of botulinum toxin just inferior to the lateral Frontalis Safety Zone, in line with the most peaked portion of the eyebrow. Figure 21-11C shows the same patient 3 weeks after receiving 1.25

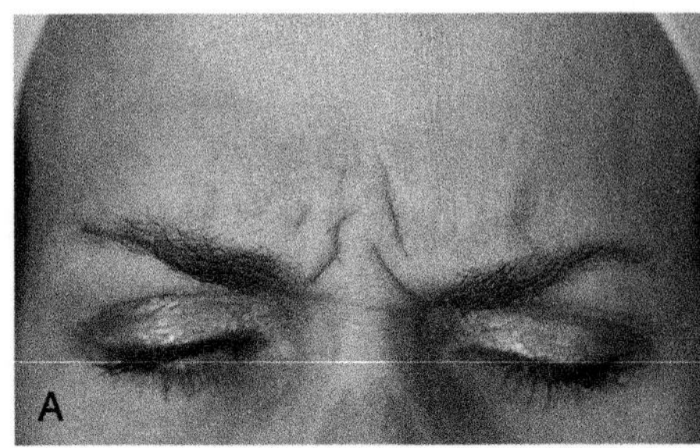

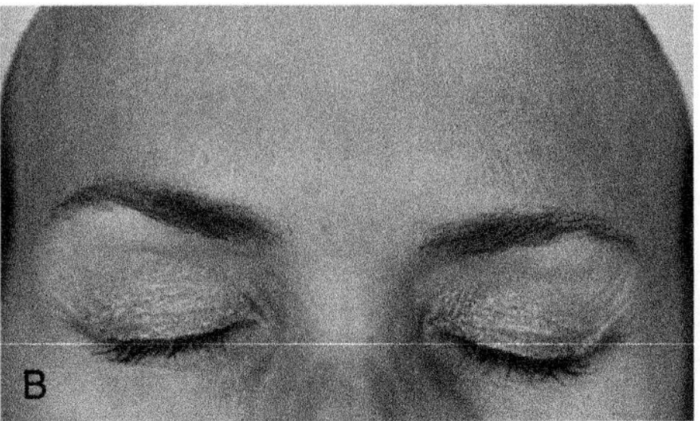

FIGURE 21-10 (A) Before botulinum toxin treatment with active frowning. (B) One month after botulinum toxin treatment with active frowning. *(Copyright Rebecca Small, MD.)*

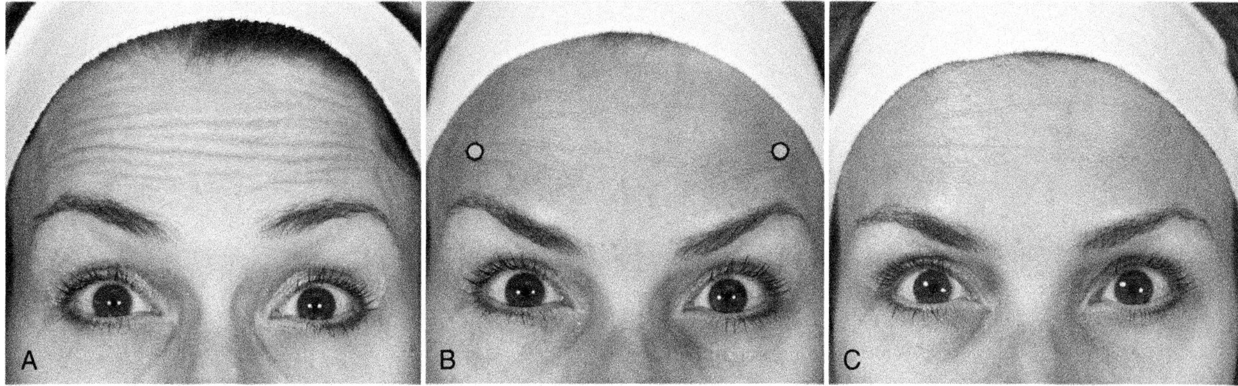

FIGURE 21-11 (A) Before botulinum toxin treatment with active eyebrow elevation. (B) One week after botulinum toxin treatment demonstrating peaked eyebrows with active eyebrow elevation. (C) Three weeks after botulinum toxin touch-up treatment with active eyebrow elevation. *(Copyright Rebecca Small, MD.)*

units of botulinum toxin above each peaked eyebrow and represents her final result. The duration of botulinum toxin effects in the frontalis muscle for reduction of horizontal forehead lines is typically 3 to 4 months.

Treatment of the lateral orbicularis oculi muscle with botulinum toxin results in reduction of crow's feet and elevates the lateral eyebrow (Figures 21-12A and B). Patients receiving botulinum toxin treatment for crow's feet should be seen in follow-up 2 weeks after treatment to evaluate for compensatory contraction of the orbicularis oculi muscle adjacent to the treated area. Adjacent orbicularis oculi contraction is treated with 1.25 to 2.5 units of botulinum toxin in the region of orbicularis oculi muscle showing excessive activity, within the Crow's Feet Safety Zone. The duration of botulinum toxin effects in the orbicularis oculi muscles for reduction of crow's feet is typically 2½ to 3 months.

AFTERCARE

On the day of treatment, instruct the patient to avoid manipulating the treated area, lying down for 4 hours immediately after treatment and activities that cause facial flushing including application of heat to the face, alcohol consumption, exercising and tanning. Avoiding these actions will help reduce the likelihood of product migration and side effects. If bruising occurs, a soft ice pack may be applied for 10 to 15 minutes to each site, every 1 to 2 hours until resolved.

COMPLICATIONS

Complications and side effects can be grouped into injection-related and botulinum toxin–related issues. Complications related to botulinum toxin occur less frequently, are usually technique dependent, and the incidence declines as injector skill improves.

Injection-Related

- Bruising
- Erythema
- Tenderness
- Swelling
- Infection
- Numbness or dysesthesia
- Headache.

Botulinum Toxin–Related

- Localized burning or stinging pain during injection
- Facial asymmetry
- Blepharoptosis (eyelid droop), 1% to 5%

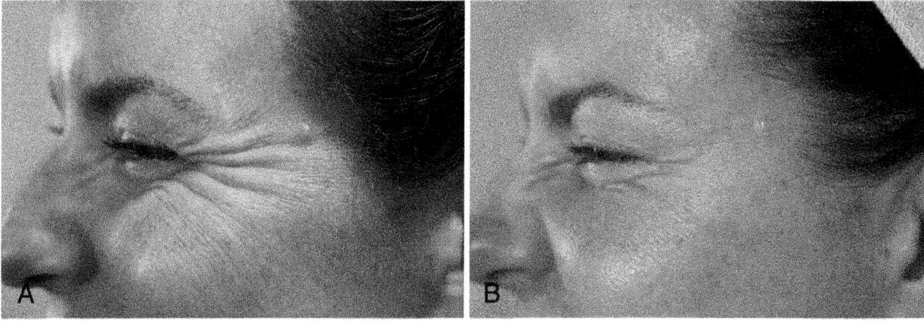

FIGURE 21-12 (A) Before botulinum toxin treatment with active squinting. (B) One month after botulinum toxin treatment with active squinting. *(Copyright Rebecca Small, MD.)*

- Diplopia, blurry vision
- Eyebrow ptosis (eyebrow droop)
- Oral incompetence with crow's feet treatment
- Ectropion
- Autoantibodies against botulinum toxin may be present or develop after treatments rendering treatments ineffective (1% to 2% of patients treated for cosmetic indications per Allergan)
- Poor aesthetic result
- Extremely rare, immediate hypersensitivity reaction with signs of urticaria, edema, and a remote possibility of anaphylaxis
- Case reports of side effects due to distant spread from the site of injection have been reported with large doses of botulinum toxin, including generalized muscle weakness, ptosis, dysphagia, dysarthria, urinary incontinence, respiratory difficulties, and death due to respiratory compromise.[18]

Temporary blepharoptosis can occur as a complication with treatment of the glabellar complex muscles for frown lines, particularly if botulinum toxin is injected inferior to the Glabellar Complex Safety Zone, too close to the supraorbital ridge at the lateral limbus. Figure 21-13 shows a patient 3 weeks after botulinum toxin treatment (not by the author) in the glabellar complex muscles with a profound right-sided blepharoptosis and mild right eyebrow ptosis. Blepharoptosis is infrequent (1% to 5%)[7] and is almost always unilateral. It results from migration of botulinum toxin through the orbital septum fascia to the upper eyelid levator muscle, levator palpebrae superioris. At the bony supraorbital margin in the mid-eyebrow, some of the levator palpebrae superioris muscle fibers pass up through the orbital septum, and botulinum toxin can more easily migrate into and relax the levator palpebrae superioris from this site. Blepharoptosis is typically seen as a 2- to 3-mm lowering of the affected eyelid, which is most marked at the end of the day with muscle fatigue. It usually resolves spontaneously within 6 weeks.

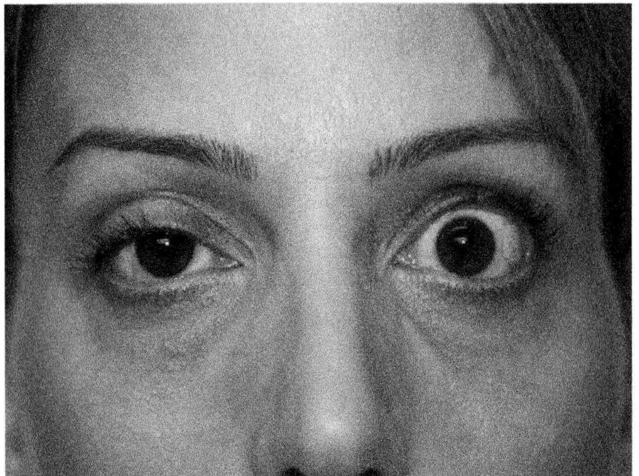

FIGURE 21-13 Right-sided blepharoptosis 3 weeks after botulinum toxin treatment for frown lines (not performed by the author). *(Copyright Rebecca Small, MD.)*

Blepharoptosis can be treated using over-the-counter alpha-adrenergic eye drops such as Naphcon-A, 1 drop four times per day in the affected eye, or prescription Iopidine (apraclonidine), 0.5% solution, 1 to 2 drops three times per day. Both of these medications cause contraction of Mueller's muscle, an adrenergic levator muscle of the upper eyelid, which results in elevation of the upper eyelid. Iopidine should be used with caution because it can exacerbate or unmask underlying glaucoma and is reserved for refractory cases.[19]

Severe complications resulting from distant spread of botulinum toxin from the site of injection such as generalized muscle weakness, ptosis, dysphagia, dysarthria, urinary incontinence, respiratory difficulties, and death due to respiratory compromise have been reported in patients receiving very large doses of botulinum toxin (e.g., 300 units in the calves[20]) and have not been reported with cosmetic use of botulinum toxin at the labeled dose of 20 units (for glabellar lines) or 100 units (for severe primary axillary hyperhidrosis). These symptoms have been reported hours to weeks after injection. The risk of symptoms is presumed to be greatest in children treated for clinical conditions such as spasticity, particularly in patients with compromised baseline respiratory function.

LEARNING THE TECHNIQUES

Begin with conservative doses and ensure botulinum toxin injection is within the defined Safety Zones. Additional botulinum toxin can be added if required at subsequent visits. Marking injection sites initially using a marker or soft white eyeliner pencil is helpful with placement, but lengthens the visit time.

Consider performing initial treatments on staff and family as feedback will be available and the evolution of botulinum toxin effects may be closely observed and touch-up procedures may be performed if necessary. Receiving a treatment is one of the best ways to gain knowledge about botulinum toxin treatments.

CURRENT DEVELOPMENTS

AbobotulinumtoxinA (trade name Dysport®, see the *Resources* section below) was FDA approved in 2009 for cosmetic use to treat glabellar frown lines. It is estimated that Dysport requires 2.5 to 3 times the number of units to achieve effects equivalent to Botox,[21] but may have a more rapid onset of action.[22]

Several new botulinum toxin products for cosmetic use are in clinical trials or in the FDA approval process. PurTox (Mentor Corporation) and Xeomin (Merz Pharmaceuticals) are injectable botulinum toxin formulations that are under investigation for cosmetic use and in clinical trials for approval in the United States.

A physician-applied topical botulinum toxin by ReVance Therapeutics shows promise for the treatment of axillary hyperhidrosis[23] and is under investigation for cosmetic applications including treatment of crow's feet. The company claims to have a novel method of delivery of topical products (TransMTS™) that allows for macromolecules such as botulinum toxin to penetrate beneath the skin and reach the neuromuscular junction.

FINANCIAL CONSIDERATIONS

Cosmetic botulinum toxin treatments are not covered by insurance. Fees for botulinum toxin injections may be based on the number of units used, or based on the number of treatment sites, where a site is the glabellar complex, frontalis or orbicularis oculi muscles. Pricing per unit has the potential for patients to request the dose that they desire for treatment, which can impact efficacy and outcomes. The author prefers pricing per site, which includes a touch-up procedure if necessary, to enhance outcomes and patient satisfaction. Prices vary according to local pricing, and range from $10 to $20 per unit or $250 to $500 per site.

CONCLUSION

Botulinum toxin is the treatment of choice for lines and wrinkles occurring in the upper one-third of the face, particularly frown lines, horizontal forehead lines, and crow's feet. Treatments in these areas offer the most predictable results, are highly effective with few side effects, and are essential procedures for providers incorporating aesthetics into office practice.

Resources

Allergan (Botox)
Phone: 800-377-7790
www.allergan.com

Medicis Pharmaceutical (Dysport)
Phone: 602-808-8800
www.medicis.com

Mentor Corporation (PurTox)
Phone: 805-879-6000
www.mentorcorp.com

Merz Pharmaceuticals (Xeomin)
Phone: 888-637-9872
www.merzusa.com

ReVance Therapeutics (topical botulinum toxin)
Phone: 510-742-3400
www.revance.com

References

1. Cosmetic Surgery National Data Bank 2008 Statistics. American Society for Aesthetic Plastic Surgery; 2008.
2. Small R. Aesthetic procedures in office practice. *Am Fam Physician.* 2009;80(11):1231–1237.
3. Carruthers JD, Fagien S, Matarasso SL. Consensus recommendations on the use of botulinum toxin type a in facial aesthetics. *Plast Reconstr Surg.* 2004;114(6 Suppl):1S–22S.
4. Training guidelines for the use of botulinum toxin for the treatment of neurologic disorders. Report of the Therapeutics and Technology Assessment Subcommittee of the American Academy of Neurology. *Neurology.* 1994;44:2401–2403.
5. Naumann MK, Lowe NJ. Botulinum toxin type A in treatment of bilateral primary axillary hyperhidrosis: randomised, parallel group, double blind, placebo controlled trial. *Br Med J.* 2001;323(7313):596–599.
6. Silberstein S, Matthew N, Saper J, *et al.* Botulinum toxin type A as a migraine preventive treatment. *Headache.* 2000;40(6): 445–450.
7. Carruthers JA, Lowe NJ, Menter MA, *et al.* A multicenter, double-blind, randomized, placebo-controlled study of the efficacy and safety of botulinum toxin type A in the treatment of glabellar lines. *J Am Acad Dermatol.* 2002;46(6):840–849.
8. Carruthers A, Carruthers J, Cohen JL. A prospective, double-blind, randomized, parallel-group, dose-ranging study of botulinum toxin type a in female subjects with horizontal forehead rhytides. *Derm Surg.* 2003;29(5):461–467.
9. Lowe NJ, Lask GP, Yamauchi PS, *et al.* Bilateral, double-blind, randomized comparison of 3 doses of botulinum toxin type A and placebo in patients with crow's feet. *J Am Acad Dermatol.* 2002;47(6):834–840.
10. Maas CS. Botulinum neurotoxins and injectable fillers: minimally invasive management of the aging upper face. *Facial Plast Surg Clin North Am.* 2006;14(3):241–245.
11. Carruthers JD, Carruthers A. The use of botulinum toxin type A in the upper face. *Facial Plast Surg Clin North Am.* 2006; 14(3):253–260.
12. Small R. Aesthetic procedures introduction. In: Mayeaux E, ed. *The Essential Guide to Primary Care Procedures.* Philadelphia: Lippincott Williams & Wilkins; 2009:195–199.
13. Fields K, Falla TJ, Rodan K, et al. Bioactive peptides: signaling the future. *J Cosm Derm.* 2009;8:8–13.
14. Zimmerman EM. Botulinum toxin. In: Pfenninger J, Fowler G, eds. *Pfenninger and Fowler's Procedures for Primary Care.* Philadelphia: Mosby/Elsevier; 2010.
15. Carruthers A, Bogle M, Carruthers JD, et al. A randomized, evaluator-blinded, two-center study of the safety and effect of volume on the diffusion and efficacy of botulinum toxin type A in the treatment of lateral orbital rhytides. *Dermatol Surg.* 2007;33(5):567–571.
16. Hexsel DM, De Almeida AT, Rutowitsch M, et al. Multicenter, double-blind study of the efficacy of injections with botulinum toxin type A reconstituted up to six consecutive weeks before application. *Derm Surg.* 2003;29(5):523–529.
17. Small R. Botulinum toxin type A for facial rejuvenation. In: Mayeaux E, ed. *The Essential Guide to Primary Care Procedures.* Philadelphia: Lippincott Williams & Wilkins; 2009:200–213.
18. Allergan Inc. *Botox cosmetic (onabotulinumtoxin A) purified neurotoxin complex package insert.* Irvine, CA: Allergan Inc.; 2010.
19. Fagien S. Temporary management of upper lid ptosis, lid malposition, and eyelid fissure asymmetry with botulinum toxin type A. *Plast Reconstr Surg.* 2004;114(7):1892–1902.
20. Nong LB, He WQ, Xu YH, et al. [Severe respiratory failure after injection of botulinum toxin: case report and review of the literature]. *Chinese J Tuberculosis Resp Dis.* 2008;31(5): 369–371.
21. Monheit GD, Carruthers A, Brandt FS, et al. A randomized, double-blind, placebo-controlled study of botulinum toxin type A for the treatment of glabellar lines: determination of optimal dose. *Derm Surg.* 2007;33(1 Spec No.):S51–S59.
22. Lowe P, Patnaik R, Lowe NJ. Comparison of two formulations of botulinum toxin type A for the treatment of glabellar lines: a double-blind, randomized study. *J Am Acad Dermatol.* 2006; 55(6):975–980.
23. Glogau RG. Topically applied botulinum toxin type A for the treatment of primary axillary hyperhidrosis: results of a randomized, blinded, vehicle-controlled study. *Derm Surg.* 2007;33(1): S76–S80.

Additional Reading

Small R, Hoang D. Botulinum toxin introduction and foundation concepts. *In:* Small R, Hoang D, eds. *A Practical Guide to Botulinum Toxin Procedures*. Philadelphia: Lippincott Williams & Wilkins, 2011.

Small R, Hoang D. Crow's feet. *In:* Small R, Hoang D, eds. *A Practical Guide to Botulinum Toxin Procedures*. Philadelphia: Lippincott Williams & Wilkins, 2011.

Small R, Hoang D. Frown lines. *In:* Small R, Hoang D, eds. *A Practical Guide to Botulinum Toxin Procedures*. Philadelphia: Lippincott Williams & Wilkins, 2011.

Small R, Hoang D. Horizontal forehead lines. *In:* Small R, Hoang D, eds. *A Practical Guide to Botulinum Toxin Procedures*. Philadelphia: Lippincott Williams & Wilkins, 2011.

22 Chemical Peels

REBECCA SMALL, MD • KATHLEEN O'HANLON, MD

Chemical peeling is a skin resurfacing procedure that utilizes topical agents to remove the outermost layers of the skin.[1] This controlled method of wounding stimulates a reparative healing response with regeneration of a healthier epidermis and dermis. Chemical peeling, also called chemexfoliation, is commonly used for skin rejuvenation to improve photodamage, reduce hyperpigmentation and acne, and smooth rough skin texture and superficial scarring.[2]

As with all skin resurfacing procedures, deeper penetration into the skin is associated with greater potential benefits. However, risks and complications also increase with greater depths of penetration into the skin. The depth of penetration achieved with chemical peels ranges from the superficial epidermis to deep dermis. Standard terminology for skin resurfacing depths is illustrated in Figure 19-12 in Chapter 19, *Aesthetic Principles and Consultation*. The focus of this chapter is *light chemical peels*, which include very superficial chemical peels that remove the stratum corneum, and superficial chemical peels that remove the entire epidermis and may extend to the upper papillary dermis.[3]

Chemical peels are one of the most common cosmetic procedures performed in the United States, ranking closely behind botulinum toxin, laser hair removal, and dermal fillers, according to data from the American Society for Aesthetic Plastic Surgery.[4] They are technically straightforward to perform and, with minimal start-up costs, they are often one of the first aesthetic procedures incorporated into office practice.[1,5] Chemical peels can be readily combined with other minimally invasive aesthetic modalities such as microdermabrasion, topical products, and nonablative lasers to enhance skin rejuvenation results.

PATIENT SELECTION

While almost any patient will derive benefit from light chemical peels, patients with mild to moderate photoaging changes such as solar lentigines, skin dullness, rough texture[6–8] (e.g., Glogau types I and II), and acneic conditions[9,10] typically derive the most noticeable benefits (see Chapter 19 for a description of Glogau types). Results with light chemical peels are slow and progressive, requiring a series of treatments for improvements to become evident. Light peels may also improve fine lines, coarse pores, and superficial atrophic scarring,[7] but results are not comparable to more aggressive forms of skin resurfacing, such as medium-depth peels or laser resurfacing. Assessment of patients' expectations at the time of consultation and commitment to a series of treatments is essential to ensure success with these treatments.

Very superficial chemical peels (e.g., glycolic acid 20%, salicylic acid 20% and retinol) can be used in all skin types (Fitzpatrick types I through VI). Patients with darker skin types (IV through VI) have increased risks with aesthetic procedures, particularly postinflammatory hyperpigmentation, and these gentle peels are one of the treatment options available to manage aesthetic skin conditions in darker skin types such as acne, enlarged pores, and hyperpigmentation (see Chapter 19 for a description of Fitzpatrick skin types).[11–14] A conservative approach for providers getting started with superficial chemical peels (e.g., glycolic acid 70%, trichloroacetic acid 20% to 30%, and Jessner's 4 to 7 layers) is to restrict use of these peels to lighter skin types (Fitzpatrick types I through III) to minimize the risk of complications.

Patients with erythematous conditions such as rosacea, telangiectasias, and poikiloderma of Civatte are also treated conservatively with light chemical peels, as aggressive chemical peels may exacerbate erythema associated with these conditions.[15]

INDICATIONS

- Photodamaged skin
- Hyperpigmentation (e.g., solar lentigines, melasma, postinflammatory hyperpigmentation)
- Dull, sallow skin color
- Comedonal acne (whiteheads and blackheads); also called clogged pores or skin congestion by laypersons
- Papulopustular conditions including acne vulgaris, acne rosacea, pseudofolliculitis barbae
- Rough skin texture
- Enlarged pores
- Fine lines
- Atrophic scars (e.g., acne and chicken pox scars)
- Keratosis pilaris
- Thickened scaling skin (e.g., ichthyosis)
- Early thin seborrheic keratoses
- Actinic keratoses
- Enhanced penetration of topical products.

While the superficial and very superficial peels discussed in this chapter are appropriate for the above indications, some subtle trends for selecting one peel over another exist with regard to indication. Salicylic and glycolic acid are often used for oily skin and acneic conditions; lactic acid for dehydration; mandelic acid for sensitive skin; and retinoids for augmenting other peels they are combined with to enhance skin sloughing.

ALTERNATIVE THERAPIES

Microdermabrasion (MDA) is comparable to a superficial chemical peel in terms of the depth of resurfacing, and is a reasonable alternative treatment for skin rejuvenation. MDA offers certain advantages over chemical peels such as greater control over the depth of exfoliation, comparatively less discomfort, and no "downtime" for skin flaking and peeling. However, MDA equipment is more costly than chemical peels. Superficial dermaplaning, which uses a specialized scalpel blade that is gently scraped across the skin, is another alternative method of exfoliation and is particularly useful for patients with erythematous conditions such as rosacea.

Deeper skin resurfacing can be achieved using more aggressive procedures such as medium-depth chemical peels or laser resurfacing. Laser resurfacing may be performed as an ablative procedure, where the epidermis is removed (e.g., with the 2940 nm wavelength), or as a nonablative procedure, where the epidermis remains intact (e.g., with the 1550 nm wavelength). Relative to light chemical peels, laser resurfacing and deeper chemical peels offer significantly greater reduction of wrinkles and improvements in photodamaged skin. However, these more aggressive resurfacing procedures have longer recovery times and greater risks of complications.

Light chemical peels will not improve deep wrinkles related to volume loss and hyperdynamic musculature, which respond to treatment with dermal fillers and botulinum toxin, respectively.

PRODUCTS CURRENTLY AVAILABLE

Numerous chemical peels are available and common agents, along with their typical depth of skin penetration, are summarized in Figure 22-1.[15–18] Many factors influence the depth of penetration with chemical peels, and although a given chemical peel may be classified as a superficial peeling agent, in practice, peels may vary in the depth of penetration. Figure 22-1 is, therefore, intended only as a general guide for chemical peel depths.

Chemical Peel Depth of Penetration

The depth achieved with light chemical peels ranges from very superficial resurfacing with removal of the stratum corneum, to superficial resurfacing with penetration to the upper papillary dermis. Although the type and concentration of chemical agent used are the main determinants of the depth of penetration in the skin, other factors also influence the depth of penetration including[19]:

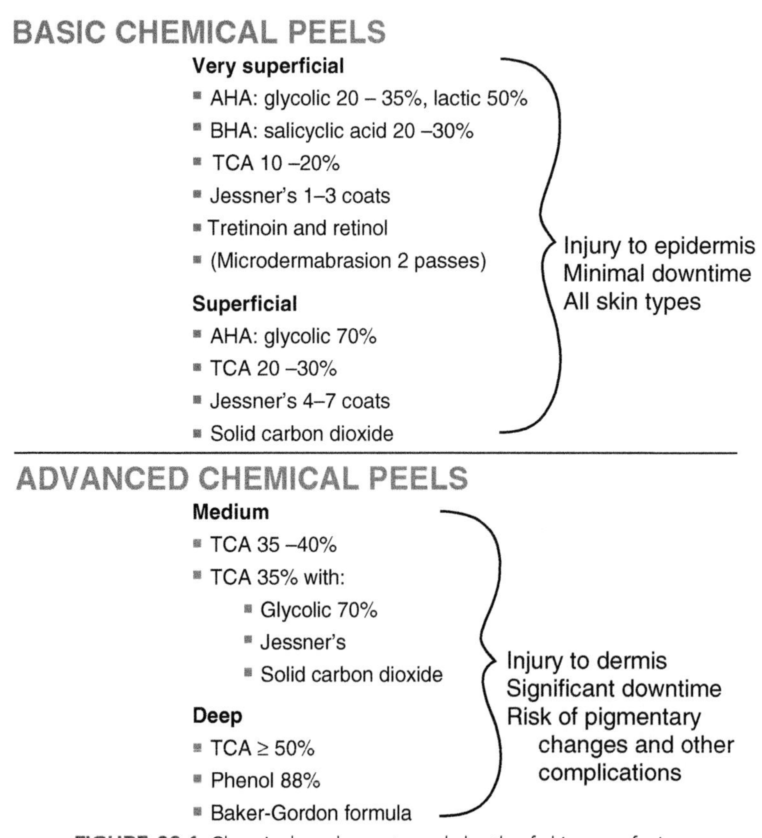

FIGURE 22-1 Chemical peel agents and depth of skin resurfacing.

- Chemical peel agent
- Concentration
- pH
- Application time (i.e., the duration for which the peel is in contact with the skin)
- Application technique (e.g., application pressure)
- Quantity (e.g., number of layers)
- Skin preparation (e.g., previous skin resurfacing procedures, topical products used at home prior to procedure)
- Skin type (e.g., thick sebaceous or thin dry skin)
- Area of the body treated (e.g., face, neck, back).

Alpha Hydroxy Acids

Alpha hydroxy acids (AHAs) are derived from organic fruit acids and include: glycolic (sugar cane), lactic (milk), malic (apples), tartaric (grapes), citric (citrus), mandelic (almonds), and phytic (rice) acids. These products are keratolytic and penetrate through the stratum corneum, causing exfoliation by disrupting corneocyte adhesion. AHAs in more acidic formulations (i.e., lower pHs) and in higher concentrations have stronger biologic effects. Glycolic acid peels typically have a pH of 2.5 to 3. Very low pHs (pH < 2) of glycolic acid, however, are associated with greater risk of necrosis and crusting, and do not offer improved results over less acidic preparations.[20] AHAs found in topical products as part of daily skin care regimes typically contain low AHA concentrations (10% or less) in less acidic formulations (pH 3.5 or greater).

Glycolic acid (GA) is the most commonly used AHA and is an agent frequently selected by providers getting started with chemical peels.[12] Glycolic acid is a small, water-soluble molecule that readily penetrates the skin. GA peels are clear colorless solutions that do not change in appearance upon application to the skin, unlike salicylic acid for example. Figure 22-2 shows GA applied to the dorsum of one hand, and salicylic acid on the other hand with its characteristic white precipitate. Because GA chemical peels do not exhibit a reliable clinical endpoint that is visible, application must be carefully monitored and timed, and the acid neutralized at the appropriate point to control the procedure. Clinical response to glycolic acid can be variable. Some patients have a brisk inflammatory response to low-strength (20% to 35%) short-duration applications (1 to 3 minutes), whereas others may tolerate higher strengths (70%) for longer duration (up to 7 minutes). The effects of GA can be terminated after application through neutralization, which raises the pH and renders the acid ineffective. Neutralization of alpha hydroxy acids may be performed with water or sodium bicarbonate solution (5% to 15%). If neutralization is not performed, AHAs will continue to be active and may penetrate deeper than intended.

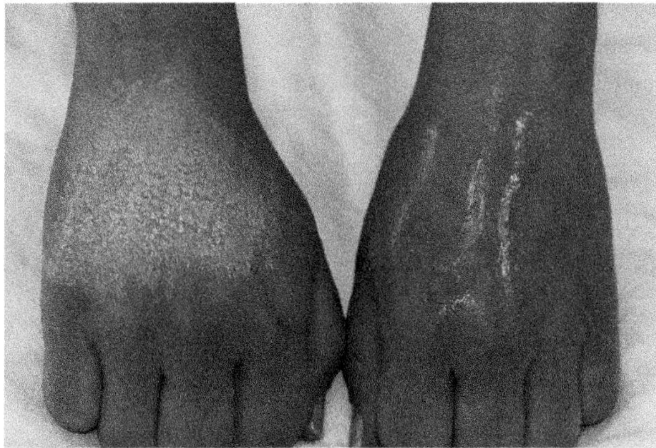

FIGURE 22-2 Salicylic acid (on the left) produces a white precipitate or pseudofrost, while glycolic acid (on the right) is clear and colorless. *(Copyright Rebecca Small, MD.)*

Beta Hydroxy Acids

Salicylic acid (SA), derived from willow bark, is a lipophilic, slower penetrating acid than GA. For the purposes of this chapter it will be classified as a beta hydroxy acid, but it should be noted that in the purest chemical terms, the hydroxyl group of beta hydroxy acids is neutral and in salicylic acid it is acidic. SA dissolves and reduces sebum, has anti-inflammatory effects, and is FDA approved as an anti-acne therapy.

The benefits of SA as compared to the AHAs include less stinging, because SA has a mild anesthetic effect; a visible clinical endpoint with a fine white precipitate ("pseudofrost"), which helps ensure even application (see Figure 22-2), and no requirement for neutralization. Once a white precipitate is formed, there is little additional penetration of the acid and water may be used to wash off the precipitate. A disadvantage of SA is more obvious post-treatment desquamation than with GA. SA peels are available as pure or combination products, and instructions for application and endpoints vary based on the product used. For example, La Roche-Posay's Biomedic SA peel 30% ends with frosting, whereas SkinCeutical's SA/Mandelic Peel (SA 20% combined with mandelic acid 10%) does not frost.

Trichloroacetic Acid

Trichloroacetic acid (TCA) is an agent familiar to many clinicians who have used it as therapy for condylomata acuminata (in highly concentrated preparations of 80% to 90%). For superficial chemical peels, it can be used as pure TCA 10% to 30%, or in combination with other peeling agents, such as TCA 15% combined with lactic acid 10%, or TCA 15% combined with SA 15% and lactic acid 15%. After application, TCA causes skin erythema and a whitish discoloration called frosting, which occurs 30 seconds to 2 minutes after application. Histologically, frosting corresponds to coagulation of epidermal proteins and keratinocytes. The intensity of frosting correlates directly with the depth of penetration (see Table 22-1).[21] The desired clinical endpoint for superficial depth peels with TCA is level I frosting, visible as patchy erythema with faint white coloration.

The technique for application of TCA is very important because the depth of penetration is dependent on

TABLE 22-1 Frosting with Trichloroacetic Acid Chemical Peels and Depth of Penetration

Frosting	Depth of Penetration	Clinical Findings
Level I	Superficial	Patchy erythema with faint patchy white color
Level II	Medium	Even white color with some erythema visible through the white
Level III	Deep	Opaque confluent white

the application *quantity*. It is usually applied in multiple consecutive applications, called layers, with a period of 2 to 3 minutes of observation for clinical endpoints between layers. Neutralization is not required with TCA, but water may be used at the end of the treatment to remove the white precipitate. Frosting usually disappears within 1 to 2 hours and erythema becomes more evident. A disadvantage of pure TCA is that it has significant post-treatment peeling and may be more painful than SA and GA peels. However, combination TCA chemical peels, as listed above, do not appear to be more uncomfortable than other superficial peel agents. A well-known TCA peel is the Obagi Blue Peel™, which has TCA 20% peel formulated with a blue-colored base containing glycerin and saponins to slow penetration and release of TCA in the skin.

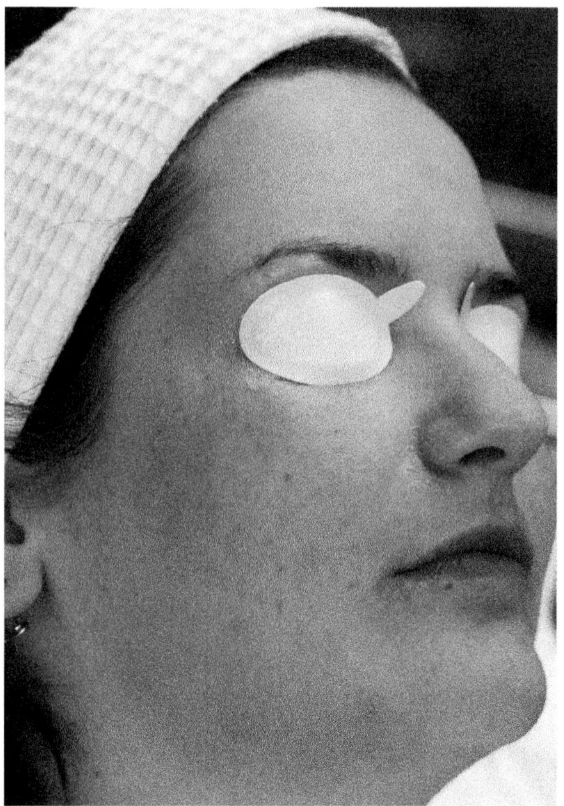

FIGURE 22-3 Jessner's peel immediately after application of six layers, showing mild erythema and faint white skin coloration from the salicylic acid precipitate. *(Copyright Rebecca Small, MD.)*

Jessner's Solution

Jessner's solution is a combination of resorcinol 14%, salicylic acid 14%, and lactic acid 14% in ethanol, which was originally developed to lower the concentration of any one agent and, hence, reduce the risk of toxicity.[22] Modified Jessner's formulations are also available that have no resorcinol, such as salicylic acid 14%, lactic acid 14%, and citric acid 8% in ethanol (e.g., PCA Peel®). Once applied, erythema is followed by a powdery whitening of the skin due to precipitation of salicylic acid. Neutralization is not required, but water may be used to remove the white precipitate. Jessner's peels are frequently applied in multiple layers, with a period of 4 to 7 minutes of observation for clinical endpoints between layers. Figure 22-3 shows a patient with mild erythema and a faint whitish coloration after application of six layers of a Jessner's peel.

Retinoids

Topical retinoids, such as *tretinoin (Retin-A)* and *tazarotene (Tazorac)*, have been principal therapies for acne and skin rejuvenation for many years as part of home skin care regimes. More recently, retinoids have been used as superficial peeling agents ranging from tretinoin peels 0.05% to 1%[23] to lower strength preparations containing retinol (e.g., retinol 15% combined with lactic acid 15%). Retinoid peels cause a yellowish discoloration after application. They are not neutralized and are typically washed off by the patient 8 hours after application. Retinol peels may be layered over other superficial peeling agents (such as glycolic and salicylic acids) to enhance desquamation. Figure 22-4 shows a patient immediately after application of six layers of Jessner's peel followed by one layer of retinol 15% peel combined with lactic acid 15% peel with characteristic yellow skin coloration.

CONTRAINDICATIONS

- Pregnancy and nursing
- Active infection, open wound or inflammation in the treatment area (e.g., herpes simplex or cellulitis)
- History of keloid or hypertrophic scar formation
- Sunburn or recent suntan
- Isotretinoin (Accutane) use within the past 6 months
- Melanoma (or lesions suspected for melanoma), basal cell or squamous cell carcinomas in the treatment area
- Bleeding abnormality
- Impaired healing (e.g., due to immunosuppression)
- Skin atrophy (e.g., chronic oral steroid use or genetic syndromes such as Ehlers-Danlos syndrome)
- Dermatoses such as vitiligo and active psoriasis, seborrheic or atopic dermatitis in the treatment area
- Deep chemical peel, dermabrasion, or radiation therapy within the preceding 6 months
- Ectropion (if treating near the lower eyelid)
- Aspirin allergy (for salicylic acid peels)

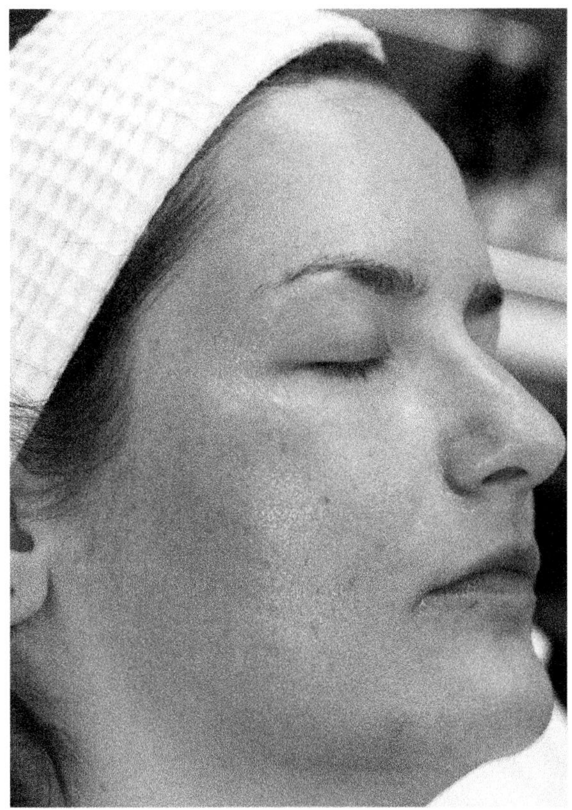

FIGURE 22-4 Retinoid peel (retinol 15% combined with lactic acid 15%) on top of a Jessner's peel (six layers) immediately after application, showing yellow skin coloration. *(Copyright Rebecca Small, MD.)*

- Obsessive picker
- Insufficient sun protection
- Severe erythema associated with conditions such as rosacea, telangiectasias, poikiloderma of Civatte
- Uncontrolled systemic condition
- Unrealistic expectations
- Body dysmorphic disorder.

Isotretinoin diminishes pilosebaceous units, which are in part responsible for re-epithelialization, and facilitates postprocedure healing. Radiation has a similar effect and causes skin atrophy. Recent isotretinoin use or radiation can result in prolonged healing and increase the risk of scarring. The presence of vellus hair can indicate adequate pilosebaceous units in previously irradiated areas.

ADVANTAGES OF SUPERFICIAL CHEMICAL PEELS

- Minimal risk of complications relative to deeper resurfacing procedures
- No anesthesia required
- Very superficial chemical peels are safe for all Fitzpatrick skin types
- May be combined with other aesthetic treatments, particularly topical products, for enhanced results
- Affordable.

DISADVANTAGES OF SUPERFICIAL CHEMICAL PEELS

- Depth of acid penetration can be unpredictable and is dependent on many factors
- Short "downtime" is required for resolution of redness and peeling
- Series of treatments is necessary for best results
- Cumulative effects for superficial peels do not equate to the effects achievable with medium-depth resurfacing procedures.

ANATOMY

With photoaging, the stratum corneum thickens while the deeper papillary dermis thins as collagen and elastin become more sparse. Pores dilate and become plugged with desquamated debris. Loss of normal vascularity causes a sallow coloring and slows transportation of nutrients to outer layers of skin. Abnormal vasculature, or telangiectasia, may proliferate and pigmentation increases and becomes irregular, forming lentigines. Atypical cells develop, resulting in preneoplastic lesions such as actinic keratoses, and neoplasia.[24]

Chemical peels can address many of the skin changes associated with photoaging. They diminish corneocyte cohesion, promoting a more rapid rate of cell turnover, which normalizes epidermal keratinization. Histologic changes in the skin are evident after chemical peels including a compacted stratum corneum, smoother epidermis, and increased dermal thickness with fibroblast production of new collagen, elastin, and glycosaminoglycans.[25–27] Chemical peels promote dispersion of melanin accumulated in the basal epidermal layer and transportation of the pigment to the skin surface for exfoliation. They reduce follicular plugging and decrease skin oiliness.

EQUIPMENT

- Head band or surgical cap for patient
- Facial wash
- Alcohol or alcohol-based astringent to degrease the skin
- Adhesive eye pads for patient eye protection
- Cotton tipped applicators (e.g., Q-tips)
- Petrolatum
- 2 × 2-inch non-woven gauze for peel application
- 4- × 4-inch non-woven gauze for cleansing
- Nonsterile gloves
- Saline eyewash in the event of eye infiltration
- Timer
- Hand towels
- Small fan (with soft blades) for patient comfort
- Chemical peel
- Small dispensing cups or ceramic bowl
- Neutralizer if indicated (e.g., sodium bicarbonate solution 5% to 15% or water for AHA peels)

- Postpeel products including moisturizer without active ingredients (e.g., SkinCeutical's Epidermal Repair) and broad spectrum sunscreen of SPF 30 or greater with zinc or titanium for postprocedure application.
- Cool compresses or wrapped ice packs.

Chemical peels are stored in containers as directed by the manufacturer as decomposition and evaporation can affect the strength. Small brushes or cotton-tipped applicators may be used instead of gauze for application of the acid; these are often brand specific and available from the chemical peel manufacturer. Moist gauze is used by some providers for patient eye protection instead of adhesive pads.

PROCEDURE PREPARATION

1. Review the patient's medical history (see Chapter 19, *Aesthetics Principles and Consultation*). Confirm that the patient has no food allergies to common chemical peel agent derivatives including: milk (lactic), apples (malic), grapes (tartaric), citrus (citric), or almonds (mandelic).
2. Perform a detailed aesthetic consultation (see Chapter 19) and complete the Skin Analysis Form (Figure 22-5), noting the patient's Fitzpatrick skin type, Glogau score, skin thickness, dryness, acne, scars, pigmentation, and vascular and pigmented lesions.
3. Obtain informed consent (see Chapter 19; also see Appendix A for an informed consent form and patient information handout titled *Skin Care Treatments*).
4. Obtain pretreatment photographs (see Chapter 19).
5. Four weeks before the procedure: Advise the patient to start preprocedure topical skin care products (see below).
6. Two weeks before the procedure: Advise the patient to avoid waxing.
7. One week before the procedure: Advise the patient to stop using products with retinoids or alpha hydroxy acids.
8. Two days before the procedure: Start the patient on a course of prophylactic antiviral medication (e.g., acyclovir or vancyclovir) for patients with a history of herpes simplex or varicella in or around the treatment areas and continue 3 days postprocedure.
9. On the day of the procedure: Advise the patient to wash the treatment area, remove any makeup and take out contact lenses.

Preprocedure Skin Care Products

Preparation of the skin prior to chemical peeling enhances chemical peel effects, facilitates postprocedure healing, and may reduce the risks of complications.[28] Topical products are typically begun 4 weeks prior to a procedure and consist of a retinoid, alpha hydroxy acid, broad-spectrum zinc or titanium sunscreen with SPF 30 or higher and sun avoidance, and for patients with darker Fitzpatrick skin types or those who are prone to hyperpigmentation, a skin-lightening agent such as hydroquinone (2% to 8%). Retinoids and exfoliants such as alpha hydroxy acids prepare the skin by decreasing stratum corneum thickness and reducing corneocyte cohesion, which allows for enhanced and more uniform penetration of the chemical peel agent. See Chapter 24, *Skin Care Products*, for a more detailed discussion of preprocedure topical products.

VERY SUPERFICIAL CHEMICAL PEELS: STEPS AND PRINCIPLES

The following procedure uses glycolic acid 20% as an example of an alpha hydroxy acid chemical peel. Techniques will vary for different peeling agents and providers are advised to familiarize themselves with protocols specific not only to the agent, but also to the exact formulation used and with the manufacturer's instructions for that chemical peel.

Patch Testing

A *patch test* may be performed prior to a chemical peel treatment to evaluate for a possible allergic reaction or adverse response to a specific chemical peel. Patients with a history of multiple allergies or sensitivity to parabens (a common preservative in over-the-counter products and local anesthetics) or perfumes may be at increased risk for allergic reactions. The patch test site is located discretely near the treatment area, such as behind the ear, or alternatively on the dorsum of the forearm. The skin is prepped as usual for peeling, and the desired peel applied, timed, and neutralized if indicated. The site is evaluated 3 days after patch testing for signs of excessive erythema, urticaria, vesiculation (i.e., epidermolysis), or reports of excessive pruritis or pain. A patch test is positive if any of these signs or symptoms are present and the chemical peel tested is avoided. A negative patch test is reassuring. However, a negative patch test does not ensure that an allergic reaction or adverse response will not occur with the peel tested. Record the date, location, and products used in the patch test, along with the date of evaluation and description of response in the chart.

General Treatment Technique

The Chemical Peel Safety Zone, which is the area within which chemical peel treatments can be safely performed on the face, is shown in Figure 22-6. Chemical peels may be applied to the full face apart from the lips and, in the periocular area, peels are applied above the eyebrows and 2 to 3 mm below the inferior eyelash margin.

Chemical peels are typically thin liquids and can pool in skinfolds and creases, which intensifies their effects. Common areas of potential pooling include the marionette lines, nasolabial folds, and lateral canthal creases. Petrolatum is applied to these areas as a barrier to protect them from overtreatment (Figures 22-6 and 22-7).

SKIN ANALYSIS FORM

Name: ______________________ DOB: ______________________

Date of last skin treatment and type: ______________________

Reported skin type: Normal Dry Combination Oily Acneic Sensitive Rosacea

Allergic to : Sulfa Milk Aloe Aspirin Grapes Apples Citrus Shellfish

Reaction: ______________________

Current Regime: ______________________

Specific Complaints: ______________________

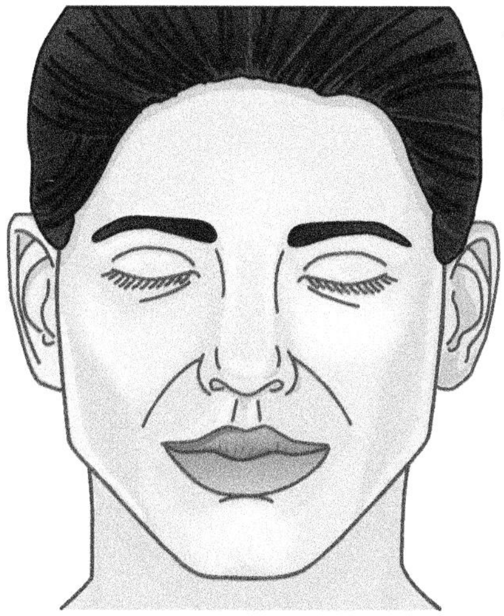

______ Fitzpatrick Skin Type

______ Glogau

W- Wrinkles
HP- Hyperpigmentation
HYP- Hypopigmentation
PP- Papules/ Pustules
T- Telangiectasias
S- Scaling
C- Comedones
ER- Erythema
LP- Large Pores
M- Milia
SC- Scarring
O- Oiliness

Observations: ______________________

Assessment: ______________________

Treatment Plan:

Topical Products: ______________________

In-Office Treatments: ______________________

- [ ] Risks, benefits, alternatives and complications of skin care treatments discussed with patient and all questions were answered
- [ ] Skin Care Consent signed and placed in the chart
- [ ] Photographs taken

Signature: ______________________ Date: ______________________

FIGURE 22-5 Skin Analysis Form. *(Copyright Rebecca Small, MD, Monterey Bay Laser Aesthetics, Capitola, CA.)*

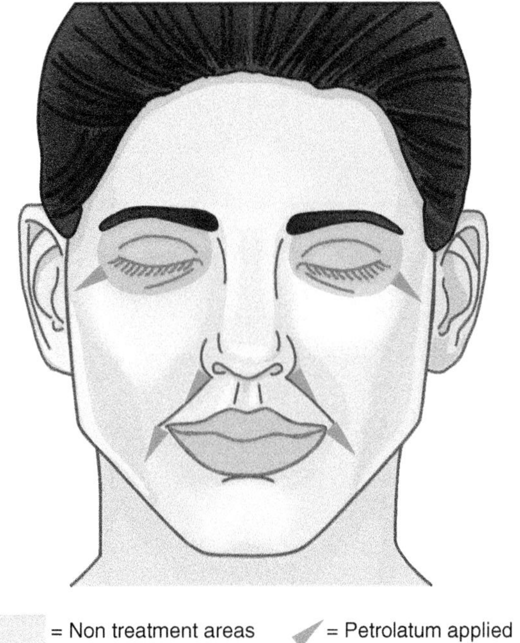

FIGURE 22-6 Chemical Peel Safety Zone for treatments on the face showing areas of petrolatum application and nontreatment areas.

Most providers develop their own systematic method for applying a chemical peel to the face. In general, the chemical peel is applied to the least reactive areas first, such as the forehead, and to the most sensitive areas, such as the upper lip, last. Figure 22-8 shows one possible sequence for applying a chemical peel to the face.

General Chemical Peel Technique

1. Apply the chemical peel using even strokes with firm pressure.
2. Extend the peel 1 cm below the jaw line and apply lightly to "feather" the edges of the treatment area so as to avoid a possible line of demarcation between treated and untreated skin.
3. If deep wrinkles are present, stretch the skin.

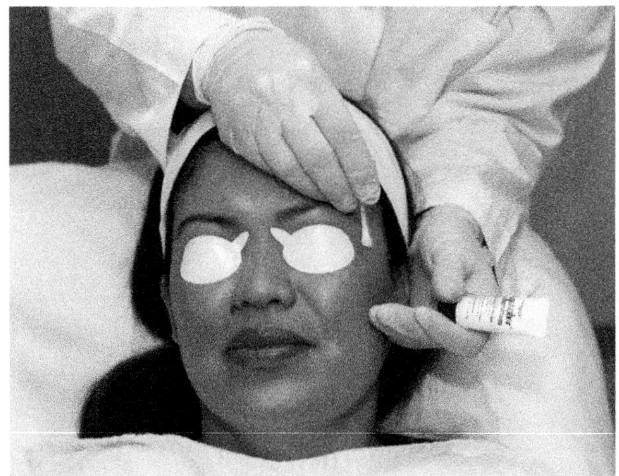

FIGURE 22-7 Application of petrolatum to areas of potential chemical peel pooling. *(Copyright Rebecca Small, MD.)*

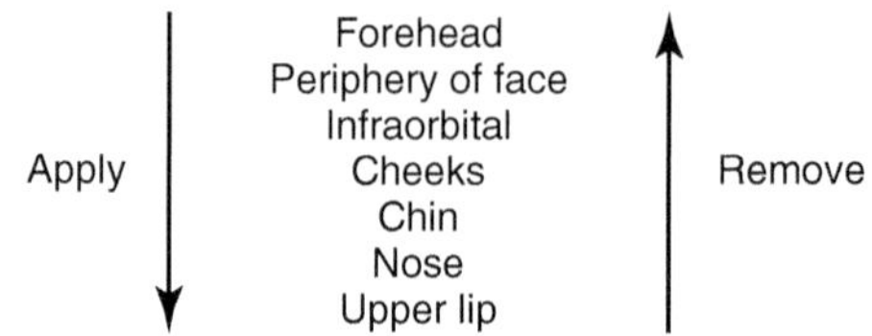

FIGURE 22-8 Sequence for chemical peel application and removal on the face.

4. Do not overlap strokes during one application.
5. Apply carefully and sparingly to areas of potential pooling, especially periocular areas.
   TIP: Certain areas of the face are oilier, such as the forehead, nose, and cheeks. These areas with greater density of sebaceous glands can tolerate more aggressive chemical peeling.

Clinical endpoints for very superficial and superficial peels depend on the agent used. In most cases mild erythema is the desired endpoint and for those peels that frost, level I frosting with patchy erythema and whitening of the skin is the endpoint. Salicylic acid may form a fine white precipitate, which is also a desired clinical endpoint. Table 22-2 summarizes key characteristics and clinical endpoints for common chemical peel agents.

Attempt to intensify chemical peel treatments over time by advancing to higher strength peel solutions and longer application times. It is recommended that only one variable, either the strength or the time, be increased at any given visit. For example, a progressive chemical peel series of glycolic acid may use a lower concentration of glycolic acid (20% to 30%) for the initial visit with a duration of 3 minutes. At the subsequent visit, the acid concentration can remain the same and the time increased to a maximum of 5 to 7 minutes. At the next visit, the acid concentration may be increased and the time reduced, and so on.

TIP: Increasing treatment intensity may not be possible at all visits.

Skin is dynamic, and characteristics such as the sebaceous quality and acne may change over the course of a series of chemical peel treatments affecting the intensity of the peel. It is advisable to carefully assess the skin and review home product use at each visit prior to application of a chemical peel.

Chemical peels may also be performed on the neck, anterior chest (also called or décolletage), hands, back, and almost any area of the body requiring exfoliation. However, *nonfacial* areas have fewer pilosebaceous units, which serve as sites of re-epithelialization. These areas have delayed healing relative to the face, a greater tendency to scar, and conservative treatment is recommended. It may not be possible to advance the strength of acid or duration of application significantly in these areas over a series of treatments. For example, a patient may advance to GA 70% by the end of a series of peels on their face, but may only tolerate GA 20% to 35% below the angle of the jaw.

TABLE 22-2 Superficial Chemical Peel Key Properties

Chemical Peel	Neutralization Required	Frosting Possible	Desquamation	Discomfort
Glycolic and lactic acid	Yes Bicarbonate	No	Inconsistent	+
Salicylic acid	No	Yes	Yes	+
Trichloroacetic acid	No	Yes	Yes	++
Jessner's	No	Yes[a]	Yes	++
Tretinoin and retinol	No	No	Yes	+

+, mild; ++, moderate.
[a]Salicylic acid forms a pseudofrost, which is crystallization of the acid rather than true coagulation of epidermal proteins and keratinocytes as seen with TCA frosting.

Planning and Designing

There are four main steps with any chemical peel procedure:

1. Skin preparation (cleansing and degreasing)
2. Chemical peel application
3. Neutralization (if indicated)
4. Soothing (topical products for hydration and protection).

Anesthesia

Preprocedure anesthesia is typically not required with superficial chemical peels.

Performing a Very Superficial Glycolic Acid 20% Chemical Peel

1. Comfortably position the patient supine flat on the treatment table.
2. Place a headband or surgical cap on the patient to pull hair away from the face. Cover the patient's eyes with adhesive pads for protection.
3. Drape a towel on the neck when treating the face.
4. Set up all products necessary for the procedure within arms' reach.
   TIP: Always have the appropriate neutralizing agent ready to be quickly applied. For GA, a bowl of water or sodium bicarbonate solution (5% to 15%) is used for neutralization.
5. Clean the treatment area with a cleanser.
6. Degrease the skin with alcohol or an alcohol-based astringent.
   TIP: Degrease the face with the same method you intend to use for application of the chemical peel so as to practice the application technique.
7. Reevaluate skin and limit treatment areas if indicated.
   TIP: Acne papules and pustules may be treated, but the acid may penetrate deeper than intended and these areas should be watched closely during the treatment and neutralized when desired clinical endpoints are reached (see below).
8. Using a cotton-tipped applicator apply petrolatum sparingly to areas of potential pooling, including lateral canthae, nasolabial folds, nasal ala, and oral commissures (see Figure 22-7).
9. Select the glycolic acid 20% peeling agent and dispense the amount indicated by the manufacturer into a dispensing cup or ceramic bowl.
10. Apply the glycolic acid 20% peel evenly to the face using a 2 × 2-inch non-woven gauze in the sequence outlined above in the *General Treatment Technique* section (Figure 22-9).
    TIP: Attempt to complete application within 30 seconds so as not to increase the treatment time in areas where first applied.
    CAUTION: Brushes can capture more product than anticipated and care should be taken to squeeze excess product on the side of a dispensing cup to minimize the risk of dripping. **An open bottle or soaked applicator should never be passed over the eyes.**
    CAUTION: If acid infiltrates into the eye, flush immediately with copious amounts of normal saline or water.

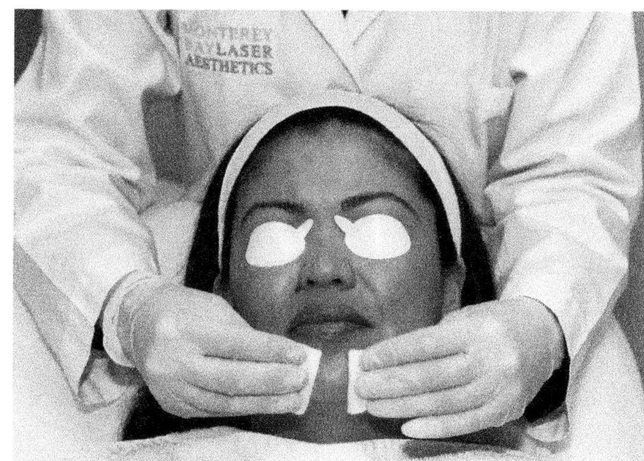

FIGURE 22-9 Technique for application of chemical peel using gauze. *(Copyright Rebecca Small, MD.)*

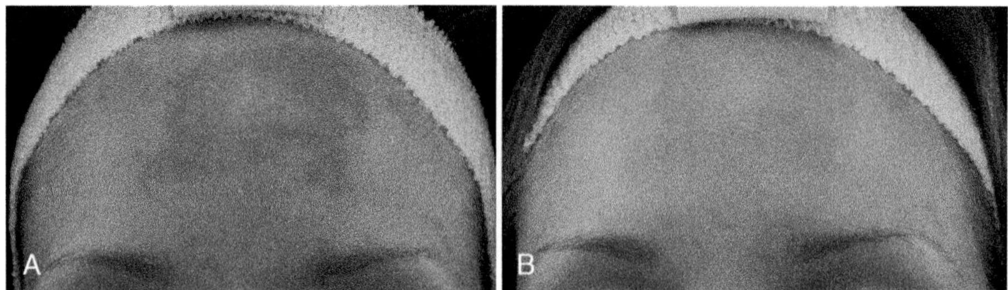

FIGURE 22-10 Melasma (A) before and (B) after three modified Jessner's chemical peels. *(Courtesy of PCA Skin, Scottsdale, AZ.)*

11. Begin the timer. The goal for a first glycolic acid 20% peel is 3 minutes.
    TIP: Providing the patient with a handheld fan to fan themselves will reduce discomfort and serve as a distraction.
12. Once the peel has been applied to the skin, observe the treatment area at all times and communicate with the patient regarding discomfort using a pain scale. Inform the patient that they will likely experience tingling/burning/stinging, which peaks at approximately 2 to 3 minutes after application and then subsides. Pain of up to 5 or 6 out of 10 is acceptable.
13. If undesired clinical endpoints are present, neutralize the peel by applying sodium bicarbonate solution 5% to 15% or water to the treatment area using a freshly saturated gauze each time the neutralizer is applied. Neutralizer may be applied two or three times or more. Undesirable clinical endpoints for *alpha hydroxy* acid chemical peels include:
    - Blanching.
    - Blistering/vesiculation, which is indicative of epidermolysis.
    - "Frosting" or whitening of the skin. Note that frosting or whitening is a desirable endpoint with salicylic acid and TCA but *not* with AHAs. Whitening or graying of the skin indicates overtreatment with AHAs.
    - Excessive patient discomfort with pain greater than 6 out of 10.
14. Observe the skin for the desired clinical endpoint of mild erythema. Once mild erythema is achieved, the procedure is terminated and the glycolic acid neutralized.
    TIP: Neutralize areas having the greatest discomfort first.
15. Many patients do not demonstrate erythema, and the glycolic acid should be neutralized once the timer indicates 3 minutes.
16. Cold gauze sponges or wrapped ice packs can be applied after neutralization for patient comfort.
17. Apply a soothing moisturizer (such as SkinCeutical's Epidermal Repair) and a broad spectrum sunscreen of SPF 30 or higher containing zinc or titanium after the treatment.

RESULTS

A single superficial or very superficial depth chemical peel typically yields subtle improvements. Multiple peels performed at 2- to 4-week intervals will provide more appreciable benefits, including enhanced skin smoothness, decreased oiliness and comedones, reduced papulopustular lesions, improved fine lines, and fading of hyperpigmentation.[2,6,8–10,19,29] In addition, chemical peel results can be enhanced with the use of rejuvenating topical products at home.

Figure 22-10 shows a patient with melasma on the forehead (A) before and (B) after three modified Jessner's peels containing lactic acid 14%, salicylic acid 14%, hydroquinone 2%, and kojic acid 3%, pH 1.5 to 1.9 (PCA Peel®). Home care products included a daily arbutin lightening agent, alpha hydroxy acids, and sunscreen.

Figure 22-11 shows a patient with papulopustular acne (A) before and (B) after four modified Jessner's peels (PCA Peel) and four salicylic acid 20% treatments.

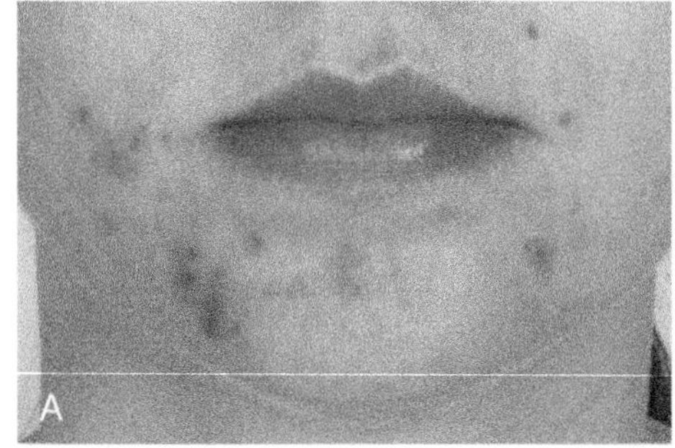
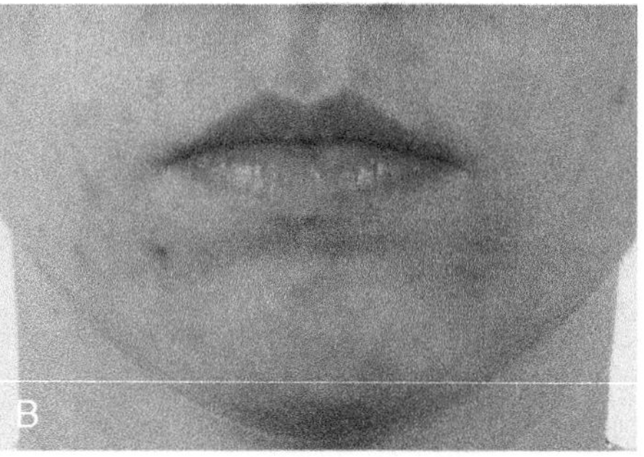

FIGURE 22-11 Papulopustular acne (A) before and (B) after four modified Jessner's peels and four salicylic acid 20% treatments. *(Courtesy of PCA Skin, Scottsdale, AZ.)*

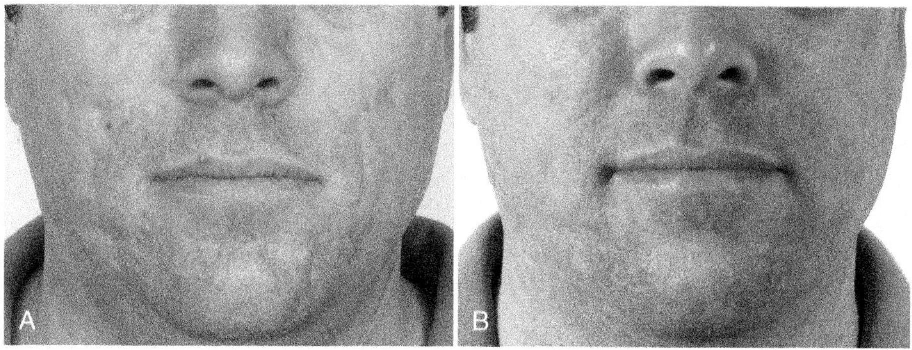

FIGURE 22-12 Acne scarring **(A)** before and **(B)** after six combination treatments of microdermabrasion followed by TCA 10% combined with lactic acid 20% chemical peels. *(Courtesy of PCA Skin, Scottsdale, AZ.)*

Home care products included daily benzoyl peroxide 5% cleanser, retinol serum 0.5% with lightening agents of kojic acid, licorice, arbutin, alpha hydroxy acid, and sunscreen.

Figure 22-12 shows a patient with acne scarring (A) before and (B) after six combination treatments of microdermabrasion followed by TCA 10% combined with lactic acid 20%, pH 0.62 to 1.02 (PCA Ultra Peel® I). Home care products included daily palmitoyl oligopeptide/tetrapeptide-7 serum (Matrixyl 3000™) for skin texture.

Figure 22-13 shows a patient with wrinkles marked in the periocular areas and erythema (A) before and (B) after one treatment with three layers of TCA 20% combined with lactic acid 10%, pH 0.62 to 1.02 (PCA Ultra Peel® Forte), followed by retinol 10% combined with lactic acid 20%, pH 3 to 3.4 (PCA Esthetique Peel®).

AFTERCARE

Erythema, dryness, and sensitivity are common in the first 1 to 2 days postprocedure. By day 3 the skin may feel tighter, texture may appear more coarse, wrinkles may be accentuated, and patients may report mild pruritis. Exfoliation usually occurs on day 3 to 5, persists for a few days, and ranges from skin flaking to skin sloughing and peeling. Figure 22-14 shows a patient with peeling on day 3 after treatment with six layers of a Jessner's chemical peel followed by a combination peel of retinol 15% with lactic acid 15%. In some instances, no flaking or peeling may be evident, particularly when very superficial chemical peels are used in patients whose skin is conditioned (i.e., who regularly exfoliate). Lack of peeling or flaking does not indicate that a peel was histologically or clinically ineffective.

The week following treatment, patients are instructed to use a gentle cleanser and topical products that are hydrating and soothing and do not contain potentially irritating ingredients such as AHAs or retinoids. An example of a postpeel regime would include daily use of a full-spectrum physical sunscreen in the day time, which may be reapplied if the skin is dry, and in the evening, a nonocclusive moisturizer. If dryness is severe, an occlusive moisturizer such as Aquaphor may be substituted in the evening. If erythema persists for more than 3 days, or for patients with darker skin types,

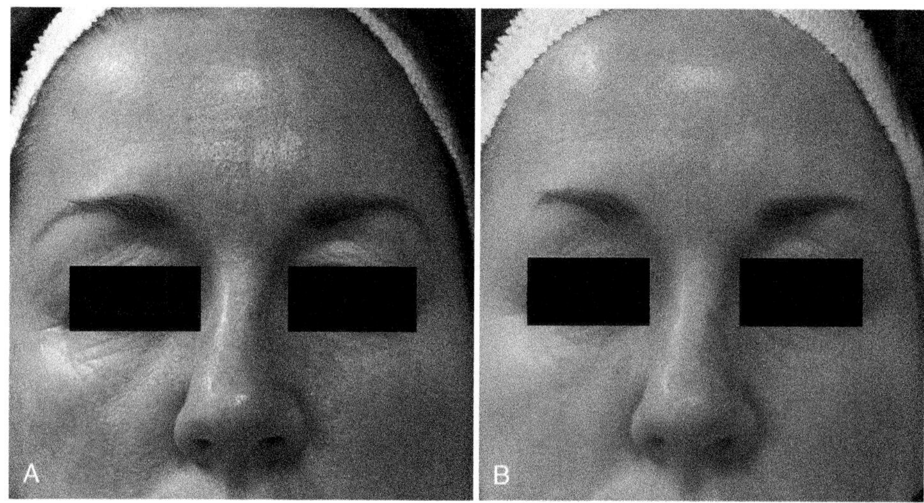

FIGURE 22-13 Periocular wrinkles and laxity **(A)** before and **(B)** after one treatment with three layers of TCA 20% combined with lactic acid 10% followed by retinol 10% combined with lactic acid 20% chemical peels. *(Courtesy of PCA Skin, Scottsdale, AZ.)*

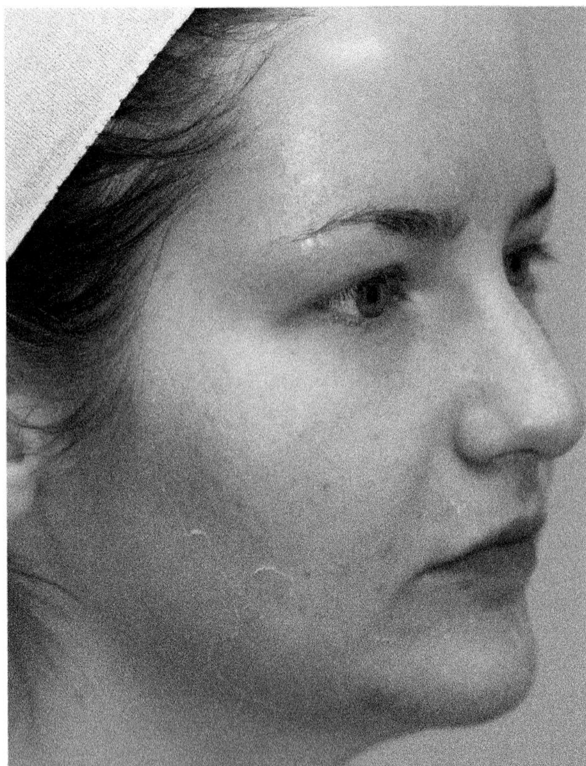

FIGURE 22-14 Desquamation 3 days after Jessner's chemical peel (six layers) and retinol 15% combined with lactic acid 15% chemical peels. *(Copyright Rebecca Small, MD.)*

hydrocortisone 1% or 2½% may be applied twice a day to prevent postinflammatory hyperpigmentation. Makeup may be worn 24 hours after the procedure and mineral products are preferable. Strict sun avoidance for 2 weeks postprocedure is important, including the use of a wide-brimmed hat.

Patients should follow up if they notice prolonged erythema for 5 days or more, severe pruritis, discomfort, pain, crusting, drainage, or other signs or symptoms that deviate from the usual postprocedure course. Regular skin care products may be resumed once the skin is no longer irritated or peeling, usually at 2 weeks postprocedure. During a peel series, prescription retinoic acid products are not recommended as the repeated stopping and starting required pre- and postprocedure can induce a cyclic retinoid dermatitis. Gentler retinol products may be resumed 2 weeks postprocedure.

FOLLOW-UP

Treatments may be performed every 2 to 4 weeks during a series of six treatments. As the intensity of treatments increases, the degree of exfoliation and, therefore, time to re-epithelialization increases. Most patients require 2 weeks between very superficial peels and 4 weeks between superficial treatments. Maintenance chemical peels after a series may be performed every 4 to 6 weeks, or as deemed necessary by the patient and provider.

ADVANCED CHEMICAL PEELING

Once providers gain experience and skill with a basic chemical peel agent, such as glycolic acid, they may choose to combine different chemical peels in a progressive treatment series to intensify treatments. For example, a chemical peel series for photodamaged skin might start with a glycolic acid 30% peel, advance to glycolic acid 70% by the third or fourth treatment, and end with a Jessner's peel using six layers on the sixth treatment. In general, very superficial peels are used in the beginning of the treatment series and superficial peels are used at the end of the series.

Microdermabrasion can be used as part of skin preparation prior to the application of chemical peels to allow for more even acid penetration, and increase the depth of penetration to enhance results.[30] Providers are advised to follow established manufacturer protocols when combining these two exfoliation modalities because acid penetration can be significantly altered by the lack of the stratum corneum barrier that is removed by microdermabrasion.

COMPLICATIONS

- Pain or temporary discomfort
- Prolonged irritation or erythema
- Hyperpigmentation
- Hypopigmentation
- Milia
- Blistering and crusting
- Infection such as activation of herpes simplex, impetigo, candidiasis
- Acne exacerbation
- Dermatitis exacerbation
- Erythema exacerbation particularly in patients with telangiectasias, rosacea, and poikiloderma of Civatte
- Allergic reactions including urticaria, papules, and the remote possibility of severe reactions such as bronchospasm and anaphylaxis
- Scarring and textural changes
- Salicylism with salicylic acid (very rare).

The risk of complications from chemical peels is primarily related to the depth of penetration in the skin. Light chemical peels (very superficial and superficial), which cause injury to the epidermis and upper papillary dermis, have a very low risk of complications. Transient hyperpigmentation in response to prolonged erythema is one of the most common complications encountered. Deeper peels, which can penetrate down to the reticular dermis, have greater potential for severe complications, such as scarring and permanent pigmentary changes, including hypopigmentation.

Pain is usually transient, present only at the time of chemical peel application. Postprocedure pain requires evaluation and may be associated with infection.

Postprocedure erythema is common and the duration depends on the inherent reactivity of the patient's skin and the depth of injury. Most erythema with superficial peels resolves spontaneously within a few days.

Prolonged erythema of more than 5 days, particularly in patients with darker Fitzpatrick skin types (IV through VI), can result in *postinflammatory hyperpigmentation* (PIH). Erythema present at 5 days post-treatment may be treated with either a medium-potency (triamcinolone 0.1%) or low-potency (hydrocortisone 2.5% or 1%) topical steroid twice daily for 3 to 5 days or until erythema resolves. Contact dermatitis should also be considered as a cause of prolonged erythema. Sun avoidance is very important to reduce the risk of PIH when erythema is present.

Hyperpigmentation can be treated with lightening agents such as hydroquinone cream (2% to 8%) or cosmeceutical agents such as kojic acid, arbutin, and licorice (see Chapter 24, *Skin Care Products*). Figure 22-15 shows a patient with hyperpigmentation in the marionette lines 1 month after receiving a Jessner's chemical peel (six layers) who did not have petrolatum applied to marionette lines, an area of potential chemical peel pooling. Hyperpigmentation usually resolves, but in rare instances, can be permanent. In darker Fitzpatrick skin types, resolution of hyperpigmentation may take several months. The risk of hyperpigmentation is greater with the use of exogenous hormones, photosensitizing medications, and sun exposure. *Hypopigmentation* is rare and occurs more commonly in darker Fitzpatrick skin types (IV through VI). Hypopigmentation usually resolves, but may be permanent.

Milia, which appear as tiny 1- to 2-mm white papules, result from occlusion of sebaceous glands. Use of occlusive moisturizers, such as petrolatum-based products, frequently cause milia. Milia may be treated by lancing with a 20-gauge needle and extracting the sebaceous plug.

Blistering or *vesiculation* is rare and signifies epidermolysis. This can occur as a result of increased depth of chemical peel penetration if the epidermis is not fully intact at the time of treatment. The epidermis may not be fully intact with retinoid use the week prior to peeling, aggressive exfoliation such as scrubbing with exfoliants or microdermabrasion prior to peel application, active acne, and seborrheic or other dermatoses. Glycolic acids with lower pHs cause more desquamation, have a greater risk of epidermolysis and do not offer improved clinical effects.[20] Vesicles typically form into crusts, which are kept moist with Bacitracin and dressed with a bandage until healed.

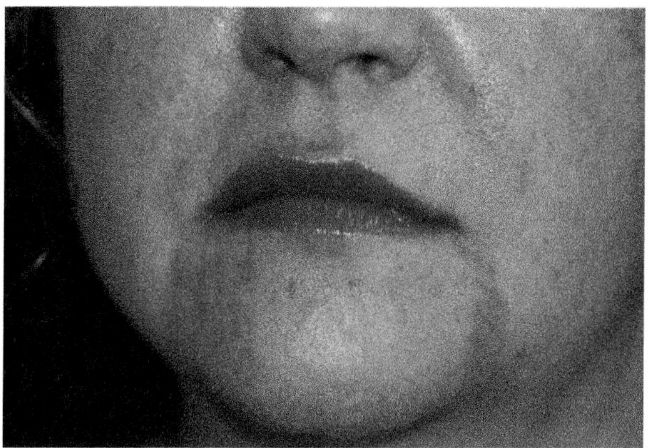

FIGURE 22-15 Postinflammatory hyperpigmentation in the marionette lines 3 weeks after Jessner's chemical peel (6 layers) without protective application of petrolatum to areas of pooling. *(Copyright Rebecca Small, MD.)*

Postpeel infections are rare with superficial peels and require treatment specific to the infection. *Acne exacerbations* are best treated with oral medications, such as doxycycline or minocycline, as postpeel skin is more sensitive and may be prone to irritation with topical acne therapies. Oral *herpes simplex activation* may occur despite adequate prophylaxis and should be treated aggressively due to the risk of spread with nonintact skin (e.g., vancyclovir 1 g twice or maximally three times per day for 7 days until the skin is fully reepithelialized). *Cutaneous candidiasis* appears as bright red patches with small surrounding erythematous macules most often in the perioral area, and may be associated with pruritis or burning. Topical antifungals or oral fluconazole may be used (150 mg daily for 3 days). It is advisable to culture infections prior to initiating therapy if there is any question of the diagnosis.

Scarring is extremely rare. The risk of scarring is increased with previous medium or deep peels, laser resurfacing, dermabrasion, isotretinoin use, radiation therapy, or facial surgery within the preceding 6 months, connective tissue diseases (e.g., Ehlers-Danlos syndrome) and other factors that impair wound healing, such as tobacco use or chronic disease states. Scarring is also more common if postprocedure infection occurs. Impending scarring is usually evident as bright red patches with textural changes and may be treated with high-potency topical steroids (e.g., Cordran tape) or pulsed dye lasers.

Systemic toxicity with salicylic acid applied to large areas is reported and extremely rare.[31]

LEARNING THE TECHNIQUES

Providers are encouraged to practice first on themselves, on the dorsum of the hand, and then on the face of staff and friends prior to treating patients. It is important to develop a systematic and stepwise approach for chemical peel application and to understand the sensations patients may describe during the chemical peel treatment (e.g., stinging or burning). One can also experience the sense of relief provided with fanning, cool compresses, and postpeel product application.

FINANCIAL CONSIDERATIONS

Chemical peeling agents can be purchased for approximately \$50 to \$80 for a 4-oz bottle, which typically yields 20 peels and can be purchased from skin care product or medical suppliers (see the *Resources* list below). Charges for chemical peels vary by geographic region, and range from \$65 to \$450 based on the type of peel. The more aggressive higher strength superficial peels tend to have higher fees. Some insurance companies cover chemical peels for indications such as acne (see Box 22-1), however, most do not and patients

BOX 22-1 *Codes for Chemical Peel Procedures*

CPT Codes

15788 Chemical peel, facial; epidermal
15789 Chemical peel, facial; dermal
15792 Chemical peel, nonfacial; epidermal
15793 Chemical peel, nonfacial; dermal

ICD-9 Codes

706.1 Acne
695.3 Rosacea
702.0 Actinic keratosis
709.00 Dyschromia, unspecified
709.09 Lentigo, melasma

pay for these procedures out of pocket. Chemical peels are often performed and charged as a series of six treatments. Committing to a series of treatments helps patients achieve the best possible results and helps to ensure high patient and provider satisfaction.

CONCLUSION

Demand for anti-aging treatments continues to rise as patients become better educated about skin health and desire to maintain a vibrant appearance. A series of light chemical peels can improve many photoaging-related changes such as hyperpigmentation and rough skin texture. They may also improve fine lines, acneic conditions, and superficial scars. Minimal risks are associated with light peels and they have short recovery times. In addition, chemical peels can be readily combined with other office-based aesthetic procedures such as microdermabrasion, laser photorejuvenation, and injectables like botulinum toxin and dermal fillers, for enhanced skin rejuvenation results.

Resources

Bioglan/Bradley Pharmaceuticals
Phone: 888-246-4526
www.bioglan.com

Biomed/LaRoche-Posay
Phone: 888-577-5226
www.laroche-posay.us/contact.html

Delasco/Dermatologic Lab and Supply
Phone: 800-831-6273
www.delasco.com

Glymed Plus
Phone: 800-676-9667
www.glymedplus.com

MD Forte (Allergan)
Phone: 800-699-6890
www.allergan.com

Neostrata
Phone: 800-628-9904
www.neostrata.com

Obagi
Phone: 800-636-7546
www.obagi.com

Physicians Choice Arizona (PCA Skin)
Phone: 877-722-7546
www.pcaskin.com

Rx Systems
Phone: 800-899-0167
www.rxsystemspf.com

SkinCeuticals
Phone: 800-811-1660
www.skinceuticals.com

SkinMedica
Phone: 866-867-0110
www.skinmedica.com

References

1. Small R. Aesthetic procedures in office practice. *Am Fam Physician.* 2009;80(11):1231–1237.
2. Kuwahara R, Rasberry R. *Chemical peels.* EMedicine; 2007.
3. Zakapoulu N, Kontochistopoulous G. Superficial chemical peels. *J Cosm Dermatol.* 2006;5(3):246–253.
4. Cosmetic Surgery National Data Bank 2010 Statistics. American Society for Aesthetic Plastic Surgery; 2010.
5. Small R. Aesthetic procedures introduction. *In:* Mayeaux E, ed. *The Essential Guide to Primary Care Procedures.* Philadelphia: Lippincott Williams & Wilkins; 2009:195–199.
6. Swinehart JM. Salicylic acid peeling of the hands and forearms. Effective nonsurgical removal of pigmented lesions and actinic damage. *J Dermatol Surg Oncol.* 1992;18:495–498.
7. Matarasso SL, Salman SM, Glogau RG, *et al.* The role of chemical peeling in the treatment of photodamaged skin. *J Dermatol Surg Oncol.* 1990;16:945–954.
8. Bergfeld WF, Tung RC, Vidimos AT. Improving the appearance of photoaged skin with glycolic acid. *J Am Acad Dermatol.* 1997;36: 1011–1013.
9. Kligman D, Kligman A. Salicylic acid as a peeling agent for the treatment of acne. *J Cosm Dermatol.* 1997;10(9):44–47.
10. Kessler E, Flanagan K, Chia C, *et al.* Comparison of alpha- and beta-hydroxy acid chemical peels in the treatment of mild to moderately severe facial acne vulgaris. *Dermatol Surg.* 2008;34(1):45–50.
11. Khunger N, Sarkar R, Jain RK. Tretinoin peels versus glycolic acid peels in the treatment of Melasma in dark-skinned patients. *Dermatol Surg.* 2004;30(5):756–760.
12. Sarkar R, Kaur C, Bhalla M, *et al.* The combination of glycolic acid peels with a topical regimen in the treatment of Melasma in dark-skinned patients: A comparative study. *Dermatol Surg.* 2002;28:928–932.
13. Lawrence N, Cox SE, Brody HJ. Treatment of melasma with Jessner's solution versus glycolic acid: a comparison of clinical efficacy and evaluation of the predictive ability of Wood's light examination. *Am Acad Dermatol.* 1977;36:589–593.
14. Grimes PE. The safety and efficacy of salicylic acid chemical peels in darker racial-ethnic groups. *Dermatol Surg.* 1999;25: 18–22.
15. Tse Y. Choosing the correct peel for the appropriate patient. *In:* Rubin M, ed. *Chemical Peels.* Philadelphia: Elsevier; 2006:13–19.
16. Khunger N. Standard guidelines for chemical peels. *Indian J Dermatol Venerol Leprol.* 2008;74:S5–S12.
17. Perkins SW, Gillum TG. Management of aging skin. In: Cummings C, ed. *Otolaryngology: Head and Neck Surgery.* Philadelphia: Elsevier; 2005.
18. Cox SE, Butterwick KJ. Chemical peels. *In:* Robinson J, Hanke W, Sengelmann RD, Siegel D, eds. *Surgery of the Skin.* Philadelphia: Mosby/Elsevier; 2005:463–482.

19. Briden ME. Alpha-hydroxyacid chemical peeling agents: case studies and rationale for safe and effective use. *Cutis.* 2004;73(2 Suppl):18–24.
20. Becker FF, Langford FPJ, Rubin MG, et al. A histological comparison of 50% and 70% glycolic acid peels using solutions with various pHs. *Dermatol Surg.* 1996;22:463–465.
21. Monheit GD. Chemical peels. *Skin Therapy Lett.* 2004;9:6–11.
22. Fulton J. Jessner's peel. *In:* Rubin M, ed. *Chemical Peels.* Philadelphia: Elsevier; 2006:57–71.
23. Cuce L, Bertino M, Scattone L, *et al.* Tretinoin peeling. *Dermatol Surg.* 2001;27:12–14.
24. Zimbler MS, Kokoska MS, Thomas JR. Anatomy and pathophysiology of facial aging. *Facial Plast Surg Clin North Am.* 2001;9(2):179–187, vii.
25. Berardesca E, Distante F, Vignoli GP, *et al.* Alpha hydroxyacids modulate stratum corneum barrier function. *Br J Dermatol.* 1997;137(6):934–938.
26. Murad H, Shamban AT, Premo PS. The use of glycolic acid as a peeling agent. *Dermatol Clin.* 1995;13:285–307.
27. El-Domyati M, Attia S, Saleh F, *et al.* Trichloroacetic acid versus chemical peeling: a histometric, immunohistochemical and ultrastructural comparison. *Dermatol Surg.* 2004;30:179–188.
28. Drake LA, Dinehart SM, Goltz RW, *et al.* Guidelines of care for chemical peeling. Guidelines/Outcomes Committee: American Academy of Dermatology. *J Am Acad Dermatol.* 1995;33:479–503.
29. Sehgal V, Luthra A, Aggerwal A. Evaluation of graded strength glycolic acid facial peel: an Indian experience. *J Dermatol.* 2003;30(758):761.
30. Briden ME, Jacobsen E, Johnson C. Combining superficial glycolic acid (alpha-hydroxy acid) peels with microdermabrasion to maximize treatment results and patient satisfaction. *Cutis.* 2007;79(1 Suppl):13–16.
31. Davies MG, Briffa DV, Greaves MW. Systemic toxicity from topically applied salicylic acid. *Br Med J.* 1979;1(6164):661.

Additional Reading

Small R, Linder J. Chemical peels. In: Small R, Linder J, eds. *A Practical Guide to Skin Care Procedures and Products.* Philadelphia: Lippincott Williams & Wilkins; 2011.

Uecker C. Chemical peels. In: Pfenninger JL, Fowler GC, eds. *Pfenninger and Fowler's Procedures for Primary Care.* 3rd ed. Philadelphia: Mosby/Elsevier; 2010.

23 Microdermabrasion

REBECCA SMALL, MD • RACQUEL QUEMA, MD

Microdermabrasion (MDA) is a superficial skin resurfacing procedure that utilizes gentle mechanical abrasion to remove the outermost layers of the epidermis.[1] Removal of outer skin layers, also called exfoliation, has been used for skin rejuvenation since 1500 BC, when the ancient Egyptians used sandpaper and sour milk baths containing lactic acid. Microdermabrasion uses refined abrasive elements, such as diamond-tipped pads or a constant flow of crystals swept across the skin, to remove the stratum corneum.[2] Due to popular marketing, patients are aware of MDA and it is often considered as an initial treatment for aesthetic rejuvenation. It is one of the most commonly performed aesthetic procedures in the United States today, with more than half a million MDA treatments performed annually, according to data from the American Society for Aesthetic Plastic Surgery,[3] and it is one of the most common aesthetic procedures incorporated into office practice.[4,5]

Mechanical exfoliation of the skin ranges in depth from very superficial microbead scrubs found over the counter, which partially remove the stratum corneum, to deep operative procedures, such as laser resurfacing and dermabrasion, which can ablate the reticular dermis. The target depth for most microdermabrasion procedures is removal of the stratum corneum; however, the depth of resurfacing achieved with MDA can vary from the stratum corneum to the upper papillary dermis.

Skin rejuvenation with microdermabrasion is based on the principles of wound healing. By wounding and removing superficial skin layers in a controlled manner, cell renewal is stimulated with regeneration of a healthier epidermis and dermis.[1] After a series of MDA treatments, histologic changes in the skin are evident. These changes include a compacted stratum corneum and smoother epidermis, increased dermal thickness with fibroblast production of new collagen and elastin,[6] and increased skin hydration with improved epidermal barrier function.[7,8] Clinical improvements can be seen in hyperpigmentation[9] and rough skin texture.[10] Some studies also show improvements in fine lines, pore size, superficial acne scars, and acne vulgaris.[7,9,11] MDA can be readily combined with other minimally invasive aesthetic procedures, such as chemical peels and nonablative laser treatments, many of which can be performed in the same visit, to enhance skin rejuvenation results.[12]

PATIENT SELECTION

While almost any patient will benefit from exfoliation with MDA, patients with mild to moderate photoaging changes of solar lentigines, rough texture, and fine lines (e.g., Glogau types I and II) typically derive the most noticeable benefits (see Chapter 19, *Aesthetics Principles and Consultation,* for a description of Glogau types). Results with MDA are slow and progressive, requiring a series of treatments for visible improvements. Assessment of patients' expectations at the time of consultation and commitment to a series of treatments is essential to the success of these treatments.

Patients of all Fitzpatrick skin types may be treated with MDA (see Chapter 19 for a description of Fitzpatrick skin types). It is advisable to treat darker skin types (IV through VI) conservatively because they have increased risks of pigmentary changes such as postinflammatory hyperpigmentation. Elderly patients with thin and friable skin and patients with erythematous conditions such as rosacea, telangiectasias, and poikiloderma of Civatte are also treated conservatively, because they have greater risks of abrasion and worsening of erythema respectively.

COSMETIC INDICATIONS[1]

- Photodamaged skin
- Rough skin texture
- Hyperpigmentation (e.g., solar lentigines, melasma, postinflammatory hyperpigmentation)
- Comedonal acne (whiteheads and blackheads); also called clogged pores or skin congestion by laypersons
- Mild to moderate papulopustular acne
- Fine lines
- Dull, sallow skin color
- Enlarged pores
- Superficial scars
- Keratosis pilaris
- Thickened scaling skin (e.g., ichthyosis)
- Dry skin (xerosis)
- Seborrheic keratoses
- Enhanced penetration of topical agents (e.g., chemical peels).

ALTERNATIVE THERAPIES

The depth of skin resurfacing with MDA is comparable to a light chemical peel, which is a reasonable alternative treatment for skin rejuvenation. MDA offers certain advantages over chemical peels such as greater control over the depth of exfoliation, comparatively less discomfort, and no "downtime" for skin flaking and peeling. Superficial dermaplaning, performed with a specialized scalpel blade gently scraped across the skin, is a good alternative to MDA for patients with erythematous conditions such as rosacea, because there is no vacuum suction with this procedure to potentially exacerbate erythema. Dermaplaning requires greater treatment times and takes longer to acquire proficiency than MDA.

For more aggressive skin resurfacing, procedures such as medium-depth chemical peels, dermabrasion, or laser resurfacing are required. Dermabrasion involves the use of a high-speed rotating brush to abrade the skin and can penetrate to the reticular dermis. Laser resurfacing can also penetrate to the reticular dermis, and may be performed as an ablative procedure, where the epidermis is removed (e.g., with 2940 nm wavelength), or as a nonablative procedure, where the epidermis remains intact (e.g., with 1550 nm wavelength). Relative to MDA, these more aggressive resurfacing procedures offer significantly greater reduction of wrinkles and improvements in photodamaged skin. However, deeper resurfacing procedures such as these have longer recovery times and can be associated with complications such as scarring, dyspigmentation, and infection.

Microdermabrasion will not improve deep wrinkles and folds related to volume loss or hyperdynamic musculature, which respond to treatment with dermal fillers and botulinum toxin, respectively.

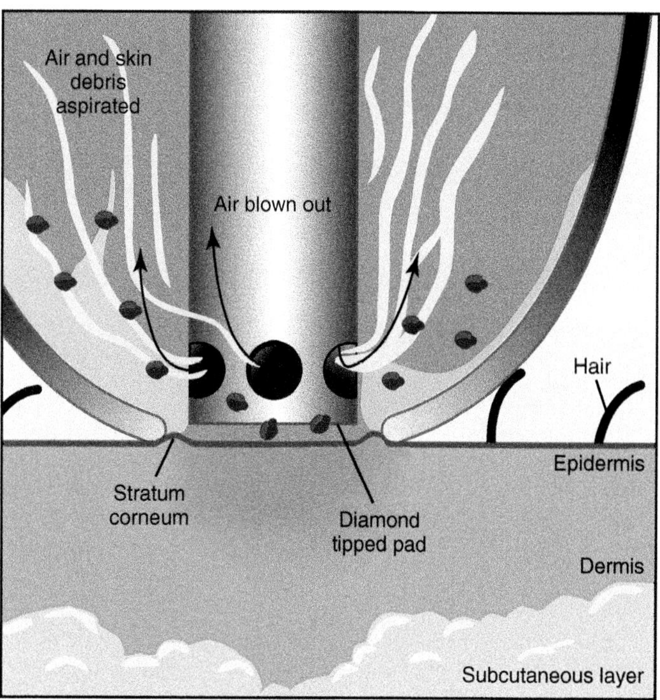

FIGURE 23-1 Microdermabrasion exfoliation process. *(SilkPeel™ Envy Medical, Los Angeles, CA.)*

MICRODERMABRASION DEVICES CURRENTLY AVAILABLE

Most MDA devices utilize a closed-loop vacuum system, which draws the skin up to an abrasive element on the handpiece tip. The handpiece is passed across the skin and cellular debris is removed and suctioned up into a collection container and disposed of after treatment. The process of MDA exfoliation using a diamond-tipped device is shown in Figure 23-1. Abrasive elements used by MDA devices vary and the most commonly used elements are:

- Crystals
- Diamonds
- Bristles.

Aluminum oxide (typically 100 μm in diameter) is the crystal most often used for MDA. It is inert, very hard, water insoluble, and its crystalline structure has multiple sharp edges, making it good for abrasion. Other types of crystals less commonly used include sodium chloride, sodium bicarbonate, and magnesium oxide. Most crystal devices blow crystals across the skin and aspirate them along with skin debris into a closed container. Some devices use crystal covered pads rather than aerosolized crystals. Aerosolized crystal devices have the disadvantage of leaving a dust residue, and have risks of ocular injury and dust inhalation. Crystals are not reusable but their expense is modest.

Crystal-free MDA devices have become popular because they lack these ocular and inhalation risks. Common crystal-free abrasive elements include diamond-tipped pads and bristles. Figure 23-2 shows a MDA handpiece with diamond-tipped treatment heads of various coarseness. Most of these devices have reusable treatment heads that can be sterilized following treatment. Some crystal-free devices combine simultaneous application of topical solutions during exfoliation, called *infusion*. The intent is to deliver topical products more effectively to the skin by taking advantage of the transient disruption of the epidermal barrier. Selection of topical solutions is based on the presenting condition. For example, hydroquinone or cosmeceuticals such as kojic acid and decapeptide-12 may be used for patients with hyperpigmentation; erythromycin and salicylic acid for acne and rosacea; and hyaluronic acid and glycerin for dehydrated skin.

MDA devices are classified by the FDA as type I devices, which do not require the manufacturer to establish performance standards or perform clinical

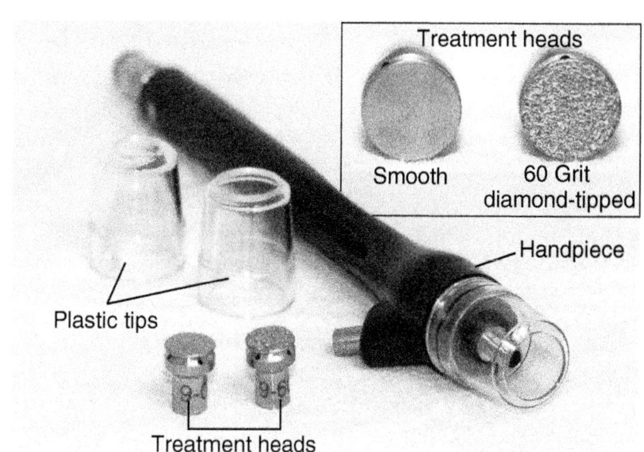

FIGURE 23-2 Microdermabrasion handpiece and diamond-tipped treatment heads. *(SilkPeel Envy, copyright Rebecca Small, MD.)*

trials to demonstrate efficacy. With more than 30 MDA devices available, this presents a challenge to providers when selecting a device. Most MDA machines are either manufactured for estheticians ("esthetician grade") or for clinical providers ("medical grade"), with the latter capable of deeper exfoliation with higher vacuum pressures and more abrasive treatment heads. Commonly used MDA devices are listed in the *Resources* section at the end of the chapter.

CONTRAINDICATIONS[1]

- Pregnancy or nursing
- Active infection or open wound in the treatment area (e.g., herpes simplex or cellulitis)
- Keloidal or hypertrophic scarring
- Isotretinoin (Accutane) use within the past 6 months
- Melanoma (or lesions suspected for melanoma), basal cell or squamous cell carcinoma in the treatment area
- Bleeding abnormality (e.g., thrombocytopenia or anticoagulant use)
- Impaired healing (e.g., due to immunosuppression)
- Skin atrophy (e.g., chronic oral steroid use or genetic syndromes such as Ehlers-Danlos syndrome)
- Dermatoses such as vitiligo, active psoriasis, or atopic dermatitis in the treatment area
- Uncontrolled systemic condition
- Deep chemical peel, dermabrasion, or radiation therapy in the treatment area within the preceding 6 months
- Severe forms of erythematous conditions such as rosacea, telangiectasias, or poikiloderma of Civatte
- Severe pustular acne
- Excessive laxity and skinfolds
- Insufficient sun protection
- Unrealistic expectations
- Body dysmorphic disorder.

ADVANTAGES OF MICRODERMABRASION

- Controlled depth of exfoliation
- Safe for all Fitzpatrick skin types (I through VI)
- Minimal to no discomfort during the procedure
- No anesthesia required
- Minimal risk of complications
- No recovery time postprocedure (e.g., for skin flaking and peeling as with chemical peels)
- May be combined with other aesthetic treatments, particularly topical products, for enhanced results.
- Procedural proficiency rapidly acquired.

DISADVANTAGES OF MICRODERMABRASION

- MDA devices are relatively costly (compared to chemical peels).
- There are costs associated with the disposable crystals and topical solutions.
- A series of treatments is necessary for best results.

ANATOMY

Histologic evaluation of skin immediately after treatment with MDA demonstrates smoothing of the stratum corneum.[13] Each pass of an aluminum oxide crystal MDA handpiece removes approximately 10 to 15 µm of skin, two passes fully remove the stratum corneum, and four passes penetrate to the stratum granulosum layer of the epidermis.[14] The epidermal barrier function is transiently disrupted for 2 to 3 days after treatment with increased transepidermal water loss. These effects, however, are reversed 1 week after treatment, and a more compacted stratum corneum is regenerated with improved barrier function and increased skin hydration compared to pretreatment skin.[15,16]

In addition to short-term improvements in epidermal barrier function, longer term improvements have also been demonstrated in the epidermis and dermis following repeated MDA treatments. Epidermal thickness increases by up to 40% due to increased cellularity,[7] and dermal collagen and elastin deposition increase, which can be seen clinically as a reduction of coarse pores and fine lines.[6]

EQUIPMENT

- MDA device with abrasive element
- Facial wash
- Alcohol or alcohol-based astringent to degrease the skin
- Headband or surgical cap for patient
- Towel to drape the patient
- Protective eye shields (e.g., adhesive eye pads or extraocular goggles)
- Nonsterile gloves
- 4- × 4-inch nonwoven gauze pads
- Clear goggles for provider (with crystal MDA)
- Mask for provider to reduce particle inhalation (with crystal MDA)
- Postprocedure products including a soothing moisturizer (e.g., SkinCeutical's Epidermal Repair) and broad-spectrum sunscreen (SPF 30 or greater) with zinc or titanium
- Saline eyewash (with crystal MDA).

PROCEDURE PREPARATION

1. Review the patient's medical history (see Chapter 19, *Aesthetic Principles and Consultation*).
2. Perform a facial aesthetic consultation (see Chapter 19).
3. Perform a detailed skin evaluation noting the patient's Fitzpatrick skin type, skin thickness, wrinkles, dryness, acne, scars, pigmentation, and vascular and other skin conditions. An example of a form

that may be used for skin evaluation is shown in Figure 22-5 in Chapter 22, *Chemical Peels*.

4. Obtain informed consent (see Chapter 19; also see Appendix A for an informed consent form and patient information handout titled *Skin Care Treatments*).
5. Pretreatment photographs are advised (see Chapter 19).
6. Broad-spectrum sunscreen containing zinc or titanium (SPF 30 or higher) is used daily throughout the treatment series.
7. Two weeks prior to procedure: Advise patients to avoid chemical peels, depilatory creams, electrolysis, and to refrain from tanning and direct sun exposure.
8. One week prior to procedure: Advise patients to discontinue products containing retinoids or hydroxy acids.
9. Two days prior to procedure: Start the patient on a prophylactic antiviral medication (e.g., acyclovir or vancyclovir) for patients with a history of herpes simplex or varicella in or around the treatment area, and continue for 3 days postprocedure.
10. The day of the procedure: Advise patients to wash the treatment area, remove any facial jewelry, and take out contact lenses.

MICRODERMABRASION: STEPS AND PRINCIPLES

The following recommendations are guidelines for microdermabrasion treatments on the face using the SilkPeel (manufactured by Envy), which is a crystal-free device that utilizes diamond-tipped pads as the abrasive element with simultaneous infusion of topical solutions. Comparisons and recommendations for crystal and bristle MDA devices are also included where possible. Recommended treatment parameters vary according to the device used, and specific manufacturer guidelines should be followed at the time of treatment.

General Treatment Technique

- MDA may be performed as a very superficial or superficial skin resurfacing procedure (see Chapter 19 for definitions of resurfacing terminology). Greater depths of penetration have greater potential for improvements. Although MDA has few risks, greater depths of penetration with any exfoliation procedure can be associated with a greater risk of complications.
- Certain factors increase the exfoliation depth for all MDA devices:
  - Higher vacuum pressure
  - Greater number of passes, where a pass is defined as contiguous coverage of the treatment area.
- For *crystal MDA devices*, increased exfoliation depth is also related to slower handpiece speed, more acute angle of impaction, larger crystal size, and higher crystal flow rate.
- For *diamond-tipped MDA* devices, increased exfoliation depth is also related to grit coarseness and downward pressure on the skin (if the tip is not recessed). Note that the SilkPeel has a recessed treatment tip. Treatment heads range from smooth (no diamond chips) to fine (120 grit) to coarse (30 grit), as shown in Figure 23-2.
- For *bristle MDA devices*, increased depth of exfoliation is also related to bristle stiffness and downward pressure on the skin.
- In general, the clinician can assume that two passes with most medical-grade MDA devices using aggressive treatment parameters will exfoliate the stratum corneum, and four passes will exfoliate the lower epidermis. For example:
  - *Crystal (aluminum oxide) MDA devices* fully exfoliate the stratum corneum after two passes at a vacuum setting of 4 psi (200 mm Hg) using crystals of at least 20 μm.
  - *Diamond-tipped MDA devices*, such as the SilkPeel, fully exfoliate the stratum corneum after two passes at a vacuum setting of 5 psi (260 mm Hg) using a 60-grit treatment head.
- Devices utilizing infusion of topical solutions are associated with less discomfort, hence, patient feedback may be a less reliable indicator of treatment intensity. For example, patients may experience superficial abrasions without reporting pain during treatment. Observation of tissue response is, therefore, particularly important in determining treatment parameters with infusion MDA devices.
- Bleeding is a sign that the papillary dermis has been breached. This is to be avoided, due to increased risks of scarring with dermal injury.
- Conservative treatment settings are advised for patients with thin skin or erythematous conditions and for patients with higher Fitzpatrick skin types (IV through VI) to reduce the risks of prolonged erythema and pigmentary changes.

Planning and Designing

Microdermabrasion *treatment intensity* is selected based on the presenting skin condition and treatment area, as outlined below:

- *Mild treatments* (two passes, mild abrasive element, low vacuum settings) are used for pustular acne, conditions with facial erythema such as rosacea, telangiectasias, or poikiloderma of Civatte, and patients with thin skin.
- *Moderate treatments* (two to four passes, moderate abrasive element, moderate vacuum settings) are used for treatment of hyperpigmentation, rough skin, fine lines, coarse pores, comedonal acne, keratosis pilaris, skin maintenance treatments, and when an MDA procedure is followed by application of a chemical peel.
- *Aggressive treatments* (four or more passes, coarse abrasive element, high vacuum settings) are used for treatment of superficial acne scars and nonfacial

hyperkeratotic areas such as elbows/knees and pedal calluses.

Anesthesia

Preprocedure anesthesia is not required with MDA.

Safety Zone

The area within which MDA treatments can be safely performed on the face, called the Microdermabrasion Safety Zone, is shown in Figure 23-3. All areas of the face may be treated, apart from the area within the bony orbital rim and, for most devices, the lips. Some MDA devices have nonabrasive smooth treatment tips that may be used on the lips (Figure 23-2). MDA can be used on the face, neck, chest, hands, back, and almost any area of the body requiring exfoliation.

Performing Microdermabrasion

1. Comfortably position the patient supine on the treatment table.
2. Place a headband or surgical cap on the patient to pull hair away from the face. Cover the patient's eyes with protective eye shields. If using crystal MDA, the provider should also wear protective eyewear and a mask.
3. Clean the treatment area with a cleanser and then degrease with alcohol or an alcohol-based astringent. Wait for the skin to dry completely before starting the procedure.
4. Select the size of the treatment head based on the treatment location, use larger heads for most body treatment areas, and smaller heads for the face.

TABLE 23-1 Treatment Parameters for SilkPeel Microdermabrasion

Treatment Intensity	Tip Coarseness	Vacuum Pressure (psi)
Mild	140 grit	3.0–4.0
Moderate	120 grit	3.5–4.3
Aggressive	100 grit	4.4–5.0

- With the SilkPeel, use the 6-mm head for face, neck, chest and hands, and 9-mm head for other body areas.

5. For devices with abrasive treatment heads, such as diamond-tipped heads, select the coarseness of the head based on the aggressiveness of treatment. Recommended treatment parameters using the SilkPeel are shown in Table 23-1.
6. Select the vacuum setting by inverting the handpiece and occluding the tip with a gloved finger (Figure 23-4). The strength of the vacuum affects the depth of resurfacing, and small adjustments in this parameter can fine-tune the intensity of a treatment. Vacuum pressures are device dependent and the manufacturer's recommended settings should be used. In general, conservative vacuum settings should be selected for initial treatments.
   TIP: Reduce vacuum pressure in the thin-skinned periorbital areas.
7. If using a device that infuses solutions, select a topical product appropriate for the presenting condition, then select a flow rate of infusion per the manufacturer's guidelines.
   - For hyperpigmentation, use lightening agents such as hydroquinone, kojic acid, arbutin, or brightening peptides (e.g., decapeptide-12).

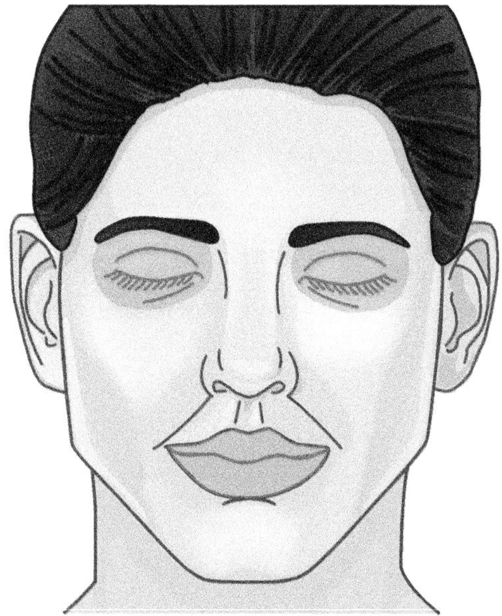

FIGURE 23-3 Microdermabrasion Safety Zone for facial treatments.

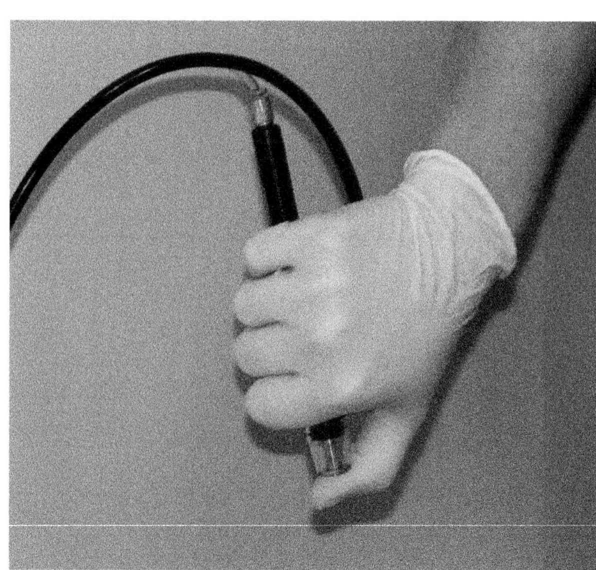

FIGURE 23-4 Handpiece occlusion for selection of microdermabrasion vacuum settings. *(SilkPeel Envy, copyright Rebecca Small, MD.)*

- For dehydration and fine lines, use hyaluronic acid, allantoin, and glycerin.
- For photodamage, use vitamin C.
- For acne, use erythromycin and salicylic acid.

TIP: Two topical solutions may be infused during a treatment to address two conditions. For example, hyaluronic acid may be used with the first pass and to improve dehydration and decapeptide-12 for hyperpigmentation with the second pass.

8. The direction of handpiece strokes on the face are from the medial face toward the periphery (Figure 23-5). Begin at the forehead, then proceed down the nose, cheeks, chin, and lastly, around the mouth.
9. Stretch the skin between two fingers, hold the handpiece perpendicular to the skin and bring the tip gently in contact with the skin. Move the handpiece smoothly and slowly across the skin with even pressure, parallel to the tension line between the fingers (Figure 23-6).

TIP: Exfoliation with the SilkPeel will not occur unless the tip is moving across the skin.

CAUTION: With crystal MDA, do not leave the handpiece in one spot because this will increase the abrasion depth.

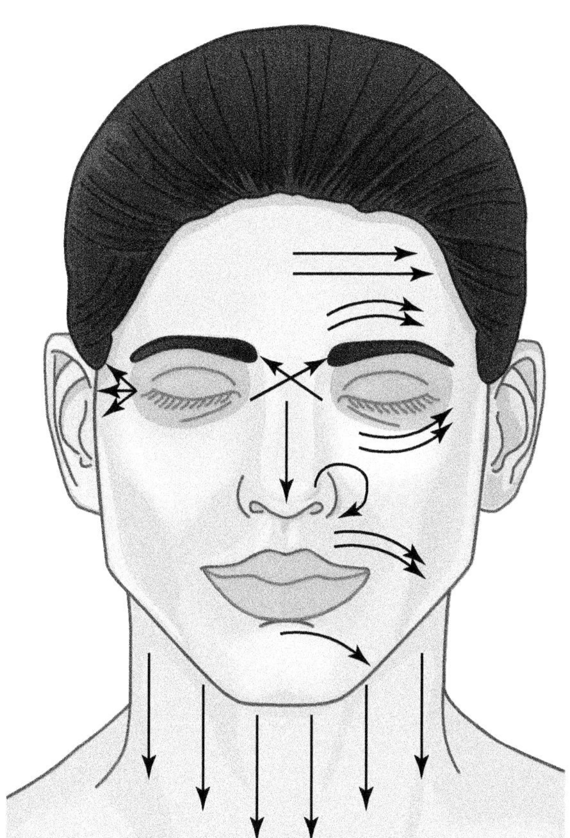

FIGURE 23-5 Direction guide for microdermabrasion treatment of the face and neck.

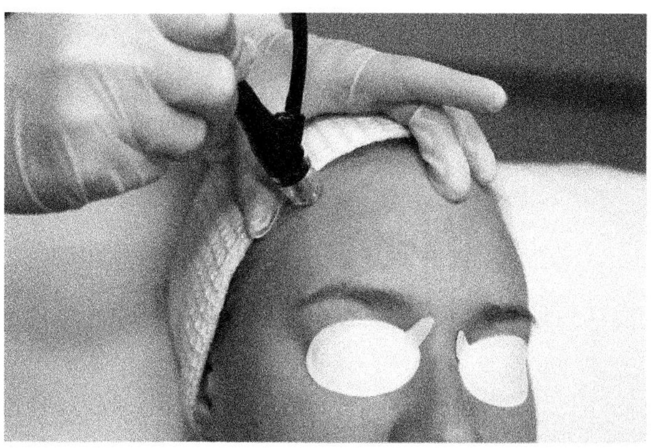

FIGURE 23-6 Technique for microdermabrasion first pass. *(Copyright Rebecca Small, MD.)*

CAUTION: With crystal MDA and devices with nonrecessed abrasive treatment heads, avoid excessive downward pressure because this increases the abrasion depth.

10. Observe the skin for the desired clinical endpoint of mild erythema.
11. Overly aggressive treatment is indicated by:
    - Petechiae and purpura
    - Patient intolerance (pain of 6/10 or more)

    If either of these occur, settings should be promptly modified by reducing vacuum pressure and other parameters affecting treatment intensity.
12. After completing treatment of the entire area, a second pass to the same treatment area may be performed by moving the handpiece perpendicular to the previous stroke direction (Figure 23-7).
13. Other treatment areas:
    - *Neck:* Patient should lift the chin to extend the neck. Perform only one pass using vertical strokes with mild treatment parameters.
    - *Chest:* Perform two passes with strokes from the midline to the periphery.
    - *Hands:* Have the patient make a fist while holding a soft ball or rolled towel. Perform the first pass with strokes parallel to the axis of the forearm and a second pass with perpendicular strokes.

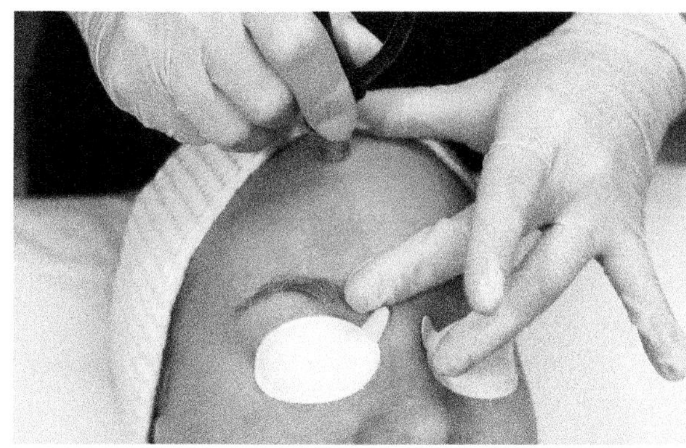

FIGURE 23-7 Technique for microdermabrasion second pass. *(Copyright Rebecca Small, MD.)*

14. At subsequent visits, parameters may be increased to intensify treatments. In general, either the number of passes or the grit coarseness is changed to intensify treatments in any given visit. It is advisable to change only one parameter during a treatment to safely escalate treatment intensity.
    TIP: It is important to reassess the skin at each visit prior to treatment, because the condition of the skin is dynamic and may vary between treatments.
15. Apply a soothing topical moisturizer (e.g., Epidermal Repair by SkinCeuticals) and a zinc or titanium sunscreen with SPF 30 or higher (e.g., products by Solar Protection, SkinCeuticals, and Skin Medica) after the treatment. If using a crystal device, ensure that all crystal debris is removed with moist gauze, especially in the periorbital area prior to application.
16. Sanitize and sterilize reusable equipment parts between treatments per the manufacturer guidelines. This is commonly performed by circulating a disinfectant solution through the machine. Dispose of used crystals and topical solutions. Diamond-tipped and other reusable abrasive heads require debridement with a brush and enzyme bath, followed by autoclaving after procedures.

RESULTS

Microdermabrasion is a progressive treatment. A slight improvement in skin texture or skin brightness after a single treatment may be evident. However, for more marked results and improvements in pigmentation, acne, fine lines, and other conditions, a series of six treatments is usually necessary.

Figure 23-8 shows a patient demonstrating signs of moderate photodamage with solar lentigines, dullness, and fine lines (A) before and (B) after a series of six treatments with a bristle MDA using an infusion of topical solutions containing glycolic and lactic acid, and cosmeceutical lightening agents of kojic and azelaic acids, bearberry, and licorice.

Figure 23-9 shows a patient with papulopustular acne (A) before and (B) after a series of six MDA treatments with a diamond-tipped MDA using an infusion of topical solutions containing salicylic, glycolic and kojic acids and arbutin.

Figure 23-10 shows a patient with darker Fitzpatrick skin type with solar lentigines and dullness (A) before and (B) after a series of six MDA treatments with a diamond-tipped MDA using an infusion of topical solutions containing a lightening peptide, decapeptide-12 (Lumixyl™).

AFTERCARE

Patients may experience mild erythema, dryness, and/or tingling for 1 to 3 days after treatment, more so with crystal MDA and devices without infusion of topical solutions. A nonocclusive moisturizer (e.g., SkinCeutical's Epidermal Repair) may be applied as frequently as needed for dryness during this time. Patients are instructed to avoid irritating products including retinoids, astringents, depilatories, and exfoliants such as glycolic acid, for 2 weeks, or until the skin has no more signs of irritation. Botulinum toxin treatment may be performed on the same day, immediately following MDA if desired. Patients are instructed to avoid direct sun exposure for 4 weeks and use a daily sunscreen with SPF 30 or higher (containing zinc or titanium)

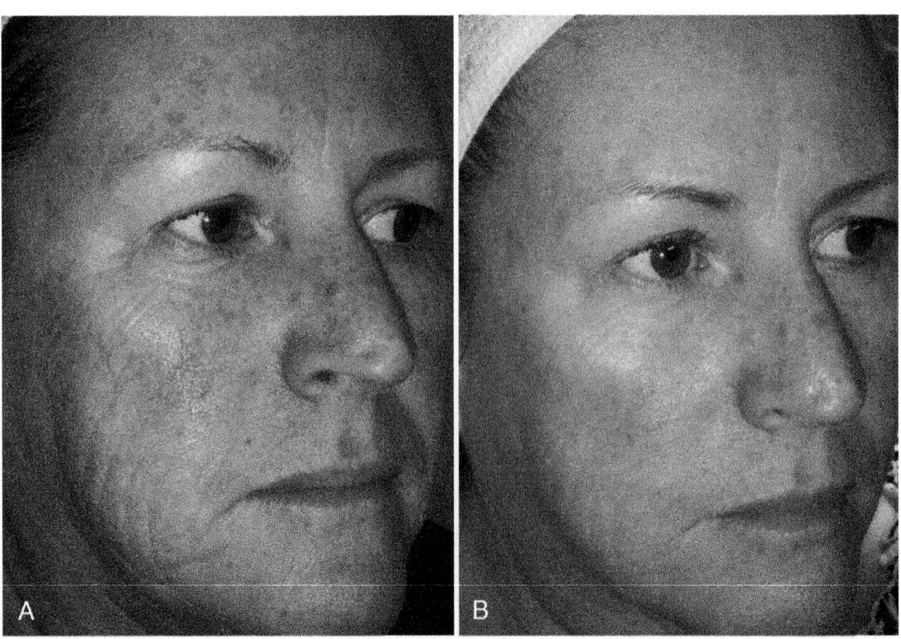

FIGURE 23-8 Moderate photodamage changes of solar lentigines, dullness, and fine lines before **(A)** and after **(B)** six bristle (DermaSweep™) microdermabrasion treatments. *(Courtesy of CosMedic R&D, Inc., Roseville, CA.)*

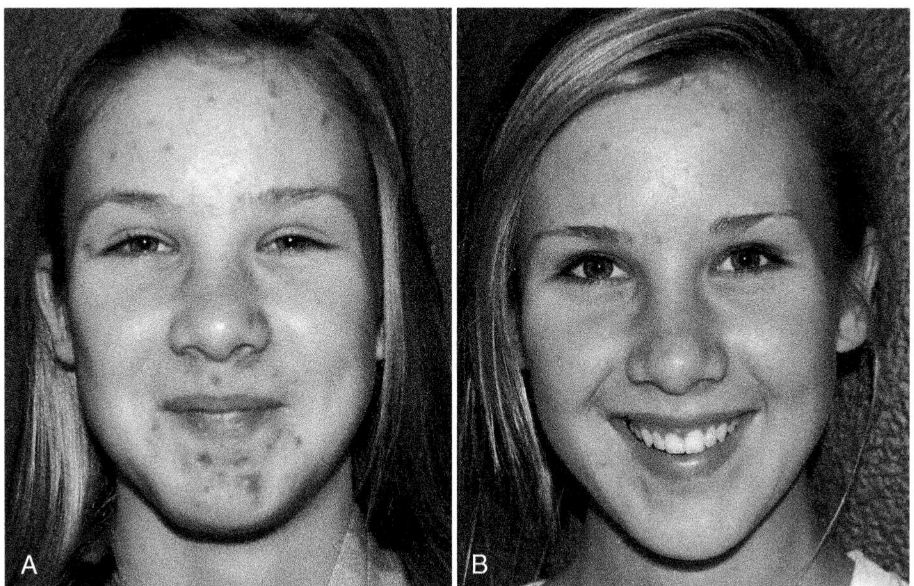

FIGURE 23-9 Acne vulgaris (**A**) before and (**B**) after six diamond-tipped (SilkPeel) microdermabrasion treatments. *(Courtesy of Envy Medical, Los Angeles, CA.)*

during the course of their treatments. If a scab or abrasion occurs, a topical antibiotic ointment (e.g., Bacitracin) may be used daily until healed and patients are advised to avoid picking, as this can increase the risk of scarring and other complications.

FOLLOW-UP

Treatments may be performed every 2 to 4 weeks during a series of six treatments. Maintenance treatments thereafter may be done every 4 to 6 weeks, or as deemed necessary by the provider.

ADVANCED MICRODERMABRASION

As providers gain experience and skill with microdermabrasion, they may choose to broaden its applications and combine it with other procedures to increase treatment intensity. Microdermabrasion can be used as part of skin preparation prior to the application of certain

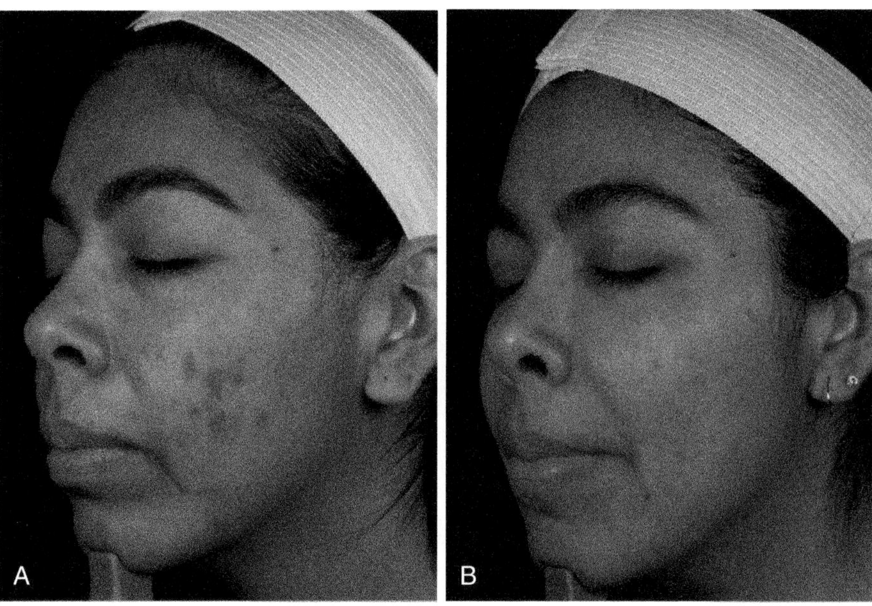

FIGURE 23-10 Postinflammatory hyperpigmentation and acne in a patient with darker Fitzpatrick skin type (**A**) before and (**B**) after six diamond-tipped (SilkPeel) microdermabrasion treatments. *(Courtesy of A. Bhatia, MD, using SilkPeel, Envy Medical, Los Angeles, CA.)*

chemical peels to allow for more even peel penetration and to enhance the depth of penetration into the skin. Providers are advised to use established manufacturer protocols when combining these two exfoliation modalities because peel penetration can be significantly altered by the lack of the stratum corneum barrier that is removed by microdermabrasion.[12]

Microdermabrasion may also be used as part of photodynamic therapy (PDT), an FDA-approved treatment for nonhyperkeratotic actinic keratoses of the face and used off label to enhance photorejuvenation treatments with lasers (see Chapter 27, *Photorejuvenation with Lasers*, for more information about PDT). Prior to application of topical photosensitizing medications, such as 5-aminolevulinic acid (Levulan®), MDA can be performed which enhances product penetration and increases intensity of the treatment.[17]

COMPLICATIONS

- Pain
- Superficial abrasion
- Infection such as herpes simplex, impetigo, or candidiasis
- Prolonged irritation or erythema
- Petechiae or purpura
- Urticaria
- Postinflammatory hyperpigmentation
- Exacerbation of erythema in patients with telangiectasias, rosacea, and poikiloderma of Civatte
- Remote possibility of scarring
- Ocular injury with crystals.

MDA has minimal risks of side effects and complications.[1] One study of more than 100 patients receiving MDA during a 2-year period reported no instances of infection, long-term hyperpigmentation, or scarring.[18] However, complications are possible with any procedure, and knowledge of these is important to help ensure the best possible outcomes.

Postprocedure erythema is common and the duration depends on the aggressiveness of the procedure and inherent reactivity of the patients' skin. Most erythema resolves spontaneously within a few hours to 1 day. Prolonged erythema of more than 5 days, particularly in patients with darker Fitzpatrick skin types (IV through VI), can result in postinflammatory hyperpigmentation (PIH). If erythema is marked immediately after treatment, ice can be applied to the skin for 15 minutes every hour followed by a topical steroid cream. A high-potency topical steroid cream may be used in the office (e.g., triamcinolone 0.5%) and the patient sent home with a low-potency steroid (e.g., hydrocortisone 2.5% or 1%) to be used twice daily for 3 to 5 days or until erythema resolves. Sun avoidance is very important to reduce the risk of PIH when erythema is present.

Excessive dryness or pruritis can be managed with application of moisturizers. Use of highly occlusive moisturizers, such as Aquaphor, will reduce these symptoms but can be associated with development of acne and milia. Therefore, thinner, less occlusive moisturizer formulations (e.g., Epidermal Repair by SkinCeuticals) with frequent application is preferable to manage dryness and pruritis.

Superficial abrasions can occur with deeper MDA penetration. These are usually erythematous immediately after treatment and can either hyperpigment or crust slightly. Superficial abrasions are also referred to as *striping*, due to the appearance of lines on the skin. Abrasions may also be circular if the tip has dwelled too long or excessive downward pressure was applied in one spot. Crusting is managed with moist wound care using a topical antibiotic ointment (e.g., Bacitracin) as needed daily until healed.

Hyperpigmentation can be treated with lightening agents such as hydroquinone or cosmeceutical agents such as kojic acid, arbutin, and licorice (see Chapter 24, *Skin Care Products*). In darker Fitzpatrick skin types, resolution of hyperpigmentation typically takes several months. Hyperpigmentation usually resolves, but in rare instances can be permanent.

Urticaria has been reported as a rare complication after MDA,[19] and is presumed to be dermatographic or pressure-induced. Products applied during treatment may also trigger an allergic response. Ice may be applied, an oral antihistamine (e.g., cetirizine 10 mg) given to the patient, and a high-potency topical steroid applied to the treatment area. Although extremely unlikely, it is also advisable to assess patients for signs and symptoms of more severe allergic responses such as bronchospasm or anaphylaxis if an allergic reaction occurs.

Petechiae and *purpura* can occur with overly aggressive vacuum settings, particularly in older patients with thin skin or if using anticoagulants. If petechiae occur, vacuum settings should be decreased and the affected area avoided for the remainder of treatment. Petechiae resolve more rapidly than purpura, which can take up to 2 weeks to clear.

Scarring is a remote possibility and can occur if treatment parameters are aggressive, and is more likely if infection occurs or crusts are excoriated. *Hypopigmentation* is also a rare possibility, with greater risks in darker Fitzpatrick skin types. Hypopigmentation can be a temporary or permanent complication.

Ocular injury due to crystal adherence to the conjunctiva or punctuate keratopathy can occur with crystal MDA devices. Symptoms include ocular pain, photophobia, and conjunctival erythema.[11] Protective eye shields or moist gauze is advised with crystal MDA to cover patients' eyes, appropriate eyewear and masks for providers, and removal of all crystals from the face following treatment.

TREATING SPECIFIC LESIONS

- *Seborrheic keratoses*. MDA can reduce the hyperkeratosis of these lesions but the lesions do not typically resolve.
- *Actinic keratoses (AKs)*. MDA can reduce the hyperkeratosis of AKs, but it is not a treatment for AKs. Rather, reducing hyperkeratosis may obscure the presence of AKs, because the rough texture of these

lesions is often their only presenting sign. Given that AKs have a small potential for conversion to squamous cell carcinoma, treatment of AKs with appropriate therapies is recommended.

- *Nevi.* Nevi should be avoided with MDA so as not to cause depigmentation.
- *Erythematous conditions such as rosacea, telangiectasia, and poikiloderma of Civatte.* Poikiloderma of Civatte is a pattern of erythema and mottled pigmentation commonly seen on the sides of the neck, face, and chest due to photodamage (Figure 23-11). Treatment of erythematous conditions is controversial with MDA. Clearly, excessive vacuum pressures can accentuate superficial vasculature, making erythema worse. However, in rosacea patients, for example, who have impaired barrier function, mild MDA treatments performed at low vacuum settings, may ultimately strengthen the epidermal barrier, reducing erythema.[20] Some providers, therefore, do perform MDA on patients with erythematous conditions using reduced vacuum settings in areas of high vascularity such as the midface and chin, and higher settings around the periphery of the face (Figure 23-12). Patients intolerant of MDA may alternatively receive superficial dermaplaning.
- *Acne vulgaris.* MDA can be used for mild to severe noninflammatory acne (comedonal) and mild to moderate papulopustular acne. MDA is not feasible with extensive pustules as seen with severe papulopustular acne, and alternative treatments such as oral medications and/or chemical peels are preferred treatment options.

LEARNING THE TECHNIQUES

Providers are encouraged to practice first on themselves, on the anterior thigh, and then on the face of staff and friends prior to treating patients.

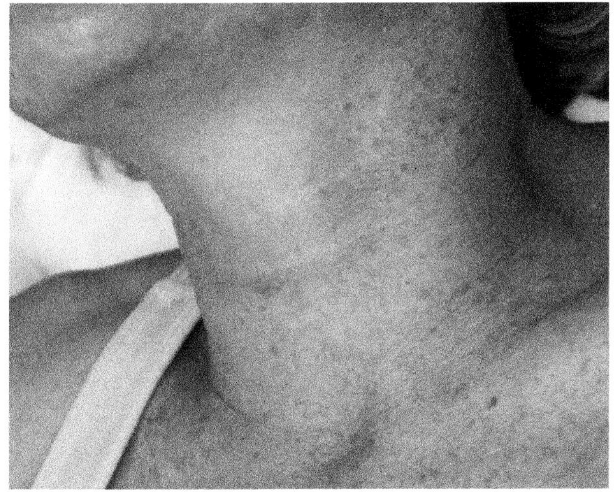

FIGURE 23-11 Poikiloderma of Civatte. *(Copyright Rebecca Small, MD.)*

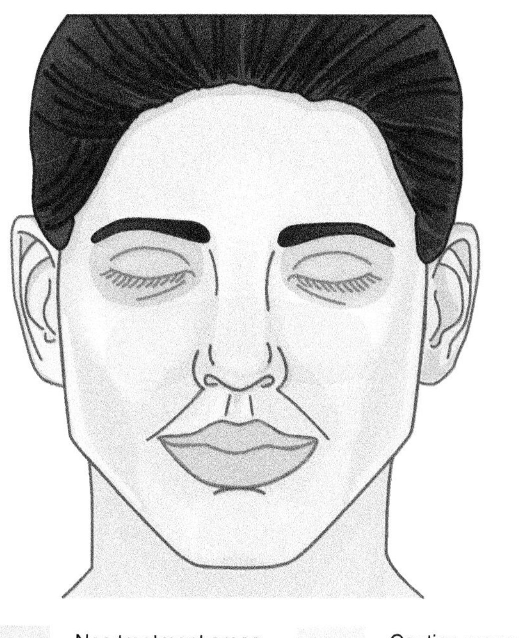

FIGURE 23-12 Caution areas for microdermabrasion treatments in patients with facial erythema and rosacea.

CURRENT DEVELOPMENTS

Ultrasonic MDA Devices

Some MDA devices utilize dull spatula blades with ultrasonic oscillation to disrupt and exfoliate the stratum corneum. The treatment area is kept cool by applying water to the skin during treatment, and these procedures are associated with splatter of skin debris and water. No studies are available regarding this new modality, and manufacturers claim that these devices are more gentle and penetrate less deeply than standard MDA devices.

Light-Emitting Diodes with MDA

Some newer devices combine light-emitting diodes (LEDs) with MDA. Blue-light LEDs are used as enhancements for treatment of acne, and red-light LEDs are used to enhance treatment of photodamaged skin and stimulate collagen and elastin deposition.[21]

FINANCIAL CONSIDERATIONS

Medical-grade MDA devices, capable of more aggressive treatments, are priced higher than esthetician-grade MDA devices. Crystal MDA machines need continuous replacement of crystals, because these are not recyclable. Diamond-tipped MDA machines use either disposable or reusable diamond treatment heads. The use of disposables should always be kept in mind when purchasing a system. Solutions for infusion are one such disposable.

Insurance does not reimburse for microdermabrasion procedures. The charges for treatments vary and are

BOX 23-1 *Codes for MDA Procedures*

CPT Codes

17999 Unlisted skin procedure
A9270 Noncovered service (for non-Medicare carriers)
Note: In 2008, the American Academy of Dermatology Association clarified that CPT code 15783 (dermabrasion, superficial, any site) is not appropriate to use for MDA.

ICD-9 Codes

706.1 Acne, comedones
709.09 Melasma
709.0 Dyschromia, unspecified
701.8 Wrinkling of skin
709.2 Scarring
695.3 Rosacea

largely determined by local prices. Patients may pay for individual treatments, which generally range from $75 to $100. However, MDA is most effective as a series of treatments, and packages of treatments (usually six) may be offered so that patients achieve the best possible results and satisfaction with the procedure. Box 23-1 lists codes for MDA procedures.

CONCLUSION

Microdermabrasion is a popular cosmetic procedure for aesthetic skin rejuvenation. From a patient perspective, it is safe, noninvasive, has relatively no recovery time, has minimal adverse effects, and is reasonably priced. From a provider perspective, it is technically straightforward and easily integrated into a practice. Microdermabrasion may be safely combined with skin care treatments, such as topical products, and with other minimally invasive aesthetic procedures such as chemical peels, lasers, or injectables, to enhance results.

Resources

Microdermabrasion Devices

Aesthetic Technologies (Parisian Peel)
Phone: 408-464-8893
www.mmizone.com

Altair Instruments (DiamondTome)
Phone: 866-325-8247
www.diamondtome.com

Bella Products (Bellamed)
Phone: 877-550-5655
www.bellaproducts.com

Bio-Therapeutic (Bio-Brasion)
Phone: 800-976-2544
www.bio-therapeutic.com

DermaMed International (MegaPeel)
Phone: 888-789-6342
www.megapeel.com

DermaSweep
Phone: 916-632-9134
www.dermasweep.com

DermaTone USA
Phone: 800-289-1574
www.dermatoneusa.com

DermaVista
Phone: 800-333-5773
www.dermavista.com

Dynatronics
Phone: 800-874-6251
www.dynatronics.com

Edge Systems
Phone: 800-603-4996
www.edgesystem.net

Envy Medical (SilkPeel)
Phone: 888-848-3633
www.silkpeel.com

ExcellaDerm
Phone: 877-969-7546
www.excelladerm.com

Lumenis
Phone: 408-764-3000
www.lumenis.com

Marketech International (Dermagrain)
Phone: 877-452-4910
www.dermagrain.com

Mattioli Engineering (Ultrapeel)
Phone: 703-312-6000
www.mattioliengineering.com

Med-Aesthetic Solutions
Phone: 877-733-7627
www.medaestheticsolutions.com

RAJA Medical
Phone: 877-880-4184
www.rajamedical.com

Refine USA (MicroGem)
Phone: 866-491-7546
www.refineusa.com

Silhouet-Tone USA
Phone: 800-463-2710
www.silhouet-tone.com

Sybaritic
Phone: 800-445-8418
www.sybaritic.com

Syneron
Phone: 866-259-6661
www.syneron.com

Crystal Supplier

NeedCrystals.com (wholesale aluminum oxide crystals)
Phone: 619-422-7576
www.needcrystals.com

References

1. Grimes PE. Microdermabrasion. *Derm Surg*. 2005;31(9 Pt 2):1160–1165.
2. Small R. Microdermabrasion. *In:* Mayeaux E, ed. *The Essential Guide to Primary Care Procedures*. Philadelphia: Lippincott Williams & Wilkins; 2009:265–277.
3. Cosmetic Surgery National Data Bank 2010 Statistics. American Society for Aesthetic Plastic Surgery; 2010.
4. Small R. Aesthetic procedures in office practice. *Am Fam Physician*. 2009;80(11):1231–1237.
5. Small R. Aesthetic procedures introduction. In: Mayeaux E, ed. *The Essential Guide to Primary Care Procedures*. Philadelphia: Lippincott Williams & Wilkins; 2009:195–199.
6. Rubin MG, Greenbaum S. Histologic effects of aluminum oxide microabrasion on facial skin. *J Aesthet Dermatol Cosm Surg*. 2000;1(4):237–239.
7. Coimbra M, Rohrich RJ, Chao J, *et al.* A prospective controlled assessment of microdermabrasion for damaged skin and fine rhytides. *Plast Reconstr Surg*. 2004;113(5):1438–1443.
8. Karimipour DJ, Kang S, Johnson TM, *et al.* Microdermabrasion with and without aluminum oxide crystal abrasion: a comparative molecular analysis of dermal remodeling. *J Am Acad Dermatol*. 2006;54(3):405–410.
9. Shim EK, Barnette D, Hughes K, *et al.* Microdermabrasion: a clinical and histopathologic study. *Derm Surg*. 2001;27(6): 524–530.
10. Hernandez-Perez E, Ibiett EV. Gross and microscopic findings in patients undergoing microdermabrasion for facial rejuvenation. *Derm Surg*. 2001;27(7):637–640.
11. Tsai RY, Wang CN, Chan HL. Aluminum oxide crystal microdermabrasion. A new technique for treating facial scarring. *Derm Surg*. 1995;21(6):539–542.
12. Briden ME, Jacobsen E, Johnson C. Combining superficial glycolic acid (alpha-hydroxy acid) peels with microdermabrasion to maximize treatment results and patient satisfaction. *Cutis*. 2007;79(1 Suppl):13–16.
13. Koch RJ, Hanasono MM. Microdermabrasion. *Facial Plast Surg Clin North Am*. 2001;9(3):377–382.
14. Blome D. Microdermabrasion. *In:* Pfenninger JL, Fowler GC, eds. *Pfenninger and Fowler's Procedures for Primary Care*. 3rd ed. Philadelphia: Mosby/Elsevier; 2010.
15. Freedman BM, Rueda-Pedraza E, Waddell SP. The epidermal and dermal changes associated with microdermabrasion. *Derm Surg*. 2001;27(12):1031–1033.
16. Rajan P, Grimes PE. Skin barrier changes induced by aluminum oxide and sodium chloride microdermabrasion. *Derm Surg*. 2002;28(5):390–393.
17. Nootheti PK, Gold MH, Goldman MP. Photodynamic therapy for photorejuvenation. *In:* Goldman MP, ed. *Photodynamic Therapy*. Philadelphia: Saunders/Elsevier; 2008:125–135.
18. Freeman MS. Microdermabrasion. *Facial Plast Surg Clin North Am*. 2001;9(2):257–266.
19. Farris P, Rietschel R. An unusual response to microdermabrasion. *Dermatol Surg*. 2002;28:606–608.
20. Desai T, Moy RL. Evaluation of the SilkPeel system in treating erythematotelangectatic and papulopustular rosacea. *Cosm Dermatol*. 2006;19:51–57.
21. Taub A. Photodynamic therapy: other uses. *Dermatol Clin*. 2007;25(1):101–109.

Additional Reading

Hantash BM. Microdermabrasion and dermal infusion. *In:* Pfenninger JL, Fowler GC, eds. *Pfenninger and Fowler's Procedures for Primary Care*. 3rd ed. Philadelphia: Mosby/Elsevier; 2011.

Small R, Linder J. Microdermabrasion. *In:* Small R, Linder J, eds. *A Practical Guide to Skin Care Procedures and Products*. Philadelphia: Lippincott Williams & Wilkins; 2011.

24 Skin Care Products

REBECCA SMALL, MD • BARBARA GREEN, RPH, MS

Skin care is an essential component of aesthetic medicine. Topical skin care products are used for treatment of photoaging, such as fine lines, rough texture, and dyschromia, and are particularly beneficial in patients with darker Fitzpatrick skin types, where more aggressive treatments may be contraindicated. Visible changes with most topical products are subtle and slow, and typically require regular use over a 3- to 6-month period. Another key role for topical products in aesthetic practice is supporting and enhancing the results of minimally invasive aesthetic procedures. They are used preprocedure to condition and prepare the skin, postprocedure to promote healing and soothe skin, and are helpful in the management of complications.[1,2]

The three main categories of topical products, based on their regulatory status, are:

- Prescription medications
- Over-the-counter (OTC) medications
- Cosmeceuticals.

Prescription and OTC medications contain ingredients that are regulated by the Food and Drug Administration (FDA). Cosmeceuticals, defined as topical products that contain active ingredients in sufficient concentrations to deliver perceptible skin benefits, are not regulated by the FDA.

Patients seek advice from and expect physicians practicing aesthetics to be familiar with topical products, particularly those used for skin rejuvenation. A plethora of topical products exist, and incorporating them into treatment plans can be a daunting task. This chapter provides a basic foundation in cosmeceutical ingredients and offers an integrated approach to management of common aesthetic skin conditions using cosmeceutical and prescription topical products. Topics covered include treatment of dry skin, prevention and management of photoaging, and preprocedure and postprocedure products.

DRY SKIN (XEROSIS)

Xerosis, scaling, winter itch, and *flaking* are all terms used to describe dry skin. To understand treatment options for dry skin, one must first consider how the skin naturally maintains moisture. Skin is comprised of the epidermis, dermis, and subcutaneous layers (see Figure 19-3 in Chapter 19, *Aesthetic Principles and Consultation*). The outermost layer of the epidermis, the stratum corneum, forms the *epidermal barrier*. It functions as an evaporative barrier, maintaining skin hydration and suppleness, and as a protective physical barrier against microbes, trauma, and chemical irritants, and it reduces the harmful effects of ultraviolet (UV) light.[3]

Photoaged skin has sluggish, disorganized keratinocyte maturation, which leads to corneocyte retention and disruption of the epidermal barrier. Water escapes more freely from the skin causing dehydration and dryness, which can be measured as increased transepidermal water loss.[4] Environmental insults such as harsh topical chemicals, temperature and humidity extremes, and genetic abnormalities (e.g., ichthyosis) can also damage the integrity of the skin barrier contributing to dryness.

Treatment of Dry Skin

Moisturizers used to treat dry skin increase hydration by binding and trapping water in the epidermis, and by enhancing epidermal barrier function to reduce evaporative water loss. Skin is rendered more supple and healthy, and clinically demonstrates improvements in smoothness and wrinkles.[5] These effects can be temporary, such that once the moisturizer is removed the effects are gone. Effects can also be long-lasting when the integrity of the skin barrier is strengthened following repeated use.

Moisturizers contain three main types of ingredients, each of which serves a unique function[6–8]:

- Occlusives trap water in the skin and enhance the lipid component of the epidermal barrier.
- Humectants attract water from the dermis and bind it at the epidermis.
- Emollients smooth uneven corneocytes and improve tactile roughness.

Most moisturizers are composed of all three ingredient types (occlusives, humectants, and emollients) to create a product that is both effective and cosmetically elegant and does not feel oily to the touch. Although the term *emollient* is sometimes used interchangeably with *moisturizer*, it is truly one of three components that can be found in moisturizers. Table 24-1 lists common ingredients found in moisturizers.

Moisturizers are formulated in oil-in-water emulsions as creams or lotions, and their heaviness depends on the relative amounts of oil and water. Ointments contain nearly all oil, creams contain more oil relative to water, and lotions contain more water relative to oil. Creams and lotions tend to be less irritating and drying than gels and solutions. The following list shows product formulations from most to least hydrating:

TABLE 24-1 Common Moisturizing Agents and Their Function[4,12]

Moisturizer Types	Functions	Ingredients
Occlusive	Trap water on the skin surface and enhance lipid component of epidermal barrier.	Oils (petrolatum, mineral oil) Cholesterol, squalene Waxes (beeswax, carnauba wax, liquid wax) Silicones (dimethicone, cyclomethicone) Stearic acid, cetyl alcohol, stearyl alcohol Lanolin, lanolin alcohol
Humectant	Attract water from the dermis.	Glycerin Urea Hyaluronic acid Sorbitol Propylene glycol
Emollient	Smooth roughened epidermis.	C12-15 alkyl benzoate Cetyl stearate Glyceryl stearate Octyl octanoate Decyl oleate Isostearyl alcohol

- Ointment (most hydrating)
- Cream
- Lotion
- Gel
- Solution (least hydrating).

Barrier repair creams are a newer class of moisturizer that contain occlusive and humectant ingredients at ratios that closely mimic the content of normal, healthy stratum corneum: ceramides (50%), fatty acids (30%), and cholesterol (30%). They enhance barrier function, reduce transepidermal water loss, and increase the skin's resistance to environmental irritants.[9] These products may be used by patients with compromised barriers, such as those exposed to cleansers and chemicals, and conditions such as atopic dermatitis. Barrier repair products include nonprescription CeraVe® and TriCeram®, and prescription Mimyx®, Atopiclair®, and EpiCeram®.

Dry skin may also be associated with hyperkeratosis as seen with ichthyosis, keratosis pilaris, and callouses. Topical hydroxy acids such as lactic acid 5% to 12% (e.g., generic ammonium lactate available in the brand names of Lac-Hydrin® and AmLactin®) and urea 10% to 40% (e.g., Carmol® and Vanamide®) are keratolytic and function to reduce stratum corneum thickness and increase hydration.[10]

Exfoliation treatments, which superficially resurface the skin by removing the topmost layers of the epidermis, can also be used to treat dry skin. Exfoliation stimulates the keratinocyte maturation process with regeneration of a healthier epidermis. This results in a compacted stratum corneum and increased production of ceramides, which improves epidermal barrier function and skin hydration.[11,12] Exfoliation, where the outermost layers of skin are removed, can be achieved using mechanical methods (e.g., microdermabrasion) with gentle abrasion, or using chemical methods (e.g., chemical peels) with application of topical products such as acids (see Chapter 23, *Microdermabrasion*, and Chapter 22, *Chemical Peels*, respectively).

PHOTOAGING

Most of the changes seen with skin aging are due to years of cumulative UV exposure, referred to as photoaging.[13,14] Skin is affected by ultraviolet A radiation (UVA, 320 to 400 nm), long-wavelength solar radiation that penetrates into the dermis, and ultraviolet B (UVB, 290 to 320 nm), shorter wavelength radiation that is absorbed by the epidermis.

Skin Rejuvenation Products

Skin rejuvenation products are aimed at preventing and treating cosmetic issues associated with photoaging, which include textural changes, dyschromia, and vascular ectasias. A simple three-part regime of topical products can be used to cleanse, treat, and protect the skin, whereby each product provides a specific benefit.

Products used for the treatment of photoaging must address several aspects of the aging process, including increasing skin exfoliation and stimulating epidermal renewal, increasing synthesis of collagen and other dermal matrix components, reducing hyperpigmentation, and increasing hydration. Products used for skin protection are aimed at preventing damage from UV exposure and free-radical oxidation. Skin care regimes usually consist of multiple topical products, including prescription medications and cosmeceuticals, to address these various aspects of skin aging. Table 24-2 lists topical products commonly used for skin rejuvenation and their functions.[15]

TABLE 24-2 Skin Rejuvenation Products and Their Functions[16–19]

CLEANSE	
Cleanser selected based on skin oiliness/dryness	
TREAT	
Textural changes Fines lines Rough skin	Retinoids, hydroxy acids, N-acetyl glucosamine, growth factors, kinetin, peptides, moisturizers
Dyschromia Solar lentigines Postinflammatory hyperpigmentation	Retinoids, hydroquinone, kojic acid, azelaic acid, arbutin, and others (Tables 24-3 and 24-4)
Vascular ectasias Telangiectasias Rosacea	Bisoprolol, allantoin, aloe, algae extract, borage and evening primrose oil, vitamin C, chamomile, green tea extracts
PROTECT	
Antioxidants	Vitamin C, vitamin E, ferulic acid, coffee berry, idebenone, gluconolactone, polyhydroxy acids, resveratrol, tea and red wine extracts
Sunscreens	Zinc oxide, titanium dioxide, and others (Figure 24-1)

Prevention of Photoaging

Antioxidants

UV light generates free radicals in skin which oxidize nucleic acids, proteins, and lipids, leading to the development of skin cancers and signs of photoaging.[13] The skin protects itself by preventing free-radical damage with endogenous antioxidants consisting primarily of vitamin C in the aqueous compartment, and vitamin E in the lipid compartment such as cell membranes and stratum corneum. Vitamins C and E can be applied topically to enhance antioxidant protection.[16,17] These two antioxidants act synergistically. Ferulic acid is another antioxidant that can improve the protective effects of vitamins E and C.[17] In addition to antioxidant properties, vitamin C also directly increases collagen synthesis and clinically reduces fine lines.[20] The greatest percutaneous absorption of topical vitamin C is obtained with L-ascorbic acid in acidic formulations at pH 3.5 or less, with concentrations of 10% to 20%.[17]

Sunscreens

Sunscreens protect the skin by reducing UV exposure. There are two main types of sunscreen ingredients each of which has a different mechanism of action. Physical sunscreens, composed of inorganic compounds, reflect and scatter UV light, whereas chemical sunscreens, composed of organic sunscreens, absorb UV light.[18] To achieve broad-spectrum UVA and UVB coverage, multiple sunscreens are often combined. Figure 24-1 shows common sunscreen ingredients and their UV blocking capabilities. Certain sunscreen combinations offer greater photostability. For example, avobenzone alone has poor photostability; however, the addition of oxybenzone (HelioPlex®) renders it highly photostable. Sunscreens with broad-spectrum UVA and UVB coverage with an SPF 30 are generally recommended for daily use. Because sunscreens do not block all UV radiation, maximal protection from UV damage is provided by using an antioxidant in addition to a sunscreen.[17]

SPF stands for sun protection factor (soon to be renamed as sunburn protection factor by the FDA) and represents the ability of a sunscreen to delay erythema on sun-exposed skin, primarily by blocking UVB. For example, if erythema develops after 10 minutes of sun exposure in a given individual with unprotected skin, after application of an SPF 30 sunscreen, the individual will develop the same degree of erythema in 10 × 30 or 300 minutes (5 hours) of sun exposure. The standard SPF testing dose for sunscreens on human skin, and the basis for a sunscreen product's SPF designation, is 2 mg/cm^2, regardless of the formulation (cream, lotion, spray, powder, makeup, etc.), which equates to ⅓ tsp for the face and 1 oz for the body of cream sunscreens.

Treatment of Photoaging

Retinoids

Topical retinoids are used to treat virtually all cosmetic aspects of photoaged skin, including: fine lines, dry and rough skin, hyperpigmentation, as well as acne.[19,21,22]

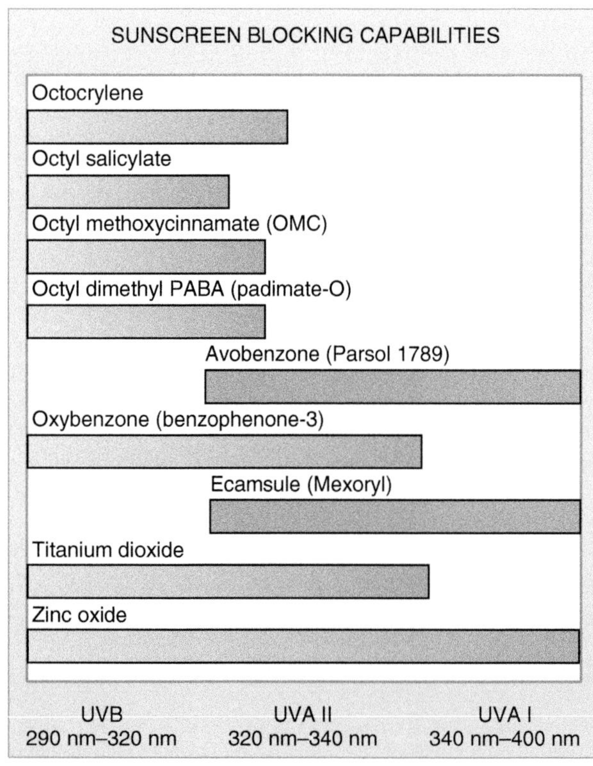

FIGURE 24-1 Sunscreens and their ultraviolet light blocking capabilities.

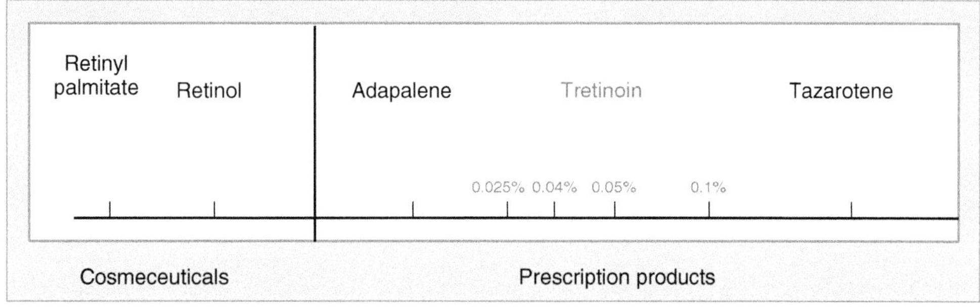

FIGURE 24-2 Topical retinoids.

Retinoids are vitamin A derivatives, which range from potent prescription products such as tretinoin and synthetic tretinoin derivatives such as tazarotene, to less active cosmeceutical products such as retinol (Figure 24-2). Two topical retinoid products are FDA approved to treat photoaging: Renova® (tretinoin) and Avage® (tazarotene). Several other topical prescription retinoids approved to treat acne are also used off-label to treat photoaging such as Retin-A® (tretinoin), Retin-A® Micro (a less irritating formulation of tretinoin), Differin® (adapalene), and other generic versions of these.

Prescription retinoids have an associated local skin reaction of erythema, sensitivity, peeling, and flaking, called a *retinoid dermatitis*, which usually occurs within a week of initiating therapy. While this irritative response spontaneously resolves for most patients in 4 to 6 weeks, it can persist for the duration of use. The rejuvenating effects of prescription retinoids are more rapid than cosmeceuticals. Results are usually apparent by 1 month, with improved texture due to compaction of the stratum corneum, and by 3 months reduction of hyperpigmentation and fine lines are evident. Combining prescription retinoids with other aesthetic procedures such as lasers and chemical peels can be challenging, because retinoids must be discontinued 1 week prior to treatment and restarted 2 weeks after these treatments. This repeated initiation and termination of therapy can cyclically induce a retinoid dermatitis. For this reason, some providers use prescription retinoids as a stand-alone intervention for photoaged skin. Prescription retinoids are a particularly useful treatment option for skin rejuvenation in patients with darker Fitzpatrick skin types (IV through VI), where more aggressive procedures may be contraindicated.

Cosmeceutical retinoids include retinol (vitamin A), retinal (vitamin A aldehyde), and retinol storage forms (retinyl acetate and retinyl palmitate).[23] They are less irritating than prescription retinoids and, when used in recommended doses, do not cause a retinoid dermatitis. However, they are much less effective than prescription retinoids in reducing the signs of photoaging.

Matrix Metalloproteinase Inhibitors

Matrix metalloproteinases (MMPs) are naturally occurring enzymes that degrade the skin's extracellular matrix to facilitate recycling of collagen, elastin, and glycoaminoglycans.[24] In young, healthy skin, production of matrix components exceeds destruction caused by MMPs. In photoaged skin, matrix degradation is accelerated because UV light upregulates MMPs. Enhanced matrix degradation combined with age-related decline in collagen synthesis, decreases the structural integrity of the skin's matrix and contributes to the formation of wrinkles, skin laxity, and telangiectasias.[25] Products that inhibit MMPs, such as zinc, calcium, idebenone, and lactobionic acid (polyhydroxy acid) reduce destruction of dermal matrix, increase dermal collagen and elastin, and clinically improve textural changes in photoaged skin.[26,27]

Human-Derived Growth Factors

Endogenous growth factors are regulatory proteins that initiate wound healing by mediating signaling pathways within and between cells.[28] Multiple growth factors migrate to wounds and interact synergistically to promote wound healing and tissue regeneration including synthesis of new dermal matrix components. Topical application of growth factor products, such as Nouricel-MD®, which is derived from human fibroblast cultures, twice daily for 3 months has been shown to improve skin hydration and reduce roughness, hyperpigmentation, and wrinkles in photoaged skin.[29,30] Growth factors are large protein molecules and their size may limit penetration through an intact epidermis. Combining them with skin resurfacing procedures that thin or disrupt the skin's barrier, such as laser resurfacing, chemical peels, and microdermabrasion, or topical exfoliants such as hydroxy acids, may improve penetration of these active proteins.[31]

Peptides

Peptides are short-chain amino acids that act as protein mimics to stimulate repair processes in photoaged skin.[32] Peptides, rather than their parent proteins, are used topically because these smaller compounds have greater skin penetration. Palmitoyl pentapeptide-3 (e.g., Matrixyl® by Sederma, StriVectin® by Klein Becker) is a sequence from procollagen that has been found to stimulate the production of collagens. Palmitoyl oligopeptide (by Sederma) is derived from elastin and stimulates growth of fibroblasts and angiogenesis.[33]

Another peptide, acetyl hexapeptide-8 (e.g., Argireline® by Lipotec), is derived from the SNAP-25 protein, which is designed to reduce the effects of acetylcholine in producing muscle contraction and purported to have "botulinum toxin–like effects." One report suggests that 10% acetyl hexapeptide-8 used for 30 days reduces wrinkle depth by 30%.[33] Additional studies are necessary to support this finding and its proposed mechanism of action. Novel peptide research is a growing area of cosmeceutical development. Significant effects with many peptides can be demonstrated *in vitro*, where target receptors are easily accessed, and the challenge for peptides, as with all topical products, is to demonstrate penetration through the skin barrier and good clinical efficacy *in vivo*, when the biologic target is less accessible.

Plant Hormones

Kinetin (N^6-furfuryladenine) is a plant cytokinin that functions as a natural antioxidant and is used as an ingredient in rejuvenation skin care products.[34,35] It has reported rejuvenation effects on cultured human fibroblast cells (*in vitro*),[36] but no studies are currently available *in vivo* to assess for clinical efficacy.

Hydroxy Acids

Alpha hydroxy acids (AHAs) are part of almost any skin rejuvenation topical product regime, and they include glycolic, lactic, citric, and mandelic acids. AHAs stimulate epidermal cell production, exfoliation, and even out the distribution of melanin in photodamaged skin.[10,37,38] AHA histologic effects include increased deposition of glycosaminoglycans, improved elastin fiber quality, and increased collagen synthesis.[37–39] When formulated in more acidic preparations with higher concentrations, AHAs are commonly used as chemical peel agents. Polyhydroxy acids (such as gluconolactone) and bionic acids (such as lactobionic acid and maltobionic acid) are second-generation hydroxy-acids that have AHA-like effects but are less irritating. They also function as humectant moisturizers and antioxidants.[40–42]

Amino Sugars

N-acetylglucosamine is a naturally occurring amino sugar compound that is a building block of hyaluronic acid (a glycosaminoglycan). Topical application stimulates synthesis of hyaluronic acid in fibroblasts and keratinocytes, increases skin thickness,[43,44] and enhances exfoliation.[45] Clinically, N-acetylglucosamine has been found to reduce wrinkles, increase hydration, and improve hyperpigmentation.[46–48]

In summary, prescription retinoid products can address many aspects of skin aging and offer significant improvements for photodamaged skin. For patients intolerant of prescription retinoids, alternative cosmeceutical therapies are available. These rejuvenation skin care regimes typically contain a combination of three to four cosmeceutical products that address fine lines and rough skin texture, improve skin brightness, and offer protection from UV damage. Box 24-1 lists topical products that can be used for a rejuvenation skin care regime (or as a preprocedure skin care regime).

BOX 24-1 *Rejuvenation Skin Care Regime*

Cleanse

Cleanser selected based on skin oiliness/dryness

Treat

Prescription retinoid *or*
Retinol
Hydroxy acids
Human-derived growth factors
Peptides
Moisturizer

Protect

Vitamins C and E
Zinc oxide or titanium dioxide sunscreen

HYPERPIGMENTATION

Hyperpigmentation is a common aesthetic complaint and typically presents as solar lentigines, postinflammatory hyperpigmentaion or melasma. Solar lentigines are apparent in photoaged skin as small brown macules that increase in size and number with chronic sun exposure. Postinflammatory hyperpigmentation can be seen in susceptible individuals, especially darker Fitzpatrick skin types (IV through VI), as brown discoloration commonly arising at sites of previously inflamed acne lesions or sites of wound healing. Melasma presents as hyperpigmented reticular patches and brown macules, typically on the cheekbones, upper lip, forehead, and/or chin (Figure 24-3). Melasma is frequently observed following a change in female hormonal status such as during pregnancy (chloasma) or with use of oral contraceptives.[49]

Hyperpigmentation results from increased melanin synthesis and deposition in the epidermis and dermis. An understanding of the melanin synthesis and distribution pathways is helpful in selecting treatments for hyperpigmentation. The key regulatory step in melanin synthesis is the enzymatic conversion of tyrosine to melanin by tyrosinase in melanocytes. Melanin is packaged into melanosomes in the melanocytes and then distributed to surrounding epidermal keratinocytes (Figure 24-4). One of the physiologic roles of melanin in the skin is to shield keratinocyte nuclei by absorbing harmful UV light. Upregulation of melanin synthesis is thus a physiologic protective mechanism against UV damage. Many other factors, however, can also upregulate melanin synthesis contributing to unwanted hyperpigmentation (see Figure 24-4).[50]

Treatment of Hyperpigmentation

Assessment pigmentation depth in the skin can be helpful prior to initiating treatment for hyperpigmentation, because epidermal pigment is more responsive to topical products compared to dermal pigment. Pigmentation depth can be evaluated using a Wood's lamp. Illuminated epidermal pigment typically enhances

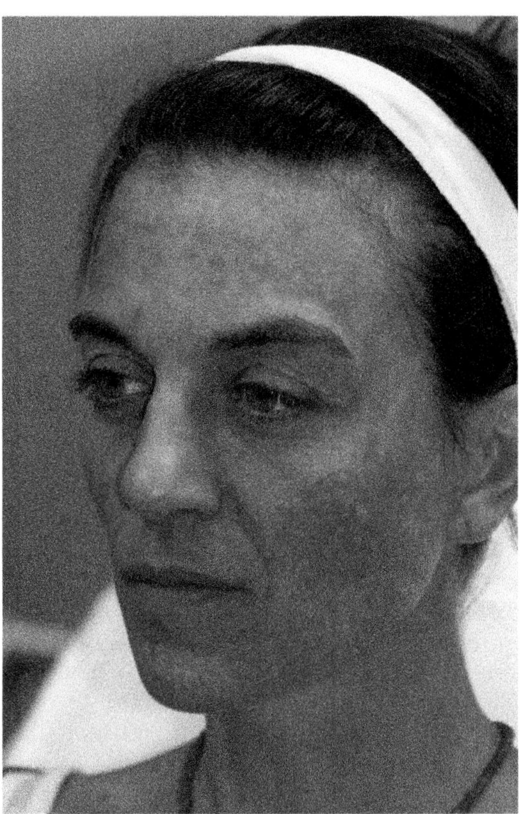
FIGURE 24-3 Melasma. *(Copyright Rebecca Small, MD.)*

under a Wood's lamp, whereas dermal pigment does not.

Treatment of hyperpigmentation with topical products is aimed at suppressing melanin synthesis and deposition in the skin and at removing pigment that is already present. Topical products for hyperpigmentation, commonly called lightening, brightening, or bleaching agents, include prescription products and cosmeceuticals. Most topical lightening agents act by inhibiting tyrosinase, the key enzymatic step in melanin production (Figure 24-4).

Hydroquinone, a tyrosinase inhibitor, is the most potent topical lightening agent. It is available as an OTC drug in 2% formulations and may be prescribed as a 4% cream or formulated by compounding pharmacies in strengths of 6% to 8%. Combination products containing hydroquinone and retinoids are commonly used, and some of these often have steroids added to reduce the irritation associated with their use. Tri-Luma® is one such combination product that is FDA approved for treatment of melasma. Other prescription topical products commonly used for hyperpigmentation are summarized in Table 24-3.[51]

Cosmeceutical skin lightening agents, such as kojic acid and arbutin, are also tyrosinase inhibitors. Although not as effective as hydroquinone, their efficacy can be improved by combining them with products that enhance penetration into the skin such as hydroxy acid exfoliants or retinoids, such as retinol. Copper metal

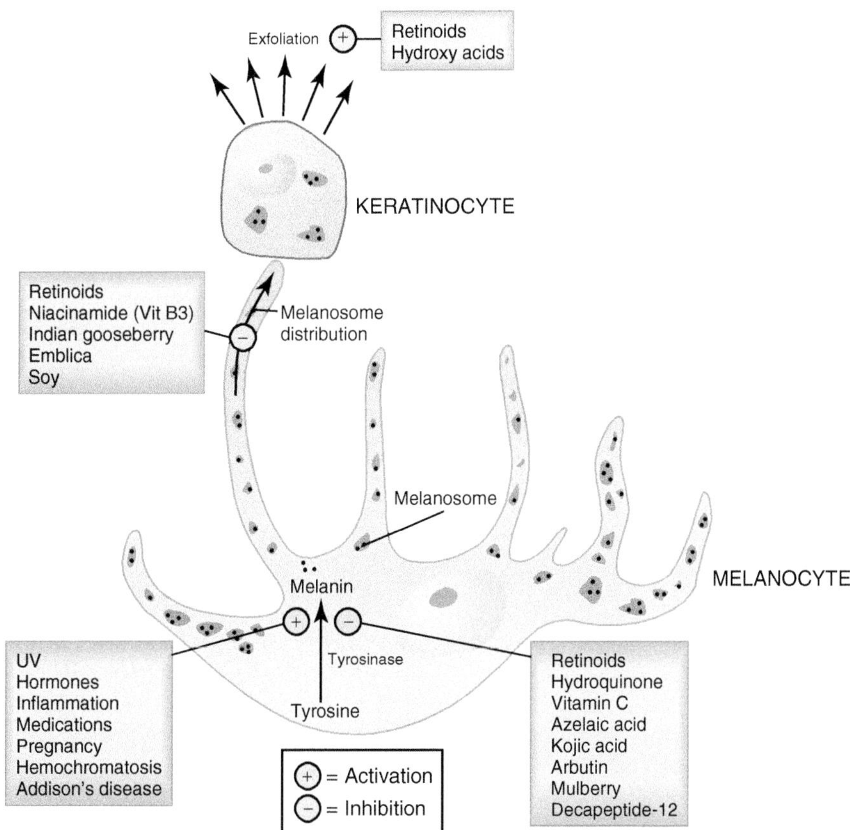

FIGURE 24-4 Melanin synthesis and cellular distribution.

TABLE 24-3 Prescription Topical Products for Hyperpigmentation[51]

Product Brand Name	Lightening Ingredient	Retinoid	Sun Protectant	Other Components
Azelex®	AZ 20%	None	None	
Claripel®	HQ 4%	None	Sunscreen	
Eldopaque Forte®	HQ 4%	None	Sunscreen	
Eldoquin Forte®	HQ 4%	None	None	
EpiQuin®	HQ 4%	Retinol 0.15%	None	Vitamins C and E
Finacea®	AZ 15%	None	None	
Glyquin®	HQ 4%	None	Sunscreen	Vitamins C and E Glycolic acid 10%
Glyquin XM®	HQ 4%	None	Sunscreen	Vitamins C and E Hyaluronic acid
Lustra®	HQ 4%	None	None	Vitamins C and E Glycolic acid 2%
Lustra AF®	HQ 4%	None	Sunscreen	Vitamins C and E Glycolic acid 2%
Lustra Ultra®	HQ 4%	None	Sunscreen	Petrolatum
Alustra®	HQ 4%	Retinol	None	
Melquin®	HQ 4%	None	None	Petrolatum
Nuquin®	HQ 4%	None	Sunscreen	Petrolatum
Obagi NuDerm Clear®	HQ 4%	None	None	Vitamins C and E Lactic acid
Obagi-C Night Therapy®	HQ 4%	None	None	Vitamins C and E Lactic acid Salicylic acid
Solage®	Mequinol 2%	Tretinoin 0.01%	None	
Solaquin Forte®	HQ 4%	None	Sunscreen	
Tri-Luma®	HQ 4%	Tretinoin 0.05%	None	Fluocinolone acetonide 0.01%

AZ, azelaic acid; HQ, hydroquinone.

chelators can also be used to help reduce pigment production, because copper is an essential cofactor necessary for synthesis of melanin. Common cosmeceuticals used for treatment of hyperpigmentation are summarized in Table 24-4.

Reduction of hyperpigmentation with topical products typically requires 3 months of daily application. Figure 24-5 shows a patient with lentigines and mottled hyperpigmentation of the lower face (A) prior to treatment and (B) after 3 months with daily use of 0.05% tretinoin, 4% hydroquinone, hydroxy acid, 20% vitamin C, and broad spectrum sunscreen. Figure 24-6 shows a patient with melasma and postinflammatory hyperpigmentation (A) before and (B) after 3 months of twice daily use of four main products containing 0.5% retinol, an exfoliant (lactic acid), brightening agents (2% hydroquinone, 3% kojic acid and 5% azelaic acid, licorice extract, and arbutin), anti-inflammatory ingredients (borage and evening primrose oils), and a broad-spectrum sunscreen.

Reduction of hyperpigmentation can also be achieved with procedures that exfoliate and remove melanin-laden keratinocytes in the epidermis. Various methods of exfoliation can be used in combination with topical products, such as chemical peels, microdermabrasion, and superficial laser skin resurfacing. Certain lasers (e.g., Q-switched 1064 nm) treat hyperpigmentation by targeting and reducing melanosomes in the dermis. Combination therapy with minimally invasive aesthetic procedures such as these and topical products can achieve the most rapid and effective reduction in hyperpigmentation.

PREPROCEDURE AND POSTPROCEDURE PRODUCTS

Proper selection and use of skin care products before and after aesthetic procedures, such as chemical peels and laser treatments, contributes to successful and sustainable clinical results and may reduce procedure risks such as hyperpigmentation.

Preprocedure topical regimens often contain the same products as rejuvenation skin care regimes and

TABLE 24-4 Cosmeceutical Topical Products for Hyperpigmentation[16,37,52–55]

Product	Occurrence
Acetyl glucosamine	Chitin
Arbutin, methyl arbutin	Bearberry extract, certain herbs, pear trees
Decapeptide-12 (Lumixyl®)	Synthetic
Emblica	Indian gooseberry
Glycolic acid	Sugar cane
Kojic acid	Fungi
Licorice extract (glabridin)	Licorice root
Mulberry extract	Roots of the broussonetia papyrifera tree
Niacinamide	Amide form of vitamin B_3
Retinoids (retinol, retinal, retinyl acetate, retinyl palmitate)	Vitamin A
Soy isoflavones	Soybean
Vitamin C	Citrus fruits

usually consist of retinoids, hydroxy acids, antioxidants, sunscreens, and skin lightening agents (see Box 24-1).[56] The goal for using these products is to condition the skin and create a healthier baseline epidermis and dermis. This allows for more even penetration of products, as with chemical peels, and promotes more rapid postprocedure healing. Preprocedure skin care regimens are ideally started 1 month prior to cosmetic procedures and discontinued 1 week prior to the procedure, to ensure a fully intact epidermis at the time of treatment. In persons prone to hyperpigmentation, a topical lightening agent is also used, such as hydroquinone 4% to 8%, which may reduce the risk of postinflammatory hyperpigmentation postprocedure.

Selection of postprocedure products depends on the type of cosmetic procedure performed. Ablative procedures, which disrupt the epidermis, require use of an occlusive ointment moisturizer without active ingredients immediately postprocedure. Common occlusive postprocedure products are shown in Table 24-5. This product is used for approximately 4 to 7 days postprocedure, until re-epithelialization occurs. There is some evidence that certain nonocclusive products, such as Biafine® (see Table 24-6), may be used as alternatives to occlusive topical products during this phase of wound healing.[57] Because sunscreen is not used during this time, sun avoidance is critical.

Once the skin has fully re-epithelialized, postprocedure occlusive products may be discontinued and products that are soothing and reparative used. Some common non-occlusive reparative products are listed in Table 24-6. A broad-spectrum sunscreen (SPF 30 or greater) containing zinc and/or titanium is used daily. At 1 month postprocedure, when skin is no longer sensitive, patients' preprocedural rejuvenation products may be resumed. If postinflammatory hyperpigmentation is a concern or if the procedure is targeting pigment reduction, skin-lightening products are also resumed.

Procedures that leave the epidermis intact, such as nonablative laser treatments and superficial resurfacing treatments like chemical peels and microdermabrasion, require nonocclusive postprocedure products for 2 weeks with resumption of routine rejuvenation skin care products thereafter.

CONCLUSION

Topical products are an essential part of aesthetic practice. They are effective therapies for treatment of dry skin, rough texture, hyperpigmentation, and fine lines seen with photoaging. In addition, topical products are readily integrated with other minimally invasive aesthetic procedures, supporting and enhancing skin rejuvenating results.

Resources

Allergan
Phone: 800-433-8871
www.allergan.com

Beiersdorf
www.eucerinus.com

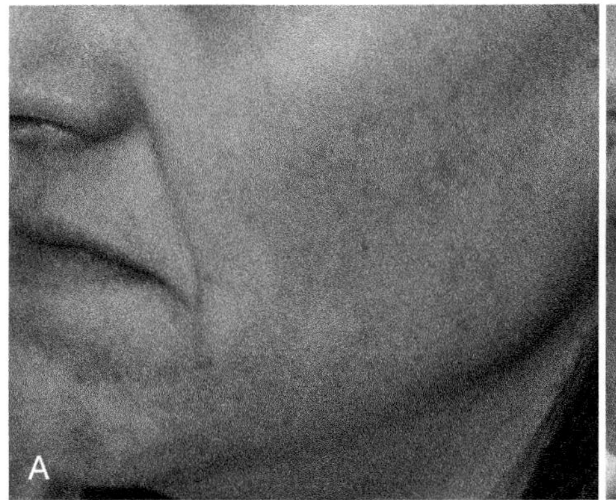

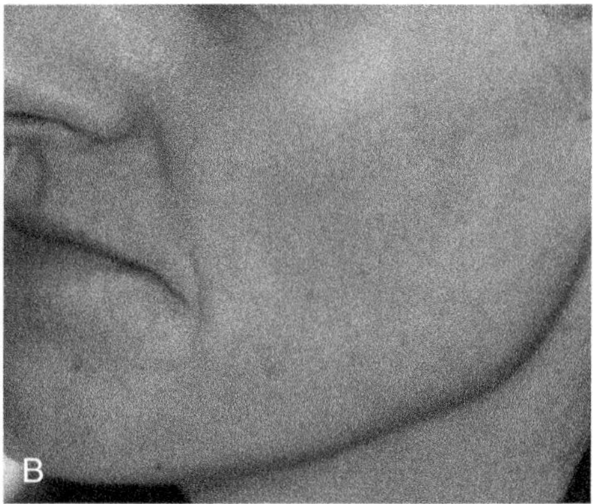

FIGURE 24-5 Hyperpigmentation (**A**) before and (**B**) after daily use for 3 months of 0.05% tretinoin, 4% hydroquinone, and lactic acid. *(Copyright Rebecca Small, MD.)*

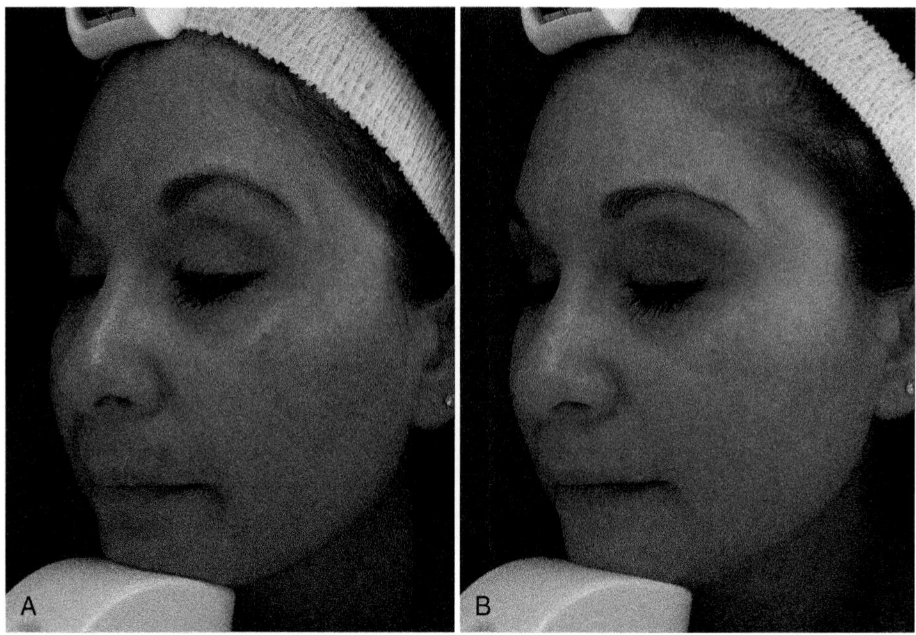

FIGURE 24-6 Melasma and postinflammatory hyperpigmentation **(A)** before and **(B)** after twice daily use for 3 months of 0.5% retinol, lactic acid, 2% hydroquinone, 3% kojic acid, and 5% azelaic acid. *(Courtesy of PCA Skin, Scottsdale, AZ.)*

BiO2 Cosmeceuticals
Phone: 800-599-8885
www.oxymist.com

Biopelle
Phone: 866-424-6735
www.biopelle.com

Clinique Laboratories
Phone: 212-572-3829
www.clinique.com

Coria Laboratories
Phone: 800-441-8227
www.corialabs.com

Del-Ray Dermatologicals
Phone: 800-334-4286
www.bluelizard.net

Dermablend
Phone: 877-900-6700
www.dermablend.com

Dermik
Phone: 800-207-8049
www.dermik.com

Dusa Pharmaceuticals
Phone: 978-657-7500
www.dusapharma.com

TABLE 24-5 Occlusive Postprocedure Products[58,57]

Product Brand Name (Manufacturer)	Hydrating Ingredients	Other Ingredients
Aquaphor® (Beiersdorf)	Mineral oil Lanolin	Panthenol (vitamin B5) Bisoprolol (chamomile)
Catrix 10® (Lescarden)	Petrolatum Beeswax Paraffin	10% Bovine mucopolysaccharide cartilage
Primacy® (SkinCeuticals)	Petrolatum Squalene Oat kernel oil Rose oil	Bisoprolol (chamomile) Aloe Vitamin E
Protective Recovery Balm® (BiO2 Cosmeceuticals)	Mineral oil Petrolatum Paraffin Dimethicone	
Puralube® (Nycomede)	Light mineral oil White petrolatum	

TABLE 24-6 Nonocclusive Postprocedure Products[57,59,60]

Product Brand Name (manufacturer)	Reparative Ingredients (intended effect)
Epidermal Repair® (SkinCeuticals)	Beta glucan *Centella asiatica* (collagen synthesis)
TNS Ceramide Treatment Cream® (SkinMedica)	Hydroxypropyl bispalmitamide MEA (ceramide for barrier enhancement) NouriCel-MD® (growth factors) Palmitoyl oligopeptide and palmitoyl tetrapeptide-7 (matrix synthesis)
Biafine® (Ortho-McNeil)	Trolamine and sodium alginate (wound healing)

EltaMD Skincare
Phone: 800-633-8872
www.eltamd.com

Fallene
Phone: 800-332-5536
www.fallene.com

Ferndale Laboratories
Phone: 248-548-0900
www.ferndalelabs.com

Galderma Laboratories
Phone: 817-961-5000
www.galdermausa.com

Graceway Pharmaceuticals
Phone: 800-447-4537
www.gracewaypharma.com

Intendis
Phone: 866-463-3634
www.intendis.us.com

Iredale Mineral Cosmetics
Phone: 413-644-9900
www.janeiredale.com

Jan Marini Skin
Phone: 800-347-2223
www.janmarini.com

Johnson and Johnson
Phone: 800-526-3967
www.aveenoprofessional.com

Kao Brands
Phone: 800-742-8798
www.kaobrands.com

La-Roche Posay
Phone: 800-LRP-LABO
www.laroche-posay.us

Lescarden
Phone: 212-687-1050
www.catrix.com

L'Oreal Paris
www.lorealparisusa.com

Medicis
Phone: 602-808-8800
www.medicis.com

Mentholatum
Phone: 716-677-2500
www.mentholatum.com

Merz Pharmaceuticals
Phone: 877-MERZUSA
www.merzusa.com

Neostrata Company
Phone: 800-225-9411
www.neostrata.com

Neutrogena
Phone: 310-642-1150
www.neutrogena.com

NIA 24
Phone: 866-NIADYNE
www.nia24.com

Nu Skin Enterprises
Phone: 800-487-1000
www.nuskinusa.com

Obagi
Phone: 562-628-1007
www.obagi.com

OrthoMcNeil Pharmaceutical
Phone: 800-526-7736
www.ortho-mcneil.com

Osmosis Skincare
Phone: 877-777-2305
www.osmosisskincare.com

Physicians Choice Arizona (PCA Skin)
Phone: 877-722-7546
www.pcaskin.com

Procter and Gamble
Phone: 513-983-2697
www.pgdermatology.com

Promius Pharma
Phone: 908-429-4507
www.promiuspharms.com

Revision Skincare
Phone: 800-385-6652
www.revisionskincare.com

SkinCeuticals
Phone: 800-811-1660
www.skinceuticals.com

SkinMedica
Phone: 866-867-0110
www.skinmedica.com

Stiefel Laboratories
Phone: 800-724-1565
www.stiefel.com

Topix Pharmaceuticals
Phone: 800-445-2595
www.topixpharm.com

Unilever
Phone: 201-567-8000
www.unileverusa.com

Valeant Pharmaceuticals
Phone: 949-461-6100
www.valeant.com

Vichy Laboratories
www.vichyusa.com

Warner Chilcott
Phone: 800-424-5202
www.wcrx.com

Young Pharmaceuticals
Phone: 860-529-7919
www.youngpharm.com

References

1. Small R. Aesthetic procedures introduction. *In:* Mayeaux E, ed. *The Essential Guide to Primary Care Procedures.* Philadelphia: Lippincott Williams and Wilkins; 2009:195–199.
2. Small R. Aesthetic procedures in office practice. *Am Fam Physician.* 2009;80(11):1231–1237.
3. Proksch E, Folster-Holst R, Jensen JM. Skin barrier function, epidermal proliferation and differentiation in eczema. *J Dermatol Sci.* 2006;43(3):156–169.
4. Del Rosso JQ. Moisturizers: function, formulation and clinical applications. *In:* Draelos Z, Dover JS, Alam M, eds. *Procedures in Cosmetic Dermatology: Cosmeceuticals.* Philadelphia: Saunders/Elsevier; 2009:97–101.
5. Loden M. The clinical benefit of moisturizers. *J Eur Dermatol Venereol.* 2005;19(6):672–688.
6. Draelos ZD. Therapeutic moisturizers. *Dermatol Clin.* 2000;18(4):597–607.
7. Flynn TC, Petros J, Clark RE, *et al.* Dry skin and moisturizers. *Clin Dermatol.* 2001;19(4):387–392.
8. Del Rosso JQ. Moisturizers: function, formulation and clinical applications. In: Draelos Z, Dover JS, Alam M, eds. *Procedures in Cosmetic Dermatology: Cosmeceuticals.* Philadelphia: Saunders/Elsevier; 2009:97–101.
9. Elias PM, Feingold KR. Does the tail wag the dog? Role of the barrier in the pathogenesis of inflammatory dermatoses and therapeutic implications. *Arch Dermatol.* 2001;137:1079–1081.
10. Van Scott EJ, Yu RJ. Hyperkeratinization, corneocyte cohesion and alpha hydroxy acids. *J Am Acad Dermatol.* 1984;11:867–879.
11. Rawlings AV, Davies A, Carlomusto M. Effect of lactic acid isomers on keratinocyte ceramide synthesis, stratum corneum lipid levels and stratum corneum barrier function. *Arch Dermatol.* 1996;288:383–390.
12. Draelos Z. Dry skin. *In:* Draelos Z, Dover JS, Alam M, eds. *Procedures in Cosmetic Dermatology: Cosmeceuticals.* Philadelphia: Saunders/Elsevier; 2009:174.
13. Haywood R, Wardman P, Saunders R, *et al.* Sunscreens inadequately protect against ultraviolet-A-induced free radicals in skin: implications for skin aging and melanoma? *J Invest Dermatol.* 2003;121:862–868.
14. Lowe NJ, Meyers DP, Wieder JM. Low doses of repetitive ultraviolet A induce morphologic changes in human skin. *J Invest Dermatol.* 1995;105:739–743.
15. Draelos Z. The latest cosmeceutical approaches for anti-aging. *J Cosm Derm.* 2007;6:2–6.
16. Placzek M, Gaube S, Kerkmann U, *et al.* Ultraviolet B-induced DNA damage in human epidermis is modified by the antioxidants ascorbic acid and D-α-tocopherol. *J Invest Dermatol.* 2005;124:304–307.
17. Lin FH, Lin JY, Gupta RD, *et al.* Ferulic acid stabilizes a solution of vitamins C and E and doubles its photoprotection of skin. *J Invest Dermatol.* 2005;125:826–832.
18. Sayre RM, Kollias N, Roberts RL, *et al.* Physical sunscreens. *J Soc Cosmet Chem.* 1990;41:103–109.
19. Kligman A, Grove GL, Hirose E, *et al.* Topical tretinoin for photoaged skin. *J Am Acad Dermatol.* 1986;15:836–859.
20. Farris PK. Cosmeceutical vitamins: vitamin C. *In:* Draelos Z, Dover JS, Alam M, eds. *Procedures in Cosmetic Dermatology: Cosmeceuticals.* Philadelphia: Saunders/Elsevier; 2009:51–56.
21. Singh M, Griffiths CE. The use of retinoids in the treatment of photoaging. *Dermatol Ther.* 2006;19(5):297–305.
22. Del Rosso JQ. Topical retinoids in the management of acne: the best path to clear results. *Cutis.* 2004;74(4 Suppl):2–3.
23. Kafi R, Kwak HS, Schumacher WE, *et al.* Improvement of naturally aged skin with vitamin A (retinol). *Arch Dermatol.* 2007;143(5):606–612.
24. Ratzinger G, Stoitzner P, Ebner S, *et al.* Matrix metalloproteinases 9 and 2 are necessary for the migration of Langerhans cells and dermal dendritic cells from human and murine skin. *J Immunol.* 2002;168:4361–4371.
25. Thibodeau A. Metalloproteinase inhibitors. *Cosmet Toil.* 2000;115(11):75–76.
26. Ryan ME, Ramamurthy S, Golub LM. Matrix metalloproteinases and their inhibition in periodontal treatment. *J Current Opin Periodont.* 1996;3(1):85–96.
27. Upadhya GA, Strasberg SM. Glutathione, lactobionate, and histidine: cryptic inhibitors of matrix metalloproteinases contained in the University of Wisconsin and histidine/tryptophan/ketoglutarate liver preservation solutions. *Hepatology.* 2000;31(5):1115–1122.
28. Fitzpatrick RE, Rostan EF. Reversal of photodamage with topical growth factors: a pilot study. *J Cosmet Laser Ther.* 2003;5(1):25–34.
29. Fitzpatrick RE. Endogenous growth factors as cosmeceuticals. *Derm Surg.* 2005;31:827–831.
30. Mehta RC, Smith SR, Grove GL, *et al.* Reduction in facial photodamage by a topical growth factor product. *J Drugs Dermatol.* 2008;7(9):864–871.
31. Small R. Microdermabrasion. *In:* Mayeaux E, ed. *The Essential Guide to Primary Care Procedures.* Philadelphia: Lippincott Williams and Wilkins; 2009:265–277.
32. Lupo MP. Cosmeceutical peptides. *Derm Surg.* 2005;31:832–836.
33. Fields K, Falla TJ, Rodan K, *et al.* Bioactive peptides: signaling the future. *J Cosm Derm.* 2009;8:8–13.
34. Rattan SI. N6-furfuryladenine (Kinetin) as a potential anti-aging molecule. *J Anti-Aging Medicine.* 2002;5(1):113–116.
35. Rattan SI, Sodagam L. Gerontomodulatory and youth-preserving effects of zeatin on human skin fibroblasts undergoing aging *in vitro. Rejuvenation Res.* 2005;8(1):46–57.
36. Minorsky PV. Kinetin: the elixir of life? *Plant Physiol.* 2003;132(3):1135–1136.

37. Ditre CM, Griffin TD, Murphy GF, *et al.* Effects of alpha hydroxyacids on photoaged skin: a pilot clinical, histological and ultrastructural study. *J Am Acad Dermatol.* 1996;34:187–195.
38. Bernstein EF, Underhill CB, Lakkakorpi J, *et al.* Citric acid increases viable epidermal thickness and glycosaminoglycan content of sun-damaged skin. *Derm Surg.* 1997;123(8):689–694.
39. Bernstein EF, Lee J, Brown DB, *et al.* Glycolic acid treatment increases type I collagen mRNA and hyaluronic acid content of human skin. *Derm Surg.* 2001;27(5):429–433.
40. Berardesca E, Distante F, Vignoli GP, *et al.* Alpha hydroxyacids modulate stratum corneum barrier function. *Br J Dermatol.* 1997;137(6):934–938.
41. Bernstein EF, Green BA, Edison BL, *et al.* Poly hydroxy acids (PHAs): clinical uses for the next generation of hydroxy acids. *Skin and Aging.* 2001;9(Suppl):4–11.
42. Green BA, Briden ME. PHAs and bionic acids: next generation hydroxy acids. In: Draelos Z, Dover JS, Alam M, eds. *Procedures in Cosmetic Dermatology: Cosmeceuticals.* Philadelphia: Saunders/Elsevier; 2009:209–215.
43. Sayo T, Sakai S, Inoue S. Synergistic effect of N-acetylglucosamine and retinoids on hyaluronan production in human keratinocytes. *Skin Pharmacol Physiol.* 2004;17:77–83.
44. Breborowicz A, Kuzlan-Pawlaczyk M, Wieczorowska-Tobis K, *et al.* The effect of N-acetylglucosamine as a substrate for in vitro synthesis of glycosaminoglycans by human peritoneal mesothelial cells and fibroblasts. *Adv Perit Dial.* 1998;14:31–35.
45. Mammone T, Gan D, Fthenakis C, *et al.* The effect of N-acetylglucosamine on stratum corneum desquamation and water content in human skin. *J Cosmet Sci.* 2009;60:423–428.
46. Briden ME. Alpha-hydroxyacid chemical peeling agents: case studies and rationale for safe and effective use. *Cutis.* 2004;73(2 Suppl):18–24.
47. Bissett DL, Robinson LR, Raleigh PS, *et al.* Reduction in the appearance of facial hyperpigmentation by topical N-acetyl glucosamine. *J Cosm Derm.* 2007;6:20–26.
48. Bissett DL. Glucosamine: An ingredient with skin and other benefits. *J Cosm Derm.* 2006;5:309–315.
49. Yamaguchi Y, Brenner M, Hearing VJ. The regulation of skin pigmentation. *J Biol Chem.* 2007;282(38):27557–27561.
50. Pugliese PT. Physiology of the skin: pigmentation revisited. *Skin Inc.* 2009;21(3):68–76.
51. Rendon MI, Gaviria JI. Review of skin-lightening agents. *Derm Surg.* 2005;31:886–889.
52. Fisher GJ, Kang S, Varani J, *et al.* Mechanisms of photoaging and chronological skin aging. *Arch Dermatol.* 2002;138:1462–1470.
53. Rabe JH, Mamelak AJ, McElgunn PJS, *et al.* Photoaging: mechanisms and repair. *J Am Acad Dermatol.* 2006;55:1–19.
54. Zhai H, Cordoba-Diaz M, Wa C, *et al.* Determination of the antioxidant capacity of an antioxidant complex and idebenone: an *in vitro* rapid and sensitive method. *J Cosm Derm.* 2008;7:96–100.
55. Thornfeldt CR. Cosmeceutical botanicals: part 2. In: Draelos Z, Dover JS, Alam M, eds. *Procedures in Cosmetic Dermatology: Cosmeceuticals.* Philadelphia: Saunders/Elsevier; 2009:77–85.
56. Weinstein GD, Nigra TP, Pochi PE, *et al.* Topical tretinoin for treatment of photodamaged skin: a multicenter study. *Arch Dermatol.* 1991;127:659–665.
57. Rendon MI, Cardona L, Benitez A. The safety and efficacy of trolamine/sodium alginate topical emulsion in postlaser resurfacing wounds. *J Drugs Dermatol.* 2008;7(5):S23–S28.
58. Tanzi EL, Perez M. The effect of a mucopolysaccharide-cartilage complex healing ointment on Er:YAG laser resurfaced facial skin. *Dermatol Surg.* 2002;28:305–308.
59. Maquart FX, Chastang F, Simeon A, *et al.* Triterpenes from Centella asiatica stimulate extracellular matrix accumulation in rat experimental wounds. *Eur J Dermatol.* 1999;9(4):289–296.
60. Atkin DH, Trookman NS, Rizer RL, *et al.* Combination of physiologically balanced growth factors with antioxidants for reversal of facial photodamage. *J Cosmet Laser Ther.* 2010;12(1):14–20.

Additional Reading

Small R, Linder J. Skin care products. *In:* Small R, Linder J, eds. *A Practical Guide to Skin Care Procedures and Products.* Philadelphia: Lippincott Williams and Wilkins; 2011.

Smeltzer W. Cosmeceutical skin care. *In:* Pfenninger JL, Fowler GC, eds. *Pfenninger and Fowler's Procedures for Primary Care.* 3rd ed. Philadelphia: Mosby/Elsevier; 2011.

25 Dermal Fillers

REBECCA SMALL, MD

Soft-tissue augmentation, commonly referred to as *dermal filler treatment*, reduces facial lines and improves contour defects by temporarily restoring volume to the dermis and soft tissues through the use of injectable products.[1] With the use of appropriate techniques and volumes, dermal filler treatments can enhance appearance in a subtle, natural way. Treatments require short recovery times and can be safely performed in the outpatient setting.[2,3]

Dermal filler treatments have become the second most commonly performed minimally invasive cosmetic procedure in the United States, according to statistics from the American Society for Aesthetic Plastic Surgery.[4] The popularity of this procedure is largely due to increased patient demand for less invasive cosmetic treatment options and to recent product innovations that have prolonged treatment results.

Numerous dermal fillers (DFs) are available, each varying in composition, duration of action, palpability, ease of administration, complications, and other factors.[5] In addition to the provider's knowledge of DF products and injection skill, an appreciation for aesthetic facial proportions and symmetry is required to achieve desirable outcomes. Injection of dermal fillers has a steeper learning curve than botulinum toxin injections and requires practice to achieve desirable results.[6] This chapter is intended to assist aesthetic providers in getting started with products and techniques that consistently achieve good results and have a low risk of complications. The focus is on the use of hyaluronic acid DF products for the FDA-approved treatment of nasolabial folds (NLFs).

COSMETIC INDICATIONS

- Dermal filler treatments with hyaluronic acid are approved by the U.S. Food and Drug Administration (FDA) for injection in the mid to deep dermis for correction of moderate to severe facial wrinkles and folds, such as nasolabial folds.
- Dermal filler treatment for lip enhancement, marionette lines, oral commissures, cheek augmentation, acne and chicken pox scars, and other cosmetic areas are off label.

ALTERNATIVE THERAPIES

Alternative therapies for the treatment of facial lines and wrinkles include botulinum toxin for dynamic wrinkles, and skin resurfacing procedures such as microdermabrasion, chemical peels, and laser (nonablative and ablative) treatments for static lines. Severe wrinkling with laxity may be better addressed with surgical treatments, such as face-lifts, than with dermal fillers.

PRODUCTS CURRENTLY AVAILABLE

Dermal filler products can be categorized based on their duration of action as either short acting (less than 4 months), long acting (6 months to 1 year), semipermanent (1 to 2 years), and permanent (2 years or more) (see Table 25-1).[7–9]

Injectable hyaluronic acid (HA) products are one of the most versatile dermal fillers currently available. HA is a naturally occurring glycosaminoglycan in the dermal extracellular matrix that provides structural support and nutrients and, through its hydrophilic capacity, adds volume and fullness to the skin. Commercially available HAs vary in formulation, concentration, and degree of cross-linkage, which affects their duration of action as well as postprocedure risks of swelling and bruising.[10,11]

CONTRAINDICATIONS

- Pregnancy or nursing
- Active infection (e.g., herpes simplex and pustular acne) or inflammation in the treatment area
- Hypertrophic or keloidal scar formation
- Bleeding abnormality (e.g., thrombocytopenia or anticoagulant use)
- Accutane use in the previous 6 months due to impaired healing
- Skin atrophy (e.g., chronic steroid use or conditions such as Ehlers-Danlos syndrome)
- Impaired healing (e.g., due to immunosuppression)
- Dermatoses such as vitiligo and active psoriasis or eczema in the treatment area
- Uncontrolled systemic condition
- Previous anaphylactic reaction to anything at any time
- Multiple severe allergies
- Previous allergic response to dermal filler products or gram-positive bacterial proteins (which are commonly found in hyaluronic dermal fillers)
- Body dysmorphic disorder
- Unrealistic expectations, intolerance of bruising.

ADVANTAGES OF DERMAL FILLERS

- Immediate results.
- Most undesirable outcomes spontaneously resolve with temporary fillers.

TABLE 25-1 Dermal Fillers in Common Use[7–9]

Agent	Company	Common Treatment Areas	Component	Duration
Short-Acting				
CosmoPlast®	Allergan	Lips Fine lines, scars	Collagen with lidocaine	2–4 months
Prevelle Silk®	Johnson & Johnson	Lips Fine lines, scars	Hyaluronic acid with lidocaine	2–3 months
Long-Acting				
Hydrelle®	Coapt	NLF, ML	Hyaluronic acid with lidocaine	6–12 months
Juvederm®	Allergan	Lips NLF, ML	Hyaluronic acid with or without lidocaine	6–12 months
Perlane®	Medicis	NLF, ML	Hyaluronic acid with or without lidocaine	6–12 months
Restylane®	Medicis	Lips NLF, ML	Hyaluronic acid with or without lidocaine	6–12 months
Semipermanent				
Radiesse®	Bioform	Cheek augmentation NLF, ML	Calcium Hydroxylapatite	1–1.5 years
Sculptra®	Dermik	Lipoatrophy NLF, ML	Poly-L-lactic acid	1–2 years
Permanent				
ArteFill®	Artes	NLF, ML	PMMA with collagen	Permanent

PMMA, polymethyl methacrylate; NLF, nasolabial folds; ML, marionette lines.

DISADVANTAGES OF DERMAL FILLER

- Post-treatment swelling and bruising is common.
- Repeat treatments are necessary to maintain results.

ANATOMY

Facial wrinkles and folds of the lower two-thirds of the face commonly treated with dermal fillers are shown in Figure 25-1. Arterial and venous supply for these areas is shown in Figure 25-2. The lateral nasal artery is a noteworthy vessel for NLF treatments. It is found at the junction of the facial artery and angular artery, and is the main vascular supply for the nasal tip and ala. It is located 2 to 3 mm superior to the nasal alar groove.[12]

EQUIPMENT

Anesthesia

- 3.0- and 5.0-mL Luer-Lok™ tip syringes
- Lidocaine HCl 2% with epinephrine 1:100,000
- 18-gauge, 1.5-inch needles
- 30-gauge, 1-inch needles
- Benzocaine/lidocaine/tetracaine (20:6:4) ointment
- Ice packs.

Dermal Filler Treatment

- Dermal filler prefilled syringes
- 30-gauge, 0.5-inch needles
- 3- × 3-inch nonwoven gauze
- Alcohol wipes
- Surgical marker or soft white eyeliner pencil for marking the treatment area
- Hyaluronidase (e.g., Vitrase®) at least 30 units, and sterile saline with which to make a to 1:1 dilution for management of vascular occlusion.

HANDLING AND STORAGE

Hyaluronic acid dermal fillers are supplied in individual prepackaged syringes ranging from 0.4 to 0.8 mL based on the manufacturer. Syringes are typically stored at room temperature (up to 25°C or 77°F) prior to use, and the specific manufacturer package insert guidelines should be followed. Shelf-life ranges from 6 months to 1 year.

PROCEDURE PREPARATION

1. Review the patient's medical history and perform an aesthetic evaluation and consultation (see Chapter 19, *Aesthetic Principles and Consultation*).

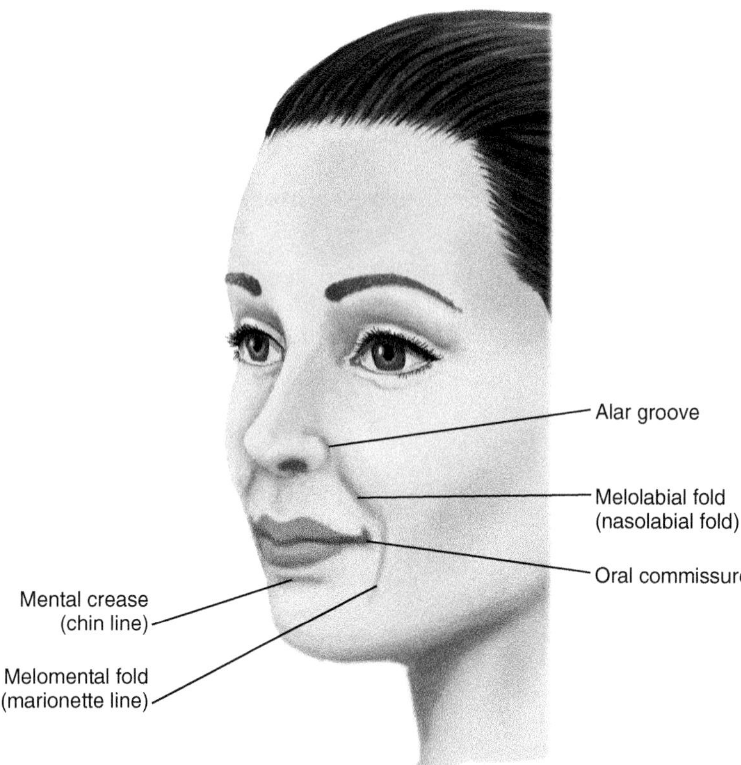

FIGURE 25-1 Wrinkles and folds of the face.

2. Obtain informed consent (see Chapter 19; also see Appendix A for an informed consent form and patient information handout titled *Dermal Filler Treatments*).
3. Pretreatment photographs at rest and with the patient actively contracting muscles in the intended treatment area are advisable (see Chapter 19).

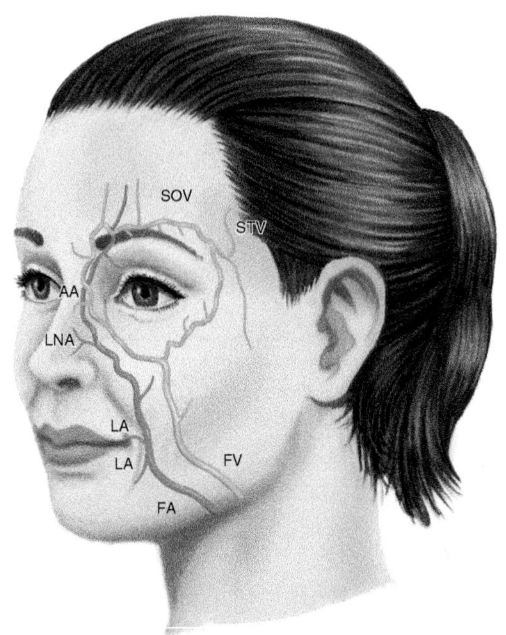

FIGURE 25-2 Arterial and venous supply of the face. AA, angular artery; FA, facial artery; FV, facial vein; SOV, supraorbital vein; STV, superficial temporal vein; LA, labial artery; LNA, lateral nasal artery.

4. Document and discuss any notable asymmetries prior to treatment.
5. Schedule treatment well in advance of social events.
6. Minimize bruising by discontinuation of aspirin, vitamin E, St. John's wort, and other dietary supplements including ginkgo biloba, evening primrose oil, garlic, feverfew, and ginseng for 2 weeks prior to treatment. Discontinue other nonsteroidal anti-inflammatory medications and alcohol consumption 2 days prior to treatment.
7. Prophylactic antiviral medication (e.g., valacyclovir 500 mg 1 tablet twice daily) may be given 2 days prior to procedure and continued for 3 days post-procedure for a history of labial or facial herpes simplex, or varicella zoster.
8. Discuss the estimated volume of dermal filler necessary for treatment and cost with patient prior to treatment.

DERMAL FILLER TREATMENT FOR NASOLABIAL FOLDS: STEPS AND PRINCIPLES

The following recommendations are guidelines for treatment using hyaluronic acid dermal fillers.

General Treatment Technique

1. All injections are placed in the mid to deep dermis. Figure 25-3 shows a cross section of skin illustrating appropriate filler placement in the dermis.

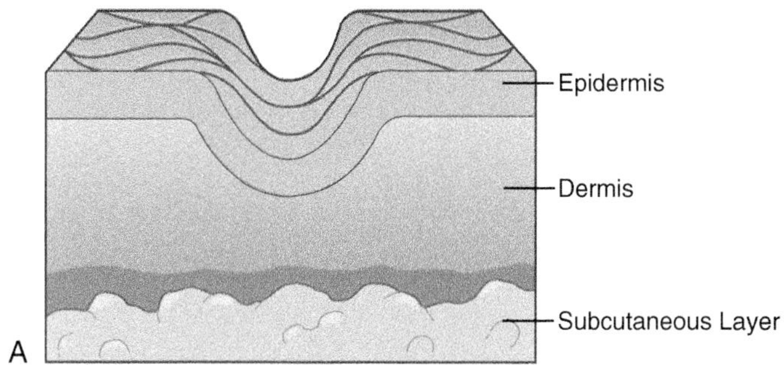

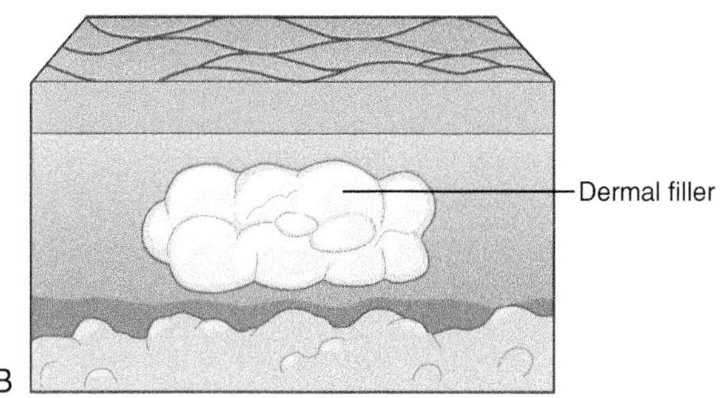

FIGURE 25-3 Dermal filler placement in the skin: (A) before and (B) after filler treatment.

Placement of DF in the desired level of the skin is one of the challenges with DF treatments and is a skill that takes time and practice to acquire. The depth of injection can be determined by several factors:

- Feel of the needle moving through tissue
- Plunger resistance during injection
- Visibility of the needle tip.

When *injecting in the dermis,* slight resistance is felt as the needle advances through the tissue, some plunger resistance will be felt during injection, and the needle tip is not visible.

When *injecting too deeply in the subcutaneous layer,* minimal to no resistance is felt when advancing the needle or against injection, and the needle tip is not visible.

When *injecting too superficially in the epidermis or superficial dermis,* significant resistance is felt when advancing the needle and during injection, and the gray needle tip is visible in the skin.

TIP: If injecting at the incorrect level, withdraw the needle to the skin insertion and retry.

2. Dermal fillers are injected using firm, constant pressure on the syringe plunger as the needle is withdrawn in a linear thread (called retrograde injection). *Pressure on the plunger is released just prior to pulling the needle out of the skin, to avoid tracking product in the epidermis.*

   CAUTION: Blanching during injection indicates that blood flow to the treatment site has been compromised, either by injecting too much filler into the dermis or injecting intravascularly. Discontinue injecting, massage the area until the tissue appears pink, and institute other measures outlined in the *Complications* section later in the chapter if indicated.
3. Complete treatment in one area to the satisfaction of the provider and patient before moving on to the next area for treatment.

Methods for Dermal Filler Injection

The two main methods for injecting dermal filler in the dermis are (Figure 25-4):

- *Fanning technique.* This technique utilizes a single needle insertion point to inject a series of adjacent linear threads. Upon completion of fanning, product is placed in a triangular area. Fanning is commonly used for treatment of NLFs, particularly in the superior NLFs near the ala of the nose.
- *Cross-hatching technique.* This technique utilizes multiple insertion points with placement of linear threads

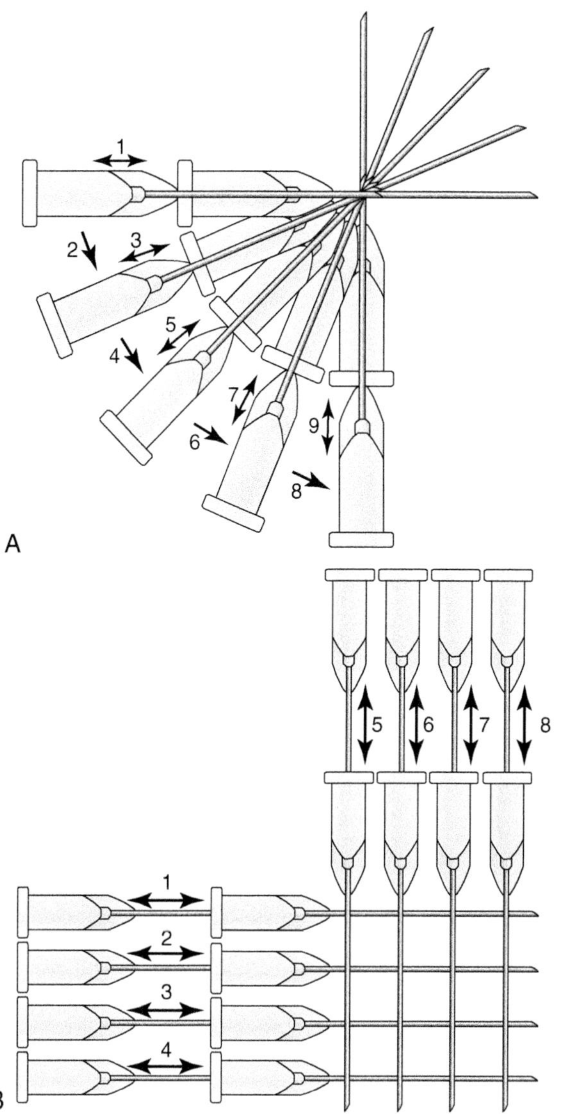

FIGURE 25-4 Dermal filler injection techniques: (A) fanning; (B) cross-hatching.

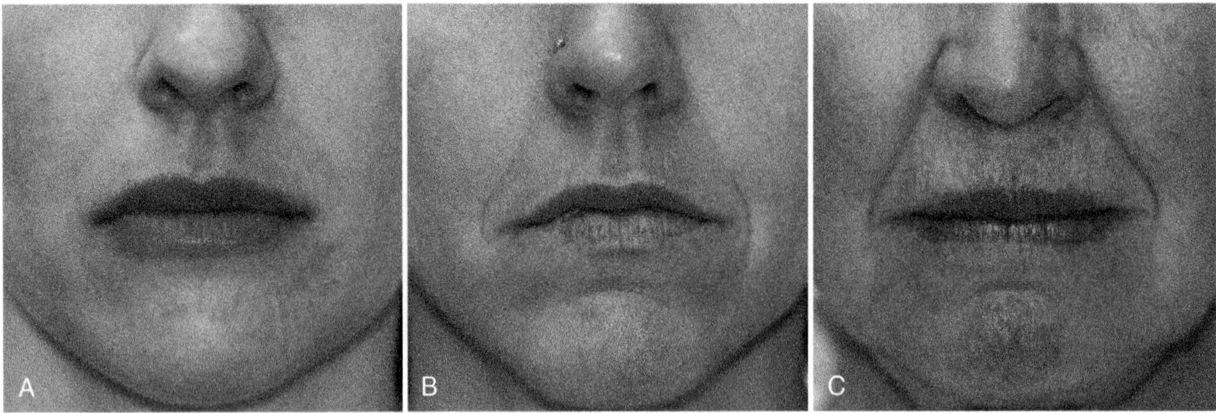

FIGURE 25-5 Nasolabial fold grading scale of (A) mild, (B) moderate, and (C) severe. *(Copyright Rebecca Small, MD.)*

in a grid pattern. Upon completion of cross-hatching, product is placed in a square area.

Planning and Designing

The goal of NLF treatment with dermal fillers is to soften NLFs without full effacement. The NLF is a natural facial contour and full effacement gives a simian appearance and is not aesthetically pleasing. In addition, undertreatment with small volumes may not yield a visible change to the NLF.

Figure 25-5 shows a grading scale for the severity of NLFs. Patients with mild, moderate, and severe NLFs are candidates for dermal filler treatments. Deep folds with excess laxity may have less satisfactory outcomes with dermal filler treatments and may require surgical interventions for significant improvement.

Dermal filler is placed within the Nasolabial Fold Safety Zone, which is bounded laterally by the nasolabial fold superiorly by the edge of the nasal ala and extends to the inferior-most portion of the nasolabial fold (Figure 25-6).

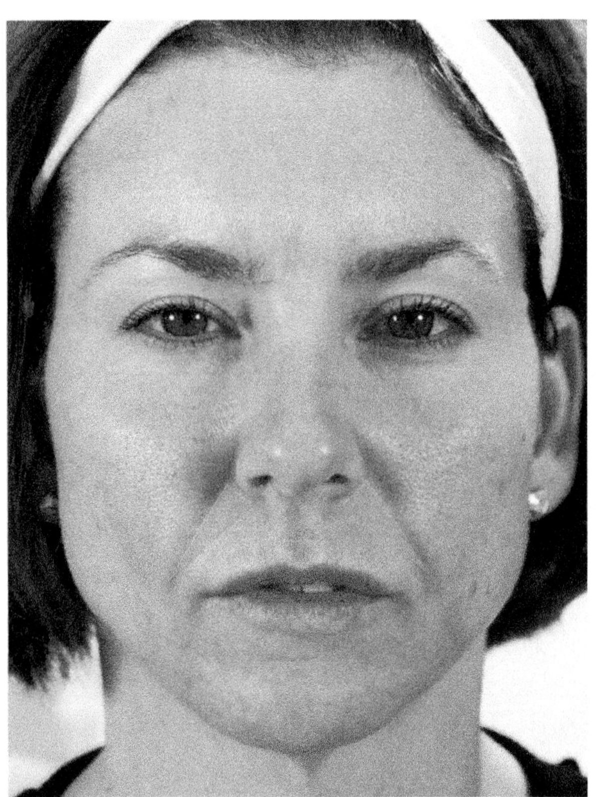

FIGURE 25-6 Nasolabial Fold Safety Zone. *(Copyright Rebecca Small, MD.)*

CAUTION: Injection superior-lateral to the NLF Safety Zone can accentuate the folds and can result in dermal filler placement in the angular artery (see Figure 25-2).

CAUTION: Injection inferior to the NLF Safety Zone, or placement of too much DF product in the NLF, can add heaviness to tissues and turn down the corners of the mouth, accentuating oral commissures and marionette lines.

An overview of injection points for treatment of NLFs using an HA dermal filler is shown in Figure 25-7. All injections are placed medial to the NLFs. Injections proceed superiorly from number 1 to 3, with the filler product fanned medially at the nasal ala.

The estimated HA dermal filler volume necessary for treatment is based on patients' observed facial anatomy and volume loss in the treatment area (see Figure 25-5):

- Mild NLFs typically require 0.5 syringe (0.4 mL) per side of the face.
- Moderate NLFs typically require one syringe (0.8 mL) per side of the face.
- Severe NLFs typically require 1.5 syringes (1.2 mL) per side of the face.

Maximum doses of dermal filler vary by manufacturer and are reported in the product package insert. For example, the maximal dose for Juvederm is 20 mL/year and for Restylane 6.0 mL per patient per treatment.

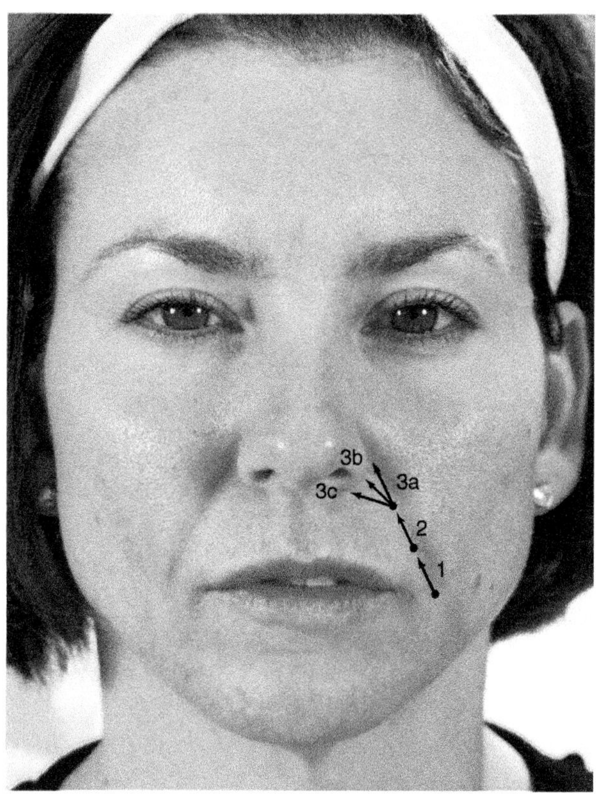

FIGURE 25-7 Overview of nasolabial fold injection points and technique. *(Copyright Rebecca Small, MD.)*

Anesthesia

Providing adequate anesthesia is an essential part of dermal filler treatments. Minimizing discomfort improves provider injection precision and offers the patient a better experience. The goal for anesthesia with dermal filler treatments is to achieve maximal anesthesia while minimizing tissue distortion of the treatment area to preserve the baseline anatomy.

The four main methods for providing anesthesia to the nasolabial folds are as follows:

1. *Local infiltration adjacent to the NLFs.* Figure 25-8 shows an overview of injection points and doses for local infiltration of anesthetic for treatment of NLFs. After preparing the skin with alcohol, 0.1 mL of 2% lidocaine with epinephrine 1:100,000 is injected subcutaneously at each injection site, superior to the NLFs. The injection sites are compressed to minimize edema from the anesthetic.
   CAUTION: Placing anesthetic into the nasolabial fold may blunt the fold and make filler treatment volumes more difficult to determine.
   TIP: Sensitivity increases with proximity to the nose, and injections are started at the inferior portion of the NLF and advance superiorly toward the nose.
2. *Infraorbital nerve block.* Nerve blocks are recommended instead of local infiltration when several facial regions are being treated simultaneously. For example, when treating lips and NLFs in the same visit, an infraorbital nerve block can be used to anesthetize both treatment areas. See Chapter 20, *Anesthesia for Cosmetic Procedures,* for details of performing nerve blocks.
3. *Topical anesthetic.* In-office application of a topical anesthetic, such as benzocaine : lidocaine : tetracaine (BLT), with a maximum dose of ½ g applied for 15 minutes, may be used prior to treatment of NLFs. See Chapters 3 and 20 for additional information on topical anesthetics.
   TIP: Topical anesthetics reduce discomfort associated with needle insertion but do not reduce the burning sensation that frequently accompanies HA fillers during the injection. Less burning sensation is reported by patients with HAs formulated with lidocaine.
4. Ice may be used as an alternative to or adjunctively with the methods listed above. Anesthesia is achieved by applying ice to the skin immediately before the injection until the skin is erythematous but not blanched.

Performing the Dermal Filler Injection

1. Position the patient comfortably in a semireclined position for the procedure, at about 65 degrees.
2. Prepare the skin with alcohol.
3. Anesthetize the treatment area using the minimal necessary anesthetic volume to reduce tissue distortion (see earlier *Anesthesia* section).

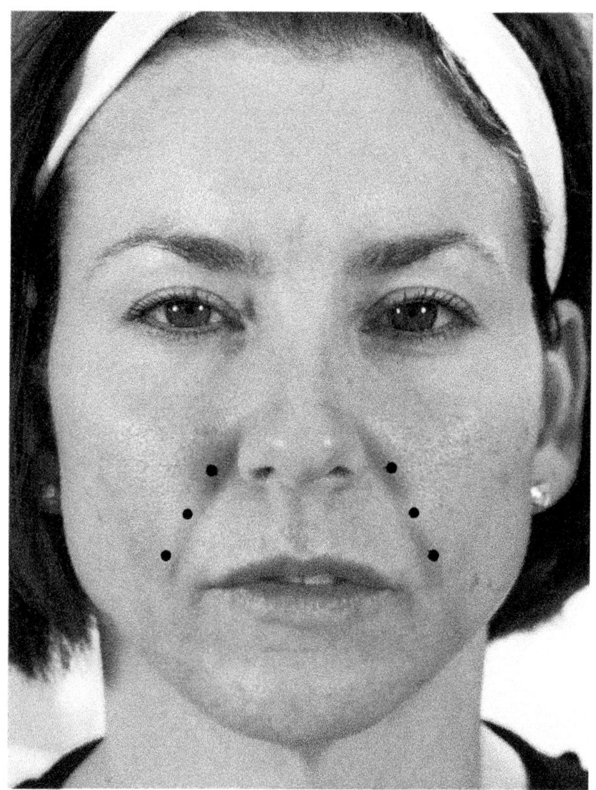

FIGURE 25-8 Nasolabial fold anesthesia. *(Copyright Rebecca Small, MD.)*

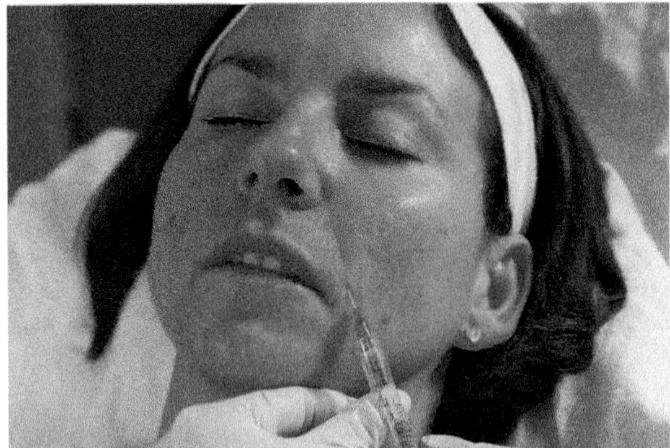

FIGURE 25-9 First injection point for nasolabial fold dermal filler treatment. *(Copyright Rebecca Small, MD.)*

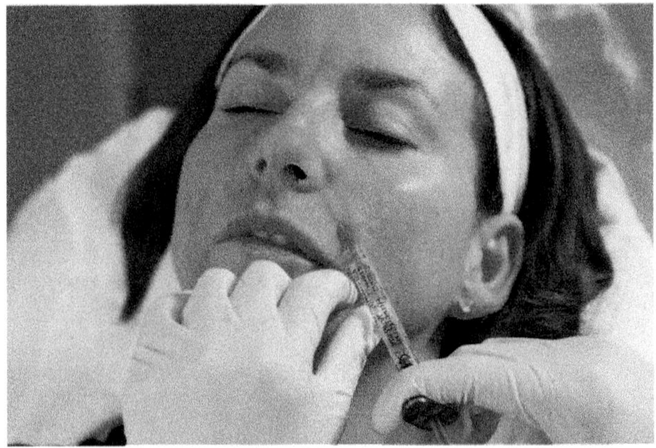

FIGURE 25-10 Second injection point for nasolabial fold dermal filler treatment. *(Copyright Rebecca Small, MD.)*

4. A soft white eyeliner pencil or surgical marker may be used to draw on top of the NLFs prior to administering anesthesia to better define the area for treatment.
5. Attach a 30-gauge, 0.5-inch needle to the prefilled dermal filler syringe.
6. Prime the needle by depressing the syringe plunger until a small amount of dermal filler extrudes from the needle tip. Ensure that the needle is tightly affixed to the dermal filler syringe to prevent the needle popping off when plunger pressure is applied.
7. The first injection is medial to the NLFs at the inferior portion of the fold (Figure 25-9). Insert the needle at a 30-degree angle to the skin and advance to the needle hub. Apply firm and constant pressure on the syringe plunger while gradually withdrawing the needle to inject a linear thread of filler in the mid to deep dermis.
8. The second injection point is approximately 1 cm superior to the first injection point (Figure 25-10).
9. The third injection point is 1 cm superior to the second injection point closer to the nose (Figures 25-11A and B). Use the fanning technique: Advance the needle to the hub and inject filler in a linear thread; without fully withdrawing the needle from the skin, redirect the needle counterclockwise and advance the needle to the hub again, and repeat.
10. Repeat injections 1 to 3 for the contralateral side of the face.
11. Compress the treatment area with thumb and first finger to smooth any visible or palpable bumps of filler product by placing the thumb on the skin and the first finger intraorally. If bumps do not easily compress, the area may be moistened with water and stretched between the provider's fingers. The more the filler product is compressed and manipulated, the more swelling and bruising may occur.

CAUTION: Avoid placing filler product in the superficial dermis because this may result in an undesirable visible ridge of filler that does not readily compress.

CAUTION: Avoid overfilling the treatment area because this may eliminate the nasolabial folds altogether resulting in an unnatural appearance.

RESULTS

Immediate correction of lines and contour defects are seen with dermal filler injections. Figure 25-12 shows

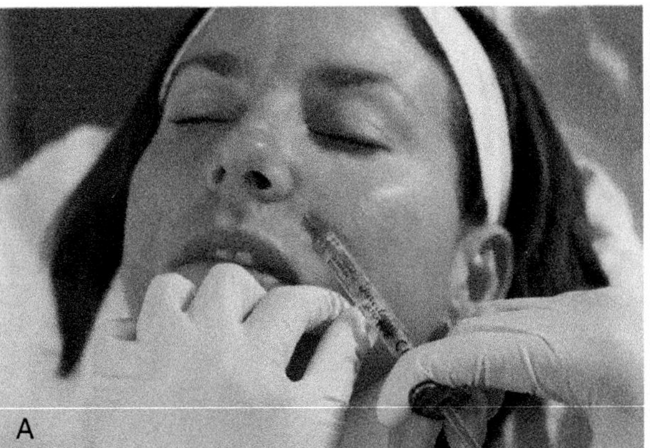

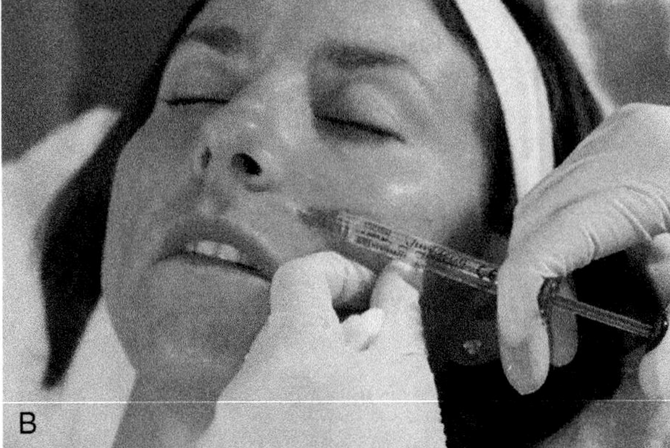

FIGURE 25-11 Third injection point for nasolabial fold dermal filler treatment with fanning from **(A)** superior to **(B)** inferior. *(Copyright Rebecca Small, MD.)*

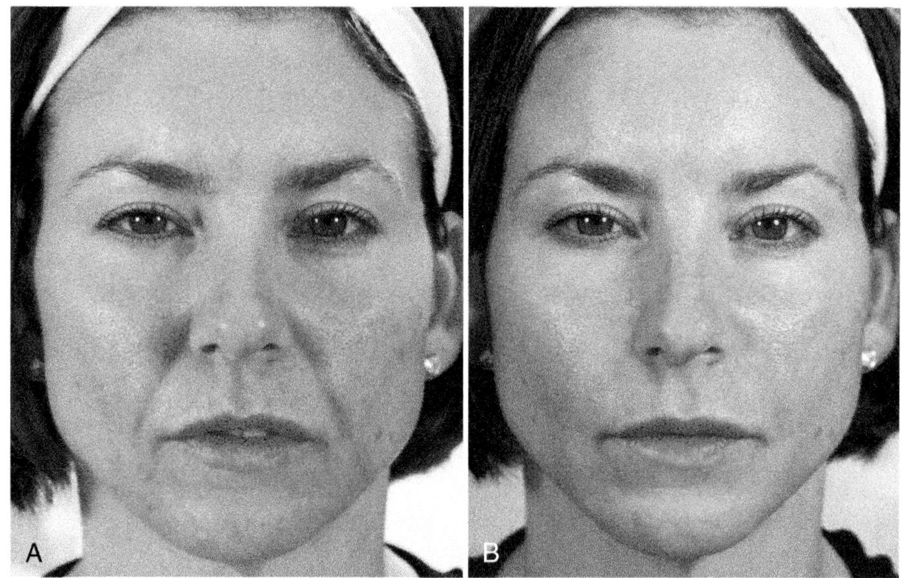

FIGURE 25-12 (A) Before and (B) after hyaluronic acid dermal filler treatment of the nasolabial folds. *(Copyright Rebecca Small, MD.)*

a 38-year-old patient with moderate nasolabial folds (A) before and (B) 1 week after treatment with an HA dermal filler, Juvederm Ultra Plus®, using 0.8 mL (one syringe) in each nasolabial fold for a total volume of 1.6 mL.

Figure 25-13 shows a 46-year-old patient with severe nasolabial folds (A) before and (B) 4 weeks after layering treatment with 1.5 mL of a calcium hydroxylapatite filler, Radiesse®, and 0.8 mL of a hyaluronic acid filler, Juvederm Ultra Plus®, in the nasolabial folds.

AFTERCARE

Ice is applied to treatment area for 10 to 15 minutes every 1 to 2 hours and continued for 1 to 3 days, or until swelling and bruising resolve. Patients are instructed to avoid activities that can cause facial flushing, such as application of heat, alcohol consumption, exercising, and tanning, until swelling resolves. Patient self-massage of the filler in the treatment areas is not recommended. Acetaminophen may be used if needed for discomfort.

FOLLOW-UP

The longevity of visible tissue filling with dermal fillers depends on several factors including: the type of product and volume used, the patient's metabolism, degree of motion in the treatment area, and facial expressivity. Hyaluronic acid dermal filler effects typically last 6 months to 1 year. To maintain the desired results, subsequent treatment is recommended at about 6 to 9 months, when the volume of dermal filler product visibly diminishes but is still palpable. Maintenance

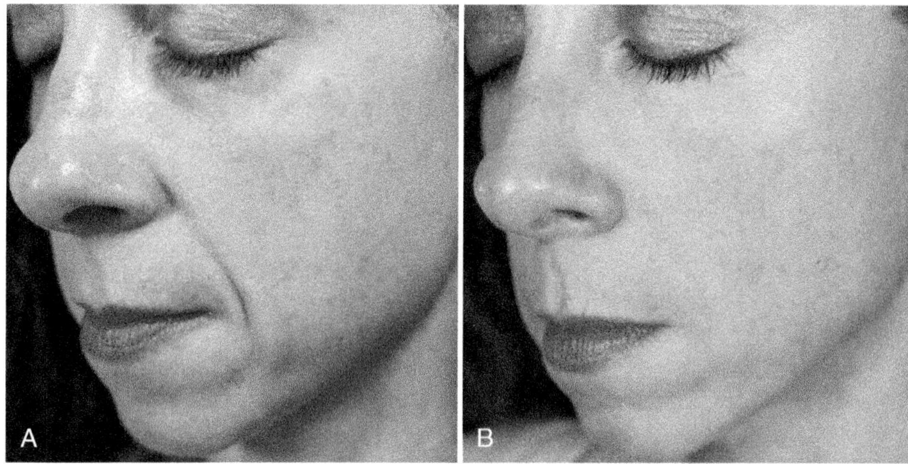

FIGURE 25-13 (A) Before and (B) after calcium hydroxylapatite and hyaluronic acid dermal filler treatment of the nasolabial folds. *(Copyright Rebecca Small, MD.)*

treatments usually require less product volume, particularly if some volume from the initial treatment is still present.

COMPLICATIONS

- Bruising or, rarely, hematoma
- Visible filler lumpiness
- Prolonged swelling
- Extremely rare: allergic hypersensitivity reaction with signs of urticaria, angioedema, and a remote possibility of anaphylaxis
- Prolonged erythema
- Hyperpigmentation (and rare possibility of hypopigmentation)
- Infection
- Erythematous tender bumps and nodules
- Granulomatous nodules
- Tyndall effect (bluish discoloration) with HAs placed superficially in thin-skinned areas
- Tissue ischemia, skin necrosis
- Blindness
- Asymmetry, overcorrection, or undercorrection
- Migration or extrusion of filler
- Unpredictable persistence of filler, either shorter or longer than anticipated.
- Keratoacanthomas
- Scarring

Some degree of transient postinjection *bruising, swelling, erythema* and *tenderness* is common and expected with any dermal filler treatment. These typically resolve within a few days to a few weeks.[13,14] Specific side effects are associated with each filler product[15] and the following discussion focuses on complications reported with hyaluronic acid fillers and their management.

Visible filler lumpiness occurring at the time of, or shortly after treatment, can usually be treated with aggressive compression by the provider. This may require local anesthetic infiltration prior to compression for patient comfort, and a bruise may form as a result of compression. In addition, hyaluronidase has been used by some providers for treatment of HA bumps, but it is not FDA approved for this use (see below).[16] Some providers report lancing large filler collections with a scalpel and expressing the product.[17]

Prolonged or excessive swelling can be treated with regular use of ice, as described above, and oral antihistamines (e.g., cetirizine 10 mg, 1 tablet daily until swelling resolves). *Severe swelling* and *allergic hypersensitivity reactions,* such as *angioedema,* have been reported, and oral or intramuscular steroids are indicated in these rare cases.[18]

Prolonged erythema is often due to tissue hypervascularity above the dermal filler. Discrete telangiectasias may be present with the erythema. Hypervascularity may be due to vascular congestion from filling the tissue, or an inherent tissue response to the dermal filler product.[19] Lasers or intense pulsed light devices specific for reduction of vascularities are useful treatment modalities to reduce erythema associated with hypervascularity. Prolonged erythema may also be due to irritation and/or inflammation in the treatment area, particularly when treatments are performed in highly mobile areas, such as the oral commissures.

Prolonged erythema may stimulate *postinflammatory hyperpigmentation,* which can be treated with topical lightening products such as hydroquinone (see Chapter 24, *Skin Care Products*).

Infection, such as reactivation of herpes simplex, can occur and may be prevented with prophylactic antiviral medications. Any time the skin barrier is breached, bacterial or fungal infection is possible.

Erythematous tender bumps and *nodules* (also called inflammatory nodules) are treated as bacterial infections. These can occur immediately after treatment or be delayed, up to a year or more.[19] Management consists of empiric antibiotics with a macrolide (e.g., clarithromycin 500 mg BID) or tetracycline (e.g., minocycline 100 mg BID).[20,21] A 6-week course of antibiotics is common; however, the duration of treatment depends on the intensity of infection. If fluctuant, it is advisable to incise, drain, and culture the nodule. HA fillers may be degraded by injecting *hyaluronidase* into the nodular area (10 to 30 units, based on the volume to be removed). New evidence is emerging to suggest that late-onset inflammatory nodules (and perhaps *granulomas*) may be due to biofilms, which are aggregates of microorganisms within adhesive protective coverings that commonly adhere to foreign bodies, and can be elusive to standard culture methods and highly resistant to antibiotics. Once the dermal filler foreign body is gone, the biofilm is presumed to resolve.[20]

Granulomas are a delayed complication, appearing 6 months to 2 years after dermal filler treatment, which are much more common with permanent and certain semipermanent fillers such as poly-L-lactic acid. A minority of granulomas spontaneously resolve, however, intralesional steroid injection or excision is often required.[15]

A *Tyndall effect* with bluish skin discoloration may occur with superficial placement of HA dermal fillers in thin-skinned areas.[17] Product can either be reduced using compression, hyaluronidase, or expressed as described above.[22]

Tissue ischemia, due to reduced blood supply to tissue, although rare, is a potentially serious complication. Blood flow can be compromised by overfilling tissue with filler product or injecting intravascularly.

Ischemia with possible impending tissue necrosis may present with pain or painlessly, and may be visible as a violaceous reticular pattern or white blanching. With NLF treatments, intravascular injection of the angular artery may occur (see Figure 25-2), with ischemic signs visible on the nose and/or nasolabial fold. Ischemia is managed urgently because it can rapidly progress to tissue necrosis. If ischemia occurs, attempt to revascularize by massaging the ischemic area, and if intravascular injection of the artery is suspected, apply heat packs, inject 10 to 30 units of hyaluronidase in the area, and administer aspirin 2 tablets of 325 mg orally. In addition, reports of applying of a vasodilator such as nitropaste to the affected area have also been used successfully.[12,23] It is advisable to contact the local emergency room and/or plastic surgeon if ischemia does not rapidly resolve.

Blindness due to retinal artery embolization has been reported with dermal filler treatment in the glabella.

Asymmetry, overcorrection, and *undercorrection* relate to the volume of product injected and their incidence usually decreases as injector skill improves. It is important to discuss these possible outcomes with patients prior to treatment, and inform them that additional product, incurring additional expense, may be required to correct an asymmetry or for undercorrection. A similar pretreatment discussion about the *duration of correction* (or persistence of the product) is also important because a product may not last as long as its FDA-approved duration, particularly if small product volumes are used, treatment areas are highly mobile, or the patient has a high metabolism. *Overcorrection,* as with product lumpiness, can often be corrected with compression to mechanically break down the product. *Migration* of filler product adjacent to the treatment area can occur if the treatment area is compressed shortly after treatment. For this reason it is advisable to instruct patients not to massage their filler product after treatment. If filler is tracked into the epidermis or superficial dermis upon withdrawal of the needle during injection, rarely, product may *extrude* spontaneously.

Keratoacanthomas, benign epithelial tumors, can arise in response to trauma and have been reported with DF treatments. These lesions can be refractory to treatment and it may be advisable to seek consultation for management.

Scarring is very rare with DF treatments, but may occur with any injection, particularly if treatment is complicated by an infection. Patients with a history of hypertrophic or keloidal scarring are also at increased risk of scarring.

LEARNING THE TECHNIQUES

Dermal filler injection requires practice to obtain proficiency. Providers can practice the linear thread, fanning, and cross-hatching techniques using clear silicon packs or synthetic skin models (which dermal filler manufacturers may provide). However, to place filler in the correct level of the skin, providers must acquire a "feel" for intradermal injection, which can only be obtained by injecting patients. Initially, it is advisable to start with treatment of the nasolabial folds of staff and family, using small volumes. Additional volume for further correction may be added subsequently.

CURRENT DEVELOPMENTS

Many hyaluronic acid dermal fillers are being formulated with lidocaine to reduce treatment discomfort and the need for anesthesia. Advanced techniques involving layering of fillers in different levels of the skin may improve outcomes with wrinkle reduction. In addition, new approaches to facial rejuvenation focusing on restoration of facial contours, in combination with the traditional approach of filling wrinkles, are increasing the applications of dermal fillers in facial aesthetics.

BOX 25-1 ***CPT Codes for Dermal Filler Procedures***

11950 Subcutaneous injection of filling material, ≤1.0 mL
11951 Subcutaneous injection of filling material, 1.1–5.0 mL
11952 Subcutaneous injection of filling material, 5.1–10 mL

FINANCIAL CONSIDERATIONS

Cosmetic dermal filler treatments are generally not covered by insurance. In rare instances, coverage for filler treatments to scars may be possible. Dermal filler fees are based on the type of filler used, size and number of syringes, injector skill, and vary according to local prices in different geographic regions. Prices range from $500 to $650 per syringe of hyaluronic acid filler (0.8 mL). Box 25-1 lists CPT codes for DF procedures.

CONCLUSION

Treatment of facial lines and wrinkles with dermal fillers is well tolerated by patients and can reliably achieve good results in the nasolabial fold area. Dermal fillers are an integral part of aesthetic care and are the treatments of choice for wrinkles in the lower two-thirds of the face. Once proficiency has been achieved with treatment of nasolabial folds, providers may choose to expand dermal filler use to other facial areas and aesthetic applications.

Resources

Dermal Fillers

Allergan
Phone: 800-377-7790
www.allergan.com

Bioform Medical/Merz
Phone: 650-286-4000
www.bioform.com

Coapt Systems
Phone: 650-461-7600
www.coaptsystems.com

Johnson and Johnson
Phone: 732-524-6678
www.JNJ.com

Medicis Aesthetics
Phone: 866-222-1480.
www.medicis.com

Mentor
Phone: 866-250-5115
www.mentorcorp.com

Sanofi Aventis
Phone: 800-981-2491
www.sanofi-aventis.us

Hyaluronidase

Ista Pharmaceuticals
Phone: 949-788-6000
www.istavision.com/products/vitrase.html

References

1. Small R. Aesthetic procedures in office practice. *Am Fam Physician.* 2009;80(11):1231–1237.
2. Wise JB, Greco T. Injectable treatments for the aging face. *Facial Plast Surg.* 2006;22(2):140–146.
3. Small R. Aesthetic procedures introduction. *In:* Mayeaux E, ed. *The Essential Guide to Primary Care Procedures.* Philadelphia: Lippincott Williams & Wilkins; 2009:195–199.
4. Cosmetic Surgery National Data Bank 2008 Statistics. American Society for Aesthetic Plastic Surgery; 2008.
5. Eppley BL, Dadvand B. Injectable soft-tissue fillers: clinical overview. *Plast Reconstr Surg.* 2006;118(4):98e–106e.
6. Small R. Dermal fillers for facial rejuvenation. *In:* Mayeaux E, ed. *The Essential Guide to Primary Care Procedures.* Philadelphia: Lippincott Williams & Wilkins; 2009:214–233.
7. Goldman MP. Optimizing the use of fillers for facial rejuvenation: the right tool for the right job. *Cosm Dermatol.* 2007;20(7 S3): 14–26.
8. Johl SS, Burgett RA. Dermal filler agents: a practical review. *Curr Opin Ophthalmol.* 2006;17(5):471–479.
9. Sadick NS. Soft tissue augmentation: selection, mode of operation, and proper use of injectable agents. *Cosm Dermatol.* 2007;20(5 S2):8–13.
10. Monheit GD, Coleman KM. Hyaluronic acid fillers. *Dermatol Ther.* 2006;19(3):141–150.
11. Green MS. Not all hyaluronic acid dermal fillers are equal. *Cosm Dermatol.* 2007;20(11):724–729.
12. Grunebaum LD, Allemann IB, Dayan S, *et al.* The risk of alar necrosis associated with dermal filler injection. *Derm Surg.* 2009;35:1635–1640.
13. Lowe NJ, Maxwell CA, Patnaik R. Adverse reactions to dermal fillers: review. *Derm Surg.* 2005;31(11 Pt 2):1616–1625.
14. Gladstone HB, Cohen JL. Adverse effects when injecting facial fillers. *Semin Cutan Med Surg.* 2007;26(1):34–39.
15. Zielke H, Wolber L, Wiest L, *et al.* Risk profiles of different injectable fillers: results from the Injectable Filler Safety Study (IFS Study). *Derm Surg.* 2008;34(3):326–335.
16. Brody HJ. Use of hyaluronidase in the treatment of granulomatous hyaluronic acid reactions or unwanted hyaluronic acid misplacement. *Derm Surg.* 2005;31(8 Pt 1):893–897.
17. Cohen JL. Understanding, avoiding, and managing dermal filler complications. *Derm Surg.* 2008;34(Suppl 1):S92–S99.
18. Geisler D, Shumer S, Elson M. Delayed hypersensitivity reaction to Restylane. *Cosm Dermatol.* 2007;20(12):784–786.
19. Narins RS, Jewell M, Rubin M, *et al.* Clinical conference: Management of rare events following dermal fillers—focal necrosis and angry red bumps. *Derm Surg.* 2006;32(3):426–434.
20. Narins RS, Coleman III WP, Glogau RG. Recommendations and treatment options for nodules and other filler complications. *Derm Surg.* 2009;35(Suppl 2):1667–1671.
21. Sclafani AP, Fagien S. Treatment of injectable soft tissue filler complications. *Derm Surg.* 2009;35(Suppl 2):1672–1680.
22. Cox SE. Clinical experience with filler complications. *Derm Surg.* 2009;35:1661–1666.
23. Hirsch RJ, Cohen JL, Carruthers JD. Successful management of an unusual presentation of impending necrosis following a hyaluronic acid injection embolus and a proposed algorithm for management with hyaluronidase. *Derm Surg.* 2007;33(3):357–360.

Additional Reading

Elson M. Dermal fillers. *In:* Pfenninger JL, Fowler GC, eds. *Pfenninger and Fowler's Procedures for Primary Care.* 3rd ed. Philadelphia: Mosby/Elsevier; 2011.

Small R, Hoang D. Nasolabial folds. *In:* Small R, Hoang D, eds. *A Practical Guide to Dermal Filler Procedures.* Philadelphia: Lippincott Williams & Wilkins; 2011.

Small R, Hoang D. Dermal Filler Introduction and foundation concepts. In: Small R, Hoang D, eds. *A Practical Guide to Dermal Filler Procedures.* Philadelphia: Lippincott Williams & Wilkins; 2011.

Small R, Hoang D. Anesthesia. In: Small R, Hoang D, eds. *A Practical Guide to Dermal Filler Procedures.* Philadelphia: Lippincott Williams & Wilkins; 2011.

Small R, Hoang D. Complications. In: Small R, Hoang D, eds. *A Practical Guide to Dermal Filler Procedures.* Philadelphia: Lippincott Williams & Wilkins; 2011.

26 Hair Reduction with Lasers

REBECCA SMALL, MD • JIMMY CHEN, MD

Since the first FDA-approved laser hair reduction (LHR) device was introduced in 1995, LHR has become one of the most commonly performed cosmetic procedures with over 1 million treatments annually, according to statistics from the American Society for Aesthetic Plastic Surgery.[1] Much of the popularity surrounding LHR can be attributed to its efficacy and excellent safety profile, with minimal discomfort and downtime.[2]

Unwanted hair growth affects both men and women, although the sites of concern and causes may vary. For men, body areas typically sought for treatment are the chest, back, shoulder, neck and ears, whereas for women, the face, chest, axilla, bikini line, and legs are usual areas of concern. Moreover, some individuals may choose to remove undesired hair for cosmetic, psychosocial, or cultural reasons; others may suffer from hirsutism due to medical conditions. In either case, undesired hair growth, if left untreated, can lead to significant distress for affected individuals and negatively influence self-image and self-esteem.

This chapter provides a basic foundation in laser principles as they relate to hair removal and a practical approach to the treatment of unwanted hair.

LASER PRINCIPLES

Laser hair removal is based on the principle of selective photothermolysis, which is the conversion of laser energy to heat, to selectively destroy hair follicles without damaging the surrounding skin tissues. To achieve this effect, laser energy is first absorbed by melanin, the target chromophore in hair. The energy absorbed by melanin is then converted into heat, which subsequently damages the hair growth structures. The surrounding skin, which minimally absorbs energy, remains unaffected.[3,4]

Several device parameters affect the safety and efficacy of LHR. These parameters include wavelength, fluence, pulse duration, and spot size (see *Laser Parameters* in Chapter 19, *Aesthetic Principles and Consultation*).

To target the hair follicle, *wavelength selection* should be specific for melanin, which preferentially absorbs laser energy between 650 and 1100 nm (Figure 26-1). These longer wavelengths also penetrate deeper into the skin to better target the hair follicles and facilitate hair removal. Four main lasers fall within this wavelength spectrum: ruby (694 nm), alexandrite (755 nm), diode (810 nm), and Nd:YAG (1064 nm) (see Figure 26-1). Whereas lasers emit single wavelengths of light energy, intense pulsed light (IPL) devices emit polychromatic light in a broad wavelength spectrum, typically between 400 and 1400 nm. Both lasers and IPL devices (collectively referred to as lasers*) used for hair reduction operate under the principle of selective photothermolysis.[5]

Fluence describes the amount of energy delivered per unit area (J/cm^2). In general, the higher the fluence utilized, the better the hair removal results. However, higher fluences are also associated with a greater risk of complications.

Pulse duration is the amount of time the laser pulse is applied to the skin (typically in milliseconds). To confine thermal damage due to laser light energy to the desired target hair follicle, the pulse duration must be shorter than or equal to the thermal relaxation time of the follicle, typically between 10 and 100 ms (see *Laser Parameters* in Chapter 19 for a discussion of thermal relaxation time). Longer pulse durations are used with coarse (i.e., thick), dark hairs and for areas with high hair density. Shorter pulse durations are used for fine (i.e., thin), light hairs and areas with low hair density. Figure 26-2 summarizes the fluences and pulse durations that are used based on hair characteristics. In addition, longer pulse widths penetrate deeper into the skin and are safer for the epidermis. Therefore, darker skin types are treated with longer pulse widths and lighter skin types are treated with shorter pulse widths.

Spot size, or the diameter of the laser beam emitted (mm), correlates with energy absorption and penetration into the skin. Larger spot sizes are associated with better LHR results because larger spots have higher absorption and deeper penetration compared to small-diameter spots. Furthermore, the larger the spot size, the more body area covered per pulse, which translates to shorter treatment times.

By manipulating these various factors of wavelength, fluence, pulse width, and spot size, maximal efficacy and safety can be achieved with laser hair reduction treatments.

PATIENT SELECTION

Proper patient selection based on an individual's Fitzpatrick skin type, hair color, coarseness, and density is crucial for achieving successful treatments. (Refer to Chapter 19 for a review of Fitzpatrick skin types.) The ideal candidate for LHR possesses fair skin and dark, coarse hair. Fair-skin individuals (Fitzpatrick skin types I to III) have little to no epidermal melanin, which, if present, can serve as a competing target for laser energy. Thus, darker skin types (IV to VI) are at greater risk of epidermal injury with LHR treatments. Patients with Fitzpatrick skin types VI pose the greatest challenge to treatment and have the highest risk of complications,

*Refers to laser and light-based technologies.

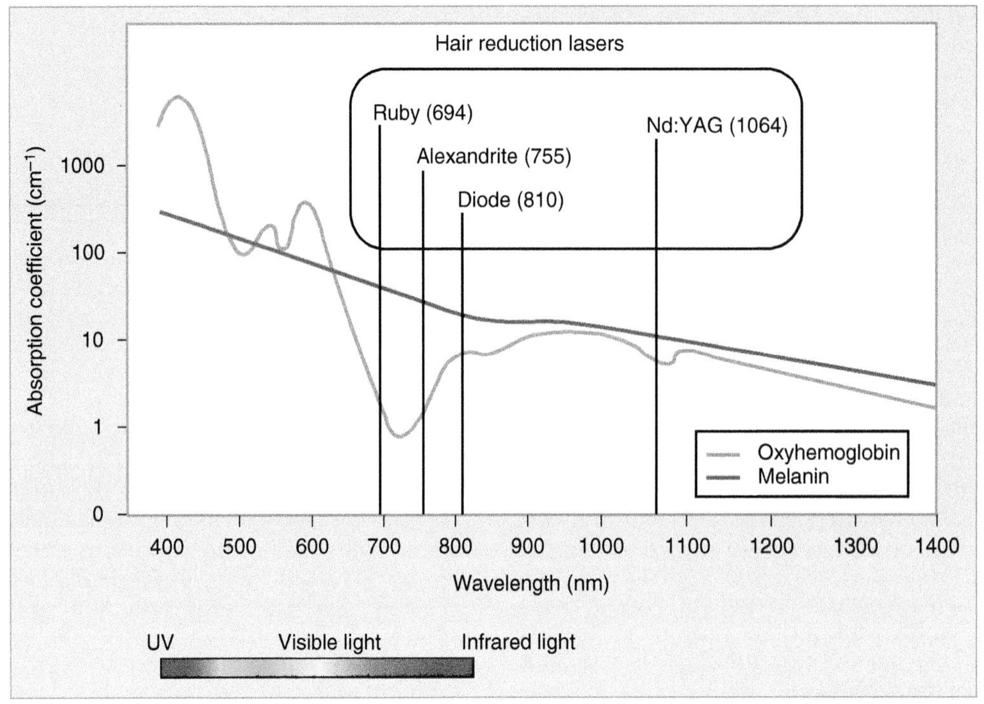

FIGURE 26-1 Chromophore absorption spectrum and common hair reduction lasers.

and recommendations for treatment are outside the scope of this chapter. White, light-colored (i.e., gray, blonde), and fine vellus hair lack melanin target in the hair follicle, and patients with these hair characteristics are poor candidates for LHR.

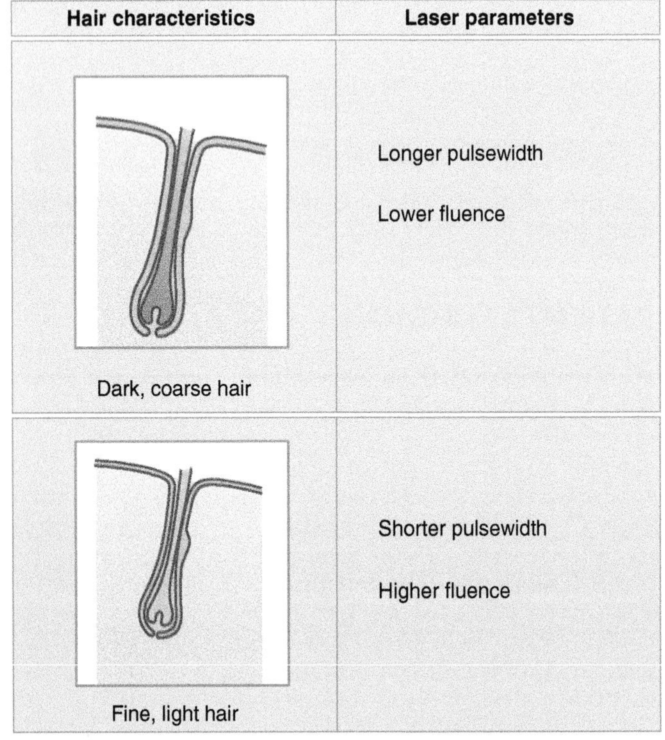

FIGURE 26-2 Hair characteristics and laser parameters.

INDICATIONS

- Permanent hair reduction (FDA approved)
- Pseudofolliculitis barbae
- Pseudofolliculitis pubis
- Hirsutism
- Hypertrichosis.

Hirsutism is excessive hair growth due to medical conditions associated with hyperandrogenic states, such as polycystic ovarian syndrome. *Hypertrichosis* is excessive hair growth that is not androgen dependent and, although generally idiopathic and genetic, can be due to thyroid disease, malnutrition, and medications (e.g., phenytoin, corticosteroids, and cyclosporine).

PATIENT EXPECTATIONS

Addressing patient expectations is fundamental to ensuring patient satisfaction. First, it is important to clarify a common misconception that laser hair reduction results in complete permanent hair loss. According to the FDA, LHR is approved for permanent hair reduction, which is defined as "long-term, stable reduction in the number of hairs re-growing after a treatment regime." Patients may experience a range of different outcomes, such as fewer, thinner, slower hair regrowth, or lighter hairs, all of which are still clinically significant and desirable.

Candidates for LHR should expect to undergo several treatments in order to achieve optimal results. Because hair growth is asynchronous and LHR is most effective for hair follicles in the anagen phase (see below), patients can expect, on average, 20% to 30% permanent hair reduction after one treatment and up to 60% to 90% reduction after completing a treatment series.[6] Typically, individuals with Fitzpatrick skin types I to III require a series of six sessions, whereas skin types IV and V require eight sessions or more because treatment fluences are increased more slowly and conservatively over time with darker skin types to minimize the risk of complications.[7]

ALTERNATIVE THERAPIES

Common alternative treatment options to LHR include temporary hair removal methods, such as shaving, chemical depilatories, waxing, and tweezing. Currently, the only other FDA-approved method of permanent hair reduction is electrolysis, which utilizes a high-frequency electric current, via a fine-wire electrode, to destroy the hair follicle. Electrolysis is most effective for treating finer hair and may be used for nonpigmented hair including white, blonde, and gray hair. However, electrolysis is associated with more pain and longer treatment times than LHR.

PRODUCTS CURRENTLY AVAILABLE

A wide selection of hair removal lasers and IPL devices are available and vary by their emitted wavelengths, peak fluences, pulse durations, spot size, and cooling methods (see the *Resources* section at the end of the chapter for a list of suppliers).

Ruby lasers (694 nm) were one of the first lasers used for hair reduction. Although this wavelength is effective for hair reduction, it has a significant risk of complications given the high melanin absorption with this wavelength and short device pulse widths; therefore, it is not in general use today.

Alexandrite lasers (755 nm) for hair reduction are commonly used for lighter skin types (I through III).[8] Relative to ruby lasers, this wavelength is safer, because it is less strongly absorbed by melanin and penetrates deeper into the epidermis. However, it is still a shorter wavelength than others used for LHR and complications such as postinflammatory hyperpigmentation can occur with darker skin types. Alexandrite devices have the advantage of being easy to use with flexible fiber-optic arms. These devices typically use cryogen spray or cool air as a means of cooling the epidermis.

Diode lasers (810 nm) are popular LHR devices that are highly effective on coarse dark hair. Darker skin types can be treated more safely than with alexandrite lasers due to the longer wavelength with deeper penetration, longer pulse widths and contact cooling of the laser tip.[6] These devices also have the advantage of not having disposable parts and are small enough to sit on a tabletop.

Neodymium-doped yttrium aluminum garnet or *Nd:YAG lasers* (1064 nm) can be used for LHR in all skin types and are the safest devices for darker skin types (V and VI). This long wavelength is deeply penetrating, which aids in hair reduction. It has relatively poor melanin absorption and, while this protects the skin from epidermal injury, reduced melanin absorption is a disadvantage for LHR treatments. This can be overcome with the use of high fluences, coupled with intense epidermal cooling, to adequately damage hair growth structures.[9]

Q-switched Nd:YAG lasers, previously thought to provide only for temporary hair reduction, have recently been found to achieve permanent reduction of fine dark hair.[10] The short pulse widths of these lasers (in the nanosecond range) cause mechanical oscillation of the target, also known as photoacoustic vibration. Damage to the hair follicle results from both photothermolysis and photoacoustic vibration. These lasers are most useful for the treatment of fine dark hairs, particularly on the face, and can be used with all skin types.

Intense pulsed light devices emit noncoherent, multi-wavelength light ranging from 400 to 1200 nm. Cutoff filters are used to eliminate short wavelengths and allow for peaks of emission at certain desired wavelengths. For example, IPLs used for hair reduction will often use a filter that cuts off all wavelengths below 590 nm and allows for a wavelength peak between 600 and 800 nm. In this way, IPL devices can target the melanin chromophore and penetrate deeply into the skin.[11] IPL devices have either single or multipulse modes (see Chapter 19). One head-to-head study showed similar clinical efficacy in hair reduction with diode, alexandrite, and IPL devices.[12] Some devices are now available that combine IPL and 1064 nm to allow for treatment of a wide spectrum of skin types and hair characteristics.

Electro-optical synergy (ELOS) devices utilize radio-frequency (RF) and optical (laser or IPL light) energy together. The electrical RF energy heats the hair bulb and bulge, and the optical energy heats the hair shaft. One disadvantage of this device is that RF tends to be a more painful method of delivering energy to the skin.

In summary, different laser wavelengths are best suited to different skin types and different hair characteristics. The preceding discussion provides general guidelines; however, the indications for treatment of different skin types are device specific and are determined by the FDA. For example, most IPL devices are approved for LHR in skin types I through IV, however, certain IPL manufacturers' devices are also approved for treatment of skin type V. The specifics about a particular device should be sought from the laser manufacturer.

CONTRAINDICATIONS

General Laser Contraindications

The following contraindications apply to LHR and the laser treatments discussed in Chapters 27 through 30:

- Active infection in the treatment area (e.g., herpes simplex, pustular acne, cellulitis)

- Dermatoses such as vitiligo and active psoriasis or eczema in the treatment area
- Uncontrolled systemic condition
- Cardiac pacemaker
- Recent sun exposure, tanned skin in the treatment area, or insufficient sun protection
- Self-tanning product use in the previous 2 weeks
- Photosensitive disorder (e.g., systemic lupus erythematosus)
- Isotretinoin (Accutane) use in the previous 6 months
- Pregnancy or nursing
- Melanoma or lesions suspected for melanoma in the treatment area
- Gold therapy (an arthritis treatment)
- Seizures
- Treatment inferior to the eyebrows or any area inside the orbit
- History of livido reticularis, a rare autoimmune vascular disease associated with mottled skin discoloration of the arms or legs exacerbated by heat exposure with laser treatments
- History of erythema ab igne, a rare acquired reticular erythematous rash related to heat exposure with lasers
- Deep chemical peel, dermabrasion, or radiation therapy within the preceding 6 months (for hair removal on the face)
- Use of products containing retinoids in the treatment area 1 week prior to treatment
- Hypertrophic or keloidal scarring
- Bleeding abnormality (e.g., thrombocytopenia or anticoagulant use)
- Impaired healing (e.g., due to immunosuppression)
- Peripheral vascular disease
- Skin atrophy (e.g., chronic oral steroid use or genetic syndromes such as Ehlers-Danlos syndrome)
- Photosensitizing medications (e.g., tetracyclines, St. John's wort, thiazides)
- Unrealistic patient expectations
- Body dysmorphic disorder.

Contraindications Specific to LHR

- Hair removal by waxing, tweezing, or electrolysis during the previous month
- Use of bleaching or depilatory cream during the previous 2 weeks
- Recent, undiagnosed increase in hair growth.

ADVANTAGES OF LHR

- Permanent hair reduction
- Relatively brief treatment sessions
- Mild to moderate discomfort
- Good safety profile for devices with built-in cooling
- Useful for large body areas, such as backs and legs
- Minimal to no recovery time.

DISADVANTAGES OF LHR

- Not effective for permanent reduction of white, gray, or blond hair
- Must be used cautiously on darker skin types (types V and VI)
- Requires eye protection
- Possible risk of burns, infection, or skin discoloration.

ANATOMY

Hair follicles are composed of the *bulb* (which consists of the matrix and dermal papilla), *outer root sheath, bulge,* and *hair shaft* (Figure 26-3). The hair matrix depth in the skin ranges from 2 to 7 mm, depending on the body location, and the hair bulge is approximately 1.5 mm. Hair growth occurs in three phases with distinct changes below the skin in the hair bulb: (1) *anagen,* the active growth phase during which the hair bulb is most darkly pigmented; (2) *catagen,* the regression phase when cell division ceases and the follicle begins to involute; and (3) *telogen,* the resting phase during which the hair bulb is minimally pigmented (Figure 26-4). The hair shaft visible on the surface of the skin, however, is indistinguishable throughout these phases.

Hair growth is initiated by epithelial stem cells located in the "bulge," a protrusion near the attachment of the arrector pili muscle, and also occurs from the rapidly dividing matrix cells of the hair bulb. Hairs are most susceptible to laser treatment during the early anagen phase when the melanin content of the matrix is greatest. The percentage of hairs in anagen varies for different parts of the body (Table 26-1), and those areas with the greatest percentage in anagen, such as the scalp, respond most rapidly to laser treatments. The duration of the telogen phase serves as a rough

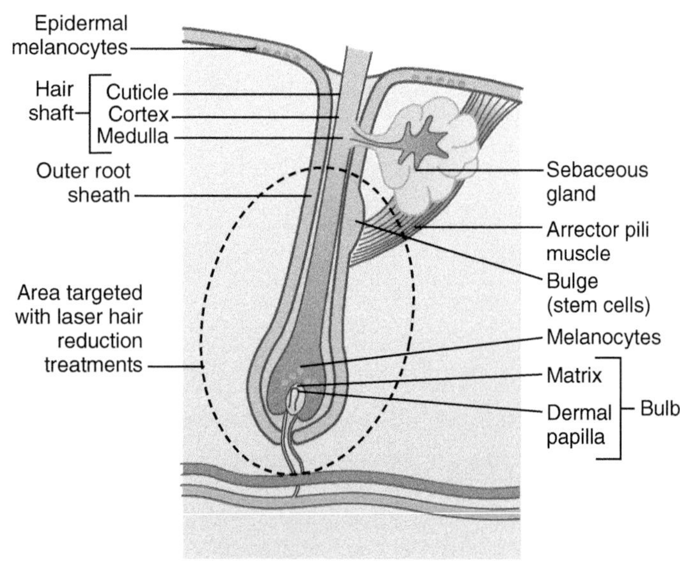

FIGURE 26-3 Hair anatomy.

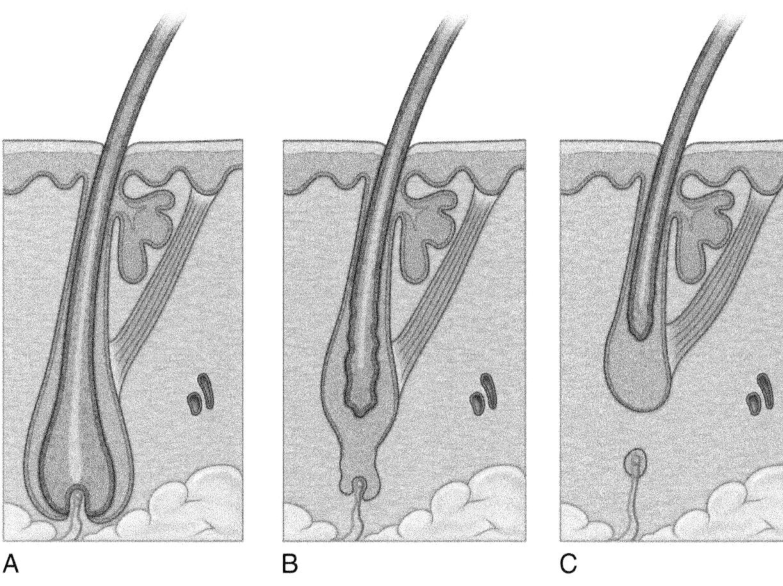

FIGURE 26-4 Three phases of hair growth: **(A)** anagen, **(B)** catagen, and **(C)** telogen. *(From Robinson J, Hanke W, Sengelmann R, Siegel D.* Surgery of the Skin: Procedural Dermatology, *2nd ed. Philadelphia: Mosby; 2010.)*

guideline for the interval between treatments. For example, the lower legs, which have a long telogen phase, require intervals of approximately 3 months between treatments, whereas the upper lip, which has a short telogen phase, requires approximately 1 month between treatments (Table 26-1).

EQUIPMENT

- Laser device appropriate for hair reduction treatments
- Eyewear for the patient and provider that is specific to the laser used
- Nonalcohol wipes to cleanse the treatment area
- Topical anesthetic such as EMLA, ELA-Max, or benzocaine:lidocaine:tetracaine (BLT)
- Clear colorless gel (e.g., clear ultrasound gel)
- Gauze, 4 × 4 inches
- Ice packs
- Sunscreen that is broad spectrum with SPF 30 or greater for application after treatment
- Hydrocortisone cream, 1% and 2.5%
- Alcohol wipes for cleaning the laser tip
- Germicidal disposable wipes for sanitizing the laser
- Soft white eyeliner pencil to mark treatment areas.

TABLE 26-1 Percentage of Hairs in Anagen and Duration of Telogen Phase for Different Body Areas

Body Area	Anagen Hair (%)	Telogen Duration (months)
Scalp	85	3 to 4
Beard	70	2.5
Upper lip	65	1.5
Axillae	30	3
Pubic area	30	3
Arms	20	4.5
Lower legs	20	6

PROCEDURE PREPARATION

1. Perform an aesthetic consultation and review the patient's medical history (see Chapter 19, *Aesthetic Principles and Consultation*) including recent onset of unexplained hair growth; medications that may cause hypertrichosis, such as hormone therapy, corticosteroids, immunosuppressives; conditions that cause hirsutism such as polycystic ovarian syndrome and tumors; history of herpes genitalis, which is particularly important when treating the bikini area; previous hair reduction methods and success.[13]
2. Determine the Fitzpatrick skin type (see Chapter 19)
3. Obtain informed consent (see Chapter 19; also see Appendix A for an informed consent form and patient information handout titled *Laser Hair Reduction*).
4. Take pretreatment photographs (see Chapter 19).
5. Examine the treatment area, and document the density, coarseness, and color of hair in the treatment area.
6. If the patient has a prior history of herpes simplex or varicella in or near the treatment area, provide prophylactic antiviral medication (e.g., valacyclovir 500 mg 1 tablet twice daily) for 2 days prior to the procedure, and continue for 3 days postprocedure.

7. Consider lightening the skin for darker Fitzpatrick skin types (IV and V). Use a skin-lightening topical product daily or twice daily for at least 1 month prior to treatment. Products include hydroquinone or a cosmeceutical such as kojic acid, arbutin, niacinamide, or azelaic acid (see the *Hyperpigmentation* section of Chapter 24, *Skin Care Products*).
8. Advise strict sun avoidance for 1 month and daily use of a full-spectrum sunscreen (see Chapter 24 for sunscreen product recommendations).
9. Perform test spots for skin types III with high-risk ethnic backgrounds (Mediterranean, Latino, and Asian) and skin types IV and V prior to initial treatment. Select appropriate test spot parameters based on the patient's Fitzpatrick skin type and hair characteristics using the manufacturer's guidelines for spot size, fluence, and pulse width. Test spots are placed discretely near the desired treatment area (such as under the chin, behind or inferior to the ear) with 20% overlap of pulses. Evaluate test spots 3 to 5 days after placement for evidence of erythema, burn, or other adverse effect. Inform patients that lack of an adverse reaction with test spots does not ensure that a side effect or complication will not occur with any treatment.
10. Instruct patients to shave the treatment area 1 to 2 days prior to treatment. Hair should be barely visible (approximately 1 to 2 mm above the skin) at the time of treatment.

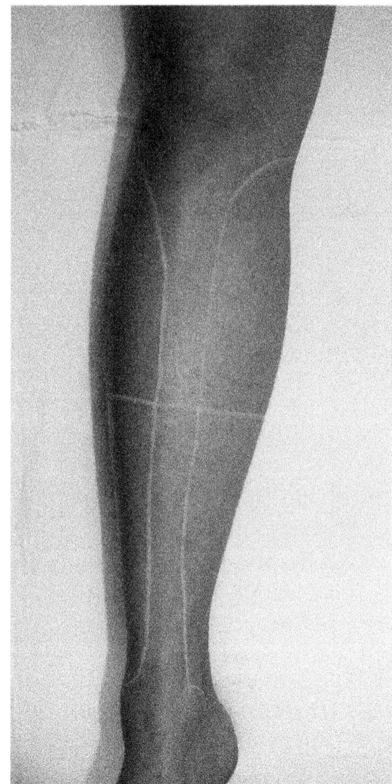

FIGURE 26-5 Grid pattern for laser hair treatments. *(Copyright Rebecca Small, MD.)*

LASER HAIR REDUCTION: STEPS AND PRINCIPLES[7]

The following recommendations are guidelines for hair reduction treatments using an intense pulsed light (IPL) device (Palomar StarLux 500 using the LuxRs handpiece). Manufacturer's guidelines for the specific device used should be followed at the time of treatment.

General Treatment Technique

1. The IPL tip is placed firmly on the skin, with the entire tip in contact with the skin and surrounded by gel.
2. The IPL handpiece is moved toward the provider to allow for maximal visibility of the treatment area. The degree of recommended overlap with pulses varies for different devices, but in general, there should be 20% overlap.
   CAUTION: Incomplete coverage of the treatment area will result in noticeable stripes of hair regrowth 1 to 2 weeks after treatment and is associated with patient dissatisfaction.
3. Fluence is decreased over bony areas and prominences, because increased reflection off the bone can intensify treatments and result in overtreatment.

Planning and Designing

A grid pattern may be drawn on the skin using a soft white pencil to help ensure complete coverage of the treatment area (Figure 26-5). This is particularly useful when treating large areas such as the leg and back.

Anesthesia

Discomfort associated with LHR treatment is usually likened to the snap of a rubber band. Because of the rich sensory nerve supply around hair follicles, LHR treatments are rarely free from pain. Anesthesia requirements vary according to the equipment used, patients' tolerance, and treatment area. Many LHR devices have built-in cooling mechanisms, such as a cooled sapphire window, that maintain the tip of the laser at a constant temperature. This provides epidermal contact cooling, which increases safety and provides some anesthesia. Some patients may require a topical anesthetic such as EMLA (prilocaine 21/2%:lidocaine 21/2%), ELA-Max (lidocaine 4%), or BLT (benzocaine 20%:lidocaine 6%:tetracaine 4%) (see Chapter 3, *Anesthesia*, and Chapter 20, *Anesthesia for Cosmetic Procedures*). All topical anesthetics are applied in the office for safety reasons.

The use of ice or cold packs is an excellent method of anesthesia and may be used for pretreatment and post-treatment cooling. A cryogen cooling spray or forced cool air is used by some devices for epidermal cooling during treatment, and these may also provide some pain reduction. Pneumatic skin flattening is a newer method of anesthesia whereby the tip of the laser compresses the skin using vacuum pressure, thereby reducing pain sensation (see Chapter 20).

Performing Laser Hair Reduction

1. Shave the treatment area if it is unshaven.
   CAUTION: If hair is too long at the time of treatment, singed hair on the skin surface may result in epidermal injury.
2. Anesthetize the treatment area if necessary (see *Anesthesia* section above).
3. Provide appropriate laser-safe eye protection for the patient and all people in the treatment room prior to beginning treatment.
   TIP: Always angle the laser tip away from the eyes during treatment.
4. Cover tattoos and permanent makeup with wet gauze and perform treatments at least 2 inches away from them.
   CAUTION: Full-thickness burns may result from treating over tattoos.
5. Always operate the device in accordance with your clinic's safety policies and procedures and the manufacturer's guidelines.
6. Select the pulse width based on the patient's Fitzpatrick skin type, using the manufacturer's guidelines. Darker Fitzpatrick skin types (IV and V) require longer pulse widths due to their greater risk of epidermal injury. For example, the manufacturer may recommend 40- to 100-ms pulse widths initially for a Fitzpatrick skin type IV versus 20- to 30-ms pulse widths for a Fitzpatrick skin type II.
7. Refine the pulse width selection and the fluence using the manufacturer's guidelines by assessing the hair characteristics in the treatment area including color, coarseness, and density. Coarse, dark hairs and areas with high hair density require longer pulse widths and lower fluences. For example, an initial treatment for a patient with Fitzpatrick skin type IV having black, coarse hair with high density may require a pulse width of 100 ms and fluence of 24 to 26 J/cm^2. The same patient with black, fine hairs with a sparse distribution may require a 40-ms pulse width and fluence of 30 to 32 J/cm^2.
8. Apply a clear colorless gel to the skin. Place the tip firmly on the skin, making certain that the entire tip is in contact with the skin and is surrounded by gel.
9. Perform a single pulse in the treatment area and assess for patient tolerance and clinical endpoints (see below). In general, there should be subtle endpoints with initial treatments and pain should be less than or equal to 6 on a scale of 1 to 10.
   TIP: Ice may be used immediately prior to treatment to reduce discomfort. Application of ice to the treatment area after treatment also reduces the incidence of paradoxical hair growth.[14]
10. Desirable clinical endpoints for LHR treatments include:
    - Singed hair smell
    - Erythema (Figures 26-6, 26-7 and 26-8)
    - Perifollicular edema (PFE) (see Figure 26-7)
    - Singed hair (see Figures 26-6 and 26-8)
    - Hair extrusion (see Figure 26-8).

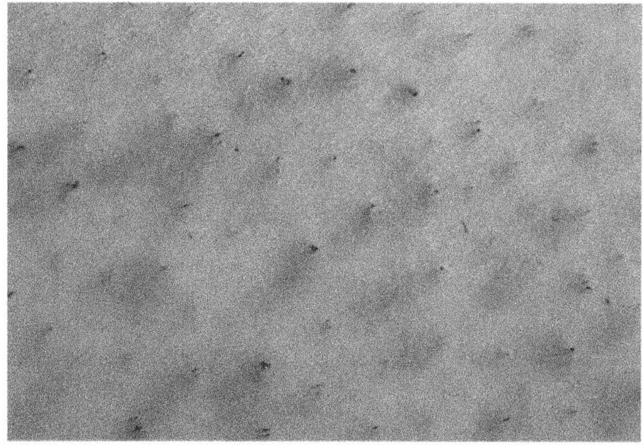

FIGURE 26-6 Laser hair treatment clinical endpoints of erythema and singed hair. *(Copyright Rebecca Small, MD.)*

11. Figure 26-7 shows the desired clinical endpoints of erythema, which develops rapidly, and perifollicular edema (PFE), which typically develops a few minutes after the pulse and indicates that the hair bulb has been effectively treated. PFE is more commonly seen with longer pulse widths.
12. Figure 26-8 shows the desired clinical endpoints of erythema, perifollicular edema, singed and extruded hair.
    TIP: Clean the IPL tip between pulses with moist gauze to reduce the buildup of singed hair.
13. Continually assess laser/tissue interactions and clinical endpoints throughout the treatment and adjust settings accordingly.
14. For subsequent treatments, fluence is increased and pulse width decreased according to the manufacturer's guidelines to target finer, lighter hairs. In general, only one parameter is changed to intensify treatments in any given visit. Typically, the fluence is increased initially for a few treatments to achieve desired clinical endpoints, and pulse width is decreased in later treatments.
    TIP: Finer, lighter hairs are the most challenging to treat. It is important to inform patients that once

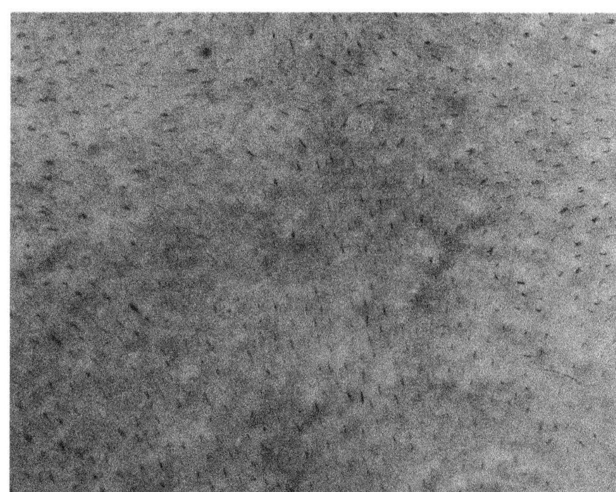

FIGURE 26-7 Laser hair treatment clinical endpoints of perifollicular edema and erythema. *(Copyright Rebecca Small, MD.)*

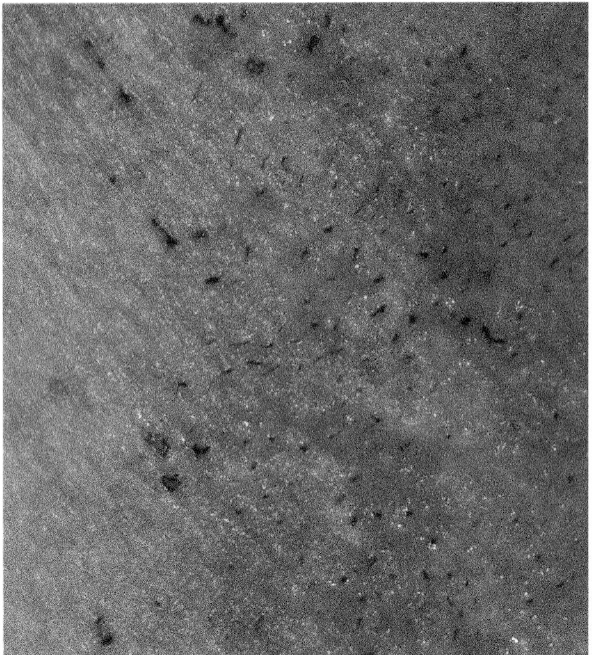

FIGURE 26-8 Laser hair treatment clinical endpoints of erythema, perifollicular edema, and hair singeing and extrusion. *(Copyright Rebecca Small, MD.)*

hair becomes very fine and light, the efficacy limits of the laser may be reached. Subsequent, more aggressive treatments may not be of therapeutic benefit and may be associated with greater risks from high fluences.

15. The entire treatment area is covered at each laser hair treatment session.
16. Ice may be applied immediately after treatment to soothe the treatment area and reduce PFE.
17. A topical steroid may be applied to erythematous areas, such as 1% to 2.5% hydrocortisone cream.
18. A full-spectrum sunscreen (SPF 30 with zinc or titanium) is applied to sun exposed areas.

RESULTS

After the first treatment, patients may experience a prolonged delay in hair regrowth from 1 to 3 months. This is temporary hair reduction, and although patients are usually very pleased with the lack of growth, they should be forewarned that regrowth will occur. Hair regrowth may appear in some parts of the treatment area and not others. This patchy regrowth is normal and indicates that a group of hairs in the anagen phase was effectively treated.

The greatest efficacy with permanent hair reduction is achieved with use of high fluences, a greater number of treatments, and adequately long intervals between treatments that approximate the telogen phase for the treatment area.[6]

Figure 26-9 shows hair reduction results for the anterior neck and chin (A) before and (B) after six treatments using an IPL (Starlux, Palomar).

Figure 26-10 shows hair reduction results for fine dark upper lip hair in a darker Fitzpatrick skin type (A) before and (B) after a series of treatments using a Q-switched 1064 nm laser. This is one of the only laser devices that can reduce fine hairs (RevLite, HOYA ConBio).

Figure 26-11 shows hair reduction results for the jawline and sideburns (A) before and (B) after completion of a series of treatments using a 755 nm laser (GentleLase, Candela).

Figure 26-12 shows hair reduction results for the axilla (A) before and (B) after completion of a series of treatments using a 755 nm laser (GentleLase, Candela).

Figure 26-13 shows hair reduction results for pseudofolliculitis barbae in a patient with Fitzpatrick skin type VI (A) before and (B) after a series of treatments using a 1064 nm long-pulse laser (ClearScan YAG, Sciton).

AFTERCARE

Erythema and perifollicular edema usually resolve within a few hours to 1 week after treatment and can

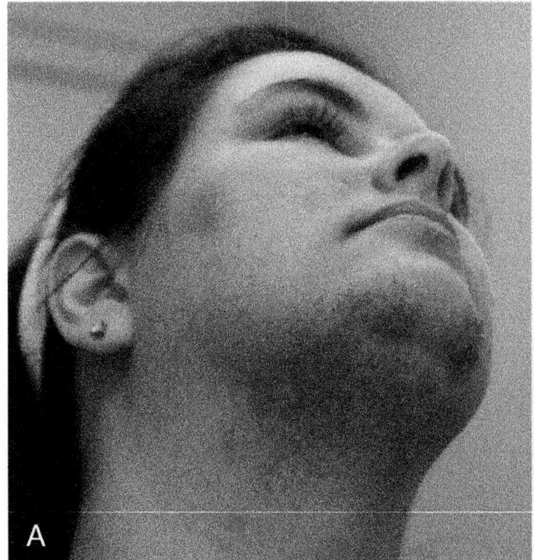

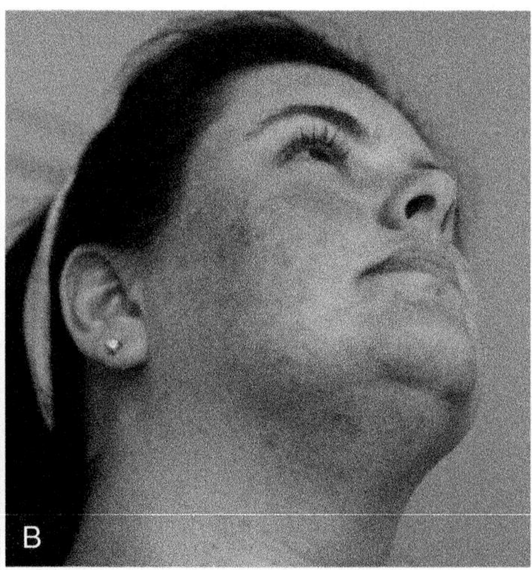

FIGURE 26-9 Anterior neck and chin hair (A) before and (B) after completion of six hair reduction treatments with intense pulsed light. *(Copyright Rebecca Small, MD.)*

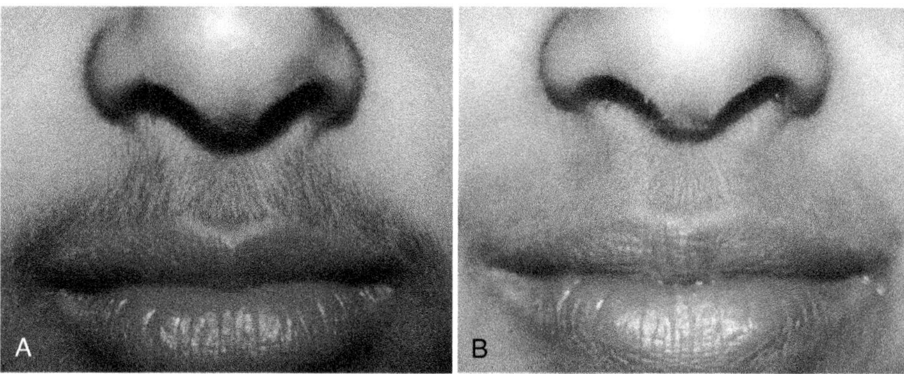

FIGURE 26-10 Upper lip hair **(A)** before and **(B)** after completion of a series of hair reduction treatments with a Q-switched 1064 nm laser. *(Courtesy of HOYA ConBio, Fremont, CA; J. Garden, MD, using laser.)*

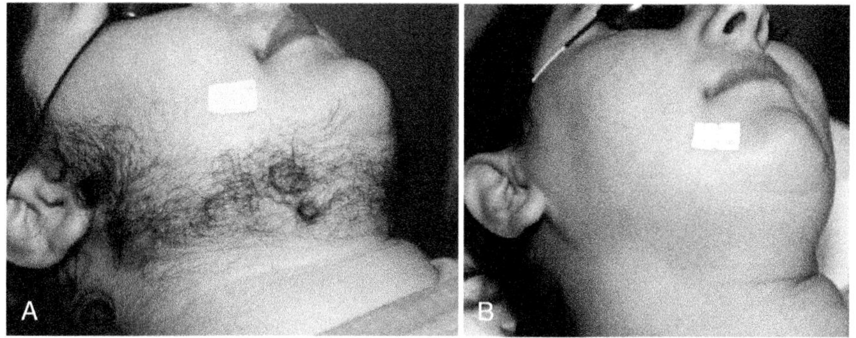

FIGURE 26-11 Jawline and sideburn hair **(A)** before and **(B)** after completion of a series of hair reduction treatments with a 755 nm laser. *(Courtesy of Candela, Wayland, MA; M. Ercan, MD, using laser.)*

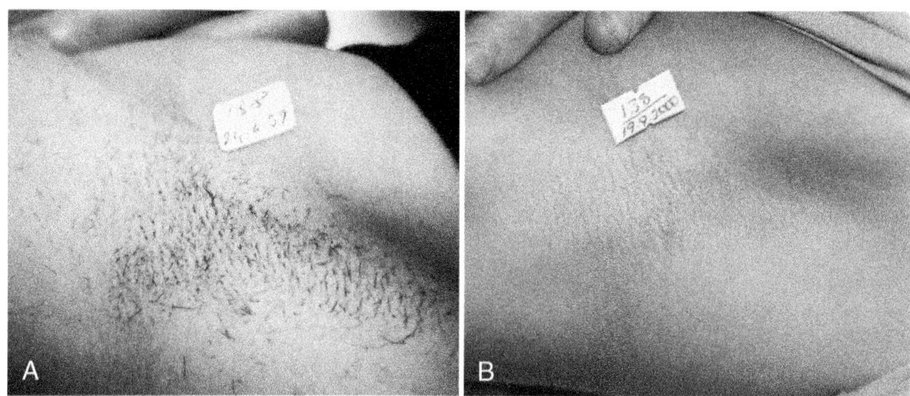

FIGURE 26-12 Axilla hair **(A)** before and **(B)** after completion of a series of hair reduction treatments with a 755 nm laser. *(Courtesy of Candela, Wayland, MA; M. Ercan, MD, using laser.)*

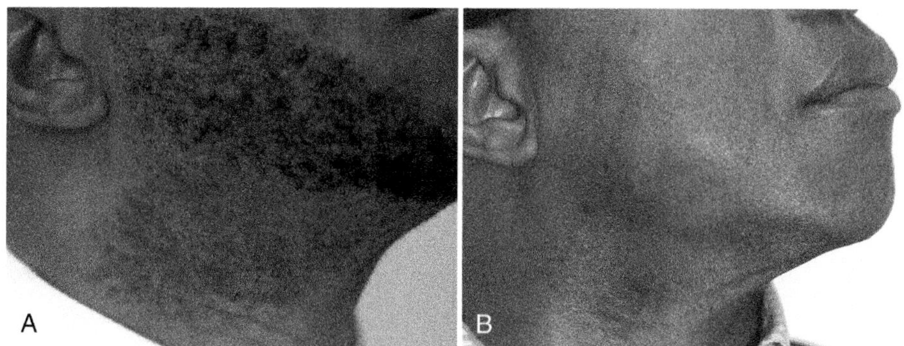

FIGURE 26-13 Pseudofolliculitis barbae **(A)** before and **(B)** after completion of 12 hair reduction treatments with a 1064 nm long-pulse laser. *(Courtesy of Sciton, Palo Alto, CA; L. Haney, RN, using laser.)*

be managed with application of ice for 15 minutes every 1 to 2 hours and 1 to 2½% hydrocortisone cream two to three times per day for 3 to 4 days or until resolved. Singed hairs may be evident immediately after treatment, and treated hairs may extrude 1 to 2 weeks after treatment. A washcloth may be used to wipe these hairs off in the direction of the hair follicles. Postinflammatory hyperpigmentation can occur with prolonged erythema, and patients are instructed to contact their provider if erythema persists for more than 5 days. Daily use of a full-spectrum sunscreen (SPF 30 with zinc or titanium) and sun avoidance for 4 weeks after treatment helps minimize the risk of pigmentary changes. If blistering and/or crusting occur, manage with moist wound care using bacitracin and a bandage until healed.

FOLLOW-UP

Typical hair reduction treatment intervals include:

- 4 to 6 weeks for the face
- 8 to 10 weeks for the upper body
- 12 weeks for the lower body.

After completion of a treatment series, patients may require a touch-up treatment for dormant hairs that have entered the active growth cycle approximately 6 months to 1 year after completion of their series.

COMPLICATIONS

- Pain
- Hyperpigmentation
- Hypopigmentation
- Burn
- Infection
- Failure to reduce the number of hairs or hair coarseness
- Reduction of hair adjacent to the treatment area
- Damage or alteration to tattoos and permanent makeup
- Eye injury.

Rare and Idiosyncratic Complications

- Scarring
- Paradoxical hair growth
- Erythema ab igne, a rare reticular erythematous rash related to heat exposure with laser treatments
- Livedo reticularis, a rare autoimmune vascular disease associated with mottled skin and discoloration of the legs or arms exacerbated by heat exposure with laser treatments
- Urticaria, bruising, pruritus.

Pain is unavoidable with LHR because all hairs are innervated. Epidermal cooling methods and topical anesthetics can reduce discomfort, but most patients will complain of discomfort during treatment which significantly improves once the laser pulse ceases. Certain areas such as the upper lip, axillae, and genitalia are more sensitive than other areas.

Pigmentary complications are most commonly seen in darker Fitzpatrick skin types (IV and V) and in patients with a recent tan. These complications typically occur with short pulse widths and/or high fluences and poor epidermal cooling. Hyperpigmentation and hypopigmentation are usually transient, lasting on the order of months, and rarely may be permanent. The use of a lightening agent such as hydroquinone for 1 month prior to treatment and after treatment may reduce hyperpigmentation, particularly in darker skinned patients (see Chapter 24, *Skin Care Products*, for additional information).

A *burn* can result from aggressive treatment parameters of short pulse widths and high fluences with inadequate epidermal cooling. Figure 26-14 shows an erythematous area with crusting on the back 1 week after a laser hair reduction treatment. Routine moist wound care is performed with application of an antibiotic ointment and bandage until healed. *Scarring* is highly unlikely, but may occur with overaggressive treatments and with treatments complicated by infection.

Herpes simplex and *varicella zoster* may be reactivated in the treatment area, and pretreatment prophylactic

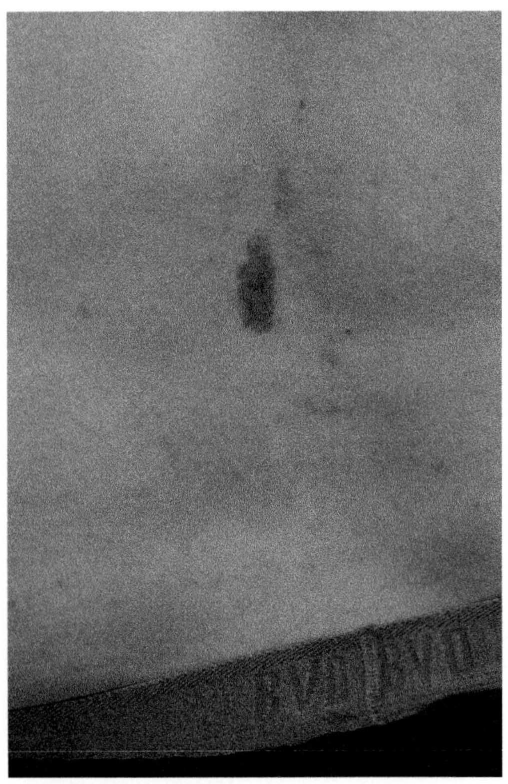

FIGURE 26-14 Area of overtreatment with erythema and crust on the back after laser hair reduction treatment in a patient with Fitzpatrick skin type IV. *(Copyright Rebecca Small, MD.)*

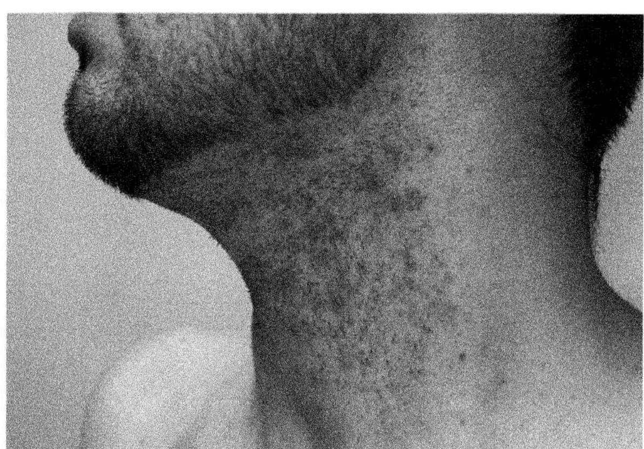

FIGURE 26-15 Neck folliculitis after laser hair reduction treatment. *(Copyright Rebecca Small, MD.)*

antiviral medication can reduce this risk (see the *Procedure Preparation* section above). *Impetigo* may occur, particularly with treatments around the mouth. *Folliculitis* may also occur, particularly after vigorous exercise, swimming or hot tub use immediately after treatments (Figure 26-15).

Failure to reduce unwanted hair can be the result of undiagnosed hyperandrogenic conditions such as polycystic ovarian syndrome, suboptimal laser parameters, or intervals between treatment sessions that are too short. For example, if lower extremity LHR treatments are performed at monthly intervals, a large number of hairs will not have cycled out of telogen into anagen and treatments will be less effective.

Hair grows at an angle to the skin and it is possible to *unintentionally reduce hair growth* adjacent to the treated area. Providers are cautioned against treating near the eyebrows for this reason. *Paradoxical hair growth* has been described, whereby LHR treatments stimulate hair growth. In this case, LHR may cause conversion of vellus hairs to coarse terminal hairs in the treatment area, or stimulate fine hair growth adjacent to the treatment area. Most cases are reported in skin types IV through VI, particularly with treatment of fine hairs in the lateral face.[14] One study found that immediate application of ice around the treatment area and two passes of the laser in the treatment area reduced the risk of paradoxical hair growth.[15]

Tattoos and permanent makeup have concentrated ink pigments and treatment over these may result in epidermal injury. *Ocular injury* can be avoided by wearing appropriate laser-safe eyewear at all times during treatment, directing the laser tip away from the eye, and treating outside of thc cyc orbit.

Erythema ab igne and *livedo reticularis* are extremely rare, as is *bruising, pruritus,* and *urticaria.*

SPECIAL POPULATIONS

- Pregnant and nursing women are not treated due to the discomfort associated with the procedure.
- For patients with darker Fitzpatrick skin types (IV and V) it is advisable to use conservative settings with long pulse widths and low fluences, and to increase treatment parameters gradually, so as to reduce the risk of complications.
- Hirsute adolescents may be treated with parental consent after hormonal evaluation for hirsutism.
- Patients with polycystic ovarian syndrome commonly have excessive hair growth that is distressing and seek LHR treatments. If androgen excess is untreated, LHR treatments will not provide permanent hair reduction and will only offer temporary results.

LEARNING THE TECHNIQUES

Providers may initially perform laser hair reduction treatments on patients with light Fitzpatrick skin types (I through III) who have dark, coarse hair to minimize the risk of side effects and for ease of visualizing clinical endpoints. Axillae are a preferred area to start with as they are usually minimally sun exposed and have coarse hair.

CURRENT DEVELOPMENTS

Some of the newer laser hair reduction devices have larger treatment heads to shorten treatment times. Analgesic devices, such as pneumatic skin-flattening tips are available for LHR devices to reduce the discomfort associated with treatment[16] (see Chapter 20, *Anesthesia for Cosmetic Procedures*). Recently, laser hair reduction devices have become available for use at home. One such device, Tria (by TriaBeauty), is a diode laser (810 nm) that has a long pulse width of 400 ms and low fluences of 7 to 20 J/cm^2. Another device, Silk'n (by Home Skinovations), is an IPL with a pulsewidth of less than 1 ms and low fluences of 3-5 J/cm^2. Data is limited on these devices and they will likely provide temporary hair reduction given their limited treatment parameters.

FINANCIAL CONSIDERATIONS

LHR is not reimbursable by insurance. The charges for treatments are usually based on the size of the treatment area and are largely determined by local prices. Patients may pay for individual treatments. However, because LHR is only effective with a series of treatments, packages of treatments (usually six) may be offcrcd so that patients achieve the best possible results and have the greatest satisfaction. Box 26-1 lists applicable codes for LHR procedures.

CONCLUSION

Lasers and intense pulsed light devices can effectively reduce unwanted hair. A series of treatments is required,

BOX 26-1 *Codes for Laser Hair Removal Procedures*

CPT Code

17380 Epilation (hair reduction)

ICD Codes

256.4 Polycystic ovarian syndrome
704.1 Hirsutism
704.8 Pseudofolliculitis barbae

typically six for lighter Fitzpatrick skin types (I through III) and eight or more for darker skin types (IV and V). Laser hair reduction is generally well tolerated and has a low risk of side effects and complications with proper use of these devices and appropriate selection of treatment parameters.

Resources

See the *Aesthetics Buyers Guide* (www.miinews.com/productcharts.php) for specific laser technologies made by laser companies.

Alma Lasers
Phone: 866-414-2562
www.almalasers.com

Asclepion Lasers
www.asclepion.com

CoolTouch
Phone: 877-858-COOL
www.cooltouch.com

Cutera
Phone: 888-4-CUTERA
www.cutera.com

Cynosure
Phone: 800-886-2966
www.cynosure.com

Ellipse
www.ellipse.org

Energist
Phone: 845-348-4900
www.energisint.com

Fotona
Phone: 888-550-4113
www.fotonamedicallasers.com

HOYA ConBio
Phone: 800-532-1064
www.conbio.com

IRIDEX
Phone: 650-940-4700
www.iridex.com

Lumenis
Phone: 408-764-3000
www.lumenis.com

Lutronic
Phone: 888-588-7644
www.lutronic.com

Palomar
Phone: 800-725-0628
www.palomarmedical.com

Quantel Medical
Phone: 888-660-6726
www.quantelmedical.com

Radiancy
Phone: 888-661-2220
www.radiancy.com

Sciton
Phone: 888-646-6999
www.sciton.com

SharpLight Technologies
Phone: 905-337-7797
www.sharplightech.com

Syneron (formerly Candela)
Phone: 866-259-6661
www.syneron.com

References

1. Cosmetic Surgery National Data Bank 2010 Statistics. American Society for Aesthetic Plastic Surgery; 2010.
2. Small R. Aesthetic procedures in office practice. *Am Fam Physician.* 2009;80(11):1231–1237.
3. Altschuler GB, Anderson RR, Manstein D, *et al.* Extended theory of selective photothermolysis. *Lasers Surg Med.* 2001;29:416–432.
4. Anderson RR, Parrish JA. Selective photothermolysis: precise microsurgery by selective absorption of pulsed radiation. *Science.* 1983;220(4596):524–527.
5. Dierickx CC. Hair removal by lasers and intense pulsed light sources. *Semin Cutan Med Surg.* 2000;19(4):267–275.
6. Lou WW, Quintana AT, Geronemus RG, *et al.* Prospective study of hair reduction by diode laser (800 nm) with long-term follow-up. *Dermatol Surg.* 2000;26(5):428–432.
7. Small R. Laser hair removal. *In:* Mayeaux E, ed. *The Essential Guide to Primary Care Procedures.* Philadelphia: Lippincott Williams & Wilkins; 2009:234–248.
8. Gorgu M, Aslan G, Akoz T, *et al.* Comparison of alexandrite laser and electrolysis for hair removal. *Dermatol Surg.* 2000;26:37–41.
9. Battle EF, Hobbs LM. Laser-assisted hair removal for darker skin types. *Dermatol Ther.* 2004;17:177–183.
10. Bakus AD, Garden JM, Yaghmai D, Massa MC. Long-term fine caliber hair removal with an electro-optic Q-switched Nd:YAG Laser. *Laser Surg Med.* 2010;42:706–711.
11. Gold MH, Bell MW, Foster TD, *et al.* One-year follow-up using an intense pulsed light source for long-term hair removal. *J Cutan Laser Ther.* 1999;1(3):167–171.
12. Amin SP, Goldberg DJ. Clinical comparison of four hair removal lasers and light sources. *J Cosmet Laser Ther.* 2006;8(2):65–68.
13. Small R. Aesthetic procedures introduction. *In:* Mayeaux E, ed. *The Essential Guide to Primary Care Procedures.* Philadelphia: Lippincott Williams & Wilkins; 2009:195–199.

14. Alajlan A, Shapiro J, Rivens J, *et al*. Paradoxical hypertrichosis after laser epilation. *J Am Acad Dermatol*. 2005;53:85–88.
15. Willey A, Torrontegui J, Azpiazu J, *et al*. Hair stimulation following laser and intense pulsed light photo-epilation: review of 543 cases and ways to manage it. *Lasers Surg Med*. 2007;39:297–301.
16. Bernstein EF. Pneumatic skin flattening reduced pain during laser hair reduction. *Lasers Surg Med*. 2008;40:183–187.

Additional Reading

Page G. Lasers and pulsed-light devices: hair removal. *In:* Pfenninger JL, Fowler GC, eds. *Pfenninger and Fowler's Procedures for Primary Care*. 3rd ed. Philadelphia: Mosby/Elsevier; 2011.

Small R. Laser hair reduction. *In:* Small R, ed. *A Practical Guide to Cosmetic Lasers*. Philadelphia: Lippincott Williams & Wilkins; 2012.

27 Photorejuvenation with Lasers

REBECCA SMALL, MD • DALANO HOANG, DC

Cumulative damage to the skin over time from ultraviolet light results in photoaging. Photoaging changes are clinically evident as benign pigmented lesions, such as solar lentigines, freckles (ephelides), hyperpigmentation, melasma, and as benign vascular lesions, such as telangiectasias, poikiloderma of Civatte, rosacea, and cherry angiomas.[1] *Photorejuvenation* refers to the cosmetic treatment of photoaged skin with nonablative lasers and light-based technologies (collectively referred to as lasers*).[2] Treatments are most commonly performed on the face, neck, chest, and hands, but may be performed on almost any photodamaged area of the body.[3] Photorejuvenation treatments reliably achieve improvements, have short postprocedure recovery times and minimal risks of complications, and are associated with high patient satisfaction.[4,5]

LASER PRINCIPLES

Laser treatments are based on the principle of selective photothermolysis. Light-absorbing pigments in the skin, called chromophores, selectively absorb light energy and convert it to heat in the targeted lesions. The lesions are heated, damaged, and eliminated, while the surrounding skin is left unaffected. Photorejuvenation treatment of benign pigmented and vascular lesions is achieved through selectively targeting two main chromophores in the skin, oxyhemoglobin, which is found in red blood, and melanin, which is found in pigmented lesions.[6]

When treating *red vascular lesions*, laser energy is absorbed by the oxyhemoglobin chromophore. The vessel is heated, causing injury to the vessel wall and perivascular collagen damage, which results in vessel closure and obliteration. Oxyhemoglobin absorbs light between 510 and 600 nm (Figure 27-1). Lasers used for the treatment of red vascular lesions produce light in this range and include argon (510 nm), potassium titanyl phosphate or KTP (532 nm), and pulsed dye (585 nm) lasers.

When treating *benign pigmented lesions*, such as lentigines, light energy is absorbed by the target chromophore melanin that is contained within the melanosomes of epidermal melanocytes and keratinocytes. The melanosome is heated, ruptured, and the melanin eliminated. Melanin preferentially absorbs light between 650 and 1100 nm (see Figure 27-1). Lasers used for treatment of epidermal pigmented lesions produce light in this range and include ruby (694 nm), alexandrite (755 nm), diode (810 nm), and neodymium-doped yttrium aluminum garnet or Nd:YAG (1064 nm) lasers. The light from KTP (532 nm) and argon (510 nm) lasers has high absorption by both melanin and oxyhemoglobin and can be used to treat both pigmented and vascular lesions.

Intense pulsed light (IPL) devices emit a spectrum of wavelengths, and certain desired wavelengths can be selected with the use of filters. For example, some IPL filters have an emission peak from 500 to 670 nm and a second emission peak from 870 to 1200 nm. Melanin and oxyhemoglobin are targeted with these wavelengths. In addition, lesions at different depths are also targeted because the shorter wavelengths target more superficial lesions and the longer wavelengths target deeper lesions. In this way, a single IPL device can be used to target both vascular and pigmented lesions at a variety of depths in the skin.

Several device parameters affect the safety and efficacy of photorejuvenation treatments. These parameters include wavelength, fluence, pulse duration, and spot size (see *Laser Parameters* in Chapter 19, *Aesthetic Principles and Consultation*).

- The wavelength used for treatment is determined by the chromophore in the targeted lesion, as well as the desired depth of penetration into the skin.
- For treatment of red vascular lesions, selection of laser parameters is based on the size and depth of the vessels. Smaller superficial red vessels are treated with shorter pulse widths. Larger vessels are treated with longer pulse widths, and larger spot sizes.
- For treatment of benign pigmented lesions, short pulse durations are effective, because most pigmented lesions seen with photoaging are located superficially in the epidermis (Figure 27-2). Q-switched lasers (see Chapter 19 for a definition), which include 532 nm, ruby (694 nm), alexandrite (755 nm), and Nd:YAG (1064 nm) lasers, have very short pulse durations—in the nanosecond range—and are highly effective for the reduction of unwanted pigmentation.

PATIENT SELECTION

Patients with fair skin (Fitzpatrick skin types I through III) are the best candidates for photorejuvenation treatments because this population presents with the greatest contrast between background skin and target lesions. Both benign vascularities and hyperpigmentation are common complaints in patients with light skin types. Photodamaged skin characteristically shows midface erythema and peripheral lentigines (see Figure 19-1 in Chapter 19).

Patients with darker skin (Fitzpatrick skin types IV through VI) have increased risks of complications such as hyperpigmentation, hypopigmentation, and burns

*Refers to laser and light-based technologies.

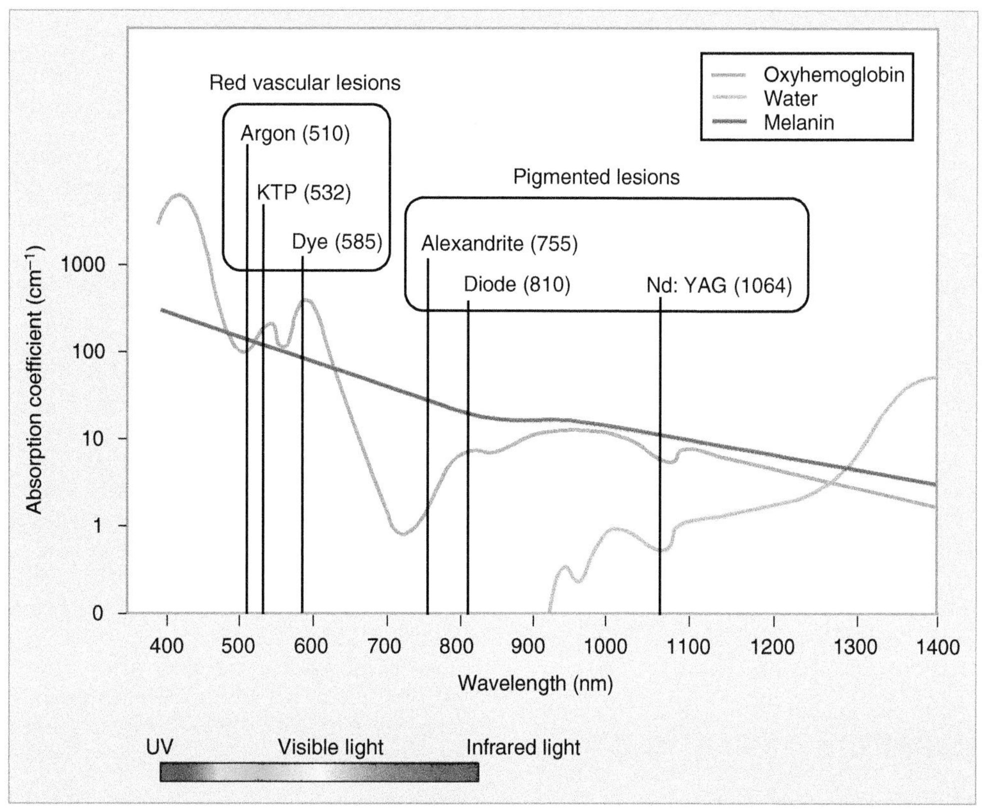

FIGURE 27-1 Absorption spectra of tissue chromophores and lasers commonly used for photorejuvenation.

due to melanin in the background skin competing with chromophores in the target lesions. Hyperpigmentation and melasma are common complaints in patients with darker skin types. The safest devices for treatment of hyperpigmentation in these patients are Q-switched Nd:YAG (1064 nm) lasers, and it is advisable for treatments to be performed by providers experienced with darker skin types.

INDICATIONS

- Lentigines (brown sun spots)
- Ephelides (freckles)
- Mottled pigmentation
- Postinflammatory hyperpigmentation
- Melasma
- Poikiloderma of Civatte (a pattern of erythema and mottled pigmentation seen most often on the sides of the face, neck, and chest; see Figure 23-11 in Chapter 23, *Microdermabrasion*)
- Telangiectasias
- Erythema
- Cherry angiomas
- Rosacea.

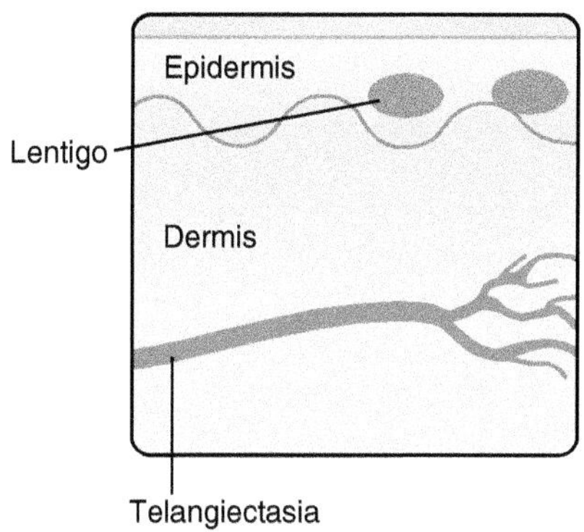

FIGURE 27-2 Common benign lesions in photoaged skin.

PATIENT EXPECTATIONS

Photorejuvenation of benign pigmented and vascular lesions may be performed on virtually any body region where photodamage is present. The face, neck, chest, and hands are some of the most commonly treated areas. Noticeable results are evident with a single treatment in properly selected candidates, but typically a series of three to five IPL treatments is required for dramatic improvements.[4] Treatment with lasers may require a fewer number of treatments than with IPL devices. Larger red facial vessels, which have more chromophore target, usually respond more dramatically than smaller lacy red vessels or diffuse erythema. Discreet lesions such as cherry angiomas typically resolve with no recurrence after one or two treatments.

ALTERNATIVE THERAPIES

Nonlaser treatment options for benign pigmented lesions include *liquid nitrogen*, exfoliation treatments such as *microdermabrasion* and *chemical peels*, and topical skin-lightening products such as *hydroquinone*. Liquid nitrogen can achieve reduction in pigmentation, however, it is frequently associated with hyperpigmentation and hypopigmentation and it is advisable to restrict use to lighter skin types for this reason. Exfoliation and topical therapies are slower to achieve improvements and results are rarely comparable to those seen with lasers. More aggressive laser treatments with longer recovery times and greater risks of complications, such as ablative carbon dioxide and erbium lasers (fractionated and nonfractionated), are also indicated for pigmented lesions. Electrosurgery may be used for some vascular lesions, although this may scar (see Chapter 14, *Electrosurgery*). *Photodynamic therapy* (PDT), utilizing topical photosensitizing medication activated by light, has also been used for photorejuvenation (see the *Current Developments* section below).

PRODUCTS CURRENTLY AVAILABLE[7–11]

Lasers commonly used for treatment of red vascular lesions include the following:

- 585 nm and 595 nm pulsed dye lasers
- 532 nm KTP lasers
- 500- to 1200 nm IPL devices.

Lasers commonly used for treatment of pigmented lesions include these:

- 755 nm alexandrite lasers
- 810 nm diode lasers
- 1064 nm Nd:YAG lasers
- 532 nm KTP lasers
- 500- to 1200 nm IPL devices
- 532, 755, and 1064 nm Q-switched lasers.

Ruby (694 nm) and argon (510 nm) lasers were some of the first lasers used for photorejuvenation, but due to their short wavelengths and high melanin absorption, they have a high incidence of hypopigmentation and are rarely used today. Q-switched ruby lasers are still used for tattoo removal.

See the *Resources* section at the end of this chapter for laser manufacturers.

CONTRAINDICATIONS

See Chapter 26, *Hair Reduction with Lasers*, for general laser contraindications. Other contraindications include:

- Vascular malformations or tumors
- Skin types V and VI with most IPL devices.

ADVANTAGES OF PHOTOREJUVENATION

Laser photorejuvenation offers dramatic improvements in a relatively short amount of time compared to topical products such as retinoids or hydroquinone. Compared to more aggressive treatments such as fractional and nonfractional ablative carbon dioxide and erbium lasers, the recovery time is minimal and the risks of complications such as hyperpigmentation, hypopigmentation, scarring, or infection are minimal. Although liquid nitrogen is a less expensive option for treating hyperpigmentation, it has a greater risk of hypopigmentation than photorejuvenation lasers.

DISADVANTAGES OF PHOTOREJUVENATION

Proper precautions need to be taken during laser treatments to avoid alteration to tattoos and permanent makeup. Photorejuvenation treatments for patients with darker Fitzpatrick skin types (IV and higher) have increased risks of hyperpigmentation, hypopigmentation, and scarring. The initial cost of laser technologies is a disadvantage.

ANATOMY

Benign pigmented lesions, such as lentigines, and benign vascular lesions, such as telangiectasias, are some of the most common lesions evident in photodamaged skin. Figure 27-2 shows the relative location of these lesions in the skin, with lentigines in the epidermis and telangiectasias in the dermis.

Telangiectasias are these cutaneous vessels that range in size from 0.1 to 1.0 mm. The three main types linear, arborizing and spider, are shown in Figure 27-3. Telangiectasias that arise from dilated arterioles are bright red with small diameters; those from venules are bluish in color with larger diameters; and those from capillaries are fine lacy red vessels or appear as background erythema to the naked eye.[12] Red facial telangiectasias seen with photoaging are commonly located in the midface on the nasal ala and dorsum of the nose and cheeks. Telangiectasias may also be associated with clinical conditions such as rosacea, genetic syndromes, and collagen vascular diseases (Box 27-1).

Solar lentigines are small brown macules that increase in size and number with chronic sun exposure and are typically located around the periphery of the face (see Figure 27-8A later in the chapter). *Postinflammatory hyperpigmentation* can be seen in susceptible individuals, typically darker skin types (Fitzpatrick IV through VI), as brown macules arising at sites of previously inflamed acne lesions or sites of wound healing (see Figure 24-6A in Chapter 24, *Skin Care Products*). *Melasma* presents as hyperpigmented reticulated patches and brown macules, typically on the cheekbones, upper lip, forehead, and chin (see Figure 27-13A later in this chapter). It is frequently observed following a change in female

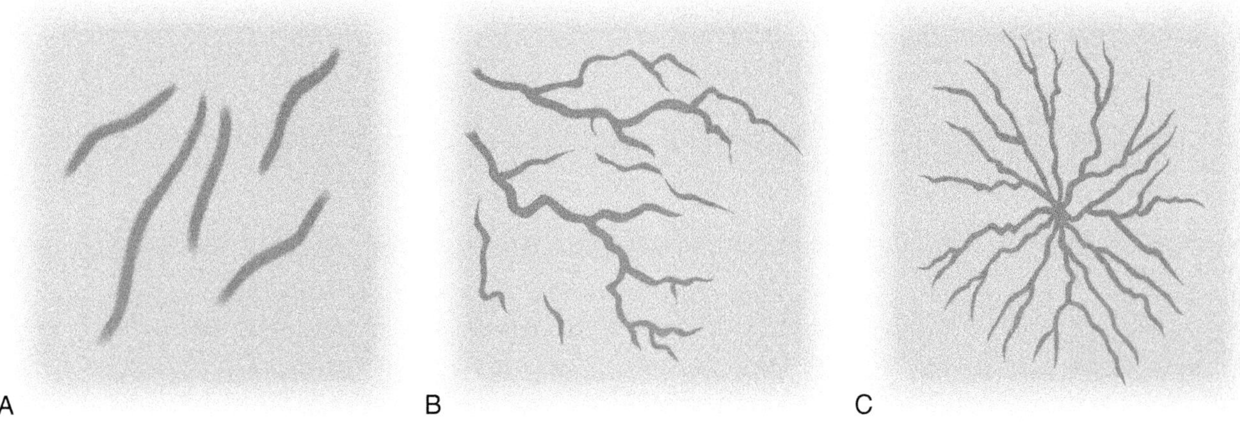

FIGURE 27-3 Telangiectasia types (**A**) linear, (**B**) arborizing and (**C**) spider.

hormonal status such as during pregnancy (chloasma) or after initiating use of oral contraceptives.

Cutaneous pigmented lesions may be located in the epidermis, dermis, or in both. Solar lentigines and ephelides (freckles) are located in the epidermis. Postinflammatory hyperpigmentation and melasma may be located in any of these levels. A Wood's lamp can be used to determine the depth of melanin pigmentation in the skin.[13] Epidermal pigmentation appears darker with more contrast against the background skin under Wood's lamp illumination, whereas dermal pigmentation has less contrast.

BOX 27-1 ***Causes of Telangiectasias***

Primary (Cause Unknown)

Ataxia telangiectasia
Generalized essential telangiectasia
Hemorrhagic hereditary telangiectasia (Osler-Weber-Rendu syndrome)
Spider angiomas
Unilateral nevoid telangiectasia syndrome

Secondary (Related to a Known Condition)

Actinically damaged skin
After cryosurgery
After laser or electrosurgery
Basal cell carcinoma
Collagen vascular disease (dermatomyositis, lupus erythematosus, scleroderma)
Cushing's syndrome
Estrogen excess (cirrhosis, oral contraceptives, pregnancy)
Metastatic carcinoma
Necrobiosis lipoidica diabeticorum
Poikiloderma of Civatte
Pseudoxanthoma elasticum
Radiation therapy injury
Rosacea
Telangiectasia macularis eruptiva perstans (generalized cutaneous mastocytosis)
Topical steroid induced
Xeroderma pigmentosa

Source: Adapted from Habif TP. *Clinical Dermatology*, 5th ed. St. Louis: Mosby; 2009.

EQUIPMENT

- Laser or IPL device appropriate for photorejuvenation treatments
- Laser-safe eyewear for the patient and provider specific to the device being used
- Nonalcohol cleansing facial wipes
- Clear colorless gel for treatments if necessary per the manufacturer
- Gauze, 4 × 4 inches
- Ice packs
- Hydrocortisone cream, 1% and 2.5%
- Alcohol wipes for cleaning laser tip
- Germicidal disposable wipes for sanitizing the laser.

PROCEDURE PREPARATION

1. Perform an aesthetic consultation and review the patient's medical history (see Chapter 19, *Aesthetic Principles and Consultation*) including hormonally induced hyperpigmentation, history of postinflammatory hyperpigmentation or abnormal scarring; medications that may worsen hyperpigmentation or erythema such as oral estrogen containing hormones or topical steroids; and any previous methods for treating photodamage and success.
2. Examine the treatment area for pigmented lesions that are suspicious for melanoma or premalignant changes and biopsy or refer if indicated. Note that basal cell carcinomas can also be pigmented. Await biopsy results before proceeding with laser treatments.
3. Obtain informed consent (see Chapter 19; also see Appendix A for an informed consent form and patient information handout titled *Photorejuvenation Treatments*).
4. Determine the Fitzpatrick skin type (see Chapter 19).
5. If the patient has a prior history of herpes simplex or varicella in or near the treatment area, provide prophylactic antiviral medication (e.g., valacyclovir 500 mg 1 tablet twice daily) for 2 days prior to the procedure, and continue for 3 days postprocedure.

6. Advise sun avoidance for 1 month and daily use of a full-spectrum sunscreen (see Chapter 24, *Skin Care Products*, for sunscreen product recommendations).
7. When treating Fitzpatrick skin type III with high-risk ethnic backgrounds (Mediterranean, Latino, and Asian) or darker Fitzpatrick skin types (IV), consider using a topical skin-lightening product such as hydroquinone or a cosmeceutical such as kojic acid, arbutin, niacinamide, or azelaic acid once or twice daily for 1 month prior to treatment to lighten background skin (see Chapter 24).
8. Test spots may be performed prior to the initial treatment for patients with Fitzpatrick skin type III with high-risk ethnic backgrounds (Mediterranean, Latino, and Asian) and darker Fitzpatrick skin types (IV). Test spot parameters are based on the patient's skin type and the degree of abnormal pigmentation and/or redness in the treatment area, the laser manufacturer's guidelines for spot size, fluence, and pulse width are used. Test spots are placed discretely (under the chin, behind or inferior to the ear) near the desired treatment area. View test spots 3 to 5 days after placement for evidence of hyperpigmentation, burn, or other adverse effects. At each treatment visit, test spots may be performed using the fluence and pulse width desired for the subsequent treatment visit. Inform patients that lack of an adverse reaction with test spots does not ensure that a side effect or complication will not occur with any treatment.

LASER PHOTOREJUVENATION: STEPS AND PRINCIPLES

The following recommendations are guidelines for photorejuvenation treatments using an IPL device (Palomar StarLux 500 using the LuxG handpiece) for Fitzpatrick skin types I through IV. Manufacturer's guidelines for the specific device used should be followed at the time of treatment.

General Treatment Technique

1. The appropriate IPL handpiece is selected based on the patient's Fitzpatrick skin type and treatment indication.
2. Laser treatment parameters are further tailored to the patient's clinical presentation through selection of fluence and pulse width. More conservative treatments are achieved using longer pulse widths and lower fluences (e.g., 20-ms pulse width and 34 J/cm^2) and more aggressive treatments with shorter pulse widths and higher fluences (e.g., 15 ms and 38 J/cm^2).
   TIP: Darker Fitzpatrick skin types require more conservative settings
   TIP: Greater degrees of abnormal pigmentation (such as dark lentigines or a high density of lentigines or freckles) or greater intensity of erythema in the treatment area require more conservative settings.

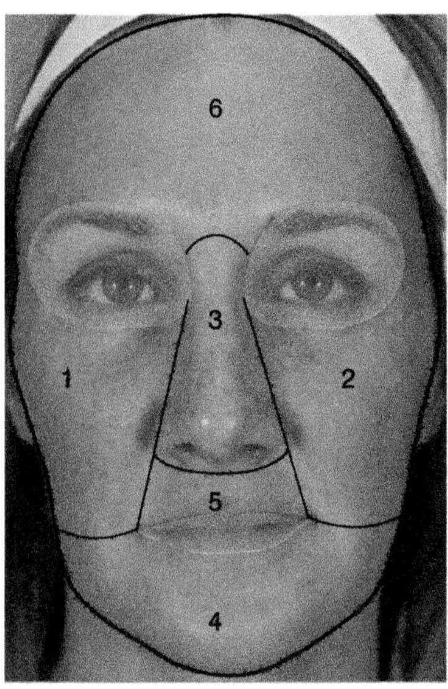

= Non treatment areas

FIGURE 27-4 Treatment sequence for IPL photorejuvenation of the face. *(Copyright Rebecca Small, MD.)*

Planning and Designing

Figure 27-4 shows a recommended sequence for IPL treatment of the full face, starting with area 1 and progressing to area 6. The direction of IPL pulses is toward the provider as shown in Figure 27-5, with approximately 20% overlap of each pulse. The amount of pulse overlap may vary with different laser devices.

TIP: The laser tip is always angled away from the eyes during treatment.
TIP: The most sensitive areas are the upper lip (philtrum) and lateral to the nose. To reduce discomfort

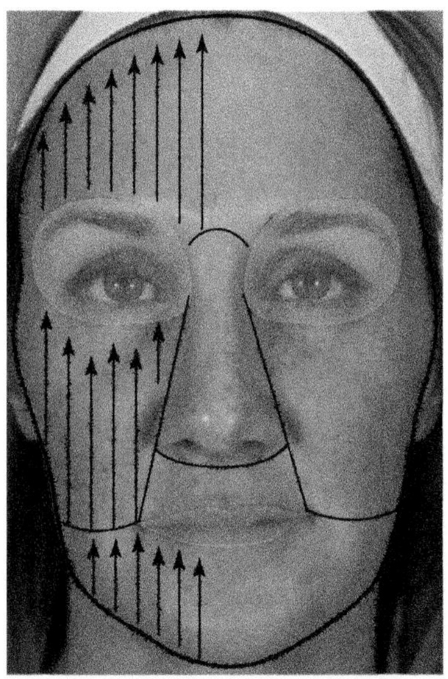

= Non treatment areas

FIGURE 27-5 Handpiece direction for IPL photorejuvenation treatment of the face. *(Copyright Rebecca Small, MD.)*

when treating the upper lip have the patient place his or her tongue over the teeth while keeping the lips closed.

CAUTION: It is advisable to avoid dark coarse facial hair, such as men's beards. Treating over darkly colored hair will singe hair and may permanently reduce hair growth or result in overtreatment of the epidermis with blistering.

Anesthesia

Anesthesia is not typically required for photorejuvenation treatments. Topical anesthetics may be used, but some contain vasoconstrictive agents which minimize vascular targets and can reduce treatment efficacy. Anesthesia may also interfere with patient feedback, an important component for selecting appropriate treatment parameters.

Safety Zone

The Laser Photorejuvenation Safety Zone for treatment of the face is shown in Figure 27-4. Laser treatments are performed outside of the ocular area: above the supraorbital ridge (above the eyebrows) and below the inferior orbital rim. When getting started with IPL treatments it is advisable to avoid the lips. As skill improves, providers may choose to treat the lip area for lesions such as lentigines.

Performing the Photorejuvenation Procedure

1. Inquire about sun exposure and sunscreen use at every visit. If the patient is recently sun exposed or has tanned skin in the treatment area, it is advisable to wait 1 month before treating to reduce the risk of complications.
2. Position the patient supine on a flat procedure table.
3. Cleanse the skin with a nonalcohol wipe.
4. Provide appropriate laser-safe eye protection for the patient and all personnel in the treatment room prior to beginning treatment
5. Cover tattoos and permanent makeup with wet gauze and keep the laser tip at least 1 inch away from the tattoo during treatment.
6. Operate the laser in accordance with your clinic's laser safety policies and procedures and the manufacturer's guidelines.
7. Apply a clear colorless laser gel to the skin, spreading to a thin 1- to 2-mm layer or as directed per the manufacturer's guideline.
8. Place the laser tip firmly on the skin, making certain that the entire tip is in contact with the skin.
   TIP: When treating vascular lesions, avoid excessive downward pressure on the skin because this will blanch vessels, diminishing the target for the laser and may reduce treatment efficacy.
9. Perform a single pulse at the lateral margin of the treatment area and assess for patient tolerance and clinical endpoints (see below). In general, there should be subtle endpoints during initial treatments with a pain score less than or equal to 6 on a scale of 1 to 10.
10. Desirable clinical endpoints for *pigmented lesions*, such as lentigines, include:
    - Darkening of the lesion and enhanced demarcation against the background skin (Figure 27-6B)
    - Mild perilesional erythema (Figure 27-6B)
    - Gray or black discoloration of the lesion, which can occur with aggressive treatment.

    TIP: Endpoints evolve rapidly with more aggressive settings of shorter pulse widths and higher fluences. Longer pulse widths typically have a delayed appearance of endpoints of up to several minutes.

    TIP: Clinical endpoints are more evident with lighter Fitzpatrick skin types (I through III) than darker skin types (IV).

    Figure 27-6A shows a patient's chest immediately after laser treatment of lentigines on the right half of the chest. The close-up view of the treated chest area (Figure 27-6B) shows endpoints of lesion darkening, demarcation, and perilesional erythema, as compared to the untreated areas (Figure 27-6C).
11. Desirable clinical endpoints for red vascular lesions, such as telangiectasias, include:
    - Spontaneous blanching
    - Darkening with a grayish discoloration
    - Mild surrounding erythema
    - No apparent change. If no change is apparent, compress the vessel and observe for blanching and refilling. An adequately treated vessel will not blanch, whereas partially treated vessels will refill sluggishly.
    - Purpura/bruise (see Figure 27-16 later in the chapter). In rare instances, short pulse widths and high fluences may cause a vessel to rupture, resulting in purpura. Purpura is an aggressive endpoint with IPL. Patients must be reassured and informed that resolution can take up to 2 weeks.
12. Desirable clinical endpoints for *cherry angiomas* include:
    - Purplish discoloration. These lesions gradually regress and fade in size and color over time.
13. Adjust laser settings based on observations of laser/tissue interaction, clinical endpoints, and patient discomfort throughout treatment.
14. The entire treatment area is covered with laser pulses, using the appropriate amount of overlap.
15. At subsequent visits, fluence is increased and pulse width decreased, according to the manufacturer's guidelines, to target lighter pigmentation and finer vessels. Typically, only one parameter is changed to intensify treatments at any given visit.
    TIP: Delay treatment by 2 weeks if microcrusts from the previous treatment are visible.
16. After treatment, apply ice for 15 minutes to minimize erythema, edema, and reduce discomfort.
17. If the treatment area is erythematous, 1% to 2.5% hydrocortisone cream may be applied.
18. A full-spectrum sunscreen (SPF 30 with zinc or titanium) is applied to sun-exposed areas.

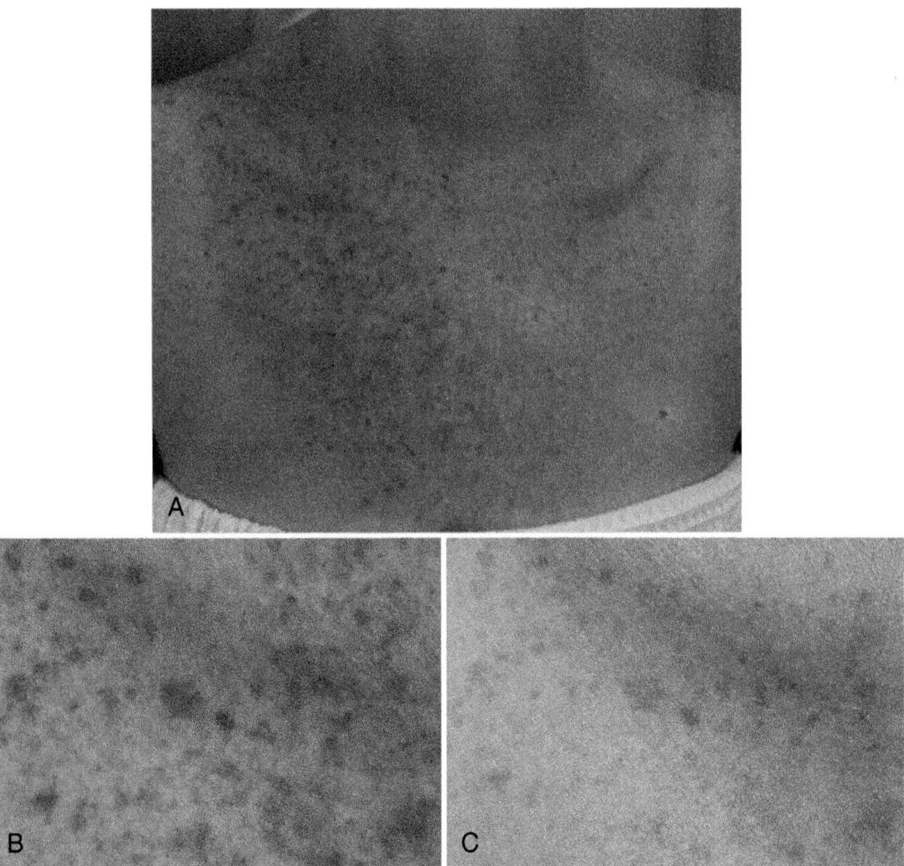

FIGURE 27-6 IPL photorejuvenation of the right chest **(A)** immediately after treatment. Close-up views show **(B)** lentigo clinical endpoints of lesion darkening, border demarcation and perilesional erythema, as compared to **(C)** the untreated area. *(Copyright Rebecca Small, MD.)*

RESULTS

Results of an initial photorejuvenation treatment with IPL for lentigines on the chest of a 36-year-old patient are shown in Figure 27-7. The patient's chest is shown prior to treatment in (A) 1 week after treatment in (B), and 2 weeks after treatment in (C). Note in (B) the darkened and flaking appearance of the lentigines 1 week after treatment due to microcrust formation and the significant improvement in pigmentation at 2 weeks.

Figure 27-8 shows the results of photorejuvenation treatments for lentigines and mottled pigmentation on the face of a 75-year-old patient (A) before and (B) after a series of five IPL treatments (Starlux, Palomar).

Figure 27-9 shows the results of photorejuvenation treatments for lentigines and mottled pigmentation on the face (A) before and (B) after a Q-switched 532 nm treatment (Laser Peel™, Medlite HOYA ConBio).

Figure 27-10 shows the results of photorejuvenation treatments for solar lentigines and under-eye pigmentation for a 48-year-old patient (A) before and (B) after two Q-switched 532 nm treatments (RevLite, HOYA ConBio).

Figure 27-11 shows the results of photorejuvenation treatments for solar lentigines on the hands of a 55-year-old patient (A) before and (B) after five IPL treatments (Starlux, Palomar).

Figure 27-12 shows the results of photorejuvenation treatment for hyperpigmentation in a patient with Fitzpatrick VI skin type (A) before and (B) after Q-switched 1064 nm treatments (MedLite, HOYA ConBio).

Figure 27-13 shows the results of photorejuvenation treatment for melasma for a 41-year-old patient (A) before and (B) after Q-switched 1064 nm treatments (RevLite, HOYA ConBio).

Figure 27-14 shows the results of photorejuvenation for nasal telangiectasias (A) before and (B) after 532 nm treatments (Gemini, Iridex).

Figure 27-15 shows the results of photorejuvenation treatments for rosacea for a 57-year-old (A) before and (B) after a series of five IPL treatments (Starlux, Palomar).

AFTERCARE

Mild swelling and *redness* are expected and usually resolve within a few hours to a few days after treatment. Application of a wrapped ice pack for 15 minutes every 1 to 2 hours and 1 to 2½% hydrocortisone cream two times per day for 3 to 4 days or until redness resolves are recommended. *Pigmented lesions typically continue to darken* 1 to 2 days after treatment, forming microcrusts

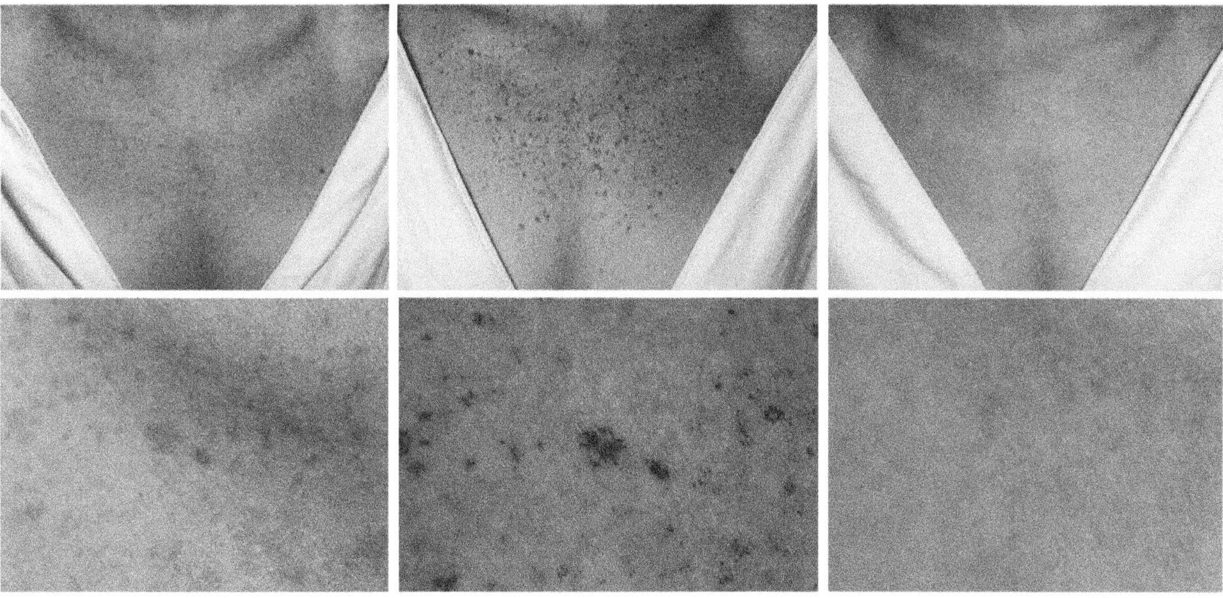

FIGURE 27-7 Chest lentigines **(A)** before, **(B)** 1 week after, and **(C)** 2 weeks after one photorejuvenation treatment with intense pulsed light. *(Copyright Rebecca Small, MD.)*

that flake off over 1 to 2 weeks, exposing lightened or resolved lesions. *Vascular lesions* that have turned grayish or darkened at the time of treatment usually fade over 1 to 2 weeks. Patients are instructed to contact their provider if erythema persists for more than 5 days because postinflammatory hyperpigmentation (PIH) can occur with prolonged erythema. Patients are also instructed to avoid intense, direct sun exposure and use a full-spectrum sunscreen (SPF 30 with zinc or titanium) daily for 4 weeks after treatment to help minimize the risk of undesired pigmentary changes.

FOLLOW-UP

Photorejuvenation of *benign epidermal pigmented* lesions typically requires a series of three to five IPL treatments at monthly intervals for dramatic improvements. Lasers

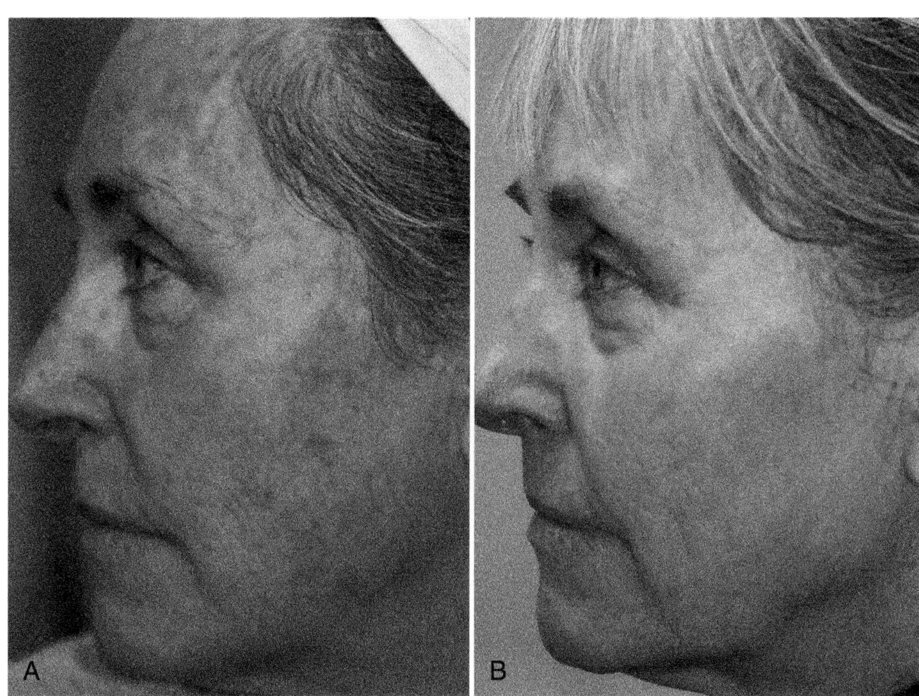

FIGURE 27-8 Lentigines **(A)** before and **(B)** after photorejuvenation treatments with intense pulsed light. *(Copyright Rebecca Small, MD.)*

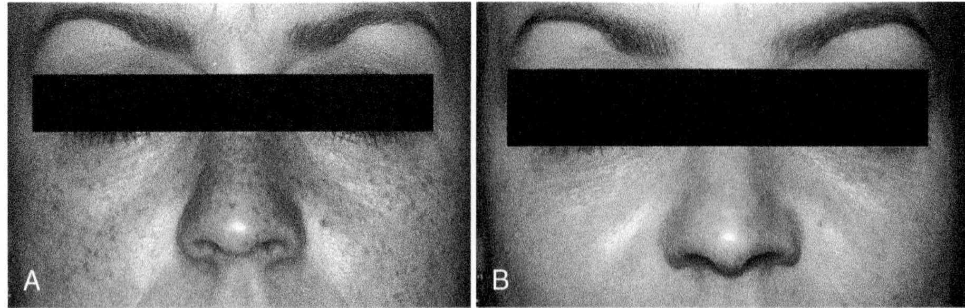

FIGURE 27-9 Lentigines and ephelides (**A**) before and (**B**) after photorejuvenation treatments with a Q-switched 532 nm laser. *(Courtesy of HOYA ConBio, Fremont, CA; B. Saal, MD, using laser.)*

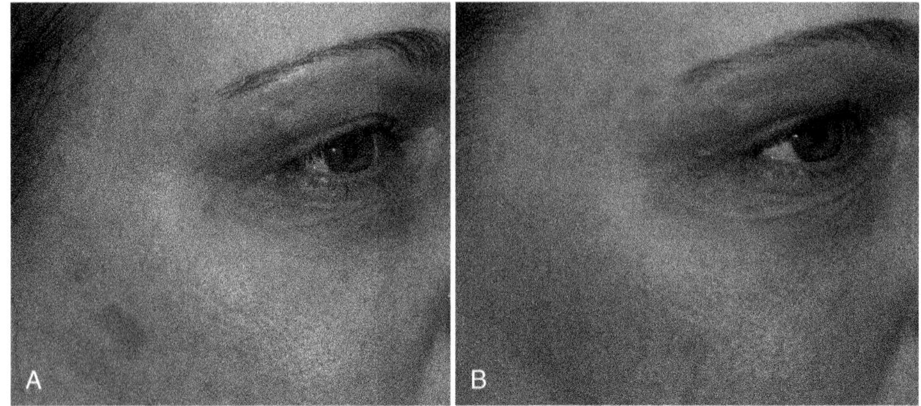

FIGURE 27-10 Hyperpigmentaion (**A**) before and (**B**) after photorejuvenation treatments with a Q-switched 532 nm laser. *(Copyright Rebecca Small, MD.)*

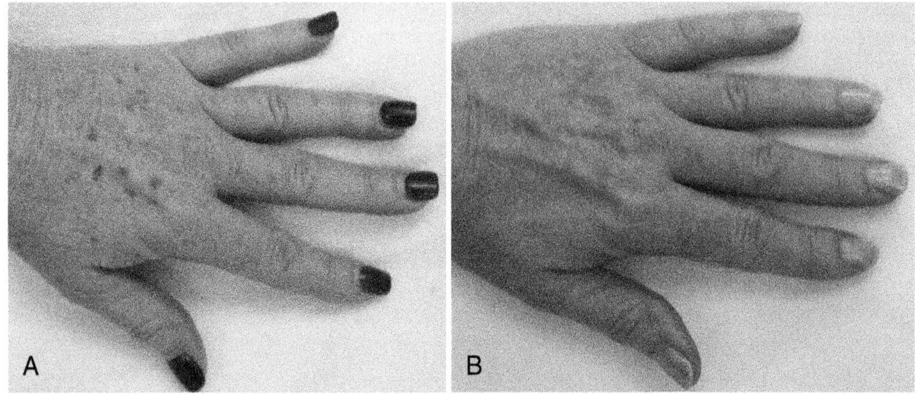

FIGURE 27-11 Hand lentigines (**A**) before and (**B**) after photorejuvenation treatments with intense pulsed light. *(Copyright Rebecca Small, MD.)*

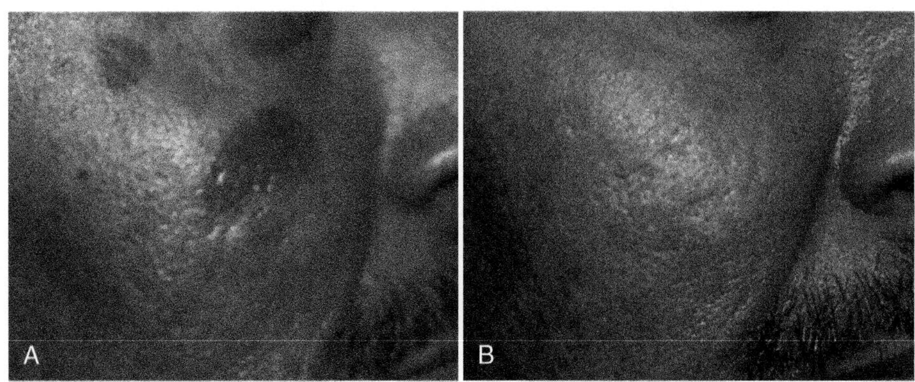

FIGURE 27-12 Hyperpigmentation in a patient with darker Fitzpatrick skin type (**A**) before and (**B**) after photorejuvenation treatments with a Q-switched 1064 nm laser. *(Courtesy of HOYA ConBio, Fremont, CA; J. Garden, MD, using laser.)*

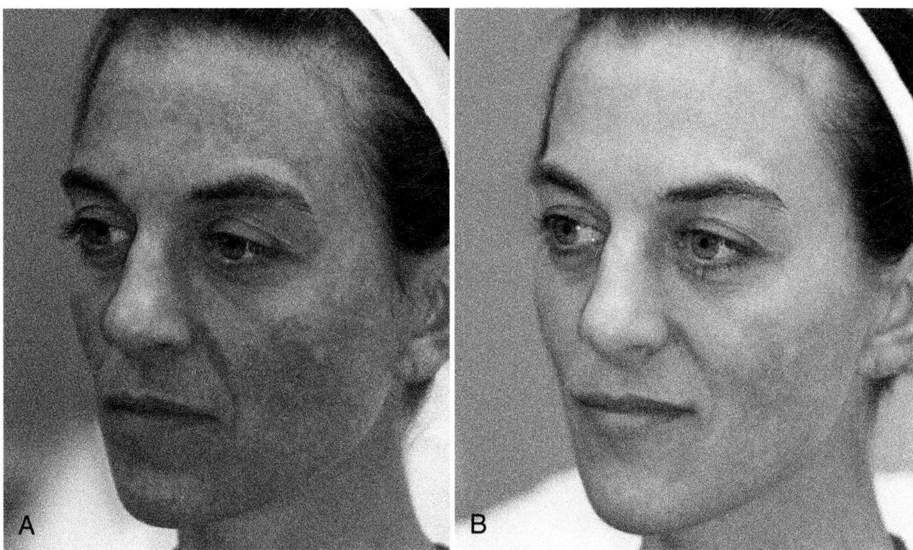

FIGURE 27-13 Melasma (**A**) before and (**B**) after photorejuvenation treatments with a Q-switched 1064 nm laser *(Copyright Rebecca Small, MD.)*

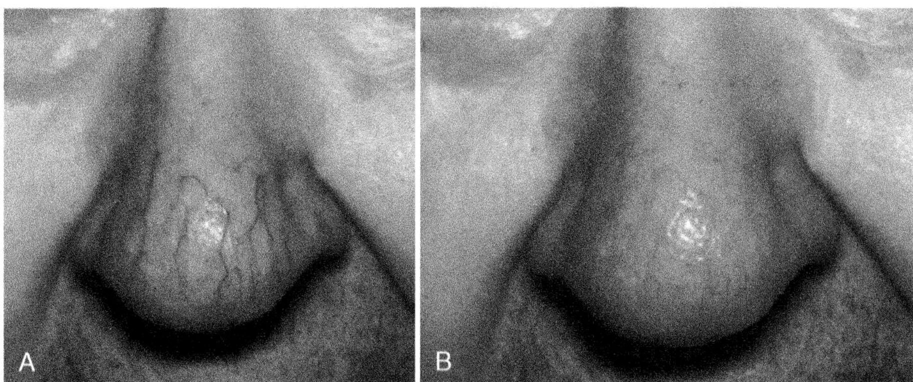

FIGURE 27-14 Nose telangiectasias (**A**) before and (**B**) after photorejuvenation treatments with a 532 nm laser. *(Courtesy of Iridex, Mount View, CA; B. Berger, MD, using laser.)*

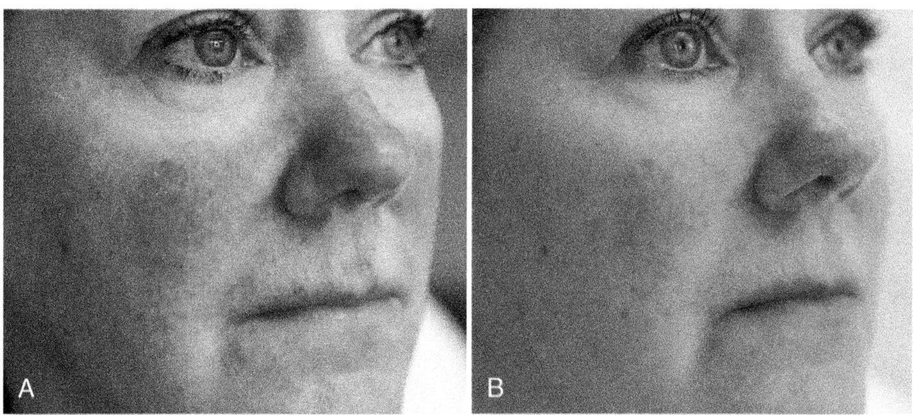

FIGURE 27-15 Rosacea (**A**) before and (**B**) after photorejuvenation treatments with intense pulsed light. *(Copyright Rebecca Small, MD.)*

may require fewer treatments. Nonfacial areas are slower to exfoliate and heal, and usually require longer intervals between treatments, up to 8 weeks. One annual follow-up treatment is recommended for patients to maintain their results.

Photorejuvenation of *benign vascular lesions* also requires three to five IPL treatments at more frequent, bimonthly intervals, for optimal results. Again, lasers may require fewer treatments. Some vascular lesions, such as telangiectasias, can gradually recur over time, particularly in patients with rosacea, active lifestyles, or regular activities that cause flushing such as sauna and hot tub use. Annual or biannual follow-up treatments are recommended to maintain results. Discreet lesions such as cherry angiomas typically resolve without recurrence after one or two treatments.

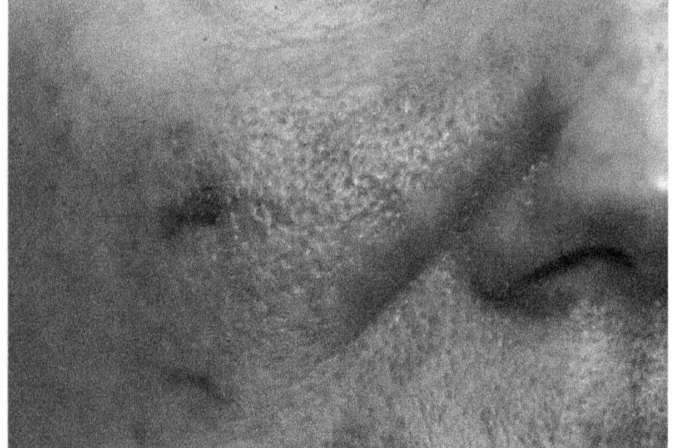

FIGURE 27-16 Purpura of the cheek immediately after a photorejuvenation treatment with IPL for rosacea. *(Copyright Rebecca Small, MD.)*

COMPLICATIONS

- Pain
- Swelling
- Purpura/bruising
- Urticaria
- Visible skin patterns or striping
- Hypopigmentation
- Hyperpigmentation, including worsening of melasma
- Burn with blistering and scabbing
- Infection
- Inadequate clearance of unwanted pigmentation or vascularities, or recurrence
- Damage or alteration to tattoos and permanent makeup
- Hair reduction in or adjacent to the treatment area
- Scarring (extremely rare)
- Ocular injury.

Temporary redness and *mild sunburn-like* discomfort after treatment are common, which may last for a few hours to several days, and are not considered complications.

Pain is usually mild to moderate and only reported during treatment. Analgesic medications are not typically required.

Swelling may occur, particularly with aggressive treatment of the cheeks. Cold compresses are recommended as described above.

Rarely, *urticaria* may be seen. A daily oral antihistamine (e.g., cetirizine 10 mg) may be used until resolved, along with cold compresses and, once identified, these patients may be pretreated with an antihistamine 1 hour prior to procedures.

Purpura is due to localized rupture of superficial blood vessels and can occur when aggressive treatment parameters are used with superficial vessels. Utilizing longer pulse widths and lower fluences will usually avoid this complication. There is no specific treatment for this and purpuric lesions usually resolve in 1 to 2 weeks. Figure 27-16 shows an example of purpura immediately after an IPL photorejuvenation treatment on the cheek.

Visible skin patterns or *striping* may be seen during the course of a series of treatments, particularly in patients with severely sun-damaged skin with background brown discoloration, called actinic bronzing. These patterns are usually the result of careful treatments with appropriate overlap of pulses, where the dark stripes represent the regions of overlap. Subsequent treatments usually blend skin patterns and striping; however, as with any pigmentary change, there is a small risk that these patterns may be permanent.

Pigmentary complications of *hyperpigmentation* and *hypopigmentation* are most commonly seen in darker Fitzpatrick skin types (IV)[14] and in patients with a recent tan. These complications are more common with short pulse widths, high fluences, and poor epidermal cooling. Hyperpigmentation is usually transient (and rarely may be permanent), lasting in the order of months. The use of a lightening agent such as hydroquinone for 1 month prior to treatment and after treatment can reduce hyperpigmentation, particularly in darker skinned patients (see Chapter 24, *Skin Care Products*, for additional information). Hypopigmentation is a more significant complication. This may be temporary or permanent. Figure 27-17 shows stripes of hypopigmentation resulting from an overly aggressive IPL treatment for lentigines (not performed by the authors) on a patient with a darker skin type.

A *burn* may result from aggressive treatment parameters of short pulse widths and high fluences with inadequate epidermal cooling. Routine moist wound care is performed with application of an antibiotic ointment and bandage until healed. Tattoos and permanent makeup have concentrated ink pigments and treatment over these may result in full-thickness skin burns.

Postprocedure infections are rare with laser photorejuvenation treatments and require treatment specific to the infection. Infections such as *herpes simplex* and *varicella zoster* may be reactivated in the treatment area, and pretreatment prophylactic oral antiviral medication can reduce this risk (see the *Procedure Preparation* section above). *Impetigo* may occur, particularly with treatments around the mouth. *Folliculitis* may also

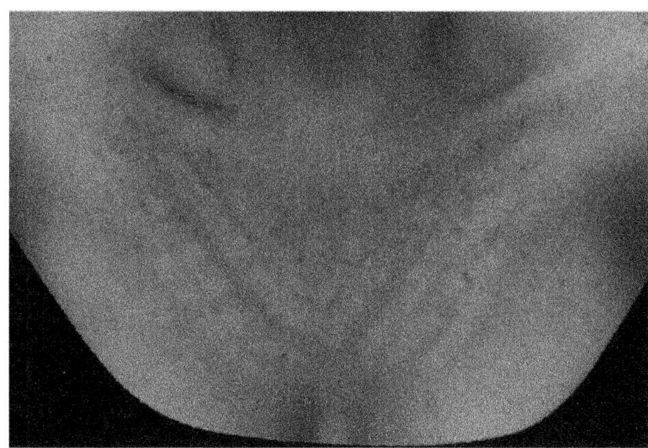

FIGURE 27-17 Hypopigmentation of the chest in a patient with darker Fitzpatrick skin type 6 weeks after IPL treatment (not performed by the author) for lentigines. *(Copyright Rebecca Small, MD.)*

occur, particularly after vigorous exercise, swimming or hot tub use immediately after treatments.

Scarring is very rare, but may occur with overaggressive treatments or with treatments complicated by infection.

Reduced hair growth in or adjacent to the treatment area may occur. This risk should be fully discussed if treating over men's facial hair.

Ocular injury can be avoided by wearing appropriate laser-safe eyewear at all times during treatment, directing the laser tip away from the eye, and treating outside of the eye orbit.

TREATING SPECIFIC LESIONS/AREAS

Melasma

Laser treatments of melasma may be variable, and in some cases hyperpigmentation may be worsened, particularly with repeated IPL treatments.

Nonfacial Areas

Nonfacial areas have fewer pilosebaceous units, which serve as sites of re-epithelialization that facilitate healing. For this reason, these areas have delayed healing relative to the face, with a greater risk of overtreatment and scarring and conservative settings are advised for treatment of non-facial areas.

LEARNING THE TECHNIQUE

Providers may initially perform treatments on the face using conservative laser parameters with longer pulse widths and lower fluences in patients with light Fitzpatrick skin types (I through III). When getting started with IPL photorejuvenation treatment, conservative clinical endpoints for pigmentation are sought including darkening with minimal perilesional erythema, and for vascular lesions, sluggish refilling after compression.

CURRENT DEVELOPMENTS

Some of the new *fractional laser technologies* used for nonablative skin resurfacing show promise as photorejuventation treatments[15] (see Chapter 29, *Skin Resurfacing with Ablative Lasers*). The fractionated 1550 nm wavelength has been shown to reduce red vascularities[16,17] and benign pigmented lesions[18,19] as well as improve skin texture[20] and scars (see Chapter 28, *Wrinkle Reduction with Nonablative Lasers*). Some newer devices combine chromophore-specific modalities with other modalities that are not chromophore specific to target pigmentation, vascularities, and skin texture, such as *IPL with radio-frequency*.[21] Lasers with longer wavelengths, such as *940 nm*, have been used for red vascular lesions and recently, a *980 nm wavelength laser*[22] has been used for targeting larger red facial vessels.

Photodynamic therapy (PDT) has also been used for photorejuvenation. PDT involves the use of a topical photosensitizing medication activated by light (usually LEDs or IPLs) . Commonly used photosensitizers include 5-aminolevulinic acid (ALA) and methyl ALA (mALA). ALA is selectively absorbed and concentrated in proliferating cells and pilosebaceous units where it is converted to protoporphyrin (PpIX). Upon activation with a light source, such as an IPL, laser (e.g., 585 nm), or LED, PpIX forms free radicals, which selectively destroy the target. PDT using ALA, activated by blue light, is currently FDA approved for treatment of nonhyperkeratotic actinic keratoses of the face and is also used off-label for photorejuvenation.[23] PDT has a greater cost to the patient than laser alone, more downtime with erythema and crusting, and requires strict patient avoidance of ambient sunlight post-treatment for 48 hours, because sun exposure can lead to extended ALA activation and associated complications.

FINANCIAL CONSIDERATIONS

Laser photorejuvenation is generally not reimbursable; however, some insurance companies may reimburse for treatment of rosacea. The charges for treatments vary and are largely determined by local prices. Individual treatment prices range from $350 to $600 for a single treatment to a large area such as the face or chest, and $150 to $300 for a small area such as the hands or neck. However, because photorejuvenation treatments are most effective with a series of treatments, packages of treatments (usually three or five) may be offered so that patients achieve the best possible results.

When covered by insurance, Box 27-2 lists the applicable ICD-9 codes for photorejuvenation procedures.

CONCLUSION

Photorejuvenation laser treatments effectively and safely reduce benign pigmented and vascular lesions associated with photoaging. Treatments have minimal discomfort, little to no recovery time, and high patient

BOX 27-2 *ICD-9 Codes for Photorejuvenation Procedures*

695.3	Rosacea
709.09	Other dyschromia (solar lentigo, melasma, poikiloderma of Civatte)
709.1	Vascular disorder of the skin (cherry angioma, telangiectasia)

satisfaction and may be readily integrated into office-based aesthetic care.

Resources

Laser Safety Training Courses

American Society for Laser Medicine and Surgery (ASLMS)
Phone: 715-845-9283
www.aslms.org

Photorejuvenation Lasers and IPL Device Suppliers

Alma Lasers
Phone: 866-414-ALMA
www.almalasers.com

Asclepion Laser Technologies
www.asclepion.com

CoolTouch
Phone: 877-858-COOL
www.cooltouch.com

Cutera
Phone: 888-4-CUTERA
www.cutera.com

Cynosure/Deka
Phone: 800-886-2966
www.cynosure.com

DermaMed USA
Phone: 888-789-6342
www.dermamedusa.com

Fotona USA
Phone: 888-550-4113
www.fotonamedicallasers.com

HOYA ConBio
Phone: 800-532-1064
www.conbio.com

Iridex Corporation
Phone: 650-940-4700
www.iridex.com

Lumenis
Phone: 408-764-3000
www.lumenis.com

Lutronic
Phone: 888-588-7644
www.lutronic.com

Palomar
Phone: 800-725-6627
www.palomarmedical.com

Quantel Medical
Phone: 888-660-6726
www.quantelmedical.com

Sciton
Phone: 888-646-6999
www.sciton.com

SharpLight Technologies
Phone: 905-337-7797
www.sharplightech.com

Solta Medical
Phone: 888-437-2935
www.fraxel.com

Sybaritic
Phone: 800-445-8418
www.sybaritic.com

Syneron (formerly Candela)
Phone: 866-259-6661
www.syneron.com

References

1. Small R. Aesthetic procedures introduction. In: Mayeaux E, ed. *The Essential Guide to Primary Care Procedures*. Philadelphia: Lippincott Williams & Wilkins; 2009:195–199.
2. Small R. Aesthetic procedures in office practice. *Am Fam Physician*. 2009;80(11):1231–1237.
3. Weiss RA, Weiss MA, Beasly KL. Rejuvenation of photoaged skin: 5 years results with intense pulsed light of the face, neck and chest. *Dermatol Surg*. 2002;28:1115–1119.
4. Bitter PH. Noninvasive rejuvenation of photodamaged skin using serial, full-face intense pulsed light treatments. *Dermatol Surg*. 2000;26:835–843.
5. Kligman DE, Zhen Y. Intense pulsed light treatment of photoaged facial skin. *Dermatol Surg*. 2004;30(8):1085–1090.
6. Small R. Laser photo rejuvenation. *In:* Mayeaux E, ed. *The Essential Guide to Primary Care Procedures*. Philadelphia: Lippincott Williams & Wilkins; 2009:249–264.
7. Uebelhoer NS, Bogle MA, Stewart B, *et al*. A split-face comparison study of pulsed 532-nm KTP laser and 595-nm pulsed dye laser in the treatment of facial telangiectasias and diffuse telangiectatic facial erythema. *Dermatol Surg*. 2007;33(4):441–448.
8. Kilmer SL. Diode laser treatment of pigmented lesions. *Lasers Surg Med*. 2000;12(Suppl):23.
9. Ross EV, Uebelhoer NS, Domankevitz Y. Use of a novel pulse dye laser for rapid single-pass purpura-free treatment of telangiectases. *Dermatol Surg*. 2007;33(12):1466–1469.
10. Ross EV, Smirnov M, Pankratov M. Intense pulsed light and laser treatment of facial telangiectasias and dyspigmentation: some theoretical and practical comparisons. *Dermatol Surg*. 2005;31(9 Pt 2):1188–1198.
11. Kilmer SL, Wheeland RG, Goldberg DJ, *et al*. Treatment of epidermal pigmented lesions with the frequency-doubled Q-switched Nd:YAG laser. A controlled, single-impact, dose-response, multicenter trial. *Arch Dermatol*. 1994;130(12):1515–1519.

12. Goldman MP, Bennett RG. Treatment of telangiectasia: a review. *J Am Acad Dermatol.* 1987;17(2 Pt 1):167–182.
13. Gilchrest BA, Fitzpatrick TB, Anderson RR, *et al.* Localization of melanin pigmentation in the skin with Wood's lamp. *Br J Dermatol.* 1977;96(3):245–248.
14. Kono T, Manstein D, Chan HH, *et al.* Q-switched ruby versus long-pulsed dye laser delivered with compression for treatment of facial lentigines in Asians. *Lasers Surg Med.* 2006;38:94–97.
15. Tierney EP, Kouba DJ, Hanke CW. Review of fractional photothermolysis: treatment indications and efficacy. *Dermatol Surg.* 2009;35(10):1445–1461.
16. Glaich AS, Goldberg LH, Dai T, *et al.* Fractional photothermolysis for the treatment of telangiectatic matting: a case report. *J Cutan Laser Ther.* 2007;9:101–103.
17. Behroozan DS, Goldberg LH, Glaich AS, *et al.* Fractional photothermolysis for treatment of poikiloderma of Civatte. *Dermatol Surg.* 2006;32:298–301.
18. Wanner M, Tanzi EL, Alster TS. Fractional photothermolysis treatment of facial and non-facial cutaneous photodamage with the 1,550-nm erbium-doped fiber laser. *Dermatol Surg.* 2007;33:23–28.
19. Jih MH, Goldberg LH, Kimyai-Asadi A. Fractional photothermolysis for photoaging hands. *Dermatol Surg.* 2008;34:73–78.
20. Manstein D, Herron GS, Sink RK. Fractional photothermolysis: a new concept for cutaneous remodeling using microscopic patterns of thermal injury. *Lasers Surg Med.* 2004;34:426–438.
21. Bitter P. Report of a new technique for enhanced non-invasive skin rejuvenation using a dual mode, pulsed light and radiofrequency energy source: selective radio-thermolysis. *J Cosm Dermatol.* 2002;1:142–145.
22. Dudelzak J, Hussain M, Goldberg DJ. Vascular-specific laser wavelength for the treatment of facial telangiectasias. *J Drugs Dermatol.* 2009;8(3):227–229.
23. Dover JS, Bhatia AC, Stewart B, *et al.* Topical 5-aminolevulinic acid combined with intense pulsed light in the treatment of photoaging. *Arch Dermatol.* 2005;141(10):1247–1252.

Additional Reading

Small R. Photo rejuvenation. *In:* Small R, ed. *A Practical Guide to Cosmetic Lasers.* Philadelphia: Lippincott Williams & Wilkins; 2012.

Van Aardt R. Lasers and pulsed-light devices: photofacial rejuvenation. *In:* Pfenninger JL, Fowler GC, eds. *Pfenninger and Fowler's Procedures for Primary Care.* 3rd ed. Philadelphia: Mosby/Elsevier; 2011.

28 Wrinkle Reduction with Nonablative Lasers

REBECCA SMALL, MD

Nonablative laser treatments for wrinkle reduction (where the term lasers* refers to both lasers and intense pulsed light devices) are aimed at heating the dermis to cause mild injury, while leaving the epidermis intact. A reparative healing process ensues after treatment with collagen shrinkage and synthesis of new collagen and extracellular matrix, referred to as dermal *collagen remodeling*.[1,2] Dermal thickness is increased and the skin is smoothed, resulting in clinical reduction of wrinkles. In addition to wrinkle reduction, collagen remodeling effects with nonablative lasers can also result in reduction of depression scars, pore size, and rough skin texture.

Nonablative lasers are most appropriate for treatment of mild to moderate wrinkles (also called *rhytids*). Relative to ablative technologies, wrinkle reduction effects are slower and more subtle with nonablative technologies. However, these treatments have the advantage of requiring little to no recovery time, they have lower risks of complications, and are easily incorporated into patients' daily lives. Common terms used for nonablative wrinkle reduction include *nonablative skin rejuvenation, noninvasive resurfacing,* and *skin toning.*

Certain nonablative laser technologies primarily target skin laxity and skin folds. Reduction of skin laxity and folds is commonly known as *skin tightening;* however, the term used by the Food and Drug Administration (FDA) is *soft tissue coagulation,* which essentially means thermal injury to the skin. Providers may want to consider using terms such as *reduction of skin laxity or crepiness* (defined as a crepey or crinkly appearance to the skin) rather than *skin tightening,* because for some patients, skin tightening may imply surgical-like results with dramatic tissue lifting.

Rejuvenation of photoaged skin typically requires reduction of wrinkles and rough texture in combination with treatment of dyschromia (such as solar lentigines and mottled hyperpigmentation) and vascular ectasias (such as telangiectasias and facial erythema). Nonablative wrinkle reduction with lasers is an important component of aesthetic care and can be readily combined with other minimally invasive aesthetic procedures into office practice to achieve global skin rejuvenation.

LASER PRINCIPLES AND DEVICES CURRENTLY AVAILABLE

The mechanism by which most nonablative lasers effect collagen remodeling and wrinkle reduction is through focal thermal injury to the dermis while avoiding epidermal injury. Thermal injury can be induced through energy absorption in the skin by melanin, oxyhemoglobin, and/or water chromophores utilizing the principle of selective photothermolysis (see Chapter 19, Aesthetic Principles and Consultation).[3] Other methods of inducing thermal injury include using radiofrequency energy, where tissue resistance to applied current heats the dermis. Some technologies utilize fractional methods of delivery that enhance the depth of laser penetration into the skin. Nonablative wrinkle reduction technologies can be broadly classified according to their clinical effects of wrinkle reduction or improvement in skin laxity, and this may be further refined based on the mechanism of action of the technology (see Table 28-1).

Wrinkle Reduction

Many of the lasers used for nonablative wrinkle reduction target the water chromophore in tissue, including infrared (IR) wavelengths of 1320, 1440, 1450, 1540, and 1550 nm (1064 nm is also an IR wavelength but has less affinity for water). Figure 28-1 shows these wavelengths superimposed on the water absorption curve. By heating water, thermal energy is conducted to the dermal tissue, which stimulates the collagen remodeling process. All of these wavelengths have demonstrated clinical improvements in wrinkles.[4–7]

Some of the *infrared lasers* employ a fractional method of delivery (see Table 28-1), of which 1550 nm has the most data.[8] Fractional lasers treat a portion or "fraction" of the skin by delivering laser energy in microscopic columns, called *microthermal zones.* Figure 19-10 in Chapter 19, *Aesthetic Principles and Consultation,* shows the pattern in the skin made by fractional laser devices. The untreated tissue between microthermal zones serves as a regenerative reservoir, which facilitates rapid wound healing.[9] This type of treatment is termed *nonablative fractional resurfacing.* In addition to the collagen remodeling effects of wrinkle and scar reduction, fractional resurfacing with 1550 nm has also shown promise with reduction of dyschromic conditions such as melasma and poikiloderma of Civatte.[10–12]

Lasers that target oxyhemoglobin, melanin, and to a lesser degree water, such as 532 nm pulsed dye lasers (585 and 595 nm), and intense pulsed light devices (IPLs) have also been found to effect collagen remodeling and wrinkle reduction.[13–15] However, the primary indication for these chromophore dependent lasers is reduction of vascular ectasias and/or pigmented lesions.

The *Q-switched 1064 nm neodymium-doped yttrium aluminum garnet (Nd:YAG) laser* was one of the first lasers to demonstrate nonablative reduction of wrinkles. Long-pulse 1064 nm Nd:YAG lasers are also used for reduction of wrinkles and results may be enhanced when combined with 532 nm.[16–18] The long 1064 nm wavelength, as with other infrared lasers, allows for deep penetration to the dermis, which is desirable for collagen remodeling and, because it has little absorption

*Refers to laser and light-based technologies.

TABLE 28-1 Classification of Nonablative Lasers and Light Devices for Wrinkle Reduction

Clinical Effects and Mechanism of Action	*Wrinkles*			*Laxity*	
	Tissue Target			*Tissue Target*	
	Oxyhemoglobin and/or Melanin	**Water**	**Photomodulation**	**Tissue Resistance**	**Water**
Laser Devices	532 nm (KTP, frequency-doubled Nd:YAG)	1320 nm (Nd:YAG)	LEDs	RF	Broadband IR
	585 and 595 nm (pulsed dye)	1440 nm[a] (Nd:YAG)	—	—	—
	1064 nm Q-switched (Nd:YAG)	1450 nm (diode)	—	—	—
	1064 nm long pulse (Nd:YAG)	1540 nm[a] (erbium glass)	—	—	—
	Intense pulsed light	1550 nm[a] (erbium)	—	—	—

[a]Devices using fractional method of delivery.

by epidermal pigment, this wavelength is safe for all skin types. Studies with Q-switched 1064 nm lasers demonstrate histologic[19,20] and clinical reduction of wrinkles, as well as other collagen remodeling effects, such as reduction of pore size, rough skin texture,[21] and superficial acne scarring.[22-24] Dermal collagen remodeling effects are due to both photothermal and photoacoustic vibration, which results from the inherent rapid, short (nanoseconds) pulses of Q-switched lasers.[25] In addition to dermal remodeling, Q-switched 1064 nm lasers are also commonly used for tattoo removal,[26] reduction of dermal pigmentation such as melasma,[27-29] and reduction of fine dark hair.[30] The diverse applications of Q-switched 1064 nm and other chromophore-dependent lasers offer a means to address many aesthetic skin complaints simultaneously.

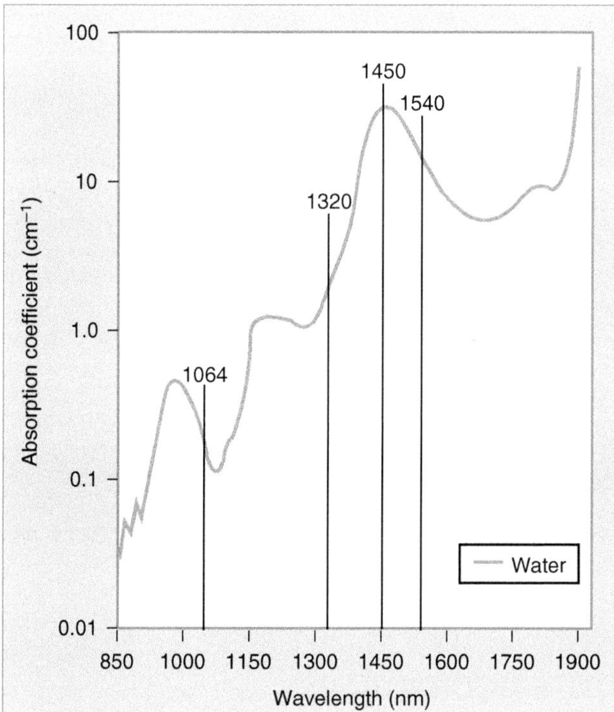

FIGURE 28-1 Water absorption spectrum and common nonablative wrinkle reduction lasers.

Light-emitting diodes (LEDs) are a newer type of light-based device that emit a narrow range, or band, of wavelengths. They do not operate based on the theory of selective photothermolysis, but are instead based on the principle of photomodulation, whereby cellular activity is modulated through illumination with particular wavelengths of light.[31] These devices have been used for mild wrinkle reduction[32] and treatment of acne. Several LEDs are available that vary in wavelength and pulsing modes such as blue light devices (400 to 500 nm) which have superficial penetration, and red light devices (570 to 670 nm) which have deeper penetration. The main advantage of LEDs is their ease of use.

LEDs have also been used for skin rejuvenation as part of *photodynamic therapy* (PDT). PDT refers to selective tissue destruction through the use of a photosensitizing medication that is activated by a laser or light-based device (such as an LED or IPL).[33] A topical photosensitizing medication such as aminolevulinic acid (Levulan®) is concentrated in particular tissues, such as sebaceous glands and actinically damaged cells. The photosensitizer is activated by a light source resulting in a cytotoxic reaction and destruction of the targeted areas.[34] PDT is currently FDA approved for treatment of nonhyperkeratotic actinic keratoses, but is used off label to enhance the results with nonablative lasers for photorejuvenation and wrinkle reduction.[35-37]

Reduction of Skin Laxity

Skin laxity is treated with two main types of technologies: broadband infrared and radio-frequency (RF) devices.[38] The improvements in laxity are believed to be due to collagen contraction initially, and later to collagen synthesis.[39] *Broadband infrared devices* (such as the Cutera Titan™) emit wavelengths ranging from 1100 to

1800 nm with long pulse widths (of several seconds). *Radio-frequency devices* (such as Solta Thermage™) employ rapidly alternating current that creates heat when applied to the skin because of the skin's resistance to the flow of current. Tissue heating with RF devices is controlled by several factors, including the type of electrodes used (e.g., monopolar or bipolar), fluence, and cooling times. These technologies have been shown to improve laxity in many areas of the body including the periocular region, nasolabial folds, jowls, neck, and abdomen.[40–45] In addition to treatment of wrinkles and skin laxity, RF devices are also used for cellulite reduction.[46] RF treatments have traditionally been associated with more discomfort than IR treatments, however, new techniques utilizing multiple passes with lower fluences have improved tolerability.[47]

Epidermal Cooling

Cooling of the skin is an important consideration with nonablative wrinkle reduction treatments. Adequate cooling is required to protect the epidermis, but overcooling can reduce clinical effects. In addition, overcooling can induce epidermal injury, particularly in darker Fitzpatrick skin types, resulting in postinflammatory hyperpigmentation. Some nonablative lasers utilize cryogen spray coolants (e.g., 1320 nm) or contact cooling through the tip of the device (e.g., broadband IR). The shorter wavelength devices (e.g., 532 nm and pulsed dye lasers) also employ larger spot sizes with lower fluences to further reduce the risk of epidermal injury. IPL devices have large spot sizes and typically use contact cooling. Due to minimal epidermal energy absorption by 1064 nm and the relatively lower fluences used for wrinkle reduction treatments (compared to leg veins, for example), these devices do not typically utilize cooling.

PATIENT SELECTION

Patient selection for wrinkle reduction treatments with nonablative lasers is based on the degree of wrinkling present and patient expectations. Patients with mild to moderate static wrinkles and laxity (Glogau types I through III) are appropriate candidates (see Chapter 19, *Aesthetic Principles and Consultation*, for a description of Glogau types). Patients with deep static wrinkles and/or severe laxity (Glogau type IV) and those who desire more rapid and dramatic results may be better candidates for more aggressive procedures such as ablative laser resurfacing or surgery.

In patients presenting with wrinkling as well as significant dyschromia and vascular ectasias, the dyschromia and vascularities are typically treated first, using technologies/therapies most appropriate for the predominant presenting issue. Improvements in texture and wrinkles will be more apparent after these other issues have been addressed.

Results with nonablative wrinkle reduction treatments occur slowly, usually 2 to 3 months after the initial laser treatment, and improvements may continue to be seen 6 months post-treatment. A series of five to six treatments is usually required at monthly intervals. Some improvements may be seen immediately post-treatment; however, this is likely due to transient tissue edema. Assessment of patients' expectations at the time of consultation and commitment to a series of treatments is essential to ensure success with these treatments.

Patients with darker skin Fitzpatrick skin types (IV through VI) have increased risks of complications, such as hyperpigmentation and hypopigmentation, and are best suited to treatment with nonablative lasers that target water (e.g., 1320 nm) and those with longer wavelengths (e.g., 1064 nm). Lighter Fitzpatrick skin types (I through III) may be treated with any of the nonablative laser technologies including those with shorter wavelengths (e.g., 532 nm and pulsed dye lasers).

INDICATIONS

- Mild to moderate rhytids
- Mild to moderate skin laxity and crepiness (with RF and broadband IR devices).

ALTERNATIVE THERAPIES

Ablative skin resurfacing, with carbon dioxide and erbium lasers, is the gold standard for reduction of wrinkles. Although the fractional method of delivery has reduced the associated recovery time and risk of complications, ablative laser treatments create an open wound and are considered aggressive treatments. Although more aggressive procedures offer greater potential for wrinkle reduction, they require longer recovery times and have greater risks of complications.

Nonlaser treatment options for wrinkle reduction include superficial skin resurfacing with *light chemical peels* or *microdermabrasion*, and *topical skin care products* such as retinoids and exfoliants. More aggressive resurfacing can be performed with *deeper chemical peels* and operative procedures such as *dermabrasion*, which utilizes a motorized rotating wire-bristle brush to abrade the skin.

PRODUCTS CURRENTLY AVAILABLE

See the *Resources* section at the end of the chapter for a list of laser manufacturers.

CONTRAINDICATIONS

See *General Laser Contraindications* in Chapter 26, *Hair Reduction with Lasers*.

ADVANTAGES OF NONABLATIVE LASERS FOR WRINKLES

- Relative to more aggressive resurfacing procedures, such as ablative treatments with carbon dioxide and erbium lasers, there is minimal recovery time and minimal risk of complications.
- Treatments are readily incorporated into patients' daily lives and easily combined with other minimally invasive aesthetic procedures.
- Many technologies used for nonablative wrinkle reduction are appropriate for darker skin types (IV and V) and some are even safe with Fitzpatrick skin type VI. More aggressive resurfacing procedures (e.g., ablative laser resurfacing and medium-depth chemical peels) are typically restricted to Fitzpatrick skin types I through III.

DISADVANTAGES OF NONABLATIVE LASERS FOR WRINKLES

- Clinical results are variable and not all patients will show demonstrable improvements.
- Wrinkle reduction is slow and may require months before becoming clinically evident.
- Subtle results may not be captured photographically.

ANATOMY

Wrinkles result from many factors including skin changes with epidermal hypocellularity, loss of dermal matrix components including collagen, glycosaminoglycans, elastin, and atrophy of subcutaneous adipose tissue. Thinning of the skin combined with repetitive contraction of underlying musculature can etch wrinkles into the skin to form static lines.[48]

Nonablative laser treatments are aimed at reducing mild to moderate static wrinkles. Most of these technologies do so by producing papillary dermal injury, at an approximately 100 to 200 μm (0.1 to 0.2 mm) depth in the skin.[49,50] Fractional nonablative laser treatments for wrinkles (e.g., fractional 1550 nm) penetrate up to 300 to 400 μm (0.3 to 0.4 mm).[9] Nonablative lasers for laxity (e.g., RF lasers) penetrate to the reticular dermis, up to 1 to 3 mm.[51]

EQUIPMENT

- Laser or IPL device appropriate for wrinkle reduction treatments
- Eyewear for the patient and provider specific to the device being used
- Nonalcohol cleansing facial wipes
- Clear colorless gel for treatments if necessary per the manufacturer
- 4 × 4 inch gauze
- Ice packs
- Soothing nonocclusive topical product (e.g., SkinCeuticals Epidermal Repair™)
- Broad-spectrum sunscreen (SPF 30 with zinc or titanium)
- Hydrocortisone cream 1% and 2.5%
- Alcohol wipes for cleaning laser tip
- Germicidal disposable wipes for sanitizing the laser.

PROCEDURE PREPARATION

1. Perform an aesthetic consultation and review the patient's medical history (see Chapter 19, *Aesthetics Principles and Consultation*) including history of postinflammatory hyperpigmentation, abnormal scarring, photosensitizing medications or isotretinoin, and previous dermal fillers in the treatment area.
2. Examine the treatment area including assessment of the degree of wrinkling (see Chapter 19 for a discussion of Glogau types). Consider referral for ablative skin resurfacing or surgical intervention in patients with excessive laxity and severe wrinkling (e.g., Glogau type IV).
3. Obtain informed consent (see Chapter 19; also see Appendix A for an informed consent form and patient information handout titled *Nonablative Laser Treatments for Wrinkle Reduction*).
4. Take pretreatment photographs (see Chapter 19).
5. Determine the Fitzpatrick skin type (see Chapter 19).
6. If the patient has a prior history of herpes simplex or varicella in or near the treatment area, provide prophylactic antiviral medication (e.g., valacyclovir, 500 mg, 1 tablet twice daily) for 2 days prior to the procedure, and continue for 3 days postprocedure.
7. Consider performing test spots prior to the initial treatment for patients with darker Fitzpatrick skin types (types IV through VI). Laser manufacturer's guidelines for spot size, fluence, and pulse width should be followed. Test spots are placed discretely (under the chin, behind or inferior to the ear) near the desired treatment area and viewed 3 to 5 days after placement for evidence of erythema, burn, or other adverse effect. Inform patients that lack of an adverse reaction with test spots does *not* ensure that a side effect or complication will not occur with any treatment.
8. Pretreatment skin care products, other than a daily sunscreen, are not required; however, patients will derive added benefit from using rejuvenation skin care products (see Chapter 24, *Skin Care Products*).

NONABLATIVE LASERS FOR WRINKLES: STEPS AND PRINCIPLES

The following guidelines are based on treatment of mild to moderate facial wrinkling using a Q-switched 1064 nm laser (Hoya ConBio RevLite™), which is indicated for all Fitzpatrick skin types. Manufacturer's guidelines for the specific device used should be followed at the time of treatment.

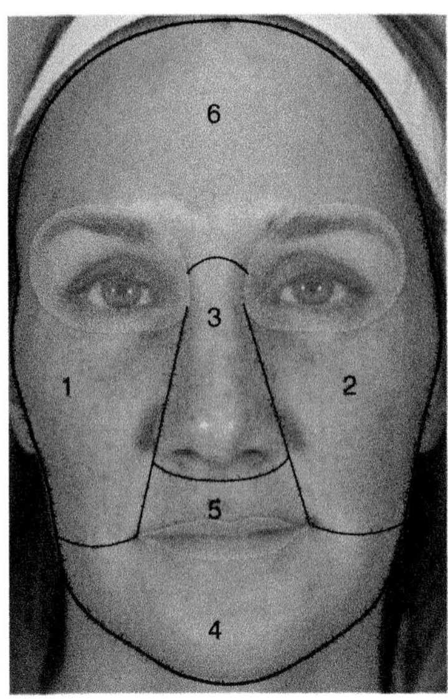

FIGURE 28-2 Nonablative Laser Safety Zone and sequence for wrinkle reduction treatments on the face. *(Copyright Rebecca Small, MD.)*

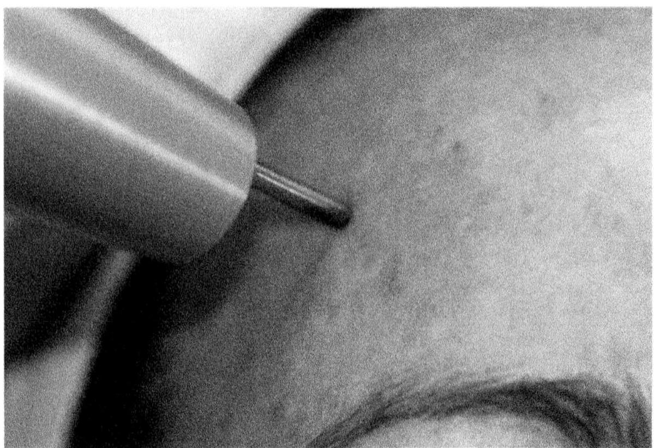

FIGURE 28-3 Technique for nonablative wrinkle reduction treatments using a Q-switched 1064 nm laser. *(Copyright Rebecca Small, MD.)*

General Treatment Technique

1. Treatment is performed on the full face within the safety zone (see below for safety zone region).
2. Laser treatment parameters are based on the patient's Fitzpatrick skin type. Darker skin types require more conservative settings with the Q-switched 1064 nm laser of larger spot sizes and lower fluences:
   - *Fitzpatrick skin type VI:* 8 mm spot size, 1.4 to 2.0 J/cm^2
   - *Fitzpatrick skin types IV–V:* 8 mm spot size, 2.0 to 3.0 J/cm^2 (PTP mode 3.5 J/cm^2; see *Tip* below for PTP mode description)
   - *Fitzpatrick skin types I–III:* 6 mm spot size, 2.5 to 3.5 J/cm^2 (PTP mode 6.9 J/cm^2).

   TIP: Certain Q-switched devices have stacked-pulse modes that allow for higher fluencies (e.g., *photo-acoustic technology pulse* (PTP) mode with the Q-switched RevLite). Once fluences are maximized in the non-PTP mode, the PTP mode may be used. Due to the method of delivery, high fluences used in the PTP mode typically do not cause additional patient discomfort. For example, a 6-mm spot size with 3.5 J/cm^2 in non-PTP mode results in the same patient discomfort as a 6-mm spot with 6.9 J/cm^2 in the PTP mode.
3. It is advisable to start at the periphery of the face and progress medially, because the central face is more sensitive. Figure 28-2 shows a recommended sequence for treating the face in regions, starting with area 1 and progressing to area 6.

   TIP: The most sensitive facial areas are the upper lip (philtrum) and lateral to the nose.
4. The handpiece for Q-switched 1064 nm lasers is held approximately 1 inch above the skin, which is determined by the handpiece depth guide (Figure 28-3). It is moved in a painting motion across the face using long switchback strokes (Figure 28-4). The direction of the laser handpiece is toward the provider, with approximately 20% overlap of each pulse. The laser tip should always be angled away from the eyes during treatment.

Planning and Designing

- Q-switched 1064 nm lasers are chromophore dependent and this wavelength is selectively absorbed by melanin. In addition to collagen remodeling effects which include reduction of wrinkles, acne scars, rough texture, and coarse pores, they are also used for:
  - Dermal hyperpigmentation (such as melasma)
  - Temporary reduction of fine dark hair.
- If these lesions are present in the area for wrinkle reduction, fluences at the lower recommended range

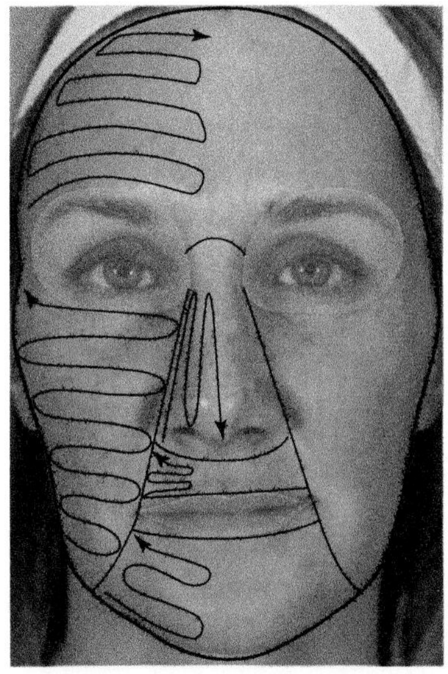

FIGURE 28-4 Handpiece direction for nonablative wrinkle reduction treatments using a Q-switched 1064 nm laser. *(Copyright Rebecca Small, MD.)*

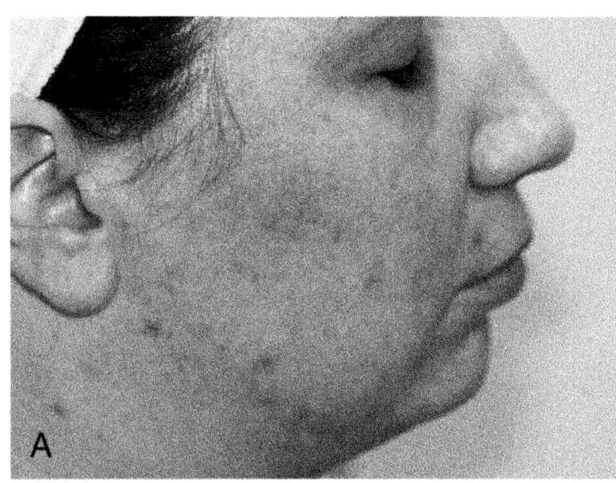

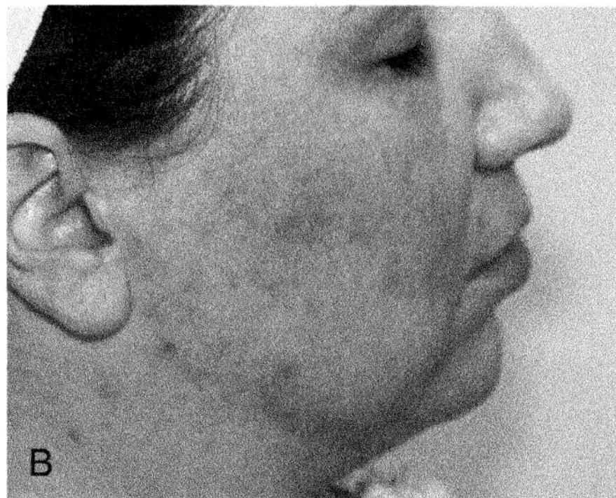

FIGURE 28-5 Clinical endpoint of mild erythema **(A)** before and **(B)** immediately after a nonablative wrinkle reduction treatment using a Q-switched 1064 nm laser. *(Copyright Rebecca Small, MD.)*

(see above) should be used due to the greater amount of target in the skin.

- A 1064 nm wavelength can also reduce fine darkly pigmented hairs. This is an advantage for women with facial hair. However, facial hair reduction may not be desirable in men and this should be discussed prior to treatment.

Anesthesia

Anesthesia is not required for nonablative wrinkle reduction treatments.

Safety Zone

The area within which lasers may be used for wrinkle reduction treatments on the face is called the Nonablative Laser Safety Zone (Figure 28-2). Laser treatments are performed outside of the orbit: above the supraorbital ridge (above the eyebrows) and below the inferior orbital rim, to reduce the risk of ocular injury.

Performing the Procedure

1. Inquire about sun exposure and sunscreen use at every visit. If the patient is recently sun exposed or tan, wait 1 month before treating to reduce the risk of complications.
2. Position the patient supine on a flat treatment table.
3. Cleanse the skin with a nonalcohol wipe.
4. Provide appropriate laser-safe eye protection for the patient and all personnel in the treatment room prior to beginning treatment.
5. Always operate the laser in accordance with your office's laser safety policies and the manufacturer's guidelines.
6. Tattoos and permanent makeup should be covered with wet gauze and the laser tip kept at least 1 inch away from them during treatment.
7. Perform a single pulse at the lateral margin of treatment area 1 and assess for patient tolerance and clinical endpoints (see below). In general, there are subtle endpoints with initial treatments, and pain should be less than or equal to 5 on a scale of 1 to 10.
8. Desirable clinical endpoints include:
    - Fitzpatrick skin types I–III: mild to moderate erythema (Figure 28-5)
    - Fitzpatrick skin types IV–VI: mild or no erythema
    - Pigmented lesion darkening (especially dermal lesions, such as melasma) with enhanced demarcation against the background skin (Figure 28-6)
    - Papular acne lesions: mild to moderate erythema
    - Vaporization of sebum in sebaceous facial areas such as the nose and chin, and areas with coarse pores and comedonal acne (Figure 28-7)
    - Audible snapping sound with laser pulses, loudest over sebaceous areas.
9. Petechiae (see Figure 28-15 later in this chapter) may be seen with aggressive treatment parameters. If these occur during treatment, the fluence should be reduced or the spot size increased to reduce treatment intensity. The treatment may be continued but the petechial area should not receive additional passes.
10. Perform one pass (where a pass is full coverage of the treatment area) to the entire face. If there is mild to no erythema, perform a second pass to the treatment area. In areas with wrinkles, hyperpigmentation, papular acne, or coarse pores, perform up to three to four additional passes, or until the desired endpoints have been reached.
11. Adjust laser settings based on observations of laser/tissue interaction, clinical endpoints, and patient discomfort throughout treatment.
12. At subsequent visits, the intensity of treatments may be increased by either:
    - Increasing the fluence
    - Decreasing the spot size
    - Increasing the number of passes.

    In general, only one parameter is changed to intensify treatments in any given visit. Typically, the fluence or number of passes is increased initially for a few treatments to achieve desired clinical endpoints, and spot size is decreased in later treatments.
13. After treatment, apply a soothing topical nonocclusive product (e.g., SkinCeuticals Epidermal Repair) and broad-spectrum sunscreen (SPF 30

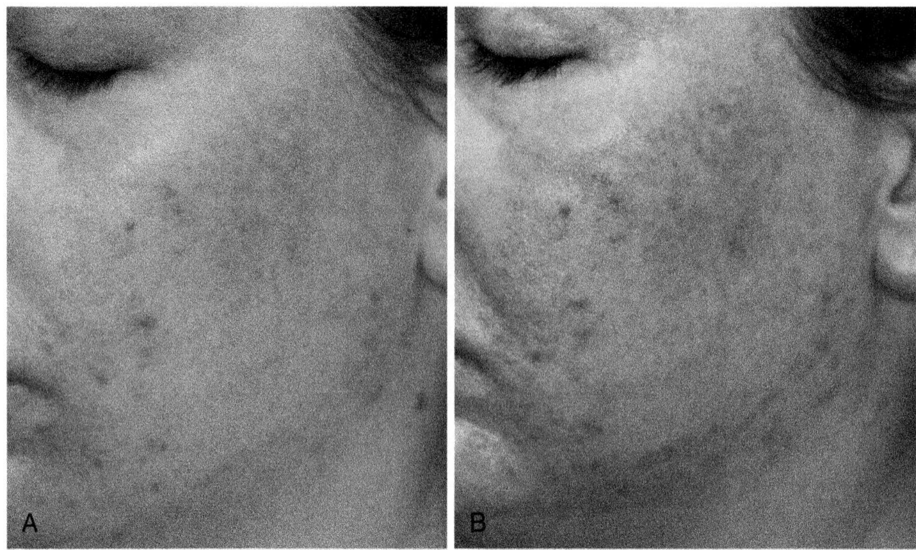

FIGURE 28-6 Clinical endpoint of hyperpigmentation darkening **(A)** before and **(B)** immediately after a nonablative wrinkle reduction treatment using a Q-switched 1064 nm laser. *(Copyright Rebecca Small, MD.)*

with zinc or titanium). If the treatment area is significantly erythematous, hydrocortisone cream 1% to 2.5% may also be applied. Ice is generally not necessary unless there is a reported area of discomfort and should not be used unless needed, because the desired thermal reaction in the skin continues for a short while after treatment and it is terminated upon application of ice.

RESULTS

Treatments are performed in a series, and most nonablative wrinkle reduction lasers show improvements approximately 3 months after the initial treatment, with continued improvements up to 6 months following the last treatment. It is extremely important to inform patients that reduction of mild to moderate wrinkles with nonablative lasers is slow and results vary based on the technology used and with individual patients. Studies of nonablative lasers consistently show histologic improvements with increased numbers of fibroblasts and collagen deposition.[23,52] However, clinical improvements are less predictable and do not always correlate with histologic changes. Figures 28-8 through 28-14 show before and after photos for some of the nonablative wrinkle reduction technologies discussed in the chapter.

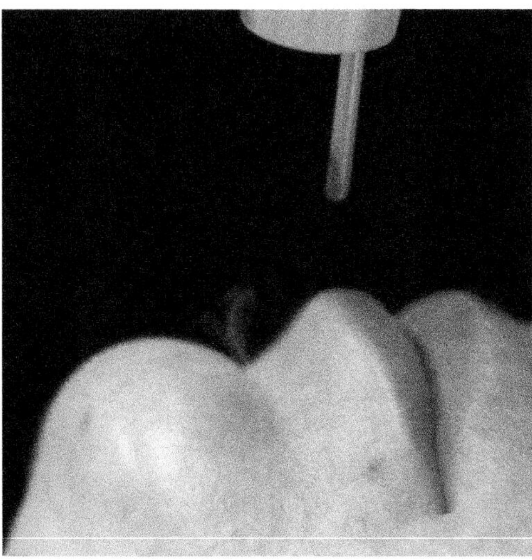

FIGURE 28-7 Clinical endpoint of sebum vaporization on the chin during a nonablative wrinkle reduction treatment using a Q-switched 1064 nm laser. *(Copyright Rebecca Small, MD.)*

Figure 28-8 shows results of nonablative wrinkle reduction treatments for facial rhytids (A) before and (B) after a series of six treatments with a long-pulse 1064 nm Nd:YAG laser (Cutera Laser Genesis™).

Figure 28-9 shows results of nonablative wrinkle reduction treatments for infraocular rhytids (A) before and (B) after a series of treatments with a Q-switched 1064 nm Nd:YAG laser (HOYA ConBio RevLite™).

Figure 28-10 shows wrinkle reduction treatments for cheek rhytids and crow's feet, as well as hyperpigmentation reduction (A) before and (B) after fractional resurfacing treatments using a 1550 nm laser (Solta Fraxel Re:store™).

Figure 28-11 shows results of nonablative collagen remodeling treatments for acne scars (A) before and (B) after fractional resurfacing treatments using a 1550 nm laser (Solta Fraxel Re:store™).

Figure 28-12 shows results of nonablative skin laxity reduction treatments of the lower face (A) before, (B) after 6 months, and (C) after 3 years following a series of RF treatments (Solta Thermage™).

Figure 28-13 shows results of nonablative skin laxity reduction treatments of the neck (A) before and (B) after a series of RF laser treatments (Solta Thermage™).

Figure 28-14 shows results of nonablative skin laxity reduction treatments of the abdomen (A) before and

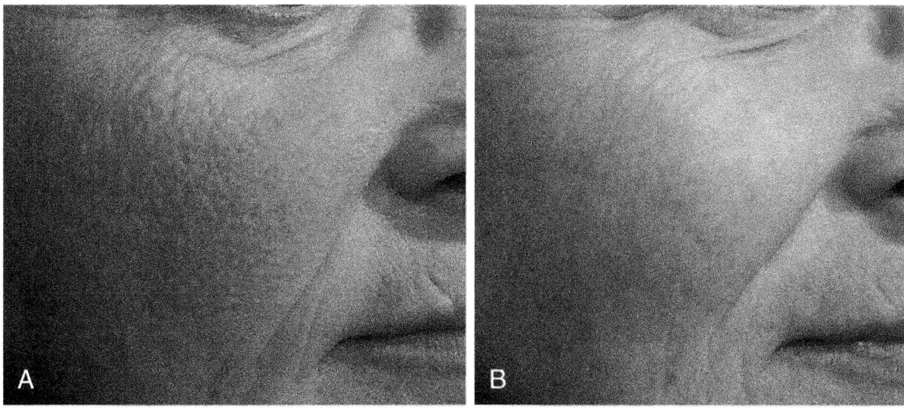

FIGURE 28-8 Facial wrinkles (**A**) before and (**B**) after a series of six treatments with a long-pulse 1064 nm Nd:YAG laser. *(Courtesy of Cutera, Brisbane, CA; laser genesis; photograph by K. Smith.)*

(B) after a series of broadband infrared treatments (Cutera Titan™).

AFTERCARE

Mild swelling and *mild erythema* are expected and usually resolve within 15 minutes to 1 hour after treatment. If patients report areas that feel hot, or have more significant erythema, a wrapped ice pack may be applied for 15 minutes every 1 to 2 hours and hydrocortisone cream 1 to 2½% two times per day for 3 to 4 days or until redness resolves. Patients are instructed to contact their provider if erythema persists for more than 5 days because *postinflammatory hyperpigmentation* (PIH) can occur with prolonged erythema (see complications below). Patients should avoid direct sun exposure for 1 to 2 days after treatment to help minimize the risk of pigmentary changes and use a broad-spectrum sunscreen (SPF 30 with zinc or titanium) daily.

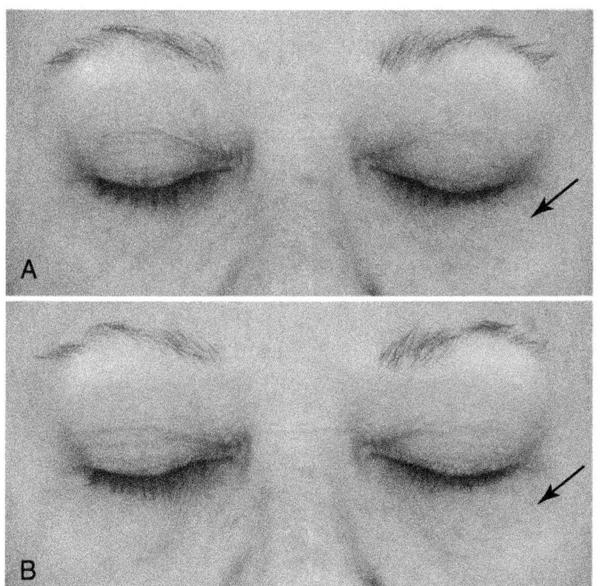

FIGURE 28-9 Infraocular wrinkles (**A**) before and (**B**) after a series of treatments with a Q-switched 1064 nm Nd:YAG laser. *(Courtesy of HOYA ConBio, Fremont, CA; laser toning by D. Goldberg, MD, using RevLite.)*

FOLLOW-UP

Nonablative laser treatments for wrinkle reduction typically require a series of six treatments at monthly intervals for demonstrable improvements, although fewer treatments may be required for fractional lasers. It is generally accepted that results persist for 1 to 2 years. Figure 28-12 shows recurrence of lower face laxity 3 years after RF treatment. Patients may, therefore, want to consider repeating a treatment series every 2 years. Alternatively, because these treatments are so well tolerated and results are cumulative, some providers recommend performing nonablative laser treatments as part of regular skin maintenance at monthly to quarterly intervals.

COMPLICATIONS

- Erythema
- Swelling
- Pain
- Petechiae/purpura (Figure 28-15)
- Urticaria (Figure 28-16)
- Hyperpigmentation
- Hypopigmentation
- Burn with blistering and scabbing
- Scarring (extremely rare)
- Inadequate collagen remodeling effects including lack of reduction of: wrinkles, folds, skin crepiness, laxity, scars, or recurrence after completion of treatments
- Damage or alteration to tattoos and permanent makeup
- Infection (e.g., herpes simplex)
- Hair reduction in or adjacent to the treatment area
- Alteration to dermal filler
- Ocular injury.

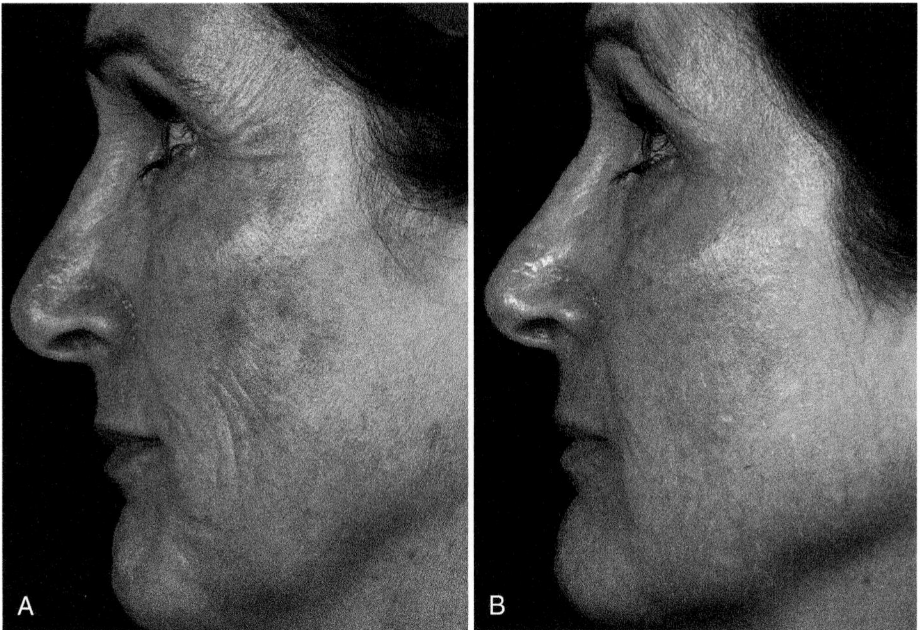

FIGURE 28-10 Cheek wrinkles, crow's feet, and hyperpigmentation (**A**) before and (**B**) after nonablative fractional resurfacing treatments using a 1550 nm laser. *(Courtesy of Solta, Hayward, CA; Z. Rahman, MD, using Fraxel Re:store™.)*

Nonablative laser treatments for wrinkle reduction and skin crepiness have minimal risks of side effects and complications. However, complications are possible with any laser procedure, and knowledge of these is important to help ensure the best possible outcomes.

Mild erythema and *swelling* are to be expected, as mentioned earlier. Prolonged erythema for 5 days or more may result from contact dermatitis, which can occur in response to topical products, and can be managed with a topical steroid such as triamcinolone cream 0.025% two times per day for 1 week and discontinuation of the offending product. Swelling may occur, particularly with aggressive treatment of the cheeks. Cold compresses are recommended as described above and a daily oral antihistamine (e.g., cetirizine 10 mg) until resolved.

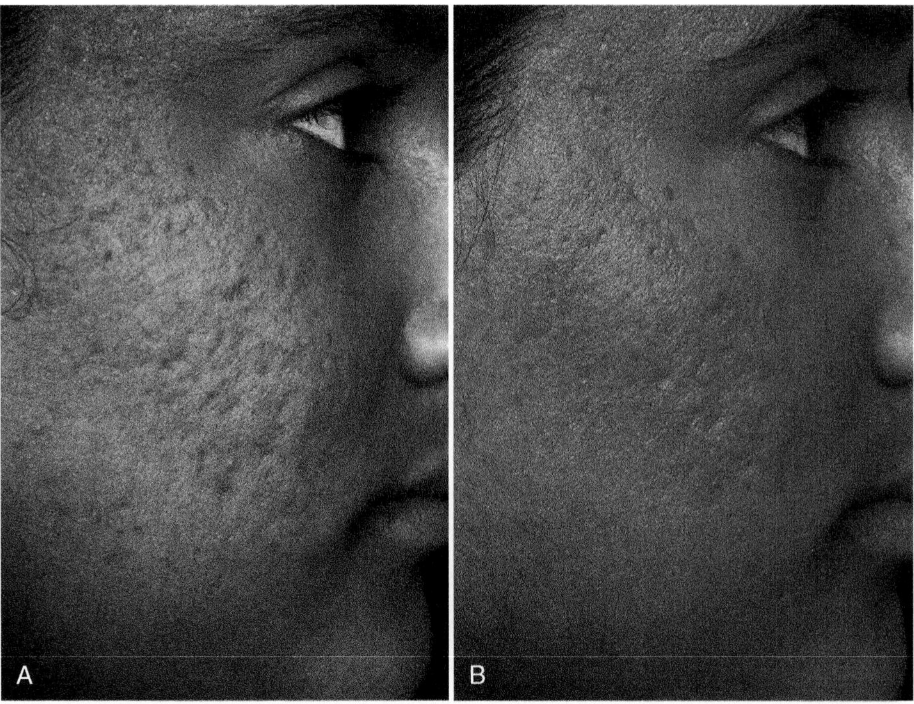

FIGURE 28-11 Acne scars (**A**) before and (**B**) after nonablative fractional resurfacing treatments using a 1550 nm laser. *(Courtesy of Solta, Hayward, CA; Z. Rahman, MD, using Fraxel Re:store™.)*

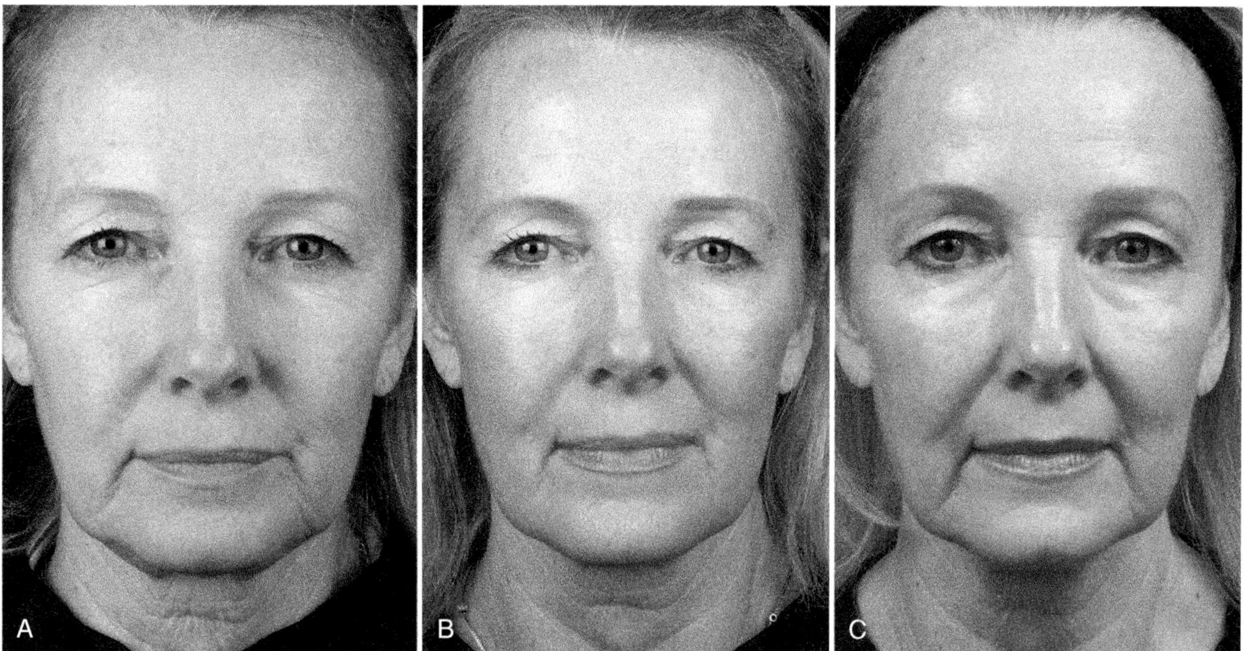

FIGURE 28-12 Skin laxity of the lower face **(A)** before, **(B)** 6 months after, and **(C)** 3 years after a series of RF laser treatments. *(Courtesy of Solta, Hayward, CA; F. Mayoral, MD, using Thermage™.)*

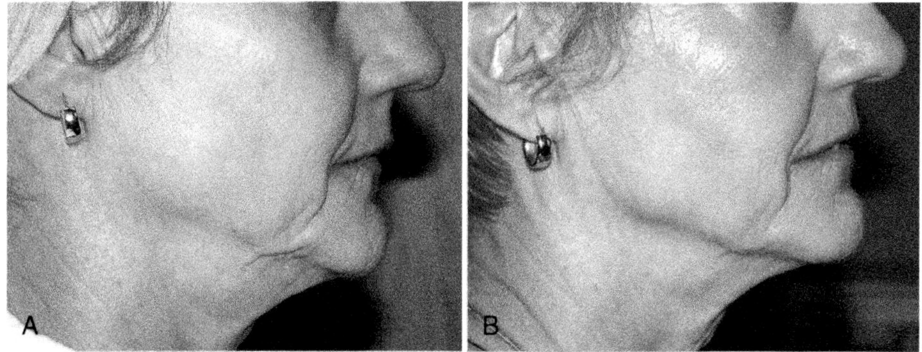

FIGURE 28-13 Skin laxity of the neck **(A)** before and **(B)** after a series of RF laser treatments. *(Courtesy of Solta, Hayward, CA; R. Euwer, MD, using Thermage™.)*

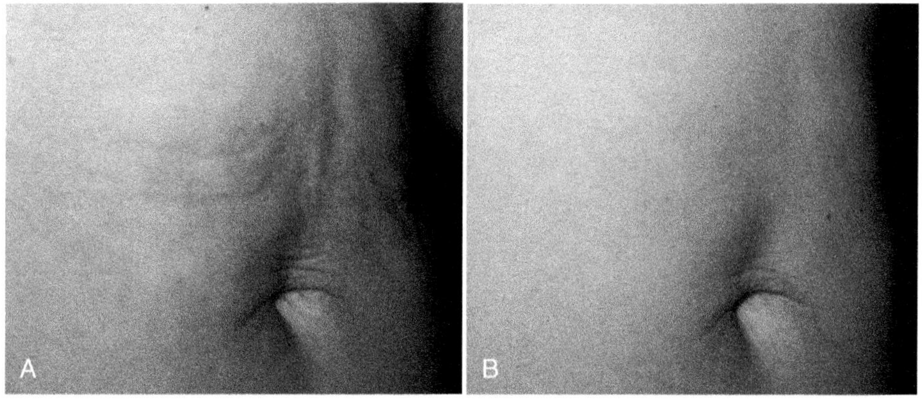

FIGURE 28-14 Skin laxity of the abdomen **(A)** before and **(B)** after a series of broadband IR laser treatments. *(Courtesy of Cutera, Brisbane, CA; J. Calkin, MD, using Titan™.)*

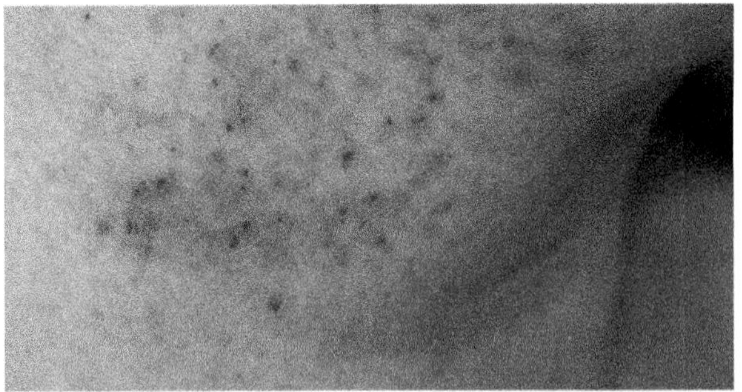

FIGURE 28-15 Petechiae of the neck with a nonablative laser wrinkle reduction treatment. *(Copyright Rebecca Small, MD.)*

Pain is mild and rarely reported to be greater than 4 or 5 (on a standard pain scale of 1 to 10) during treatment; however, RF treatments tend to be uncomfortable and may require premedication with an analgesic such as hydrocodone (Vicodin).

Petechiae may be seen with high fluences particularly in thin-skinned areas such as the neck (Figure 28-15). *Purpura* may occur with shorter wavelength lasers, particularly pulsed dye lasers, and when short pulse widths and/or high fluences are utilized during treatment.[53] Petechiae typically take 3 to 5 days to resolve and purpura can take up to 2 weeks. Utilizing larger spot sizes, lower fluences, and skin compression can reduce the incidence of purpura with devices that are prone to purpura formation.[54]

Rarely, *urticaria* may be seen with lasers (Figure 28-16).[55] This may be treated with cold compresses and an oral antihistamine (e.g., cetirizine 10 mg), which may be continued daily until resolved. Once identified, these patients may be pretreated for subsequent treatments with an antihistamine 1 hour prior to procedure.

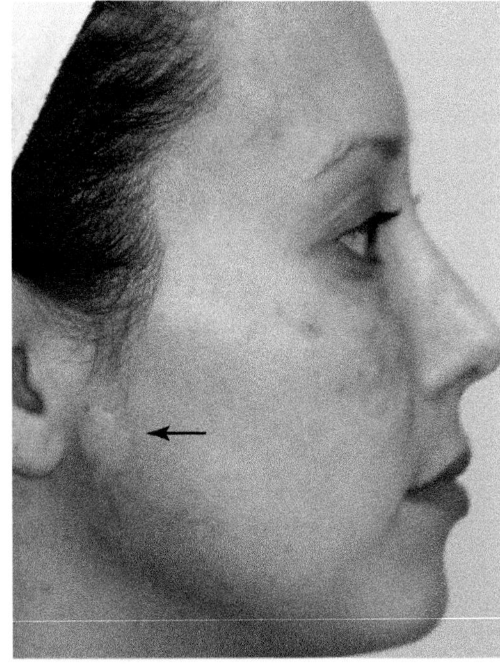

FIGURE 28-16 Preauricular urticaria with a nonablative laser wrinkle reduction treatment. *(Copyright Rebecca Small, MD.)*

Pigmentary complications of *hyperpigmentation* and *hypopigmentation* are rare, but may be seen in darker Fitzpatrick skin types (IV through VI) and patients with a recent tan. These complications are more common with devices that utilize short wavelengths (e.g., 532 nm and pulsed dye lasers) and with laser parameters of short pulse widths and/or high fluences. Inadequate epidermal cooling as well as overly aggressive cooling can also result in pigmentary changes. Hyperpigmentation is usually transient (and rarely may be permanent), lasting on the order of months. Postinflammatory hyperpigmentation has been reported with nonablative fractional devices[56,57] and has been observed as a result of epidermal injury due to overcooling by the cryogen sprays used with some infrared devices.[58] If PIH occurs, patients may use a topical lightening agent such as hydroquinone (4 to 8%) twice daily along with an exfoliating product (such as lactic or glycolic acid) and/or a retinoid. (See Chapter 24, *Skin Care Products*, for more about treatment of PIH.) The use of a lightening agent for 1 month prior to treatment may reduce the risk of PIH, particularly in darker Fitzpatrick skin types. Hypopigmentation is a more significant complication and, although often temporary, may be permanent.

A *burn* and/or *scar* may also occur, particularly with devices that utilize short wavelengths (e.g., 532 nm and pulsed dye lasers),[59,60] aggressive treatment parameters of short pulse widths, and high fluences or inadequate epidermal cooling. In addition, overtreatment can occur when treating above bony prominences because these areas are more prone to the buildup of heat, particularly with the lasers for skin laxity. Routine moist wound care should be used for these complications with application of an antibiotic ointment and bandage until healed. *Tattoos* and *permanent make-up* have concentrated ink pigments and treatment over these may result in a full-thickness skin burn.

Herpes simplex and *varicella zoster* may be reactivated in the treatment area. Pretreatment prophylaxis with an oral antiviral medication can reduce this risk (see the *Procedure Preparation* section earlier in this chapter).

Reduced hair growth in or adjacent to the treatment area may occur. This risk should be fully discussed if treating over men's facial hair.

Alteration to dermal filler is controversial. Although some evidence suggests that lasers do not affect dermal fillers in tissue,[61] other studies recommend using lasers as a treatment for undesired collections of dermal fillers to render them more moldable and reduce their appearance in the skin.[62,63] The author does treat over facial areas with fillers using nonablative lasers but not with ablative lasers.

Ocular injury can be avoided by wearing appropriate laser-safe eyewear at all times during treatment, directing the laser tip away from the eye, and treating outside of the eye orbit.

TREATING SPECIFIC LESIONS/AREAS

Melasma

Laser treatments of melasma may have variable results and in some cases, hyperpigmentation may become worse.

Nonfacial Areas

Nonfacial areas, such as the neck and chest, have fewer pilosebaceous units have delayed healing relative to the face. They have a greater risk of overtreatment and scarring, and it is advisable to treate conservatively in nonfacial areas.

LEARNING THE TECHNIQUE

Initial treatments may be performed on the face with one pass using conservative laser parameters of larger spot sizes and lower fluences in patients with light Fitzpatrick skin types (I through III).

CURRENT DEVELOPMENTS

Combination therapy utilizing nonablative lasers with other minimally invasive aesthetic procedures in the same visit is emerging as a new approach to skin rejuvenation[64] (see Chapter 31, *Combination Cosmetic Treatments*). For example, the author combines a Q-switched 1064 nm nonablative laser treatment for dermal collagen remodeling, with superficial exfoliating procedures such as microdermabrasion and superficial chemical peels, on the same day to enhance wrinkle reduction results without increasing downtime or side effects.

Recent technological improvements in Q-switched devices, such as flat-topped beam profiles, have reduced tissue "hot spots" and the associated risk of petechiae. In addition, novel pulsing modes (e.g., photoacoustic technology pulse) have been developed that allow for greater peak power without additional patient discomfort.[23]

Fractional delivery of energy is a very promising new method of nonablative laser treatments. In addition to reduction of wrinkles and improvements in dyschromia, fractional 1550 nm skin resurfacing treatments have also demonstrated good success with scar reduction.[12,65,66] Modifications to some of the newer 1550 nm fractional devices may reduce the incidence of postinflammatory hyperpigmentation.[8]

Newer approaches to reduction of skin laxity combine monopolar with bipolar radio-frequency, where the RF current travels more superficially in the skin.[67] Some devices combine radio-frequency with light-based technologies for nonablative skin rejuvenation (termed ELOS™, *electro-optical synergy*).[68]

Photomodulation with LEDs is a relatively new, non–thermally mediated method of mild skin rejuvenation. Studies have yet to determine which pulsing modes are most efficacious and compare the different wavelengths. Combining LEDs, or other nonablative laser and light-based modalities, with photosensitizing medications for photodynamic therapy enhances rejuvenation results.[36,69] Combination therapy with PDT and exfoliation treatments, such as microdermabrasion, to enhance penetration of photosensitizing medications may further improve results.[70]

FINANCIAL CONSIDERATIONS

Nonablative laser treatments for wrinkles are not reimbursable by insurance companies. The charges for treatments vary, and are largely determined by local prices. Individual treatment prices range from $200 to $500 for a single treatment to a large area such as the face, and $150 to $300 for a small area such as the neck. However, because wrinkle reduction treatments are most effective with a series of treatments, packages of treatments (usually six) may be offered so that patients achieve the best possible results. Box 28-1 lists the applicable ICD-9 codes.

CONCLUSION

Nonablative wrinkle reduction laser technologies are a heterogeneous group, but are all similar in that they induce dermal collagen remodeling with collagen synthesis while maintaining an intact epidermis. They are gentle enough to be combined with other minimally invasive procedures and can be readily integrated into office-based aesthetic care. With advances in the methods of delivery and greater energies delivered to the skin, nonablative lasers continue to improve and expand their role in rejuvenation of photodamaged skin.

Resources

Aerolase
Phone: 877-379-2435
www.aerolase.com

Alma Lasers
866-414-ALMA
www.almalasers.com

Asclepion Laser Technologies
www.asclepion.com

BOX 28-1 *ICD-9 Codes*

695.3	Rosacea
701.8	Wrinkling of skin
706.1	Acne, comedones
709.0	Dyschromia, unspecified
709.09	Melasma
709.2	Scarring

CoolTouch
Phone: 877-858-COOL
www.cooltouch.com

Cutera
Phone: 888-4-CUTERA
www.cutera.com

Cynosure/Deka
Phone: 800-886-2966
www.cynosure.com

DermaMed USA
Phone: 888-789-6342
www.dermamedusa.com

Dinona
Phone: +82-2-578-0810
www.dinonainc.com

Energist
www.energist-international.com

Enlyten Medical Technologies
Phone: 877-365-9836
www.enlyten-mt.com

Focus Medical
Phone: 866-633-5273
www.focusmedical.com

HOYA ConBio
Phone: 800-532-1064
www.conbio.com

Iridex
Phone: 650-940-4700
www.iridex.com

Lasering
Phone: 866-471-0469
www.laseringusa.com

Light BioScience
Phone: 803-409-8025
www.gentlewaves.com

Lumenis
Phone: 408-764-3000
www.lumenis.com

Lutronic
Phone: 888-588-7644
www.lutronic.com

Med-Aesthetic Solutions
Phone: 760-942-8815
www.medaestheticsolutions.com

Novalis
Phone: 866-627-4475
www.novalismedical.com

Palomar
Phone: 800-725-6627
www.palomarmedical.com

Sciton
Phone: 888-646-6999
www.sciton.com

Solta Medical
Phone: 877-782-2286
www.solta.com

Syneron (formerly Candela)
Phone: 866-259-6661
www.syneron.com

References

1. Liu H, Dang Y, Wang Z, *et al.* Laser induced collagen remodeling: a comparative study in vivo on mouse model. *Lasers Surg Med.* 2008;40(1):13–19.
2. Goldberg DJ. Nonablative resurfacing. *Clin Plast Surg.* 2000; 27(2):287–292, xi.
3. Anderson RR, Parrish JA. Selective photothermolysis: precise microsurgery by selective absorption of pulsed radiation. *Science.* 1983;220(4596):524–527.
4. Lloyd JR. Effect of fluence on efficacy using the 1440 nm laser with CAP technology for the treatment of rhytids. *Lasers Surg Med.* 2008;40(6):387–389.
5. Goldberg DJ. Full-face nonablative dermal remodeling with a 1320 nm Nd:YAG laser. *Dermatol Surg.* 2000;26(10):915–918.
6. Fournier N, Dahan S, Barneon G, *et al.* Nonablative remodeling: a 14-month clinical ultrasound imaging and profilometric evaluation of a 1540 nm Er:glass laser. *Dermatol Surg.* 2002;28(10): 926–931.
7. Paithankar DY, Clifford JM, Saleh BA, *et al.* Subsurface skin renewal by treatment with a 1450-nm laser in combination with dynamic cooling. *J Biomed Opt.* 2003;8(3):545–551.
8. Narurkar VA. Nonablative fractional resurfacing for total body rejuvenation. *J Drugs Dermatol.* 2008;7(4):352–355.
9. Manstein D, Herron GS, Sink RK. Fractional photothermolysis: a new concept for cutaneous remodeling using microscopic patterns of thermal injury. *Lasers Surg Med.* 2004;34:426–438.
10. Rahman Z, Alam M, Dover JS. Fractional laser treatment for pigmentation and texture improvement. *Skin Therapy Lett.* 2006;11(9):7–11.
11. Tannous Z. Fractional resurfacing. *Clin Dermatol.* 2007;25(5): 480–486.
12. Tierney EP, Kouba DJ, Hanke CW. Review of fractional photothermolysis: treatment indications and efficacy. *Dermatol Surg.* 2009;35(10):1445–1461.
13. Zelickson BD, Kilmer SL, Bernstein E, *et al.* Pulsed dye laser therapy for sun damaged skin. *Lasers Surg Med.* 1999;25(3): 229–236.
14. Goldberg DJ. New collagen formation after dermal remodeling with an intense pulsed light source. *J Cutan Laser Ther.* 2000;2(2):59–61.
15. Carniol PJ, Farley S, Friedman A. Long-pulse 532-nm diode laser for nonablative facial skin rejuvenation. *Arch Facial Plast Surg.* 2003;5(6):511–513.
16. Dayan SH, Vartanian AJ, Menaker G, *et al.* Nonablative laser resurfacing using the long-pulse (1064-nm) Nd:YAG laser. *Arch Facial Plast Surg.* 2003;5(4):310–315.
17. Dayan S, Damrose JF, Bhattacharyya TK, *et al.* Histological evaluations following 1,064-nm Nd:YAG laser resurfacing. *Lasers Surg Med.* 2003;33(2):126–131.
18. Lee MW. Combination visible and infrared lasers for skin rejuvenation. *Semin Cutan Med Surg.* 2002;21(4):288–300.
19. Goldberg DJ, Silapunt S. Histologic evaluation of a Q-switched Nd:YAG laser in the nonablative treatment of wrinkles. *Dermatol Surg.* 2001;27(8):744–746.

20. Cisneros JL, Rio R, Palou J. The Q-switched neodymium (Nd):YAG laser with quadruple frequency. Clinical histological evaluation of facial resurfacing using different wavelengths. *Dermatol Surg.* 1998;24(3):345–350.
21. Lee MC, Hu S, Chen MC, *et al.* Skin rejuvenation with 1,064-nm Q-switched Nd:YAG laser in Asian patients. *Dermatol Surg.* 2009;35(6):929–932.
22. Goldberg DJ, Silapunt S. Q-switched Nd:YAG laser: rhytid improvement by non-ablative dermal remodeling. *J Cutan Laser Ther.* 2000;2(3):157–160.
23. Berlin AL, Dudelzak J, Hussain M, *et al.* Evaluation of clinical, microscopic, and ultrastructural changes after treatment with a novel Q-switched Nd:YAG laser. *J Cosmet Laser Ther.* 2008;10(2): 76–79.
24. Friedman PM, Jih MH, Skover GR, *et al.* Treatment of atrophic facial acne scars with the 1064-nm Q-switched Nd:YAG laser: six-month follow-up study. *Arch Dermatol.* 2004;140(11): 1337–1341.
25. Yaghmai D, Garden JM, Bakus AD, *et al.* Photodamage therapy using an electro-optic Q-switched Nd:YAG laser. *Lasers Surg Med.* 2009;42(8):699–705.
26. Kilmer SL, Lee MS, Grevelink JM, *et al.* The Q-switched Nd:YAG laser effectively treats tattoos. A controlled, dose-response study. *Arch Dermatol.* 1993;129(8):971–978.
27. Cho SB, Kim JS, Kim MJ. Melasma treatment in Korean women using a 1064-nm Q-switched Nd:YAG laser with low pulse energy. *Clin Exp Dermatol.* 2009;34(8):e847–850.
28. Cho SB, Park SJ, Kim JS, *et al.* Treatment of post-inflammatory hyperpigmentation using 1064-nm Q-switched Nd:YAG laser with low fluence: report of three cases. *J Eur Dermatol Venereol.* 2009;23(10):1206–1207.
29. Anderson RR, Margolis RJ, Watenabe S, *et al.* Selective photothermolysis of cutaneous pigmentation by Q-switched Nd:YAG laser pulses at 1064, 532, and 355 nm. *J Invest Dermatol.* 1989;93(1):28–32.
30. Bakus AD, Garden JM, Yaghmai D, Massa MC. Long-term fine caliber hair removal with an electro-optic Q-switched Nd:YAG laser. *Laser Surg Med.* 2010;42(8):706–711.
31. Weiss RA, McDaniel DH, Geronemus RG, *et al.* Clinical experience with light-emitting diode (LED) photomodulation. *Dermatol Surg.* 2005;31(9 Pt 2):1199–1205.
32. Goldberg DJ, Amin S, Russell BA, *et al.* Combined 633-nm and 830-nm LED treatment of photoaging skin. *J Drugs Dermatol.* 2006;5(8):748–753.
33. Kennedy JC, Pottier RH, Pross DC. Photodynamic therapy with endogenous protoporphyrin IX: basic principles and present clinical experience. *J Photochem Photobiol B.* 1990;6(1–2):143–148.
34. Dover JS, Bhatia AC, Stewart B, *et al.* Topical 5-aminolevulinic acid combined with intense pulsed light in the treatment of photoaging. *Arch Dermatol.* 2005;141(10):1247–1252.
35. Uebelhoer NS, Dover JS. Photodynamic therapy for cosmetic applications. *Dermatol Ther.* 2005;18(3):242–252.
36. Alster TS, Tanzi EL, Welsh EC. Photorejuvenation of facial skin with topical 20% 5-aminolevulinic acid and intense pulsed light treatment: a split-face comparison study. *J Drugs Dermatol.* 2005;4(1):35–38.
37. Bjerring P, Christiansen K, Troilius A, *et al.* Skin fluorescence controlled photodynamic photorejuvenation (wrinkle reduction). *Lasers Surg Med.* 2009;41(5):327–336.
38. Kaufman J. Lasers and light devices. *In:* Baumann L, ed. *Cosmetic Dermatology.* New York: McGraw-Hill; 2009:212–220.
39. Dierickx CC. The role of deep heating for noninvasive skin rejuvenation. *Lasers Surg Med.* 2006;38(9):799–807.
40. Carniol PJ, Dzopa N, Fernandes N, *et al.* Facial skin tightening with an 1100–1800 nm infrared device. *J Cosmet Laser Ther.* 2008;10(2):67–71.
41. Goldberg DJ, Hussain M, Fazeli A, *et al.* Treatment of skin laxity of the lower face and neck in older individuals with a broad-spectrum infrared light device. *J Cosmet Laser Ther.* 2007;9(1):35–40.
42. Chan HH, Yu CS, Shek S, *et al.* A prospective, split face, single-blinded study looking at the use of an infrared device with contact cooling in the treatment of skin laxity in Asians. *Lasers Surg Med.* 2008;40(2):146–152.
43. Sukal SA, Geronemus RG. Thermage: the nonablative radiofrequency for rejuvenation. *Clin Dermatol.* 2008;26(6):602–607.
44. Sadick NS, Makino Y. Selective electro-thermolysis in aesthetic medicine: a review. *Lasers Surg Med.* 2004;34(2):91–97.
45. Alam M, Dover JS. Nonablative laser and light therapy: an approach to patient and device selection. *Skin Therapy Lett.* 2003;8(4):4–7.
46. Manuskiatti W, Wachirakaphan C, Lektrakul N, *et al.* Circumference reduction and cellulite treatment with a TriPollar radiofrequency device: a pilot study. *J Eur Dermatol Venereol.* 2009;23(7): 820–827.
47. Dover JS, Zelickson B. Results of a survey of 5,700 patient monopolar radiofrequency facial skin tightening treatments: assessment of a low-energy multiple-pass technique leading to a clinical end point algorithm. *Dermatol Surg.* 2007;33(8):900–907.
48. Branson DF. Dermal undermining (scarification) of active rhytids and scars: enhancing the results of CO(2) laser skin resurfacing. *Aesth Surg J.* 1998;18(1):36–37.
49. Goldberg DJ, Whitworth J. Laser skin resurfacing with the Q-switched Nd:YAG laser. *Dermatol Surg.* 1997;23(10):903–906.
50. Chernoff WG. Nonexfoliating laser rejuvenation of facial rhytids. *In:* Keller GS, Lacombe VG, Lee PK, Watson JP, eds. *Lasers in Aesthetic Surgery.* New York: Thieme; 2001:139–148.
51. Zelickson B, Ross EV, Strasswimmer J. Definition and proposed mechanisms of non-invasive skin tightening. *In:* Alam M, Dover J, eds. *Non-Surgical Skin Tightening and Lifting.* Philadelphia: Elsevier; 2009:3–7.
52. Goldberg DJ. Non-ablative subsurface remodeling: clinical and histologic evaluation of a 1320-nm Nd:YAG laser. *J Cutan Laser Ther.* 1999;1(3):153–157.
53. Travelute AC, Carniol PJ, Hruza GJ. Laser treatment of facial vascular lesions. *Facial Plast Surg.* 2001;17(3):193–201.
54. Galeckas KJ, Ross EV, Uebelhoer NS. A pulsed dye laser with a 10-mm beam diameter and a pigmented lesion window for purpura-free photorejuvenation. *Dermatol Surg.* 2008;34(3): 308–313.
55. England R. Immediate cutaneous hypersensitivity after treatment of tattoo with Nd:YAG laser: a case report and review of the literature. *Ann Allergy Asthma Immunol.* 2002;(89):215–217.
56. Chan HH, Manstein D, Yu CS, *et al.* The prevalence and risk factors of post-inflammatory hyperpigmentation after fractional resurfacing in Asians. *Lasers Surg Med.* 2007;39(5):381–385.
57. Fisher GH, Geronemus RG. Short-term side effects of fractional photothermolysis. *Dermatol Surg.* 2005;31(9 Pt 2):1245–1249.
58. Lee SJ, Park SG, Kang JM, *et al.* Cryogen-induced arcuate shaped hyperpigmentation by dynamic cooling device. *J Eur Dermatol Venereol.* 2008;22(7):883–884.
59. Gaston DA, Clark DP. Facial hypertrophic scarring from pulsed dye laser. *Dermatol Surg.* 1998;24(5):523–525.
60. Wlotzke U, Hohenleutner U, bd-El-Raheem TA, *et al.* Side-effects and complications of flashlamp-pumped pulsed dye laser therapy of port-wine stains. A prospective study. *Br J Dermatol.* 1996; 134(3):475–480.
61. Shumaker PR, England LJ, Dover JS, *et al.* Effect of monopolar radiofrequency treatment over soft-tissue fillers in an animal model: part 2. *Lasers Surg Med.* 2006;38(3):211–217.
62. Lemperle G, Rullan PP, Gauthier-Hazan N. Avoiding and treating dermal filler complications. *Plast Reconstr Surg.* 2006;118 (3 Suppl):92S–107S.
63. Hirsch RJ, Narurkar V, Carruthers J. Management of injected hyaluronic acid induced Tyndall effects. *Lasers Surg Med.* 2006;38(3):202–204.
64. Effron C, Briden ME, Green BA. Enhancing cosmetic outcomes by combining superficial glycolic acid (alpha-hydroxy acid) peels with nonablative lasers, intense pulsed light, and trichloroacetic acid peels. *Cutis.* 2007;79(1 Suppl Combining):4–8.
65. Alster TS, Tanzi EL, Lazarus M. The use of fractional laser photothermolysis for the treatment of atrophic scars. *Dermatol Surg.* 2007;33(3):295–299.
66. Behroozan DS, Goldberg LH, Dai T, *et al.* Fractional photothermolysis for the treatment of surgical scars: a case report. *J Cosmet Laser Ther.* 2006;8(1):35–38.
67. Mayoral FA. Skin tightening with a combined unipolar and bipolar radiofrequency device. *J Drugs Dermatol.* 2007;6(2): 212–215.

68. Hammes S, Greve B, Raulin C. Electro-optical synergy (ELOS) technology for nonablative skin rejuvenation: a preliminary prospective study. *J Eur Dermatol Venereol.* 2006;20(9):1070–1075.
69. Gold MH, Bradshaw VL, Boring MM, *et al.* Split-face comparison of photodynamic therapy with 5-aminolevulinic acid and intense pulsed light versus intense pulsed light alone for photodamage. *Dermatol Surg.* 2006;32(6):795–801.
70. Nootheti PK, Gold MH, Goldman MP. Photodynamic therapy for photorejuvenation. *In:* Goldman MP, ed. *Photodynamic Therapy.* Philadelphia: Saunders/Elsevier; 2008:125–135.

Additional Reading

Costello G. Lasers and pulsed-light devices: skin tightening (Chap 51). *In:* Pfenninger JL, Fowler GC, eds. *Pfenninger and Fowler's Procedures for Primary Care.* 3rd ed. Philadelphia: Mosby/Elsevier; 2011.

Small R. Non-ablative modalities for wrinkles. *In:* Small R, ed. *A Practical Guide to Cosmetic Lasers.* Philadelphia: Lippincott; 2012.

Stampar M. Non-ablative radiowave skin tightening (Chap 52). *In:* Pfenninger JL, Fowler GC, eds. *Pfenninger and Fowler's Procedures for Primary Care.* 3rd ed. Philadelphia: Mosby/Elsevier; 2011.

29 Skin Resurfacing with Ablative Lasers

KEN YU, MD • REBECCA SMALL, MD • COREY MAAS, MD

Ablative laser resurfacing is one of the most effective therapies available for wrinkle reduction. This is an aggressive method of skin resurfacing whereby water in the skin is heated and vaporized by laser energy, causing a controlled injury to the epidermis and dermis. It is most commonly performed using either carbon dioxide (CO_2) or erbium:yttrium aluminum garnet (Er:YAG) lasers. Traditional ablative laser resurfacing deeply penetrates the skin (up to 300 μm), and because the epidermis is fully ablated, it is associated with prolonged recovery times, and may have serious complications of infection, hypopigmentation, and scarring[1] and, hence, is rarely performed today. Less aggressive superficial ablative treatments (ranging in depth from 20 to 50 μm) are still commonly performed, particularly for reduction of dyschromia and mild wrinkles.[2] Superficial ablative laser resurfacing is also referred to as a *laser peel*.

In 2004, a novel method of *fractional* resurfacing, which involves treating only a portion or "fraction" of the skin, was introduced.[3] Fractional devices deliver laser energy to the skin in microscopic columns, also called *microthermal zones*. This delivery method allows for very deep penetration in the skin (up to 1.5 μm). Figure 29-1 shows a comparison between deep fractional microthermal zones and "conventional" horizontal plane resurfacing.

The untreated adjacent tissue between microthermal zones serves as a reservoir of regenerative cells that migrate into the treatment area and facilitate rapid wound healing. Fractional ablative resurfacing has been shown to effectively reduce wrinkles and improve dyschromia in photoaged skin and has the advantages of reduced recovery time and reduced risks compared to conventional ablative laser resurfacing.[4–6]

LASER PRINCIPLES

Ablative lasers achieve wrinkle reduction through the use of water as the target chromophore to heat and vaporize tissue. The two main laser wavelengths used for ablative resurfacing, 2940 nm (Er:YAG) and 10,600 nm (carbon dioxide), are well absorbed by water. A third, less frequently used wavelength is 2790 nm (yttrium scandium gallium garnet or YSGG). Figure 29-2 shows the water absorption spectrum and these three ablative resurfacing lasers. Note that the erbium 2940 nm wavelength is at a water absorption peak and is approximately 15 times more highly absorbed by water than CO_2.

Absorbed laser energy has two main effects on tissue: (1) removal of tissue, called *ablation*, and (2) heat transference to surrounding tissue, called *coagulation*. Coagulation clinically results in tissue tightening. A controlled amount of coagulation with treatments is, therefore, desirable but too much thermal injury can be associated with complications such as hypopigmentation and scarring. Due to a greater absorption by water, Er:YAG lasers ablate tissue at lower fluences (approximately 1 J/cm^2), compared to CO_2 lasers, which require higher fluences to achieve similar ablation (approximately 5 J/cm^2). Er:YAG lasers, therefore, cause less thermal damage to the surrounding tissues and have smaller zones of coagulation than CO_2 lasers. Figure 29-3 shows the zones of coagulation around a region of ablation with a CO_2 versus an erbium laser. The amount of ablation and coagulation is controlled by *laser fluence* and *pulse width* (see Chapter 19, *Aesthetic Principles and Consultation*, for a discussion of laser parameters). Ablation is most effectively achieved with short pulse widths and high fluences, whereas coagulation is achieved with longer pulse widths and lower fluences (Figure 29-4). By varying these two parameters, ablative laser devices can independently control the amounts of ablation and coagulation achieved.

Laser *fluence* is also a major determinant of the depth of injury with fractional ablative devices, where higher fluences penetrate deeper. *Density* settings control the percentage of skin that is treated. More aggressive fractional ablative treatments are, therefore, achieved with high fluences and high density parameters. Some fractional devices utilize scanners and computer software to "randomly" deliver pulses within a set pattern so that the pulses are not adjacent to one another. Changing the energy delivery pattern from sequential to nonadjacent pulses allows for high energies to be delivered without the effects of bulk heating.[7] This is particularly useful with CO_2 devices which cause greater thermal injury.

In summary, fractional ablative laser devices have variable fluences, spot sizes, spot densities, and pulse widths, all of which affect the depth of penetration as well as the degree of ablation and coagulation achieved.[8] Because these devices are still relatively new, clinical correlation is required to determine how these different parameters impact results, downtime, and side effects.

PATIENT SELECTION

Fitzpatrick skin type classification is an important factor in assessing patients for laser resurfacing (see Chapter 19, *Aesthetic Principles and Consultation*, for skin type classification). The ideal patient has a fair complexion (Fitzpatrick types I through III) with lesions responsive to laser ablation (see the *Indications* section below). Patients with darker complexions (Fitzpatrick types IV and V) may be treated as well, but must be informed about their higher risk for pigmentary complications and the need for more cautious treatment parameters, which

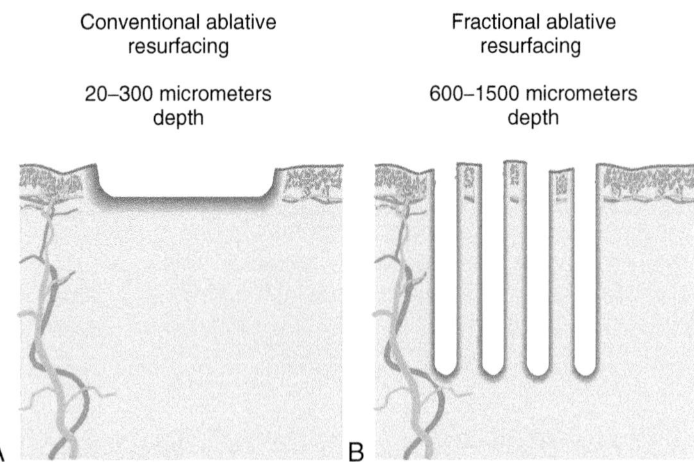

FIGURE 29-1 Ablative laser patterns of injury: (A) conventional "horizontal plane" and (B) fractional.

may limit results. Although patients with Fitzpatrick skin type V may be candidates, in reality these patients rarely present with the facial aging signs that patients with lighter skin types complain of, and one rarely encounters such a patient seeking facial resurfacing. It is advisable for providers getting started with fractional ablative resurfacing to limit treatments to lighter skin types (I through III).

It is also very important that patients have realistic expectations regarding results. Fractional ablative laser resurfacing can generally improve wrinkles, however, significant skin laxity and sagging jowls may be better addressed with surgery, such as a facelift. Patients must fully understand the ablative laser postoperative recovery course and agree to comply with the postprocedure instructions. Re-epithelialization following fractional ablative laser treatments typically requires 5 to 7 days. Patients must be able to tolerate this recovery period, and anticipated professional and social obligations should be considered with patient selection and timing of the procedure.

Patients often seek laser resurfacing to improve wrinkles near the lower eyelids and significant improvements may be achieved in this area. However, there are certain contraindications to treatment in this area including prior lower blepharoplasty and poor lower eyelid skin elasticity.

INDICATIONS[9,10]

- Static rhytids (wrinkles)
- Acne scars
- Atrophic scars
- Benign pigmented lesions (e.g., lentigines)
- Certain epidermal and dermal lesions including actinic keratoses, seborrheic keratoses, sebaceous hyperplasia, syringomas.

Ablative laser resurfacing has traditionally been used for patients with more advanced signs of facial aging (Glogau stage IV) including generalized static wrinkles, keratoses, severe dyschromia, sallow color, and coarse pores (see Chapter 19 for a discussion of the Glogau photoaging scale). With the advent of fractional technologies that have more rapid recovery times and fewer

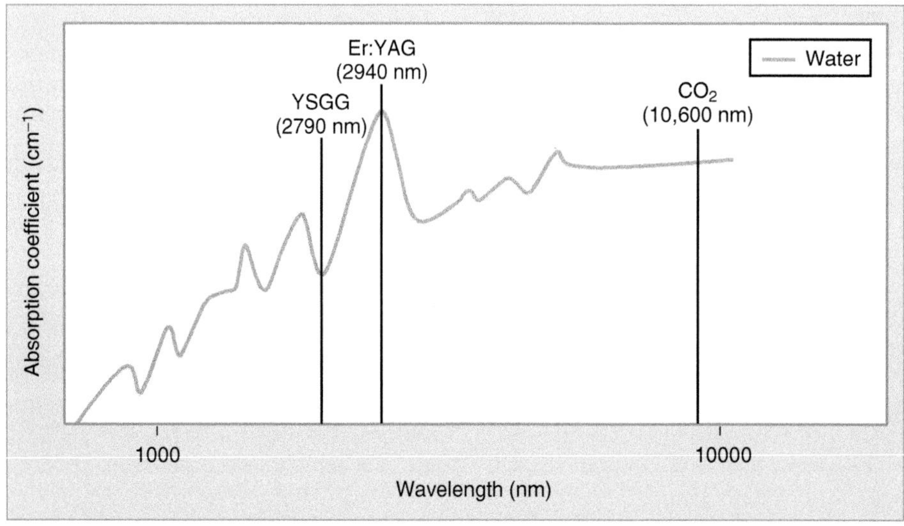

FIGURE 29-2 Water absorption spectrum and common ablative skin resurfacing lasers.

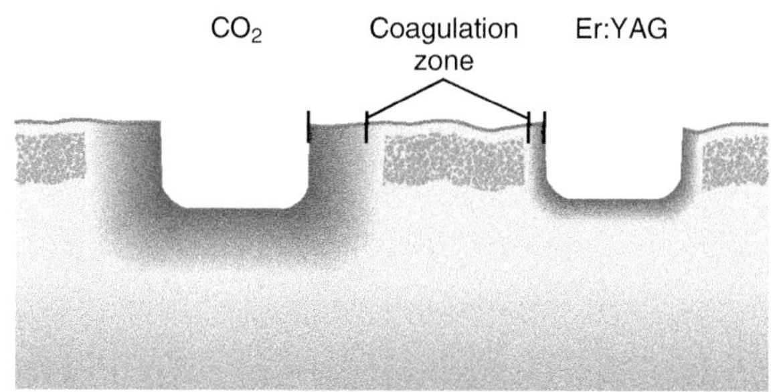

FIGURE 29-3 CO_2 and Er:YAG coagulation zones around ablated skin.

risks, ablative laser procedures are being performed in patients with less severe photoaging. Nonetheless, the most common indication today for fractional ablative laser resurfacing is still moderate to severe wrinkles as well as scars.

Although ablative lasers are indicated for treatment of pigmentation, patients presenting with only pigmented lesions without concerns about wrinkles and textural changes, may benefit from other less aggressive options, such as nonablative lasers, which maintain an intact epidermis, have minimal risks and little to no recovery time.

ALTERNATIVE THERAPIES

Skin resurfacing can also be accomplished by mechanical exfoliation procedures such as *microdermabrasion* and *chemical peeling* treatments which typically penetrate to the epidermis or upper reticular dermis (see Chapter 22, Chemical Peels and Chapter 23, Microdermabrasion). *Dermabrasion* is a mechanical, "cold steel" method of removing epidermis, papillary, or upper reticular dermis. Dermabrasion and chemical peeling have the advantage of being less expensive than laser resurfacing. However, extensive hands-on experience in a preceptor environment is required in order to learn the art of dermabrasion.[11]

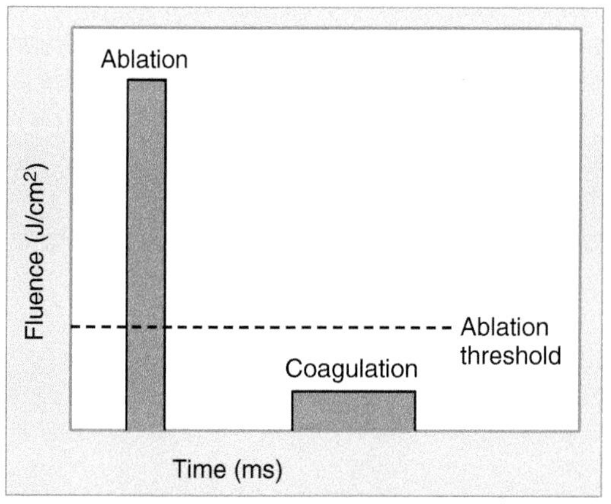

FIGURE 29-4 Ablation and coagulation with ablative lasers.

PRODUCTS CURRENTLY AVAILABLE

Fractional ablative lasers are a relatively new class of lasers. Three main wavelengths are used for these technologies:

1. 10,600 nm: carbon dioxide (CO_2)
2. 2940 nm: erbium: yttrium aluminum garnet (Er:YAG)
3. 2790 nm: yttrium scandium gallium garnet (YSGG).

See the *Resources* section at the end of the chapter for a list of manufacturers of devices that have these wavelengths.

CONTRAINDICATIONS

See the *General Laser Contraindications* section in Chapter 26, *Hair Reduction with Lasers.* Additional contraindications include the following:

- Fitzpatrick skin type VI
- Prior aggressive skin resurfacing within 1 year (e.g., dermabrasion or deep chemical peel)
- Prior radiation therapy in the treatment area
- Unwilling to adhere to preprocedure and/or postprocedure instructions (e.g., unwilling to perform post-procedure wound care)
- Resurfacing treatments near the lower eyelid are contraindicated in the presence of ectropion, significant eyelid laxity (indicated by an abnormal lower eyelid "snap test"), or prior lower blepharoplasty.

ADVANTAGES OF LASER RESURFACING

- Multiple conditions treated simultaneously with high efficacy
- Ongoing improvements post-treatment with continued collagen remodeling and wrinkle reduction.

DISADVANTAGES OF LASER RESURFACING

- Significant recovery time relative to nonablative laser treatments
- Greater potential for infection, hypopigmentation, and scarring complications compared to nonablative lasers
- Expensive.

ANATOMY

Superficial nonfractionated ablative laser treatments typically wound and remove the epidermis (up to 50 μm or 0.05 mm). *Deep nonfractionated* ablative laser treatments typically wound the papillary and upper reticular dermis (up to 300 µm or 0.3 mm) and remove the entire epidermis. *Fractional* ablative lasers penetrate into the deep reticular dermis (up to 1500 µm or 1.5 mm) and remove a portion of the epidermis.

EQUIPMENT

Anesthesia—Intraoral Nerve Blocks

- 3.0- and 5.0-mL Luer-Lok tip syringes
- Lidocaine HCl 2% with epinephrine 1:100,000
- 18-gauge 1.5-inch needles
- 30-gauge 1-inch needles.

Anesthesia—Topical

- Alcohol wipes
- Benzocaine/lidocaine/tetracaine (20:6:4) ointment or other topical anesthetic.

Anesthesia—Assistive External Device

- Cool air blower (optional but recommended).

See Chapter 20, *Anesthesia for Cosmetic Procedures*, and Chapter 3, *Anesthesia*, for more information.

Procedure

- Fractional ablative laser
- Smoke evacuator with tubing
- Gloves
- Gauze
- Alcohol wipes to prep the skin
- Laser-safe eyewear for patient, provider, and all other personnel in the room
- Mask with eye shield for provider and all personnel in the room.

Postprocedure

- Gauze
- Tap water or normal saline, 1000 mL
- Bowl
- Gloves
- Large soft ice packs
- Fan
- Towels (soft, thin muslin are preferable)
- Petrolatum-based topical product (e.g., Aquaphor or SkinCeutical's Primacy).

PROCEDURE PREPARATION

The following guidelines are based on fractional ablative laser resurfacing treatments for Fitzpatrick skin types I through III. Manufacturer guidelines for the specific device used should be followed at the time of treatment.

One Month Prior

1. Perform an aesthetic consultation and review the patient's medical history (see Chapter 19, *Aesthetic Principles and Consultation*) including history of postinflammatory hyperpigmentation, hypertrophic or keloidal scarring, blepharoplasty, previous skin resurfacing and when.
2. Patients should receive thorough counseling regarding proper post-treatment care and potential adverse effects. (See Appendix A for a patient information handout titled *Fractional Ablative Laser Resurfacing*.)
3. Determine the Fitzpatrick skin type (see Chapter 19).
4. Perform a lower eyelid "snap test" to assess for skin elasticity if planning resurfacing near the lower eyelid. Resurfacing over inelastic skin in the lower eyelid area is associated with ectropion.[12]
   - A skin "snap test" is performed by pulling the lower eyelid skin down and assessing skin recoil. If the lower eyelid skin does not briskly return to its normal resting position within 3 seconds after its release, then laser resurfacing near the lower eyelid margin should be avoided.
5. Begin use of topical products to prepare the skin (see next section) and sun avoidance.

Preprocedure Skin Care Products

Preprocedure products typically contain retinoids, alpha hydroxy acids, antioxidants such as vitamin C, sunscreens, and, for patients prone to hyperpigmentation, skin lightening agents such as hydroquinone or a cosmeceutical such as kojic acid, arbutin, niacinamide, or azelaic acid are also used.[13] The goal for using these products is to condition the skin and create a healthier pretreatment epidermis and dermis, thereby promoting more rapid healing postprocedure. Although prescription-strength retinoids have traditionally been used preprocedure,[14] some physicians recommend using less irritating retinoids such as retinol or retinaldehyde.[15]

Preprocedure skin care for ablative laser treatments should be started 1 month prior to the procedure and discontinued 1 week prior to the procedure to ensure a fully intact epidermis at the time of treatment. In darker Fitzpatrick skin types (III or higher), topical lightening agents, such as hydroquinone 4% to 8%, are commonly used pretreatment (see Chapter 24, *Skin Care Products*, for preprocedure treatment regimes).

One Week Prior

1. Obtain informed consent (see Chapter 19; also see Appendix A for an informed consent form and patient information handout titled *Fractional Ablative Laser Resurfacing*).
2. Review written postprocedure wound care *instructions* and products and encourage patient to obtain all necessary supplies (see the *Resources* section at the end of the chapter).
3. Take pretreatment photographs (see Chapter 19).
4. Schedule postprocedure appointments.
5. Give the patient prescriptions for medications to be taken prior to the procedure. These medications may include:
   - An antiviral if the patient has a prior history of herpes simplex or varicella in or near the

treatment area (e.g., valacyclovir 500 mg 1 tablet twice daily) for 2 days prior to the procedure continued for 3 to 10 days postprocedure.
- An anxiolytic or analgesic (see below) to be taken on the day of treatment if needed.

6. Patients are instructed to discontinue use of aspirin, vitamin E, St. John's wort and other dietary supplements including ginkgo biloba, evening primrose oil, garlic, feverfew, and ginseng for 2 weeks prior to treatment to reduce the risk of bleeding. Other nonsteroidal anti-inflammatory medications and alcohol consumption should also be discontinued 2 days prior to treatment.
7. Remind the patient to bring sun-protective clothing (wide-brimmed hat and scarf) on the day of the procedure.

Day of Treatment

Ask the patient to:

1. Remember to take pretreatment medications 1 hour prior to the procedure.
2. Eat a snack 1 hour before the procedure. *Note:* If the patient has not eaten prior to the procedure offer food to help sustain blood sugar.
3. Remove contact lenses.
4. Wash the face and remove all makeup.

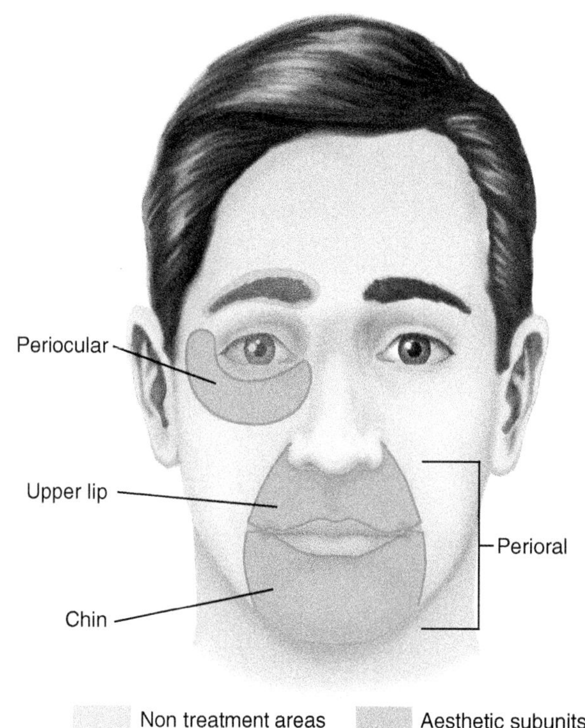

FIGURE 29-5 Fractional Ablative Laser Resurfacing Safety Zone and common facial aesthetic subunits treated.

FRACTIONAL ABLATIVE LASER RESURFACING: STEPS AND PRINCIPLES

The following guidelines are based on treatments of the full face using a fractional ablative erbium 2940 nm laser (Hoya ConBio DermaSculpt™), which is indicated for Fitzpatrick skin types I through III. Manufacturer guidelines for the specific device used should be followed at the time of treatment.

General Treatment Technique

1. Uniform coverage of the treatment area is important so as not to leave any untreated "skip" areas. This can be achieved by performing treatment to the entire area (called one pass) and ensuring that pulses are adjacent. The degree of recommended overlap and number of passes vary according to the specific device used.
2. The laser tip distance guide should be in contact with the skin when pulsing the laser.
3. Thin-skinned areas such as the periocular region require more conservative settings with lower density and lower fluence than the other areas of the face.

Planning and Designing

Ablative laser resurfacing may be performed to a region of the face or to the entire face. Figure 29-5 shows three of the most commonly treated facial aesthetic subunits (modified from Gonzales-Ulloa[16]). The *periocular subunit* is bounded inferiorly by the crest of the zygoma and superiorly by the orbital rim. The *upper lip subunit* extends laterally to the nasolabial folds and superiorly to the nose. The chin subunit extends along the line of the nasolabial fold inferiorly, below the jaw line. The *perioral subunit* includes the upper lip and chin subunits.

Anesthesia

Significant pain is associated with fractional ablative resurfacing and patients complain of a buildup of heat which is maximal at the end of the treatment. Adequate anesthesia will not only give the patient a more pleasant experience, but also assists the provider in reaching the goals settings for a given treatment.

Types of anesthesia used for fractional ablative resurfacing include:

- *Topical anesthetics* with the stronger formulations such as BLT (benzocaine 20% : lidocaine 6% : tetracaine 4%) under occlusion or Pliaglis (lidocaine 7% and tetracaine 7%) for 45 minutes.
  CAUTION: Take care in the periocular area to avoid intraocular inoculation. If this occurs, flush copiously with saline.[17]
- *Regional nerve block.* An infraorbital nerve block is helpful when treating the sensitive upper lip area. If using this block, topical anesthesia does not need to be applied to the upper lip area.

- *Analgesic devices.* A noncontact cool air blower can be used in addition to these other methods and is most useful toward the end of the treatment when patients are most uncomfortable.
- *Oral anxiolytic* and/or *analgesic medication.* In some patients, it may be helpful to give one dose 1 hour prior to the procedure of:
  - An anxiolytic, such as diazepam (Valium) 10 mg and/or
  - An analgesic, such as tramadol (Ultram), 50 to 100 mg 1 tablet, or hydrocodone with acetaminophen (Vicodin 5/500).

  CAUTION: Patients taking any opioids or anxiolytics will require a driver to take them home after completing the procedure

See Chapter 20, *Anesthesia for Cosmetic Procedures,* for more information.

Safety Zone

The Fractional Ablative Laser Safety Zone for treatments on the face includes the entire face apart from the area within the orbital rims, eyebrows, and the lips (Figure 29-5). Providers with advanced ablative laser skills may choose to treat over the eyelids with conservative settings using intraocular lead eye shields. However, it is recommended that providers getting started with this procedure restrict their treatment to the area outside of the orbital rim.

Performing Fractional Ablative Laser Resurfacing

1. Position the patient supine with the treatment table flat. The physician should be seated in a comfortable position relative to the patient.
2. Remove all topical anesthetic.
3. Prepare the skin with an alcohol or astringent.
4. Provide appropriate laser eye protection for the patient and all personnel in the treatment room prior to beginning treatment.
5. Always operate the laser in accordance with your office's laser safety policies and the manufacturer's guidelines.
6. Before treatment, direct a test spot to a tongue depressor to confirm laser functioning as well as desired treatment pattern and density.
7. Have the assistant position the smoke evacuator near the area to be treated, approximately 3 to 4 inches above the skin (Figure 29-6).

   TIP: Take care to avoid contacting the skin with the smoke evacuator because this makes a loud noise and can be startling. Also take care not to bump the laser.
8. Perform a single pulse near the lateral margin of the treatment area and assess for patient tolerance and clinical endpoints (see below).
9. Desirable clinical endpoints include:
   - White dots in the shape selected (Figure 29-6)
   - Background erythema (Figure 29-6)
   - Pain level less than or equal to 6 on a scale of 1 to 10.
10. Pinpoint bleeding (Figure 29-7) may be evident with aggressive treatments.

    TIP: Lasers used with pure ablation and no coagulation are more likely to cause bleeding.

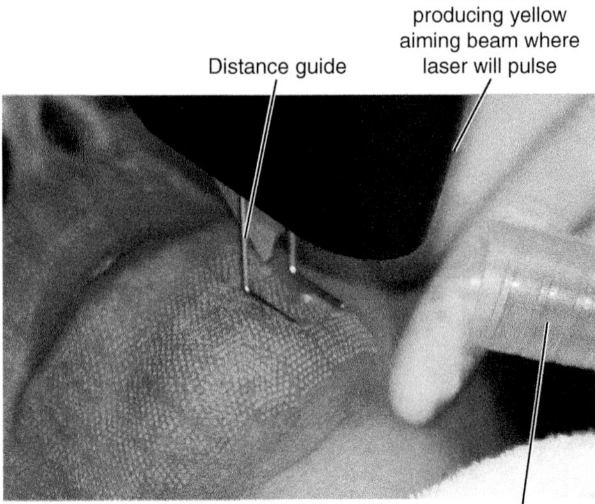

FIGURE 29-6 Clinical endpoints for fractional ablative resurfacing with crisp white laser spots and background erythema. Smoke evacuator postition is also shown. *(Copyright Rebecca Small, MD.)*

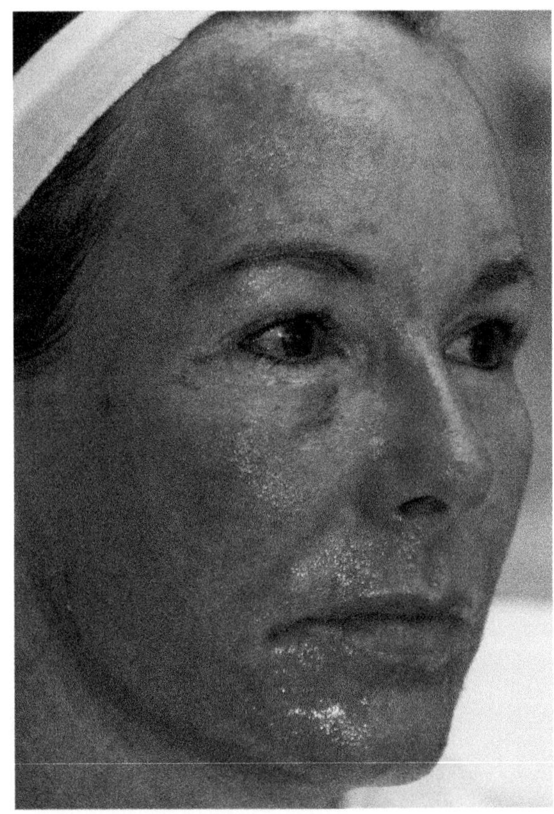

FIGURE 29-7 Clinical endpoints for fractional ablative resurfacing of pinpoint bleeding and erythema. *(Copyright Rebecca Small, MD.)*

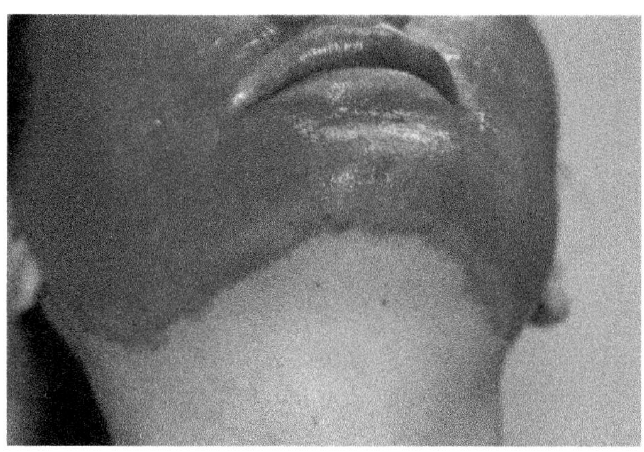

FIGURE 29-8 Ablative laser treatments on the lower face extend under the jaw line. *(Copyright Rebecca Small, MD.)*

11. Adjust laser settings based on observations of laser/tissue interaction, clinical endpoints, and patient discomfort throughout treatment.
12. Perform treatment of the entire area.
13. When treating near the jaw line, extend treatment under the jaw (Figure 29-8).
14. Blend the treatment area with adjacent untreated areas by reducing settings around the periphery of the treated area.
15. Upon completion of the treatment, patients are often uncomfortably hot and it is important to cool them down rapidly. Carefully apply wrapped ice packs to the face and/or use a cool air blower.
16. Apply an occlusive topical ointment to the treatment area (such as SkinCeutical's Primacy).

RESULTS

Fractional ablative lasers (CO_2 and Er:YAG) can significantly improve wrinkles and hyperpigmentation in photoaged skin.[4,5,18–20] Wrinkle reduction can be seen in the immediate post-treatment period, once re-epithelialization occurs, and continues to improve up to 6 months after treatment. The presumed mechanism for textural improvement is through thermally induced collagen denaturation and shrinkage immediately after treatment, with delayed fibroblast proliferation and synthesis of new collagen, also called *dermal collagen remodeling*.[21]

Laser resurfacing also plays an important role in reduction of scars. Blending scar borders with the surrounding skin, and improving pigment changes in the scar can help achieve excellent camouflage. Fractional ablative lasers have showed success with scar reduction, primarily atrophic acne scars.[22,23]

Figure 29-9 shows the results of deep ablative laser resurfacing for facial wrinkles (A) before and (B) after one treatment using an erbium laser to a 120 μm depth (Sciton Contour TRL™).

Figure 29-10 shows the results of fractional ablative laser resurfacing for facial wrinkles (A) before and (B) after one treatment using a carbon dioxide laser (Fraxel Re:pair™).

Figure 29-11 shows the results of fractional ablative laser resurfacing for facial wrinkles and pigmentation (A) before and (B) after one treatment using a carbon dioxide laser (Fraxel Re:pair™).

Figure 29-12 shows the results of fractional ablative laser resurfacing for perioral wrinkles (A) before and (B) after one treatment using a carbon dioxide laser (Lumenis TotalFX™).

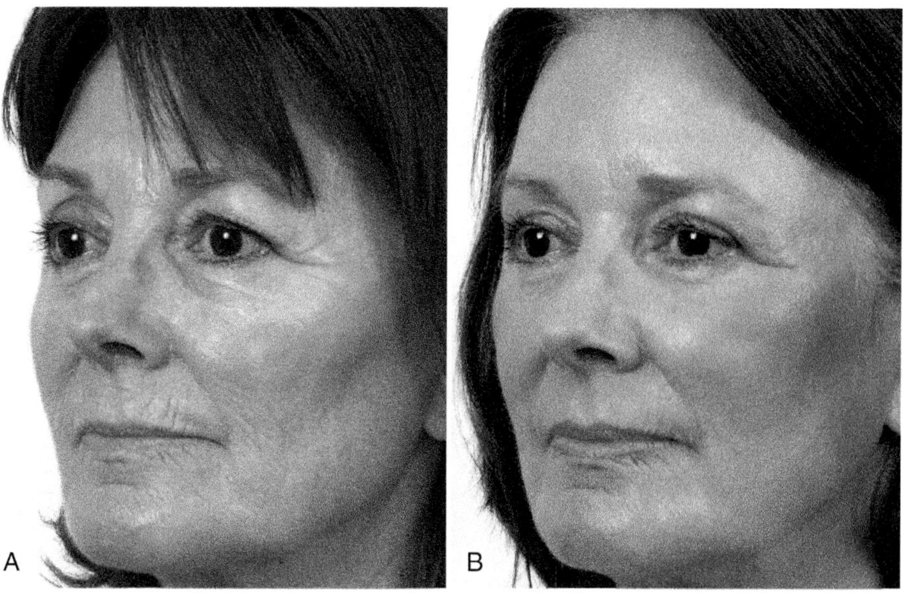

FIGURE 29-9 Deep ablative laser resurfacing for facial wrinkles **(A)** before and **(B)** after one treatment to a 120-μm depth with an erbium laser. *(Courtesy of L. Apostolakis, MD, using Sciton Contour TRL™.)*

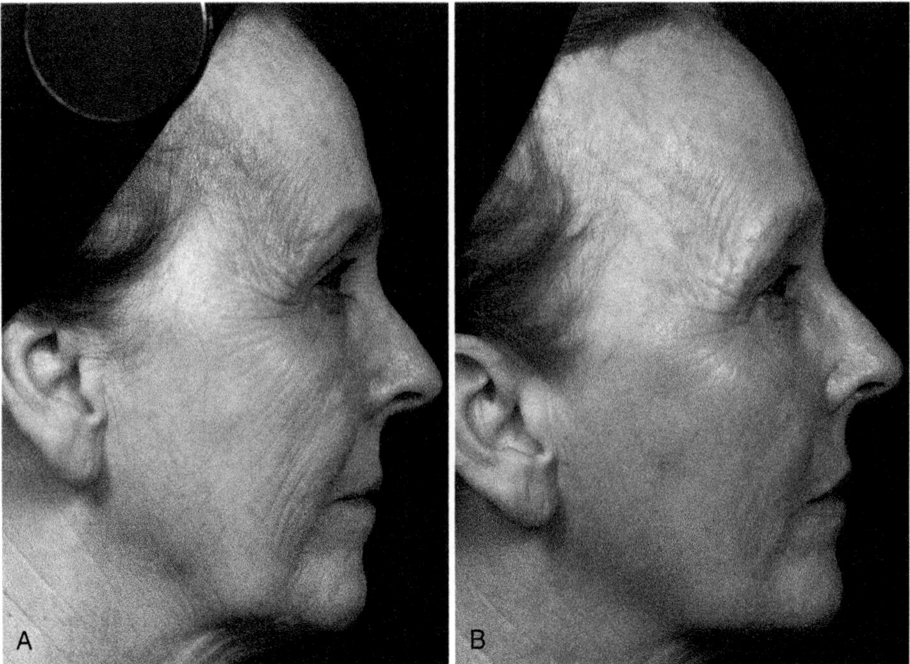

FIGURE 29-10 Fractional ablative laser resurfacing for facial wrinkles (**A**) before and (**B**) after one treatment with a carbon dioxide laser. *(Courtesy of Z. Rahman, MD, using Fraxel Re:pair™.)*

Figure 29-13 shows the results of fractional ablative laser resurfacing for facial wrinkles (A) before and (B) after one treatment using an erbium laser (Sciton Profractional-XC™).

Figure 29-14 shows the results of fractional ablative laser resurfacing for periocular wrinkles (A) before and (B) after one treatment using an erbium laser (Palomar Lux2940™).

Figure 29-15 shows the results of fractional ablative laser resurfacing for acne scarring (A) before and (B) after five treatments using an erbium laser (Sciton Profractional-XC™).

Figure 29-16 shows the results of fractional ablative laser resurfacing for actinic keratoses (A) before and (B) after two treatments using an erbium laser (Sciton Profractional™).

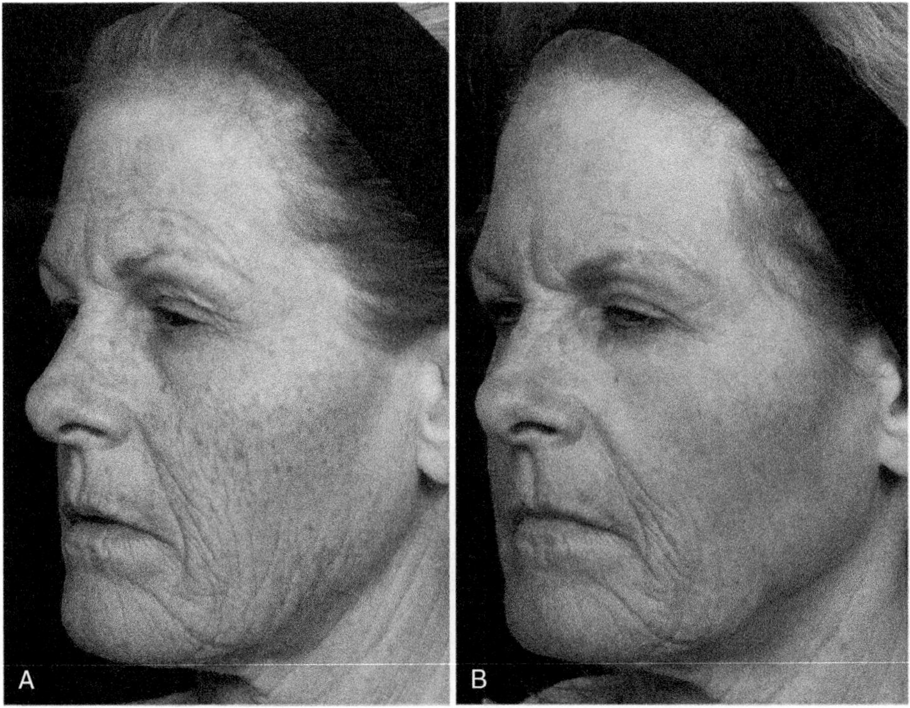

FIGURE 29-11 Fractional ablative laser resurfacing for facial wrinkles and pigmentation (**A**) before and (**B**) after one treatment with a carbon dioxide laser. *(Courtesy of Z. Rahman, MD, using Fraxel Re:pair™.)*

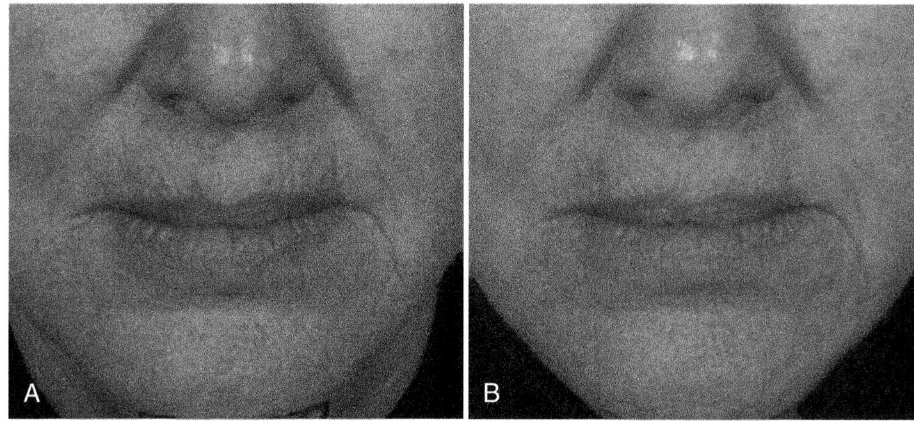

FIGURE 29-12 Fractional ablative laser resurfacing for perioral wrinkles **(A)** before and **(B)** after treatment with a carbon dioxide laser. *(Courtesy of G. Munavalli, MD, using Lumenis TotalFX™.)*

Figure 29-17 shows the results of superficial ablative laser resurfacing for solar lentigines (A) before and (B) after one treatment using an erbium laser to a 50-µm depth (Sciton Contour TRL™ MicroLaserPeel™).

Figure 29-18 shows the results of precision ablative laser resurfacing for seborrheic keratoses (A) before and (B) after one treatment using an erbium laser (HOYA ConBio Dermasculpt™ Chisel Touch™).

AFTERCARE

Fractional ablative laser treatments have *two distinct phases of healing:*

- Open wound, lasting 4 to 7 days
- Postepithelialization, lasting 3 weeks.

The open wound stage starts from the time of treatment and persists until full re-epithelialization takes place. This typically takes 4 to 7 days, with erbium lasers trending toward shorter recovery times.[24] Figure 29-19 shows the recovery process for a fractional ablative erbium laser resurfacing treatment on the face of a 41-year-old woman 1 day postprocedure (Figure 29-19A), where the treatment area is an open wound with intense erythema, some serous oozing, crusting, and pinpoint bleeding. By the fourth postprocedure day (Figure 29-19B), the treatment area is almost fully re-epithelialized, showing mild erythema with a few open areas. On day 5, this patient had fully re-epithelialized.

Open wound care consists of gentle rinsing of the treatment area with dilute acetic acid (vinegar) soaks several times a day (see the patient information handout titled *Fractional Ablative Laser Resurfacing* in Appendix A). Some providers alternatively use gentle facial rinsing with warm soapy water several times a day. Figure 29-20 shows a patient the day after fractional ablative erbium resurfacing (A) prior to and (B) immediately after a vinegar cleanse. Note the devitalized, brown tissue and crusting has been removed to reveal healthy pink tissue after cleansing. Pinpoint bleeding may occur during the cleansing process, which is not undesirable. Cleansing is followed by application of an occlusive ointment such as Aquaphor, Crisco,[25] or Primacy to promote moist wound healing. Some providers use nonocclusive products that promote wound healing, such as Biafine, during this phase.[26] Excessive or prolonged use of occlusive topical products may increase the risk of milia, folliculitis, acne, and bacterial or candidal infections, whereas too little product may result in crusting and delayed re-epithelialization. During the

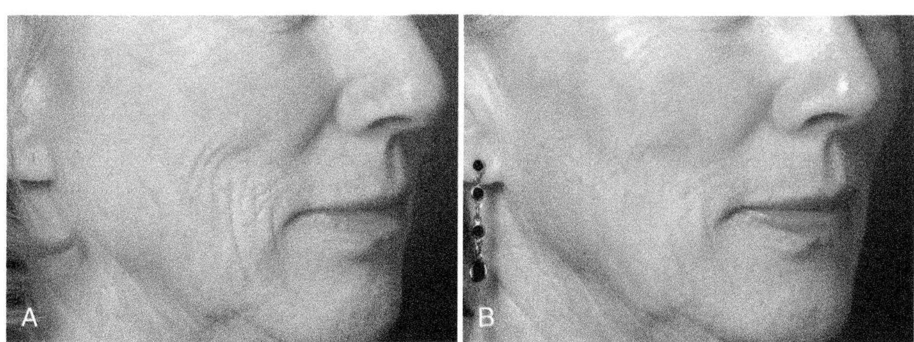

FIGURE 29-13 Fractional ablative laser resurfacing for facial wrinkles **(A)** before and **(B)** after one treatment with an erbium laser. *(Courtesy of K. Remington, MD, using Sciton Profractional-XC™.)*

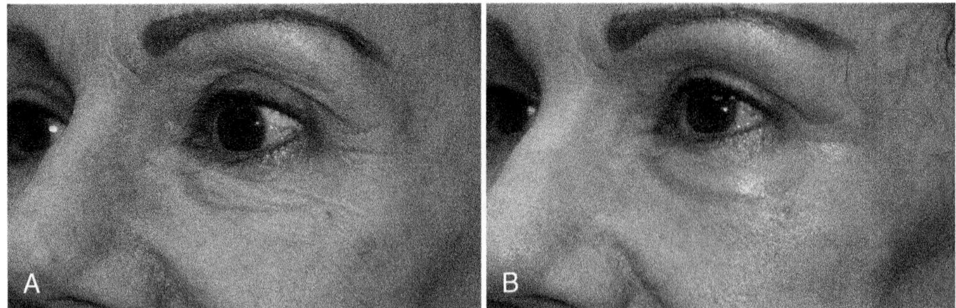

FIGURE 29-14 Fractional ablative laser resurfacing for periocular wrinkles **(A)** before and **(B)** after one treatment with an erbium laser. *(Copyright Rebecca Small, MD, using Palomar Lux2940™.)*

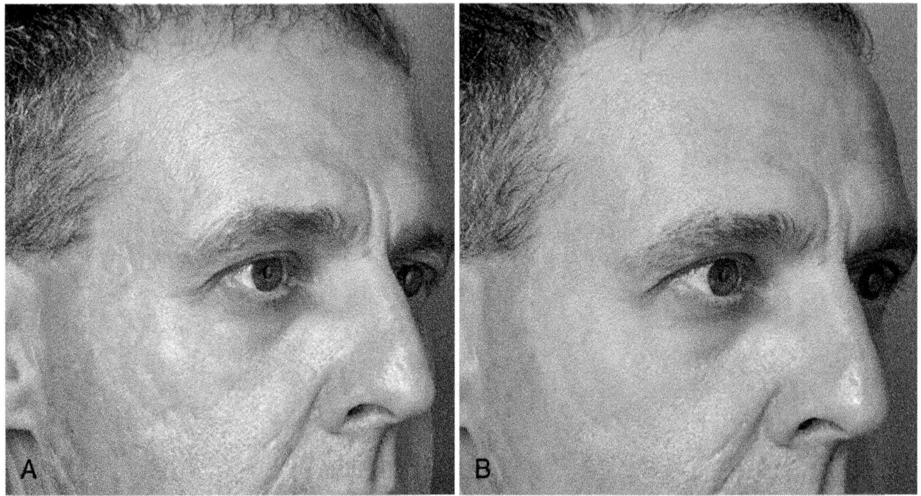

FIGURE 29-15 Fractional ablative laser resurfacing for acne scarring **(A)** before and **(B)** after five treatments with an erbium laser. *(Courtesy of K. Remington, MD, using Sciton Profractional-XC™.)*

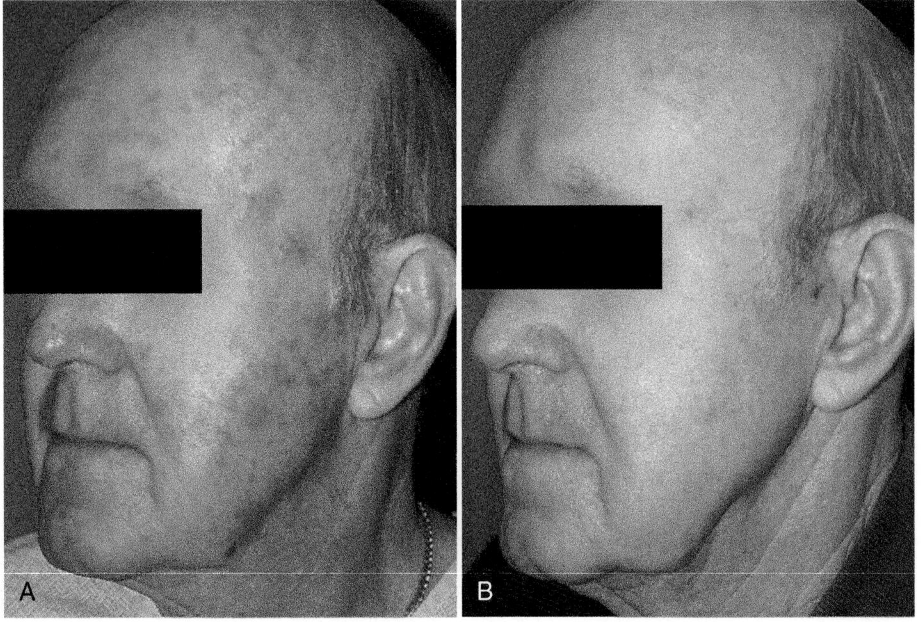

FIGURE 29-16 Fractional ablative laser resurfacing for actinic keratoses **(A)** before and **(B)** after two treatments with an erbium laser. *(Courtesy of R. Koch, MD, using Sciton Profractional™.)*

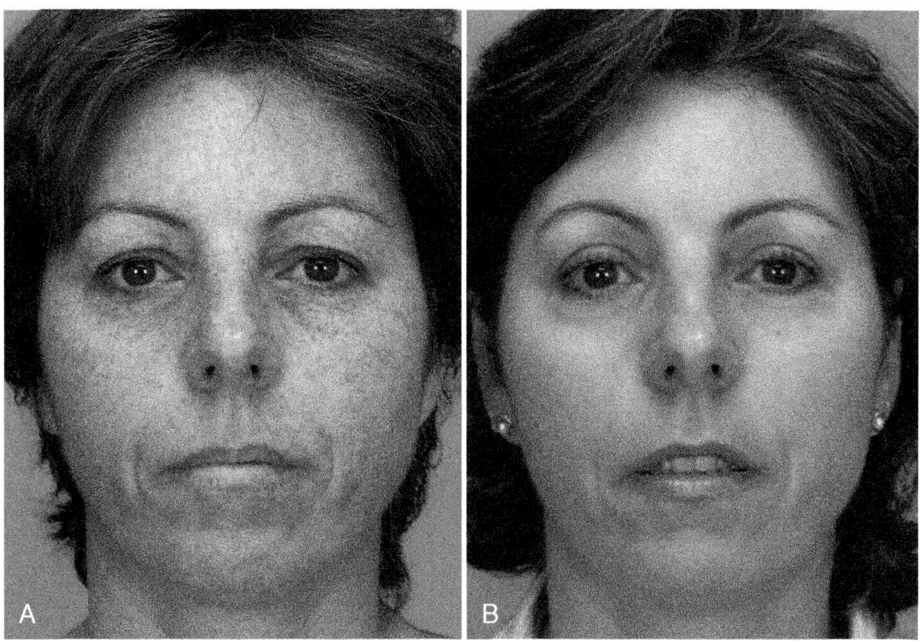

FIGURE 29-17 Superficial ablative laser resurfacing for solar lentigines **(A)** before and **(B)** after one treatment to a 50-μm depth with an erbium laser. *(Courtesy of J. Pozner, MD, using Sciton Contour TRL™ MicroLaserPeel™.)*

open wound phase, no sunscreen or makeup is worn and strict sun avoidance is imperative to reduce the risk of hyperpigmentation.

The postepithelialization stage commences once the open wound has healed and the epidermis is fully intact. This stage typically starts 1 week postprocedure and persists for 3 weeks. Skin is mildly erythematous and more sensitive than at baseline. Occlusive products are discontinued and products that are nonirritating and reparative, such as SkinCeutical's Epidermal Repair, may be used in addition to sunscreen. Mineral makeup may be applied at this time to camouflage any remaining erythema.

It is advisable to avoid aesthetic procedures such as chemical peels, microdermabrasion, dermaplaning, waxing, and lasers for 2 months after the initial treatment, unless necessary for management of a complication such as hyperpigmentation. Dermal filler treatments

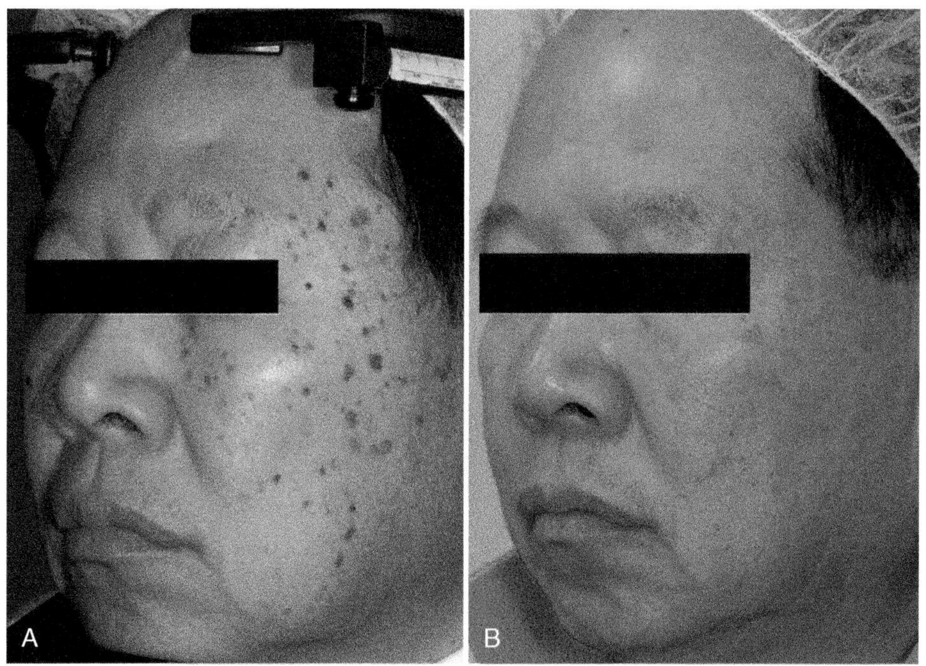

FIGURE 29-18 Ablative laser resurfacing for seborrheic keratoses **(A)** before and **(B)** after one treatment with an erbium laser microtip. *(Courtesy of K. Khatri, MD, using HOYA ConBio Dermasculpt™ Chisel Touch™.)*

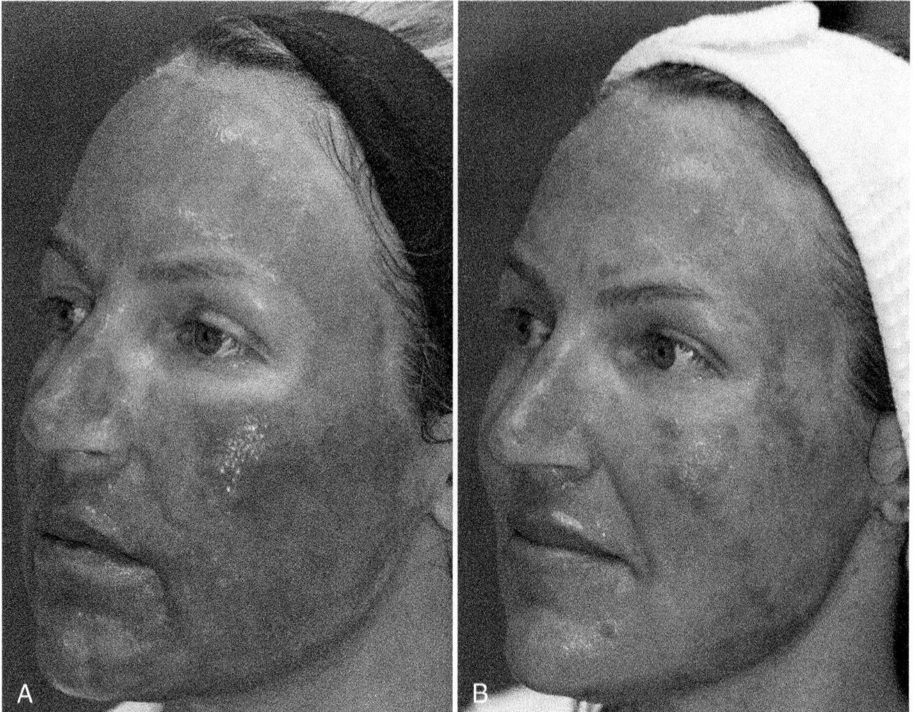

FIGURE 29-19 Recovery process for fractional ablative erbium laser resurfacing on **(A)** the first postprocedure day and **(B)** the fourth postprocedure day. *(Copyright Rebecca Small, MD.)*

may be performed 1 month after resurfacing and botulinum toxin treatments 2 weeks after resurfacing. When skin is no longer sensitive, patients' preprocedural rejuvenation products may be resumed.

See the *Preprocedure and Postprocedure Products* section in Chapter 24, *Skin Care Products*, for more information about postprocedure skin care.

FOLLOW-UP

Regular, frequent follow-up is advised initially to monitor the healing progress as well as to identify any early complications.[27] During the open wound phase in the first week, it is recommended that the patient be seen on postprocedure day 1 or 2, to evaluate the wound and ensure adherence to proper home care. A visit at 1 week is recommended to assess for full re-epithelialization, and once this is observed, the post-epithelialization stage has begun and the patient may be transitioned to nonocclusive postcare topical products. If recovery is uneventful, the follow-up schedule may be 1 month and 3 months postprocedure. Any concerns or problems warrant more frequent visits.

COMPLICATIONS

- Pain
- Bleeding
- Prolonged erythema
- Contact dermatitis
- Acne
- Milia
- Damage or alteration to tattoos and permanent make-up

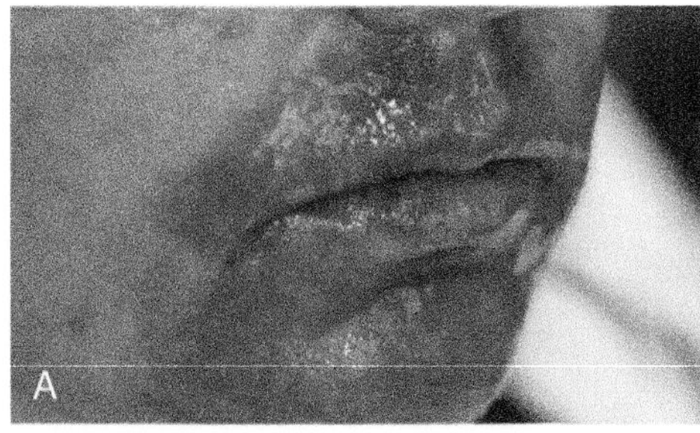

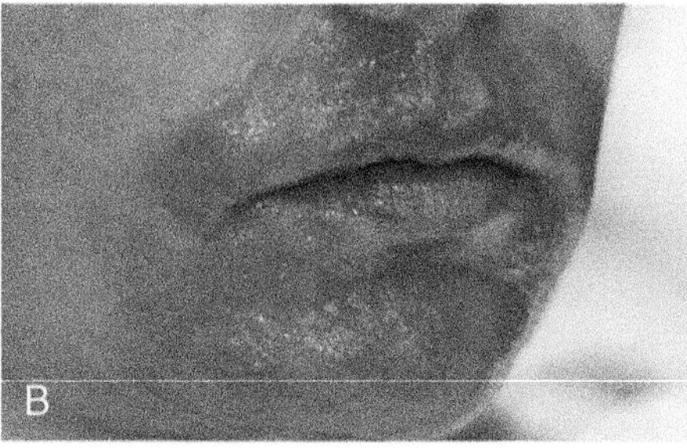

FIGURE 29-20 Perioral fractional ablative resurfacing on the first postprocedure day **(A)** prior to and **(B)** immediately after cleansing with vinegar solution. *(Copyright Rebecca Small, MD.)*

- Alteration to dermal filler
- Local infection such as activation of herpes simplex, impetigo, candidiasis
- Disseminated infection (very rare)
- Inadequate collagen remodelling effects including lack of reduction of wrinkles, scars or recurrence after treatment
- Inadequate clearance of unwanted pigmentation
- Hyperpigmentation
- Hypopigmentation
- Scarring and textural changes
- Ectropion
- Ocular injury

Despite the advances of fractional technologies that have increased safety and shortened recovery with ablative lasers, clinicians must remember that fractional ablative lasers *can be associated with complications*. An open wound is created with these treatments and complications such as infection and scarring can and do occur. Most of the complications with fractional ablative lasers to date have been reported in thin-skinned areas, such as under the eye, and in nonfacial areas, such as the neck.[27] Early recognition of complications allows the physician to initiate appropriate treatments that can help reduce the risk of permanent damage. The following discussion reviews complications and management of complications reported with ablative laser treatments, with fractional and nonfractional devices.

Adverse effects after ablative laser resurfacing range from mild to severe. Prolonged erythema, acne or milia formation, contact dermatitis, and pruritus are examples of mild reactions. Moderate complications include infections and postinflammatory hyperpigmentation. More serious complications include hypertrophic scarring, delayed onset hypopigmentation, ectropion, and disseminated infection.

Pain is usually transient, present only during treatment or for 20 to 30 minutes afterwards. Delayed postprocedure pain requires evaluation and may be associated with infection.

Bleeding may be apparent with cleansing during the open wound stage and resolves within 1 to 2 days postprocedure. It is usually evident as tiny pinpoint hemorrhages that rapidly become hemostatic and do not require bandaging.

Erythema and *edema* are normal signs after laser resurfacing and are considered abnormal if they persist longer than the expected period. Postprocedure erythema after re-epithelialization is usually mild in intensity and is resolved by 1 month. By comparison, nonfractional deep ablative lasers routinely resulted in prolonged erythema for 3 to 6 months after treatment. In general, postoperative erythema following CO_2 laser treatments lasts longer than with erbium lasers, due to the greater thermal damage from CO_2. Prolonged erythema lasting past 1 month and intense erythema lasting past 1 week should be considered unusual and addressed. Persistent erythema may indicate impending scar formation or may be due to contact dermatitis to topical compounds used during the recovery phase. If an impending scar is suspected, a strong class I topical corticosteroid should be applied[12] (see the discussion of hypertrophic scarring later in this section for additional scar therapies). If contact dermatitis is suspected, all topical medications should be discontinued and topical corticosteroids used. A history of rosacea may predispose to persistent postoperative erythema.[12,28]

Postoperative *contact dermatitis* is usually irritant in nature.[31–33] Newly resurfaced skin is vulnerable to irritation from various substances found in topically prescribed ointments, preservatives, sunscreens, and fragrances. In addition, topical antibiotics such as bacitracin, Neosporin (bacitracin zinc, neomycin sulfate, and polymyxin B sulfate), and Polysporin (bacitracin zinc and polymyxin B combinations) are common sources of irritation after laser resurfacing. Thus, their use should be avoided in the immediate postoperative period. Finally, many patients may self-prescribe various over-the-counter herbal and vitamin remedies, including vitamin E or aloe products, which can contribute to the problem. Contact dermatitis should be suspected if a patient develops worsening erythema or pruritus after treatment. To decrease this risk, moisturizers without active ingredients should be used during the first postoperative month. If contact dermatitis is suspected, all topical agents should be stopped and mild topical corticosteroids and cool, wet compresses applied regularly. In severe cases, oral antihistamines or short courses of oral corticosteroids may be necessary to control inflammation and reduce fibrosis risk.

Acne flare-ups are relatively common after laser resurfacing due to application of occlusive ointments, especially in patients who are acne prone.[29–31] These usually develop within the first few weeks in patients with a strong history of acne, and in other patients may be delayed. Often, no treatment is necessary since the flare-ups are usually mild and resolve once ointments are discontinued. If acne persists despite the discontinuation of occlusive ointments, an oral antibiotic such as doxycycline or minocycline may be used or topical antibiotics such as clindamycin may be used with fully re-epithelialized skin.

Milia, which appear as tiny 1 to 2-mm white papules, result from occlusion of sebaceous glands. Use of occlusive moisturizers, such as petrolatum-based products, frequently cause milia. Milia may be treated one skin is intact skin, by lancing with a 20-gauge needle and extracting the sebaceous plug, 1 to 2 months postprocedure.

Alteration of dermal filler may occur after ablative laser treatment, particularly with hyaluronic acid fillers. It is advisable to avoid treatment over facial areas that have hyaluronic acid fillers.

Infections can be viral, bacterial, or fungal and usually develop during the first postoperative week.[34] The appearance of infections in nonintact resurfaced skin does not always have the characteristic signs seen with intact skin. It is advisable for providers to have a low threshold for culturing areas suspected of infection.

The most frequent infectious complication following ablative laser resurfacing is reactivation of *herpes simplex virus* (HSV), reported in 2% to 7% of patients, even in those who receive antiviral prophylaxis.[35,36] Because there is a high incidence of latent HSV infection, many providers use prophylaxis with all patients undergoing facial laser resurfacing with oral antiviral medications. Acyclovir, famciclovir, or valacyclovir is routinely given 2 days before laser treatment and continued for another 3 to 10 days. Symptoms of HSV infection include tingling, burning, or discharge from isolated areas in the treated areas. Characteristic grouped vesicles may be difficult to recognize in the early postoperative period because there is no intact epithelium. Instead, one may see small superficial erosions. If a herpetic outbreak occurs despite prophylaxis, consider switching to a different antiviral medication or increase the dosage to maximal herpes zoster doses (acyclovir 800 mg 5 times a day, or famciclovir/valacyclovir 500 mg 3 times a day).

Bacterial and *fungal infections* can also occur because the moist environment of resurfaced skin presents an ideal medium for overgrowth of opportunistic pathogens. The most common bacterial infections are streptococcal, staphylococcal, or *Pseudomonas aeruginosa*. Fungal infections can be difficult to diagnose because they may resemble acne or milia in nonintact skin. Pain, increased erythema, purulent discharge, crusting, or delayed wound healing should alert one to possible bacterial or fungal infections. It is advisable to obtain wound cultures and initiate antibiotics against the common pathogens prior to obtaining culture results. Infections must be treated aggressively since local spread can lead to permanent scarring, significant morbidity and in severe cases can become *disseminated infections*. Some providers routinely use antibiotics as part of their perioperative regimen. However, there is no evidence supporting this practice, and indiscriminate antibiotic use may favor drug resistance and promote superinfection by other opportunistic pathogens.[37]

Postinflammatory hyperpigmentation may develop as postprocedure erythema resolves. It is usually seen within the first month postprocedure and spontaneously resolves during the next several months. Various treatments can be initiated to speed this resolution. Topical agents such as retinoic, azelaic, and glycolic acid compounds, hydroquinone preparations, or light glycolic acid peels (e.g., 30% to 40%) can be used after the first postoperative month.[12] It is also important to continue application of a broad-spectrum sunscreen (SPF 30 or higher) to help prevent and limit hyperpigmentation worsening.

Delayed onset hypopigmentation is a potentially serious and permanent complication that has been reported with ablative laser resurfacing.[38] Figure 29-21 shows a patient with hypopigmentation 20 years after receiving nonfractional deep ablative CO_2 resurfacing of the face. Hypopigmentation usually does not present until 6 to 12 months after ablative laser resurfacing. While relative hypopigmentation in certain areas such as the jaw line may be seen infrequently, true hypopigmentation is rare and occurs more often in patients receiving other forms of aggressive resurfacing such as dermabrasion or phenol peeling. To date, there are no reports of isolated hypopigmentation with fractional ablative resurfacing unless scarring has occurred.[27]

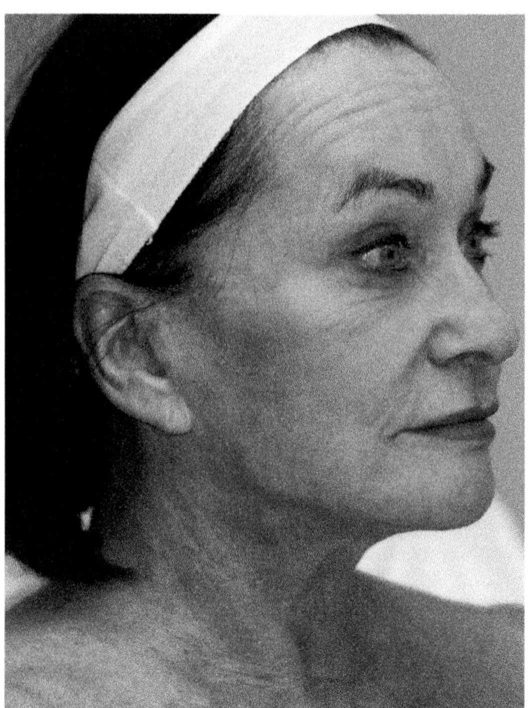

FIGURE 29-21 Hypopigmentation complication 20 years after ablative CO_2 resurfacing of the face. *(Copyright Rebecca Small, MD.)*

The treatment strategy for hypopigmentation is to reduce the contrast between the hypopigmented treatment area and adjacent skin by using chemical peels or nonablative lasers to decrease the surrounding skin's relative hyperpigmentation. Opaque makeup may be used for camouflage.

Hypertrophic scarring is an uncommon but serious complication. Factors increasing the risk for hypertrophic scarring include poor technique with overly aggressive laser parameters including high fluences, pulse stacking, excessive pulse overlapping, and high number of passes. Certain locations such as the lower eyelids, mandible, anterior neck, and chest are more susceptible to scarring and should be treated cautiously.[27,39] Postoperative contact dermatitis or wound infection can also lead to scarring if not treated appropriately. Finally, recent use of isotretinoin, previous irradiation, and a history of keloid formation can increase scarring risk.[40] Scarring is heralded by focal areas of intense erythema and induration. Early intervention is critical to avoid permanent scarring. Strong class I topical corticosteroids should be applied. Intralesional corticosteroid injections, silicone gel sheeting, and use of the pulsed dye lasers (585 nm) are other treatment options.

Ectropion is another serious complication following laser resurfacing. Prior lower blepharoplasty increases this risk, as does lower lid laxity, which must be ruled out with a "snap test" (see the *Procedure Preparation* section earlier in this chapter) prior to laser resurfacing. If lower lid laxity exists, it is advisable to avoid laser resurfacing near the lower lid. In general, conservative laser settings and fewer laser passes are employed when treating the lower lids due to the thin nature of the skin. Although topical corticosteroid application, massage, and temporary taping may be tried if ectropion results, often surgical correction is required.

Ocular injury can be avoided by wearing appropriate laser-safe eyewear at all times during treatment, directing the laser tip away from the eye, and treating outside of the eye orbit.

TREATING SPECIFIC LESIONS/AREAS

Neck, Chest, and Hands

Photoaged skin of the neck, chest and hands can be treated with fractional ablative laser resurfacing. More conservative settings are advised in these areas because the skin contains fewer adnexal glands than the face and, therefore, does not heal as well. These areas have a greater risk of complications and should be considered advanced treatment areas, to be performed by experienced laser providers.

LEARNING THE TECHNIQUES

The technique for placement of fractional ablative pulses can be practiced on an eggplant because the white pulse pattern will be clearly visible.

FINANCIAL CONSIDERATIONS

Ablative laser resurfacing is not reimbursable by insurance. The charges for treatments vary and are mainly determined by local prices. For example, fees for fractional ablative laser resurfacing in the Northern California Bay Area range from $1800 to $4500 for full face and $800 to $1200 for periocular or perioral areas. Box 29-1 lists applicable codes for ablative laser procedures.

CONCLUSION

In properly selected patients, fractional ablative laser resurfacing is an excellent choice for the treatment of moderate to severe photoaged skin, particularly for static rhytids. This novel method of delivering laser energy to the skin has resulted in dramatically reduced recovery times and minimal postprocedure complications relative to other ablative technologies. This technology offers the clinician great flexibility in skin resurfacing with its customizable treatment parameters. Fractional ablative lasers are a relatively new class of laser, and as knowledge of tissue effects with specific laser parameters expands, the performance and side effect profiles of these devices are likely to continue improving.

BOX 29-1 *Codes for Ablative Laser Procedures*

CPT Codes

17000–17111	Treatment of premalignant skin lesions or benign skin lesions

ICD-9 Codes

701.8	Other specified hypertrophic and atrophic conditions of skin (includes elastosis senilis)
702.0	Actinic keratosis
702.1	Seborrheic keratosis
709.00	Dyschromia, unspecified
709.2	Scar conditions and fibrosis of skin (i.e. cicatrix, scar NOS)

Resources

Smoke Evacuator

Buffalo Filter (e.g., Porta PlumeSafe 604 Smoke Evacuation System)
Phone: 800-343-2324
www.buffalofilter.com

Anesthesia Supplies

See Chapters 3 and 20.

Ablative Laser Companies

Alma (Er:YAG)
Phone: 866-414-ALMA
www.almalasers.com

Cutera (YSGG)
Phone: 415-657-5500
www.cutera.com

DEKA Laser Technologies (CO2)
Phone: 877-303-5273
www.dekalasers.com

Ellipse (CO2)
Phone: +45-4576-8808
www.ellipse.org

Lasering USA (CO2)
Phone: 866-471-0469
www.laseringusa.com

Lumenis (CO2)
Phone: 408-764-3000
www.lumenis.com

Lutronic (CO2)
Phone: 888-588-7644
www.lutronic.com

Palomar (Er:YAG)
Phone: 800-725-6627
www.palomarmedical.com

Sciton (Er:YAG)
Phone: 888-646-6999
www.sciton.com

Solta (CO2)
Phone: 888-437-2935
www.fraxel.com

References

1. Alster TS. Cutaneous resurfacing with CO2 and erbium:YAG lasers: preoperative, intraoperative, and postoperative considerations. *Plast Reconstr Surg.* 1999;103(2):619–632.
2. Hantash BM, De CE, Liu H, *et al.* Split-face comparison of the erbium micropeel with intense pulsed light. *Dermatol Surg.* 2008;34(6):763–772.
3. Manstein D, Herron GS, Sink RK. Fractional photothermolysis: a new concept for cutaneous remodeling using microscopic patterns of thermal injury. *Lasers Surg Med.* 2004;34:426–438.
4. Munavalli G. Single pass fractionated CO_2 laser resurfacing of lower eyelid rhytides. Presented at American Society for Laser Medicine and Surgery Conference, April 2008.
5. Lapidoth M, Yagima Odo ME, Odo LM. Novel use of erbium:YAG (2,940-nm) laser for fractional ablative photothermolysis in the treatment of photodamaged facial skin: a pilot study. *Dermatol Surg.* 2008;34(8):1048–1053.
6. Pozner JN, Glanz S, Goldberg DJ. Fractional erbium resurfacing: histologic and early clinical experience. *Lasers Surg Med.* 2007;39:S19–S73.
7. Clementoni MT, Gilardino P, Muti GF, *et al.* Non-sequential fractional ultrapulsed CO_2 resurfacing of photoaged facial skin: preliminary clinical report. *J Cosmet Laser Ther.* 2007;9(4):218–225.
8. Trelles MA, Velez M, Mordon S. Correlation of histological findings of single session Er:YAG skin fractional resurfacing with various passes and energies and the possible clinical implications. *Lasers Surg Med.* 2008;40(3):171–177.
9. Mehregan A. Actinic keratosis and actinic squamous cell carcinoma: a comparative study of 800 cases observed in 1968 and 1988. *Cutan Aging Cosmet Dermatol.* 1988;2:151.
10. Tierney EP, Kouba DJ, Hanke CW. Review of fractional photothermolysis: treatment indications and efficacy. *Dermatol Surg.* 2009;35(10):1445–1461.
11. Mandy SH, Monheit GD. Dermabrasion and chemical peels. *In:* Papel I, ed. *Facial Plastic and Reconstructive Surgery.* New York: Thieme; 2009:301–320.
12. Alster TS, Lupton JR. Treatment of complications of laser skin resurfacing. *Arch Facial Plast Surg.* 2000;2(4):279–284.
13. Weinstein GD, Nigra TP, Pochi PE, *et al.* Topical tretinoin for treatment of photodamaged skin: a multicenter study. *Arch Dermatol.* 1991;127:659–665.
14. Lowe NJ, Lask G, Griffin ME. Laser skin resurfacing. Pre- and posttreatment guidelines. *Dermatol Surg.* 1995;21(12):1017–1019.
15. Sachsenberg-Studer EM. Tolerance of topical retinaldehyde in humans. *Dermatology.* 1999;199(Suppl 1):61–63.
16. Gonzales-Ulloa M. [Selective regional plastic restoration by means of esthetic unities.] *Rev Bras Cir.* 1957;33(6):527–533.
17. Eaglstein NF. Chemical injury to the eye from EMLA cream during erbium laser resurfacing. *Dermatol Surg.* 1999;25(7):590–591.
18. Waibel J, Beer K, Narurkar V, *et al.* Preliminary observations on fractional ablative resurfacing devices: clinical impressions. *J Drugs Dermatol.* 2009;8(5):481–485.
19. Weiss R, Weiss M, Beasly KL. Prospective split face trial of a fixed spacing array computed scanned fractional CO_2 laser versus hand scanned 1550-nm fractional for rhytides. Abstract presented at American Society for Lasers Medicine and Surgery Conference, April 2008.
20. Ross V, Swann M, Barnette D. Use of a micro-fractional 2940-nm laser in the treatment of wrinkles and dyspigmentation. Abstract presented at American Society for Lasers Medicine and Surgery Conference, April 2008.
21. Liu H, Dang Y, Wang Z, *et al.* Laser induced collagen remodeling: a comparative study in vivo on mouse model. *Lasers Surg Med.* 2008;40(1):13–19.
22. Ortiz A, Elkeeb L, Truitt A, *et al.* Evaluation of a novel fractional resurfacing device for the treatment of acne scarring. Abstract presented at American Society for Lasers Medicine and Surgery Conference, April 2008.
23. Chapas AM, Brightman L, Sukal S, *et al.* Successful treatment of acneiform scarring with CO_2 ablative fractional resurfacing. *Lasers Surg Med.* 2008;40(6):381–386.
24. Lomeo G, Cassuto D, Scrimali L, et al. Er:YAG versus CO_2 ablative fractional resurfacing: a split face study. Abstract presented at American Society for Lasers Medicine and Surgery Conference, April 2008.
25. Speyer MT, Reinisch L, Cooper KA, *et al.* Erythema after cutaneous laser resurfacing using a porcine model. *Arch Otolaryngol Head Neck Surg.* 1998;124(9):1008–1013.
26. Rendon MI, Cardona L, Benitez A. The safety and efficacy of trolamine/sodium alginate topical emulsion in postlaser resurfacing wounds. *J Drugs Dermatol.* 2008;7(5):S23–S28.
27. Fife DJ, Fitzpatrick RE, Zachary CB. Complications of fractional CO_2 laser resurfacing: four cases. *Lasers Surg Med.* 2009;41(3):179–184.
28. Ruiz-Esparza J, Barba Gomez JM, Gomez de la Torre OL, *et al.* Erythema after laser skin resurfacing. *Dermatol Surg.* 1998;24(1):31–34.
29. Graber EM, Tanzi EL, Alster TS. Side effects and complications of fractional laser photothermolysis: experience with 961 treatments. *Dermatol Surg.* 2008;34(3):301–305.
30. Nanni C. Handling complications of laser treatment. *Dermatol Ther.* 2000;13:127–139.
31. Nanni C. Postoperative management and complications of laser dioxide laser resurfacing. *In:* Alster TS, Apfelberg D, eds. *Cosmetic Laser Surgery: A Practitioner's Guide.* New York: Wiley-Liss; 1999:37–55.
32. Nanni CA, Alster TS. Complications of carbon dioxide laser resurfacing. An evaluation of 500 patients. *Dermatol Surg.* 1998;24(3):315–320.
33. Ratner D, Tse Y, Marchell N, *et al.* Cutaneous laser resurfacing. *J Am Acad Dermatol.* 1999;41(3 Pt 1):365–389.
34. Sriprachya-Anunt S, Fitzpatrick RE, Goldman MP, *et al.* Infections complicating pulsed carbon dioxide laser resurfacing for photoaged facial skin. *Dermatol Surg.* 1997;23(7):527–535.
35. Alster TS, Nanni CA. Famciclovir prophylaxis of herpes simplex virus reactivation after laser skin resurfacing. *Dermatol Surg.* 1999;25(3):242–246.
36. Monheit GD. Facial resurfacing may trigger the herpes simplex virus. *Cosm Dermatol.* 1995;8:9–16.
37. Walia S, Alster TS. Laser resurfacing infection rate with and without prophylactic antibiotics. *Dermatol Surg.* 1999;25:857–861.
38. Weinstein C. Carbon dioxide laser resurfacing. Long-term follow-up in 2123 patients. *Clin Plast Surg.* 1998;25(1):109–130.
39. Alster TS. Side effects and complications of laser surgery. In: Alster TS, ed. *Manual of Cutaneous Laser Techniques.* Philadelphia: Lippincott Williams & Wilkins; 2000:175–187.
40. Katz BE, MacFarlane DF. Atypical facial scarring after isotretinoin therapy in a patient with previous dermabrasion. *J Am Acad Dermatol.* 1994;30(5 Pt 2):852–853.

Additional Reading

Buford G. Lasers and pulsed-light devices: skin resurfacing (Chap 53). *In:* Pfenninger JL, Fowler GC, eds. *Pfenninger and Fowler's Procedures for Primary Care.* 3rd ed. Philadelphia: Mosby/Elsevier; 2011.

Small R. Ablative modalities for wrinkles. *In:* Small R, ed. *A Practical Guide to Cosmetic Lasers.* Philadelphia: Lippincott; 2012.

30 Tattoo Removal with Lasers

WILLIAM KIRBY, DO, FAOCD • FRANCISCA KARTONO, DO • REBECCA SMALL, MD

The growing trend of tattooing has led to increased numbers of patients seeking tattoo removal. Studies note that 40% of Americans between the age of 26 and 40 currently have tattoos and 17% of these people are seeking removal.[1,2] With more than 20,000 tattoo studios in the United States placing tattoos, the demand for removal is likely to continue to increase in the coming years.[3]

Multiple techniques can be used for tattoo removal. Early removal methods used mechanical destruction such as dermabrasion, chemical peels, and continuous-wave lasers. These methods left patients with unsatisfactory results and were associated with suboptimal removal and scarring (Figure 30-1). The current standard of using Q-switched lasers has revolutionized tattoo removal and offers patients a safe and effective means for removing tattoo ink.

In this chapter, we describe the physiology of a tattoo, the latest tattoo removal technology, and the current standard practice recommendations for tattoo removal with Q-switched lasers.

TATTOO ANATOMY

During the tattooing process, tattoo ink is injected intradermally. The epidermis and upper papillary dermis are homogenized and ink particles (ranging in size from 2 to 400 nm) are deposited intracellularly and extracellularly. After 2 to 3 months, the skin layers are reestablished and ink is concentrated in the dermis within fibroblasts, beneath a layer of fibrotic scar tissue (Figure 30-2).

Numerous chemicals and inks are used in the tattoo industry and the component ink compounds in a given tattoo are usually unknown by the patient at the time of presenting for tattoo removal. The Food and Drug Administration (FDA) does not regulate tattoo inks and, therefore, tattoo inks are not evaluated for safety. In general, *amateur tattoos* are often carbon based such as burnt wood or pen ink, and there is a lower density of pigment particles. *Professional tattoos* are typically composed of organic dyes mixed with metallic elements that give the color: red is often made from mercury; yellow from cadmium; green from chromium; blue from cobalt; white from titanium dioxide; and flesh color from iron oxide. Tattoo inks are usually combinations of colors, so a green, red, or light blue tattoo may also contain darker colors such as black ink.

LASER PRINCIPLES

Tattoo ink serves as a cutaneous chromophore for lasers. Certain wavelengths of light are selectively absorbed by different ink colors.[4] In this way, colored inks can be targeted and removed by laser light with minimal damage to surrounding tissues. The chromophore absorption spectrum of the tissue chromophores, melanin and oxyhemoglobin, as well as wavelengths used for tattoo removal, are shown in Figure 30-3. Wavelength selection for different tattoo colors is shown in Figure 30-4 and is as follows:

- Black and dark blue inks are best treated with a 1064 nm wavelength.
- Red ink (and variations of red such as orange and yellow) is best treated with a 532 nm wavelength.
- Green ink is best treated with 650, 694, or 755 nm wavelengths.
- Sky blue is best treated with a 585 nm wavelength.
- Purple is a combination color and can be treated with 585 and 532 nm wavelengths.

Laser parameters including wavelength, pulse duration, and fluence can be tailored to maximize tattoo ink destruction and minimize thermal damage to surrounding tissue. Short pulsed, Q-switched lasers further employ photoacoustic vibration to fragment tattoo ink into smaller particles. These smaller ink particles are eliminated through epidermal extrusion, lymphatic drainage, and macrophage phagocytosis. In addition, laser-treated ink particles have altered optical properties that render the ink remaining in the skin less visible to the eye.[5]

Laser Parameters and Tattoo Treatments

- *Pulse width*, or pulse duration (measured in nanoseconds) is the length of time that laser light is in contact with the skin. Q-switched lasers have fixed nanosecond pulse widths and this parameter cannot be adjusted for treatments.
- The *thermal relaxation time* (measured in seconds) is defined as the time required for the absorbed energy within the target chromophore to cool to one-half its original value immediately after irradiation. To specifically target the chromophore ink and reduce unwanted thermal damage to surrounding tissues,

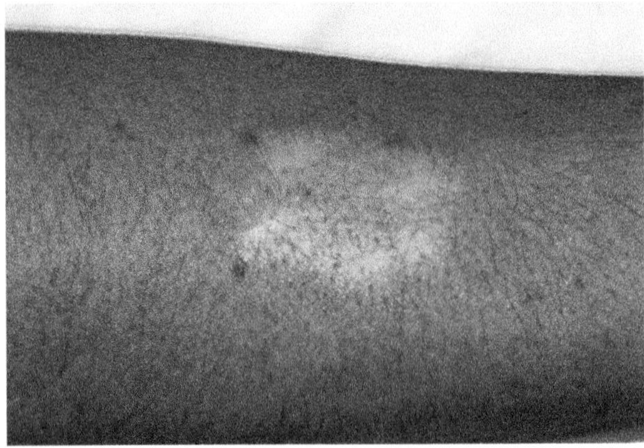

FIGURE 30-1 Dermabrasion results for tattoo removal showing scarring, hypopigmentation, and residual ink. *(Copyright Rebecca Small, MD.)*

very short pulse widths (shorter than the target thermal relaxation time) are used to heat and ablate the ink faster than heat is conducted to the surrounding tissue.

- *Spot size* (measured in millimeters) is the diameter of the laser beam on the skin surface. Use of a larger spot size results in less scatter of the photons and deeper laser beam penetration. This maximizes the distribution of laser light to the dermal ink and reduces epidermal injury. Larger spot sizes should be used as long as sufficient fluence can be obtained to achieve the desired clinical endpoint. A smaller spot size (e.g., 2 to 3 mm) has greater scattering of photons, delivers energy less efficiently, and causes

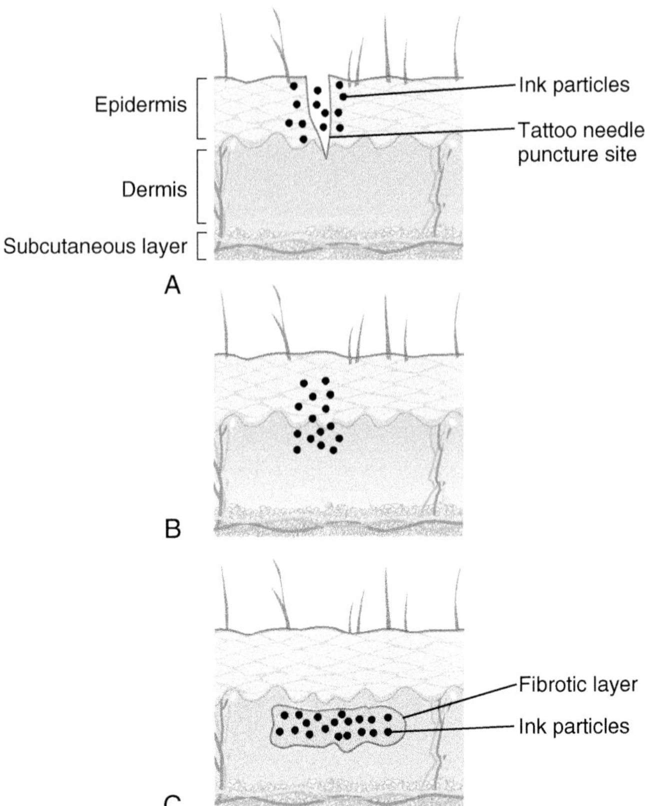

FIGURE 30-2 Tattoo placement and dermal incorporation of ink (A) immediately after tattooing, (B) 1 month, and (C) 2 to 3 months after.

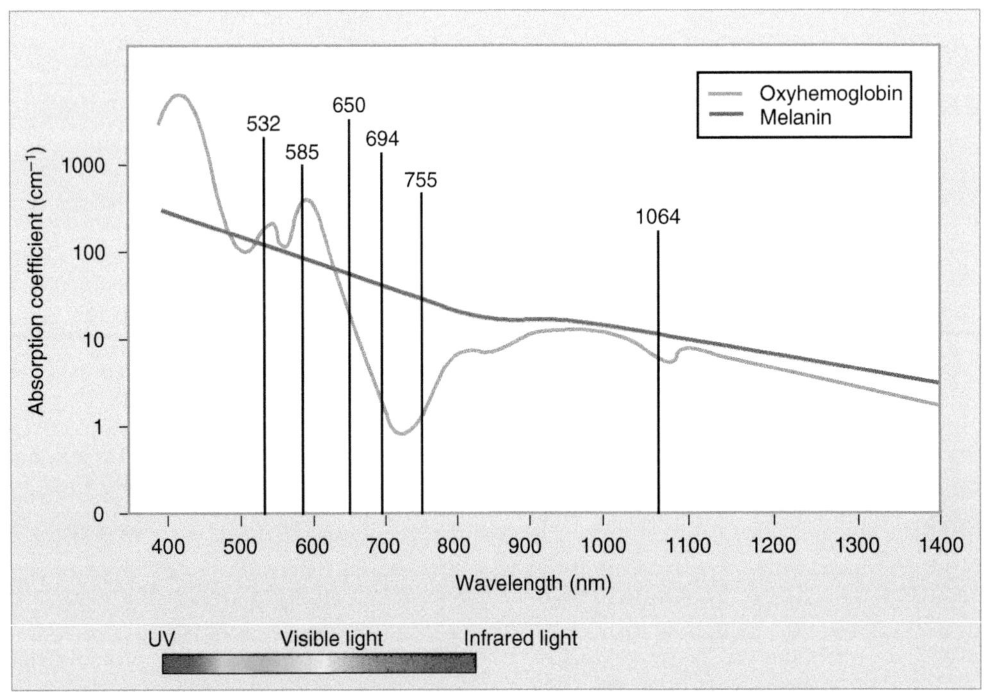

FIGURE 30-3 Chromophore absorption spectra and tattoo removal lasers.

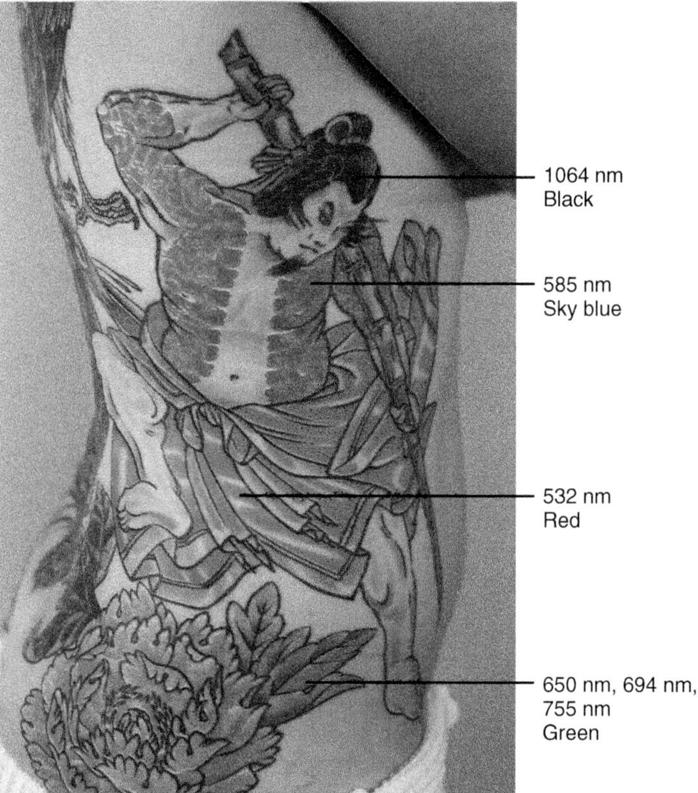

FIGURE 30-4 Laser wavelengths used for different tattoo colors. *(Copyright Rebecca Small, MD.)*

more epidermal injury than larger spot sizes (e.g., 6 to 8 mm).

- *Wavelength* (measured in nanometers) is chosen based on the tattoo ink color. In general, as the wavelength increases, so does the depth of penetration.
- The energy output is known as *fluence* (measured in joules per square centimeter). More specifically, fluence is defined as the amount of energy delivered per unit area. Fluence should be sufficient to produce immediate whitening with tattoo treatment without bleeding or blistering. The fluence emitted with a given spot size is dependent on the device used. Adequately powered tattoo laser devices can maintain high fluences (e.g., more than 4.5 J/cm^2) with large spot sizes (e.g., 6 mm).

PATIENT AND TATTOO SELECTION

Lasers may be used for tattoo removal in patients of all skin types (Fitzpatrick types I through VI). However, patients with darker skin types (IV through VI) are at greater risk for side effects, specifically hypopigmentation and hyperpigmentation. Topical hydroquinone (2% to 8%) can be used preprocedure, and resumed once the skin is healed postprocedure, to reduce the risk of postinflammatory hyperpigmentation in patients with darker skin types. Additionally, patients of Asian or African descent have a greater predisposition to hypertrophic and keloidal scarring. In general, Fitzpatrick skin type VI patients have the greatest risk of complications with any aesthetic procedure, and providers should consider treatment of this skin type an advanced laser application.

Almost any tattoo is indicated for laser tattoo removal. Multiple treatments are needed to achieve satisfactory results. Due to great variation in tattoo ink depth, density, composition, and techniques used for placement, the number of treatments needed for removal can be difficult to estimate accurately. In general, professionally placed tattoos have a high ink density and require 9 to 14 treatments, whereas amateur tattoos typically require 4 to 8 treatments. Several other factors can affect the number of treatments necessary for removal: faded, older tattoos on paler skin types in more proximal locations tend to resolve with fewer treatments than intense, multicolored tattoos on darker skin types in distal locations.[6] Patients should be questioned about other tattoo removal methods used previously. Methods that create scar tissue, such as burning or abrasion, can make tattoo removal with lasers less successful.

Certain types of tattoos are considered advanced, and treatment should not be undertaken until the provider is fully confident in his or her skill with artistic tattoo removal. Advanced tattoos include cosmetic tattoos, such as those used for permanent eyeliner or lip liner, flesh-colored inks, and traumatic tattoos.

INDICATIONS

Laser tattoo removal is indicated for the treatment of ectopic skin pigment. This pigment is usually from purposefully placed ink in tattoos (both professional and amateur artistic tattoos) as well as tattoos associated with medical procedures (e.g., radiation therapy tattoos). In rare cases ectopic pigment may be the result of trauma (traumatic tattoos) where materials such as asphalt are trapped in the dermis.

ALTERNATIVE THERAPIES

The following alternatives to Q-switched laser tattoo removal methods are not recommended:

- Dermabrasion (not to be confused with microdermabrasion)
- Salabrasion
- Cryotherapy (liquid nitrogen)
- Continuous-wave lasers
- Chemical acids
- Thermal injury (electrocautery).

The results of using these alternative modalities are often unsatisfactory to both patients and health care professionals. These techniques significantly increase the risk of adverse effects including scarring, hypopigmentation, hyperpigmentation, depigmentation, incomplete resolution of ink, pain, prolonged healing time, infection, textural changes, and unpredictable outcomes. The advantage of these techniques is that they are relatively inexpensive and may offer faster ink resolution when compared to laser tattoo removal treatments. Some providers use surgical excision as a method of tattoo removal.

PRODUCTS CURRENTLY AVAILABLE

Q-switched lasers are now widely regarded as the gold standard for laser tattoo removal. Current Q-switched lasers available include:

- Q-switched Nd:YAG laser (1064 nm)
  - Frequency doubled (532 nm)
  - Dye modules (650 nm and 585 nm)
- Q-switched alexandrite laser (755 nm)
- Q-switched ruby laser (694 nm).

The Q-switched Nd:YAG (neodymium-doped yttrium aluminum garnet) produces a 1064 nm wavelength of light that is ideal for treating black ink. A primary disadvantage is its limited efficacy in removing yellow and green inks. With some devices, through a process called *frequency doubling*, an Nd:YAG laser can also produce light with a wavelength of 532 nm to treat red, orange, and yellow inks.[20] The Nd:YAG laser has an advantage of treating darker skinned patients with less risk of hypopigmentation, hyperpigmentation, and textural changes.[7] This can be attributed to the increased dermal penetration of this longer wavelength and the lower melanin absorption. The wavelength of the light emitted by the Q-switched alexandrite laser is 755 nm. This wavelength has excellent absorption by black, good absorption by green and blue, but poor absorption by red ink. The ruby laser was one of the first Q-switched lasers, and it emits a 694 nm wavelength. It works well for darker colors (black, blue-black, and some green), but poorly on yellow and red ink. Although more effective for green ink than the Nd:YAG, the ruby laser commonly causes hypopigmentation and hyperpigmentation and, although usually transient, may be permanent.[5]

Recently, a number of lower cost, Q-switched devices have become available. Although considerably less expensive, these units have little to no long-term track records and are of unknown quality. Choosing a device with a more established company is recommended.

CONTRAINDICATIONS[8]

- Ink allergy.

Also see Chapter 26, *Hair Reduction with Lasers*, for additional laser contraindications.

ADVANTAGES OF LASER TATTOO REMOVAL

- Considered the "gold standard" for tattoo removal.
- Individual treatments are relatively quick.
- Provides the best cosmetic result when compared to other forms of tattoo removal.

DISADVANTAGES OF LASER TATTOO REMOVAL

- Expensive.
- Painful.
- Multiple treatments are required.
- The procedure has risks of hyperpigmentation, hypopigmentation, depigmentation, and textural changes.

EQUIPMENT

- Q-Switched laser device
- Topical anesthetic
- Tongue depressors to apply anesthetic
- Gauze pads to remove anesthetic
- Sterile wipes or alcohol wipes to cleanse the treatment area
- Protective eyewear for patient and laser operator and any other personnel in the room
- Appropriate door sign indicating laser usage
- Ice packs
- Nonsterile gloves
- Face shield for laser operator (optional)
- Masks for laser operator (optional).

Although relatively reliable, Q-switched lasers, like any laser device, are made of sensitive components. Q-switched lasers should not be transported from location to location and all measures should be taken to move the device as little as possible. To ensure that calibration and mirror alignment within the laser arm are adequate, one can aim the laser on a wooden tongue depressor and observe the formation of concentric circles with a laser pulse. If this pattern does not appear, the equipment is due for a calibration. When not in use, the foot pedal should be properly stored and the key removed. Always take care to not damage the laser arm.

Q-switched lasers can rupture blood vessels and aerosolize tissue, so a laser operator may choose to use a plastic shield or a cone device on the laser tip to protect from tissue and blood contact as well as a face shield and mask.

PROCEDURE PREPARATION

1. Review the patient's medical history to ensure there are no contraindications to treatment (see *Contraindication* section). If there is a history of herpes simplex in or near the treatment area, prophylactic antiviral medication is used 2 days prior and 3 days after the treatment. If the risk of herpes is low, antivirals may instead be started on the day of treatment.
2. Review the tattoo history: amateur/professional/cosmetic/traumatic, years present, flesh-colored or

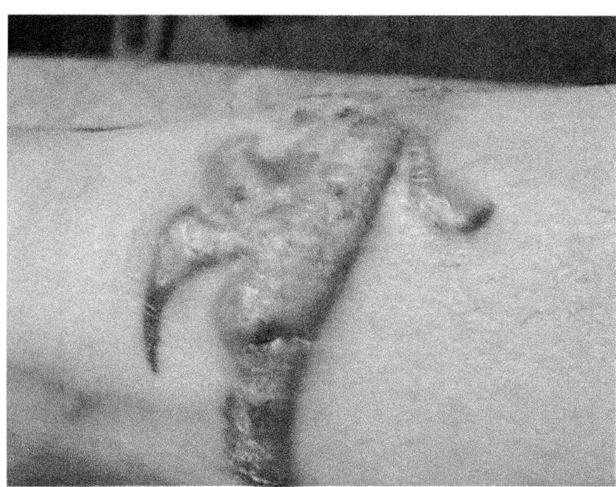

FIGURE 30-5 Red tattoo ink dermatitis, prior to laser treatment. *(Courtesy of W. Kirby, MD.)*

white ink, "cover-up" tattoo, previous methods used for removal and scarring at the tattoo site.

3. Determine the patient's Fitzpatrick skin type (see Chapter 19, *Aesthetic Principles and Consultation*).
4. Perform a brief and focused physical examination to rule out ink allergy. Ink allergy presents with signs of an allergic contact dermatitis (erythema, edema, induration, and discomfort in previously tattooed areas). A severe red ink dermatitis is shown in Figure 30-5. Examine the tattoo carefully for areas of scarring; document if present and inform the patient.
5. Photograph the tattoo.

LASER TATTOO REMOVAL: STEPS AND PRINCIPLES

The following guidelines are based on treatment of artistic tattoos using a Q-switched laser (HOYA ConBio RevLite), which is indicated for all Fitzpatrick skin types (I through VI). Manufacturer guidelines specific to the device used should be followed at the time of treatment.

General Treatment Technique

1. The appropriate wavelength is selected for the tattoo ink color to be treated. Colored inks are often a mixture of different colors and it is safest to use a 1064 nm wavelength for initial treatments of multicolored tattoos.
   - *Treatment 1:* Use a 1064 nm wavelength regardless of the color of the tattoo.
   - *Treatments 2 through 4:* Use a 1064 nm wavelength for multicolored tattoos in the dark areas (black, blue, purple, green), and a 532 nm wavelength for red-colored ink areas.
   - *Treatments 5 and greater:* Treat the whole tattoo with a 1064 nm wavelength first and then treat specific colored areas with the wavelength appropriate for the color. For example, the fifth treatment for a green tattoo with red and sky blue ink would be as follows: 1064 nm to the whole tattoo, followed by 650 nm to the whole tattoo, 532 nm to the red areas, and 585 nm to the sky blue areas.
2. Start with larger spot sizes (e.g., 6 to 8 mm) for initial treatments and progress to smaller spot sizes (e.g., 4 mm) over the treatment series. Larger spots penetrate deeper and are less aggressive with fewer side effects.
3. The laser tip is moved smoothly in a painting motion over the tattoo and is not in direct contact with the skin.
4. Universal precautions should be used during and after the treatment due to possible tissue splatter and bleeding.

Planning and Designing

Treatment of thinner skinned areas such as the neck, breast, and below the knees can result in adverse reactions, so conservative settings with lower fluences and larger spot sizes are advised.

For large tattoos covering an entire extremity, consider performing the dorsal area in one session and volar area in a subsequent session to avoid circumferential edema and a possible tourniqueting effect.

"Cover-up" tattoos, in which a second tattoo has been placed on top of the initial tattoo, have a greater density of ink and should be treated with very low fluences initially to reduce the risk of overtreatment.

Anesthesia

Tattoo treatments are painful but can be performed relatively quickly. Some patients may forgo anesthesia altogether, but many patients require some form of local anesthesia. A topical anesthetic cream such as benzocaine:lidocaine:tetracaine (see the *Resources* list at the end of the chapter) may be used under occlusion with plastic wrap for 30 minutes in the office prior to the laser treatment. If complete anesthesia is desired, injections of 1% or 2% lidocaine with epinephrine subdermally may be used. Local injection is discouraged by the authors because clinical experience has shown increased bleeding and edema at the time of treatment, rendering treatments less effective.

Performing the Procedure

1. Remove any reflective jewelry that may scatter laser light.
2. Apply topical anesthetic (such as benzocaine:lidocaine:tetracaine) in the office and remove after 30 minutes of contact time.

   TIP: Patients will experience discomfort in spite of analgesic measures used, and reminding patients to breathe during treatments will assist with pain management. Squeezing the treated area is also a useful distraction technique.

3. Position the patient on the treatment table in a comfortable position allowing for exposure of the tattoo.
4. Cleanse the treatment area with a sterile wipe or alcohol and allow to dry.
5. Provide wavelength-specific protective eyewear to all people in the room. If working on the face, provide the patient with lead extraocular goggles.
6. The laser operator should be positioned comfortably, often sitting, as opposed to leaning over the patient. This will allow for comfortable manipulation of the headpiece while depressing the foot pedal that is used with most laser systems.
7. The wheels on the device should be placed in the locked position to ensure that the unit does not roll during treatment.
8. Select the appropriate wavelength for the tattoo color (see the *General Treatment Technique* section earlier in this chapter).
9. Select the appropriate spot size based on the patient's Fitzpatrick skin type using the manufacturer's guidelines. In general, for initial treatments, larger spot sizes (e.g., 8 mm) should be selected for darker Fitzpatrick skin types (V and VI) and smaller spot sizes (6 mm) for lighter skin types (I through III).
10. Confirm again that everyone in the room is wearing appropriate eyewear at all times and all doors are fully closed.
11. Hold the handpiece at a 90-degree angle to the skin.
12. Instruct the patient not to move if he or she experiences discomfort and, to inform you if a short rest is needed during the treatment.
13. Perform a test spot on the darkest area of the tattoo using the 1064 nm wavelength (regardless of the tattoo ink color) and observe for clinical endpoints. The amount of ink present is highly variable and settings will be determined by the tissue response to the test spot performed. Desirable clinical endpoints include:
    - Whitening of the tattoo ink. Figure 30-6 shows whitening of a black ink tattoo using a 1064 nm Q-switched laser (HOYA ConBio RevLite).
    - Audible and palpable snapping felt during laser pulses due to photoacoustic vibration.
    - Edema.
    - Petechiae are desirable endpoints and indicate aggressive settings. This is more commonly seen with shorter wavelengths, such as 532 nm.

    TIP: If the tattoo ink appears yellowish or brown immediately after the laser pulse, increase the fluence to obtain a white spot.

    TIP: Dark tattoos with high concentrations of ink will require lower starting fluences and larger spot sizes than lighter faded tattoos.
14. Pinpoint bleeding results from vascular injury and represents an overly aggressive treatment. The fluence should be reduced if this occurs. Some of the newer tattoo laser technologies available have modified beam profiles, which have reduced the occurrence of pinpoint bleeding.
15. The initial treatment session may be performed with conservative settings and minimal endpoints to determine how a patient will respond, particularly with darker skin types and very dark tattoos.
16. At subsequent visits the tattoo ink will lighten and the fluence should be increased or spot size reduced for more aggressive treatments to achieve desired endpoints. Typically, the fluence is increased first, based on the manufacturer's recommended treatment parameters. After maximizing the fluence over several visits, the spot size is then decreased with an associated reduction in fluence.

    TIP: A test spot should be performed at each visit prior to initiating treatment to determine the appropriate settings.

    CAUTION: Watch for vasovagal signs of lightheadedness, perspiration, and fatigue and discontinue treatment if these occur.

RESULTS

Immediately after a Q-switched laser treatment, the tattoo will have a white discoloration. Figure 30-6 shows a blue-black tattoo during treatment with immediate whitening. This white color change is thought to be the result of rapid, heat-formed steam, causing dermal and epidermal vacuolization. Patients may perceive this as reduction of ink, but this positive change is only temporary and typically lasts for 20 minutes or less. Ink color will gradually fade during the month following each treatment. Results from laser treatments for removal of tattoo ink are cumulative and results from some treatments will be more noticeable than others.

Figure 30-7 shows a blue-black professional tattoo (A) before and (B) after five treatments with a Q-switched laser using 1064 nm wavelength (HOYA ConBio Medlite) demonstrating typical tattoo clearance. Figure 30-8 shows a multicolor professional tattoo (A) before, (B) midway through treatment with lightening of the black ink and hypopigmentation, and (C) after completion of treatment with a Q-switched laser

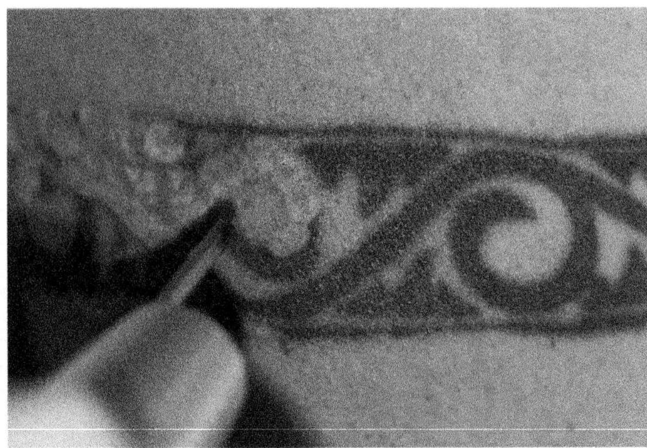

FIGURE 30-6 Laser tattoo removal treatment showing immediate clinical endpoint of whitening. *(Copyright Rebecca Small, MD, using HOYA ConBio RevLite™.)*

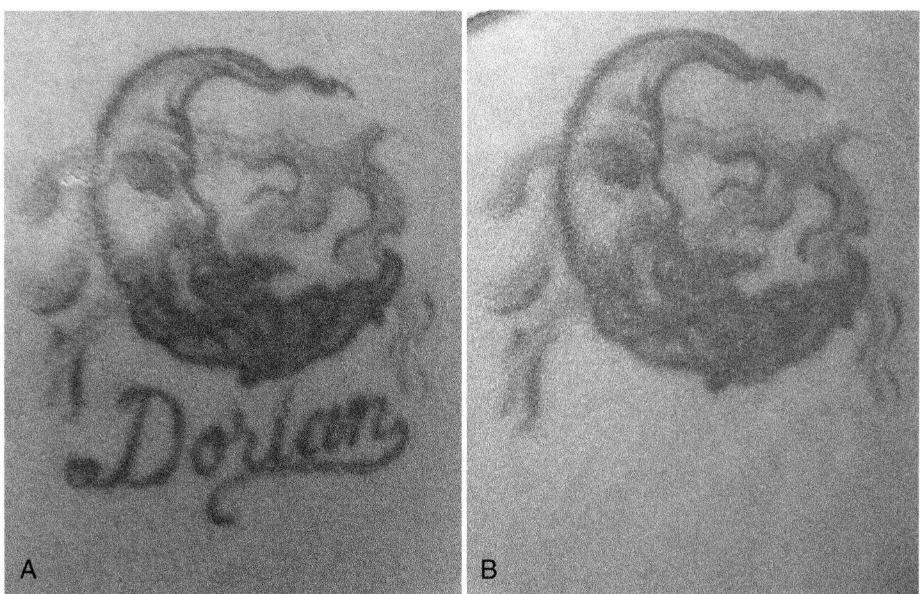

FIGURE 30-7 A blue-black professional tattoo **(A)** prior to and **(B)** after completion of five treatments with a Q-switched laser using a 1064 nm wavelength. *(Courtesy of W. Kirby, MD, using HOYA ConBio Medlite™.)*

using 1064, 532, and 585 nm wavelengths for black/blue, red/yellow, and sky blue inks, respectively (HOYA ConBio Medlite).

Occasionally colored inks may darken with treatment due to darker constituent inks. Figure 30-9A shows a red ink tattoo prior to treatment. This tattoo was initially treated with a Q-switched laser using a 1064 nm wavelength (Medlite, Hoya ConBio) and the tattoo ink darkened and became black in color (Figure 30-9B). Subsequent treatments were performed using a 1064 nm wavelength for black and a 532 nm wavelength for red ink areas.

AFTERCARE

Laser tattoo removal treatment normally results in temporary swelling, redness, and tenderness of the treated area, which may take a few hours to resolve. *Ice is applied immediately* after treatment for patient comfort and for 15 minutes every 1 to 2 hours on the day of treatment to reduce the risk of blistering.

If the treated skin is fully intact and in an area that will not be abraded, a broad-spectrum sunscreen (containing zinc or titanium) with an SPF of 30 or greater can be applied without a dressing. If the skin is not intact, an occlusive ointment, like Aquaphor, should be applied and loosely covered with a nonadherent dressing and tape that is changed once daily, for moist wound healing. Care should be taken not to macerate the treated area with excessive occlusion. Once the skin is intact, a daily broad-spectrum sunscreen should be applied for the duration of the tattoo removal treatments.

A *crust* may appear over the treated area that sloughs off at approximately 14 days post-treatment. The treated skin appears slightly shiny until the area has fully healed. Crusts or blisters should not be removed and patients cautioned against picking, which increases the risk of scarring. *Mild pruritus* is part of the healing

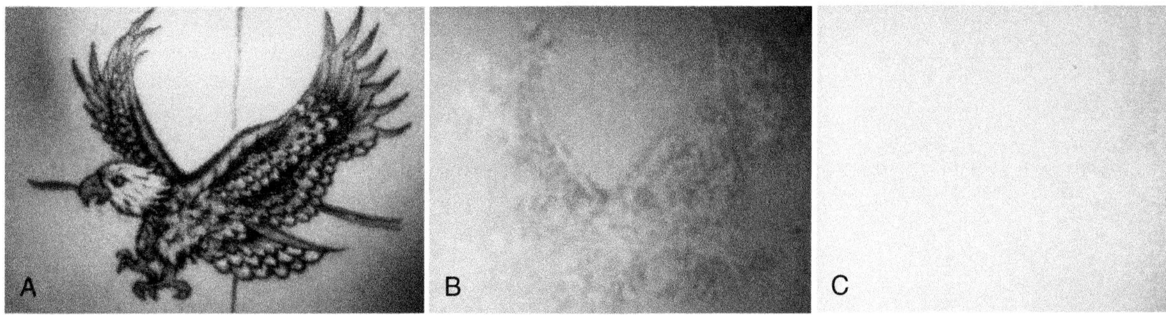

FIGURE 30-8 A multicolor professional tattoo **(A)** before, **(B)** midway through treatment with lightening of the black ink and mild hypopigmentation, and **(C)** after completion of treatment showing resolution of hypopigmentation with a Q-switched laser using 1064, 532, and 585 nm wavelengths for black/blue, red/yellow, and sky blue inks, respectively. *(Courtesy of R. Anderson, MD, and S. Kilmer, MD, using HOYA ConBio Medlite™.)*

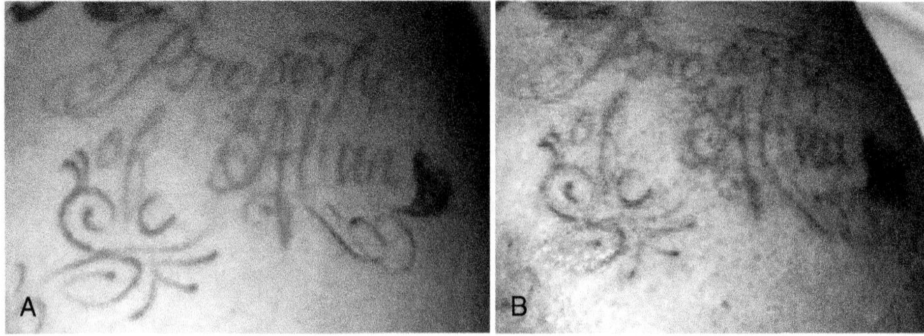

FIGURE 30-9 Red tattoo ink **(A)** prior to and **(B)** after treatment with a Q-switched laser using a 1064 nm wavelength demonstrating paradoxical darkening. *(Courtesy of W. Kirby, MD, using HOYA ConBio Medlite™.)*

process and is common during the first few weeks following treatment.

Strenuous exercise and exposure to water should be avoided until the skin is intact. Elevation of treated extremities can reduce edema.

FOLLOW-UP

A 6 to 8 week interval between treatments is necessary to allow the skin to heal completely. This interval may be extended without any reduction in efficacy and, in fact, treated tattoo ink may continue to fade slightly over time. The tattoo is appropriate for retreatment once the skin is fully intact, without a crust and the shiny appearance to the skin has resolved. Patients often request more frequent treatment sessions as they are usually highly motivated to remove their tattoos. However, treating too frequently, such as every 4 weeks, may increase the chances of textural changes, scarring, and hypopigmentation.

COMPLICATIONS

- Hyperpigmentation
- Hypopigmentation/depigmentation
- Blistering
- Bleeding
- Textural changes
- Scarring (including hypertrophic and keloids)
- Prolonged healing
- Infection (e.g., herpes simplex, varicella zoster)
- Paradoxical tattoo darkening (flesh-colored ink or permanent makeup)
- Allergic reactions with local dermatitis/nodules or systemic allergic response (rare).

A fine line exists between expected side effects and true complications from laser tattoo removal treatments. For example, discomfort, swelling, blistering, and itching are commonly associated with the treatment[8] but extreme pain, limb edema, bulla, and intractable pruritus are rare and indicate treatment complications.

About half of the patients treated with Q-switched lasers for tattoo removal will show some transient changes in the normal skin pigmentation (*hyperpigmentation* or *hypopigmentation*).[5,9] These changes usually resolve in 6 to 12 months but rarely may be permanent.[7,10] The risk of hyperpigmentation and hypopigmentation is greatest with skin types IV, V, and VI, regardless of the wavelength used. Areas that blister and bleed are more likely to have pigmentary and textural changes.[11] Twice daily treatment with hydroquinone and broad-spectrum sunscreens on fully healed skin usually resolve hyperpigmentation within a few months, although in some patients resolution can be prolonged. Shorter wavelengths, such as 532 nm, are more commonly associated with blistering and hypopigmentation than longer wavelengths.

Transient textural changes are common and typically resolve within a few months; however, permanent textural changes and scarring can occur.[10] If a patient is prone to pigmentary or textural changes, longer treatment intervals are recommended. Additionally, patients with a history of hypertrophic scarring need to be warned of their increased risk of scarring.

Local allergic responses to tattoo pigments have been reported at the time of tattoo placement, and allergic reactions to tattoo pigment can also occur after Q-switched laser treatment.[13–18] For example, photoallergic reactions have been reported to yellow cadmium sulfide, a pigment commonly added to tattoos to brighten red or yellow inks. This reaction is also reported with red ink, which may contain cinnabar (mercuric sulfide), green (chromium), and blue (cobalt).[21,22] Erythema, pruritus, and even inflamed nodules, verrucose papules, or granulomas may occur. The reaction is confined to the site of the red/yellow ink. Treatment consists of strict sunlight avoidance, use of sunscreen, intralesional steroid injections, or in some cases, surgical removal.[22] Q-switched lasers mobilize the ink through the lymphatic system and systemic allergic responses are extremely rare complications. Oral antihistamines and anti-inflammatory steroids may also be used to treat allergic reactions to tattoo ink.[23]

TREATING SPECIFIC LESIONS

Caution should be used with cosmetic ink appearing pink, flesh colored, or peach because these may contain iron oxide or titanium oxide pigments.[25] These pigments, when treated with a Q-switched laser, may turn brown or black in a phenomenon known as *paradoxical darkening*.[9] Although this brown or black color usually responds well to continued treatment, it can be disconcerting to patients as the effect of early treatment will often leave the tattoo looking darker than it did prior to treatment. If tattoo darkening does occur, after 8 weeks, the newly darkened tattoo can be treated as if it were black pigment with 1064 nm.

One of the newest forms of tattoo ink is an *iridescent pigment* that is only observable under a black light. Patients refer to these tattoos as "glow-in-the-dark." These patients should not be treated because their ink contains no chromophore for selective absorption.

Occasionally patients will present with tattoos that are slightly raised. Prior to laser treatment, if a tattoo is palpable, it will still be palpable when the treatment series is completed. It is important to remember that Q-switched lasers only treat ectopic pigment and are not intended to improve the texture of the skin.

Traumatic tattoos resulting from asphalt or "road rash" can be effectively treated with laser tattoo removal methods.[24] Obtaining a proper history is imperative when treating any traumatic tattoo because case reports of laser ignition from flammable debris have been reported.[12,26]

LEARNING THE TECHNIQUES

Practice by drawing an image on a large grapefruit or orange using a black permanent marker. This will serve as an excellent model for practitioners new to Q-switched laser techniques. As comfort level increases, practitioners can experiment with other colors until they feel their skill level warrants treatment on a patient.

CURRENT DEVELOPMENTS

A recent development is the advent of a specific type of tattoo ink called Infinitink™. The pigment in this ink is stored in transparent, biocompatible capsules, which according to the company that produces it (Freedom 2™), require fewer treatments with Q-switched lasers for removal. No studies confirming this claim are available. Furthermore, because tattoos are meant to be permanent, it is questionable whether or not the tattoo artist community will embrace the use of this ink.

FINANCIAL CONSIDERATIONS

Although tattooing of skin may be considered medically necessary when performed as part of a therapeutic intervention (e.g., radiation therapy, or with breast reconstruction), tattoo removal is considered cosmetic and is not reimbursed by insurance providers. Most providers base their fee for tattoo removal on the size of the tattoo and the presence or absence of multiple colors. For example, fees for black tattoos less than or equal to 9 in.^{2} may be \$200; 10 to 25 in.^{2}, \$350; and 26 to 49 in.^{2}, \$500; with an additional \$100 added for tattoos containing red, sky blue, or green.

CONCLUSION

Tattoo removal has advanced greatly in the past decade with the advent of highly selective Q-switched laser technologies compared to early, nonspecific tattoo removal modalities that relied on thermal and mechanical destruction. Through the process of selective photothermolysis and photoacoustic vibration, Q-switched lasers can specifically target inks of all different colors while minimizing damage to the surrounding tissues and are now considered the gold standard for patients seeking tattoo removal.

Resources

Tattoo Removal Lasers

Alma Lasers
Phone: 866-414-2562
www.almalasers.com

Asclepion Laser Technologies
www.asclepion.com

Cynosure
Phone: 800-866-2966
www.cynosure.com

HOYA ConBio
Phone: 800-532-1064
www.conbio.com

Light Age
Phone: 723-563-0600
www.light-age.com

Lumenis
Phone: 408-764-3000
www.aesthetic.lumenis.com

Syneron (formerly Candela)
Phone: 800-821-2013
www.candelalaser.com

Topical Anesthetics

American Health Solutions Pharmacy (benzocaine:lidocaine:tetracaine (20:6:4) ointment)
Phone: 310-838-7422
www.AHSRx.com

References

1. Farmer S, Laumann A, Baranwal M. Epidemiology of tattooing and body piercing: National Data Set. *J Am Acad Dermatol.* 2005;52:104.
2. Harris RB. *Harris Poll.* 2003;58.
3. Mariwalla K, Dover JS. The use of lasers for decorative tattoo removal. *Skin Ther Lett.* 2006;11:8–11.

4. Kirby W, Desai A, Kartono F. Tattoo removal techniques: effective tattoo removal treatments—Part I. *Skin and Aging*. 2005; 9:50–54.
5. Kilmer SL, Lee MS, Grevelink JM, *et al*. The Q-switched Nd:YAG laser effectively treats tattoos. A controlled, dose-response study. *Arch Dermatol*. 1993;129(8):971–978.
6. Kirby W, Desai A, Desai T, *et al*. The Kirby-Desai scale: A proposed scale to assess tattoo removal treatments. *J Clin Aesthetic Dermatol*. 2009;2(3):32–37.
7. Grevelink JM, Duke D, van Leeuwen RL, *et al*. Laser treatment of tattoos in darkly pigmented patients: efficacy and side effects. *J Am Acad Dermatol*. 1996;34(4):653–656.
8. Crawford K. Laser devices: tattoo removal. In: Pfenninger JL, Fowler GC, eds. *Pfenninger and Fowler's Procedures for Primary Care*. 3rd ed. Philadelphia: Mosby/Elsevier; 2011.
9. Anderson RR, Geronemus RG, Kilmer SL, *et al*. Cosmetic tattoo ink darkening. A complication of Q-switched and pulsed-laser treatment. *Arch Dermatol*. 1993;129:1010–1014.
10. Ho WS, Ying SP, Chan PC, Chan HH. Use of onion extract, heparin, allantoin gel in prevention of scarring in Chinese patients having laser removal of tattoos: a prospective randomized controlled trial. *Dermatol Surg*. 2006;32(7):891–896.
11. Wenzel SM. Current concepts in laser tattoo removal. *Skin Therapy Lett*. 2010:15(3):3-5.
12. Fusade T, Toubel G, Grognard C, *et al*. Treatment of gunpowder traumatic tattoo by Q-switched Nd:YAG laser: an unusual adverse effect. *Dermatol Surg*. 2000;26(11):1057–1059.
13. England R. Immediate cutaneous hypersensitivity after treatment of tattoo with Nd:YAG laser: a case report and review of the literature. *Ann Allergy Asthma Immunol*. 2002;89:215–217.
14. McFadden N, Lyberg T, Hensten-Pettersen A. Aluminum-induced granulomas in a tattoo 31. *J Am Acad Dermatol*. 1989;20(5 Pt 2):903–908.
15. Bagnato G, De Pasquale R, Glacobbe O, *et al*. Urticaria in a tattooed patient. *Allergol et Immunopathol*. 1992;71:70–73.
16. Winkelmann RK, Harris RB. Lichenoid delayed hypersensitivity reactions in tattoos. *J Cutan Pathol*. 1979;6(1):59–65.
17. Bendsoe N, Hansson C, Sterner O. Inflammatory reactions from organic pigments in red tattoos. *Acta Dermatol Venereol*. 1991; 71(1):70–73.
18. Blumental G, Okun MR, Ponitch JA. Pseudolymphomatous reaction to tattoos. Report of three cases. *J Am Acad Dermatol*. 1982;6 (4 Pt 1):485–488.
19. Tazelaar DJ. Hypersensitivity to chromium in a light-blue tattoo. *Dermatologica*. 1970;141(4):282–287.
20. Kilmer SL, Anderson RR. Clinical use of the Q-switched ruby and the Q-switched Nd:YAG (1064 nm and 532 nm) lasers for treatment of tattoos. *J Dermatol Surg Oncol*. 1993;19(4):330–338.
21. Bjornberg A. Allergic reactions to chrome in green tattoo markings. *Acta Dermatol Venereol*. 1959;39(1):23–29.
22. Bjornberg A. Allergic reaction to cobalt in light-blue tattoo markings. *Acta Dermatol Venereol*. 1961;41:259.
23. Ashinoff R, Levine VJ, Soter NA. Allergic reactions to tattoo pigment after laser treatment. *Dermatol Surg*. 1995;21:291–294.
24. Agneta M. Effective treatment of traumatic tattoos with a q-switched Nd:YAG laser. *Lasers Surg Med*. 1998;22:103–108.
25. Lee CN, Bae EY, Park JG, *et al*. Permanent makeup removal using Q-swiltched Nd:YAG laser. *Clin Exp Dermatol*. 2009;34(8): e594–e596.
26. Taylor CR. Laser ignition of traumatically embedded firework debris. *Lasers Surg Med*. 1998;22(3):157–158.

Additional Reading

Small R. Tattoo removal. *In:* Small R, ed. *A Practical Guide to Cosmetic Lasers*. Philadelphia: Lippincott; 2012.

31 Combination Cosmetic Treatments

REBECCA SMALL, MD • DALANO HOANG, DC

Facial aging is a complex process of static and dynamic wrinkling, loss of soft tissue volume with formation of folds and contour defects, and vascular and dyschromic changes. Addressing these different issues often requires the use of multiple aesthetic procedures. Many of the minimally invasive aesthetic procedures in use today are complementary, and may be combined to achieve optimal treatment outcomes and high patient satisfaction.[1,2]

Treatments typically combined with one another include botulinum toxin, dermal fillers, lasers and intense pulsed light (collectively referred to as lasers* in this chapter), microdermabrasion, chemical peels, and skin care products.[3] These procedures can be incorporated into treatment plans over several visits, or some may be combined on the same day in multimodality visits. This chapter demonstrates common treatment combinations of procedures discussed in the aesthetic section of this book.

BOTULINUM TOXIN AND DERMAL FILLERS

Wrinkles (also called rhytids) usually have both a dynamic and a static component. In many regions of the face, enhanced rhytid reduction can be achieved by addressing both dynamic muscle contraction with botulinum toxin and static lines and volume loss with dermal fillers.[4,5] Botulinum toxin is commonly used in the upper face[6] and may be combined with dermal filler treatments, particularly in the glabellar frown area (Figure 31-1).[7–9]

Botulinum toxin may also be combined with dermal fillers in the lower face, which is a more advanced application for botulinum toxin. Figure 31-2 shows a patient (the author) with radial upper lip lines elicited with active contraction of the orbicularis oris muscle (A) before, (B) 2 weeks after treatment with botulinum toxin, followed by dermal filler treatment 2 weeks later (C). Figure 31-3 shows a patient with volume loss in the oral commissure and marionette line areas, with downturned corners of the mouth, (A) before and (B) after treatment with dermal filler in these areas and botulinum toxin in the depressor anguli oris muscle which were performed in the same visit.

Dermal filler and botulinum toxin combination treatments may be performed on separate days or during the same visit. If performed on separate days, it is recommended that treatment with botulinum toxin be performed first, a few weeks prior to dermal filler treatment, to reduce muscular activity in the treatment area and allow for evaluation of the static appearance of the treatment area. If performed on the same day, the botulinum toxin injection should be performed last, to reduce tissue distortion that may occur from swelling with botulinum toxin injections. If excessive edema is present after dermal filler treatment it is advisable to postpone, botulinum toxin injection and perform treatment 1 week later.[2]

Figure 31-4 shows a patient (A) before and (B) after treatment with dermal fillers and botulinum toxin to several facial areas. Upper lip radial lip lines were treated using dermal filler and botulinum toxin, and crow's feet and glabellar complex muscles were treated using botulinum toxin. She demonstrates a typical softened appearance overall after treatment (Figure 31-4B) that is very natural looking and is the desired goal of combination aesthetic treatments.

BOTULINUM TOXIN AND SKIN RESURFACING

Skin resurfacing is a global, full-face treatment that can address rhytids and irregular texture, as well as dyschromia. Methods of resurfacing range from mild treatments with superficial chemical peels and/or microdermabrasion, to nonablative fractional laser treatments (e.g., 1550 nm) to more aggressive fractional ablative laser resurfacing (e.g., 2940 nm). Botulinum toxin treatments are often performed on the same day, following mild resurfacing treatments,[10,11] and are usually performed at least 1 week prior to laser resurfacing.

The periocular area is a common region for combination therapy with botulinum toxin and laser resurfacing.[12,13] Figure 31-5 shows a patient (A) before and (B) after receiving botulinum toxin to the crow's feet muscles and ablative laser resurfacing, demonstrating reduction of crow's feet lines and dyschromia.

In addition, different methods of superficial skin resurfacing can be combined in the same visit for enhanced results. For example, microdermabrasion, which removes the stratum corneum barrier, may immediately precede chemical peel application in the same visit to allow for more even and deeper acid penetration into the skin.[14]

COMBINING TREATMENTS WITH LASERS

Nonablative lasers (e.g., IPLs) may be readily combined with other aesthetic procedures, because the skin remains fully intact after treatment. Nonablative lasers for treatment of rhytids (e.g., 1320 and 1064 nm) may be combined with superficial resurfacing procedures.

*Refers to laser and light-based technologies.

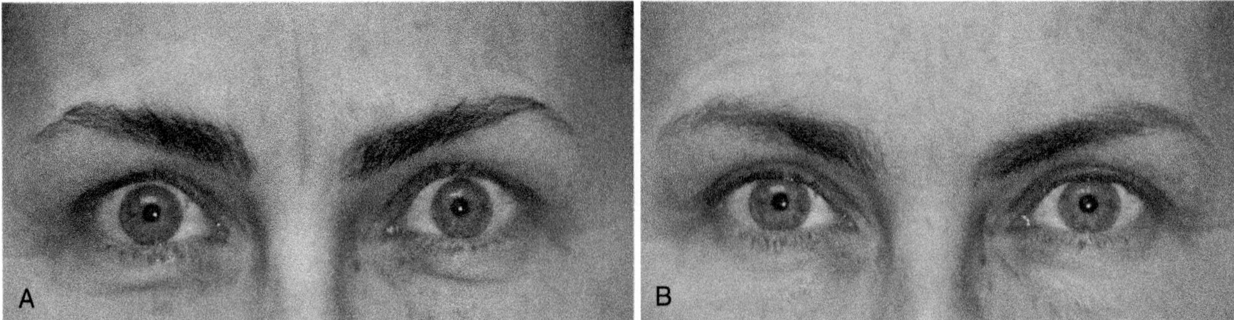

FIGURE 31-1 Frown lines **(A)** before and **(B)** after combination treatment with dermal filler (Juvederm Ultra®) to areas of volume loss and botulinum toxin (Botox®) to the glabellar complex muscles. *(Copyright Rebecca Small, MD.)*

One such technique uses a nonablative laser treatment for rhytids (Q-switched 1064 nm laser) followed by microdermabrasion and then a chemical peel—all in the same visit—to maximize collagen remodeling and reduction of fine rhytids and dyschromia.

Nonablative laser treatments for dyschromia (e.g., IPL and 532 nm lasers) may also be combined with superficial skin resurfacing procedures.[15] Following laser treatment of pigmented lesions, such as lentigines, there is microcrust formation and clinical darkening of the lesions. Resolution of these darkened lesions occurs spontaneously through exfoliation. However, improvements can be achieved more rapidly by combining superficial skin resurfacing using microdermabrasion at least 2 weeks after laser treatments for dyschromia.

Nonablative lasers of different wavelengths may be used in combination during the same visit to treat dyschromia, rhytids, and vascularities. Typically, nonablative lasers for rhytids (e.g., 1320 or 1064 nm) are performed first on the full face, and if the treatment area is not overly warm or erythematous, this may be followed by lasers that target dyschromia and vascularities (e.g., 532 nm or IPL). For example, nonablative full-face laser treatment for rhytids using a Q-switched 1064 nm laser can be immediately followed by IPL or 532 nm localized treatments in dyschromic areas and for vascularities.

When treating dyschromia, it can be useful to combine nonablative lasers that target pigmentation at different depths in the skin. Figure 31-6 shows a patient with dyschromia (A) prior to and (B) after three IPL treatments, which can target deeper pigmented lesions (based on the settings used), followed by treatment with a Q-switched 532 nm laser, which targets very superficial pigment in the skin.

Advanced facial aging changes include moderate to severe dyschromia and rhytids. These changes can be addressed by combining the more aggressive ablative resurfacing lasers (e.g., erbium and carbon dioxide lasers) for rhytid reduction with nonablative lasers that target pigmentation. Figure 31-7 shows a patient (A) before and (B) after IPL treatment for dyschromia, followed by fractional ablative laser resurfacing for textural improvement in severely photodamaged skin.

CONCLUSION

Combination therapy for rejuvenation of aging skin can be rewarding for both patients and providers by optimizing treatment outcomes in fewer visits, while improving office flow and revenue. A comprehensive aesthetic rejuvenation plan often incorporates regional treatments, such as botulinum toxin and dermal fillers, together with global treatments, such as full-face skin resurfacing or laser treatments. With a foundation in basic aesthetic principles and consultation, together with procedural proficiency using different minimally invasive procedures, providers can successfully combine aesthetic treatments to achieve subtle and natural rejuvenation results.

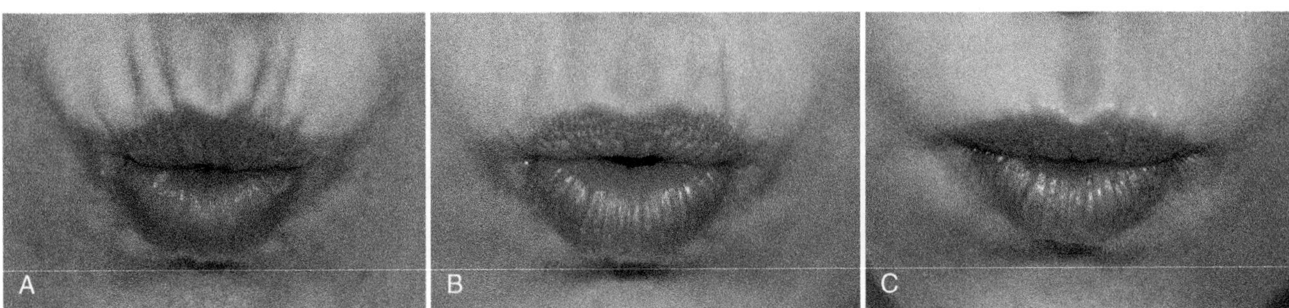

FIGURE 31-2 Dynamic and static radial lip lines **(A)** before, **(B)** after treatment with botulinum toxin (Botox) to the orbicularis oris muscle and **(C)** after dermal filler (Radiesse®) above the upper lip, during active contraction. *(Copyright Rebecca Small, MD.)*

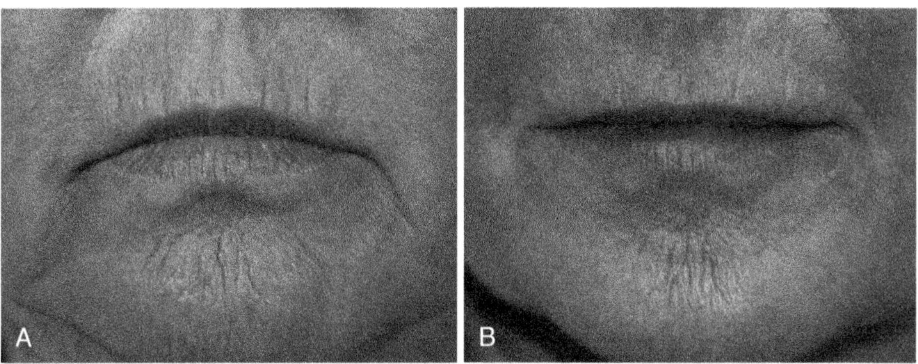

FIGURE 31-3 Oral commissures and marionette lines **(A)** before and **(B)** after combination treatment with dermal filler (Juvederm®) to areas of volume loss and botulinum toxin (Botox) to the depressor anguli oris muscle. *(Copyright Rebecca Small, MD.)*

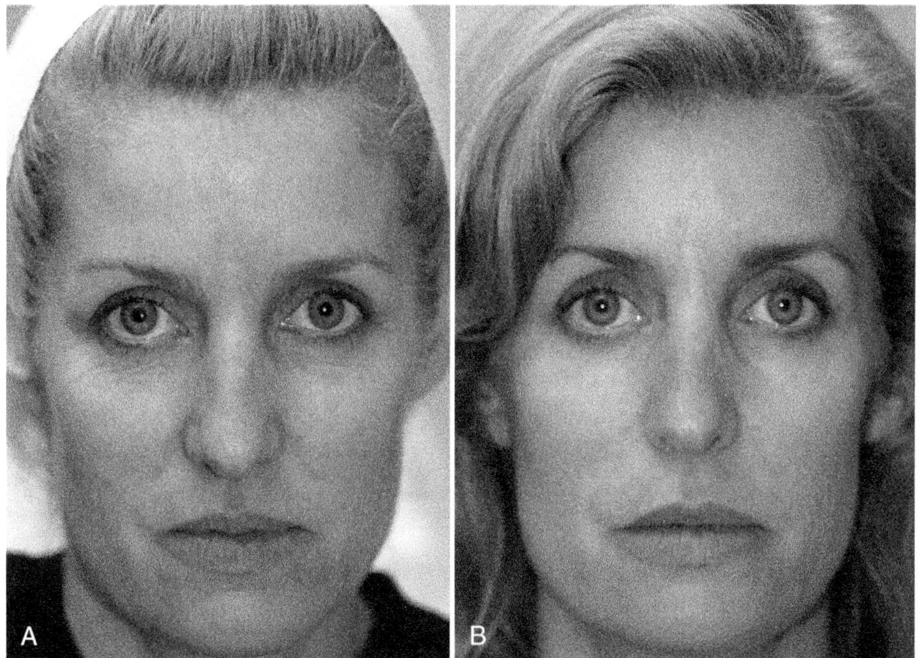

FIGURE 31-4 Overall facial rejuvenation **(A)** before and **(B)** after combination treatment with botulinum toxin (Botox) to the orbicularis oris, orbicularis oculi, and glabellar complex muscles, and dermal filler (Radiesse) above the upper lip. *(Copyright Rebecca Small, MD.)*

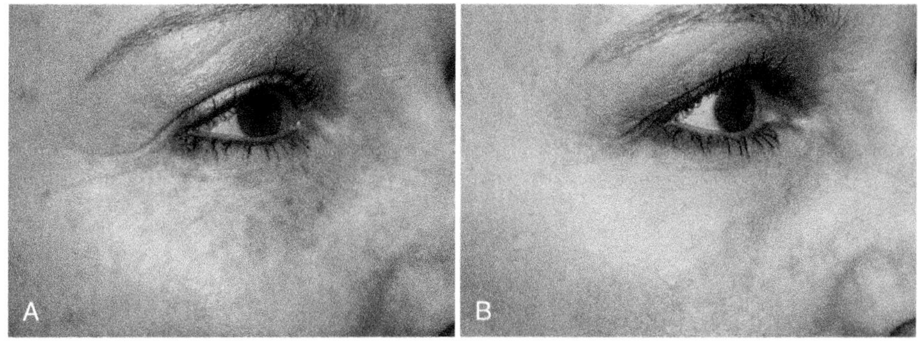

FIGURE 31-5 Periocular rhytids and lentigines **(A)** before and **(B)** after combination treatment with botulinum toxin (Botox) to the orbicularis oculi muscles and superficial ablative laser resurfacing (Polish Peel with DermaSculpt, HOYA ConBio). *(Copyright Rebecca Small, MD.)*

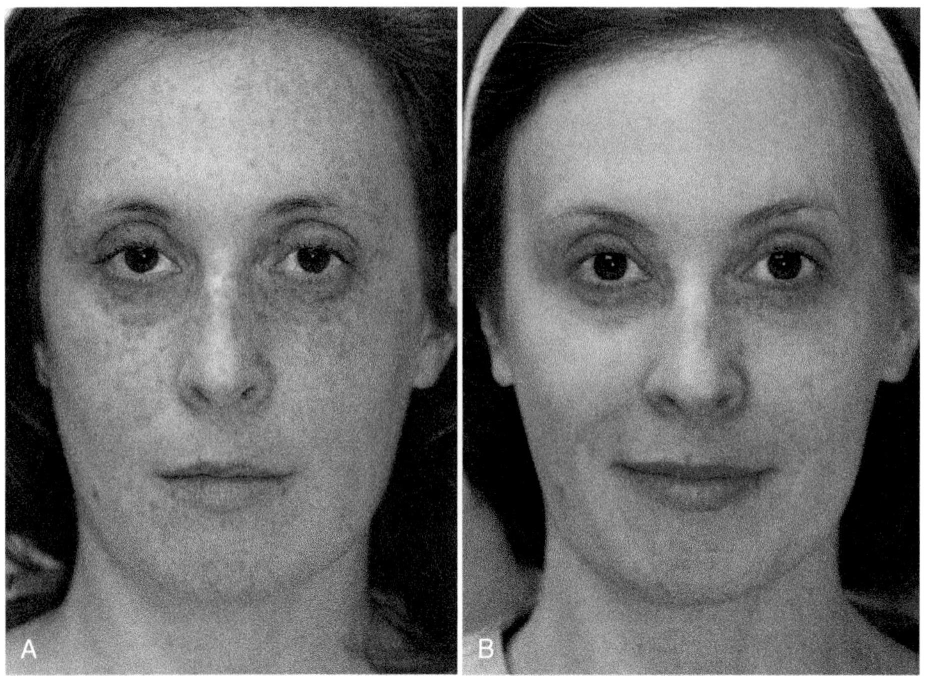

FIGURE 31-6 Dyschromia (**A**) before and (**B**) after combination treatment with intense pulsed light (LuxG with Palomar StarLux 500) and a Q-switched 532 nm laser (RevLite, HOYA ConBio). *(Copyright Rebecca Small, MD.)*

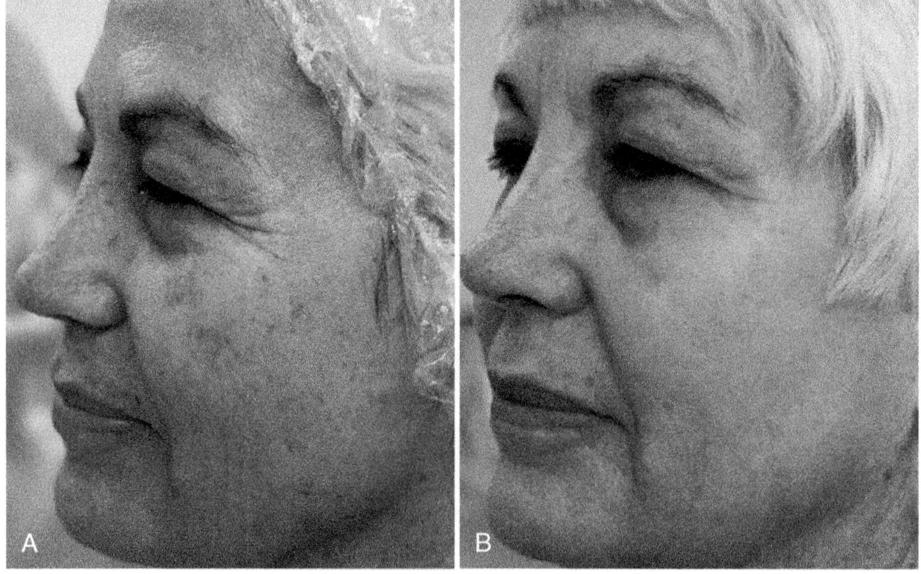

FIGURE 31-7 Severely photodamaged skin (**A**) before and (**B**) after combination treatment with intense pulsed light (560 nm filter with BBL, Sciton) for dyschromia, and fractional ablative laser treatment (ProFractional-XC, Sciton) for textural improvement. *(Courtesy of Sciton, Palo Alto, CA; and T. Bessinger, MD.)*

References

1. Small R. Aesthetic procedures introduction. *In:* Mayeaux E, ed. *The Essential Guide to Primary Care Procedures*. Philadelphia: Lippincott Williams & Wilkins; 2009:195–199.
2. Fedok FG. Advances in minimally invasive facial rejuvenation. *Curr Opin Otolaryngol Head Neck Surg*. 2008;16(4):359–368.
3. Small R. Aesthetic procedures in office practice. *Am Fam Physician*. 2009;80(11):1231–1237.
4. Carruthers JD, Glogau RG, Blitzer A. Advances in facial rejuvenation: botulinum toxin type A, hyaluronic acid dermal fillers, and combination therapies—consensus recommendations. *Plast Reconstr Surg*. 2008;121(5 Suppl):5S–30S.
5. Coleman KR, Carruthers J. Combination therapy with Botox and fillers: the new rejuvenation paradigm. *Dermatol Ther*. 2006;19(3):177–188.
6. Small R. Botulinum toxin type A for facial rejuvenation. *In:* Mayeaux E, ed. *The Essential Guide to Primary Care Procedures*. Philadelphia: Lippincott Williams & Wilkins; 2009:200–213.
7. Carruthers JD, Carruthers A. A prospective, randomized, parallel group study analyzing the effect of BTX-A (Botox) and nonanimal sourced hyaluronic acid (NASHA, Restylane) in combination compared with NASHA (Restylane) alone in severe glabellar rhytides in adult female subjects: treatment of severe glabellar rhytides with a hyaluronic acid derivative compared with the derivative and BTX-A. *Dermatol Surg*. 2003;29(8):802–809.
8. Carruthers J, Carruthers A, Maberley D. Deep resting glabellar rhytides respond to BTX-A and Hylan B. *Dermatol Surg*. 2003;29(5):539–544.
9. Maas CS. Botulinum neurotoxins and injectable fillers: minimally invasive management of the aging upper face. *Facial Plast Surg Clin North Am*. 2006;14(3):241–245.
10. Rendon MI, Effron C, Edison BL. The use of fillers and botulinum toxin type A in combination with superficial glycolic acid (alpha-hydroxy acid) peels: optimizing injection therapy with the skin-smoothing properties of peels. *Cutis*. 2007;79(1 Suppl Combining):9–12.
11. Small R. Microdermabrasion. *In:* Mayeaux E, ed. *The Essential Guide to Primary Care Procedures*. Philadelphia: Lippincott Williams & Wilkins; 2009:265–277.
12. Yamauchi PS, Lask GP, Lowe NJ. Botulinum toxin type A gives adjunctive benefit to periorbital laser resurfacing. *J Cosmet Laser Ther*. 2004;6(3):145–148.
13. Zimbler MS, Holds JB, Kokoska MS, *et al*. Effect of botulinum toxin pretreatment on laser resurfacing results: a prospective, randomized, blinded trial. *Arch Facial Plast Surg*. 2001;3(3):165–169.
14. Briden ME, Jacobsen E, Johnson C. Combining superficial glycolic acid (alpha-hydroxy acid) peels with microdermabrasion to maximize treatment results and patient satisfaction. *Cutis*. 2007;79(1 Suppl Combining):13–16.
15. Effron C, Briden ME, Green BA. Enhancing cosmetic outcomes by combining superficial glycolic acid (alpha-hydroxy acid) peels with nonablative lasers, intense pulsed light, and trichloroacetic acid peels. *Cutis*. 2007;79(1 Suppl Combining):4–8.

Additional Reading

Small R, Hoang D. Botulinum toxin introduction and foundation concepts. *In:* Small R, Hoang D, eds. *A Practical Guide to Botulinum Toxin Procedures*. Philadelphia: Lippincott Williams & Wilkins; 2011.

Small R, Hoang D. Dermal filler introduction and foundation concepts. *In:* Small R, Hoang D, eds. *A Practical Guide to Dermal Filler Procedures*. Philadelphia: Lippincott Williams & Wilkins; 2011.

Small R, Linder J. Combining therapies. *In:* Small R, Linder J, eds. *A Practical Guide to Skin Care Procedures and Products*. Philadelphia: Lippincott Williams & Wilkins; 2011.

Small R. Combining therapies. *In:* Small R, ed. *A Practical Guide to Cosmetic Lasers*. Philadelphia: Lippincott Williams & Wilkins; 2012.

SECTION FOUR

Putting it All Together

32 Dermoscopy

ASHFAQ A. MARGHOOB, MD • RICHARD P. USATINE, MD

Dermoscopy allows the clinician to observe morphologic structures below the surface of the skin that are otherwise not visible to the naked eye. Many of the dermoscopically observed structures have direct histopathology correlates. In addition, the presence or absence of dermoscopic structures, their association with each other (i.e., certain structures are often seen together such as milia and comedo openings in a seborrheic keratosis), and their distribution within a lesion often lead to a specific diagnosis. Thus, it should come as no surprise that dermoscopy improves the clinician's diagnostic accuracy. Dermoscopes are relatively inexpensive and easy to use and master. Start with this chapter and consider attending dermoscopy courses, visiting websites, and reading books on the subject once you have your dermatoscope and are ready to extend your learning.

ADVANTAGES OF AND EVIDENCE FOR DERMOSCOPY

In two separate meta-analyses, dermoscopy had significantly higher discriminating power than clinical examination for experienced users.[1–3] It is intuitively obvious that this improved diagnostic accuracy translates into improved patient management. For example, in one study, the malignant-to-benign ratio improved in dermoscopy users from 1 : 18 to 1 : 4.[4]

Primary care physicians (PCPs) who were given a 1-day training course in skin cancer detection and dermoscopic evaluation were able to improve their sensitivity for melanoma diagnosis. The study randomly assigned PCPs to the dermoscopy evaluation arm or the naked-eye (no dermoscopy) evaluation arm. The study showed that 23 malignant skin tumors were missed by PCPs performing naked-eye observation, whereas only 6 were missed by PCPs using dermoscopy ($P = 0.002$). The authors concluded that the use of dermoscopy improves the ability of PCPs to triage lesions suggestive of skin cancer without increasing the number of unnecessary expert consultations.[5]

Dermoscopy can help in the following ways:

- Allows the observer to concentrate on a lesion and formulate a logical differential diagnosis.
- Helps differentiate melanocytic from nonmelanocytic lesions.
- Helps differentiate benign from malignant lesions.
- Improves diagnostic accuracy.
- Increases the observer's confidence in his or her clinical diagnosis.
- Confirms naked-eye diagnosis (clinical-dermoscopy correlation).
- Improves malignant-to-benign biopsy ratio (hence, avoiding unnecessary biopsies).
- Helps isolate suspicious foci within lesions, allowing the clinician to give specific suggestions to the dermatopathologist for processing.
- Helps more precisely define borders of some lesions for improved presurgical margin mapping.
- Helps to reassure patients.[6]
- Helps in the surveillance of patients with many nevi.[6]

EQUIPMENT

Dermoscopes illuminate the skin via the use of light emitting diode (LED) lights with or without the use of polarizing filters. Although most units are either nonpolarized (no polarizing filters in place) or polarized (polarized filters used), a few newer units, known as hybrids, allow the operator to toggle between polarized and nonpolarized light within the same unit. Nonpolarized dermoscopes (NPDs) are manufactured by Heine and Welch Allyn (Figure 32-1A). 3Gen manufactures NPDs, polarized dermoscopes (PDs), and hybrid dermoscopes (Figure 32-1B). A number of new dermoscopes attach to smart phones for easy dermoscopic photography.

Dermoscopic images seen with and without polarization can appear quite different, often providing complementary information. During naked-eye examinations of the skin, much of the light emitted toward the skin is reflected off of the stratum corneum due to the higher reflective index of the stratum corneum as compared to that of air. This precludes the observer from seeing structures below the stratum corneum. Nonpolarized dermoscopes require direct contact between the lesion and the glass plate of the dermoscope. In addition, the presence of a liquid interface (i.e., alcohol or oil) between the lesion and the glass plate is mandatory. The elimination of the air interface and the presence of the liquid reduces the amount of light reflected off the stratum corneum, thereby allowing the observer to see structures below the stratum corneum. The requirement of a liquid interface and direct skin contact can be eliminated with the use of polarized light and a cross-polarizing filter, as utilized in polarized dermoscopes. Although both NPD and PD allow the observer to visualize similar structures below the stratum corneum, subtle differences do exist. These differences tend to provide complementary information.

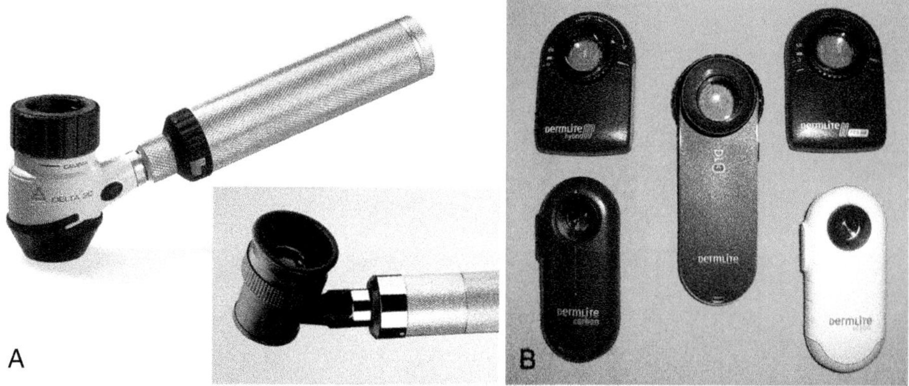

FIGURE 32-1 **(A)** Nonpolarized contact dermoscopes from Heine and Welch Allyn. **(B)** An assortment of polarized and hybrid dermoscopes from 3Gen. *(A: Courtesy of Heine, Herrsching, Germany, and Welch Allyn, Skaneateles Falls, NY; B: Courtesy of 3Gen, San Juan Capistrano, CA.)*

Nonpolarized dermoscopy works best for visualizing:

- Milia-like cysts
- Peppering due to regression
- Blue-white colors due to orthokeratosis of the stratum corneum.

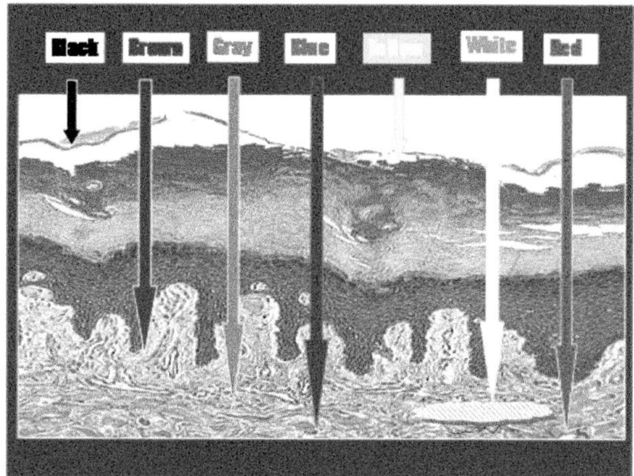

FIGURE 32-2 Colors seen on dermoscopy based on the depth of the melanin and other skin structures. *(Courtesy of Alfred W. Kopf, MD.)*

Color seen with dermoscopy	Histopathologic correlation
Yellow	Keratin in the stratum corneum devoid of blood and melanin.
Black	Melanin in stratum corneum, superficial layers of epidermis or throughout all layers of epidermis, with or without dermal involvement.
Brown	Melanin below the stratum corneum, especially if present in the dermal-epidermal junction and papillary dermis.
White	Lack of melanin and/or atrophy/fibrosis.
Gray	Free-melanin or melanophages in papillary dermis.
Red	Blood from vascularity or bleeding within the lesion.
Blue	Melanin in the deep dermis (due to Tyndall effect).

Polarized dermoscopy works best for visualizing:

- Shiny white streaks (chrysalis structures) due to altered collagen
- Blood vessels
- Red-pink colors due to increased vascular volume.

PRINCIPLES OF DERMOSCOPY

The colors seen on dermoscopy, which are based on the depth of the melanin and other skin structures, are illustrated in Figure 32-2.

Network Patterns

Pigment Network

A reticulated pigment network (Figure 32-3) has the following characteristics:

- The grid-like (honeycomb) network is composed of pigmented lines and hypopigmented "holes."
- Network lines correspond to the rete ridge pattern of the epidermis.
- Network lines are visible due to melanin pigment in keratinocytes and melanocytes along the dermal/epidermal junction.

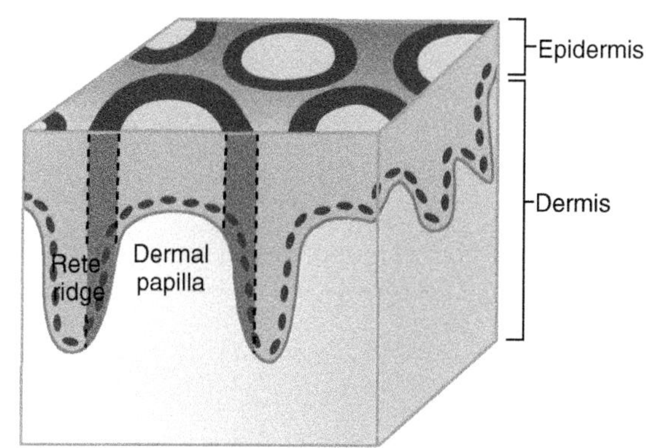

FIGURE 32-3 Pigment network is created by melanocytes along the rete ridge seen from the skin surface producing a net-like (reticulated) pattern.

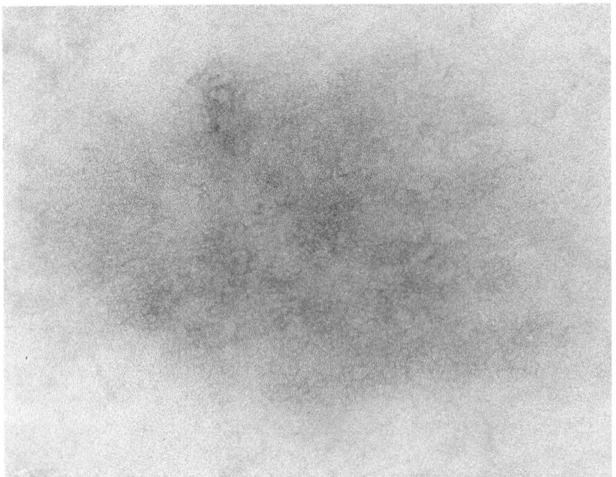

FIGURE 32-4 Typical pigment network (in a benign nevus). Note the regular line thickness and the fading of the lines at the periphery. *(Copyright Ashfaq A. Marghoob, MD.)*

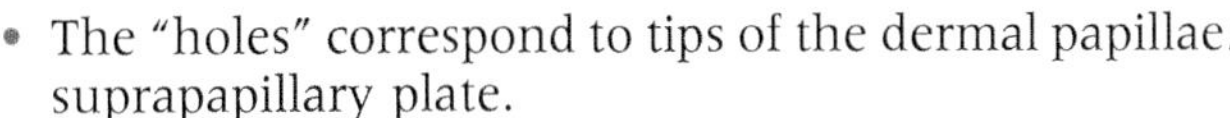

- The "holes" correspond to tips of the dermal papillae/suprapapillary plate.

A typical pigment network in a benign nevus consists of (Figure 32-4):

- A relatively uniform line thickness and color
- A regularly meshed network
- Thinning (fading) at the periphery.

For an atypical pigment network (Figure 32-5),

- The lines of the network are not uniform in thickness and color.
- The lines are darker and/or broadened compared to a typical network.
- The "holes" are heterogeneous in size.
- The lines end abruptly at the periphery.

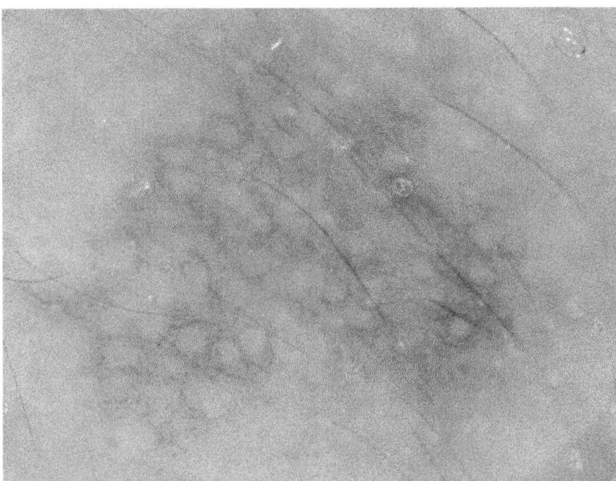

FIGURE 32-6 Pseudonetwork is the net-like pattern made by lightly-colored adnexal openings within pigmented lesions on the face. This is a solar lentigo with a typical moth-eaten border showing the adnexal openings within the pigmented lentigo. *(Copyright Ashfaq A. Marghoob, MD.)*

A *pseudonetwork* (Figure 32-6) is

- Usually seen in pigmented lesions located on the face.
- Results when the rete ridge pattern is attenuated.
- Has adnexal openings (hair follicles and sweat glands) that form the holes of the pseudonetwork.

A *negative network* is a reverse network that is seen in melanoma (Figures 32-7 and 32-8). It consists of dark, elongated, and curved globular structures surrounded by relative hypopigmentation. This results in the impression that the lines of the network appear lighter in color with an almost serpiginous pattern with holes that are darker in color (and appear sausage shaped).

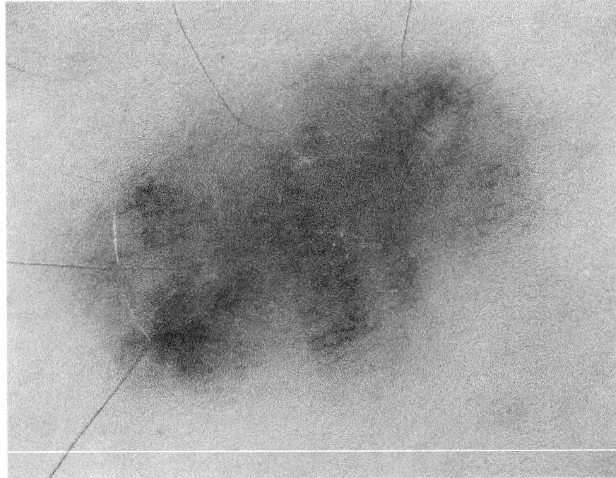

FIGURE 32-5 Atypical pigment network in a dysplastic nevus with variations in line thickness, darkness, and pattern. *(Copyright Richard P. Usatine, MD.)*

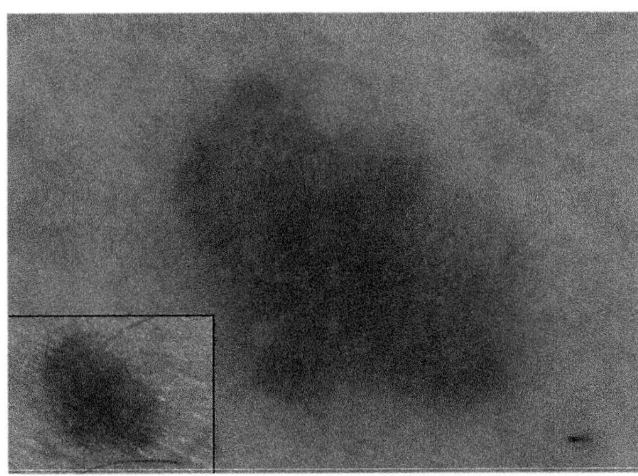

FIGURE 32-7 Negative network (reverse network) in a microinvasive melanoma. The negative network consists of dark, elongated, and curved globular structures surrounded by relative hypopigmentation. *(Copyright Ashfaq A. Marghoob, MD.)*

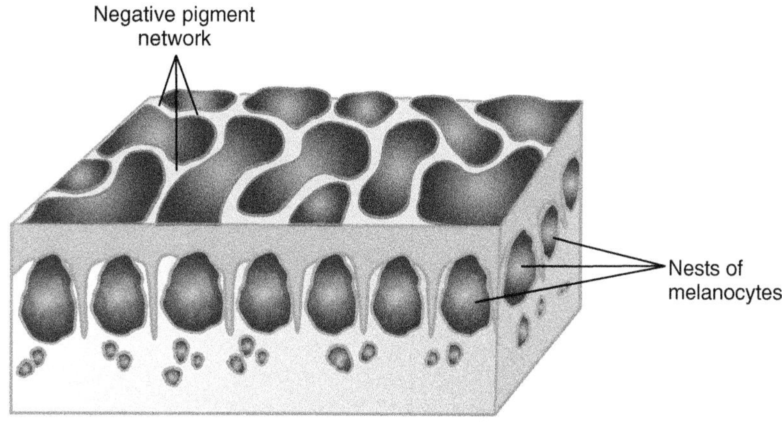

FIGURE 32-8 Negative network is created by large nests of melanocytes squeezing the rete ridges, making them into the lighter areas between the darker nests.

Other Structures

Chrysalis

- Seen only with polarized light dermoscopy.
- Consists of linear white lines/streaks that are oriented in an orthogonal fashion.
- The chrysalis structure (Figures 32-9 and 32-10) represents altered dermal collagen.

Structureless Areas

- Areas devoid of any discernible structures.
- The color is relatively hypopigmented compared to the surrounding nevus, but it is not white and it does not manifest any regression structures such as peppering.
- Results from a lack of pigment, attenuated rete ridges, or lack of contrast.

Dots

- Dots are small, round structures with a diameter of less than 0.1 mm.
- They are black, brown, blue-gray, or red in color.
- Black dots represent pigment in the stratum corneum.
- Brown dots represent small nevomelanocytic nests at the tips of the rete ridges, at the dermal/epidermal junction, or in the epidermis.
- Blue-gray dots represent free melanin in dermis or in macrophages.
- Red dots represent blood vessels.

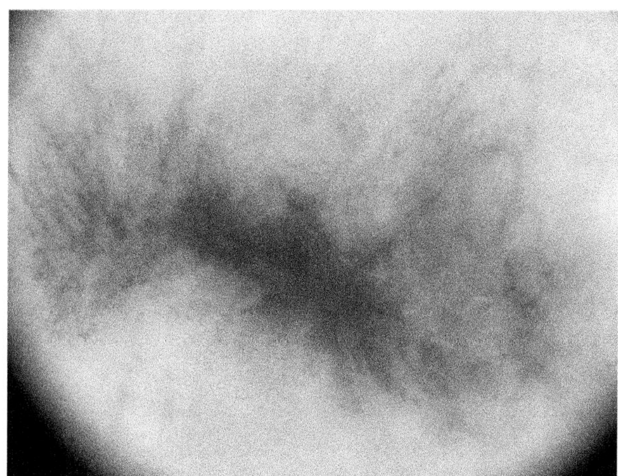

FIGURE 32-9 Melanoma with chrysalis (also known as crystalline structures) seen on the right side of the lesion. They consist of orthogonal white lines. *(Copyright Ashfaq A. Marghoob, MD.)*

Typical dots in benign melanocytic lesions are seen in Figure 32-11. Brown dots on the network appear in normal nevi (Figure 32-12). Brown dots off the network may appear in dysplastic nevi or melanoma (Figure 32-13).

Globules

- Globules are symmetrical, round to oval structures that are larger than 0.1 mm (Figures 32-13 and 32-14).
- They are brown, black, blue, or red in color.
- Brown, black, and blue globules correspond to nests of pigmented melanocytes at the dermal/epidermal junction or in the dermis.
- Red globules represent blood vessels of neovascularization.

Figure 32-14A shows typical globules evenly distributed in a benign nevus; Figure 32-14B shows atypical globules aggregated in the lower left corner of a dysplastic nevus.

Pseudopods

- Pseudopods are linear finger-like projections that radiate toward normal skin.
- They are located at the periphery of the lesion.
- They have small knobs at their tips that can make them look like tennis rackets.

Various types of pseudopods are shown in Figures 32-15 through 32-17.

Radial Streaming

The term *radial streaming* refers to radial, parallel, linear extensions that resemble pseudopods but do not have a knob at the ends (Figure 32-18). They are located at the periphery.

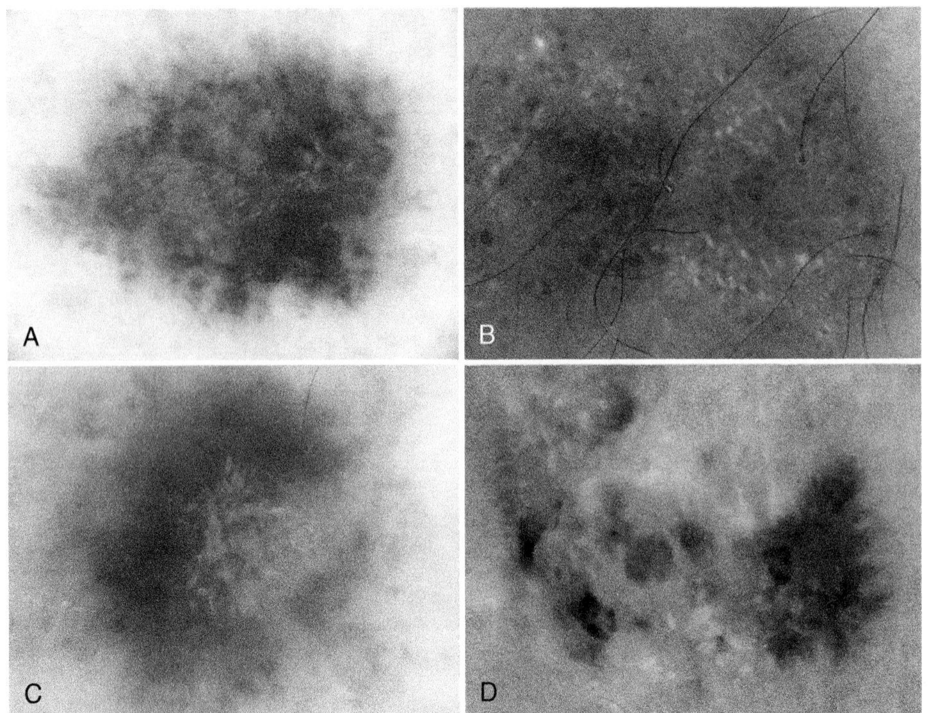

FIGURE 32-10 Chrysalis crystalline structures represent altered dermal collagen and can be seen in these four melanocytic and nonmelanocytic lesions: **(A)** melanoma; **(B)** Spitz nevus; **(C)** dermatofibroma; **(D)** basal cell carcinoma. *(Copyright Ashfaq A. Marghoob, MD.)*

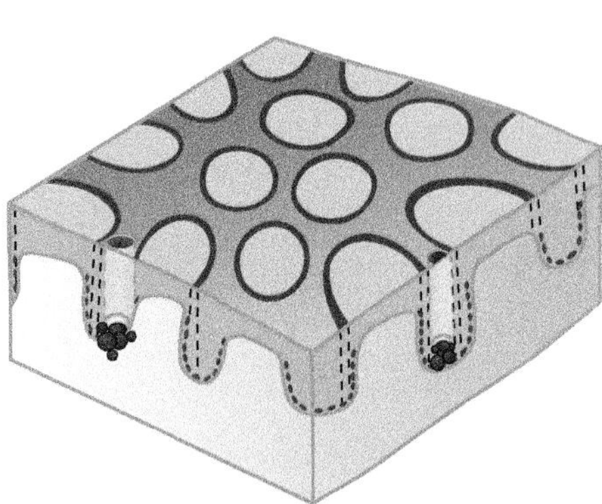

FIGURE 32-11 Typical dots in benign melanocytic lesions are seen on the pigment network and are caused by a cluster of melanocytes at the base of the rete ridge.

FIGURE 32-12 Dermoscopy of benign nevus with typical dots on the network. *(Copyright Ashfaq A. Marghoob, MD.)*

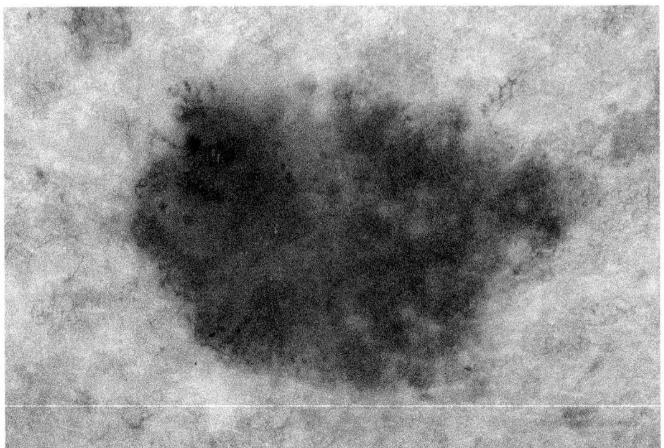

FIGURE 32-13 Invasive melanoma with atypical dots near the left edge and atypical globules in the upper left corner. *(Copyright Ashfaq A. Marghoob, MD.)*

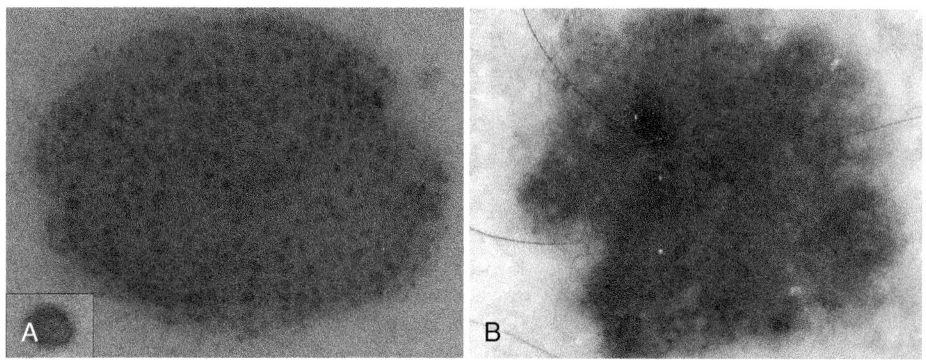

FIGURE 32-14 (**A**) Typical globules evenly distributed in a benign nevus. AM. (**B**) Atypical globules aggregated in the lower left corner of this dysplastic nevus. *(Copyright Ashfaq A. Marghoob, MD.)*

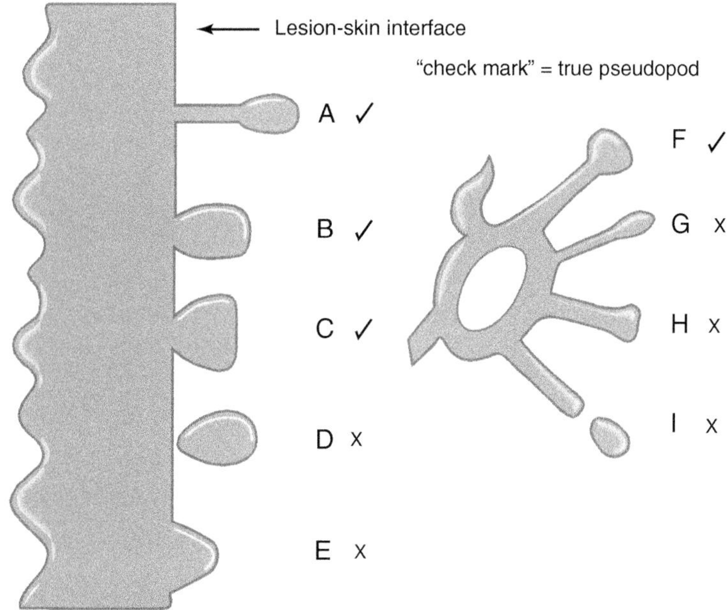

FIGURE 32-15 Pseudopods. A, B, C, and F are true pseudopods; the others are not. *(Adapted from Menzies SW, Crotty K, McCarthy W. The morphologic criteria of the pseudopod in surface microscopy. Arch Dermatol. 1995;131:436–440.)*

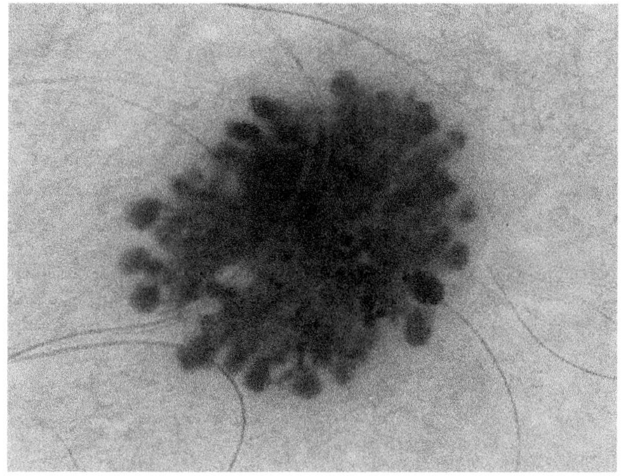

FIGURE 32-16 Pseudopods in a Spitz nevus that are nearly 360° around the nevus. *(Copyright Ashfaq A. Marghoob, MD.)*

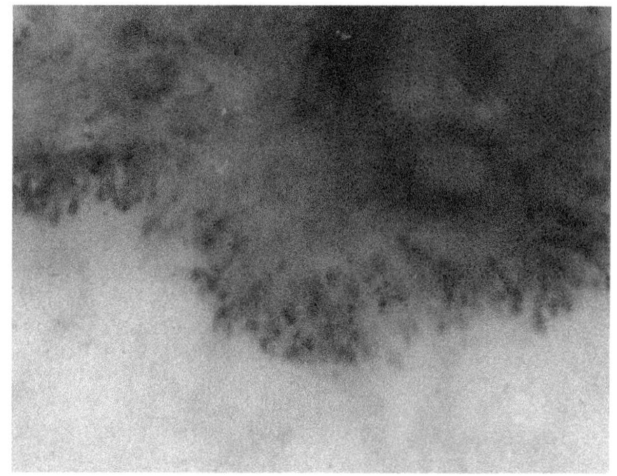

FIGURE 32-17 Pseudopods seen in a melanoma. These represent radial growth of the tumor. *(Copyright Ashfaq A. Marghoob, MD.)*

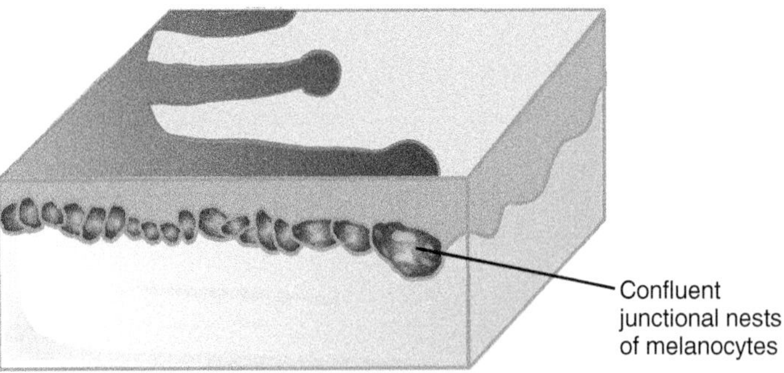

FIGURE 32-18 Radial streaming showing the radial growth pattern of nests of melanocytes in a melanoma or Spitz nevus.

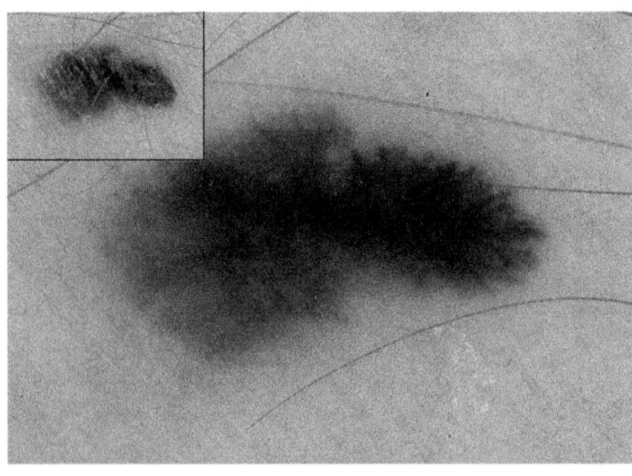

FIGURE 32-19 Streaks are visible with radial streaming on the right side of this invasive melanoma. *(Copyright Ashfaq A. Marghoob, MD.)*

Streaks

Streaks is a term that encompasses both pseudopods and radial streaming. These are seen in melanoma and Spitz nevi (Figures 32-15 through 32-19).

Blotch (Black Lamella)

- A blotch has a large concentration of melanin pigment.
- It extends throughout the epidermis and/or dermis.
- It visually obscures the underlying structures.
- A typical blotch in a benign nevus is often centrally located while an off-center blotch may be seen in a melanoma (Figure 32-20).

Blue White Veil, Raised

- Area of focal irregular, indistinct, confluent, blue pigmentation (Figure 32-21).
- Focal overlying white ground-glass haze.
- Aggregation of heavily pigmented cells/melanin in the dermis (blue color) in combination with compact orthokeratosis (anuclear keratin layer).

Figure 32-21 shows a blue-white veil over a raised area in a melanoma.

Blue White Veil, Flat

A flat blue-white veil is also called a white scar-like area with "peppering" or regression structures (Figure 32-22).

- Area of white scar-like depigmentation.
- Focal speckled multiple blue-gray granules (blue-white veil over flat area).
- Fibrosis, loss of pigmentation, epidermal thinning, effacement of the rete ridges, and melanin granules free in the dermis or in melanophages scattered in the papillary dermis.

Peppering

Also know as granularity, peppering is loose melanin in the dermis or melanin in melanophages.

Note that the blue-white veil (raised or flat) and peppering are melanoma-specific structures and should raise concern.

Structures in Nonmelanocytic Lesions

Seborrheic Keratoses

Milia-Like Cysts (Figure 32-23)

- Round whitish or yellowish structures.
- Commonly seen in seborrheic keratosis.
- They represent intraepidermal keratin-filled cysts.

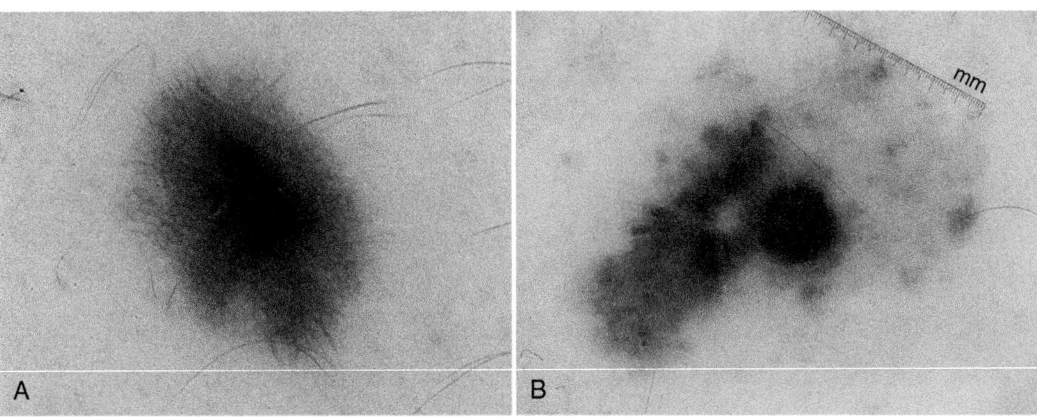

FIGURE 32-20 (A) Peripheral network with a central blotch in this benign nevus. (B) Atypical blotch (not centrally located) in a melanoma. Note the blue-white veil, atypical globules, atypical network, and the peripheral tan structureless areas. *(Copyright Ashfaq A. Marghoob, MD.)*

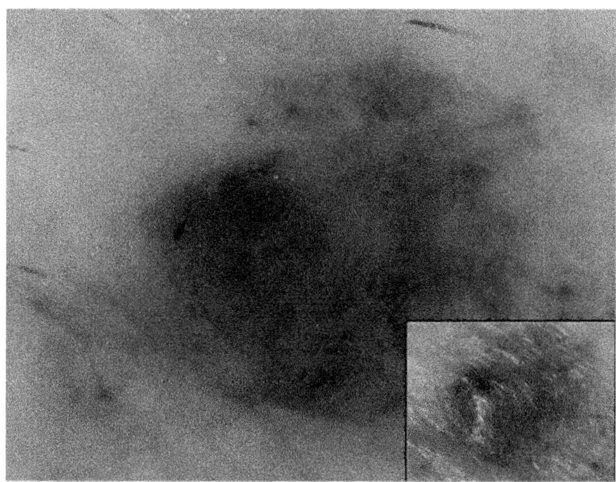

FIGURE 32-21 Blue-white veil over raised area in a melanoma. *(Copyright Ashfaq A. Marghoob, MD.)*

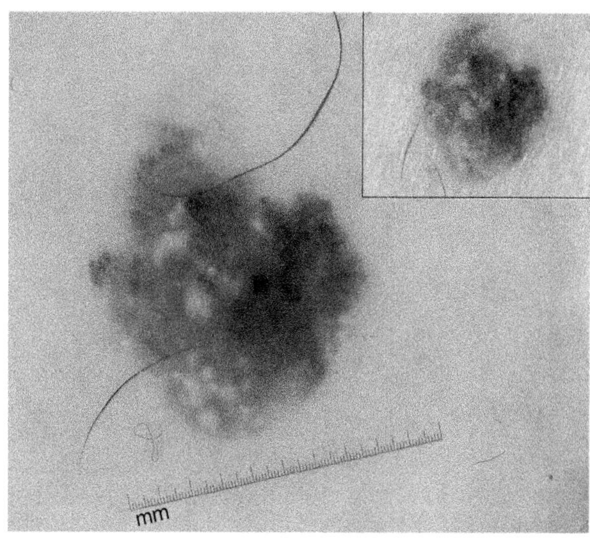

FIGURE 32-23 Seborrheic keratosis with milia-like cysts and comedo-like openings. *(Copyright Ashfaq A. Marghoob, MD.)*

Comedo-Like Openings *(Figure 32-23)*

- Commonly seen in seborrheic keratosis.
- They represent keratin-filled invaginations of the epidermis.

Gyri and Sulci *(Figure 32-24)*

- Have a cerebriform appearance.
- The gyri can sometimes resemble "fat fingers."

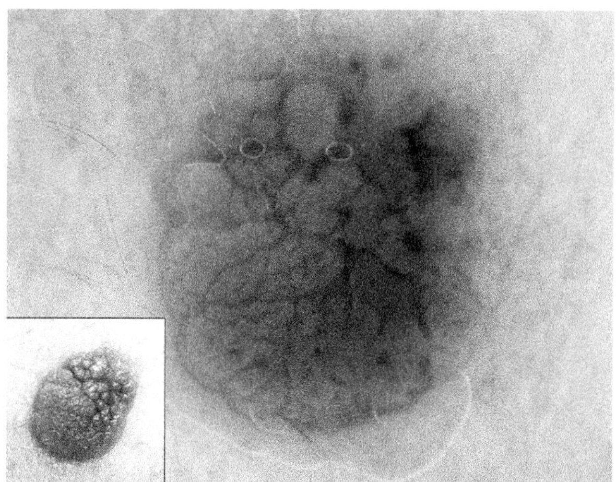

FIGURE 32-24 Cerebriform seborrheic keratosis with gyri and sulci. *(Copyright Robert Gilson, MD.)*

Basal Cell Carcinoma (BCC)

Leaf-Like Areas *(Figures 32-25 and 32-26)*

- Brown to gray-blue discrete bulbous blobs.
- "Leaf-like" pattern.

Blue-Gray Ovoid Nests *(Figure 32-27)*

- Large and well circumscribed.
- Confluent pigmented ovoid areas.

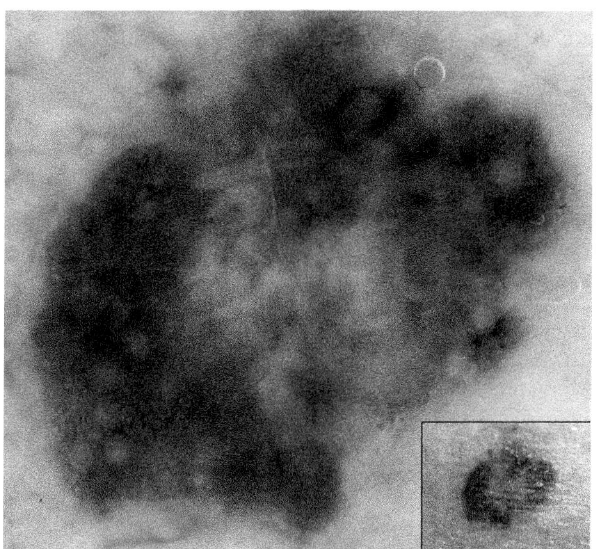

FIGURE 32-22 Blue-white veil over flat area with "peppering." These represent regression structures in a melanoma *in situ*. *(Copyright Richard P. Usatine, MD.)*

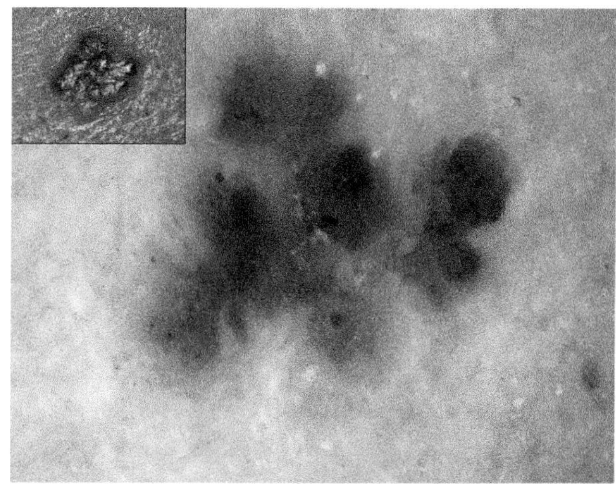

FIGURE 32-25 Leaf-like structures in a pigmented BCC. *(Copyright Richard P. Usatine, MD.)*

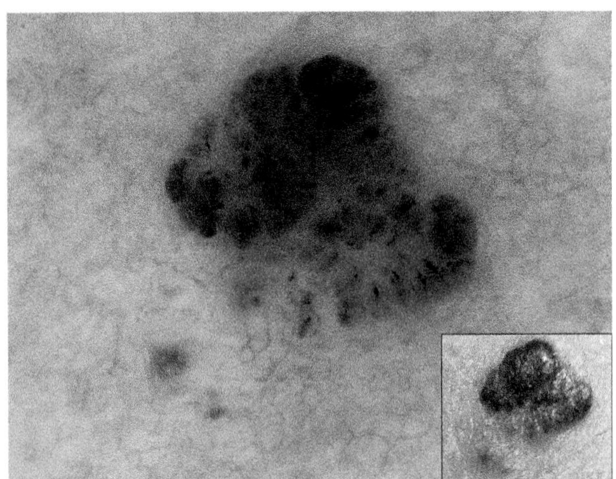

FIGURE 32-26 Leaf-like structures and blue-gray ovoid nest in bottom left-hand corner of this BCC. *(Copyright Richard P. Usatine, MD.)*

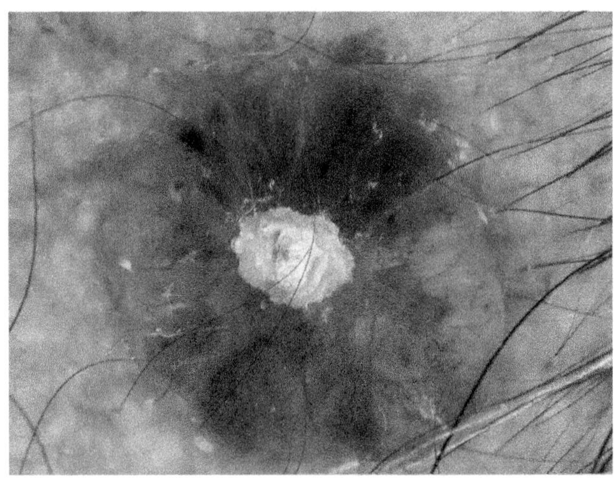

FIGURE 32-28 Arborizing blood vessels like branching trees in a BCC. *(Copyright Richard P. Usatine, MD.)*

Spoke-Wheel-Like Structures *(Figure 32-27)*

- Well circumscribed.
- Brown to gray-blue-brown.
- Radial projections.
- Meeting at a darker brown central hub.

Arborizing blood vessels are seen in BCC (Figure 32-28).

Angioma/Angiokeratoma

Angiomas have red lacunae (lagoons) (Figure 32-29). Angiokeratomas have red, maroon, blue, and black lacunae (lagoons) (Figure 32-30). Their vascular architecture is described in Figure 32-31.

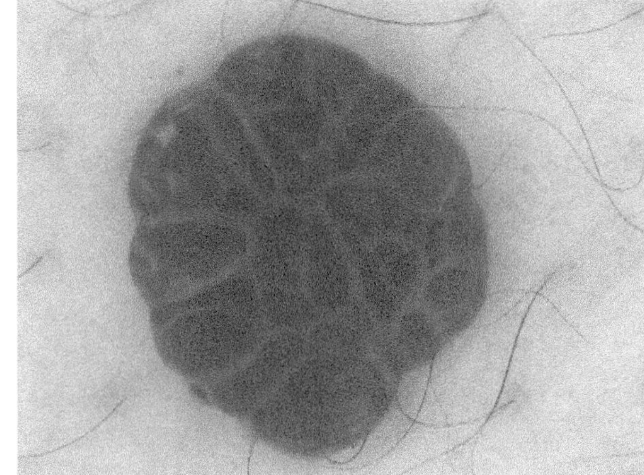

FIGURE 32-29 Hemangioma showing red lacunae (lakes or lagoons of sharply demarcated vascular tissue). *(Copyright Richard P. Usatine, MD.)*

TWO-STEP DERMOSCOPY ALGORITHM

The two-step dermoscopy algorithm forms the foundation for the dermoscopic evaluation and differentiation of skin lesions (Figure 32-32). If a lesion manifests any

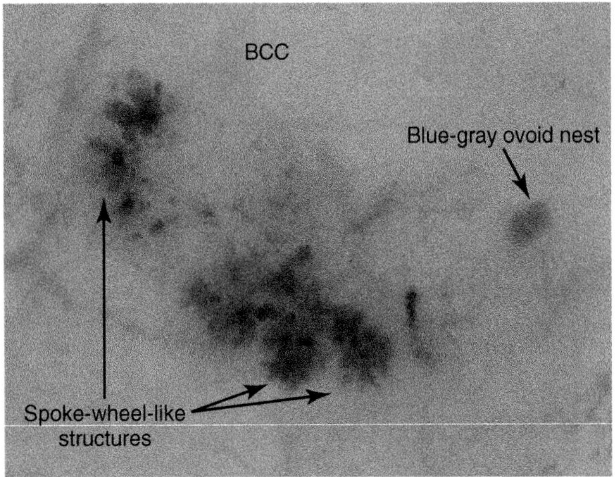

FIGURE 32-27 Spoke-wheel-like structures and isolated blue-gray ovoid nest on the left. *(Copyright Ashfaq A. Marghoob, MD.)*

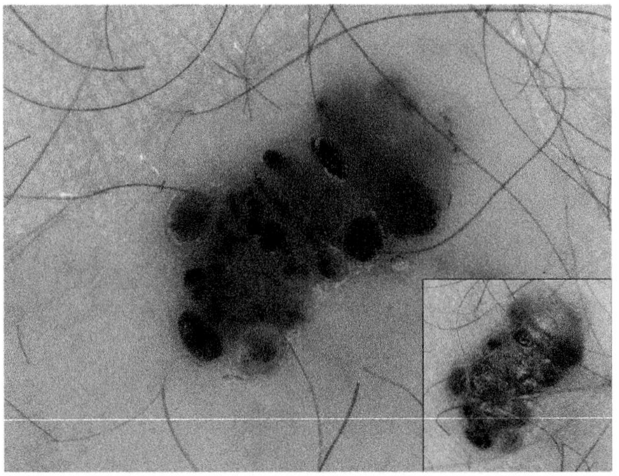

FIGURE 32-30 Angiokeratoma showing purple and black lacunae. *(Copyright Ashfaq A. Marghoob, MD.)*

Red lagoons	Sharply demarcated globular structures Colors: red, violaceous, brownish, bluish or black Absence of vessels or other pigmented structures inside the lagoons Significance: hemangiomas or angiokeratomas	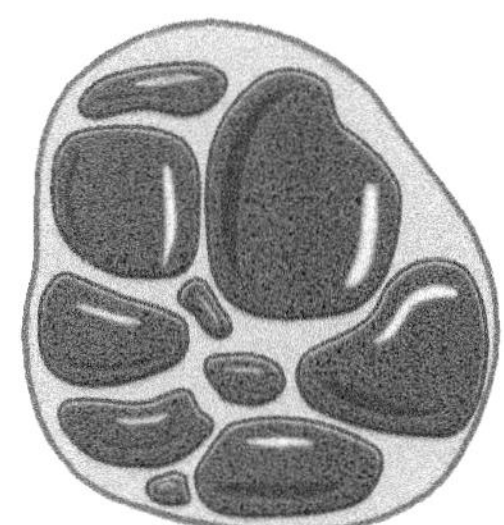
Hairpin vessels	Elongated vessels resembling hairpins Significance: when fine and surrounded by hypopigmented halo, seborrheic keratosis and other keratonizing tumors	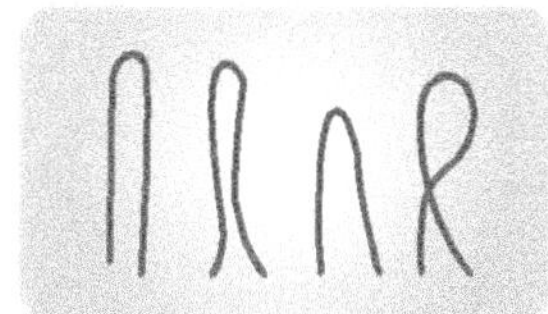
	Irregular and thick: melanoma, Spitz nevus	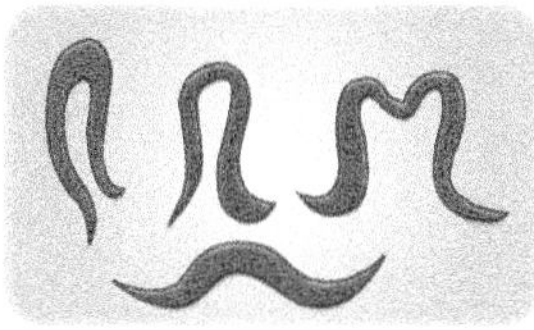
Irregular polymorphous vessels	Multiple vessels with different shapes including comma, dotted irregular lines, cork-screw, glomerular and others Significance: melanoma	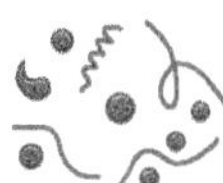
Dotted vessels	Small vessels resembling the head of a pin Significance: vertical vessels seen in Spitz nevus or melanoma. Can also be seen in other lesions such as psoriasis and squamous cell carcinoma	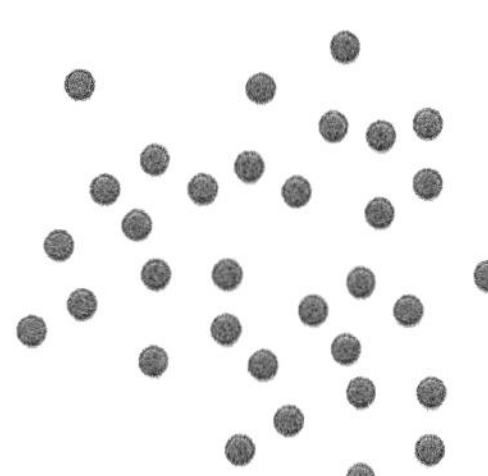

FIGURE 32-31 Vascular architecture seen by dermoscopy. *(Adapted from Malvehy J, Braun RP, Puig S,* et al. Handbook of Dermoscopy. *London: Informa Healthcare; 2006:30–31, Table 4-4.)*

Continued

Comma-like vessels	Resembling the shape of a comma Significance: compound or dermal nevus	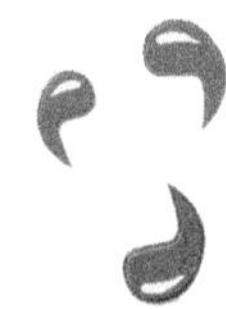
Clusters of "glomerular" vessels	Small and fine coiled vessels Significance: Bowen's disease. Can also be seen in melanoma and in stasis dermatitis	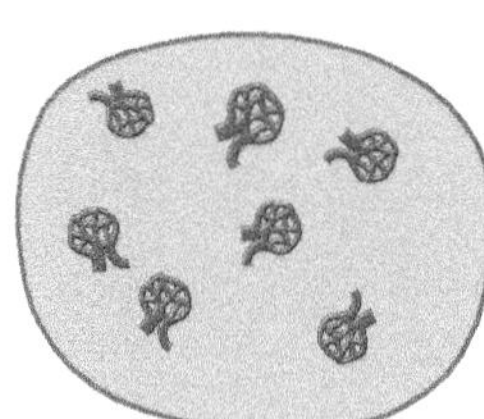
String of pearls	Globular vessels following a serpiginous distribution Significance: clear-cell acanthoma	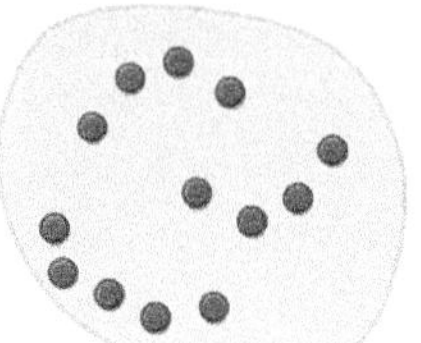
Crown vessels	Radial wreath-like or individual vessels at the periphery of the tumor. White-yellow globules, they can be seen in the center of the tumor Significance: sebaceous gland hyperplasia	
Corkscrew vessels	Irregular and thick coiled vessels Significance: melanoma including metastasis	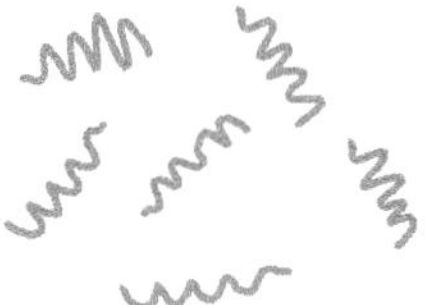
Arborizing vessels	Resembling the branches of a tree Significance: basal cell carcinoma	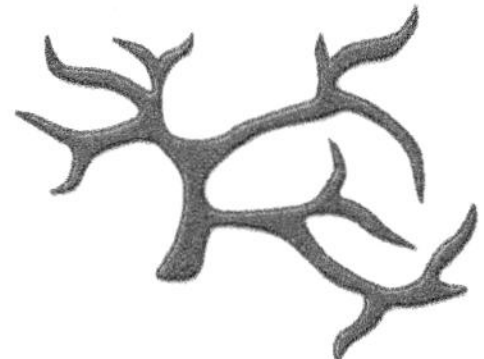

FIGURE 32-31, cont'd

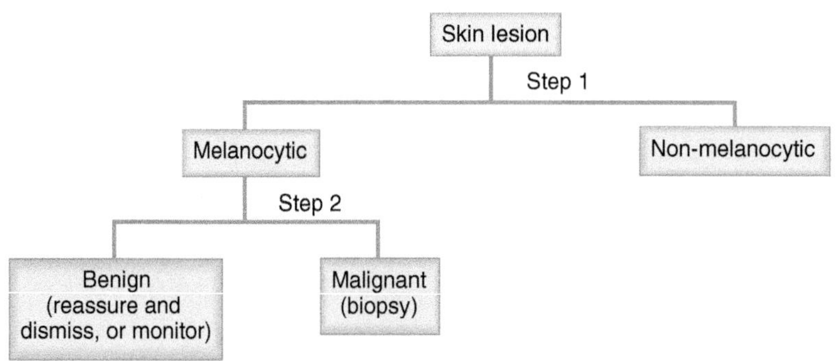

FIGURE 32-32 Two-step algorithm.

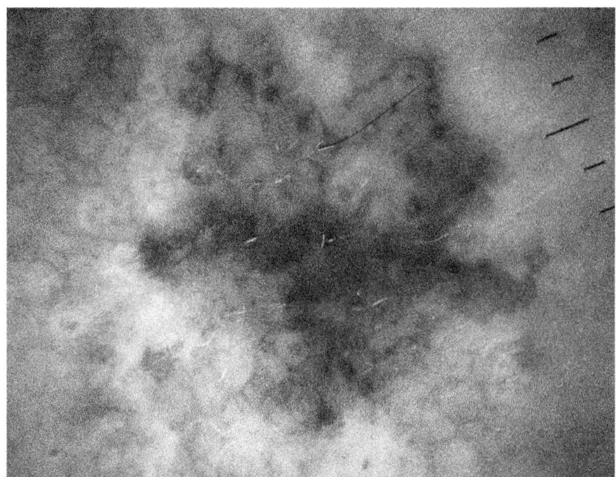

FIGURE 32-33 Atypical network in a junctional dysplastic nevus. *(Copyright Richard P. Usatine, MD.)*

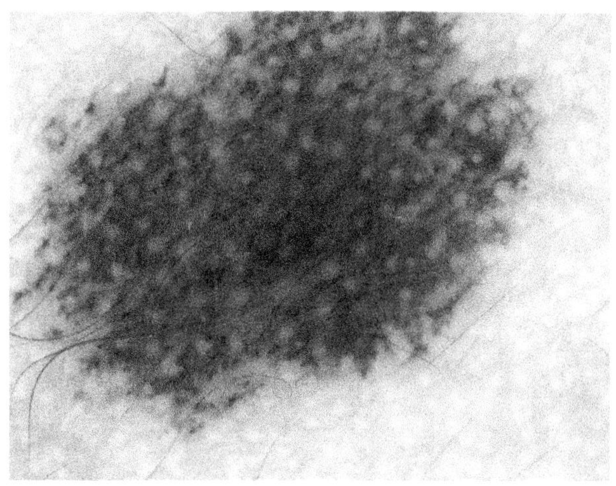

FIGURE 32-35 Pseudonetwork pattern is seen on the face in this congenital nevus. *(Copyright Richard P. Usatine, MD.)*

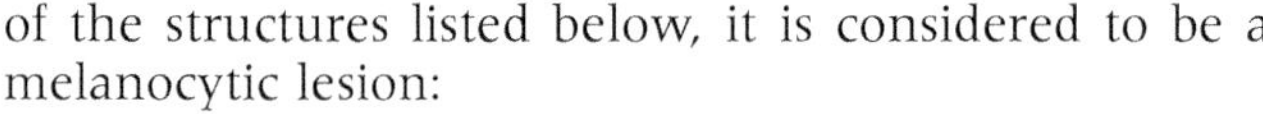

of the structures listed below, it is considered to be a melanocytic lesion:

1. Network (with one exception being the dermatofibroma), aggregated globules, streaks, homogeneous blue (Figure 32-33)
2. Parallel pattern (acral surface of palms and soles) (Figure 32-34)
3. Pseudonetwork pattern (on the face) (Figures 32-35 and 32-36).

Note, however, an exception: a pattern consisting of a delicate network surrounding a scar-like area is associated with dermatofibroma. This particular pattern trumps the presence of a network structure; thus, despite the presence of a network, this type of lesion is not considered to be melanocytic (Figures 32-37 and 32-38).

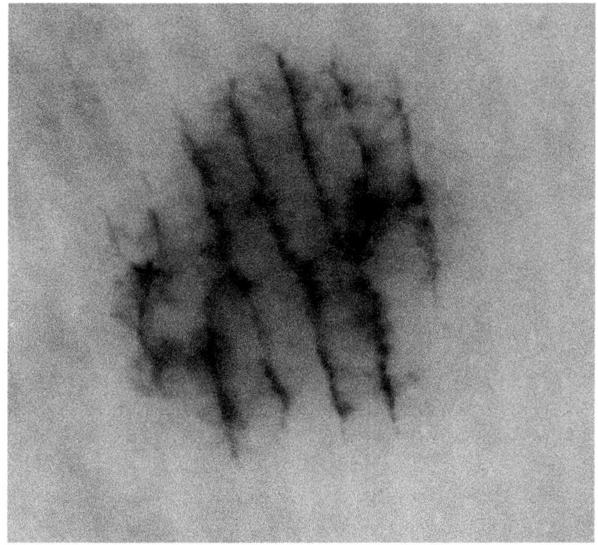

FIGURE 32-34 Nevus on the sole of the foot showing parallel network pigment in the furrows rather than the ridges. Note the white eccrine gland openings on the ridges, which are wider than the furrows. *(Copyright Richard P. Usatine, MD.)*

If the lesion does not manifest any of the structures mentioned above, look for features of:

- Dermatofibroma
- Basal cell carcinoma
- Seborrheic keratosis
- Hemangioma/angiokeratoma.

BCC has at least one of these:

- Large gray-blue ovoid nests
- Multiple gray-blue globules
- Leaf-like areas
- Spoke-wheel areas
- Arborizing tree-like telangiectasia
- Ulceration.

Seborrheic keratoses exhibits these characteristics (Figure 32-39):

- Three or more milia-like cysts
- Comedo-like openings
- Gyri and sulci (also known as fissures and ridges)
- Fingerprint-like
- Hairpin vessels with a whitish halo (Figure 32-40)
- Moth-eaten borders, especially if arising in solar lentigo.

Vascular lesions have red or blue-black lacunae (see Figures 32-29 and 32-30).

If the lesion has no melanocytic features and it has no features seen in one of the four common nonmelanocytic lesions, then search for any vascular structures/patterns as seen in Figures 32-31 and 32-41. If the lesion has no features of a melanocytic lesion, DF, BCC, SK, or hemangioma and it also lacks diagnostic vascular structures, then the lesion is considered structureless. All structureless lesions are by default considered to be melanocytic and one needs to consider the diagnosis of melanoma. These lesions should be biopsied or monitored very closely. Figure 32-42 puts this all together in one algorithm.

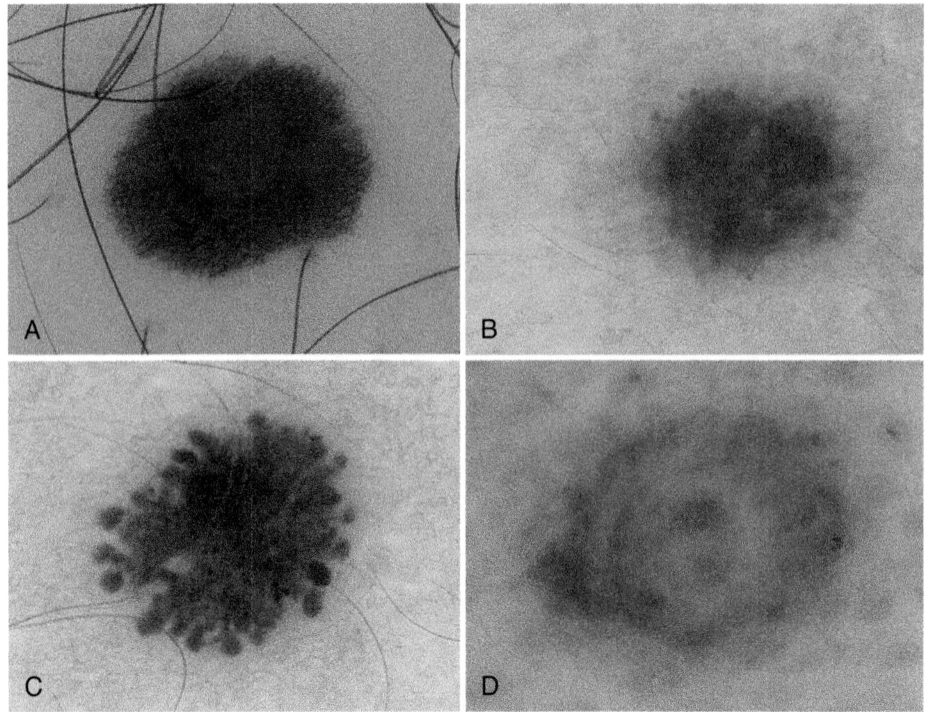

FIGURE 32-36 (A) Network, (B) aggregated globules, (C) streaks, and (D) homogeneous blue nevus are four patterns seen in melanocytic lesions. *(Copyright Ashfaq A. Marghoob, MD.)*

PATTERN ANALYSIS

Practitioners should look for the "ugly duckling" or the "Beauty and the Beast" sign. The ugly duckling is the lesion that stands out as different compared to surrounding nevi. Another way of looking at this is that the ugly lesion is the "Beast" and the other benign lesions are the "Beauty."[7]

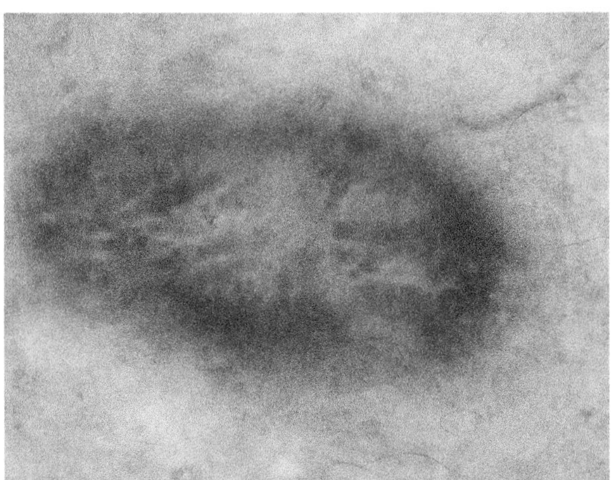

FIGURE 32-37 Pattern trumps network in this dermatofibroma. Although this appears to have a peripheral network, the central stellate scar makes this a dermatofibroma, which is not a melanocytic lesion. *(Copyright Richard P. Usatine, MD.)*

- Benign nevi tend to adhere to 1 of 10 recurrent patterns (Figure 32-43).
- These patterns all fit the definition of beauty, demonstrating symmetry of pattern, structure, and color.
- Familiarity with the dermoscopic patterns typically exhibited by benign nevi provides additional assistance in distinguishing between benign and malignant lesions.
- Melanoma, symbolized by the beast, is a melanocytic lesion that deviates from the 10 benign patterns.
- Melanomas almost invariably display some degree of asymmetry of pattern, color, and structure, which elicits a sense of unease in the viewer.

Melanoma deviates from global benign patterns and has at least one of these local features (Figure 32-44):

1. *Atypical network,* including branched streaks.
2. *Focal streaks,* that is, pseudopods and radial streaming.
3. *Atypical dots* are located at the periphery and are not overlying the pigment network lines. *Atypical globules* consist of globules of different shapes, sizes, and colors distributed in an asymmetric fashion. When reddish in color these are highly suggestive of melanoma.
4. *Focal negative pigment network.*
5. *Chrysalis-like crystalline structures* (only with polarized dermoscopy).
6. *Blotch,* a hyperpigmented area that is off center.
7. *Blue-white veil* and/or *peppering in flat lesions,* that is, regression structures.
8. *Focal blue-white veil over raised areas.*

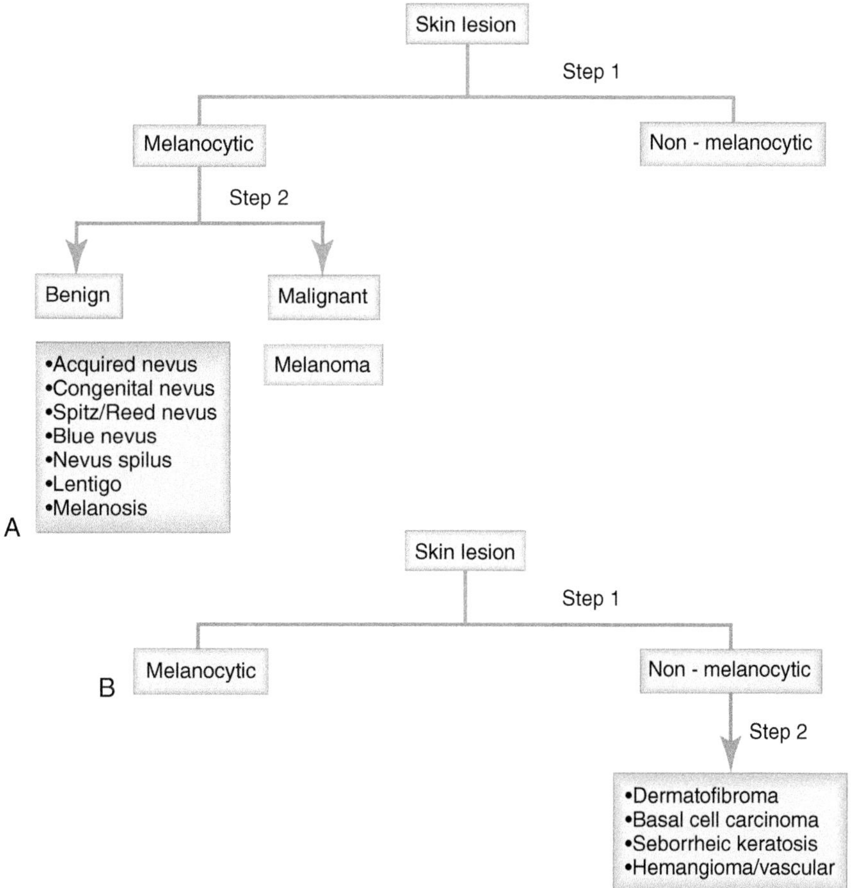

FIGURE 32-38 The first step of the two-step diagnostic algorithm requires all lesions to be separated into melanocytic (**A**) or nonmelanocytic (**B**). If the lesion is determined to be non-melanocytic (**B**) then it must manifest criteria diagnostic of basal cell carcinoma, dermatofibroma, seborrheic keratosis or hemangioma. If the lesion is determined to be melanocytic (**A**) then one needs to proceed to the second step of the two-step algorithm. The second step requires the observer to differentiate nevi from melanoma.

9. *Vascular structures,* that is, dotted, globular, irregular linear, serpentine, polymorphous, milky-red, etc., are best seen with noncontact polarized dermoscopy.
10. *Peripheral tan/brown structureless areas.*

The sensitivity and specificity of melanoma structures and features are shown in Table 32-1. A three-point checklist can be applied to pigmented lesions only:

1. *Asymmetry* in any axis taking into account colors and structures but not shape (contour or silhouette).
2. *Focal atypical network* considered when the lines of the network have differences in thickness and the sizes of the holes are nonhomogeneous. The atypical network is usually irregularly distributed.
3. *Blue-white structures* include any white or any blue color present in the lesion.

Final score and recommended treatment:

- 0–1 points: benign, but follow
- 2–3 points: suspicious; conduct a biopsy.

Special Conditions

Face

Rete ridges on the face are not prominent, especially in elderly people. Adnexal structures, hair follicles, and sweat glands are more prominent on the face and produce the pseudonetwork. Lentigo maligna is an important early melanoma that should be recognized on the face before it becomes invasive.

Three important dermoscopic features are:

1. Asymmetric pigmented follicular openings
2. Dark rhomboidal structures
3. Slate-gray dots.[12]

Schiffner et al. described the progression model for lentigo maligna that is detailed in Figure 32-45.[12] Figure 32-46 shows actual lentigo maligna with rhomboidal structures.

Acral Areas—Palms and Soles

To understand how to differentiate melanoma from other pigmented lesions on the palms or soles, the

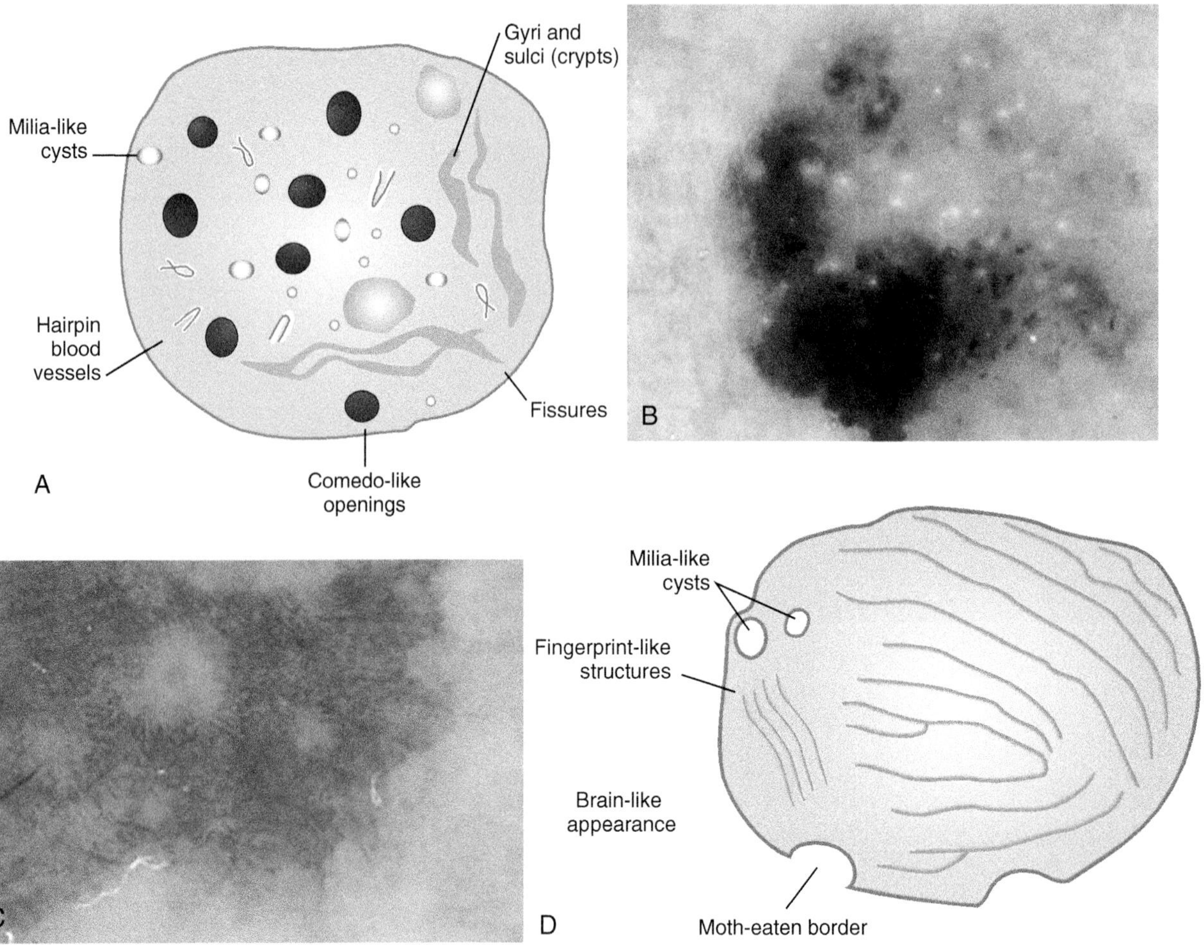

FIGURE 32-39 A seborrheic keratosis can have all or any of these structures. *(A, D: Adapted from Malvehy J, Braun RP, Puig S,* et al. Handbook of Dermoscopy. *London: Informa Healthcare; 2006:83, Figure A-21.)*

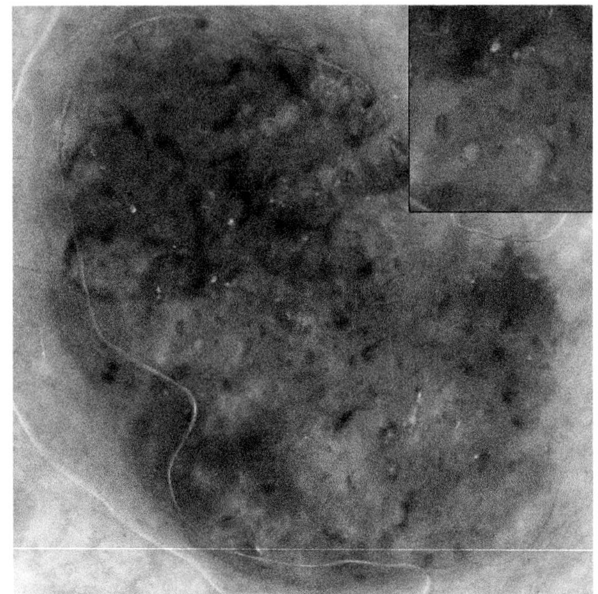

FIGURE 32-40 SK with hairpin vessels surrounded by a whitish halo. *(Copyright Richard P. Usatine, MD.)*

practitioner must understand the anatomy of the acral skin. The dermatoglyphics on acral skin consists of mountains and valleys (ridges and furrows) with eccrine sweat glands that are found on the mountains (Figure 32-47). The mountains are wider than the valleys.

Benign nevi have three common patterns:

1. Parallel furrow (pigment running along the valleys)
2. Lattice-like (pigment that creates a lattice)
3. Fibrillar (thin parallel lines that cross over the mountains and valleys).

Melanomas also have three common patterns:

1. Parallel ridge (pigment running along the mountains)
2. Diffuse pigmentation (pigment in large blotches of different shades)
3. Irregular dots and globules.

Figure 32-48 shows the pigment of a benign nevus in the furrows or valleys. There is also a lattice-like pattern

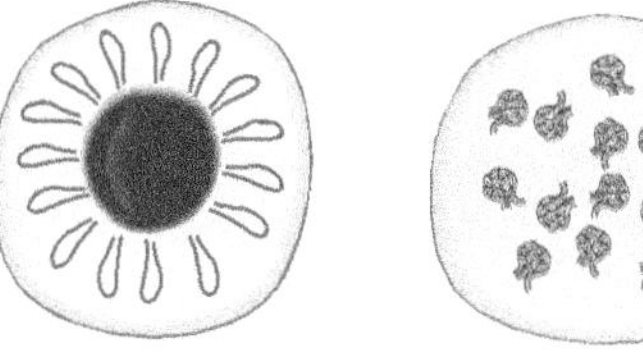
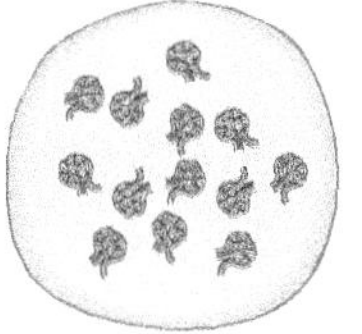
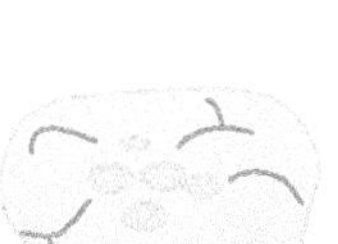
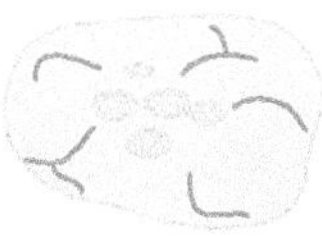
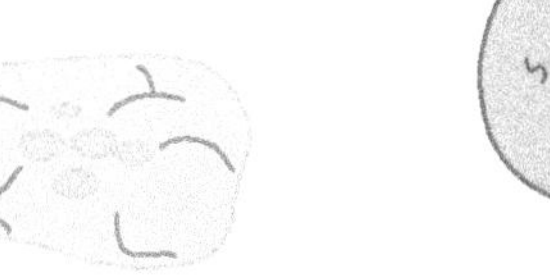
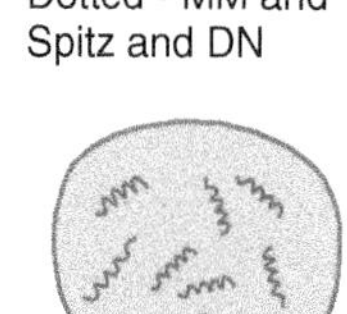
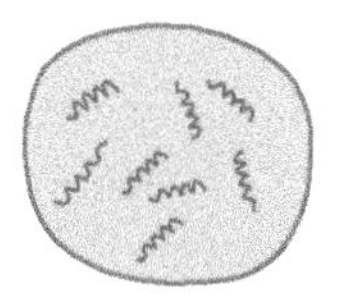
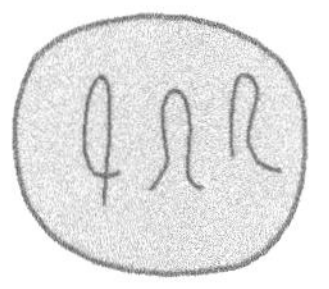
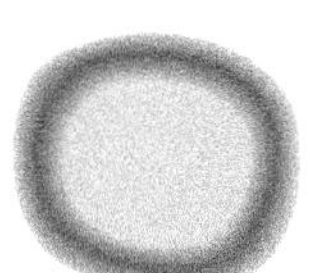

FIGURE 32-41 Benign vascular patterns.

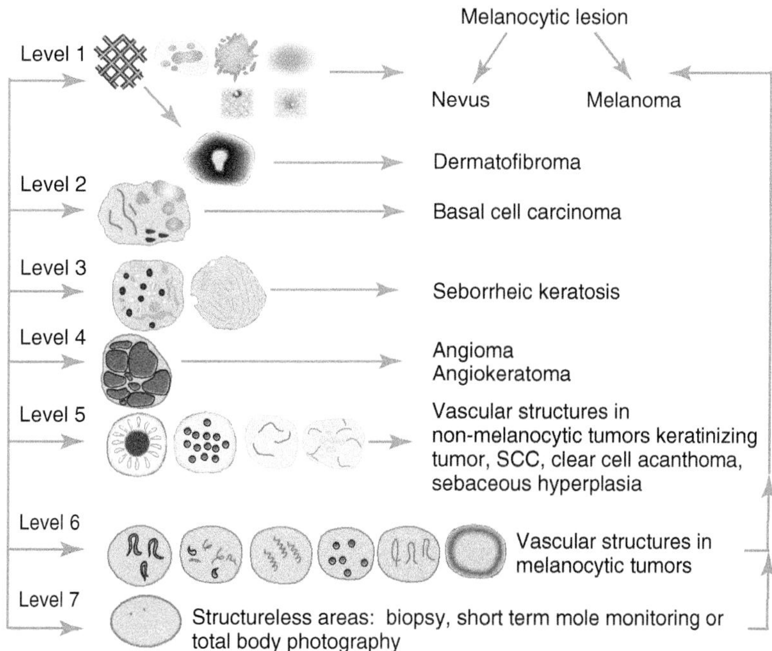

FIGURE 32-42 Putting it all together.

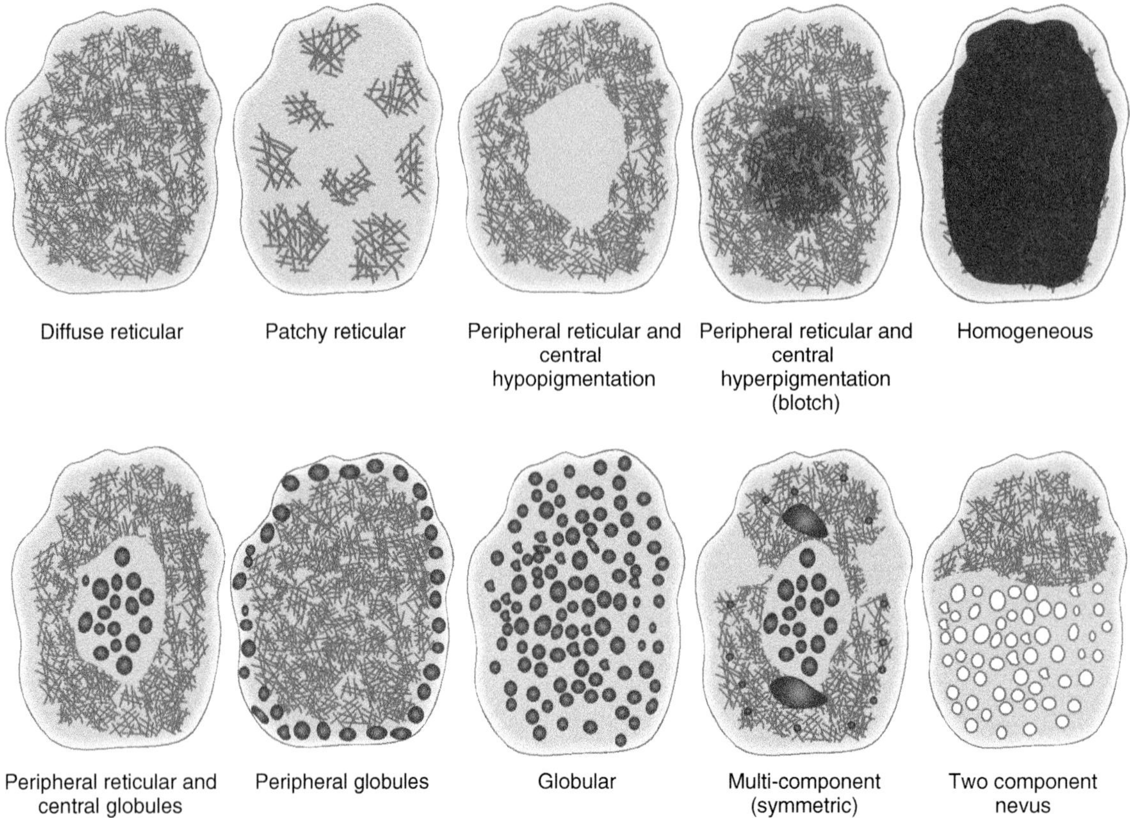

FIGURE 32-43 Benign nevi tend to adhere to 1 of 10 recurrent patterns. Melanoma is a melanocytic lesion that deviates from the 10 benign patterns. *(Adapted from Malvehy J, Braun RP, Puig S,* et al. Handbook of Dermoscopy. *London: Informa Healthcare; 2006:91, Figure A-36.)*

and the pigment is seen running in the furrows with a cross network between the furrows.

Ninety-eight percent of melanomas on the palms and soles have a parallel ridge pattern in which the pigment is on the mountains and there is hypopigmentation of the valleys. Zero percent of acral nevi have this pattern. Figure 32-49 shows an acrolentiginous melanoma on the foot with this parallel ridge pattern. Sometimes the eccrine sweat gland openings are visible in the middle of the ridges of hyperpigmentation.

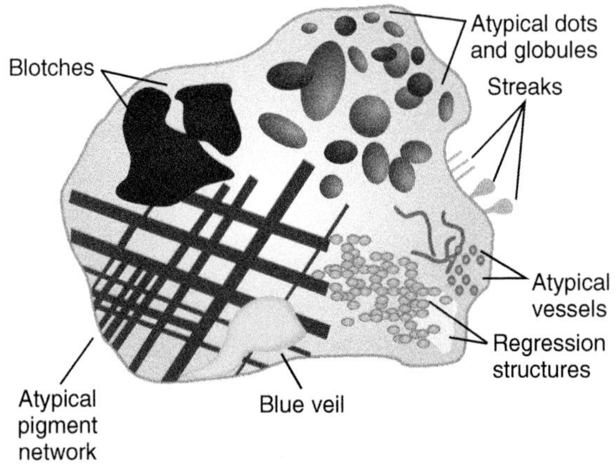

FIGURE 32-44 Melanoma-specific structures. *(Adapted from Malvehy J, Braun RP, Puig S,* et al. Handbook of Dermoscopy. *London: Informa Healthcare; 2006:75, Figure A-4.)*

It is important not to confuse hemorrhagic lesions on the palms or soles with melanoma to avoid unnecessary biopsies. Frequently the history alone will help to distinguish pigmentation caused by trauma or ill-fitting shoes from a benign or malignant pigmented lesion. These subcorneal hemorrhages can appear yellow-red to red-black in color and may have globules at the periphery or look like pebbles on the ridges. The heel and bottom of the big toe are common locations for subcorneal hemorrhages seen with sports or ill-fitting shoes. Figure 32-50 is an example of a benign subcorneal hemorrhage.

SCABIES

The dermatoscope can also be used for the diagnosis of scabies. Look for burrows in the skin and put the dermoscope over the burrow. Figure 32-51 shows scabies mites at the ends of the burrows. The mites are visible and resemble an arrowhead pointing away from the burrow (Figure 32-51). That is because the mite is in the process of burrowing through the skin using its mouth and legs to extend the tunnel. The round shape of the mite is also visible. This finding should be sufficient to confirm a suspected case of scabies. Once the mite has been identified with a dermoscope, a directed

TABLE 32-1 Sensitivity and Specificity of Melanoma Structures and Features[8–11]

Structure/Feature	Sensitivity (Highest Reported)	Specificity (Highest Reported)	Odds Ratio (Highest Reported)
Atypical network	77%	89%	9.0
Streaks	23%	99%	5.8
Negative network	22%	95%	2.0
Chrysalis	5%	99%	9.7
Atypical dots and globules	88%	97%	4.8
Atypical blotch	38%	88%	4.1
Blue-white veil	51%	99%	13
Regression structures	46%	94%	8.0
Atypical vessels	63%	96%	12.5
Peripheral brown structureless areas	63%	96%	28
Five to six colors	53%	95%	3.2

scraping may be used to see the mite, its eggs, or its feces under the microscope.

CONCLUSION

Dermoscopy is not learned overnight and this chapter is a good introduction to begin learning this important tool for diagnosis. Use the list of resources below to continue your learning.

Resources

Johr R, Stolz W. *Dermoscopy: An Illustrated Self-Assessment Guide*. New York: McGraw-Hill; 2010.

Malvehy J, Puig S, Braun RP, et al. *Handbook of Dermoscopy*. London: Taylor & Francis; 2006.

Marghoob AA, Braun R, Kopf AW, eds. *Atlas of Dermoscopy*. London: Parthenon Publishing; 2004.

Marghoob A, Braun R, Kopf A. *Interactive CD-ROM of Dermoscopy*. London: Informa Healthcare; 2007.

American Academy of Family Physicians (www.aafp.org). The AAFP's yearly fall scientific assembly now offers a dermoscopy workshop taught by the authors of this chapter. Also every summer the AAFP sponsors a course on "Skin Problems and Diseases" that includes a dermoscopy workshop taught by the authors of this chapter.

Dermoscopy website from Italy (www.dermoscopy.org); includes a free dermoscopy tutorial.

International Dermoscopy Society (www.dermoscopy-ids.org).

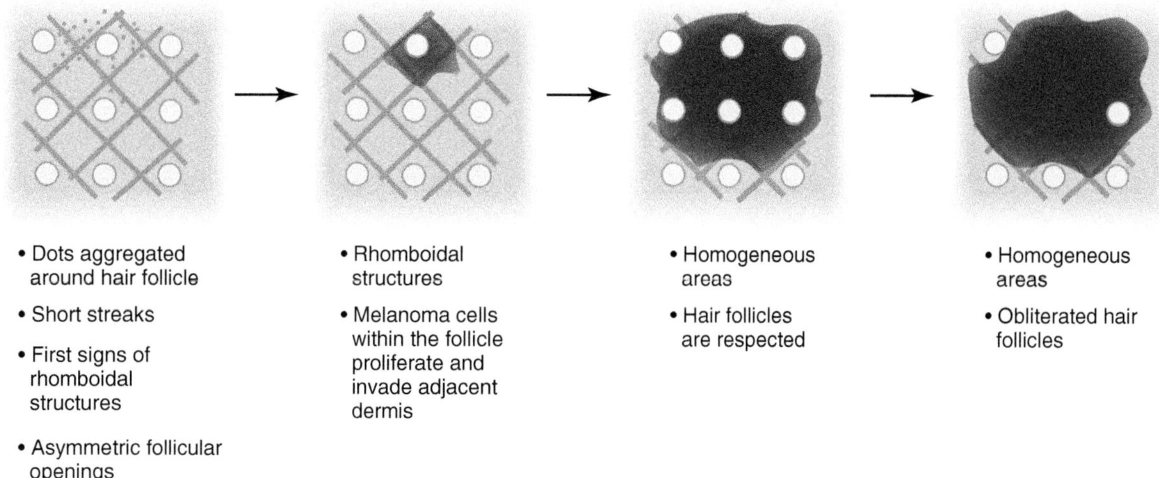

FIGURE 32-45 Lentigo maligna in the various stages of the progression model.

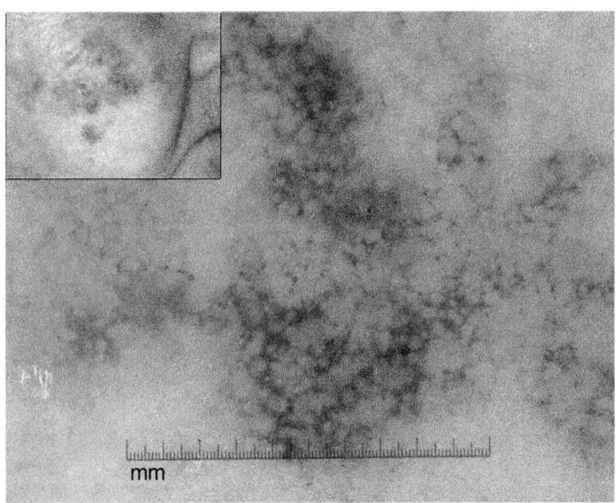

FIGURE 32-46 Lentigo maligna on the face with rhomboidal structures. *(Copyright Ashfaq A. Marghoob, MD.)*

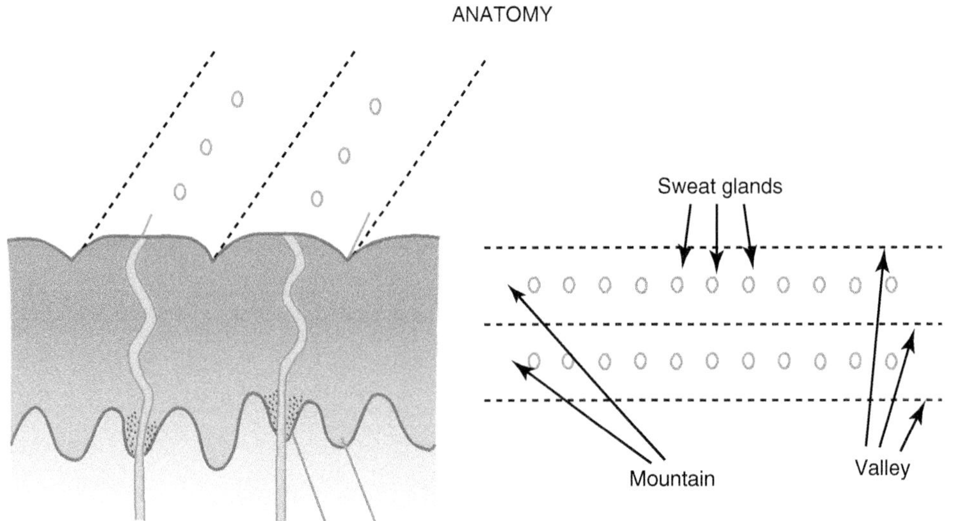

FIGURE 32-47 Acral skin consists of mountains and valleys (ridges and furrows) with eccrine sweat glands that are found on the mountains. The mountains are wider than the valleys.

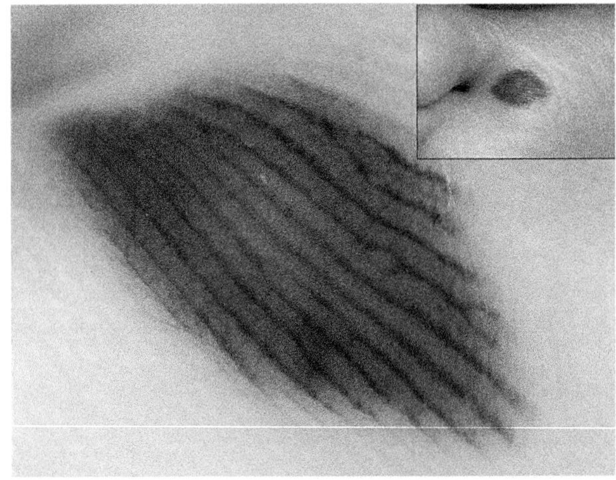

FIGURE 32-48 Pigment of a benign nevus on the sole of the foot in the furrows (valleys). *(Copyright Richard P. Usatine, MD.)*

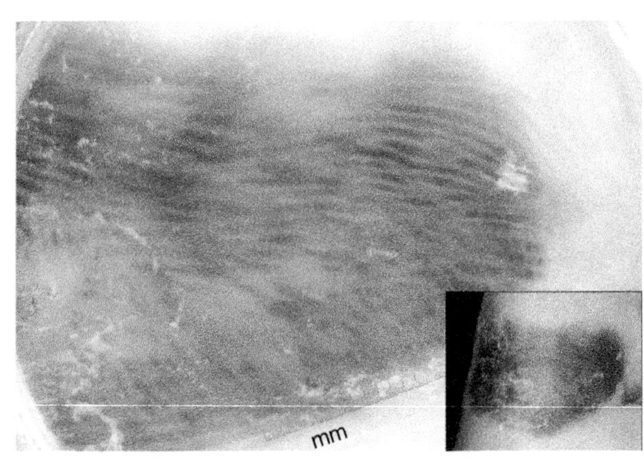

FIGURE 32-49 Acrolentiginous melanoma on the foot with a parallel ridge pattern. *(Copyright Ashfaq A. Marghoob, MD.)*

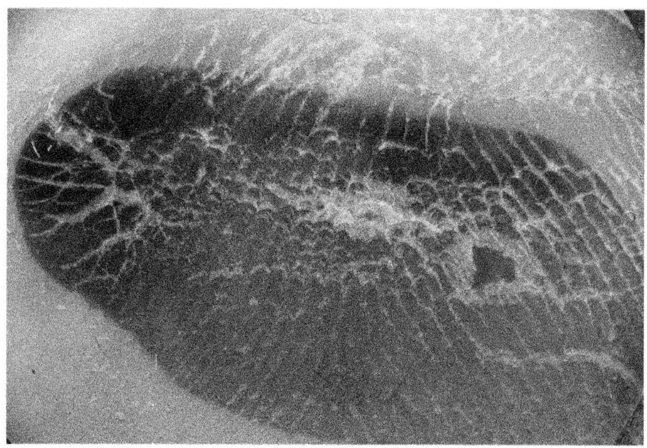

FIGURE 32-50 Benign subcorneal hemorrhage can resemble a melanoma. The subcorneal blood is sequestered on the ridges creating a pattern that mimics melanoma. *(Copyright Ashfaq A. Marghoob, MD.)*

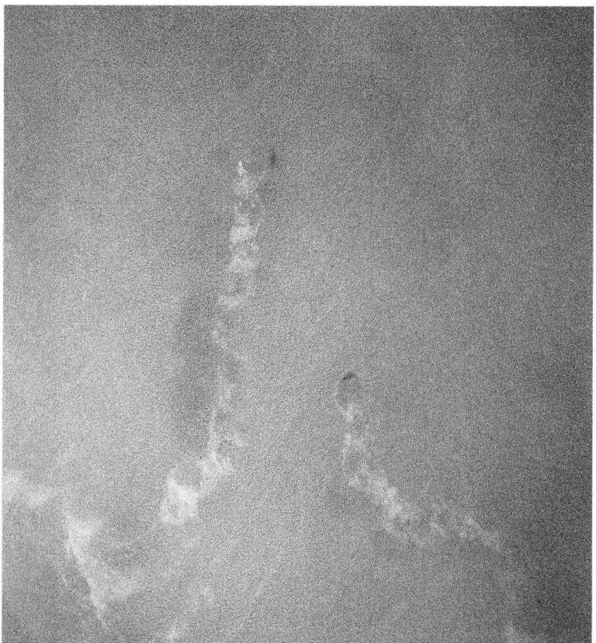

FIGURE 32-51 Two scabies mites at the end of two distinct burrows. The head and anterior legs are most visible and resemble arrowheads pointing away from the burrows. *(Copyright Richard P. Usatine, MD.)*

References

1. Bafounta ML, Beauchet A, Aegerter P, Saiag P. Is dermoscopy (epiluminescence microscopy) useful for the diagnosis of melanoma? Results of a meta-analysis using techniques adapted to the evaluation of diagnostic tests. *Arch Dermatol.* 2001;137:1343–1350.
2. Kittler H, Pehamberger H, Wolff K, Binder M. Diagnostic accuracy of dermoscopy. *Lancet Oncol.* 2002;3:159–165.
3. Vestergaard ME, Macaskill P, Holt PE, Menzies SW. Dermoscopy compared with naked-eye examination for the diagnosis of primary melanoma: a meta-analysis of studies performed in a clinical setting. *Br J Dermatol.* 2008;159:669–676.
4. Carli P, De Giorgi V, Crocetti E, *et al.* Improvement of malignant/benign ratio in excised melanocytic lesions in the 'dermoscopy era': a retrospective study 1997–2001. *Br J Dermatol.* 2004;150:687–692.
5. Argenziano G, Puig S, Zalaudek I, *et al.* Dermoscopy improves accuracy of primary care physicians to triage lesions suggestive of skin cancer. *J Clin Oncol.* 2006;24:1877–1882.
6. Venuto-Andrade C, Marghoob AA. Ten reasons why dermoscopy is beneficial for the evaluation of skin lesions. *Exp Rev Dermatol.* 2006;1:369–374.
7. Marghoob AA, Korzenko AJ, Changchien L, *et al.* The beauty and the beast sign in dermoscopy. *Dermatol Surg.* 2007;33:1388–1391.
8. Menzies SW, Kreusch J, Byth K, *et al.* Dermoscopic evaluation of amelanotic and hypomelanotic melanoma. *Arch Dermatol.* 2008;144:1120–1127.
9. Argenziano G, Soyer HP, Chimenti S, *et al.* Dermoscopy of pigmented skin lesions: results of a consensus meeting via the Internet. *J Am Acad Dermatol.* 2003;48:679–693.
10. Menzies SW, Ingvar C, McCarthy WH. A sensitivity and specificity analysis of the surface microscopy features of invasive melanoma. *Melanoma Res.* 1996;6:55–62.
11. Annessi G, Bono R, Sampogna F, *et al.* Sensitivity, specificity, and diagnostic accuracy of three dermoscopic algorithmic methods in the diagnosis of doubtful melanocytic lesions: the importance of light brown structureless areas in differentiating atypical melanocytic nevi from thin melanomas. *J Am Acad Dermatol.* 2007;56:759–767.
12. Schiffner R, Schiffner-Rohe J, Vogt T, *et al.* Improvement of early recognition of lentigo maligna using dermatoscopy. *J Am Acad Dermatol.* 2000;42:25–32.

33 Procedures to Treat Benign Conditions

DANIEL STULBERG, MD • ROBERT FAWCETT, MD •
REBECCA SMALL, MD • RICHARD P. USATINE, MD

Many skin tumors and growths are benign and can be diagnosed based on their clinical appearance and history. These lesions can arise from the epidermis, the dermis, or the subcutaneous tissues. This chapter provides a detailed discussion of the most common benign skin lesions and their treatment options. Chapter 12 covered epidermal cysts, lipomas, digital mucous cysts, and hidrocystomas so these will not be covered here.

ACNE SURGERY

Acne surgery is the name given to the removal of open comedones (blackheads) with a comedone extractor in the clinician's office. It can also be performed on actinic comedones or senile comedones. It is often performed for cosmetic reasons, but can also decrease pain around a comedone that is under pressure. Large inflammatory nodules and cysts are best treated with intralesional steroids rather than acne surgery (see Chapter 16, *Intralesional Injections*).

After informed consent, the comedones are cleaned with alcohol. No anesthesia is needed. The comedone is nicked with a No. 11 blade, a sterile needle, or the sharp end of a comedone extractor. Sebum, cells, and other debris are expressed out using pressure from a comedone extractor (Figure 33-1). If a comedone extractor is not available, one can be fashioned from a small paperclip bent to produce a homemade device. Clean the paperclip with an alcohol wipe before using it. Bill using acne surgery CPT code = 10040.

ACROCHORDONS (SKIN TAGS)

Diagnosis

- Flesh-colored, raised lesions, often pedunculated.
- Common on the neck, axillae, inguinal regions, and under the breasts.
- More common in persons with obesity, diabetes, or impaired glucose tolerance.
- Some persons develop hundreds of skin tags in conjunction with acanthosis nigricans (Figure 33-2).

Treatment

See video on the DVD for further learning. 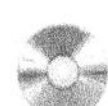

Treatment is done for cosmetic reasons or if the skin tags are getting caught in or irritated by clothing or jewelry.

Snip with Iris Scissors *(Figure 33-3)*

- Simple and quick with immediate results.
- Use lidocaine with epinephrine if skin tags have a wide base.
- Minimal bleeding for small lesions.
- Direct pressure, aluminum chloride for hemostasis if needed.

Cryo Tweezers

- Freeze with Cryo Tweezer down to normal tissue (Figure 33-4).
- Tags will necrose and fall off over 1 to 2 weeks.
- Works better for smaller skin tags and some will not fall off.
- Clean procedure, no bleeding or anesthetic.
- Great for skin tags on eyelids or around the eyes (Figure 33-4).

Electrosurgery

- Electrodesiccate to destroy or use radio-frequency (RF) loop to cut through base of lesion.
- Local anesthetic unless very small. Patients report that this hurts more without anesthesia than snipping or freezing.
- Also good for skin tags on eyelids or around the eyes because the electrosurgery minimizes bleeding and avoids the use of caustic hemostatic chemicals near the eye (Figure 33-5).

Special Considerations/Billing

- Cosmetic and not covered by insurance. Some but not all insurance will cover removal when irritated by clothing or jewelry.
- Treated lesions can recur and new ones will form.
- No need to send for pathology unless diagnosis is uncertain.
- Code 11200 once for the first 1–15 lesions destroyed by any method.
- Code 11201 in addition for each additional 10 lesions beyond 15.

ANGIOMAS/ANGIOKERATOMAS/ ANGIOFIBROMAS

Diagnosis

Cherry Angiomas

- Red papules that appear with aging.
- Dermoscopy shows red lacunae (see Figure 32-9).

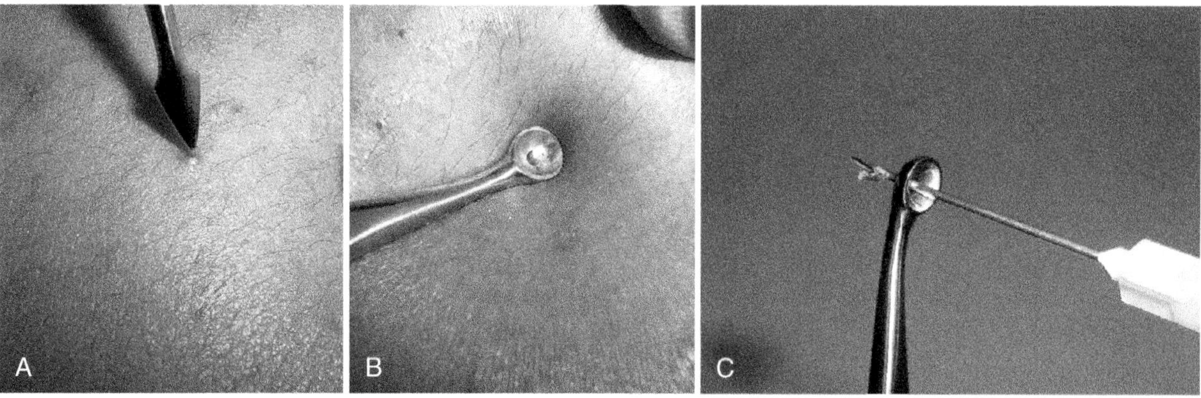

FIGURE 33-1 Acne surgery: (**A**) Pierce the comedone with the sharp side of the comedone extractor. (**B**) Press the comedone extractor against the skin and until the pilosebaceous material comes out. (**C**) The comedone extractor can be used multiple times and can be cleaned between uses with a 21-gauge needle. *(Copyright Richard P. Usatine, MD.)*

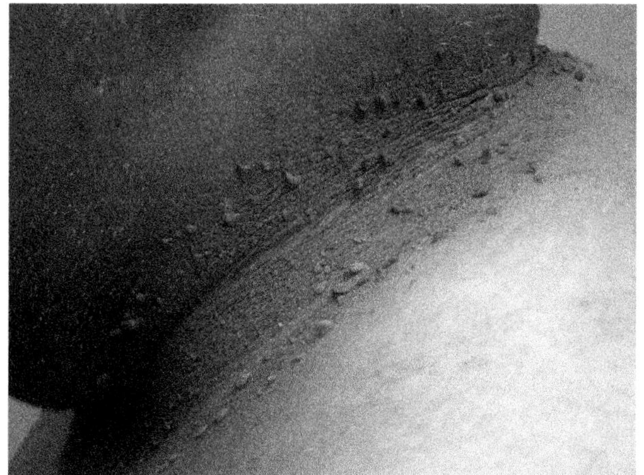

FIGURE 33-2 Multiple skin tags (acrochordons) on the neck of a man with acanthosis nigricans. *(Copyright Richard P. Usatine, MD.)*

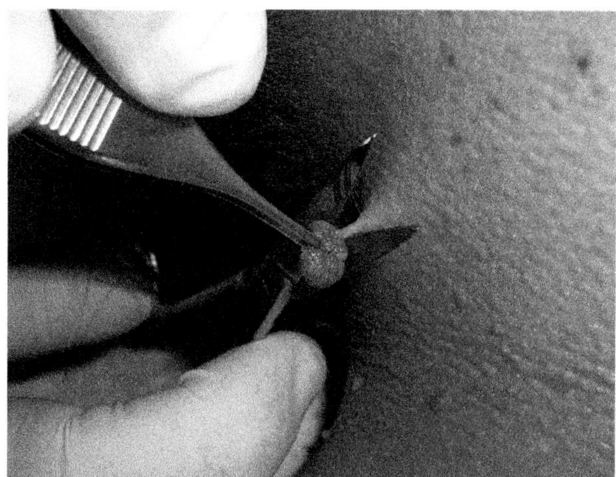

FIGURE 33-3 Snip excision of a pedunculated acrochordon. *(Copyright Richard P. Usatine, MD.)*

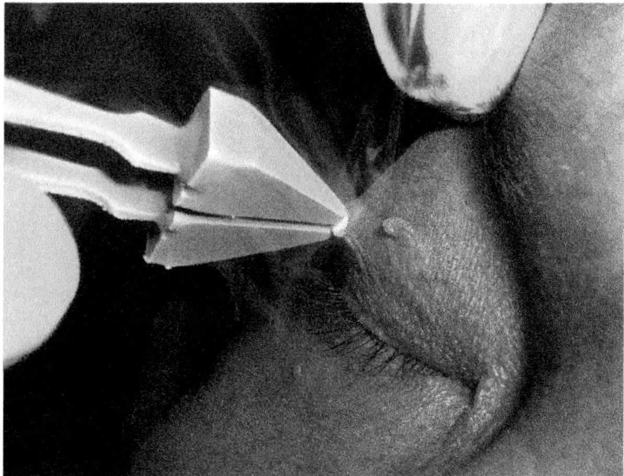

FIGURE 33-4 Cryosurgery using the Cryo Tweezer on a skin tag located on the eyelid. Grasp the acrochordon and pull the eyelid away from the globe. *(Copyright Richard P. Usatine, MD.)*

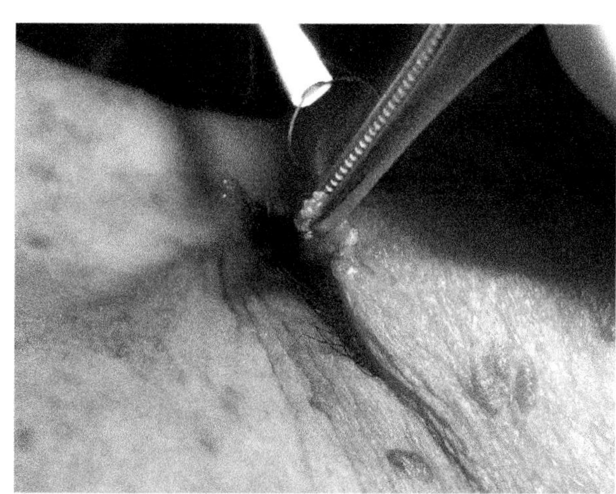

FIGURE 33-5 Removing a skin tag from the eyelid using an electrosurgical loupe. This requires local anesthetic. *(Copyright Richard P. Usatine, MD.)*

- Found most commonly on the trunk.
- Benign and can be treated if they are bleeding or for cosmetic reasons.
- Shave biopsy if diagnosis is not certain or a malignancy such as angiosarcoma is suspected.

Angiokeratomas

- Red to dark red or purple papules that appear with aging.
- Dermoscopy shows red and black lacunae (see Figure 32-10).
- Found most commonly on the scrotum or vulva.
- Benign and can be treated if they are bleeding or for cosmetic reasons.
- Shave biopsy if diagnosis is not certain or a malignancy is suspected.

Angiofibromas

- Skin-colored to pink papules found around the nose (Figure 33-6).
- Referred to as adenoma sebaceum when found in clusters around the nose in patients with tuberous sclerosis.
- Shave biopsy if diagnosis is not certain or a malignancy is suspected.

Treatment

The following treatments are used for angiomas, angiokeratomas, or angiofibromas:

Electrodesiccation for Small Lesions

See video on the DVD for further learning. 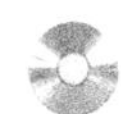

- Low power setting 2 to 3 on Hyfrecator (or similar instrument) without anesthesia. Start at 2 and only increase power if needed.
- Consider using lidocaine and epinephrine for larger angiomas, angiokeratomas in the genital area, or by patient preference (Figure 33-7).

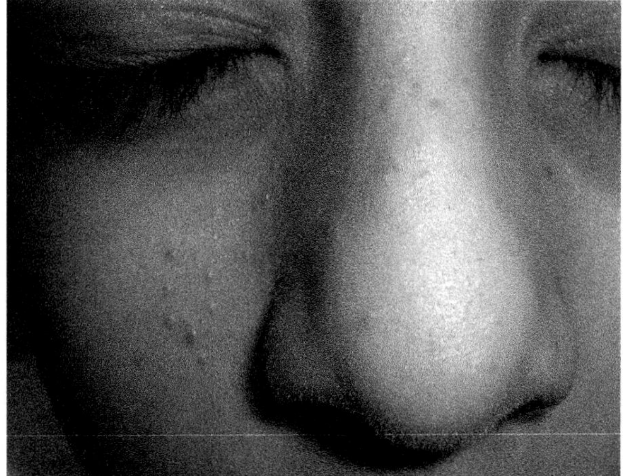

FIGURE 33-6 Multiple angiofibromas on the face of a young child. *(Copyright Richard P. Usatine, MD.)*

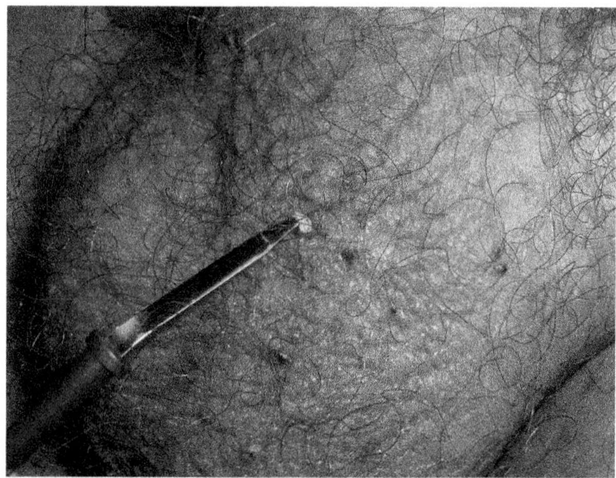

FIGURE 33-7 Multiple angiokeratomas on the scrotum. The patient requested removal, so after obtaining consent, lidocaine with epinephrine was injected for local anesthesia. The Hyfrecator was used to electrocoagulate the angiokeratomas. *(Copyright Richard P. Usatine, MD.)*

Shave Excision with Electrodesiccation of the Base for Larger Lesions

- Start with lidocaine and epinephrine and send specimen for histology if diagnosis is in doubt.

Cryosurgery

- An alternative that works best if the vascular lesion is compressed with a probe during the freeze time. Liquid nitrogen spray is not useful for cherry angiomas but may have some benefit for angiofibromas.

Lasers

- The 532-, 595-, and 980-nm lasers and intense pulsed light (IPL) devices used for treatment of red vascular ectasias are effective for angiomas (see Chapter 27, *Photorejuvenation with Lasers*).[1]
- Angiomas will darken, turning blue or black in color after a single treatment, and then regress, fading to the background skin color.

CHONDRODERMATITIS NODULARIS HELICIS

Diagnosis

- Skin-colored or erythematous firm nodule of the helix of the ear (Figure 33-8).
- Frequent shallow central scale or crust.
- Usually very tender to palpation or when trying to sleep on the affected ear.
- More common in men, and prevalence increases with age over 40. When women get this, the nodule may be on the antihelix.
- May actually be a SCC so it is best to get a tissue diagnosis with a shave biopsy or elliptical excision.

Treatment

See video on the DVD for further learning. 

Injection

- Use this treatment method only if you are certain of the diagnosis clinically or by previous biopsy.
- Triamcinolone acetonide 10 to 40 mg/mL injected into lesion can reduce the size and tenderness.
- Injections may be repeated at 2- to 4-week intervals but the overall success rate is low.

Elliptical Excision

See video on the DVD for further learning. 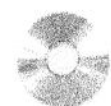

- Elliptical excision around the lesion has a high success rate (Figure 33-8).
- Draw the ellipse around the nodule and follow ear anatomy.
- Anesthetize with 1% lidocaine and epinephrine (epinephrine is not contraindicated and helps to produce a visible field).
- Curette the underlying diseased cartilage with a 3-mm curette or snip it off with a sharp scissor.
- Close the defect with a few simple interrupted sutures using 5-0 polypropylene on a small plastics needle (13 to 16 mm).
- Bill for excision of benign growth on the ear based on size.

Electrodesiccation and Curettage

- Do a shave biopsy for diagnosis (if not already done).
- Scrape off abnormal tissue with 3-mm curette.
- Use electrodesiccation to destroy any remaining abnormal tissue.
- Repeat for another cycle if needed.
- Cover with petrolatum and let heal by secondary intention.
- The remaining scar may be less cosmetic than the sutured closure done with the ellipse.
- Can only bill for destruction of a benign growth (no more than freezing a seborrheic keratosis).

Cryosurgery

- This method can be attempted but is not very effective.

Laser

- Ablate with CO_2 laser and leave open to granulate in.

CUTANEOUS HORN

Diagnosis

- Thickened keratin that grows from the skin like an animal's horn (Figure 33-9).

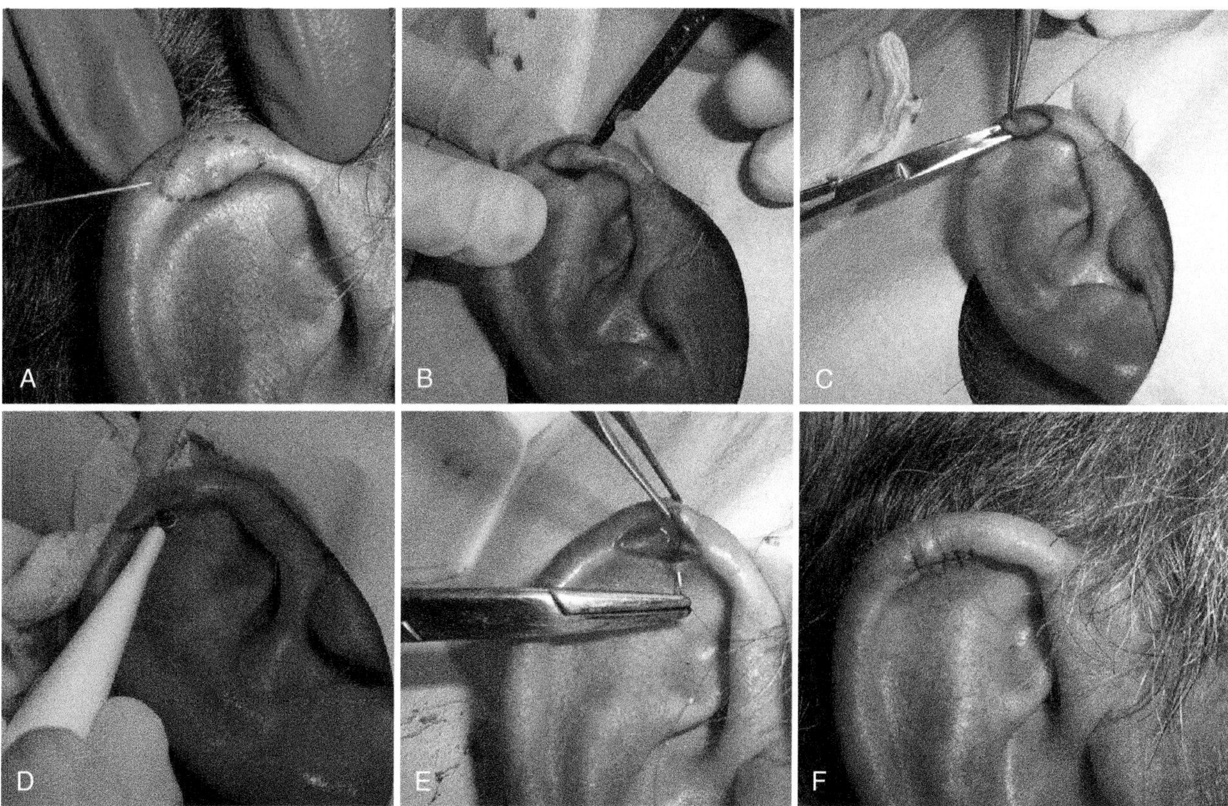

FIGURE 33-8 **(A)** 1% lidocaine with epinephrine was injected into the helical rim to excise chondrodermatitis nodularis helicis. **(B)** A 15c blade was used to cut the ellipse. **(C)** A sharp iris scissor was used to cut off the bottom of the ellipse. **(D)** A curette was used to curette away the affected cartilage. **(E)** 5-0 polypropylene was used to close the defect. **(F)** Three interrupted sutures produced an excellent closure. *(Copyright Richard P. Usatine, MD.)*

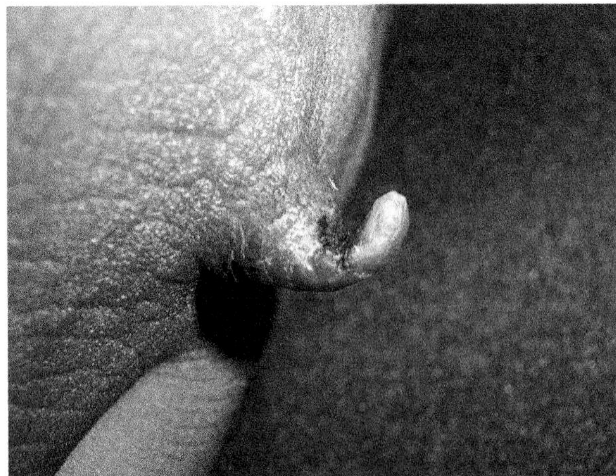

FIGURE 33-9 A cutaneous horn turned out to be a wart when it was biopsied and sent to pathology. *(Copyright Richard P. Usatine, MD.)*

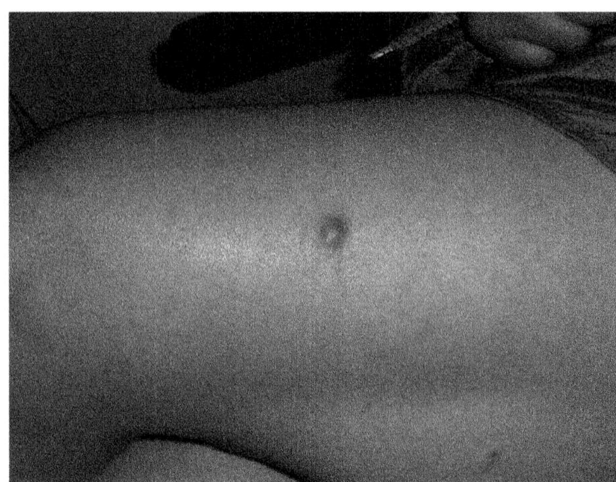

FIGURE 33-11 Large dermatofibroma on the leg that was not dermatofibrosarcoma protuberans. *(Copyright Richard P. Usatine, MD.)*

Treatment

- Shave off the horn including tissue at the base using a blade (razor or scalpel). Use electrodesiccation or aluminum chloride for hemostasis. Always send for pathology because the underlying lesion may be a skin cancer such as a SCC.
- The thick keratin itself is difficult to cut, but the biopsy should always be below the horn itself.
- Cryosurgery of the base may be performed as a second step if the original shave showed a wart, SK, or AK and some tissue is remaining.

DERMATOFIBROMAS

Diagnosis

- Firm nodular thickening of the dermis that may have a hyperpigmented halo (Figure 33-10). It can be hypopigmented, hyperpigmented, or pink.

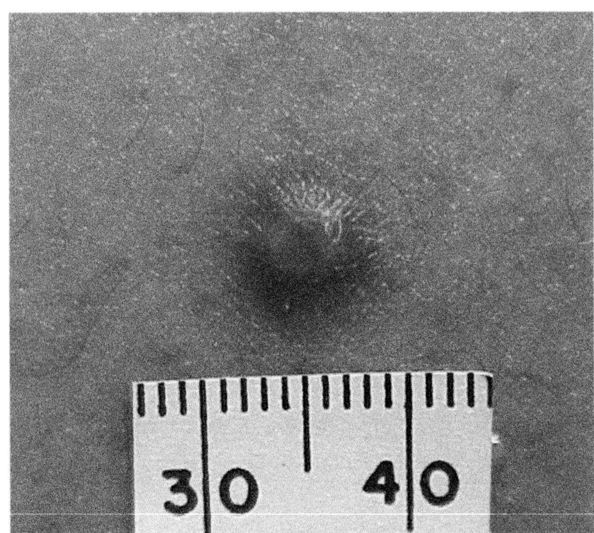

FIGURE 33-10 Typical dermatofibroma with a hyperpigmented halo and a white and pink scar at the center. *(Copyright Daniel L. Stulberg, MD.)*

- Most commonly found on the legs, particularly in women (Figure 33-11). Not unusual to see them on the arms or trunk.
- Displays retraction sign (i.e., Fitzpatrick's sign). Lesion seems to retract or dimple downward when pinching around lesion (Figure 33-12).
- Dermatofibromas have a specific dermoscopic pattern that helps with the diagnosis (see Chapter 32, *Dermoscopy*).
- Most often a clinical diagnosis.

Treatment

Discuss with the patient that a dermatofibroma is not dangerous and can be left alone. The scar from treatment may be more unsightly and more uncomfortable than the original DF. If patient insists on treatment the options consist of the following:

- Punch excision if smaller than 6 mm.
- Elliptical excision (full thickness down to SQ fat) for larger lesions (Figure 33-13).

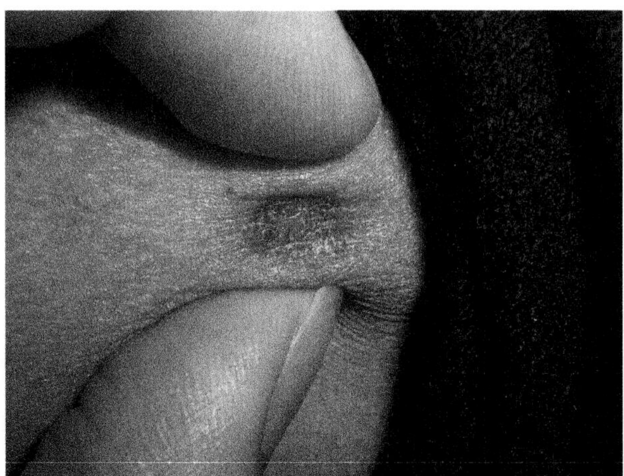

FIGURE 33-12 Positive pinch test showing how the dermatofibroma dimples down when pinched from the sides. *(Copyright Richard P. Usatine, MD.)*

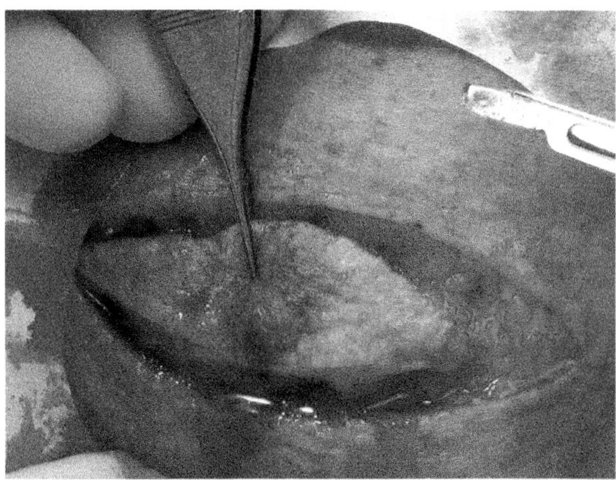

FIGURE 33-13 Elliptical excision of a dermatofibroma on the arm. *(Copyright Richard P. Usatine, MD.)*

- Always send tissue to confirm diagnosis and rule out a dermatofibrosarcoma protuberans (DFSP) (see Chapter 34, *Diagnosis and Treatment of Malignant and Premalignant Lesions*).
- A shave biopsy can be combined with cryosurgery, but this is not as effective as a complete full-thickness excision.
- Cryosurgery is less effective than surgery but can shrink the lesion if that is what the patient desires. Using liquid nitrogen (spray or probe), create a 2-mm freeze margin for a 15-second freeze time. Allow to thaw completely and consider a second freeze for another 15 seconds. Regrowth is not uncommon with this method. A closed probe may allow a deeper freeze.

Special Considerations/Billing

- Recurrence is possible.
- Send for pathology if excised.
- Bill for the excision of a benign lesion based on the size of the excision.
- If cryosurgery is used, bill for the destruction of a benign lesion.

KELOIDS AND HYPERTROPHIC SCARS

Diagnosis

- Thickened, dense proliferation at site of trauma may be pink, red or brown.
- May itch or be irritated.
- Keloids extend beyond extent of scar site in contrast to hypertrophic scar.
- More common in black skin and other dark skin types.
- More common on ear, midchest, and back.

Treatment

Cryosurgery

See video on the DVD for further learning. 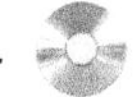

- Use a 20- to 30-second freeze with 1-mm freeze margin, then thaw. Repeat one time. In one study this was performed every 20 to 30 days until flattening with a 73% success rate.[2]
- As an adjunct before intralesional injection, wait 10 to 15 minutes to allow softening of keloids then inject.
- Cryosurgery and intralesional steroids can be combined.
- May cause hypopigmentation in addition to pain.

Injection

See video on the DVD for further learning. 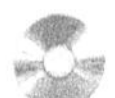

- Inject triamcinolone acetate 10 to 40 mg/mL infiltrated with a 27-gauge needle into keloids until tissue blanches (Figure 33-14).
- Start at 10 mg/mL and titrate up to 40 mg/mL as needed if no effect and no atrophy.
- Repeat every 2 to 4 weeks until nearly flat.
- May cause telangiectasias and atrophy.

Excision of Keloid

See video on the DVD for further learning. 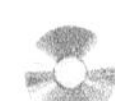

- Results in a high rate of recurrence, so this method should not be used as sole therapy.
- After excision, inject with triamcinolone 10 to 40 mg/mL into wound margins at time of surgery and every 2 to 4 weeks for 6 months. *Or* one reinjection at 4 weeks only.
- Earlobe keloids (Figure 33-15) can be shaved off, injected with triamcinolone and allowed to heal by second intent (Figure 33-16). If possible, have the patient return in 1 month for a second triamcinolone injection to prevent regrowth.
- Large keloids on the ear can be excised and sutured (Figure 33-17).
- After a keloid excision in any location (Figure 33-18), consider injections with triamcinolone to prevent keloids from recurring.

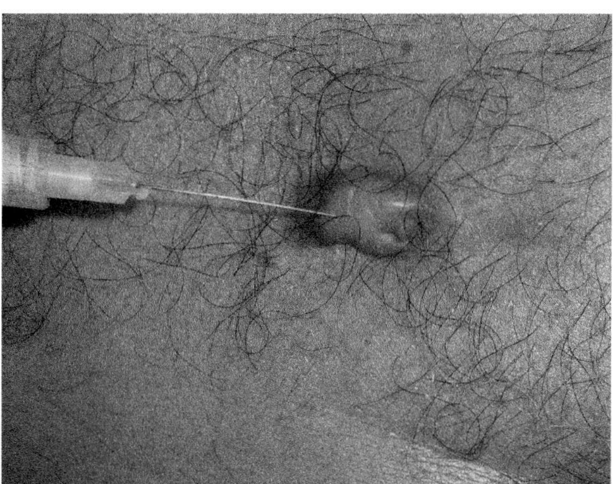

FIGURE 33-14 Injecting an acne keloid with triamcinolone using a 27-gauge needle. *(Copyright Richard P. Usatine, MD.)*

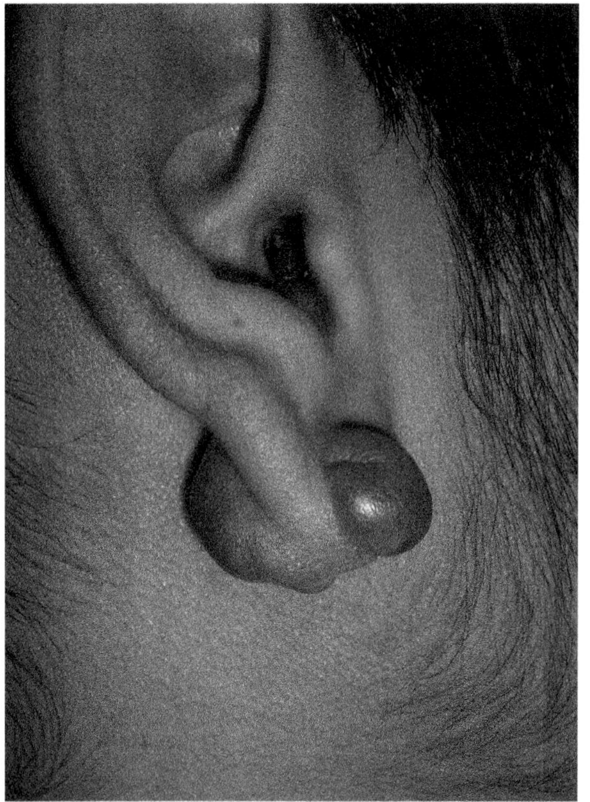

FIGURE 33-15 Keloids formed on both sides of the earlobe secondary to ear piercing. *(Copyright Richard P. Usatine, MD.)*

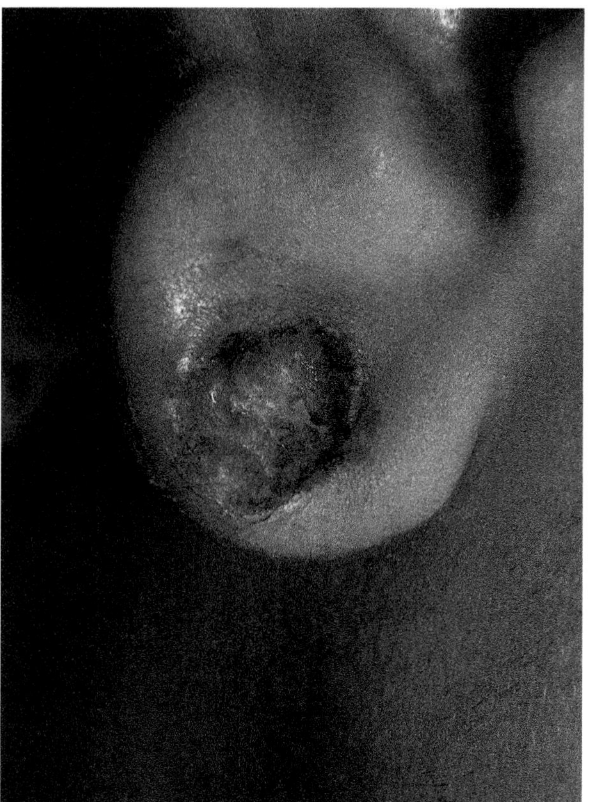

FIGURE 33-16 The front side of an earlobe after a keloid was excised. The base was electrocoagulated and steroid suspension was injected at the base. *(Copyright Richard P. Usatine, MD.)*

Lasers

- Ablative devices, including erbium and CO_2 lasers, and nonablative devices, including pulsed dye (585- and 595-nm) and fractional (1550-nm) devices, can reduce the thickness and texture of scars.[3]
- Nonablative lasers and IPL devices for treatment of red vascular ectasias can reduce the erythema associated with scars.

Other Treatments

- Use silicone sheeting or other occlusive dressings for up to 1 year.

Special Considerations/Billing

- Recurrence and future lesions are common.
- Bill for cryosurgery or intralesional injections based on treatment.
- If excised bill for the excision of a benign lesion.

LENTIGINES (SOLAR)

Diagnosis

- Pigmented macules in sun-exposed distribution (Figure 33-19).

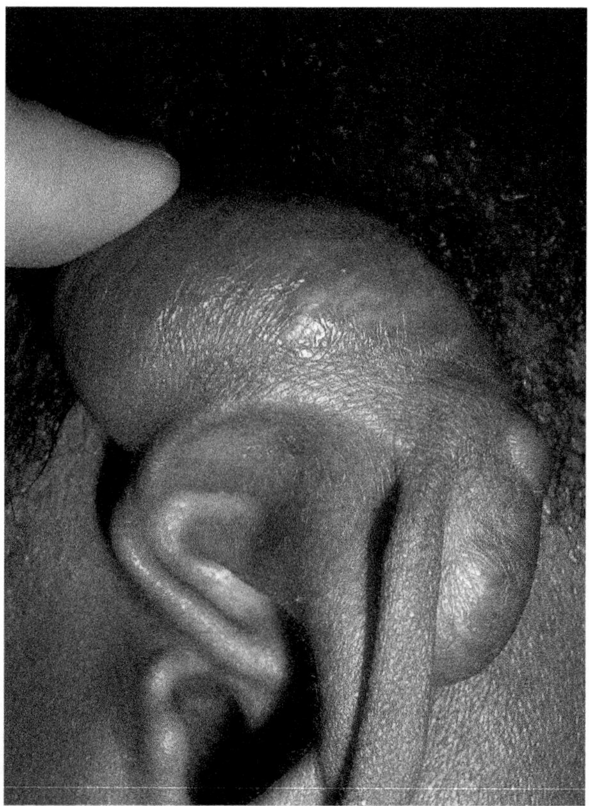

FIGURE 33-17 A large keloid developed at the site of an upper ear piercing. This was excised and the helix was sutured with an excellent cosmetic result. *(Copyright Richard P. Usatine, MD.)*

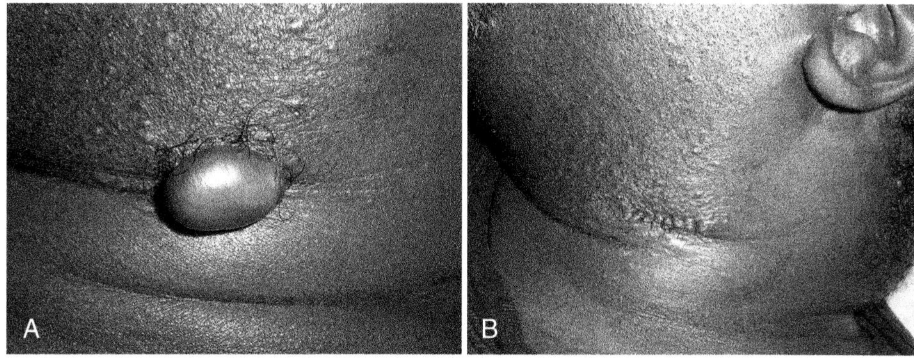

FIGURE 33-18 (A) Keloid on the neck. (B) Keloid excised and defect closed with 6-0 Prolene. The incision site was injected with triamcinolone to prevent recurrence. *(Copyright Richard P. Usatine, MD.)*

- Increased number of melanocytes.
- Single or multiple starting in adulthood and increase with age and sun exposure.
- Do not regress with sun avoidance.

Treatment

- Sunscreen and sun avoidance may decrease occurrence.
- Use makeup to cover lentigines.
- Depigmentation with cryosurgery with short superficial freezing. Warn patients that this may make the solar lentigo darker rather than produce the intended depigmentation.
- Lasers and IPL devices used for treatment of benign pigmented lesions are effective for solar lentigines (see Chapter 27).[4,5]
  - In general, devices with shorter wavelengths (e.g., 532- and 755-nm lasers and IPLs with lower cutoff filters) and Q-switched lasers are most effective for lentigines, where melanin is located superficially in the skin.
  - Lentigines typically darken immediately after treatment and spontaneously exfoliate over a few weeks.
  - One to three treatment sessions are typically needed.

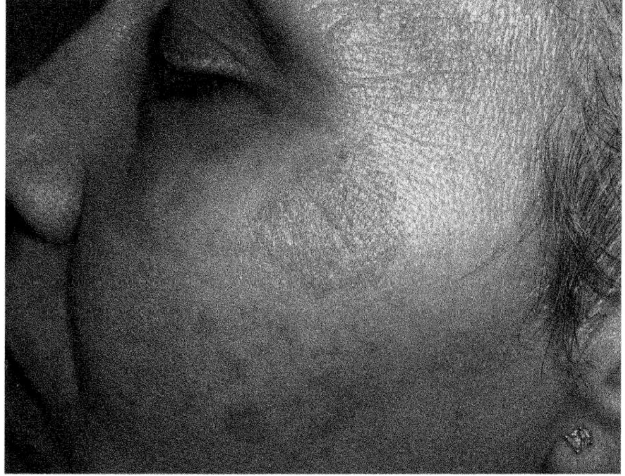

FIGURE 33-19 Large solar lentigo on the face of a 54-year-old Hispanic woman. *(Copyright Richard P. Usatine, MD.)*

- Topical retinoids may lighten lesions.
  - Tretinoin (Retin-A) nightly.
  - Adapalene 0.1% to 0.3% gel (Differin) nightly.
- Light chemical peels (see Chapter 22, *Chemical Peels*).
- Topical skin lightening agents including hydroquinone 4% to 8% (multiple brands and combinations), kojic acid, and peptides (see Chapter 24, *Skin Care Products*).

Special Considerations/Billing

- Treatment for lentigines is cosmetic, so insurance may not cover.
- Consider lentigo maligna and lentigo maligna melanoma in the differential diagnosis. Use dermoscopy to help with this differential diagnosis and if still uncertain, perform a shave biopsy.

MILIA

Diagnosis

- Superficial 1- to 3-mm white keratinized cysts (Figure 33-20).
- Common in the normal newborn, but usually regresses spontaneously.
- May occur later in children and adults where they are more persistent.
- Most common on the face and genital region.

Treatment

See video on the DVD for further learning. 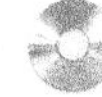

- Nick top of lesion with a No. 11 blade, sterile needle, or the sharp end of a comedone extractor (Figure 33-20B).
- Express white keratin contents by pressure with comedone extractor or paperclip (Figure 33-20C).
- This is performed without anesthesia to avoid obscuring the milia and because the small cut should be less painful than the anesthetic.
- If this does not work the first time, make a slightly larger incision. Some comedone extractors work better than others depending on the size and location

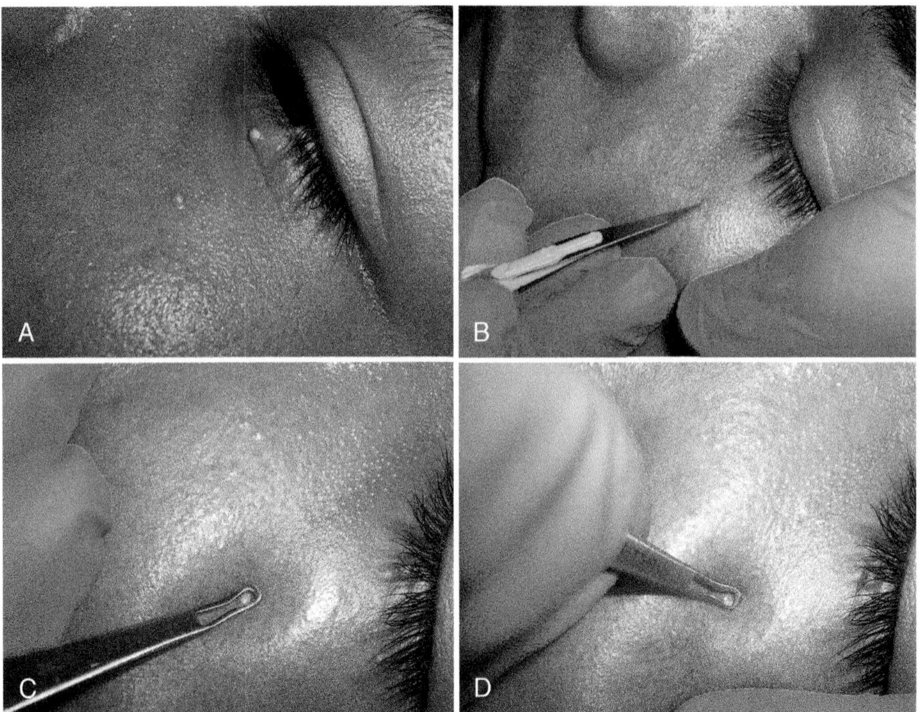

FIGURE 33-20 (A) Milia on the lower eyelid. (B) Milium incised with a No. 11 blade. (C) Milia within comedone extractor. (D) Milia removed. *(Copyright Richard P. Usatine, MD.)*

of the milia. It is therefore good to have a few types of comedone extractors in the office.

Special Considerations/ Pathology/Billing

- Bill using the CPT code for acne surgery = 10040.

MOLLUSCUM CONTAGIOSUM

Diagnosis

- Molluscum contagiosum virus infection is seen commonly in children.
- Seen as a sexually transmitted infection in adults.
- Clustered, flesh-colored epidermal papules; dome shaped often with central umbilication.

Treatment

- Spontaneous resolution, but may take months to years.
- Cryosurgery to a 1-mm freeze margin, approximately 5- to 10-second freeze, thaw, and repeat (Figure 33-21).
- Curette the papules off with a skin curette (or scrape with an 18-gauge needle).
  - Pretreat with topical anesthetic in children (EMLA or others).
  - Any bleeding may be stopped with aluminum chloride.
- Cantharidin (blister beetle extract) topically applied in office once. This method does not hurt when initially applied so it is easier to use for children who are afraid of liquid nitrogen. Apply with the wooden end of a cotton-tipped applicator (CTA). If applied carefully it can be well tolerated and effective.
- Trichloroacetic acid 20% to 30% applied in office once.
- Tretinoin (Retin-A) nightly (off label).
- Imiquimod 5% (Aldara) topically QHS three to four times per week for 2 to 4 weeks (off label). Currently relatively expensive, but less painful than destructive methods, so useful in younger children.

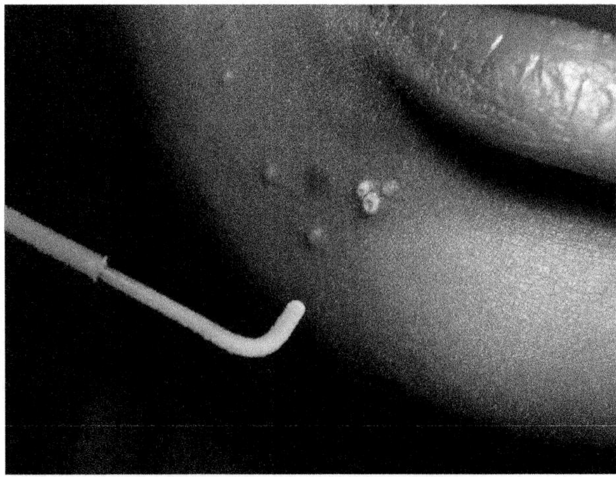

FIGURE 33-21 Molluscum contagiosum receiving cryosurgery with a bent tip spray. *(Copyright Richard P. Usatine, MD.)*

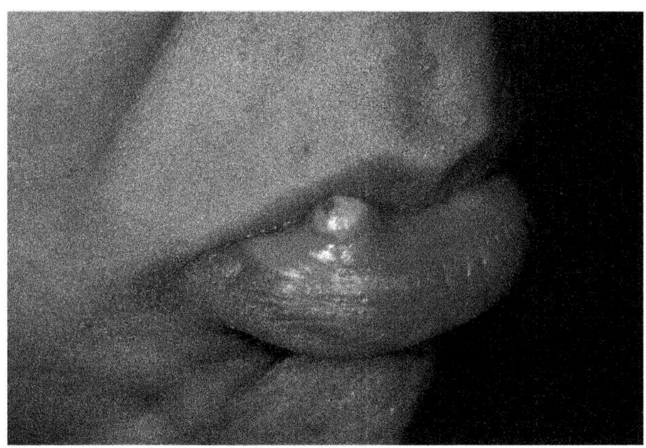

FIGURE 33-22 Mucocele on the inner lip. *(Copyright Richard P. Usatine, MD.)*

- Electrodesiccation lightly performed, no need to destroy entire lesion. The risk of scarring is probably greatest with electrodesiccation.

Billing

- 17110 used once for treatment of 1 to 14 lesions.
- 17111 used once for treatment of 15 or more lesions and these codes are mutually exclusive.

MUCOCELE

Diagnosis

- Bluish to clear or mucosal colored fluid collection, not a true cyst with epithelial lining.
- Most common on inner lower lip (Figure 33-22).
- Mucin collection due to disruption of minor salivary duct.
- Most common in children and young adults.
- Often due to biting inner lip.

Treatment

Cryosurgery

- This is an especially good technique for children old enough to permit this procedure.[6]
- Freeze the closed probe and then apply to the mucocele with pressure. A second treatment may be needed.
- Alternatively, aspirate the mucin contents and then freeze using CTAs or cryoprobe pressed against the base of the mucocele.

Shave Excision

- If the mucocele protrudes above the lip, a shave excision may be performed (Figure 33-23A). Then the base may be destroyed with cryosurgery or electrosurgery (Figure 33-23B).

Elliptical Excision

- Suture with absorbable suture or silk. Consider using buried absorbable sutures so that the ends of the sutures do not irritate the patient.[7] If a deep excision is performed be careful to not cut a labial artery. If so, ligate the artery on both ends.[7]

NEVI

Diagnosis

The three most common acquired nevi are junctional, compound, and intradermal nevi. Some nevi evolve over time from junctional to compound to intradermal nevi.

Junctional Nevi

- Flat, pigmented brown to black with nevus cells at the dermal epidermal junction.

Compound Nevi

- Have nevus cells in the epidermis and dermis.
- Slightly raised and pigmented brown to black.
- Slightly irregular surface.

Intradermal Nevi

- Raised, flesh-colored; pink or brown to black.
- Often cerebriform/variegated surface especially on scalp. The nevus cells are in the dermis.

Dysplastic Nevi (Atypical Moles)

- Have atypical features similar to an early melanoma clinically and dermoscopically.
- Based on the history and physical exam a biopsy may be needed.

There are many other types of nevi including epidermal nevi, speckled nevi, nevus sebaceous, Becker's nevi,

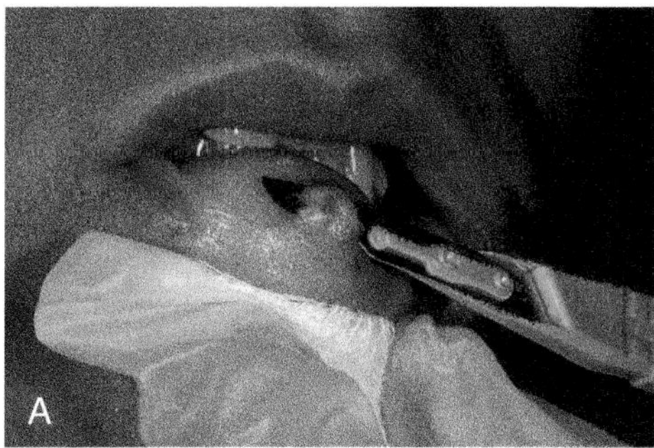

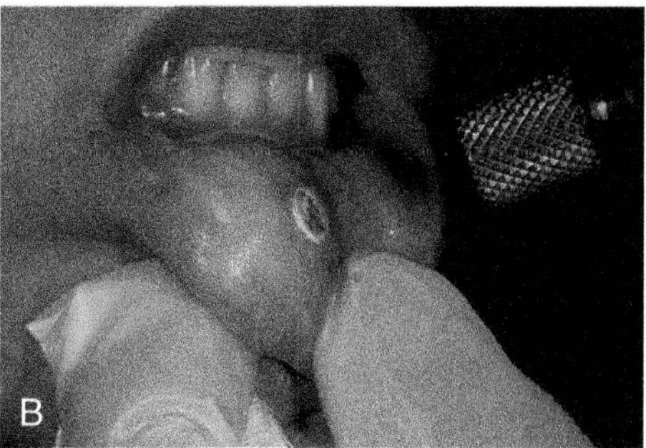

FIGURE 33-23 (A) Mucocele shaved off with scalpel. (B) Mucocele being frozen with liquid nitrogen spray. *(Copyright Richard P. Usatine, MD.)*

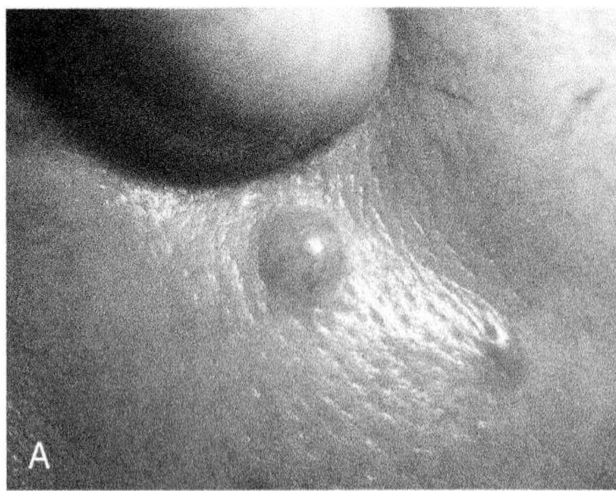

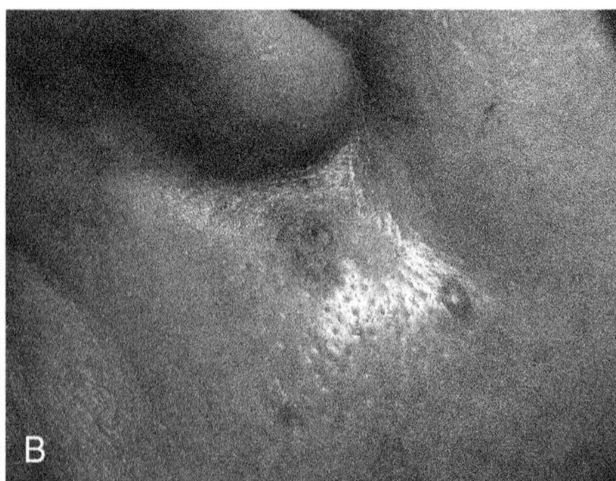

FIGURE 33-24 **(A)** Benign intradermal nevus that looks like a BCC because of its pearly nature and telangiectasias. **(B)** Intradermal nevus after a simple shave excision. *(Copyright Richard P. Usatine, MD.)*

halo nevi, Spitz nevi, nevus depigmentosus, and nevus anemicus. The most important issue is to recognize melanoma and to biopsy any suspicious nevus in a timely fashion. See Chapter 34 for further information on biopsy techniques for lesions suspicious for melanoma.

Treatment

Do not perform cryosurgery or electrodesiccation on nevi—you may be treating a melanoma inadvertently. Also if a nevus that was benign grows back a biopsy may show histology suggestive of a melanoma (pseudomelanoma). Pigmented lesions are best sent for diagnosis to avoid missing a melanoma or other skin cancer.

Shave

See video on the DVD for further learning. 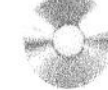

- Intradermal nevi are easily shaved flat with the surrounding surface to provide good cosmesis and adequate tissue for diagnosis (Figure 33-24). These may have features suggestive of a BCC such as telangiectasias, so a shave biopsy is a good technique to differentiate between these diagnoses.
- Scalp nevi that appear benign can easily be removed with a shave excision.
- Nevi may recur but if the pathology was normal it need not be removed again unless the patient wants it done for cosmetic reasons.
- Shave biopsy/excision may be performed with electrosurgery using an RF loop electrode (Figure 33-25)

See video on the DVD for further learning. 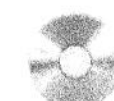

- Dysplastic nevi may be removed with a deep shave (also called *saucerization*). Shave deep enough to remove all pigmentation and a 1- to 2-mm margin. It helps to mark around the pigmented lesion before cutting (Figure 33-26).

Punch Excision

- If the nevus is less than 6 mm, it is small enough to be removed completely with a punch excision (Figure 33-27). If greater than 6 mm, an elliptical excision is preferred.
- A full-thickness excision is good for pathology and diagnostic depth if melanoma.
- Use of a VisiPunch allows the surgeon to check for good margins before starting the cutting (Figure 33-28).

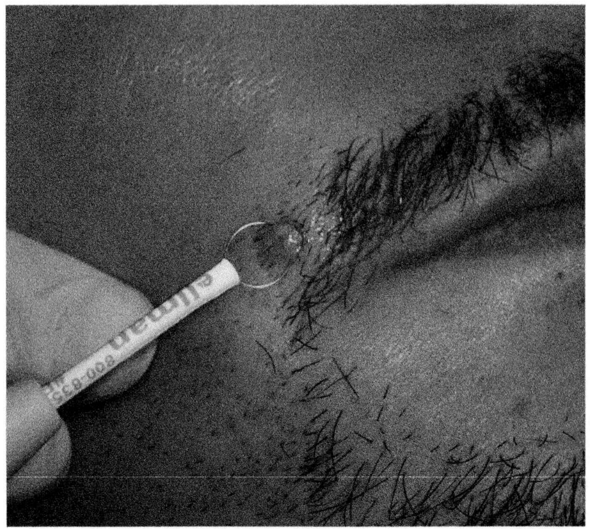

FIGURE 33-25 Excising an intradermal nevus with a radio-frequency loop. *(Copyright Richard P. Usatine, MD.)*

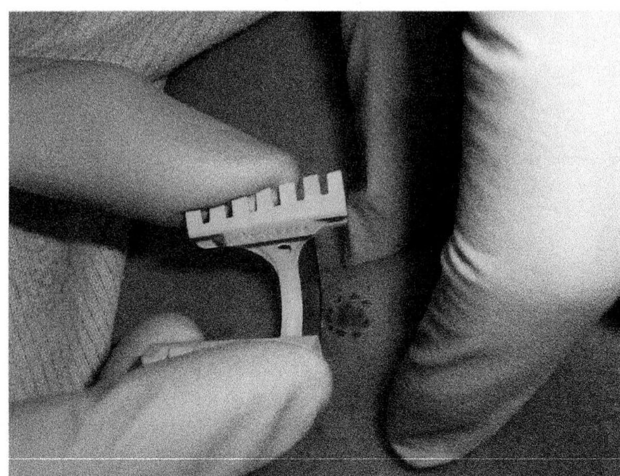

FIGURE 33-26 Physician has pinched the skin for stabilization before cutting this possible dysplastic nevus off with a shave biopsy to pathology. *(Copyright Richard P. Usatine, MD.)*

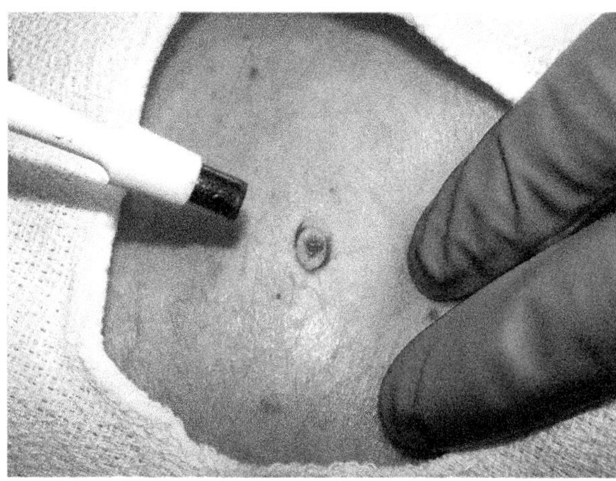

FIGURE 33-27 Punch biopsy done of a pigmented lesion. Note the elongated ellipse achieved on purpose through pulling this can away from the biopsy site using a perpendicular approach. *(Copyright Daniel L. Stulberg, MD.)*

- Junctional nevi are flat and if not suspicious for melanoma, these are best left alone. If a patient insists on removal for cosmetic purposes, a punch biopsy will give a good cosmetic result if the nevus is less than 6 mm.

Elliptical Excision

- Use for lesions greater than 6 mm when a full thickness excision is preferred.
- Nevi with hair will do better cosmetically with a full-thickness excision because most shave biopsies will not be deep enough to remove the hair follicles.
- A full-thickness excision is good for pathology and diagnostic depth if melanoma.
- Usually heals well with linear scar.
- Takes more time than other techniques.

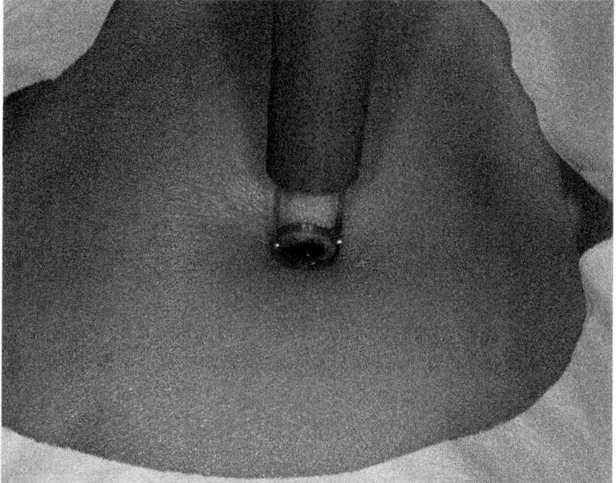

FIGURE 33-28 Punch biopsy of a dark congenital blue nevus on the dorsum of the hand of an 18-year-old girl. VisiPunch allows the surgeon to check for good visible margins. *(Copyright Richard P. Usatine, MD.)*

Dysplastic Nevus (Atypical Mole)

- Dysplastic nevi are markers for an increased risk of melanoma and if one is stable and not evolving and not suspicious for melanoma, the doctor and patient may choose to monitor it rather than excise it.
- Dysplastic nevi may be biopsied and excised using a deep shave, a punch, or an elliptical excision.
- Figure 33-29 shows how a dysplastic nevus can be fully removed with a deep shave biopsy.
- If the pathology shows severe dysplasia and the margins were not clear, it is best to go back and excise with clear margins.

Studies show that 20% to 50% of melanomas appear to arise from a preexisting nevus. The annual risk of an individual nevus transforming into a melanoma is estimated to be only 1 in 200,000.[8] The annual risk for an individual dysplastic nevus (DN) is extremely low as well but estimates are higher: 1 in 10,000 may transform into a melanoma in 1 year.[9] This raises the question of whether incompletely removed DN should be re-excised with clear margins to prevent potential evolution into melanoma. Although most physicians would agree that DN demonstrating severe dysplasia should be re-excised given the risk of early or evolving melanoma, management of incompletely excised DN demonstrating mild or moderate dysplasia has remained an open question.[10]

In one study, 271 possible DN were biopsied using the shave technique in 163 (60%), punch technique in 74 (27%), and elliptical excision in 34 (13%).[10] The authors found very low (3% to 4%) recurrence rates for both benign nevi and DN after biopsy, regardless of margin involvement, nevus subtype (junctional, compound, intradermal), or the presence of congenital features. The recurrence rates were lower than those seen in previous studies even though the follow-up period was greater than that in most of the other studies.[10] A likely explanation is that they performed deeper and broader shave biopsies of clinically atypical nevi, whereas earlier studies primarily examined recurrence of benign nevi removed for cosmetic purposes, where a more superficial shave biopsy may have been done to minimize scarring. Failure of nevi with positive margins to recur suggests that in most cases, residual nevus cells in the biopsy wound are not of sufficient number (or do not have the capacity) for regeneration and pigment production.[10]

The only statistically significant association found with nevus recurrence was the biopsy method, with the shave technique being significantly associated with recurrence.[10] One explanation for a higher recurrence rate with shave biopsies compared with punch biopsies is that nevus recurrence may be more likely to originate from a deep rather than lateral margin—which was observed in most recurrent nevi in this study.[10] Another explanation for the association between shave technique and recurrence is that lesions that are shaved tend to be much larger than those selected for punch biopsy. Larger lesions may contain more proliferative cells or be more likely to recur from residual cells for other reasons that are presently unclear.[10]

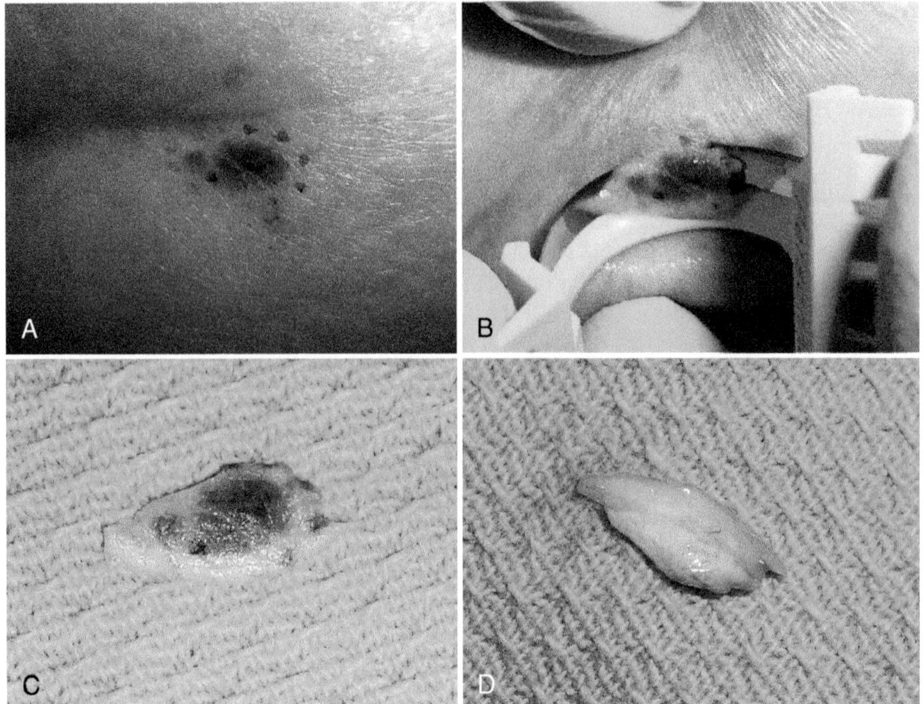

FIGURE 33-29 (A) 2-mm margins drawn around a dysplastic nevus prior to scoop shave biopsy. (B) Scoop shave being performed. (C) Specimen with adequate margins. (D) There is no remaining pigment at the depth of the shave biopsy. *(Copyright Richard P. Usatine, MD.)*

Goodson et al.'s results[10] are consistent with those of Kmetz et al.,[11] who found that no melanomas developed during a 5-year period after biopsy of 55 atypical nevi (26 lesions with at least one positive margin and 29 with clear margins) that were not re-excised.[11] Both studies suggest that lesions that demonstrate only mild or moderate dysplasia may not need to be re-excised given their low likelihood of recurrence, and can be followed clinically for evidence of recurrence or development of any concerning features.[10,11]

Congenital Nevi

Congenital nevi are frequently large and can meet all five ABCDE criteria (see page 434) as a potential melanoma. The clinical diagnosis of congenital nevus is made based on history because they have been present since birth or occurred within the first month or two of birth. Biopsy is indicated if a congenital nevus changes in color, there is a new growth within the nevus, or bleeding without trauma occurs within the nevus. It was long taught that all congenital nevi should be removed because of the potential for malignancy. Large lesions have the greatest potential to become malignant, but they may be so large as to cause major scarring if removed (>20 cm). So, they will need to be watched closely or excised by a plastic surgeon in multiple procedures. With very dark, almost black lesions, early changes will be difficult to detect. The most recent approach recommends following these lesions as with any other nevus and removing them for any observed changes or concerns.

In a prospective study of 230 medium-sized congenital melanocytic nevi (CMN) (1.5 to 19.9 cm) in 227 patients from 1955 to 1996 with average follow-up period being 6.7 years to an average age of 25.5 years, no melanomas occurred in these nevi. The authors concluded that the results of this follow-up study do not support the view that there is a clinically significantly increased risk for malignant melanoma arising in banal-appearing medium-sized CMN or that prophylactic excision of all such lesions is mandatory. Lifelong observation seems a reasonable alternative for medium-sized CMN without unusual features.[12] With the affordability of digital cameras, careful lifelong follow-up with photographs should be easy to accomplish.

Bathing Trunk Nevi

Bathing trunk nevi are very large CMN at higher risk of becoming melanoma. According to Habif,[13] 50% of the melanomas in bathing trunk nevi develop before age 5. There is a risk of neurocutaneous melanoma, which requires an MRI for diagnosis. Melanomas in these large congenital nevi can be missed by observation because they may have nonepidermal origins. In a systematic review, the risk of developing melanoma and the rate of fatal courses were by far highest in CMN ≥40 cm in diameter.[14] Although there are no evidence-based data to support this, surgical excision of bathing trunk nevi is recommended by some experts.[13] This requires multiple stages and the use of tissue expanders. This is done by plastic surgeons and the financial cost is great. The pain and suffering to the child is substantial and needs to be weighed in the decision of whether or not to recommend surgery.

Spitz Nevus

In 1947, Sophie Spitz described "juvenile melanoma" in which prognosis was frequently excellent. However, Spitz reported one patient with "juvenile melanoma" that had a fatal metastases. Currently there is still a lack of consensus about Spitz nevi but pathologists no longer use the term *juvenile melanoma.* Some experts recommend that all Spitz tumors be completely excised with clear margins.[15] Atypical Spitz nevi should be excised with wider margins up to 1 cm.[15] All patients with a history of a Spitz nevus should be carefully monitored by regular examinations for recurrence and metastasis. See Chapter 32 for dermoscopic features of the Spitz nevus.

NEUROFIBROMAS

Diagnosis

- Neurofibromas are soft fleshy papules that can feel like pushing tissue through a buttonhole when compressed downward.
- Persons without neurofibromatosis can have a few isolated neurofibromas.
- Neurofibromatosis type 1 (NF1) is associated with multiple neurofibromas.

Diagnosis of NF1 is made if an individual has two or more of the seven National Institutes of Health criteria present:

1. Multiple café au lait macules (6 or more)
2. Axillary or inguinal freckling
3. Multiple neurofibromas
4. Characteristic skeletal disorders
5. Family history of NF1
6. Iris hamartomas (Lisch nodules)
7. Optic gliomas.

Treatment

- Individual lesions can be removed if desired by the patient.
- Elliptical incision around the lesion is not usually necessary.
- Shave across the base with razor, scalpel, or electrosurgical cutting electrode (Figure 33-30A).
- Often the underlying tissue will elevate above the skin surface (pouch out).
- Cut the remaining tissue flat with the surrounding skin using a forceps to stabilize it and cut with a blade or scissors (Figure 33-30B).
- If the defect is small and flat, allow it to heal by second intention. Otherwise suture the defect with a single-layer closure. Use deep sutures only if there is tension.
- Convert to an ellipse if there are standing cones (dog ears) (see Chapter 11, *The Elliptical Excision*).

PILOMATRICOMA

Diagnosis

- Dermal or subcutaneous nodule containing calcium (also known as calcifying epithelioma of Malherbe) (Figure 33-31).
- Usually found on the head, neck or upper extremities.
- Firm to palpation.

Treatment

See video on the DVD for further learning. 

- Elliptical excision is the treatment of choice (Figure 33-31).

PYOGENIC GRANULOMA (LOBULAR CAPILLARY HEMANGIOMA)

Diagnosis

- Glistening, friable, easily bleeding vascular tissue often with a narrowed base (Figures 33-32 and Figure 14-19 in Chapter 14, *Electrosurgery*).
- Initial rapid growth and failure to heal.
- Often at site of trauma or irritation.

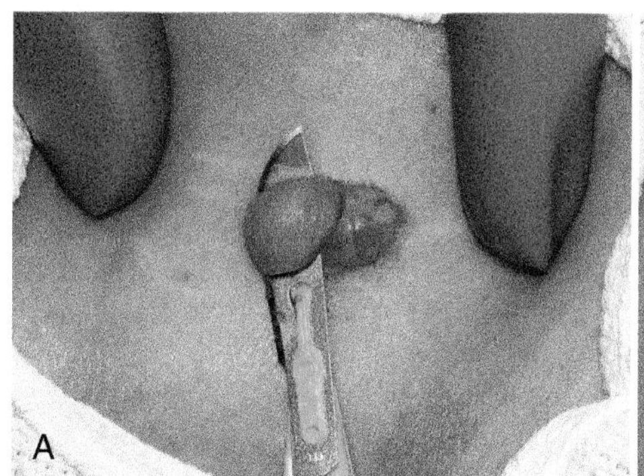

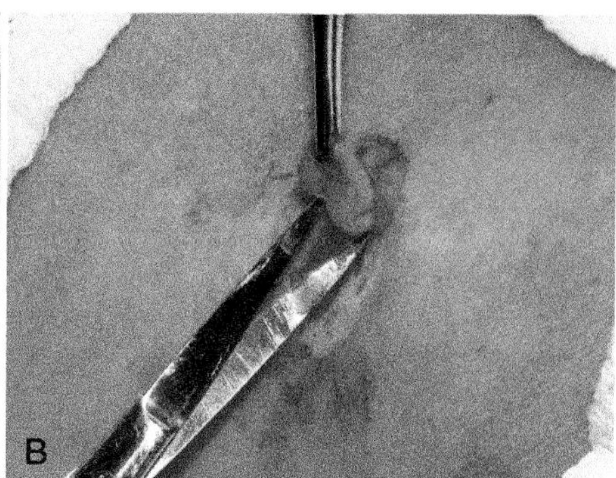

FIGURE 33-30 **(A)** Shave excision of a neurofibroma revealed an outpouching of soft tissue. **(B)** The remainder of the neurofibroma was excised with a sharp iris scissor. *(Copyright Daniel L. Stulberg, MD.)*

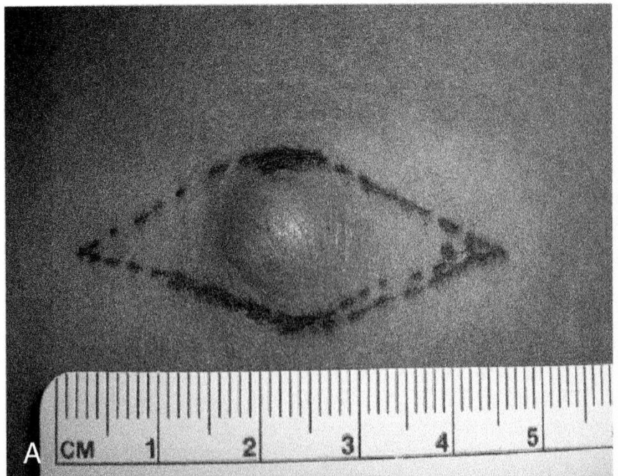

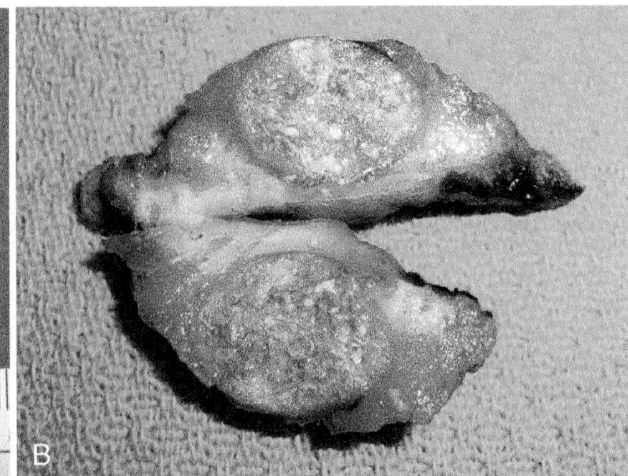

FIGURE 33-31 Pilomatricoma on the left arm of a 17-year-old girl. **(A)** The nodule is tender and she requests it to be resected. **(B)** After elliptical excision the pilomatricoma was analyzed by cutting the specimen in half. Note the white calcium granules within the tissue. *(Copyright Richard P. Usatine, MD.)*

- Common on extremities, especially fingers.
- May occur as an umbilical granuloma of the newborn or on gums of pregnant woman.

In a randomized controlled trial that compared cryotherapy with liquid nitrogen versus curettage and electrodesiccation of patients with pyogenic granuloma, the curettage and electrodesiccation had the advantage of requiring fewer treatment sessions to achieve resolution and better cosmetic results.[16] Treatment of the pyogenic granulomas resulted in complete resolution of all lesions after one to three sessions (mean 1.42) in the cryosurgery group and after one to two sessions (mean 1.03) in the curettage group ($P < 0.001$). Twenty-three patients (57.5%) in the cryotherapy group and 25 patients (69%) in the curettage group had no scar or pigmentation abnormality. From this study and personal experience, we conclude that curettage and electrodesiccation is the preferred treatment option over cryosurgery.

Treatment

Shave, Curettage, and Electrodesiccation

- Use lidocaine with epinephrine and wait at least 10 minutes for the epinephrine to work. Shave off the abnormal tissue and send this for pathology. This can be done with a razor blade, scalpel, or electrosurgical loop (Figure 33-32).
- Curette the base and use electrodesiccation to stop the bleeding (Figure 14-19 in Chapter 14). The curettage and desiccation may need to be repeated until all abnormal tissue is destroyed. If not, these have a tendency to recur.

Elliptical Excision

- Pyogenic granulomas (PGs) on the lips or face may not be adequately treated by the above method and the scarring may be unacceptable. Another option is to elliptically excise the PG. Figure 33-33 shows how the PG on the lip is excised with the ellipse running vertically for the best cosmetic result.

Cryosurgery

- Children may be afraid of needles and may not allow one to anesthetize the skin to cut off their PG. In Figure 15-26 of Chapter 15, *Cryosurgery*, a young child has a PG on the face and allowed the physician to use a Cryo Tweezer to treat her. While it is best to obtain tissue for pathology in most cases, it is safe to treat a benign-appearing PG in a child with cryotherapy.

Silver Nitrate

- Silver nitrate may be used to treat umbilical granulomas. Be careful, however, because excessive application of silver nitrate can burn and/or tattoo the surrounding skin of an infant.[17]

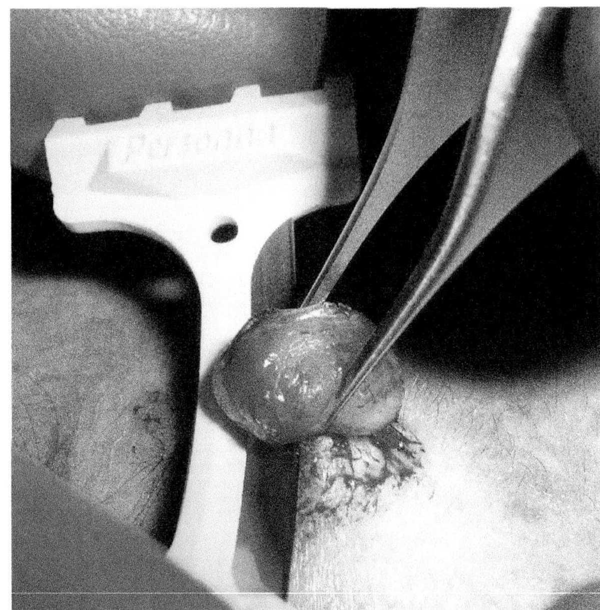

FIGURE 33-32 Shave excision of a pyogenic granuloma using a DermaBlade. The base was then curetted and electrodesiccated. *(Copyright Richard P. Usatine, MD.)*

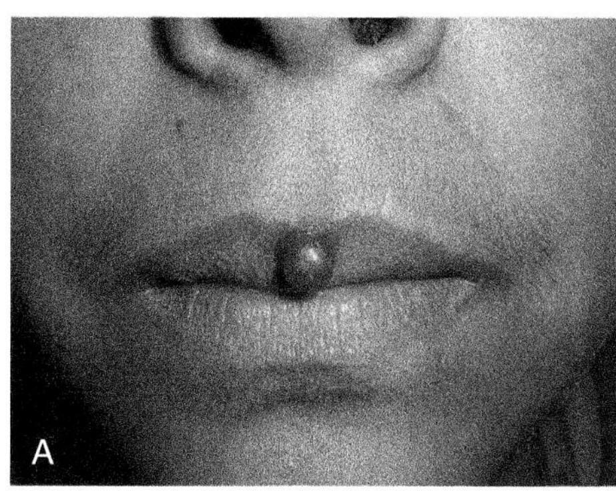

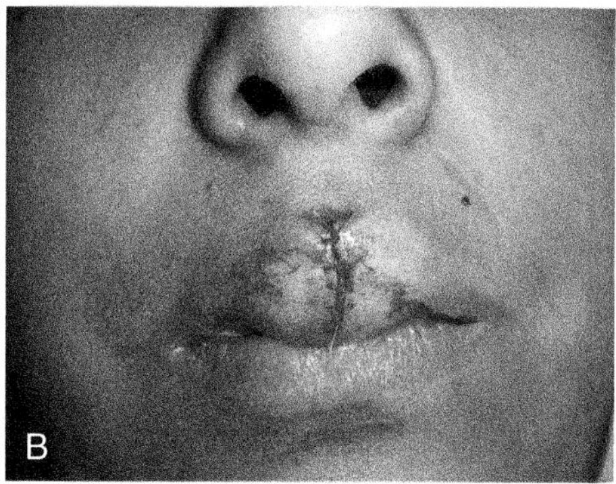

FIGURE 33-33 (A) Suspected pyogenic granuloma on the lip. (B) Pyogenic granuloma excised elliptically with direction of the ellipse being perpendicular to the vermilion border. The swelling is secondary to the anesthesia and the cosmetic result looked great the following week. *(Copyright Richard P. Usatine, MD.)*

Special Considerations/Billing

- Differential diagnosis includes amelanotic melanoma, so send tissue for pathology.
- Bill for a skin neoplasm (ICD-9 238.2) because the diagnosis is not completely certain until the pathologist reviews the slides.
- Recurrence is common so aggressive removal is prudent.

SEBACEOUS HYPERPLASIA

Diagnosis

- Flesh-colored to slightly pale papular clusters of enlarged sebaceous glands (Figure 33-34).
- Usually multiple lesions on forehead and face help to differentiate them from BCC.
- Often doughnut shaped without ulceration or bleeding.
- Telangiectasias may be present but tend to be symmetrically aligned around the doughnut like the jewels in a crown (see page 394).

Treatment

Electrodesiccation

- This is done without anesthesia using low settings as for cherry angiomas and telangiectasias (Hyfrecator 2 to 3 joules). Start at 2 and only increase power if needed.
- Lightly electrodesiccate the rim of abnormal tissue around the central pore. Using the blunt electrode can be easier than using the sharp-tipped electrode (Figure 33-34).
- Results can be seen immediately and within 1 month (Figure 33-35).
- Many lesions (especially larger lesions) will need retreatment after 1 to 2 months.
- Consider local anesthesia if lesions are large or if patients request it. Use a surgical marker before administering the anesthesia because the sebaceous hyperplasia may be hard to see afterward.

Shave Excision

- If the diagnosis is not clear and a BCC is in the differential diagnosis, a shave biopsy is a good method medically and cosmetically. Do not forget to mark the lesion with a surgical marker before administering the anesthesia.
- For sebaceous hyperplasia that has not cleared with electrosurgery, shave excisions can provide long-lasting results. The most common complication of this method is to leave a divot at the site of removal so care is needed to not shave too deeply.

Lasers

- Ablative lasers (e.g., 2940 nm and CO_2) can be used.[18,19] Certain ablative devices have microtips used for precision ablation, which is very effective for these types of small lesions.[20]
- Nonablative 1450-nm diode lasers can also be used.[22]
- A series of four to six treatments is usually necessary with nonablative lasers, whereas ablative lasers require only one or two treatments.
- Photodynamic therapy utilizes topical photosensitizing medication activated by light (lasers, LEDs, and IPL devices).[21]

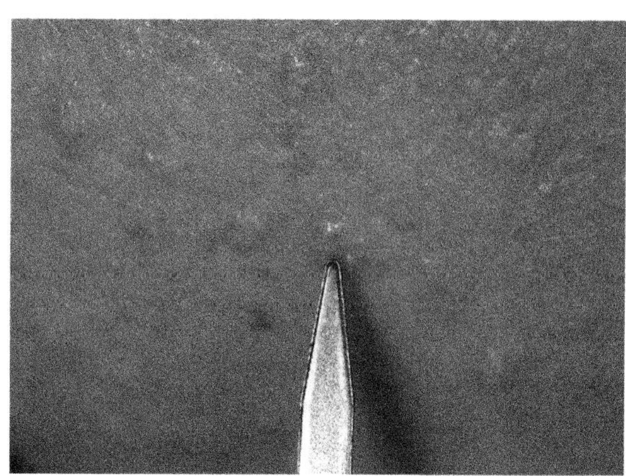

FIGURE 33-34 Blunt electrode about to electrodesiccate sebaceous hyperplasia. *(Copyright Richard P. Usatine, MD.)*

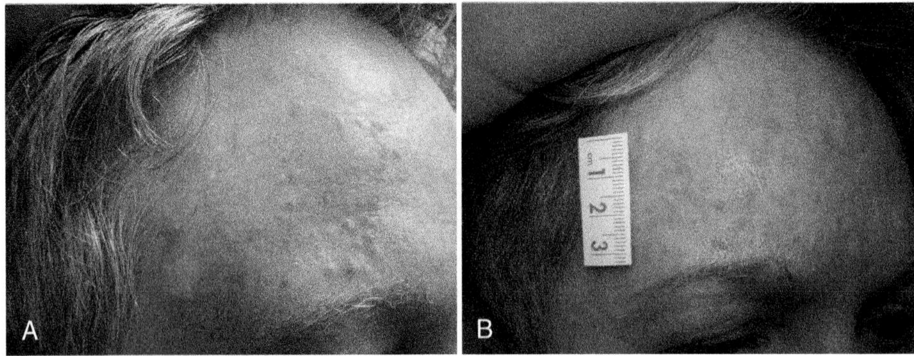

FIGURE 33-35 (A) Sebaceous hyperplasia prior to electrosurgical treatment. (B) Clearance of sebaceous hyperplasia after treatment. *(Copyright Daniel L. Stulberg, MD.)*

Special Considerations/Billing

- Often appears similar to BCC; if any question, perform the shave and send to pathology. Code these as skin neoplasms ICD-9 238.2.
- May leave depressed area/scar that over time will usually partially fill in, but may not.
- Initial diagnostic E&M (evaluation and management) service and shave biopsy if needed to rule out BCC should be covered.
- Electrosurgery or laser for cosmesis is often not covered by insurance.

SEBORRHEIC KERATOSES AND DERMATOSIS PAPULOSA NIGRA

Diagnosis

- Benign stuck-on tumors with tan, brown, or black colors
- Dermatosis papulosa nigra (DPN) is a collection of seborrheic keratoses (SKs) found on the cheeks and face—most commonly on the face of women of color and bilaterally distributed (Figure 15-22 in Chapter 15).
- Verrucous or smooth surface, often with keratin pearls (horn cysts, comedo-like openings, and milia cysts) and crevices seen on magnification and dermoscopy (see Chapter 32).
- Sharply demarcated, stuck-on appearance.
- Superficial layers peel away easily, leaving capillary bleeding at base.

Treatment

- No treatment necessary if classic appearance and asymptomatic.

  Cryosurgery of SK (Figure 33-36)

See video on the DVD for further learning. 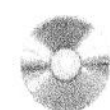

  - No anesthesia required.
  - Use a 1- to 2-mm freeze margin, 10- to 20-second freeze, thaw; consider repeating.
  - May be erythematous for weeks.
  - Can cause hypo or hyperpigmentation (especially hypopigmentation in persons of darker color).
  - Quick and clean.

Alternative treatment methods that require local anesthesia include the following:

- Shave excision with blade and aluminum chloride or electrosurgery for hemostasis (Figure 33-37). This allows tissue to be sent for pathology if diagnosis is uncertain. Even if a SK is most likely, send for pathology to avoid missing a melanoma.
- Shave excision with electrosurgical loop.
- Curettage followed by electrodesiccation or aluminum chloride for hemostasis (Figure 33-38). It may help to apply the electrodesiccation first because that will make the curettage step easier.

  Electrodesiccation with local anesthesia.
  - Desiccate the raised tissue.
  - Wipe off destroyed tissue with moistened gauze.
  - Repeat as needed until lesion is removed and flat skin remains.
- Ablative lasers (e.g., 2940 nm and CO_2) can be used.[18,19] Certain ablative devices have microtips

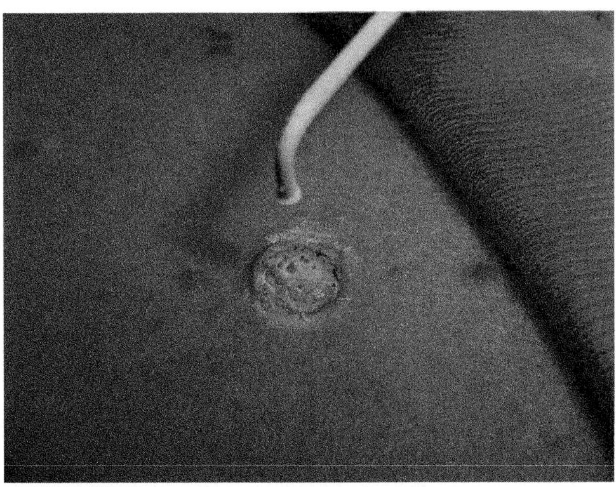

FIGURE 33-36 Cryosurgery of a seborrheic keratosis using an open spray approach with a bent-tip. The comedo-like openings can be seen. *(Copyright Richard P. Usatine, MD.)*

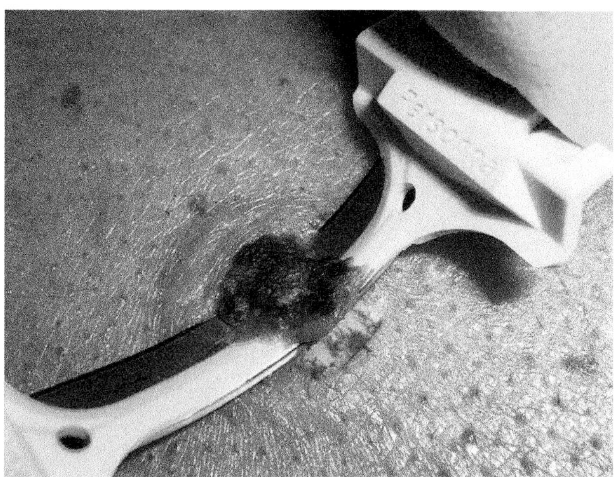

FIGURE 33-37 Shave excision of a suspicious looking seborrheic keratosis to send to pathology. *(Copyright Richard P. Usatine, MD.)*

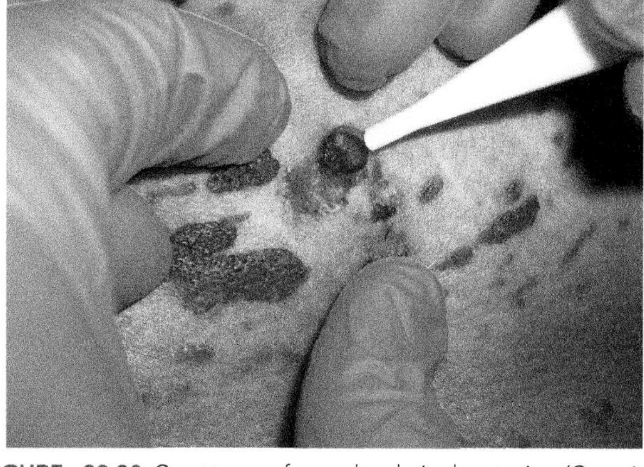

FIGURE 33-38 Curettage of a seborrheic keratosis. *(Copyright Richard P. Usatine, MD.)*

used for precision ablation, which is very effective for SKs.[20]

- Nonablative lasers and IPL devices used for treatment of benign pigmented lesions (see Chapter 27) will remove the pigmentation of SKs and DPN but not reduce lesion thickness.

Special Considerations/Billing

- Consider malignant melanoma in differential diagnosis if atypical appearance.
- Be careful when freezing SKs or DPN on the face of a darkly pigmented person—hypopigmentation can be permanent.
- 17110 used once for treatment of 1–14 lesions.
- 17111 used once for treatment of 15 or more lesions. These codes are mutually exclusive.

SYRINGOMAS

Diagnosis

- Benign periorbital adnexal tumors commonly seen on both lateral lower eyelids.
- Diagnosis is clinical based on appearance (Figure 33-39).
- Only of cosmetic concern and not a sign of any underlying illness.

Treatment

Treatment may be reassurance in many patients. If the patient insists on treatment, electrosurgery or laser treatments are most effective.

Electrodesiccation

- Apply a topical anesthetic such as EMLA. Wait for it to take effect.
- Use a Hyfrecator or other electrosurgical device using 2 to 3 W (Figure 33-39A). Use the ball electrode with the Surgitron.
- Deliver short bursts with standard electrodes or an epilation needle.[23]

Laser

- Ablative lasers (e.g., 2940 nm and CO_2) can be used.[18,19]

Cryosurgery

- This method can be used to treat syringomas without anesthesia (Figure 33-39B). It is possible that multiple sessions will be needed to produce the desired results.

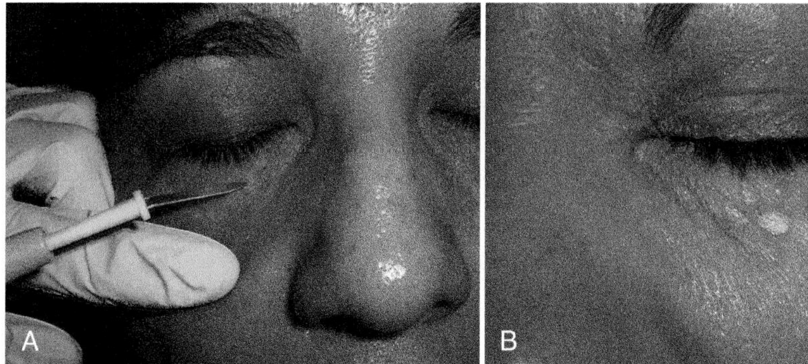

FIGURE 33-39 **(A)** Electrodesiccation of syringomas. **(B)** Cryosurgery of syringomas. *(Copyright Richard P. Usatine, MD.)*

TELANGIECTASIAS AND SPIDER ANGIOMAS

Diagnosis

- Telangiectasias are frequently found on the nose as patients age. Persons with rosacea may have many telangiectasias on the nose and face.

Treatment

Telangiectasias may be treated for cosmetic reasons using electrosurgery or laser treatments.

- Electrodesiccation is performed without anesthesia using a Hyfrecator or other electrosurgical device set at 2 to 3 W (Figure 33-40).
- Short bursts of energy are delivered with a standard electrode or epilation needle. Enough electricity should be delivered to see the vessel blanch, but to avoid leaving a burn on the skin. Epilation needles are inserted into the vessel to avoid skin scarring and provide electrodesiccation to the blood vessel.
- Telangiectasias on the legs do not respond well to electrosurgery and are best treated by lasers or sclerotherapy.
- Spider angiomas are often larger than telangiectasias and have a central feeding vessel. These are seen more commonly in patients with liver disease from viral hepatitis or alcohol addiction. In Figure 33-41 a patient with a spider angioma on the face was treated with cryosurgery using a contact probe to compress the vessel while the liquid nitrogen was used to freeze the probe. Electrosurgery and lasers are options.

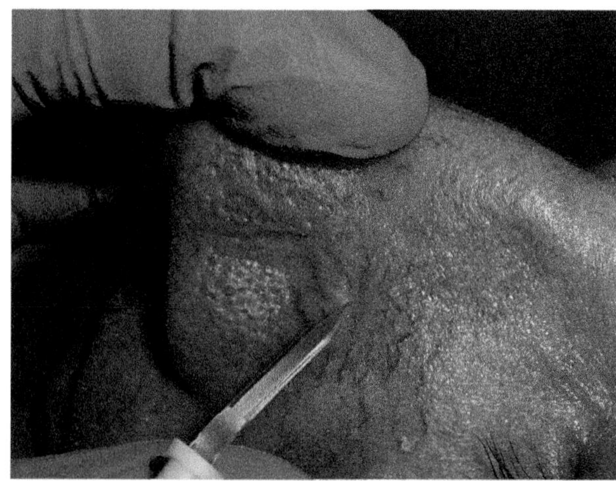

FIGURE 33-40 Electrosurgery of telangiectasias on the nose using the sharp tip electrode on the Hyfrecator. *(Copyright Richard P. Usatine, MD.)*

- Lasers (e.g., 532, 595, and 980 nm) and IPL devices used for treatment of red vascular ectasias are effective for facial telangiectasias (see Chapter 27).[24]

TRICHOEPITHELIOMA

Diagnosis

- Papular lesions most commonly of the head and upper trunk.
- May be single or multiple and may occur in childhood (Figure 33-42).

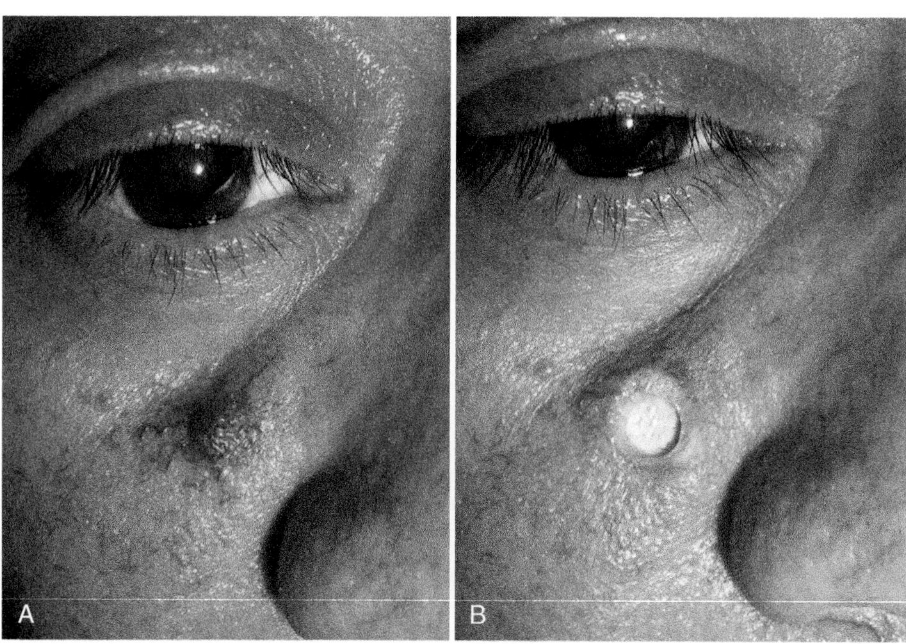

FIGURE 33-41 **(A)** Spider angioma on the face. **(B)** Cryosurgery of this angioma using the closed probe technique. *(Copyright Richard P. Usatine, MD.)*

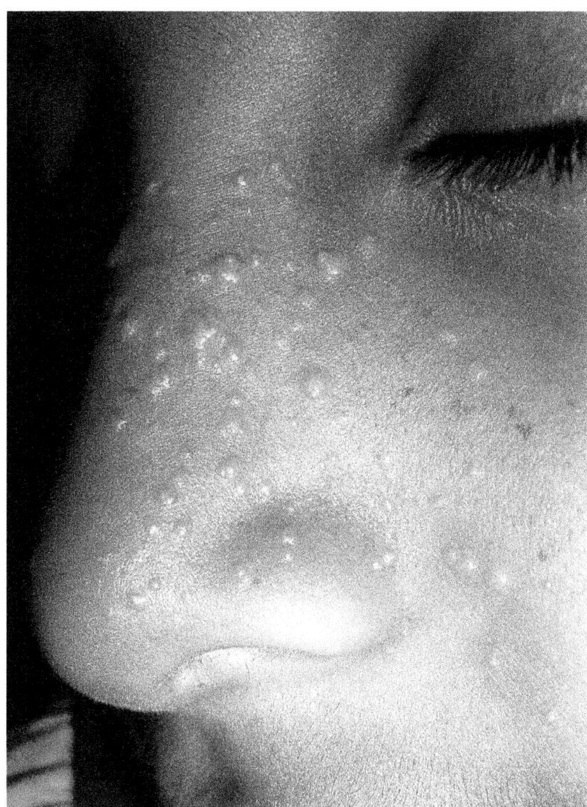

FIGURE 33-42 Multiple trichoepitheliomas are seen around the nose of a 9-year-old girl. Treatment was initiated with cryosurgery and tretinoin. *(Copyright Richard P. Usatine, MD.)*

- Shave biopsy to confirm suspected diagnosis because a single trichoepithelioma may resemble a BCC.
- Desmoplastic trichoepitheliomas are more aggressive and should be removed with clear margins. Consider Mohs surgery if this is on the face.[25]

Treatment

- Shave excision may be adequate.
- Punch or elliptical excision is an alternative.
- For multiple trichoepitheliomas on the face in children, the treatment choices include cryosurgery along with topical medications (Figure 33-42). Although no clinical trials have been done that could help guide treatment, topical imiquimod and topical tretinoin have been used alone or in combination for treatment.[26]

WARTS, COMMON

Diagnosis

- Benign human papilloma virus (HPV) infection.
- Most common on extremities.
- Range from flat to dome shaped, smooth or rough surface.

Treatment

Topical Salicylic Acid

- These preparations are up to 75% effective.[27]
- Topical liquid 17% (Compound W, Duofilm, and others) or wax-based applicator (Wart Stick) applied nightly after soaking the wart in water and debriding loose skin.
- Topical 40% salicylic acid plasters applied before bed.
- May take weeks to months.

Cryosurgery

- Use a 1- to 2-mm freeze margin and a 10- to 20-second total freeze time (may be divided into a freeze-thaw-freeze if patient can't tolerate one longer freeze).
- Repeat freeze or use longer total freeze time if warts are thick, large, or resistant to previous cryosurgery.
- Pain, erythema, possible blistering, and skin sloughing are expected.
- Damage to underlying tissues may cause hematoma or temporary local nerve damage on occasion.
- Hypopigmentation or hyperpigmentation is possible.
- Scarring is possible, but not common.

In-Office Topicals

- Cantharidin may be used as for molluscum (see page 412).
- Trichloroacetic acid 20% to 30% applied weekly after paring the wart down.
- Topical sensitizers can be used. They require inducing immune system sensitization and resultant local reaction before treatment. The dinitrochlorobenzene sensitizer has cure rates from 38% to 80%.[27]

Curettage and Desiccation

- In resistant warts, may curette or dissect out wart and electrodesiccate the base.
- Leaves large initial defect.
- Scarring is the norm.
- Electrodesiccation can aerosolize viral particles.

Immunotherapy

- Candida antigen is a useful method to treat recalcitrant warts. A detailed description of how to mix and inject candida antigen is given in Chapter 16, *Intralesional Injections* (pages 206–207).[28]

Special Considerations/Billing

- Biopsy if persistent or atypical appearance to rule out malignancy especially if patient is immunocompromised.
- 17110 used once for treatment of 1–14 lesions.
- 17111 used once for treatment of 15 or more lesions. These codes are mutually exclusive.

WARTS, FILIFORM

Diagnosis

- Finger-like projection of warty tissue.
- Common on face.

Treatment

- Due to small base can snip or shave and electrodesiccate the base.
- Electrodesiccation can aerosolize viral particles.
- Cryosurgery with Cryo Tweezers down to normal skin; thaw and repeat.

Billing

- As above for common warts.

WARTS, FLAT

Diagnosis

- Slightly raised multiple flat flesh-colored lesions, 2 to 4 mm.
- Common on face, extremities of children, and legs (if shaving legs).

Treatment

- Imiquimod (Aldara).
- Tretinoin (Retin-A) nightly.
- Topical 5-fluorouracil (Efudex) in refractory cases in adults.
- Cryosurgery to a 1-mm freeze margin; approximately 5- to 10-second freeze.

See video on the DVD for further learning 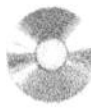

- Electrosurgery with light fulguration (use topical anesthetic first).
- Light curettement with a disposable sharp curette is effective and can be performed either without anesthesia or after topical anesthetics have been applied.

WARTS, PLANTAR

Diagnosis

- Warts on the sole of the foot (plantar surface) or palm of the hand.
- Pain with walking or pressure.
- Thickened, slightly raised.
- Differentiate from calluses by alteration of normal skin lines and thrombosed capillaries causing small black dots (Figure 33-43).

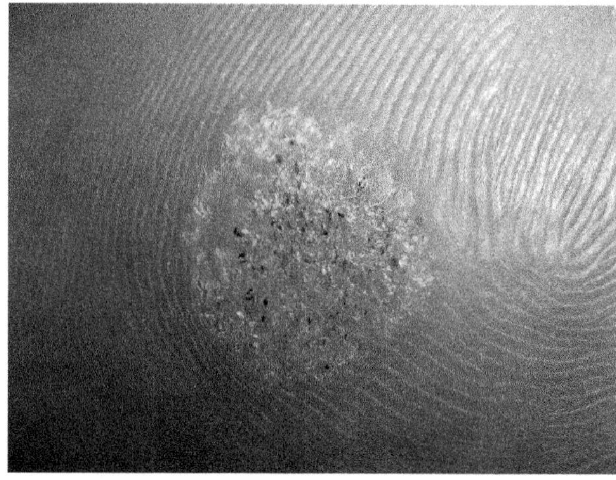

FIGURE 33-43 Plantar wart on the sole of the foot disrupting skin lines and showing black dots caused by thrombosed capillaries. *(Copyright Richard P. Usatine, MD.)*

Treatment

- As above for common warts.
- Swelling of cryosurgery and tissue destruction may cause pain with walking.
- Consider longer trial of topical therapy before more aggressive treatment.

Special Considerations/Billing

- As above for common warts.
- Resistant and recurrent warts may respond to laser treatment.

WARTS, VENEREAL (CONDYLOMA ACUMINATA)

Diagnosis

- Fleshy, polypoid, or verrucous flesh-colored raised lesions of the genital region and perirectal areas caused by HPV.

Treatment

Imiquimod 5% (Aldara)

- Topically QHS three times per week; wash off after 6 to 10 hours.
- Use up to 16 weeks.

Podofilox 0.5% Solution or Gel (Condylox)

- Apply topically BID for 3 days to lesions; repeat weekly for 1 to 4 weeks.
- Gel for perianal lesions.

Cryosurgery

- Use a 1- to 2-mm freeze margin for a 5- to 20-second total freeze time (may be divided into a freeze-thaw-freeze if patient can't tolerate one longer freeze) (Figure 33-44).

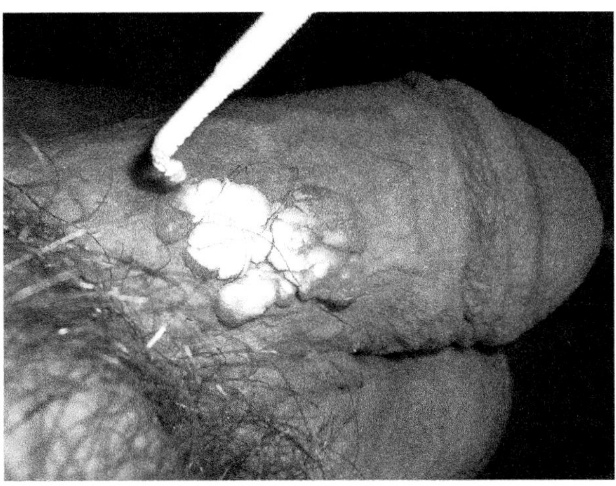

FIGURE 33-44 Cryosurgery of condyloma acuminata on the penis. *(Copyright Richard P. Usatine, MD.)*

Excision

- Large lesions can be anesthetized and excised with dissecting scissors or a scalpel with suture repair of any large defect.
- Condyloma can be excised using electrosurgery and a loop electrode (Figure 33-45). See page 170.
- Scarring is possible.

Electrodesiccation or Laser

- Electrodesiccation or laser treatment can aerosolize viral particles; use a vacuum filter.
- Use local anesthetic; general if large areas.
- Results are immediate.
- Scarring is possible.

Special Considerations/ Pathology/Billing

- Viral infection is not cleared by removal of the condyloma. Recurrence is always possible.
- Caution to not miss cervical, penile, anal, and vulvar cancer, which is often caused by HPV.
- Caution to not miss syphilitic condyloma lata.
- Use site specific codes to bill for destruction of condyloma. See Table 38-6 on page 469.

XANTHELASMA

Diagnosis

- Superficial lipid deposits around the eyes and eyelids (Figure 33-46).
- Pale, raised, rubbery.
- Fifty percent of patients have hyperlipidemia, so evaluate lipid levels and treat as appropriate.

Treatment

- Elliptical excision.
- Cryosurgery or electrosurgical destruction may be attempted.
- Ablative lasers, including erbium and CO_2, and pulsed dye lasers (585 and 595 nm).[18,29]

LESS COMMON BENIGN ADNEXAL TUMORS

- Eccrine poroma (Figure 33-47).
- Spiradenoma (Figure 33-48).

These will most likely be diagnosed when an unusual growth is removed and the pathology report comes back with one of these descriptions. Their photos are included in this chapter just as an introduction to their existence. In most cases the definitive treatment involves complete excision with clear margins.

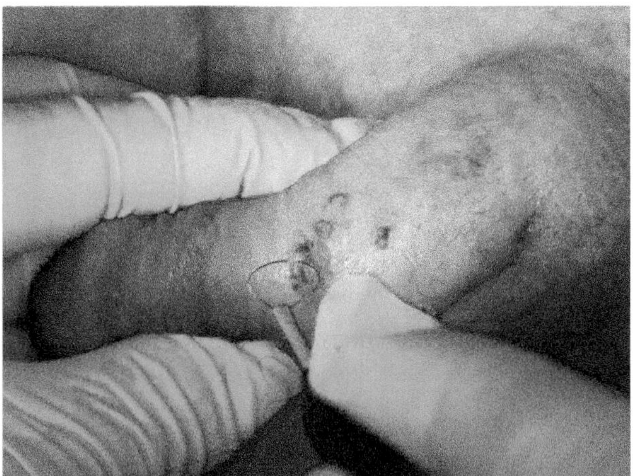

FIGURE 33-45 Electrosurgical removal of condyloma on the penis using radiofrequency and a loop electrode. Note the excellent result on the proximal penile shaft where condyloma were already shaved off with the electrosurgical loop. *(Copyright John L. Pfenninger, MD.)*

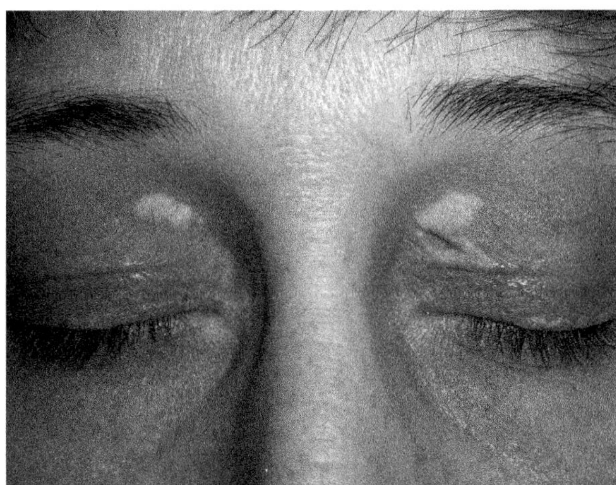

FIGURE 33-46 Xanthelasma in a woman with cholesterol over 300. *(Copyright Richard P. Usatine, MD.)*

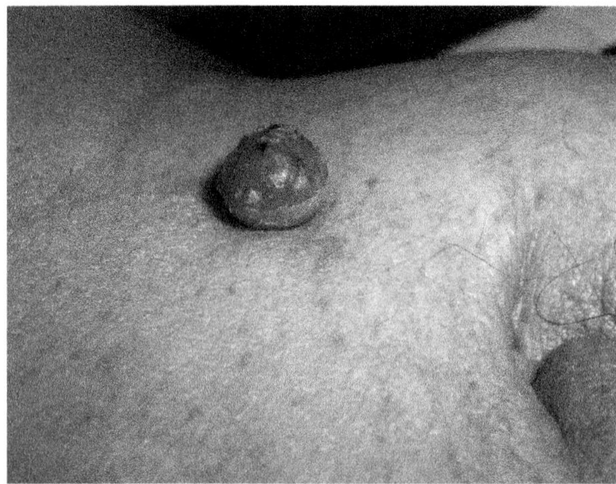

FIGURE 33-47 Eccrine poroma on the abdomen. *(Copyright Richard P. Usatine, MD.)*

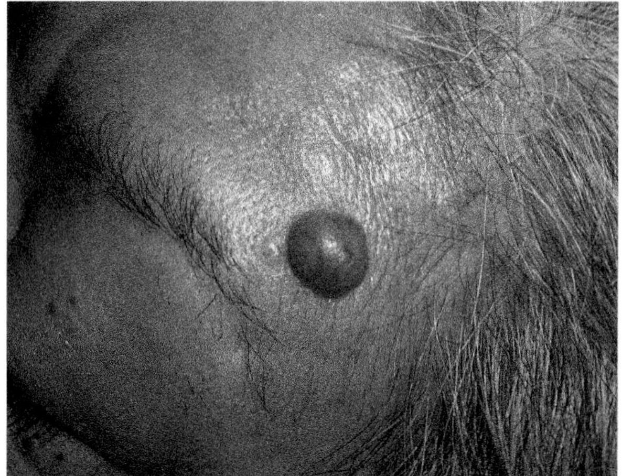

FIGURE 33-48 Spiradenoma on the forehead. *(Copyright Richard P. Usatine, MD.)*

CONCLUSION

The clinician will see multiple benign skin tumors in practice. It is important to realize that many, once diagnosed, do not require treatment or intervention. If a patient desires to have the lesion removed, there are usually multiple techniques to achieve removal with reasonable cosmetic results. Clinicians should consider their array of instruments, equipment, and their own skills and practice flow to choose the appropriate technique for the individual situation. If the diagnosis is uncertain or malignancy is high in the differential diagnosis, do not hesitate to remove the lesion and send for pathology.

References

1. Goldberg DJ, Marcus J. The use of the frequency-doubled Q-switched Nd:YAG laser in the treatment of small cutaneous vascular lesions. *Dermatol Surg.* 1996;22:841–844.
2. Rusciani L, Rossi G, Bono R. Use of cryotherapy in the treatment of keloids. *J Dermatol Surg Oncol.* 1993;19:529–534.
3. Katz TM, Glaich AS, Goldberg LH, Friedman PM. 595-nm long pulsed dye laser and 1450-nm diode laser in combination with intralesional triamcinolone/5-fluorouracil for hypertrophic scarring following a phenol peel. *J Am Acad Dermatol.* 2010;62:1045–1049.
4. Ross EV, Smirnov M, Pankratov M. Intense pulsed light and laser treatment of facial telangiectasias and dyspigmentation: some theoretical and practical comparisons. *Dermatol Surg.* 2005;31:1188–1198.
5. Small R. Aesthetic procedures in office practice. *Am Fam Physician* 2009;80:1231–1237.
6. Marcushamer M, King DL, Ruano NS. Cryosurgery in the management of mucoceles in children. *Pediatr Dent.* 1997;19:292–293.
7. Tran TA, Parlette III HL. Surgical pearl: removal of a large labial mucocele. *J Am Acad Dermatol.* 1999;40:760–762.
8. Tsao H, Bevona C, Goggins W, Quinn T. The transformation rate of moles (melanocytic nevi) into cutaneous melanoma: a population-based estimate. *Arch Dermatol.* 2003;139:282–288.
9. Naeyaert JM, Brochez L. Clinical practice. Dysplastic nevi. *N Engl J Med.* 2003;349:2233–2240.
10. Goodson AG, Florell SR, Boucher KM, Grossman D. Low rates of clinical recurrence after biopsy of benign to moderately dysplastic melanocytic nevi. *J Am Acad Dermatol.* 2010;62:591–596.
11. Kmetz EC, Sanders H, Fisher G, *et al.* The role of observation in the management of atypical nevi. *South Med J.* 2009;102:45–48.
12. Sahin S, Levin L, Kopf AW, *et al.* Risk of melanoma in medium-sized congenital melanocytic nevi: a follow-up study. *J Am Acad Dermatol.* 1998;39:428–433.
13. Habif T. *Clinical Dermatology*. 4th ed. St. Louis: Mosby; 2004.
14. Krengel S, Hauschild A, Schafer T. Melanoma risk in congenital melanocytic naevi: a systematic review. *Br J Dermatol.* 2006;155:1–8.
15. Situm M, Bolanca Z, Buljan M, *et al.* Nevus Spitz—everlasting diagnostic difficulties—the review. *Coll Antropol.* 2008;32(Suppl 2):171–176.
16. Ghodsi SZ, Raziei M, Taheri A, *et al.* Comparison of cryotherapy and curettage for the treatment of pyogenic granuloma: a randomized trial. *Br J Dermatol.* 2006;154:671–675.
17. Daniels J, Craig F, Wajed R, Meates M. Umbilical granulomas: a randomised controlled trial. *Arch Dis Child Fetal Neonatal Ed.* 2003;88:F257.
18. Krupashankar DS. Standard guidelines of care: CO_2 laser for removal of benign skin lesions and resurfacing. *Indian J Dermatol Venereol Leprol.* 2008;74(Suppl):S61–S67.
19. Riedel F, Bergler W, Baker-Schreyer A, *et al.* Controlled cosmetic dermal ablation in the facial region with the erbium:YAG laser. *HNO.* 1999;47:101–106.
20. Khatri KA. Treatment of cutaneous lesions using a novel 2.94 erbium laser with micron tips. Presented at American Society for Laser Medicine and Surgery, 2009, National Harbor, MD.
21. Richey D, Hopson B. Treatment of sebaceous hyperplasia with photodynamic therapy. *Cosm Dermatol.* 2004;17:525–529.
22. No D, McClaren M, Chotzen V, Kilmer SL. Sebaceous hyperplasia treated with a 1450-nm diode laser. *Dermatol Surg.* 2004;30:382–384.
23. Karam P, Benedetto AV. Syringomas: new approach to an old technique. *Int J Dermatol.* 1996;35:219–220.
24. Goldman MP, Bennett RG. Treatment of telangiectasia: a review. *J Am Acad Dermatol.* 1987;17:167–182.
25. Mamelak AJ, Goldberg LH, Katz TM, *et al.* Desmoplastic trichoepithelioma. *J Am Acad Dermatol.* 2010;62:102–106.
26. Urquhart JL, Weston WL. Treatment of multiple trichoepitheliomas with topical imiquimod and tretinoin. *Pediatr Dermatol.* 2005;22:67–70.
27. Gibbs S, Harvey I, Sterling JC, Stark R. Local treatments for cutaneous warts. *Cochrane Database Syst Rev.* 2003;CD001781.
28. Phillips RC, Ruhl TS, Pfenninger JL, Garber MR. Treatment of warts with Candida antigen injection. *Arch Dermatol.* 2000;136:1274–1275.
29. Karsai S, Czarnecka A, Raulin C. Treatment of xanthelasma palpebrarum using a pulsed dye laser: a prospective clinical trial in 38 cases. *Dermatol Surg.* 2010;36:610–617.

34 Diagnosis and Treatment of Malignant and Premalignant Lesions

DANIEL L. STULBERG, MD • RICHARD P. USATINE, MD

Skin cancer is the most common cancer in the United States; fortunately, however, it is not one of the most common causes of death. Skin cancers are usually divided into melanoma and nonmelanoma skin cancers. An approximate breakdown of the most common skin cancers in the United States indicates that 80% are basal cell carcinomas (BCC), 16% squamous cell carcinomas (SCC), and 4% melanomas. Some of the rare skin cancers include Merkel cell carcinoma, dermatofibrosarcoma protuberans, and cutaneous T-cell lymphoma. These account for less than 1% of skin cancers.

Nonmelanoma skin cancer typically refers to BCC and SCC. Cutaneous metastases (of nonskin cancers), human papilloma virus–related cancers, tumors arising from dermal fibroblasts, neuroendocrine cells, and cutaneous lymphomas also occur. Both BCC and SCC have an increased incidence in people with fair skin, with increased sun exposure, and with aging. Patients with xeroderma pigmentosum have a very high rate of skin cancers due to sun exposure and UVB damage because they are unable to correct errors in their sun-damaged skin, leading to multiple skin cancers. SCCs are also more frequent in skin that is exposed to carcinogens or affected by chronic wounds or burns. BCCs very rarely metastasize, but can cause severe complications and even death from local invasion if left untreated. SCCs can metastasize although this is not common in skin lesions that are not on mucosal surfaces.

For melanoma, risk factors include family history, large congenital nevi, the familial atypical mole and melanoma syndrome (FAMMS; previously dysplastic nevus syndrome) (Figure 34-1) and sun exposure, particularly blistering burns in fair-skinned individuals. After initial biopsy, Breslow's classification by depth of invasion is used to guide re-excision margins and the need for sentinel lymph node biopsy and to predict general survival rates.

In dealing with suspected skin cancer, the usual first step is to biopsy the lesion to confirm the diagnosis. For suspected melanoma, it is preferable to remove the lesion in its entirety with the initial biopsy if possible unless precluded by the size or location of the lesion. A deep shave (scoop shave) to diagnose melanoma can be done if the biopsy is deep enough to get under the entire lesion. Two or more 4- to 6-mm punch biopsies can often determine the diagnosis if the lesion is large and the clinician is not skilled at doing a deep shave. The risk of sampling error is greater with punch biopsies so a negative result may be a false negative. In SCCs and BCCs a shave biopsy is usually the easiest and least invasive way to get tissue to confirm the diagnosis. Having a histologic diagnosis can prevent a large unnecessary excision if the pathology turns out to be benign and can help guide the treatment of choice if malignancy is confirmed.

ACTINIC KERATOSES, ACTINIC CHEILITIS, AND BOWEN'S DISEASE

Actinic keratoses (AK), actinic cheilitis, and Bowen's disease (SCC *in situ*) are all caused by cumulative sun exposure and have the potential to become invasive squamous cell carcinomas. The rate of malignant transformation has been variably estimated but is probably no greater than 6% per AK over a 10-year period.[1] On a spectrum of malignant transformation, Bowen's disease is squamous cell carcinoma *in situ* before the squamous cell carcinoma becomes invasive. In one large prospective trial, the risk of progression of AK to primary SCC (invasive or *in situ*) was 0.6% at 1 year and 2.6% at 4 years. Approximately 65% of all primary SCCs and 36% of all primary BCCs diagnosed in the study group arose in lesions that had been previously diagnosed clinically as AKs.[2]

Actinic keratoses are rough scaly spots seen on sun-exposed areas that may be found by touch, as well as close visual inspection. Bowen's disease appears similar to actinic keratosis, but tends to be larger in size and thicker with a well-demarcated border (Figure 34-2). Actinic cheilitis is equivalent to AK but found on the lips (Figure 34-3).

Typical distribution of AKs and SCC *in situ* are the areas with greatest sun exposure such as the face, forearms, dorsum of hands, upper chest, lower legs of women, and the balding scalp and tops of the ears in men. Actinic keratoses that appear premalignant may be diagnosed by history and physical exam only and treated with destructive methods without biopsy. Bowen's disease requires a biopsy for diagnosis. Bowen's disease or squamous cell carcinoma should be biopsied prior to treatment. A shave biopsy should usually produce enough tissue for histopathology.

Treatment of Actinic Keratoses and Actinic Cheilitis

Cryotherapy

- Light freeze, 1-mm freeze margin.
- Treating AKs with liquid nitrogen using a 1-mm halo freeze demonstrated complete response of 39% for freeze times of less than 5 seconds, 69% for freeze times greater than 5 seconds, and 83% for freeze times greater than 20 seconds.[3]

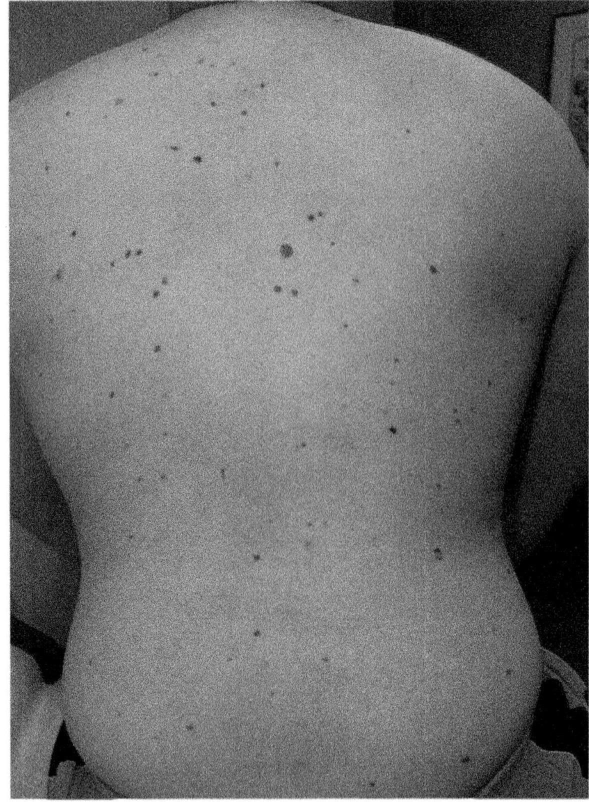

FIGURE 34-1 Young man with familial atypical mole and melanoma syndrome (FAMMS; previously called dysplastic nevus syndrome). *(Copyright Daniel L. Stulberg, MD.)*

- Considerably more hypopigmentation is caused by 20 seconds of freeze time, so base the freeze time on the size, location, and thickness of the AK.
- Excellent for a small number of lesions.
- Adjunct before and after topical therapies.

Electrodesiccation and Curettage (Single Cycle for AK)

- Use local anesthetic.
- Useful for thicker lesions (see pages 177–178).
- Adjunct after topical therapies.

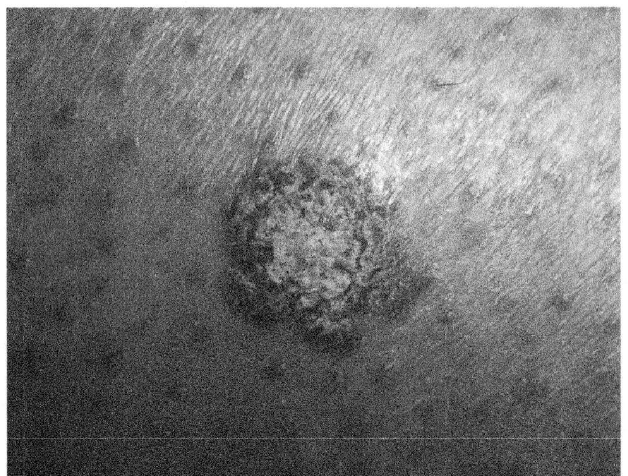

FIGURE 34-2 Bowen's disease (SCC *in situ*) on the leg. *(Copyright Richard P. Usatine, MD.)*

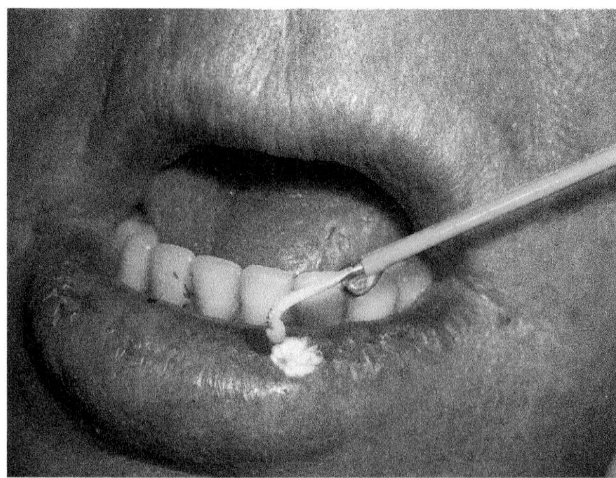

FIGURE 34-3 Actinic cheilitis undergoing cryosurgery. *(Copyright Richard P. Usatine, MD.)*

Photodynamic Therapy

- Requires special equipment (see Chapter 27, *Photorejuvenation with Lasers*).

Topical Medications

Topical medications are useful for a large area or large number of lesions in a region.

Fluorouracil

- 5% cream (Efudex), 1% cream (Fluoroplex), 0.5% microspore cream (Carac).
- Apply twice daily for 2 to 4 weeks. Usually need 4 weeks for the arms and the back of the hands. Patients should stop if the skin becomes ulcerated or infected.
- Causes marked inflammation (Figure 34-4).
- 0.5% microspore cream (Carac) may cause less inflammation.
- Treat remaining lesions with cryotherapy or curettage and electrodesiccation.

Imiquimod 5% (Aldara)

- Apply QHS 3 to 4 times per week up to 16 weeks.
- Long treatment period.
- Not as effective as fluorouracil.

Diclofenac Gel 3% (Solaraze)

- Apply twice daily for 90 days.
- Long treatment period.
- Not as effective as fluorouracil.

Treatment of Bowen's Disease

The following is based on the guidelines from Cox et al.[4]:

- The risk of progression to invasive cancer is about 3%. This risk is greater in genital Bowen's disease (BD), and particularly in perianal BD. A high risk of recurrence, including late recurrence, is a particular feature of perianal BD, and prolonged follow-up is recommended for this variant.

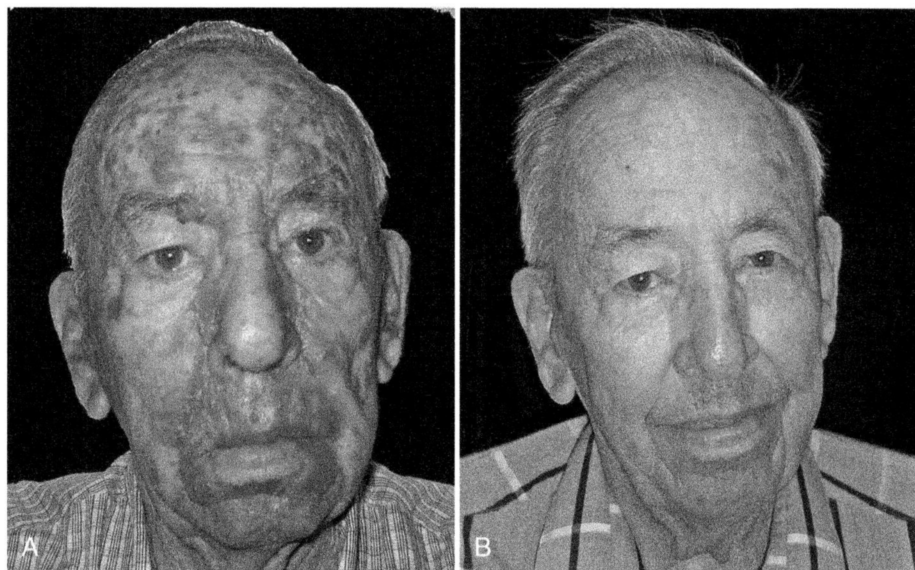

FIGURE 34-4 (A) Erythema and scaling secondary to 5-FU use to treat multiple actinic keratoses on the face. (B) The skin is much improved after the erythema resolves. *(Copyright Richard P. Usatine, MD.)*

- There is reasonable evidence to support use of 5-fluorouracil (5-FU).[4] It is more practical than surgery for large lesions, especially at potentially poor healing sites, and has been used for "control" rather than cure in some patients with multiple lesions.
- Topical imiquimod is likely to be used for BD especially for larger lesions or difficult/poor healing sites. However, it is costly and the optimum regimen has yet to be determined.[5]
- One prospective study suggests that a curettage and electrodesiccation treatment is superior to cryotherapy in treating BD, especially for lesions on the lower leg.[6] Curettage was associated with a significantly shorter healing time, less pain, fewer complications, and a lower recurrence rate when compared with cryotherapy.[6]
- Cryotherapy has good evidence of efficacy but discomfort and time to healing are inferior to photodynamic therapy (PDT) or curettage. With discretion, SCC *in situ* can be treated by cryotherapy with liquid nitrogen spray by a 30-second freeze, thaw and refreeze 30 seconds (see Chapter 15, *Cryosurgery*).
- Photodynamic therapy has been shown to be equivalent to cryotherapy and 5-FU, either in efficacy and/or in healing.[4] PDT may be of particular benefit for lesions that are large, on the lower leg, or at otherwise difficult sites, but it is costly.
- Excision should be an effective treatment with low recurrence rates, but the evidence base is limited and for the most part does not allow comment on specific sites of lesions. Lower leg excision may be limited by lack of skin mobility. Although elliptical excision with clear margins is an effective and acceptable treatment for Bowen's disease, it is too aggressive for actinic keratoses.
- Mohs surgery is recommended for BD at sites such as the digits or penis where it is important to limit removal of unaffected skin (Figure 34-5). It is useful for poorly defined or recurrent head and neck BD.
- See Table 34-1 for a summary of all recommended treatments for Bowen's disease based on location and other characteristics.

Special Considerations/Billing

- AK and actinic cheilitis treatment are coded as premalignant.
- 17000 for first lesion treated.
- 17003 repeated for each lesion 2–14.
- 17004 stand-alone code if more than 15 lesions treated.
- Treatment of Bowen's disease is coded the same as SCC (see below).

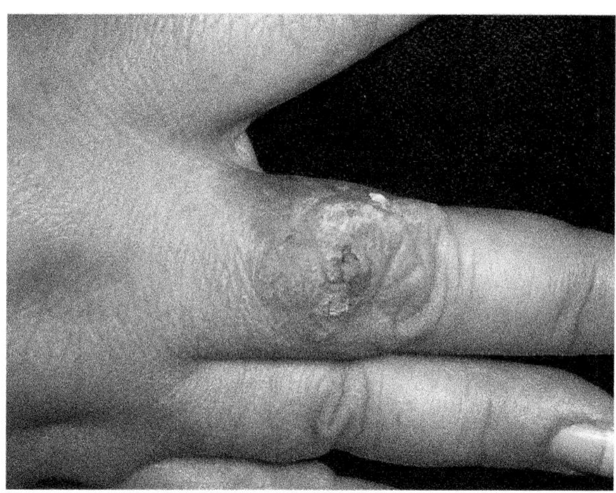

FIGURE 34-5 Bowen's disease on the finger secondary to human papilloma virus. Evidence for HPV was seen in the biopsy specimen performed with a shave. *(Copyright Richard P. Usatine, MD.)*

TABLE 34-1 Summary of the Main Treatment Options for Bowen's Disease[4]

Lesion Characteristics	Topical 5-FU	Topical Imiquimod[a]	Cryotherapy	Curettage	Excision	PDT	Radiotherapy	Laser[b]
Small, single/few, good healing site[c]	4	3	2	1	3	3	5	4
Large, single, good healing site[c]	3	3	3	5	5	2	4	7
Multiple, good healing site[c]	3	4	2	3	5	3	4	4
Small, single/few, poor healing site[c]	2	3	3	2	2	1–2	5	7
Large, single, poor healing site[c]	3	2–3	5	4	5	1	6	7
Facial	4	7	2	2	4[d]	3	4	7
Digital	3	7	3	5	2[d]	3	3	3
Perianal	6	6	6	6	1[e]	7	2–3	6
Penile	3	3	3	5	4[d]	3	2–3	3

Note: The suggested scoring of the treatments listed takes into account the evidence for benefit, ease of application or time required for the procedure, wound healing, cosmetic result and current availability/costs of the method or facilities required. Evidence for interventions based on single studies or purely anecdotal cases is not included.
5-FU, 5-fluorouracil; PDT, photodynamic therapy.
Scale: 1, probably treatment of choice; 2, generally good choice; 3, generally fair choice; 4, reasonable but not usually required; 5, generally poor choice; 6, probably should not be used; 7, insufficient evidence available.
[a]Does not have a product license for Bowen's disease.
[b]Depends on site.
[c]Refers to the clinician's perceived potential for good or poor healing at the affected site.
[d]Consider Mohs micrographic surgery for tissue sparing or if poorly defined/recurrent.
[e]Wide excision recommended.

BASAL CELL CARCINOMA

Diagnoses

- Frequent on the face, hands, upper chest, and sun-exposed skin.
- Nodular is the most common form (Figure 34-6):
  - Raised, waxy, translucent, or pearly border.
  - Central erosion, telangiectasias, and bleeding are common.
  - Usually flesh colored or pale, but may be pigmented, confusing it with melanoma.
- Superficial BCC (Figure 34-7)
  - Flat or slightly raised, often red to brown.
  - Look for a thready border that may be pearly.
  - More often on the trunk and arms than face.

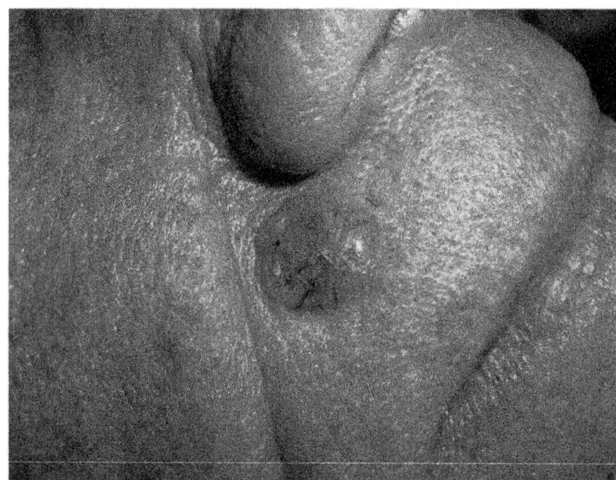

FIGURE 34-6 Typical nodular BCC on the face of a 53-year-old man. Note the pearly borders and telangiectasias. *(Copyright Richard P. Usatine, MD.)*

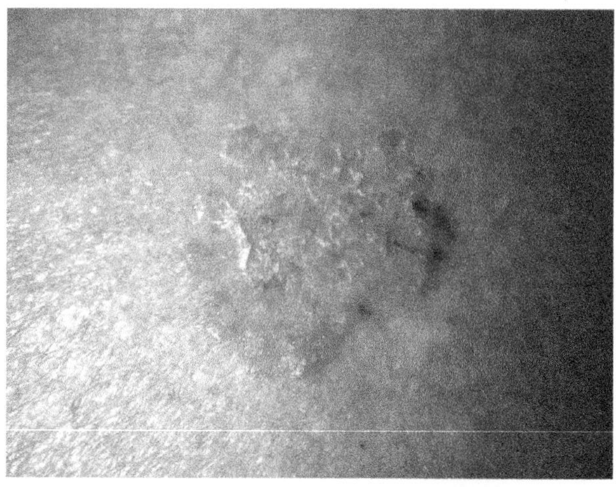

FIGURE 34-7 Superficial BCC on the back with erythema, scale, and a thready border. *(Copyright Richard P. Usatine, MD.)*

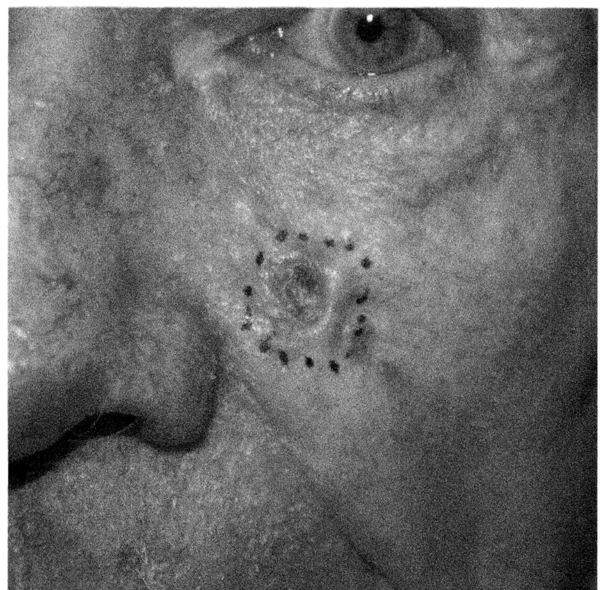

FIGURE 34-8 Sclerosing BCC that turned out to be widely invasive when removed with Mohs surgery. *(Courtesy of Ryan O'Quinn, MD.)*

- Morpheaform (also called *sclerosing*) (Figure 34-8)
  - Usually has nondiscrete margins.
  - More aggressively infiltrating.
  - Higher recurrence rate.
- Shave biopsy can confirm diagnosis.

Removal

(See Table 34-2 for cure rates of BCC treatment modalities.)

Elliptical Excision (Fusiform) (Figure 34-9)

- Remove with 3-mm surgical margin if discrete border and clinically feasible, 4 to 5 mm if indiscrete border.[7]
- Consider using a skin curette to define the margins of the BCC and redraw the ellipse as needed (Figure 34-10).
- Heals with linear scars, which can be hidden in skin lines.
- Provides immediate closure.
- Provides tissue for pathology and assurance of removal.

TABLE 34-2 Cure Rates for Different Skin Cancer Treatment Modalities

	Five-Year Cure Rate (%)	
	BCC	SCC
Surgical excision	89.9	91.9
Cryotherapy	92.5	NA
Electrodesiccation and curettage	92.3	96.3
Radiotherapy	91.3	90.0
Mohs surgery	99.0	96.9

NA, not applicable.
Source: Data from Rowe DE, Carroll RJ, Day CL. *J Dermatol Surg Oncol.* 1989;15:315–328, and *J Am Acad Dermatol.* 1992;26:976–990; and Vidimos A, Ammirati C, Poblete-Lopez C. *Dermatologic Surgery.* London: Saunders; 2008, Table 16-1.

- If you find evidence of the BCC at the base or edges (Figure 34-11) of the removed specimen, take another piece of skin or fascia at a deeper and/or wider level and put it in a second formalin container with a stitch used to mark its orientation in the body.

Electrodesiccation and Curettage

- BCC tissue is softer than the surrounding normal tissue so a skin curette can remove the BCC without taking too much normal tissue around it (Figure 34-12).
- Firmly curette in all directions then electrodesiccate and repeat to a total of three cycles at one visit (see Chapter 14, *Electrosurgery*, pages 177–178).
- Useful for smaller lesions or where closure of a full-thickness excision would be difficult.

Mohs Micrographic Surgery (Figure 34-13)

- The most effective in achieving cure with clean margins—99%.
- Specialized skin surgeon examines pathology at time of excision.
- Further resection as needed at time of surgery.
- Can minimize impact on adjacent structures.
- Useful for uncertain borders or aggressive forms of BCC (i.e., sclerosing or morpheaform).[7]

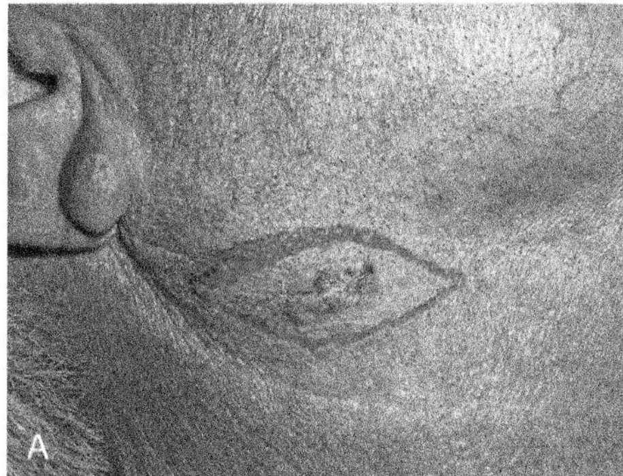

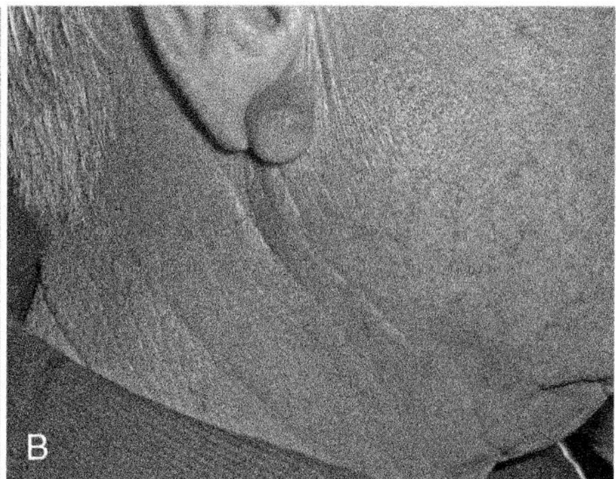

FIGURE 34-9 **(A)** Ellipse marked around a nodular BCC on the neck with a 3:1 length:height ratio. **(B)** After 1 month the scar is becoming invisible as it matches the natural skin lines of the neck. *(Copyright Richard P. Usatine, MD.)*

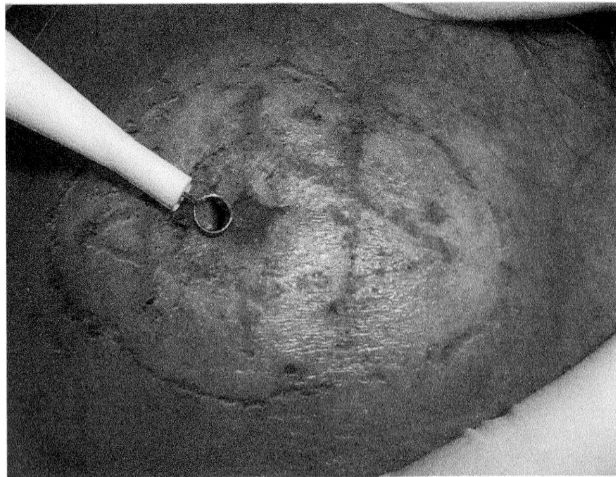

FIGURE 34-10 After marking the margins and anesthetizing the area, a curette is being used to determine the full margins of the BCC more accurately. An adjusted ellipse can then be drawn to avoid incomplete excision. *(Copyright Richard P. Usatine, MD.)*

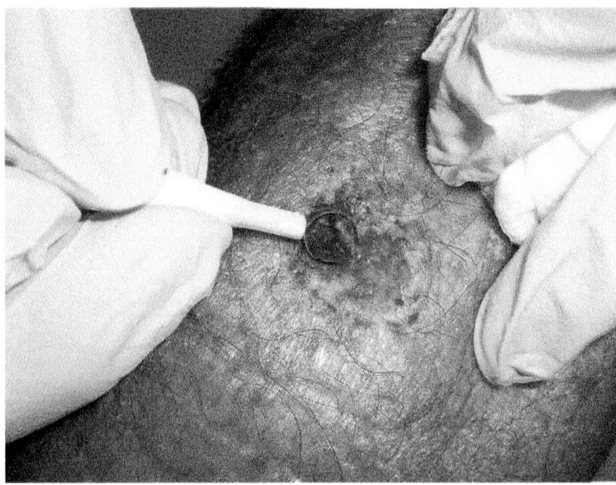

FIGURE 34-12 A curette is scooping out the abnormally soft cancer tissue from this basal cell carcinoma on the arm as the first step of an electrodesiccation and curettage. *(Copyright Richard P. Usatine, MD.)*

- Consider for H-zone on face (See Figure 37-12 on page 461), especially for recurrent BCC.[8]
- Consider referral for Mohs micrographic surgery if lesions affect sensitive structures including the eyelids, ala of the nose, and the ear canal.
- Consider referral for Mohs if aggressive lesion or if recurrent lesion.
- Basosquamous carcinoma is an aggressive subtype of basal cell cancer that has metastatic potential and high recurrence rates that should be managed by Mohs surgery.

Topical Immunotherapy

- Imiquimod (Aldara) locally boosts immune response.
- FDA approved for superficial BCC (not for other subtypes) lesions up to 2 cm in diameter. Not approved for use on the face, hands, or feet. (Note that many BCCs are on the face and hands.)

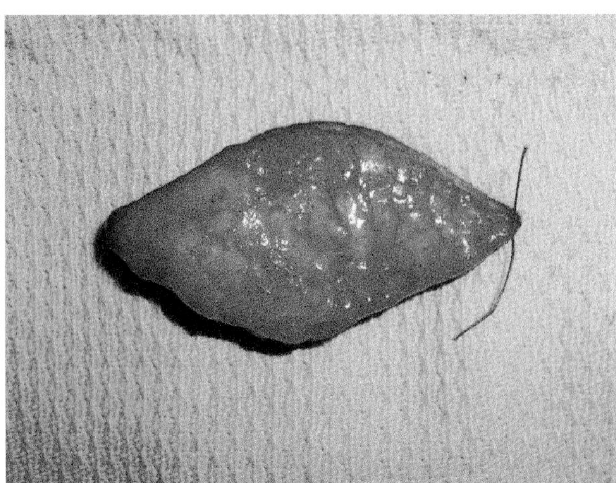

FIGURE 34-11 Basal cell carcinoma palpable and barely visible (whiter than the yellow fat) at the base of this elliptical excision. A second layer should be removed more deeply before closing up the surgical defect. *(Copyright Richard P. Usatine, MD.)*

Cryotherapy

- With discretion, superficial BCC can be treated by cryotherapy with liquid nitrogen spray by a 30- to 45-second freeze (thaw and refreeze 30 to 45 seconds) (Figure 34-14) (see Chapter 15).

Radiation Therapy

- Usually reserved for those not able to tolerate other treatments.

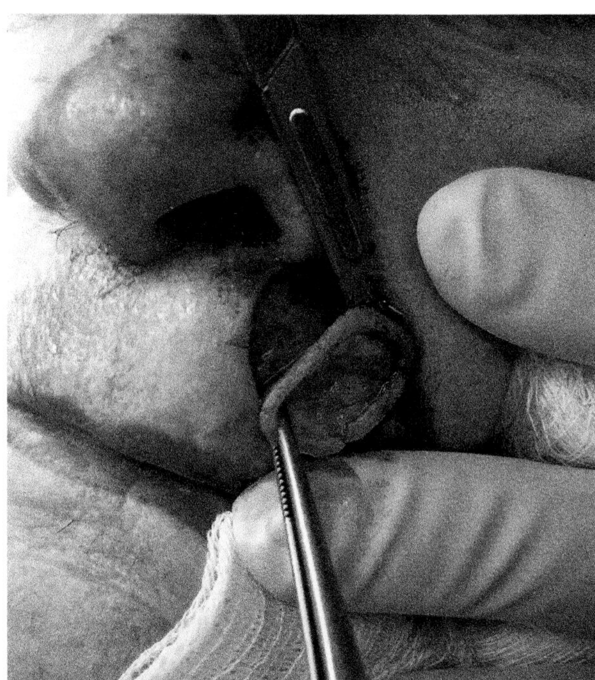

FIGURE 34-13 Mohs surgery being performed of a basal cell carcinoma of the upper lip region. First the tumor was debulked and now a thin sliver of tissue is being removed 360 degrees around the original tumor to look for adequate margin control. *(Courtesy of Ryan O'Quinn, MD.)*

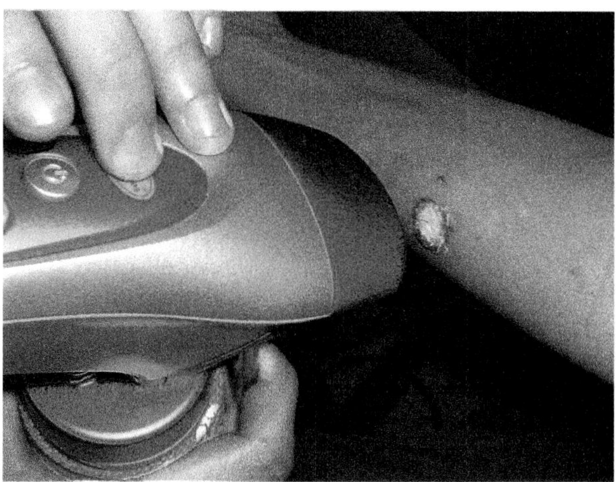

FIGURE 34-14 Cryosurgery being performed on a superficial BCC of the arm. A 5-mm margin of freeze is the goal with two freezes each of 30 seconds duration. *(Copyright Richard P. Usatine, MD.)*

Photodynamic Therapy (PDT)

- PDT has a number of limitations in the treatment of BCC.[9]

Special Considerations/Billing

- High risk of additional and future BCC and SCC, so frequent reexamination for additional lesions is required at least annually.[10]
- CPT codes for destruction or excision of malignancy should be used.

SQUAMOUS CELL CARCINOMA

Diagnoses

- Erythematous plaque with scale and/or ulceration, frequently found on the face, ears, and lower lip (Figure 34-15). May occur in any sun-exposed area or on mucous membranes of the mouth and anus.

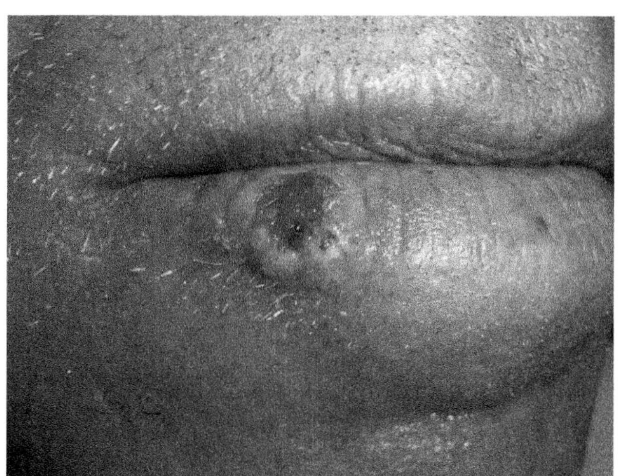

FIGURE 34-15 Squamous cell carcinoma of the lower lip related to sun exposure. *(Copyright Richard P. Usatine, MD.)*

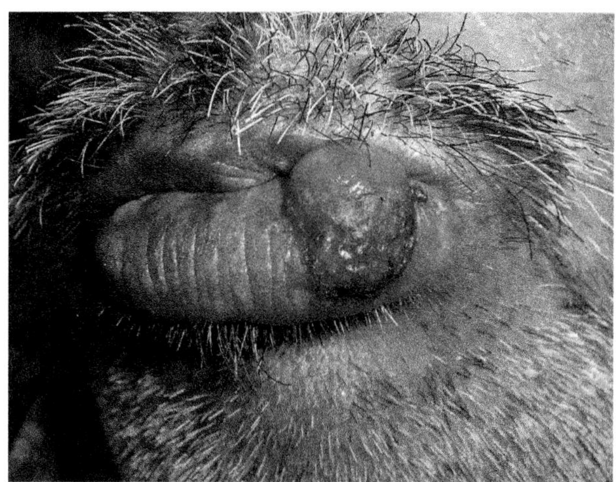

FIGURE 34-16 Large quickly growing SCC on the lip of a patient on immunosuppression after a renal transplant. *(Copyright Richard P. Usatine, MD.)*

- Transplant patients on chronic immunosuppression are at high risk to develop SCC (Figure 34-16).
- May be at the base of actinic horns or thick actinic keratoses.
- May occur in areas of chronic irritation or burns.
- A shave or punch biopsy is useful for diagnosis.

Treatment

See video on the DVD for further learning. 

(See Table 34-2 for cure rates of SCC treatment modalities.)

- Electrodesiccation and curettage (for three cycles just as in BCC) may be used for Bowen's disease and for early small SCC (see Chapter 14).
- 5-FU combined with epinephrine injected weekly has shown success in small trials.[5] This is not a mainstay of therapy.
- Removal margins for elliptical excision:
  - 4 mm if clinically feasible with SCC less than 2 cm in diameter.[11]
  - 6 mm if high-grade lesions or with SCC greater than 2 cm in diameter.[11]
- SCC can metastasize and the mainstay of treatment is surgical with assessment of the margins by conventional or Mohs micrographic surgery.
- On the trunk or extremities, SCC can be excised with an elliptical excision.

Special Considerations/Billing

- Consider referral for Mohs micrographic surgery if lesions affect sensitive structures including the eyelids, ala of the nose, and the ear canal.[11]
- Consider referral for Mohs if aggressive lesion or if recurrent lesion.
- High risk of additional and future BCC and SCC so frequent reexamination for additional lesions is required at least annually.[10]
- See Table 38-3 for ICD-9 coding and CPT coding that is specific to the procedure used to treat the malignancy.

KERATOACANTHOMA

Most pathologists and skin experts consider KA to be one type of SCC. The controversy revolves around the fact that it was considered a precancer for years, in part, because some KAs will spontaneously resolve.

Diagnosis

- Rapidly enlarging, often erythematous dome-shaped lesion (Figure 34-17).
- A central keratin plug is the classic distinguishing feature.
- Frequently on the hands or face.
- Considered a type of squamous cell cancer.
- Use a shave biopsy for pathology.
- An unknown percentage may spontaneously regress over 2 to 12 months, but it is safer to remove it than wait.

Removal

- Electrodesiccation and curettage (see pages 177–178).
- Excision by ellipse with 3 to 5 mm margins.
- Inject 5-FU, methotrexate, or interferon.
- Radiation therapy if unable to treat by measures above.

Billing

- Bill using CPT codes for destruction or excision of malignant lesions.

MELANOMA

Diagnosis

- Use the **ABCDE** guidelines for diagnosing melanoma (Figure 34-18).

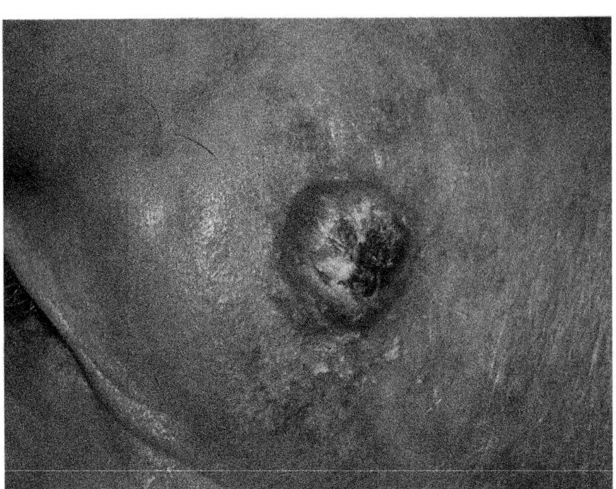

FIGURE 34-17 Keratoacanthoma-type SCC growing rapidly over the temple region of the face. The central keratin core is a distinct feature of a keratoacanthoma. *(Copyright Richard P. Usatine, MD.)*

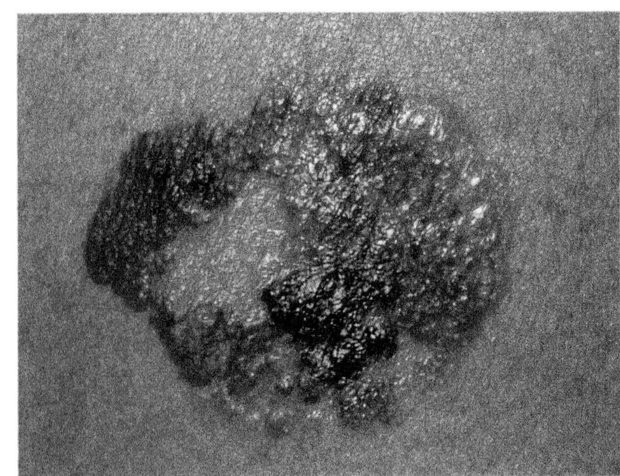

FIGURE 34-18 Superficial spreading melanoma with all features of ABCDE. *(Courtesy of Skin Cancer Foundation, New York, NY.)*

  - **A = Asymmetry.** Most melanomas are asymmetrical: a line through the middle will not create matching halves.
  - **B = Border.** The borders of melanomas are often uneven and may have scalloped or notched edges.
  - **C** = variation in **Color.** Melanomas are often varied shades of brown, tan, or black. As melanomas progress, they may appear red, white, and blue.
  - **D = Diameter** greater than or equal to 6 mm. Melanomas tend to grow larger than most nevi. (*Note:* Congenital nevi are often large.)
  - **E = Evolving or Elevated.** Any enlarging nevus is suspect for melanoma even though benign nevi may also grow. Melanoma is often elevated, at least in part, so that it is palpable.
- A prospective controlled study compared 460 cases of melanoma with 680 cases of benign pigmented tumors and found significant differences for all individual ABCDE criteria ($p < 0.001$) between melanomas and benign nevi.[12]
- Sensitivity of each criteria (percentage of melanomas that were positive for each one of the ABCDE criteria): A, 57%; B, 57%; C, 65%; D, 90%; E, 84%.[12]
- Specificity of each criteria (percentage of benign nevi that were negative for each one of the ABCDE): A, 72%; B, 71%; C, 59%; D, 63%; E, 90%.[12]
- Sensitivity of ABCDE criteria varies depending on the number of criteria needed: Using two criteria, the sensitivity was 89.3; with three criteria, 65.5% (i.e., 34.5% did not have at least three criteria positive so melanomas should not be expected to meet all criteria).
- Specificity was 65.3% using two criteria and 81% using three.[12]
- The number of criteria present was different between benign nevi (1.24 ± 1.26) and melanomas (3.53 ± 1.53; $p < 0.001$). No significant difference was found between melanomas and atypical nevi.[12]

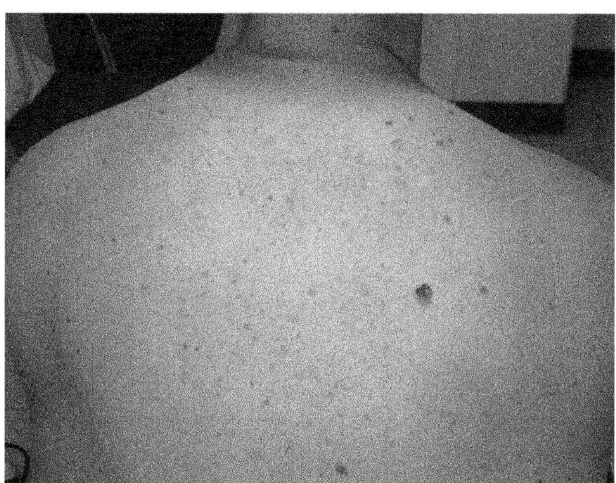

FIGURE 34-19 The "ugly duckling" sign with one pigmented lesion standing out on the upper right side of the back. This was indeed a malignant melanoma caught early by careful observation. *(Copyright Richard P. Usatine, MD.)*

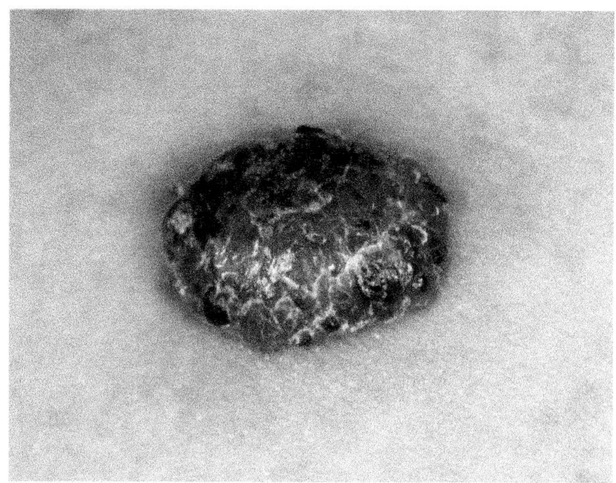

FIGURE 34-21 Nodular melanoma on the shoulder of a young woman. After being missed by a previous doctor, the nodular melanoma was excised with an elliptical excision and found to be 8.5 mm in depth. *(Copyright Richard P. Usatine, MD.)*

Clinical Appearance

- The "ugly duckling" rule: If a mole looks different than the patient's other moles, there is a higher likelihood that it is malignant (Figure 34-19).
- May be friable, ulcerating, nonhealing, or bleeding.

The four major categories of melanomas are as follows:

1. *Superficial spreading melanoma* is the most common type of melanoma, accounting for about 70% of melanomas in the United States.[13] This melanoma has a radial growth pattern before dermal invasion occurs (Figure 34-20). The first sign is the appearance of a flat macule or slightly raised discolored plaque that has irregular borders and is somewhat geometrical in form. The color varies with areas of tan, brown, black, red, blue, or white. These lesions can arise in an older nevus. The melanoma can be seen almost anywhere on the body, but is most likely to occur on the trunk in men, the legs in women, and the upper back in both. Most melanomas found in the young are of the superficial spreading type.

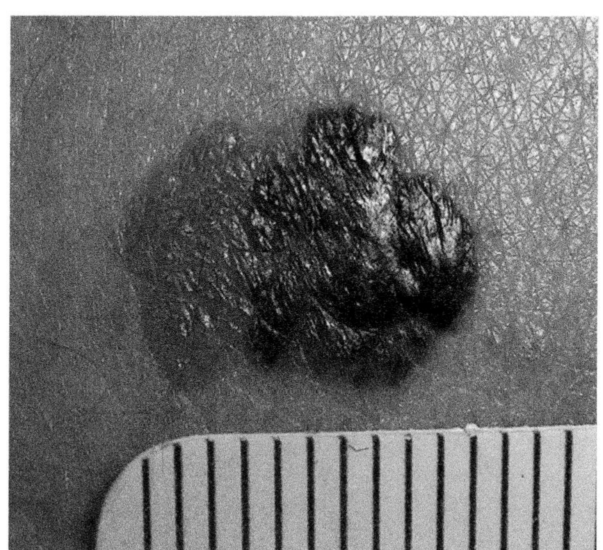

FIGURE 34-20 Superficial spreading melanoma in its radial growth phase on the back of the patient above (0.35 mm in depth). *(Copyright Richard P. Usatine, MD.)*

2. *Nodular melanoma* occurs in 15% of melanoma cases.[13,14] The color is most often black, but occasionally is blue, gray, white, brown, tan, red, or nonpigmented (Figure 34-21). It is often ulcerated and bleeding at the time of diagnosis. The nodule in Figure 34-21 is multicolored. Although it is often evolving and elevated, it may lack the ABCD criteria.
3. *Lentigo maligna melanoma* (LMM) is found most often in the elderly and arises on the chronically sun-damaged skin of the face. The term *lentigo maligna* is used for the melanoma precursor in the setting of atypical melanocytic hyperplasia alone and the term *melanoma in situ, LM type,* is used to represent the true *in situ* melanoma. LM is the precursor to LMM and not a nevus (Figure 34-22). Globally, LM/LMM is estimated to account for 4% to 15% of all melanomas, and 10% to 26% of all head and neck melanomas.[15]

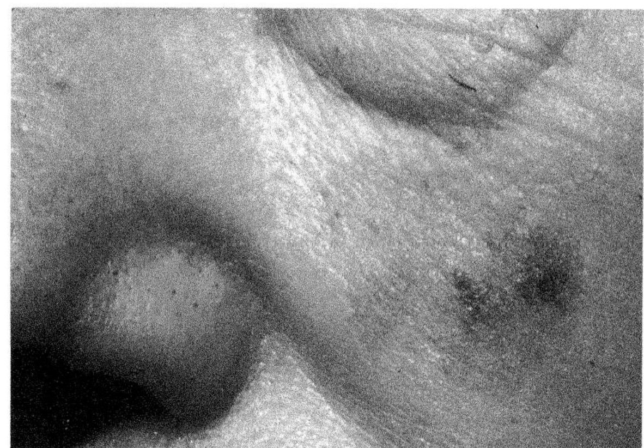

FIGURE 34-22 Lentigo maligna melanoma on the face. *(Courtesy of Skin Cancer Foundation, New York, NY.)*

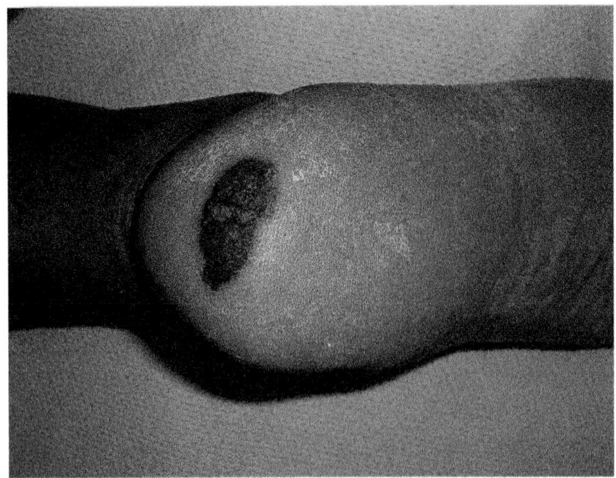

FIGURE 34-23 Acral lentiginous melanoma on the heel of a young woman. *(Copyright Richard P. Usatine, MD.)*

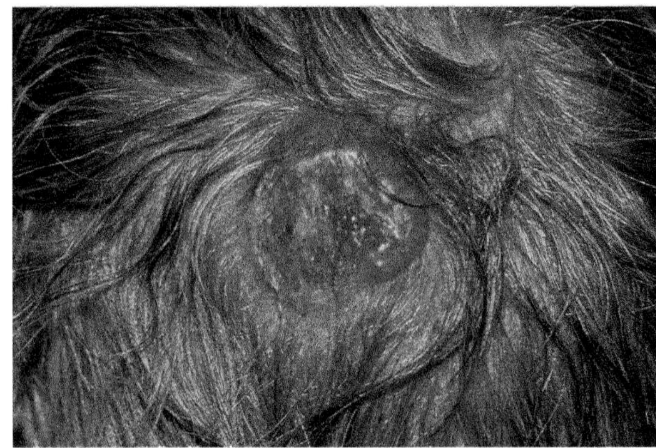

FIGURE 34-25 Amelanotic melanoma arising on the scalp. *(Courtesy of the University of Texas Health Science Center San Antonio, Division of Dermatology, San Antonio, TX.)*

4. *Acral lentiginous melanoma* is the least common subtype of melanoma and accounts for 2% to 3% of melanomas.[13] It occurs under the nail plate or on the soles or palms (Figure 34-23). Acral lentiginous melanoma has 5- and 10-year melanoma-specific survival rates of 80.3% and 67.5%, respectively, which is less than those for all cutaneous malignant melanomas overall (91.3% and 87.5%, respectively; $p < 0.001$).[13] Subungual melanoma may manifest as diffuse nail discoloration or a longitudinal pigmented band within the nail plate. When subungual pigment spreads to the proximal or lateral nail fold, it is referred to as Hutchinson's sign and is highly suggestive of acral lentiginous melanoma (Figure 34-24).

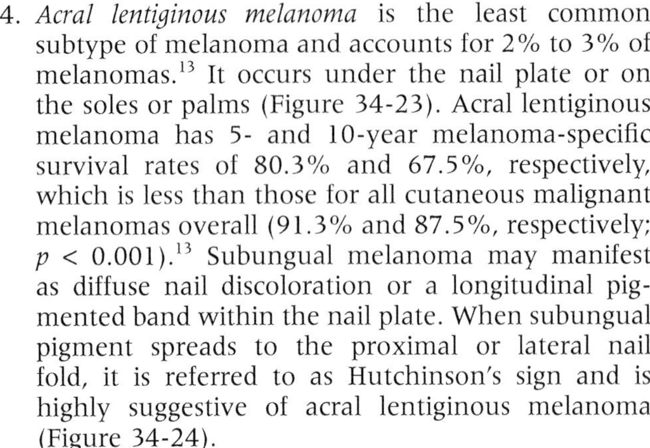

Less common types of melanomas include the following:

- *Amelanotic melanoma* (<5% of melanomas) is nonpigmented and appears pink or flesh colored, often mimicking BCC or SCC or a ruptured hair follicle. It may be a nodular melanoma subtype or melanoma metastasis to the skin, because of the inability of these poorly differentiated cancer cells to synthesize melanin pigment (Figure 34-25).
- Other rare melanoma variants include (1) desmoplastic/neurotropic melanoma, (2) mucosal (lentiginous) melanoma, (3) malignant blue nevus, and (4) melanoma arising in a giant congenital nevus.

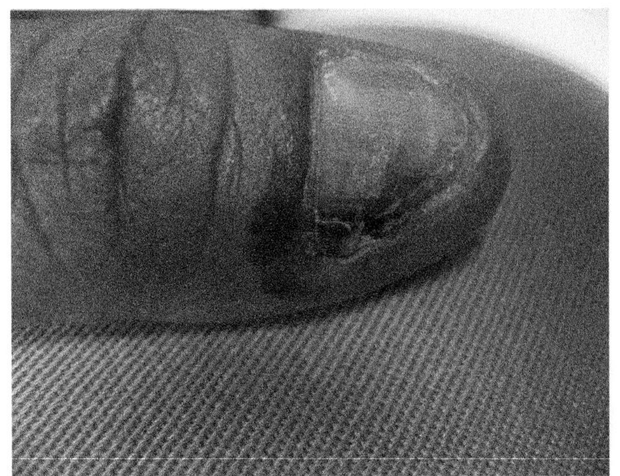

FIGURE 34-24 Subungual melanoma that has spread to the proximal nail fold producing a positive Hutchinson sign. *(Courtesy of Ryan O'Quinn, MD.)*

Diagnosis starts with history (change) and physical exam (ABCDE).

- Use dermoscopy if available (see Chapter 32, *Dermoscopy*).
- Biopsy per recommendations in Chapter 8, *Choosing the Biopsy Type*.
- It is better to give the pathologist the whole lesion or a large representative portion of the lesion rather than a few small punch biopsies.
- A broad deep shave is often better than a single punch biopsy unless the punch biopsy will remove the whole lesion.

Treatment

Definitive treatment is based on Breslow depth.

- Surgical excision is based on the recommendations given in Table 34-3.
- If depth greater than 1.0 cm, refer to surgical oncologist for excision and simultaneous sentinel node biopsy.
- When dealing with facial, acral, or anogenital melanomas, Mohs surgery may be preferable to allow reduced margins and conservation of tissue.[16,17]
- Staging of the melanoma is accomplished using the TNM system.

Oncology referral is based on staging (including if sentinel node positive or >4 mm in depth). Close clinical

TABLE 34-3 Recommended Excision Margins for Melanoma[a]

Tumor Thickness (Breslow)	Excision Margin (cm)	Sentinel Node Biopsy Suggested
In situ	0.5	No
<1.0 mm	1	No
1.0–2.0 mm	1	Yes
>2.0 mm	2	Yes

[a]These recommendations are based on both prospective, randomized studies and international consensus conferences.[16,17] Limited data suggest that margin has an effect on local or regional recurrence, but there are no data to support an impact of margin on survival.[16,17]

follow-up—at least annual complete skin examinations—is required.

CUTANEOUS T-CELL LYMPHOMAS (INCLUDING MYCOSIS FUNGOIDES)

Diagnosis

- Mycosis fungoides is the most frequent of the cutaneous T-cell lymphomas.
- Erythematous scaling plaques and patches are seen in early localized forms (Figure 34-26).
- Plaques and patches may be hyperpigmented or hypopigmented (Figure 34-27).
- Can progress to diffuse erythema (erythroderma) in later disseminated stage—Sézary syndrome.
- May present as refractory or recurrent eczema.
- Itching and photosensitivity are common.
- May develop into raised fungating lesions (see nasal lesion in Figure 34-27).

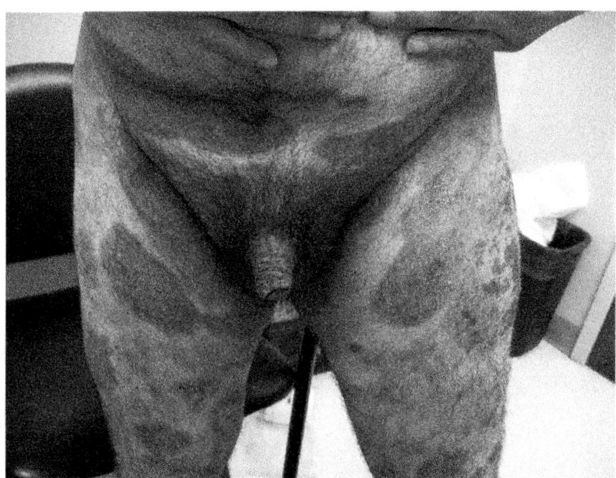

FIGURE 34-26 Plaque-type mycosis fungoides on the extremities and trunk. Biopsy a few years before this was read as atopic dermatitis only. Lack of response to medications and the suspicious appearance led to a new biopsy and the correct diagnosis. *(Courtesy of Deborah Henderson, MD.)*

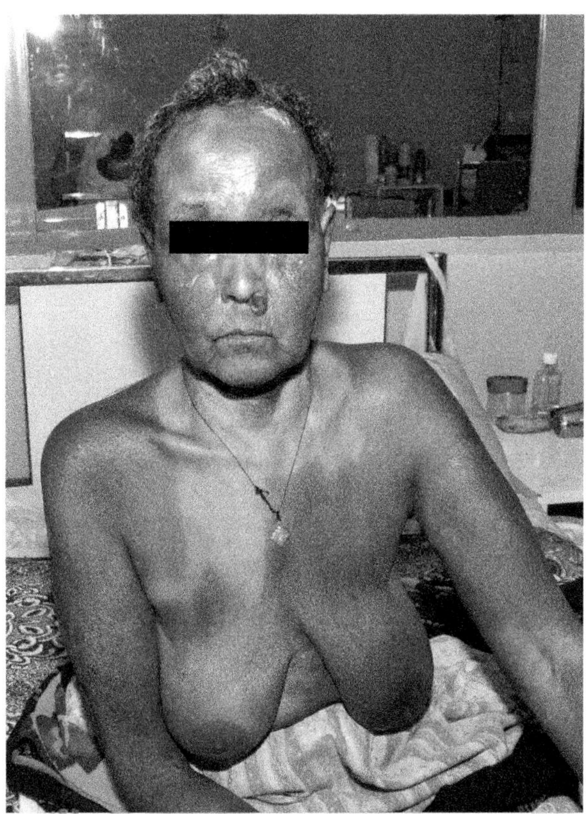

FIGURE 34-27 Cutaneous T-cell lymphoma causing large hyperpigmented patches and plaques on this Ethiopian woman. She also has a tumor under her left ala. *(Copyright Richard P. Usatine, MD.)*

Biopsy

- Perform a broad shave biopsy or a 4-mm punch biopsy of involved skin.
- Alert the pathologist that this is on your differential diagnosis so that special stains can be done.
- The first biopsy may not show the disease, so consider repeating the skin biopsies if the clinical suspicion remains high.
- Flow cytometry can be done on peripheral blood to look for abnormal lymphocytes.
- Palpate for lymph nodes and consider a lymph node biopsy if the skin biopsies and flow cytometry are not definitive.
- CT of the abdomen and pelvis can be used to look for enlarged lymph nodes and/or splenomegaly.
- Consult specialists if needed—this can be a hard diagnosis to make.

Treatment and Prognosis

- Early stages are treated locally with topical steroids, nitrogen mustards, psoralen and UVA, UVB, and others with excellent prognosis for remission and preventing progression of disease.
- More advanced disease carries a poor prognosis and is treated with a combination of topical medications as above, radiation therapy, and systemic immune system modulators and chemotherapy.

DERMATOFIBROSARCOMA PROTUBERANS

Diagnosis

- Flesh-colored gradually enlarging nodule from one to several or more centimeters in diameter. It may be shiny with a look of multiple deep nodules (Figure 34-28).
- It is of different origin than a dermatofibroma and is not a dermatofibroma becoming malignant.
- May be erythematous or occasionally pigmented.
- Site distribution is typically 45% head and neck and 55% trunk and extremities.[18]

Biopsy

- Use a 4-cm punch biopsy or larger incisional biopsy to provide adequate tissue for diagnosis.

Treatment and Prognosis

- The tumor can invade into adjacent deep structures, becoming locally invasive and highly recurrent.
- Mohs surgery is the preferred treatment to decrease the recurrence rate.
- Wide local excision with 2–4 cm margins is the alternative with lower cure rates.
- One study using pooled data from the literature reported a recurrence rate of 1.3% with Mohs surgery and 20.7% with wide local excision.[19]
- Frequent clinical follow-up is indicated for more than 5 years because 25% of recurrences occur after 5 years.[18]

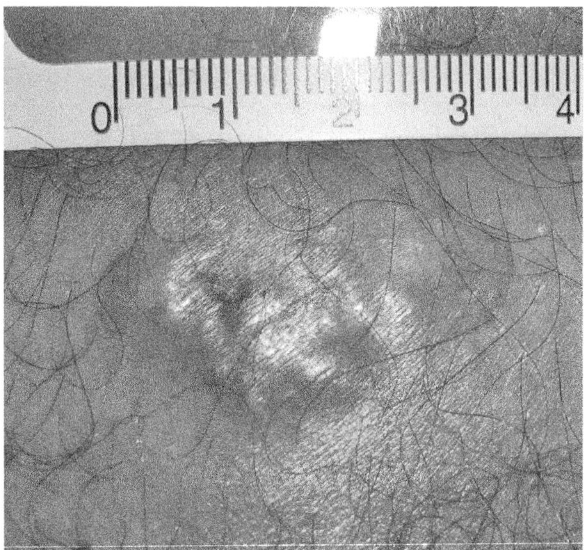

FIGURE 34-28 Dermatofibrosarcoma protuberans on the leg. *(Copyright Richard P. Usatine, MD.)*

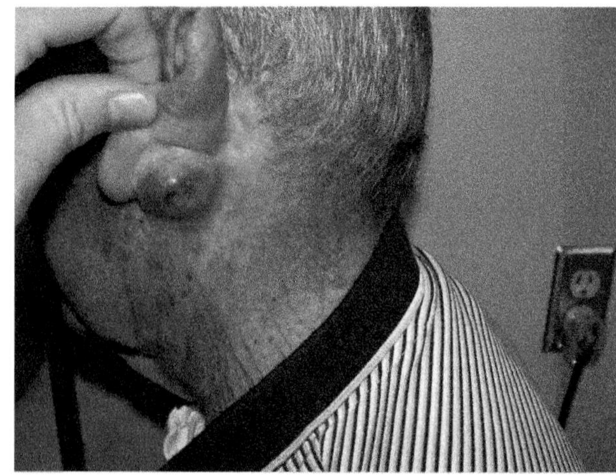

FIGURE 34-29 Merkel cell carcinoma on the ear. *(Courtesy of Frank Miller, MD.)*

MERKEL CELL CARCINOMA

Diagnoses

- Blue red nodular lesion most commonly of the head and neck (Figures 34-29 and 34-30).
- Mostly older patients and/or immunosuppressed persons.
- Rapidly growing.
- Usually in sun-exposed areas (Figure 34-30).
- Viral etiology with polyoma virus under investigation.[20]

Biopsy

- Perform a shave, 4-mm punch, or excisional biopsy.

Treatment and Prognosis

- High rate of nodal metastasis and distant metastasis even for small primary tumors.[21]
- Up to 30% have regional lymph node metastases.[20]

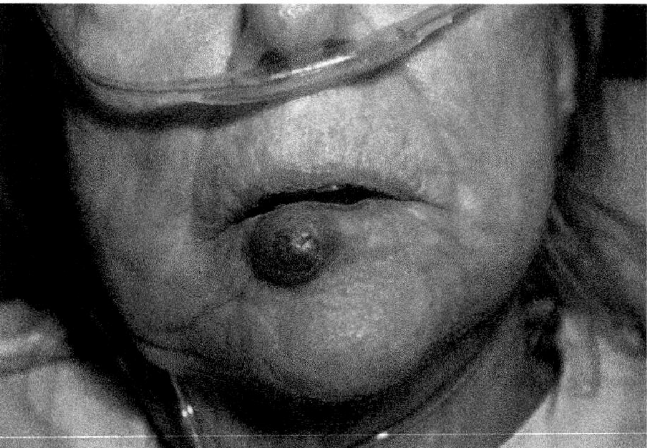

FIGURE 34-30 Merkel cell carcinoma on the lip. *(Courtesy of Jeff Meffert, MD.)*

- Chest x-ray to check for lung cancer as primary site with cutaneous metastasis.
- Wide local excision with 2- to 3-cm margins.
- Best outcome is achieved with multidisciplinary management that includes local radiotherapy and chemotherapy for distant metastases.[20–22]

CODING AND BILLING PEARLS

- Bill for malignant lesion removals after pathology is determined because malignancies have different codes and higher reimbursements.
- When calculating the size of the excised lesion, it is important to include the necessary margins. Therefore, if you are excising a 1-cm basal cell carcinoma with 4-mm margins, you would bill for an excision at 1.8 cm. Do not forget to make these measurements so that you get paid for what you do.

CONCLUSION

There are choices among the methods of removal of malignant lesions. Small lesions that are not near important structures, have distinct margins, and are not high-grade cancers can usually be managed by clinicians with good basic skills in their office. For high-risk locations and lesions, the best results of complete lesion removal are typically obtained by Mohs micrographic surgery. This chapter has provided a general guideline for malignant lesion management, but as always providers must use their best clinical judgment and adjust the specific treatment based on their individual patient's needs.

Resources

The American Cancer Society (www.cancer.org) provides information on skin cancers and brochures for patients and clinicians on the ABCDE rules for melanoma.

References

1. Anwar J, Wrone DA, Kimyai-Asadi A, Alam M. The development of actinic keratosis into invasive squamous cell carcinoma: evidence and evolving classification schemes. *Clin Dermatol.* 2004;22:189–196.
2. Criscione VD, Weinstock MA, Naylor MF, *et al.* Actinic keratoses: natural history and risk of malignant transformation in the Veterans Affairs Topical Tretinoin Chemoprevention Trial. *Cancer.* 2009;115:2523–2530.
3. Thai KE, Fergin P, Freeman M, *et al.* A prospective study of the use of cryosurgery for the treatment of actinic keratoses. *Int J Dermatol.* 2004;43:687–692.
4. Cox NH, Eedy DJ, Morton CA. Guidelines for management of Bowen's disease: 2006 update. *Br J Dermatol.* 2007;156:11–21.
5. Ridky TW. Nonmelanoma skin cancer. *J Am Acad Dermatol.* 2007;57:484–501.
6. Ahmed I, Agarwal S, Ilchyshyn A, *et al.* Liquid nitrogen cryotherapy of common warts: cryo-spray vs. cotton wool bud. *Br J Dermatol.* 2001;144:1006–1009.
7. Ricotti C, Bouzari N, Agadi A, Cockerell CJ. Malignant skin neoplasms. *Med Clin North Am.* 2009;93:1241–1264.
8. Mosterd K, Krekels GA, Nieman FH, *et al.* Surgical excision versus Mohs' micrographic surgery for primary and recurrent basal-cell carcinoma of the face: a prospective randomised controlled trial with 5-years' follow-up. *Lancet Oncol.* 2008;9:1149–1156.
9. Szeimies RM. Methyl aminolevulinate-photodynamic therapy for basal cell carcinoma. *Dermatol Clin.* 2007;25:89–94.
10. Marcil I, Stern RS. Risk of developing a subsequent nonmelanoma skin cancer in patients with a history of nonmelanoma skin cancer: a critical review of the literature and meta-analysis. *Arch Dermatol.* 2000;136:1524–1530.
11. Arora A, Attwood J. Common skin cancers and their precursors. *Surg Clin North Am.* 2009;89:703–712.
12. Thomas L. Semiological value of ABCDE criteria in the diagnosis of cutaneous pigmented tumors. *Dermatology.* 1998;197:11–17.
13. Bradford PT, Goldstein AM, McMaster ML, Tucker MA. Acral lentiginous melanoma: incidence and survival patterns in the United States, 1986–2005. *Arch Dermatol.* 2009;145:427–434.
14. Kalkhoran S, Milne O, Zalaudek I, *et al.* Historical, clinical, and dermoscopic characteristics of thin nodular melanoma. *Arch Dermatol.* 2010;146:311–318.
15. Swetter SM, Boldrick JC, Jung SY, *et al.* Increasing incidence of lentigo maligna melanoma subtypes: northern California and national trends 1990–2000. *J Invest Dermatol.* 2005;125:685–691.
16. Garbe C, Hauschild A, Volkenandt M, *et al.* Evidence and interdisciplinary consensus-based German guidelines: surgical treatment and radiotherapy of melanoma. *Melanoma Res.* 2008;18:61–67.
17. Garbe C, Peris K, Hauschild A, *et al.* Diagnosis and treatment of melanoma: European consensus-based interdisciplinary guideline. *Eur J Cancer.* 2010;46:270–283.
18. Snow SN, Gordon EM, Larson PO, *et al.* Dermatofibrosarcoma protuberans: a report on 29 patients treated by Mohs micrographic surgery with long-term follow-up and review of the literature. *Cancer.* 2004;101:28–38.
19. Paradisi A, Abeni D, Rusciani A, *et al.* Dermatofibrosarcoma protuberans: wide local excision vs. Mohs micrographic surgery. *Cancer Treat Rev.* 2008;34:728–736.
20. Zampetti A, Feliciani C, Massi G, Tulli A. Updated review of the pathogenesis and management of Merkel cell carcinoma. *J Cutan Med Surg.* 2010;14:51–61.
21. Tai P, Yu E, Assouline A, *et al.* Management of Merkel cell carcinoma with emphasis on small primary tumors—a case series and review of the current literature. *J Drugs Dermatol.* 2010;9:105–110.
22. Eng TY, Boersma MG, Fuller CD, *et al.* A comprehensive review of the treatment of Merkel cell carcinoma. *Am J Clin Oncol.* 2007;30:624–636.

35 Wound Care

LUCIA DIAZ, MD • RICHARD P. USATINE, MD

A wide variety of wound care techniques can be used depending on the type, size, and location of the wound. Sutured wounds are dealt with differently than wounds that are allowed to heal on their own through secondary intention.

Teaching wound care to the patient or family members is best done after the surgical procedure has been completed. Patients appreciate receiving written and verbal instructions after the procedure because worries prior to the procedure may prevent them from fully understanding the information. They should be encouraged to look at the wound in the office so that they will not be frightened at home; a mirror can be used when the wound is on the face. If the patient feels faint at the sight of the affected area, it can be more safely managed in the office.

Quite often, patients will not want to or cannot see the wound. In this case, wound care may be demonstrated to a family member or the person who is accompanying the patient. A follow-up examination may be appropriate if the physician wants to assess the wound and/or the patient's ability to care for it. Examples of wound care instructions are available in Appendix A.

WOUND HEALING PHASES

Inflammatory

The inflammatory phase starts immediately and lasts for 2 to 3 days. Tissue injury leads to vasodilation and extravasation of blood constituents that initiate hemostasis and healing. Platelets aggregate to stop bleeding, release vasoconstrictors, and activate the coagulation cascade. Prostaglandins and activated complement increase capillary permeability, leading to the inflammatory exudate. Platelets then release cytokines and chemotactic factors that attract neutrophils and macrophages. Neutrophils destroy bacteria immediately, while macrophages phagocytize bacteria and release collagenase.

Proliferative

The proliferative phase lasts from 2 days to 3 weeks. Macrophages, platelets, and fibroblasts release cytokines that initiate the formation of granulation tissue. Fibroblasts create a collagen bed to fill the defect and grow new capillaries. High lactate levels and low oxygen tension in the wound stimulate fibroblast proliferation and angiogenesis.[1] Keratinocytes proliferate and migrate from the intact epidermis around the wound as well as from remaining structures in the base. The rate of re-epithelialization is directly related to moistness of the wound; open, dry superficial wounds re-epithelialize significantly more slowly than occluded moist wounds.[2] One week after injury, myofibroblasts initiate contraction by pulling the wound edges closer together.

Remodeling

This phase lasts from 3 weeks to 2 years. Contraction continues, and an organized form of collagen gradually replaces the immature collagen. Wounds created by destructive techniques such as cryosurgery heal more slowly than those caused by a scalpel. Wound tensile strength is 40% at 1 month and never increases to more than 80% of the preinjury strength.[1] This demonstrates the importance of supporting wounds with buried sutures and adhesive wound-closure strips, especially at the time of suture removal.

TYPES OF WOUNDS

Two common types of skin wounds result from basic dermatologic surgery: a full-thickness wound that heals by primary intention and a partial-thickness wound that heals by secondary intention. However, even a full-thickness wound can be allowed to heal by secondary intention such as after a cancer removal on the scalp (Figure 35-1).

Full-Thickness Wounds

The epidermis and full thickness of the dermis are lost. This is usually created by a full-thickness excision. The wound heals slowly by granulation tissue formation, contracture, and re-epithelialization from the wound edges. If the edges are approximated with sutures or adhesive tape (healing by primary intention), there will be less wound contracture and therefore less scarring.

Partial-Thickness Wounds

The epidermis and part of the dermis are lost. This is usually created by shave excisions, curettage and electrodesiccation, CO_2 laser surgery, and chemical peels. If left to heal alone (healing by secondary intention), re-epithelialization from the wound edges and adnexal structures in the base of wound will quickly follow. The greater the depth of dermal injury, the more scarring there will be.

DRESSINGS

Various types of dressings are available for use depending on the type of wound and physician preference.

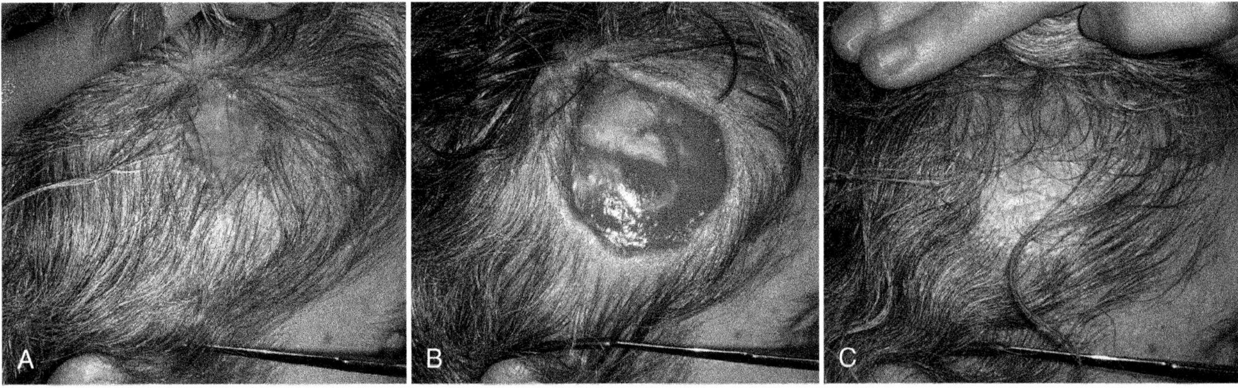

FIGURE 35-1 **(A)** Large nodular BCC on the scalp of a 37-year-old woman. **(B)** The BCC was resected in the operating room by ENT and the patient preferred to allow the wound to heal by secondary intention rather than have a large flap done. This photo was taken 2 weeks after the surgery was completed when the patient removed the dressing for a postop check. **(C)** Six months later the wound was completely re-epithelialized, and in the following year the scar retracted and shrunk in size so that it was no longer visible under her hair. *(Copyright Richard P. Usatine, MD.)*

They are generally divided into open dressings (e.g., gauze) and occlusive dressings (e.g., films, foams, gels, hydrocolloids, and alginates). The selection and use of wound dressings can be highly personalized and modified by physician experience. The purpose of a dressing is to protect a wound from trauma or contamination, absorb wound drainage that may lead to maceration, provide hemostasis through compression, and facilitate healing by providing a moist environment. There is evidence that occlusive dressings increase re-epithelialization rates by 30% to 40% and collagen synthesis by 20% to 60% over air-exposed wounds.[3] However, a randomized, controlled trial showed that there is no difference in infection between dressed and undressed clean sutured wounds.[4] For physicians who do prefer to use wound dressings, characteristics required for the ideal dressing are found in Table 35-1.

Many of the common wound dressings have three layers: a contact layer, an absorbent layer, and an outer (secondary) layer.

TABLE 35-1 Ideal Dressing Characteristics

Handling of excess exudate	Removal of toxic substances
Maintenance of moist environment	Barrier to microorganisms
Thermal insulation provided	Freedom from particulate contaminants
Removal without trauma to new tissue	Adheres well to a thin margin of surrounding skin
Does not adhere to wound	Nontoxic and nonreactive
Conforms well to body contours and motion	Promotes patient comfort and is not bulky
Readily available and inexpensive	Long shelf-life

Source: From Freitag DS. Surgical wound dressings. In: Lask G, Moy R, eds. *Principles and Techniques of Cutaneous Surgery.* New York: McGraw-Hill; 1996.

Contact Layer

The contact layer of a dressing is placed directly on the wound. It is usually selected for its nonadherent properties to limit the risk of sticking to the underlying wound. Plain gauze absorbs exudate but will readily stick to both open and sutured wounds. Nonadherent dressings may be applied either directly to the wound or after the application of an ointment to minimize the risk of adherence and facilitate dressing removal. Plain gauze may be used if petrolatum or an antibiotic ointment is applied liberally to the wound to prevent sticking. A variety of dressings are available for use as a nonadherent contact layer including petrolatum-impregnated gauze, Telfa, and a number of semipermeable dressings (e.g., Op-Site, Tegaderm, and Vigilon).

Absorbent Layer

The absorbent layer of a dressing takes up exudate extruded from the wound and cushions the wound from outside trauma. The combination of both the contact and absorbent layers is referred to as the primary dressing. Many manufacturers have produced single dressings that combine both the contact and absorbent layer. For example, the widely used Telfa dressing consists of an absorbent layer of cellulose sandwiched between two layers of nonadherent polyester film.

Outer (Secondary) Layer

The outer, or secondary, layer of dressing, usually consists of gauze or cotton wadding. This layer is also referred to as the pressure dressing and is secured in place with adhesive tape or a bandage. Pressure dressings prevent hematomas by applying pressure to the subcutaneous dead space and immobilizing the underlying wound.

Complete Dressing

The best example of a complete wound dressing involving all three layers is the ordinary household adhesive bandage (e.g., Band-Aid, Elastoplast, and Telfa Ouchless Adhesive Pad). It combines the contact, absorbent, and outer adhesive layers into a single sterile unit.

WOUND CARE

Wound Healing by Secondary Intention

Partial-thickness wounds that heal by secondary intention may be cleansed after surgery using a cotton-tipped applicator (CTA) dipped in saline. The swab is gently rolled—not rubbed—over the wound to remove any loose debris and/or crusting. Although antiseptic use is recommended prior to procedure, a review by Brown and Zitelli[5] recommended avoiding the use of antiseptics such as hydrogen peroxide or chlorhexidine in open wounds because they are toxic to epithelial cells and delay wound healing.

After cleansing, the wound should be dressed with generous amounts of ointment (Table 35-2 lists typical ointments used). Patients with an allergy to antibiotic ointments should use only petrolatum (e.g., petroleum jelly, Vaseline). Neomycin-containing ointments should be avoided because of their high potential for contact dermatitis.[6] Although data support the use of antibiotic-containing ointments in contaminated wounds, data to support their superiority to petrolatum in clean wounds is lacking.[1] The ointments have various antimicrobial properties:

- Bacitracin covers staphylococci and streptococci.
- Neomycin covers staphylococci and most gram-negative bacilli
- Bactroban covers streptococci and staphylococci resistant to methicillin.
- Polymyxin B covers gram-negative bacilli and *Pseudomonas*.[1]

White petrolatum is as safe and effective as Bacitracin with less risk for inducing allergy.[7] Furthermore, a review by Sheth and Weitzul[8] recommended using petrolatum instead of antimicrobial ointment on clean wounds given that the rate of allergic contact dermatitis from antibacterial ointments (1.6% to 2.3%) is similar to the rate of postoperative infections (1% to 2%) in dermatologic surgery.

TABLE 35-2 Types of Antibacterial Agents

Brand Name	Active Antimicrobial Ingredients
Bacitracin	Bacitracin zinc
Polysporin	Bacitracin zinc, Polymyxin B sulfate
Neosporin	Neomycin sulfate, Bacitracin zinc, Polymyxin B sulfate
Gentamicin	Gentamicin sulfate
Bactroban	Mupirocin

Note: All can cause contact dermatitis.

If the wound is small, patients are encouraged to use adhesive bandages to cover the wound. When the wound is large, it may be covered with a nonstick dressing pad, such as Telfa, and secured with a hypoallergenic tape. This approach can be used for wounds of all depths in almost all locations.

The wound should be cleaned gently with soap and water once daily, starting the day after the surgery. The dressing can subsequently be changed 1 to 2 times a day as needed with the reapplication of ointment to maintain a moist wound throughout the day. This process should be repeated until the wound has healed completely.

Occlusive Dressings

Deeper exudative or superficial slow-healing wounds such as leg ulcers can be treated with calcium alginate or hydrocolloid (e.g., DuoDERM) dressings. These dressings are used in an occlusive fashion, minimizing the air penetration to the wound site. Before applying an occlusive dressing, the wound is first cleansed with saline using a CTA. The dressing is placed onto or into the wound and then covered with a piece of Telfa followed by gauze. The dressings are cut down to the size of the wound and secured with transparent tape. Note that this dressing may produce a yellow, foul-smelling drainage that is not a sign of infection.

The dressings are changed every 3 to 4 days and can be changed less often as clinically indicated; they are usually used for approximately 2 weeks. When the occlusive dressing is discontinued, the patient is instructed to clean the wound with soap and water followed by the application of ointment and a Band-Aid until complete healing has occurred.

Wound Healing by Primary Intention

One method of caring for sutured wounds is similar to that for wounds healing by secondary intention (see recommendations above). A CTA is dipped in saline and gently rolled—not rubbed—along the suture line to remove any loose debris and/or crusting. Some physicians cover sutured wounds with ointment prior to applying a nonstick dressing pad or Band-Aid, while others leave them exposed. A recent study showed that wounds covered with paraffin ointment, Bactroban, and no ointment under occlusive dressings had similar rates of wound infection, scar, hemorrhage, or dehiscence at the time of suture removal.[9] Also, the patients indicated the same level of satisfaction with all treatments at 6 to 9 months after the surgery.[9]

Another dressing method involves using Steri-Strips and/or micropore tape over the incision site immediately after surgery. These are left in place until the sutures are removed. Suture removal time depends on many factors, but is generally 4 to 6 days for the head and neck, 7 days for upper limbs, 10 days for the trunk and abdomen, and 14 days for lower limbs. Semipermeable tape strips (e.g., Steri-Strips) may be applied transversely across the wound, providing support and reducing tension across the suture line. Spaces left between the strips allow wound exudate and blood to escape and be absorbed by the overlying dressing. Tissue adhesives (e.g., tincture of benzoin, and Mastisol) should be used to increase the adherence of tape strips to the skin. A nonadherent primary dressing may then be applied and taped in place with pressure dressing applied on top. In most situations, pressure dressings consist of bulky gauze or cotton wadding secured in place by adhesive tape.

The use of pressure dressings to reduce the risk of hematoma formation is especially important after the excision of cysts or lipomas. Patients may be instructed to remove the bulky outer pressure dressing 24 to 36 hours after surgery, leaving the underlying primary dressing undisturbed. In view of the unique local vasculature, it is not advisable to apply pressure dressings to the digits.

Hydrocolloid Dressing

All of the dressings discussed previously require varying degrees of maintenance by patients. One maintenance-free dressing for sutured wounds uses wound closure tape (e.g., Steri-Strips) or a hydrocolloid dressing (e.g., DuoDERM) cut to cover and extend beyond the suture line 5 to 10 mm in all directions. This is then covered with Tegaderm, Op-Site, or a standard pressure dressing.[10] If the wound is deep and hematoma formation is a concern, a pressure dressing can be placed. This pressure dressing consists of generous amounts of absorbent gauze taped firmly over the Tegaderm to apply pressure. Patients are instructed to remove the pressure dressing in 24 hours, leaving the DuoDERM and Tegaderm dressing in place for an additional week. Absorbable sutures below the skin are hydrolyzed and significantly weakened, whereas sutures above the surface will have melted into the DuoDERM. When the DuoDERM is removed, the absorbable sutures detach with it.[10]

Hydrocolloid dressing is unique and popular with patients because it is water resistant and maintenance free. It is ideal for wounds that are closed by 6-0 and 5-0 fast-absorbing plain or mild chromic gut sutures on the surface. Also, if there is a higher risk of infection, such as in a patient who has diabetes, hydrocolloid dressings are translucent and allow for daily observation.

POSTOPERATIVE WOUND CARE PATIENT INSTRUCTIONS

Patients should be instructed to keep their wound covered and moist to prevent the formation of any scabs and crusts. The primary dressing should neither get wet nor be removed until 24 hours postoperatively.

Showering

Specific advice on bathing and taking showers is necessary because this is a potential point of confusion for patients. Many physicians advise patients with sutured wounds to keep their dressings dry until suture removal. There is evidence, however, that there is no increased risk of infection or wound dehiscence in undressed sutured wounds washed with soap and water twice a day starting 24 hours after surgery.[11] After showering, patients should apply ointment and redress the wound. Immersion of the wound in water such as in swimming pools or hot baths should be avoided to prevent infection.

Pain

For discomfort following surgery, patients may take acetaminophen. Aspirin increases the risk of bleeding and should be avoided if possible. If the wound and patient are not at high risk of bleeding, an oral NSAID may be used. For patients who might suffer more pain after surgery, consider giving them a small prescription for acetaminophen/hydrocodone. If the patient has a problem with addiction or is a recovering addict, discuss alternative nonnarcotic methods of treating pain.

Bleeding

If bleeding occurs, the patient should apply firm pressure to the site for 5 to 10 minutes, without discontinuing the pressure to see if bleeding has stopped. A clock should be used because it is easy to overestimate the time and look for bleeding too soon. If shorter holding times do not work, it is best to hold pressure up to 20 minutes before giving up. If the bleeding does not stop, then the patient must promptly return to the office or go to the emergency department if the office is closed.

Infection

An infection should be suspected if the wound becomes painful or red or drains pus. The patient must be instructed to return to the office or go to the emergency department if the office is closed. Patients should also know that fevers and swollen lymph nodes are signs of infection.

Wound Healing

Patients should know what to expect during wound healing. Scar maturation typically lasts 6 to 12 months or even longer in children and teenagers. Often, patients complain of wound itchiness and tightness. Scar hydration and massage with aloe vera or vitamin E alleviates these symptoms by preventing the wound from cracking or peeling.

There is no evidence that any "scar cream" or topical ointment accelerates the process of wound maturation or even improves the final scar appearance. If scar hypertrophy is a concern, patients may tape the area at all times for 3 months with Micropore tape or another type of hypoallergenic nonsterile tape, because evidence suggests that this may reduce tension on the scar and reduce the tendency toward hypertrophy.[12,13]

Patients should also know that wound redness can take 6 months to 1 year to fade. Prolonged sun exposure may delay scar maturation and turn the pink scar to a darker red or purple color. To prevent these changes, patients should keep the scar covered and/or apply sunscreen during scar maturation.

SPECIAL LOCATIONS

Periorbital Wounds

Wounds that approach the cutaneous-conjunctival junction should not be cleaned with antiseptic solutions because they are potentially oculotoxic. If there is a chance that the ointment on the wound may get into the eye, a preparation specifically formulated for the eye (e.g., Polysporin ophthalmic ointment) should be used.

Ear

If cartilage is exposed, chondritis can occur with desiccation. To prevent this, antibiotic ointment should be applied liberally. Cotton should be placed in the external auditory meatus to prevent wound drainage that may lead to otitis media.

Digits

When applying dressings to a finger or toe, two main types may be used: a tubular dressing or a bandage applied obliquely and attached at the wrists. Excessive pressure should be avoided.

COMPLICATIONS AND HOW TO AVOID THEM

Factors that negatively affect wound healing include the following:

- Excessive tension
- Hemostatic agents
- Antiseptic agents
- Infection
- Hypoxia
- Reactions to ointments
- Protein deficiency
- Vitamins A and C and zinc deficiency
- Immunocompromised state
- Nicotine use
- Steroids
- Vascular disease.

Contact Dermatitis

Erosions, bullae, and bruising may be associated with the use of adhesive tapes, particularly when used with tissue adhesives (Figure 35-2). This commonly occurs on the facial skin of elderly patients and those patients on systemic steroid therapy. Avoiding the use of topical antibiotics can minimize the risk of contact dermatitis (Figure 35-3).

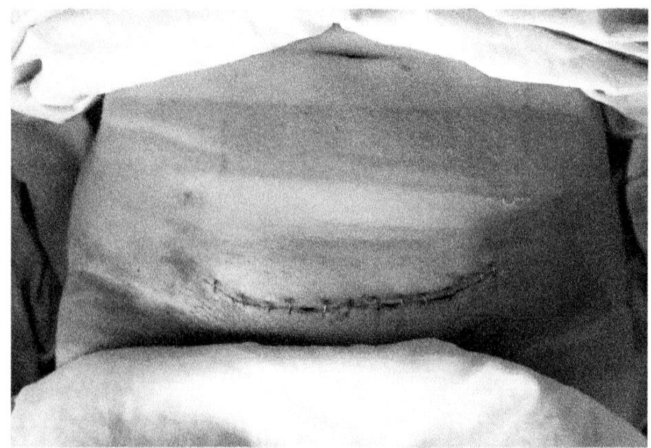

FIGURE 35-2 Contact allergy to tape placed to hold a dressing over a hysterectomy incision. *(Copyright Richard P. Usatine, MD.)*

Optimizing Outcomes

- Avoid leakage of wound by using the proper dressing.
- Keep the wound moist with topical ointment and dressing.
- Remove necrotic tissue through debridement.
- Control pain.
- Ensure patient adherence to written and verbal instructions.

CONCLUSION

There are many ways to dress a wound and obtain good wound healing. The physician can choose the wound dressing based on the characteristics of the surgery, the patient, and the availability of the needed resources. Use of the principles discussed in this chapter will help produce optimal healing with minimal pain and scarring. For further information on potential complications of surgery and wound healing, see Chapter 36, *Complications: Postprocedural Adverse Effects and Their Prevention.*

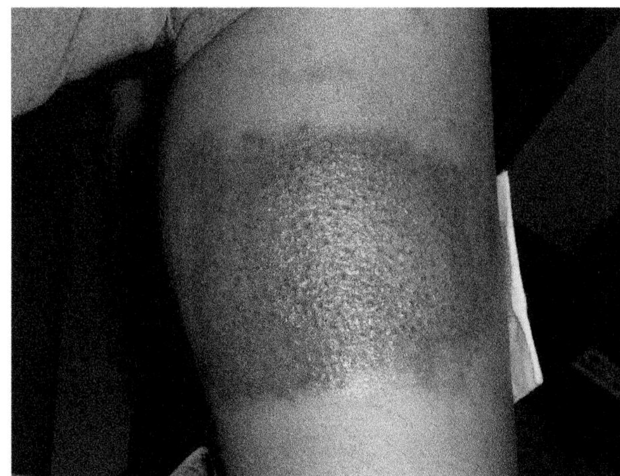

FIGURE 35-3 Contact allergy to Neosporin applied broadly over a shave biopsy wound. The erythema and inflammation match the size of the Telfa pad and a contact allergy may be to the dressing as well. *(Copyright Richard P. Usatine, MD.)*

Acknowledgments We thank Dr. Bret R. Baack for his contributions to this chapter.

References

1. Cho CY, Lo J. Dressing the part. *Dermatol Clin.* 1998;16(1): 25–47.
2. Telfer N, Moy R. Wound care after office procedures. *Dermatol Surg Oncol.* 1993;19:722–731.
3. Bolton LL, Johnson CL, Rijswijk LV. Occlusive dressings: therapeutic agents and effects on drug delivery. *Dermatol Clin.* 1992;9:573–583.
4. Merei J. Pediatric clean surgical wounds: is dressing necessary? *J Pediatr Surg.* 2004;39(12):1671–1673.
5. Brown CD, Zitelli JA. A review of topical agents for wound and methods of wounding. *J Dermatol Surg Oncol.* 1993;19:732–737.
6. Kaye ET. Topical antibacterial agents. *Infect Dis Clin N Am.* 2000;14:321–339.
7. Smack DP, Harrington AC, Dunn C, *et al.* Infection and allergy incidence in ambulatory surgery patients using white petrolatum vs bacitracin ointment: a randomized controlled trial. *JAMA.* 1996;276:972–977.
8. Sheth VM, Weitzul S. Postoperative topical antimicrobial use. *Dermatitis.* 2008;19(4):181–189.
9. Dixon AJ, Dixon MP, Dixon JB. Randomized clinical trial of the effect of applying ointment to surgical wounds before occlusive dressing. *Br J Surg.* 2006;93(8):937–943.
10. Siegel DM, Sun DK, Artman N. Surgical pearl: a novel cost-effective approach to wound closure and dressings. *J Am Acad Dermatol.* 1996;34(4):673–675.
11. Noe JM, Keller M. Can stitches get wet? *Plast Reconstr Surg.* 1988;81:82–84.
12. Atkinson JA, McKenna KT, Barnett AG, *et al.* A randomized controlled trial to determine the efficacy of paper tape in preventing hypertrophic scar formation in surgical incisions that traverse Langer's skin tension lines. *Plast Reconstr Surg.* 2005;116:1648–1658.
13. Reiffel RS. Prevention of hypertrophic scars by long-term paper tape application. *Plast Reconstr Surg.* 1995;96:1715–1718.

36 Complications: Postprocedural Adverse Effects and Their Prevention

RICHARD P. USATINE, MD

Many adverse effects can occur during and after dermatologic procedures and skin surgeries. Some are predictable and inevitable, such as some pain and erythema, and others may fall into the category of complications such as nerve damage and infections. Whatever method we use to classify these adverse effects, practitioners must be aware of the potential complications for each procedure in order to maximize prevention and early detection. Discussing possible complications with the patient is part of informed consent, but is also part of the patient education that goes along with postoperative care. Patients need to know what they can do if a complication arises and when they need to seek medical care. If postoperative patients have a concern about a possible complication, it is usually worthwhile to offer them an appointment that day. Whereas some complications can be handled over the phone, the offer of a face-to-face visit is useful and should be documented in the medical record.

Calling a patient at home the evening after or day after a large skin surgery or procedure goes a long way toward preventing complications, building good relationships, and preventing malpractice claims. It is worthwhile to make sure you have a working phone number for patients before they leave your office. Put the call on your "to do" list and take that number home with you for the evening call. If the call is not made that evening, a call the following morning is equally appreciated. This also allows you to find out if the patient was able to sleep and whether he or she is having problems with pain or bleeding. Patients are delighted that you care enough to call. In addition, this is one way to diminish your anxiety about potential complications of the procedure.

Being available to take your patients' calls is another positive way to build good relationships and deal with complications early before they become severe. If you do not have an answering service, consider giving out your cell phone number to select patients for whom your concerns are greatest. Remember, your call between 6 p.m. and 9 p.m. may eliminate their call between 9 p.m. and 6 a.m.!

The incidence of complications can be decreased with good procedural techniques and early recognition of problems before they become severe. Potential adverse effects and complications of skin procedures can be categorized by the time when they occur, as listed in Box 36-1.

An informed consent form covering the potential complications should be discussed with and signed by the patient. The informed consent form should cover the items in the list above that pertain to the surgical procedure for the specific site and patient. No absolute guarantees of cosmetic results should be made. See Chapter 1, *Preoperative Preparation*, and the sample consent form titled *Disclosure and Consent: Medical and Surgical Procedures* in Appendix A.

REVIEW OF THE LITERATURE

In a prospective study of 3788 dermatologic surgery procedures, there were 236 complications (6%).[1] Most complications were minor and bleeding was the most common (3%). Vasovagal syncope was the main anaesthetic complication (51 of 54). Infectious complications occurred in 79 patients (2%). Complications requiring additional antibiotic treatment or repeat surgery accounted for only 22 cases (1%). No statistically significant correlation was found with the characteristics of the dermatologists, especially with respect to their training or amount of surgical experience. Multivariate analysis showed that anaesthetic or hemorrhagic complications were independent factors that predicted infectious complications. Patients on anticoagulants or immunosuppressant medications, type of procedure performed and duration exceeding 24 minutes were independent factors that predicted hemorrhagic complications.[1]

Two years later, the same group published a study of 3491 dermatologic surgical procedures describing postoperative infections in 67 patients (1.9%), with superficial suppuration accounting for 92.5% of surgical site infections.[2] The incidence was higher in the excision group with a reconstructive procedure (4.3%) than in excisions alone (1.6%). Infection control precautions varied according to the site of the procedure; multivariate analysis showed that hemorrhagic complications were an independent factor for infection in both types of surgical procedures. Male gender, immunosuppressive therapy, and not wearing sterile gloves were independent factors for infections occurring following excisions with reconstruction.[2]

Dixon et al. performed a prospective study of 5091 lesions (predominantly nonmelanoma skin cancer) treated on 2424 patients.[3] None of the patients was given prophylactic antibiotics, and warfarin or aspirin was not stopped. The overall infection rate was 1.47%. Individual procedures had the following infection incidence:

- Simple excision and closure: 0.5% (16/2974)
- Curettage: 0.7% (3/412)
- Skin flap repairs: 2.9% (47/1601)
- Wedge excision of lip and ear: 8.6% (3/35)
- Skin grafts: 8.7% (6/69).

BOX 36-1 *Potential Adverse Effects and Complications of Skin Procedures*

May Occur within the First Few Weeks

- Pain
- Bleeding
- Hematoma
- Bruising and swelling
- Infection
- Dehiscence
- Suture spitting
- Flap necrosis

May Start Early and Become Permanent

- Distortion of normal anatomy around any facial feature
- Ectropion and entropion of eyelids
- Alopecia
- Nerve damage

Prolonged or Permanent

- Scarring
- Skin indentation
- Hypertrophic scars
- Keloid
- Hyperpigmentation
- Hypopigmentation
- Recurrence of the excised condition

Surgery below the knee had an infection incidence of 6.9% (31/448) and groin excisional surgery had an infection incidence of 10% (1/10). Patients with diabetes, those on warfarin and/or aspirin, and smokers showed no difference in infection incidence. In conclusion, all procedures below the knee, wedge excisions of the lip and ear, all skin grafts, and lesions in the groin had the highest rates of infection and the authors suggest considering wound infection prophylaxis in these patients.[3]

In a prospective study of hospitalized patients undergoing diagnostic skin biopsies, infection, dehiscence, and/or hematoma occurred in 29% of the patients.[4] Complications occurred significantly more frequently when biopsies were performed below the waist, in the ward compared with the outpatient operating room, in smokers, and in those taking corticosteroids.[4] In addition, elliptical incisional biopsies developed complications more frequently when subcutaneous sutures were not used.[4]

In one study of 1400 Mohs procedures, 25 infections were identified.[5] Statistically significant higher infection rates were found in patients with cartilage fenestration with second intent healing and patients with melanoma. There was no statistical difference in infection rates with all other measured variables including the use of clean, nonsterile gloves rather than sterile gloves during the tumor removal phase of surgery.[5] Sterile gloves were used by all surgeons during the repair phase.

In 2008, an advisory statement on antibiotic prophylaxis in dermatologic surgery was published.[6] Expert consensus based on a small number of studies suggests that antibiotics for the prevention of surgical site infections may be indicated for procedures on the lower extremities or groin, for wedge excisions of the lip and ear, skin flaps on the nose, skin grafts, and for patients with extensive inflammatory skin disease.[6] Also, patients with high-risk cardiac conditions, and a defined group of patients with prosthetic joints at high risk for hematogenous total joint infection, should be given prophylactic antibiotics (to prevent bacterial endocarditis) when the surgical site is infected or when the procedure involves breach of the oral mucosa.[6]

PAIN

Most skin procedures and surgeries will result in some pain when the anesthesia wears off. Explain to patients that they may safely use acetaminophen for pain relief unless they have severe liver disease or some other unusual contraindication. Ibuprofen should be safe unless the patient is anticoagulated or has another contraindication to the use of ibuprofen or other nonsteroidal anti-inflammatory drugs (NSAIDs). Aspirin should be avoided for pain control because it can increase the risk of bleeding and hematoma. Acetaminophen and hydrocodone combination products are generally not needed unless the procedure was large and particularly painful. When this is the case, it is helpful to write out that prescription before the patient leaves the office. A quick discussion about pain control can prevent unnecessary distress to the patient later and unnecessary phone calls to you at night. If a patient complains of increasing pain over time, a hematoma or infection should be considered and it is best to see the patient in the office.

BLEEDING

The most likely complication of dermatologic surgery is bleeding (accounting for half of a 6% complication rate).[1] Larger surgeries with more undermining are at highest risk of bleeding complications. Good intraoperative hemostasis, appropriate suturing techniques, and pressure dressings can help minimize bleeding complications. Aspirin can cause excessive bleeding during surgery if not stopped 2 weeks before surgery. NSAIDs can also cause excessive bleeding if not stopped 2 days before surgery. Warfarin (Coumadin) also increases the risk of bleeding intraoperatively and postoperatively (Figure 36-1). That said most clinicians would not postpone skin surgery because the patient has recently taken aspirin or an NSAID. Often the risk of stopping warfarin or aspirin is greater to the patient (such as stroke) than dealing with the bleeding issues. In fact, in a study of 2424 patients undergoing dermatologic surgery, the warfarin or aspirin was not stopped in any of these patients.[3] For further information on the risks and benefits of anticoagulation before surgery see Chapter 1 on preoperative preparation.

The risk of intraoperative bleeding can be decreased by waiting 10 minutes after injecting lidocaine and epinephrine to allow the epinephrine to have maximal vasoconstrictive effect before beginning the procedure.

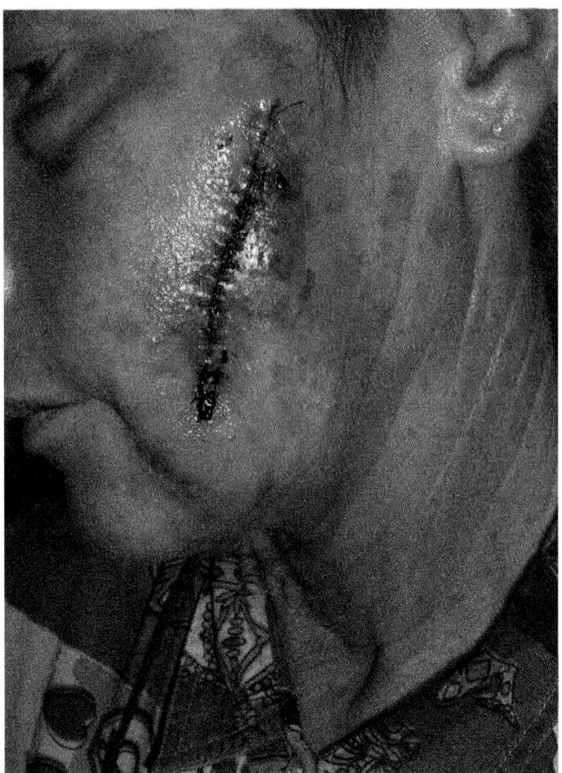

FIGURE 36-1 Bleeding and ecchymosis after the removal of a large squamous cell carcinoma on the face of a woman on Coumadin. Although this looked bad at this point in time, all healed well over time and by continuing the Coumadin, she never had a stroke. *(Courtesy of Richard P. Usatine, MD.)*

The risk of hematoma can be lessened with careful attention to hemostasis using appropriate electrocoagulation and tying off larger vessels. However, excessive electrocoagulation can cause unnecessary tissue damage, leading to impaired wound healing. Although sutures that are placed tightly can cause suture marks, they can also stop bleeding. Tighter sutures might be used in a situation where the patient seems to be oozing or bleeding excessively. If the patient has a bleeding diathesis, undermining should be kept to the absolute minimum necessary.

Pressure dressings are helpful following most skin surgeries except the majority of shave biopsies, which have little risk of bleeding. A good, firm pressure dressing will prevent many after-hour bleeding episodes. The pressure dressing may be constructed with gauze that is doubled up (or dental roll) and tape applied on top using firm pressure during the first 24 hours. Blood on the dressing is better than blood in the wound. Sending the patient home with gauze in hand along with instructions about what to do if bleeding occurs is also helpful. Although blood-soaked bandages can be one manifestation of excessive bleeding, internal bleeding can result in hematoma formation and/or ecchymosis.

Postoperative bleeding usually occurs within the first 24 hours after surgery. It will occur more often in a patient who was taking aspirin but may also occur more often in a patient who has high blood pressure or who is physically active. The usual scenario for postoperative bleeding is that the patient will call the clinician and complain of blood soaking through the bandage. The patient should be instructed to apply firm pressure for 20 to 30 minutes by the clock. This will usually stop the bleeding in a majority of situations. If not, the patient may need to come into the office or go to the emergency department.

Hematoma

Hematomas can best be prevented with good electrocoagulation, the tying off of large bleeders and large blood vessels, and the use of buried absorbable sutures to close dead space and a pressure bandage.

If the patient complains of increased pain and bulging around the surgical incision wound, the patient needs to be evaluated for a potential hematoma. If the hematoma is detected during the first 24 hours, the incision usually needs to be opened. All of the sutures should be removed, and the bleeding should be stopped with electrocoagulation. The wound can then be sutured again and the patient started on systemic antibiotics to prevent wound infection.

If the hematoma is detected more than 24 hours postoperatively and there does not seem to be active bleeding or an expanding hematoma, the wound may not need to be opened. Instead, a syringe with an 18-gauge needle may be used to extract the blood through the incision line. A pressure dressing is then applied, and the patient is started on antibiotics. Oral antibiotics are used because a hematoma is good bacterial growth media and the risk of infection is higher. The use of a needle to decrease the size of the hematoma may not work after 1 week, when the blood from the hematoma has organized and formed a clot. If the hematoma has clotted, this must resolve with time.

SWELLING AND BRUISING

Patients should be warned that surgery performed around the nose or forehead can cause swelling and bruising around the eyes (Figure 36-2). It is even possible that the eyes may swell shut. The use of ice may help prevent some of this edema if it is used during the first few hours after surgery. The lips can also stay swollen for many weeks or months after surgery.

Bruising and swelling are common adverse effects of surgery on the face, especially around the eyes. The best prevention for excessive bruising and swelling after facial surgery is to have the patient sleep with the head elevated for the first 2 to 3 days. A reclining chair can be helpful and propping the head and shoulders up with pillows on the bed is an alternative.

INFECTION

Everyone is disappointed when the site of a skin procedure becomes infected. The highest risk for infection of skin procedures is for the larger elliptical excisions

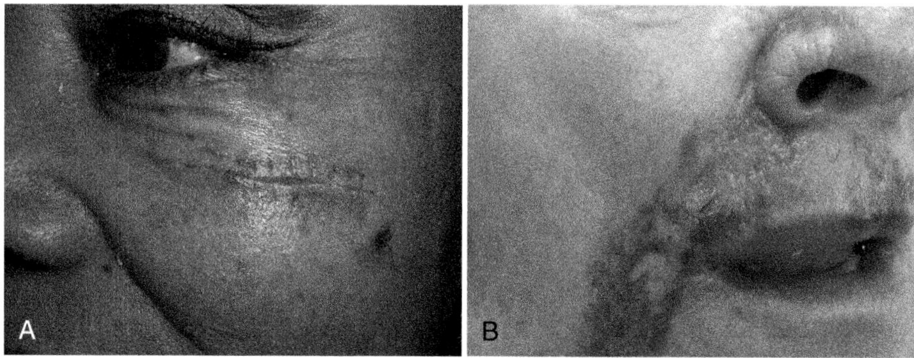

FIGURE 36-2 (A) Ecchymosis around the site of a BCC removal on the face. *(Copyright Richard P. Usatine, MD.)* (B) Ecchymosis around the site of an island pedicle flap. *(Courtesy of Ryan O'Quinn, MD.)*

and flap procedures. The more cutting, undermining, and sewing that is done, the higher the risk of infection. Shave biopsies and intralesional injections are very low risk for infections and these procedures can be performed as clean procedures without sterile gloves. All elliptical excisions and flaps should be performed with sterile technique. Unfortunately, there is little evidence-based information to guide how sterile these procedures should be. The spectrum ranges from sterile gloves and sterile equipment only to the use of hair caps, face masks, sterile gowns, and full surgical scrubs before putting on the gloves. We all need to monitor infection rates in our practice and decide how much prevention and cost we want to assume.

The highest risks for infections involve procedures below the knee or in the groin, wedge excisions of the lip and ear, and all skin flaps and grafts.[3] Patients who smoke and those taking oral corticosteroids are at higher risk of infection.[4] The 2008 AAD advisory statement states that prophylactic antibiotics may be indicated for:

- Procedures on the lower extremities or groin
- Wedge excisions of the lip and ear
- Skin flaps on the nose
- Skin grafts
- Patients with extensive inflammatory skin disease.[6]

One study describes the use of intraoperative injectable clindamycin to prevent wound infections. In a total of 1030 consecutive patients who underwent Mohs surgery, prior to reconstruction, patients were randomly assigned to receive either intraincisional buffered lidocaine with epinephrine containing clindamycin or buffered lidocaine with epinephrine without clindamycin.[7] The surgical wounds that received the clindamycin had a lower rate of infection than those that did not. The authors concluded that the results of their study support the efficacy of single-dose preoperative intraincisional antibiotic treatment for dermatologic surgery.[7]

Wound infections may initially be subtle and appear like the erythema seen around a healing incision. If you are uncertain about a possible infection, pressure applied with the gloved hand can be used to express pus hidden below the skin (Figure 36-3). If no pus is expressed but the suspicion for infection is great, consider removing a few stitches early and applying some pressure with a cotton-tipped applicator to detect pus. Send all purulent exudates for culture in this time when methicillin-resistant *Staphylococcus aureus* (MRSA) is so prevalent (Figure 36-3). The choice of antibiotic should consider MRSA as a possible cause of any wound infection.

A wound infection may present with the classic signs of redness, warmth, and pain. The patient may have a slight fever, and pus may be expressed from the wound. These symptoms usually become obvious around 5 to 7 days postoperatively or at the time of suture removal (Figure 36-4). Infections can manifest at postoperative day 2 to 4. If a patient has any complaints, it is best to examine the wound for evidence of infection. If the wound is tender and fluctuant, removal of one or more sutures to allow drainage will speed up resolution of the infection. Empirical antibiotic treatment in adults may start with cephalexin 500 mg tid–qid or clindamycin 300 mg tid in the penicillin-allergic patient. If the patient has a known history of MRSA infections, consider starting with trimethoprim/sulfamethoxazole or clindamycin. Of course, culture results in the coming days should be reviewed and may necessitate changing antibiotics.

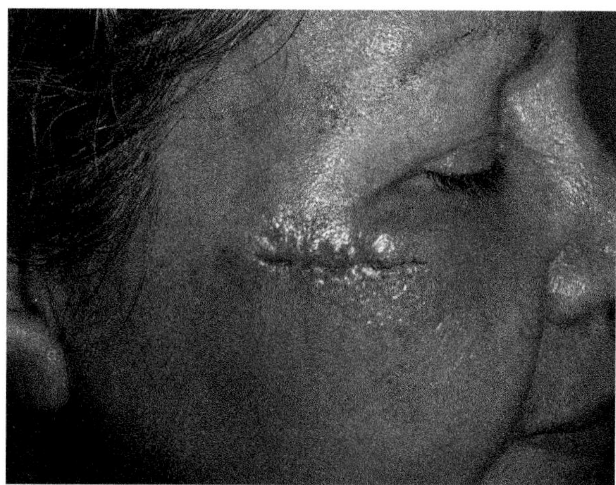

FIGURE 36-3 Erythema and swelling at the site of a wound infection caused by MRSA. *(Courtesy of Richard P. Usatine, MD.)*

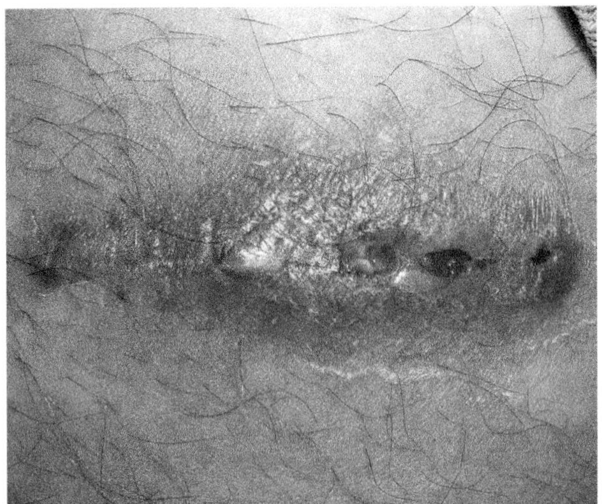

FIGURE 36-4 Purulence and erythema at the site of a wound infection near the groin. *(Courtesy of Richard P. Usatine, MD.)*

Suture Reactions

Suture reactions are frequently mistaken for infections and must be differentiated from them. These may arise in areas where buried sutures have been placed and can present as a small pustule or erosion in the suture line (Figure 36-5). The patient can complain of a "pimple" on the suture line or a piece of suture extruding from the incision line. This can occur when a buried suture is placed too close to the skin surface. Purulent material from these sites is sterile.

Suture reactions can range from mild, with only a spicule of suture "spitting," to more severe reactions in which the entire wound gets warm and boggy. These reactions are self-limited and can be calmed with intralesional injections of triamcinolone 2.5 mg/mL and warm compresses. Removal of reacting and spitting sutures can speed up resolution. Antibiotics are frequently given with severe reactions to cover the chance that there is also an element of infection. Suture reactions rarely affect the ultimate cosmetic outcome.

SCARRING

Scarring can occur in any patient operated on by any clinician. In some situations scarring is predictable and cannot be prevented. The deltoid area, the chest, and the back are prone to scarring because of either the skin tension in these areas, the thicker skin in these areas, or some unknown factor. Surgery on sebaceous skin, such as the type that appears on the nose, often leads to obvious incisional scars. The most important point is to warn the patient that in these areas excisional surgery will often result in scarring no matter who does the surgery. Therefore, on the back, chest, and deltoid areas, a shave technique should be used when it is an acceptable alternative because it can offer a better cosmetic result than an excision with sutures. If a patient is overly concerned about a scar or expresses the unrealistic desire to have absolutely no scar, it is better to recommend a plastic surgeon before the procedure than after.

Excessive or increased skin tension leads to a widened scar. This is the reason why buried sutures that decrease tension can improve cosmetic results. The increased skin tension in younger patients probably contributes to the widened scars seen in young patients compared with the narrow, fine scars seen in older patients. In Figure 36-6A, a widened scar is seen on a young woman's arm years after the wide excision of a melanoma.

Allowing sutures to remain in place for too long can also increase scarring. Complications such as infection, necrosis, or dehiscence can increase scarring (Figure 36-6B). Excessive skin tension often leads to dehiscence and scarring. Infection or necrosis often leads to dehiscence. Dehiscence may be prevented by using good excision planning, undermining when necessary, and using deep absorbable sutures to decrease skin tension across a wound. Tying sutures too tightly can also cause scarring.

Depressed scars may result from a deep shave biopsy or scarring within the dermal layer of the skin. Depressed scars can be excised or dermal fillers may be used.

The most important point when discussing potential scarring after surgery is to warn the patient about the risk of scarring or highly visible incision lines. The patient should understand that if scarring does occur, it can be treated with dermabrasion, intralesional steroids, laser resurfacing, or the yellow light laser used to treat persistent redness. See the cosmetic chapters in this book for the specifics of scar treatment.

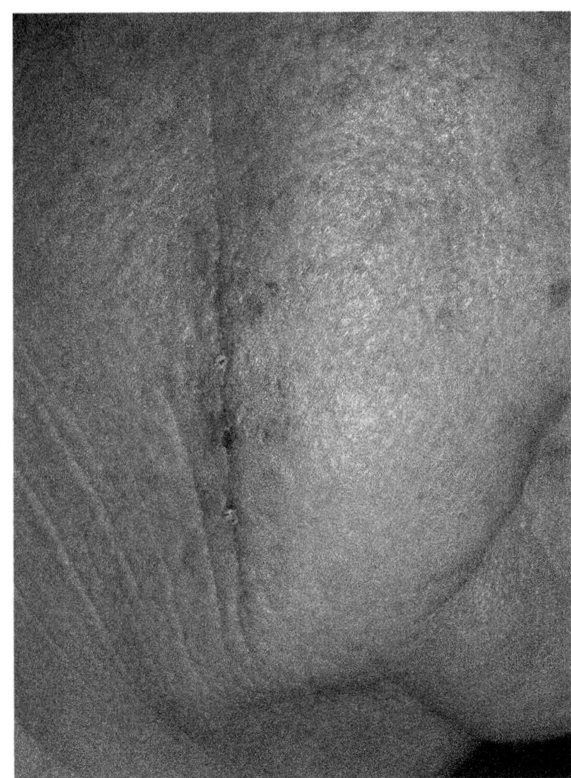

FIGURE 36-5 Spitting sutures along a facial repair. *(Courtesy of Richard P. Usatine, MD.)*

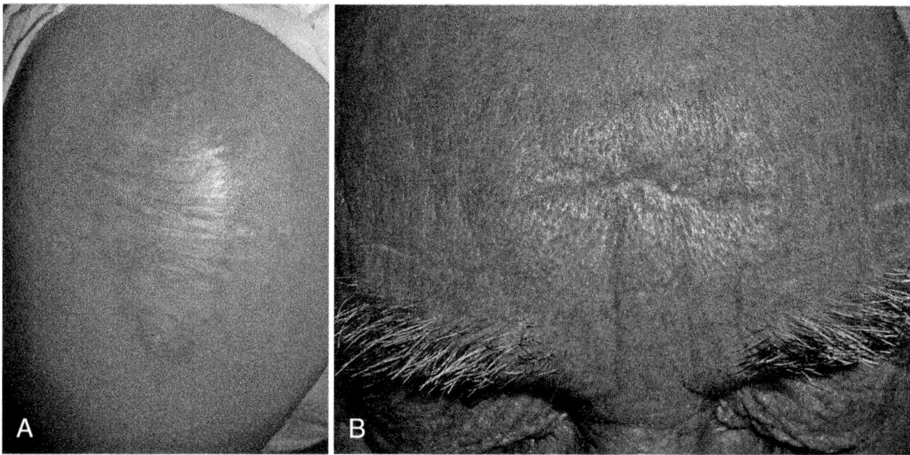

FIGURE 36-6 **(A)** Widened scar on the upper arm of a young woman with a melanoma excised years before. **(B)** Scarring that occurred after a wound infection. Note the milia seen at the wound edge, which can occur at sites of wound healing. *(Courtesy of Richard P. Usatine, MD.)*

WOUND DEHISCENCE

If a wound dehiscence occurs without evidence of infection, it might be advisable to resuture the wound with interrupted sutures and start the patient on antibiotics. The sutures may only have to be left in place for half the normal time because the fibroblasts have already initiated the wound site and the wound is partially healed. The cause of the dehiscence may need to be addressed if significant wound tension exists. A buried absorbable suture may decrease the wound tension.

If infection or a hematoma is the cause of dehiscence, the wound should be opened and irrigated, and the patient should be started on antibiotics. The wound should be cleansed daily and left to heal naturally. It will usually take at least 3 to 4 weeks before the wound healing is complete. The patient should be informed that a scar revision may be performed at a later time if desired.

HYPOPIGMENTATION

Hypopigmentation is most likely to occur with the following procedures: cryosurgery, ED&C, and shave biopsies. Although it may be cosmetically worse in darker skinned persons, it can occur in anyone. Patients must be warned of this complication, which can be permanent. Cryotherapy to treat nonmelanoma skin cancers is likely to cause hypopigmentation because of the long freeze times that are used (Figure 36-7A). Even a simple shave excision can lead to hypopigmentation (Figure 36-7B).

FLAP NECROSIS

A long, thin advancement flap in violation of the 3:1 ratio runs a high risk of distal flap tip necrosis (Figure 36-8). Patients who smoke excessively experience a much higher risk of flap tip necrosis and flap failure, and encouraging smoking cessation in the perioperative and postoperative course is helpful to achieve the best healing. The use of flaps must also be carefully weighed in those patients who may have underlying skin conditions that can lead to increased complications. Decreased flexibility and therefore impaired movement of skin can be seen in patients with extensive scarring from burns or other injuries, previous radiotherapy, or an underlying skin disease such as scleroderma. Decreased perfusion of skin leading to flap failure or infection can be

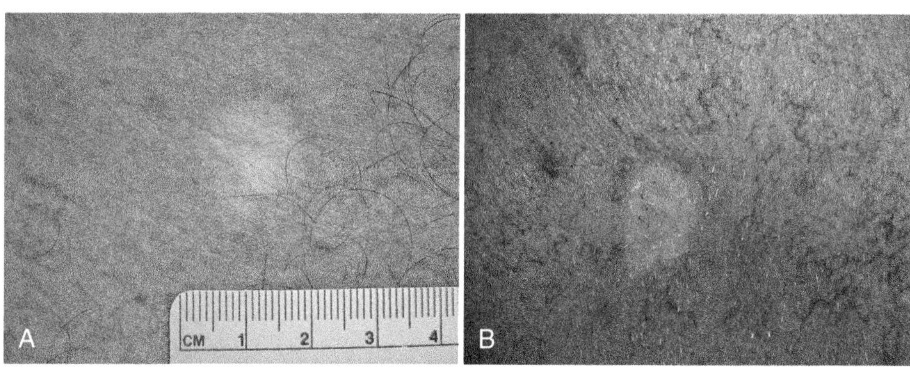

FIGURE 36-7 **(A)** Hypopigmentation that occurred after cryosurgery of a superficial BCC. **(B)** Hypopigmentation after the shave excision of a basal cell carcinoma on sun-damaged skin. *(Courtesy of Richard P. Usatine, MD.)*

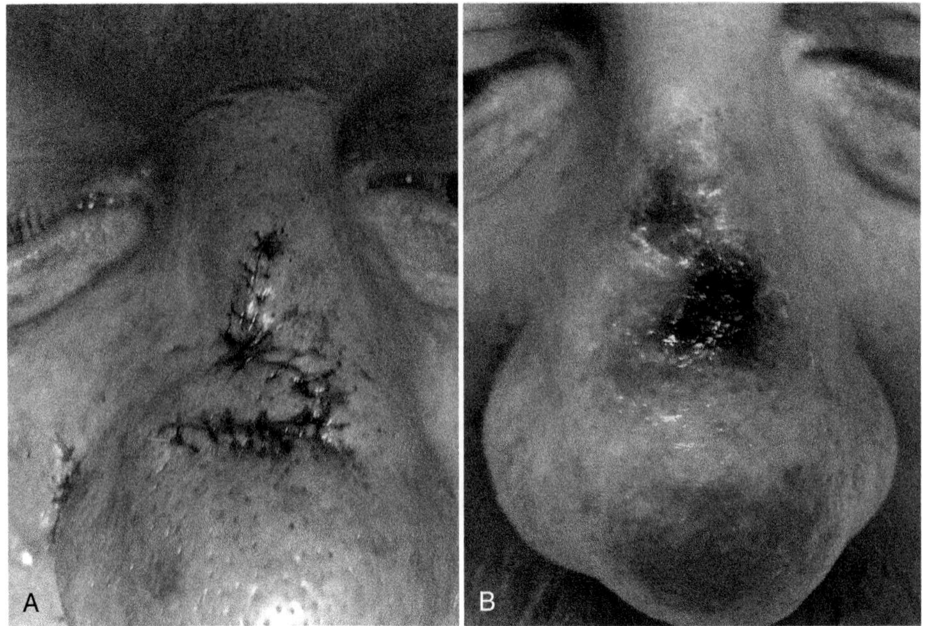

FIGURE 36-8 (A, B) Flap necrosis in a patient unable to quit smoking. *(Courtesy of Ryan O'Quinn, MD.)*

seen in conditions such as diabetes mellitus, lung disease, or poor circulation secondary to atherosclerosis, especially in peripheral areas. Finally, the use of a flap may not be possible in patients with extremely thin skin that will not bear the stresses of flap movement such as elderly patients with extreme photodamage or long-term users of corticosteroids.

NERVE DAMAGE

Numbness is a common complaint from patients after cutaneous surgery. It usually resolves in about 6 to 12 months after the nerves have regrown and arborized. The concern from cutaneous surgery is damaging a superficial motor nerve. The three motor nerves that are most vulnerable to damage are the temporal branch of the facial nerve, the spinal accessory nerve, and the marginal branch of the mandibular nerve.

The temporal branch of the facial nerve can be damaged by surgery to the temple area. The nerve lies just below the superficial musculoaponeurotic system (SMAS). It can be difficult to see, and there is enough anatomic variation that it can be unpredictable in its location. One way to locate the nerve is to draw an imaginary line from the tragus to the eyebrow and another imaginary line from the tragus to the upper forehead wrinkle area (Figure 36-9). The area between these two lines within the temple area is where the temporal branch of the facial nerve is most superficial. If this nerve is cut, the patient will not be able to wrinkle the forehead because the innervation to the frontalis muscle is lost. The patient will also have a permanent inability to raise the upper eyelid (Figure 36-10). If any surgery is performed in this area, it is important to discuss this risk with the patient in the informed consent process. Also explain that the anesthesia after surgery alone can cause a temporary paralysis of this nerve (See Figure 11-2B in Chapter 11, *The Elliptical Excision*). When electrodesiccation and curettage is an option for a superficial skin cancer in this area, it may be a good choice. Mohs surgery is also an appropriate technique in this area because the tissue is removed layer by layer by an experienced surgeon.

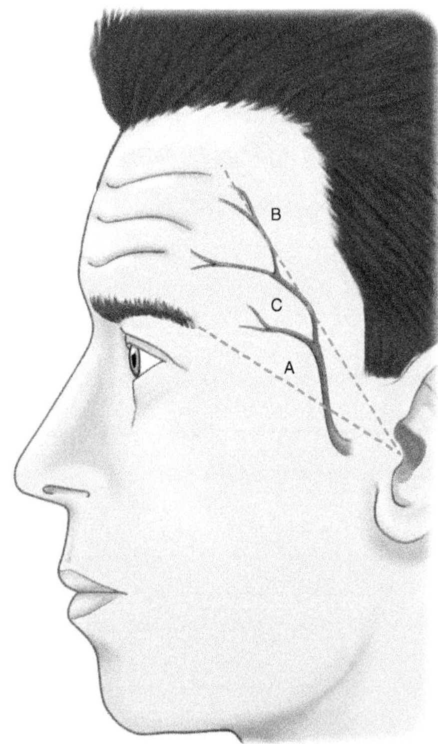

FIGURE 36-9 Drawing of the temporal branch of the facial nerve. *(From Usatine RP.* Skin Surgery: A Practical Guide. *St. Louis, MO: Mosby; 1998.)*

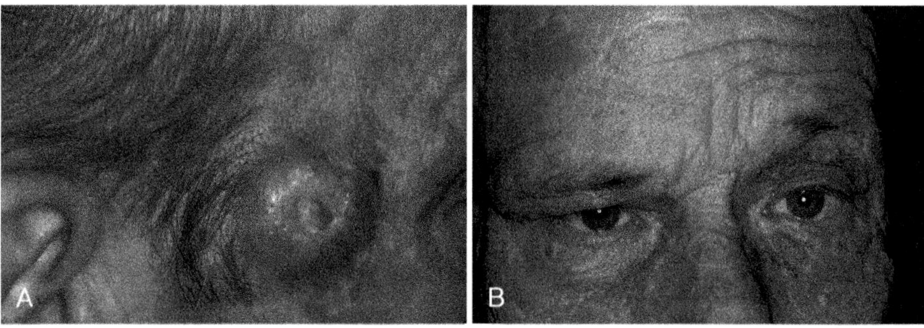

FIGURE 36-10 **(A)** BCC in the region of the temporal branch of the facial nerve. **(B)** Permanent inability to raise the eyebrow after the temporal branch of the facial nerve was cut during surgical excision of the BCC. *(From Usatine RP.* Skin Surgery: A Practical Guide. *St. Louis, MO: Mosby; 1998.)*

The spinal accessory nerve lies within the posterior triangle posterior to the sternocleidomastoid muscle (Figure 36-11). The nerve can lie very superficially posterior to the sternocleidomastoid muscle at the level of the thyroid cartilage notch. If this nerve is cut, the patient will lose major innervation to the trapezius muscle, resulting in impaired mobility of the scapula and shoulder.

The marginal branch of the mandibular nerve (Figure 36-12) is the third nerve in the head and neck area that is vulnerable to injury during surgery. If it is cut then motor innervation to the depressor anguli oris and depressor labii inferioris can be lost. This results in a cosmetic deformity and imbalance in the appearance of the mouth, especially when the mouth is opened or when the patient wants to frown. Fortunately the nerve is not that superficial but each clinician operating in the area of the lower mandible should be aware of this branch of the facial nerve.

RECURRENCE OF A LESION OR SKIN CANCER

There is almost nothing in the practice of medicine that is a 100% guarantee. Mohs' micrographic surgery for the removal of skin cancer has a cure rate of only 99% in primary skin cancers. Most other surgical techniques have cure rates of about 90%, depending on a number

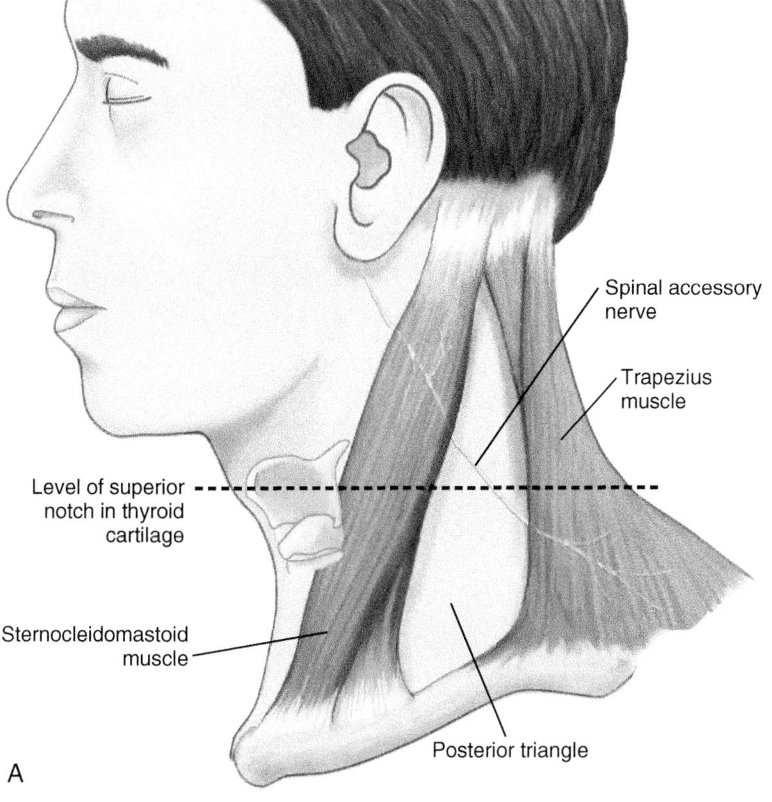

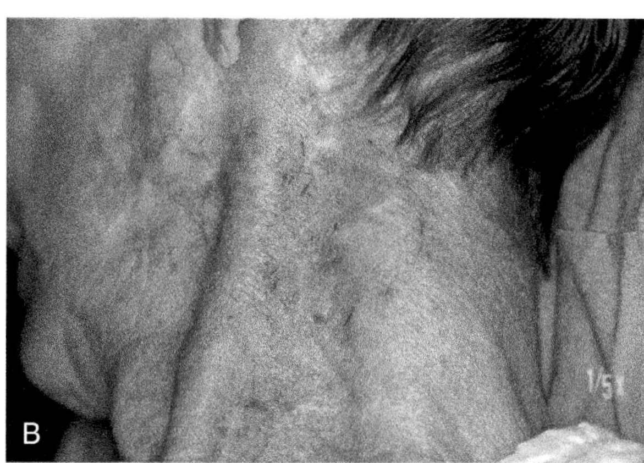

FIGURE 36-11 **(A)** Drawing of the spinal accessory nerve in the posterior triangle of the neck. **(B)** Recurrent BCC over the site of the spinal accessory nerve in the posterior triangle of the neck. Care must be taken to avoid cutting that nerve if possible. *(A: From Usatine RP.* Skin Surgery: A Practical Guide. *St. Louis, MO: Mosby; 1998.)*

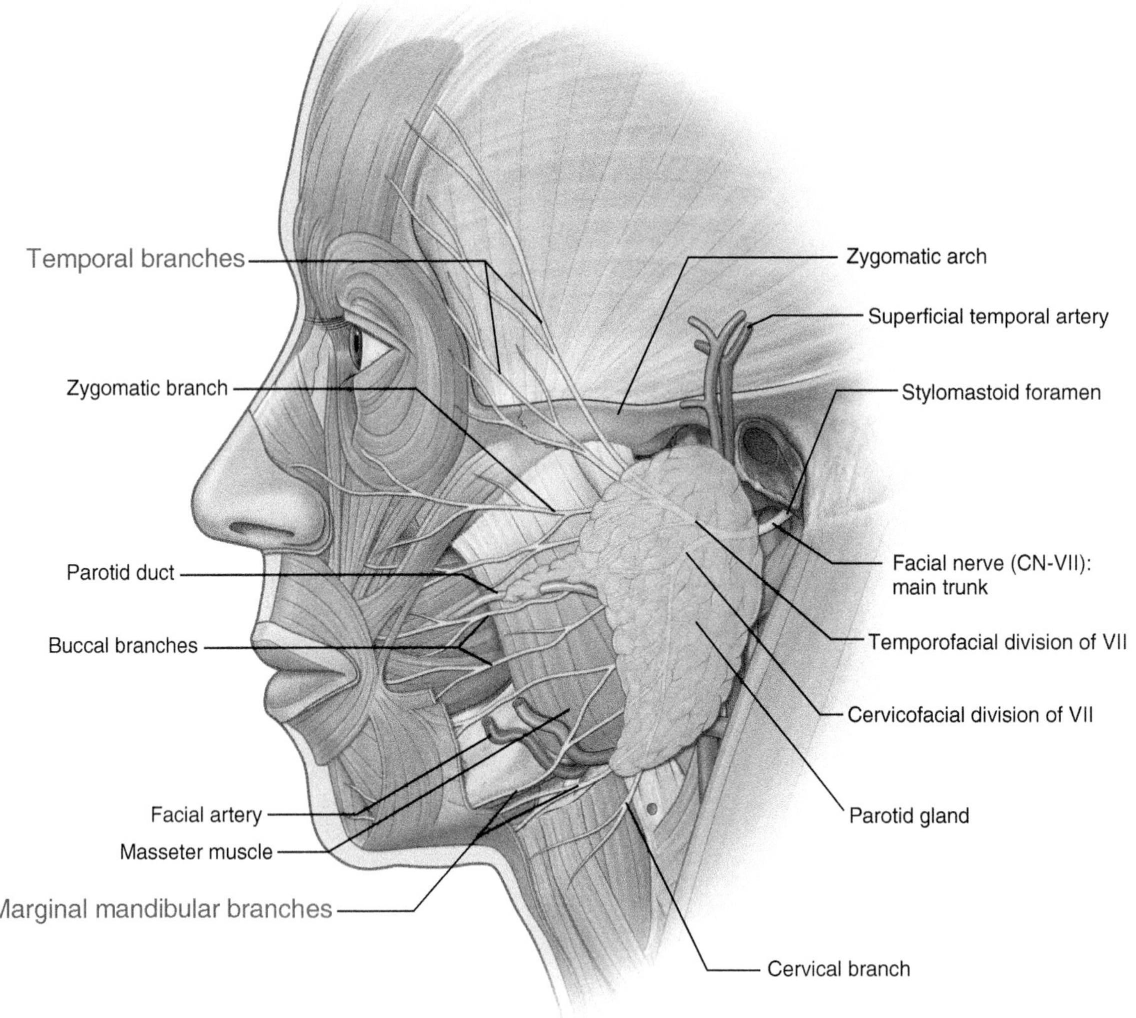

FIGURE 36-12 The branches of the facial nerve most prone to be cut during facial surgery include the temporal branches and the marginal mandibular branches. *(From Vidimos A, Ammirati C, Poblete-Lopez C.* Dermatologic Surgery. *London: Saunders; 2008.)*

of factors. Lipomas, cysts, and nevi (especially if they are removed with a shave) can all recur. Although recurrent lesions may be considered a complication, the patient and clinician should both realize that recurrences will occur in a small percentage of cases. When a recurrent lesion develops, the lesion will usually need to be excised again. In Figure 36-13, a BCC recurred in the incision line after a large flap was placed on the neck.

With regards to recurrence of BCC, one study showed that Mohs surgery had significantly fewer recurrences for the treatment of facial *recurrent* BCC than after standard surgical excision.[8] However, there was no significant difference in recurrence of *primary* BCC between Mohs surgery and surgical excision in this study.[8]

In a systematic review of treatment modalities for primary BCC, the following recurrence rates were noted:

- Mohs micrographic surgery (three studies, $n = 2660$): recurrence rate 0.8 to 1.1.
- Surgical excision (three studies, $n = 1303$): recurrence rate was 2 to 8.1. The mean cumulative 5-year rate (all three studies) was 5.3.
- Cryosurgery (four studies, $n = 796$): recurrence rate 3.0 to 4.3. The cumulative 5-year rate (three studies) ranged from 0 to 16.5.
- Curettage and desiccation (six studies, $n = 4212$): recurrence rate ranged from 4.3 to 18.1. The cumulative 5-year rate ranged from 5.7 to 18.8.[9]

Therefore, it is important to go over possible recurrence rates with patients before the final procedure is chosen. Even benign lesions like pyogenic granulomas can recur if all of the abnormal tissue is not removed at the time of surgery (Figure 36-14).

MAKING MISTAKES

As a clinician, it feels awful to make a mistake that leads to harming a patient. It may also feel bad when a

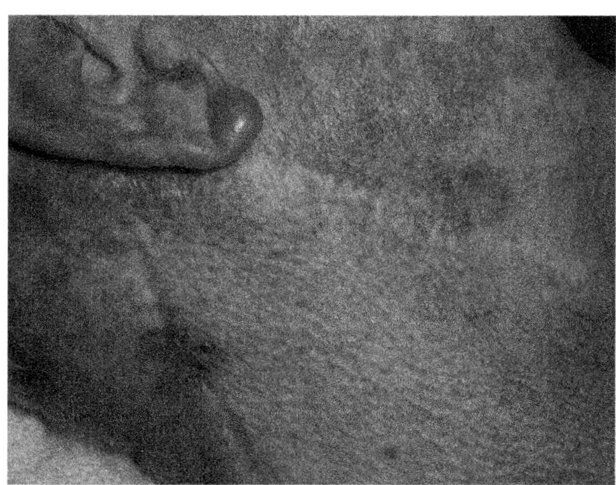

FIGURE 36-13 Recurrent BCC at two sites along the area of a large flap repair to an extensive BCC on the neck. *(Courtesy of Richard P. Usatine, MD.)*

patient gets a less than optimal cosmetic result after a surgical procedure. We all took the oath "First, do no harm." In performing skin surgery it is inevitable that you will have wounds that dehisce, scars that are larger than expected, flaps that necrose, and infections and hematomas that will occur in surgical sites. These are known complications of skin surgery and may not be caused by an error on your part. However, it is also possible for all of us to make mistakes. Postoperative infections and hematomas can occur even in the most carefully performed surgery. However, if a clinician is in a rush and uses less careful sterile technique or pays less attention to bleeders, he or she may contribute to these complications. We have presented ways to minimize complications, but poor outcomes can and do happen. In all cases, the goal will be to provide the patient with the best possible outcome.

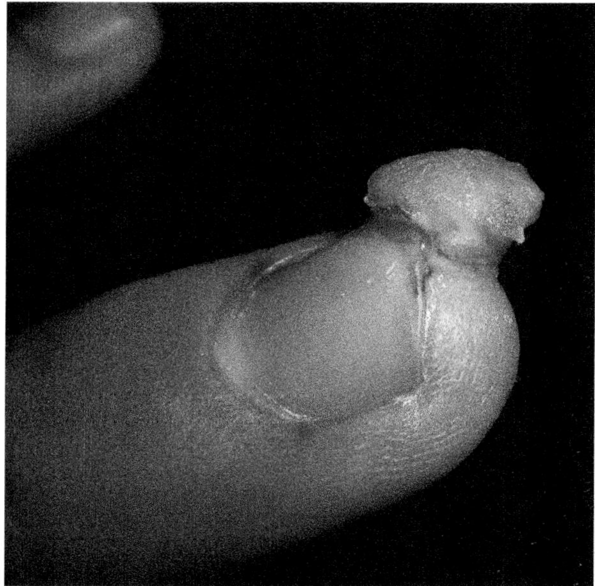

FIGURE 36-14 Recurrent pyogenic granuloma on the finger after previous excision. *(Courtesy of Richard P. Usatine, MD.)*

It is always important to express empathy to the patient and/or patient's family after an adverse surgical event. "I am sorry" is an appropriate expression of empathy that does not express fault. In the book *Sorry Works!* the authors make a strong case for using the phrase "I'm sorry" along with disclosure, apologies, and relationships to prevent medical malpractice claims.[10] They make the distinction that the phrase "I'm sorry" is an expression of empathy and "I apologize" is a communication that expresses responsibility along with empathy. They suggest to only apologize after due diligence has proven that a medical error occurred.

The authors make the case that it is better to disclose an error than to attempt to cover it up.[10] They state that "people can actually live with mistakes but they do not accept or tolerate cover-ups." They suggest the use of honesty, candor, and a real commitment to fix problems when something goes wrong. Showing empathy works by making a difficult situation a little better. To learn more about how to prevent lawsuits and improve relationships with patients during and after an adverse event, consult the book *Sorry Works!* and the website www.sorryworks.net.

CONCLUSION

Careful planning and execution of surgery can prevent most complications. Early recognition of complications and rapid treatment can minimize the potential adverse outcomes that can occur when complications are allowed to progress untreated.

References

1. Amici JM, Rogues AM, Lasheras A, *et al.* A prospective study of the incidence of complications associated with dermatological surgery. *Br J Dermatol.* 2005;153:967–971.
2. Rogues AM, Lasheras A, Amici JM, *et al.* Infection control practices and infectious complications in dermatological surgery. *J Hosp Infect.* 2007;65:258–263.
3. Dixon AJ, Dixon MP, Askew DA, Wilkinson D. Prospective study of wound infections in dermatologic surgery in the absence of prophylactic antibiotics. *Dermatol Surg.* 2006;32:819–826.
4. Wahie S, Lawrence CM. Wound complications following diagnostic skin biopsies in dermatology inpatients. *Arch Dermatol.* 2007;143:1267–1271.
5. Rhinehart MB, Murphy MM, Farley MF, Albertini JG. Sterile versus nonsterile gloves during Mohs micrographic surgery: infection rate is not affected. *Dermatol Surg.* 2006;32:170–176.
6. Wright TI, Baddour LM, Berbari EF, *et al.* Antibiotic prophylaxis in dermatologic surgery: advisory statement 2008. *J Am Acad Dermatol.* 2008;59:464–473.
7. Huether MJ, Griego RD, Brodland DG, Zitelli JA. Clindamycin for intraincisional antibiotic prophylaxis in dermatologic surgery. *Arch Dermatol.* 2002;138:1145–1148.
8. Mosterd K, Krekels GA, Nieman FH, *et al.* Surgical excision versus Mohs' micrographic surgery for primary and recurrent basal-cell carcinoma of the face: a prospective randomised controlled trial with 5-years' follow-up. *Lancet Oncol.* 2008;9:1149–1156.
9. Thissen MR, Neumann MH, Schouten LJ. A systematic review of treatment modalities for primary basal cell carcinomas. *Arch Dermatol.* 1999;135:1177–1183.
10. Wojcieszak D, Saxton W, Finklestein M. Sorry Works! Disclosure, Apology, and Relationships Prevent Medical Malpractice Claims. Bloomington, IN: Author House; 2008.

37 When to Refer/Mohs Surgery

JOHN L. PFENNINGER, MD • RICHARD P. USATINE, MD

The primary care clinician handles a multitude of problems and each person has his or her own level of comfort and expertise. There are no hard-and-fast guidelines to determine when a consultation/referral should be obtained. Some clinicians will feel very comfortable performing extensive flaps, whereas others will be anxious about doing a fairly straightforward skin biopsy. This chapter provides some general guidelines to help gauge when, and if, the expertise of another clinician is needed.

WHEN TO REFER

In general, a *referral* means that the patient is being turned over to another physician for care. A *consult* asks for direction, but the patient remains under the care of the consulting physician. In practice, these two terms are often used interchangeably. The term *verbal consult* is often used to relay the fact that the case was discussed with someone else for input and direction as to proper care but not referred formally. Although discouraged on a legal basis, it is commonly done and for simple questions such as "What should the margins of the excision be?" it functionally works well.

Medical-legal considerations are important. Hospitals may limit privileges and require that a referral be made for performing certain procedures in hospital-owned facilities. In such cases, it may not be a matter of expertise, but rather of legal restriction as to what may be done.

HMOs and insurance companies may also limit the ability of a clinician to employ the full use of his or her skills. Some restrict payment to certain specialties only. It is not a matter of competence (despite the insurers' claims), but rather a matter of rules, regulations, and "protecting turf."

It is important for clinicians to always provide *complete disclosure* to patients about their background and training. Patients must not be misled into thinking that the physician assistant, nurse practitioner, family physician, or internist is a dermatologist or plastic surgeon. The simplest procedure for professionals may appear to be very complex to the patient and can be a fearful ordeal. It is always appropriate to mention that a dermatologist, plastic surgeon, or referral to some other center is readily available should the patient so desire. A statement such as "This is a common procedure that has few complications. I perform it frequently and I would be happy to do it for you. However, if you'd like to see someone else, I understand and can easily arrange a referral" goes a long way toward putting the patient at ease. *Do not forget the family members* in the equation. Some may be extremely concerned about a scar, even though it involves an elderly parent. These issues need to be discussed and dealt with prior to performing any procedure. If the patient or the family appears to be hesitant, it is prudent to make a referral.

No clinician will ever feel totally comfortable in every situation that he or she will encounter. Sometimes, too, a straightforward diagnosis and planned treatment becomes more complicated than expected. It is important to have *lines of communication open with other specialists* so that when these "complications" do arise, the clinician has support. Whether this consultant is a plastic surgeon, dermatologist, general surgeon, or another colleague who performs the same procedure, it is important to have the backup. Immediate complications will most likely involve bleeding or the inability to close a large, gaping wound; wound dehiscence; or nonhealing of a treated site. Rarely, a nerve may be transected or the repair may leave the surrounding structures distorted. Long-term complications include scarring, missing a diagnosis, or recurrence.

Clinicians should not be hesitant to perform a skin biopsy. Multiple methods are available (see Chapters 8 through 11). Complications are so rare, and the benefits are so great, that all clinicians, especially those in primary care, should consider mastering this skill. If one wants to limit procedural acumen solely to skin biopsies, then referral would be necessary for many findings. However, the average primary care clinician should be able to evaluate and treat 95% of all dermatologic conditions that come into the office using the techniques described in this text. Cryotherapy, electrosurgery, injection techniques, laceration repair, and simple incisions/excisions will be adequate to treat the majority of conditions. When the excisions become larger and more complicated, it is then that many patients may need to be referred.

Keeping in mind all of the considerations noted above, *the clinician will individually define when a referral is indicated*. As expertise increases with training and experience, fewer consultations and referrals will be needed. General guidelines for when to consult and when to refer include the following:

1. *Lack of experience* with the method needed for diagnosis and/or treatment.
2. *Significant cosmetic concerns* with the skills for removal being beyond the practitioner's comfort level.
3. *Large lesions,* whether benign or malignant. These often need to be referred to a specialist. "Large" is relative and depends on the practitioner's expertise and the nature of the lesion (benign or malignant, location, new or recurrent, etc.).
4. *Request by the patient or the family for a referral.*
5. *A poor or questionable patient–doctor relationship.*
6. *An uncooperative patient.*
7. *Medical-legal or insurance requirements/regulations.*

8. *Advanced and/or complicated disease.* In general, the major considerations for aggressiveness of a tumor are histologic type, size, and location of the lesion.

All factors should be considered when deciding whether or not to make a referral. The skin cancers that cause the most concern for all of us can be categorized as follows by histologic type (from least to most aggressive):

Basal Cell Carcinoma (BCC)

- Superficial
- Nodular/ulcerative
- Micronodular
- Infiltrating
- Morpheaform (aggressive, sclerotic)
- Perineural invasion.

Squamous Cell Carcinoma (SCC)

- *In situ* (depending on size and location, generally does not need aggressive treatment)
- Invasive (more aggressive on mucus membranes and non-sun-exposed areas)
- Perineural invasion.

Melanoma

- *In situ*
- Superficial
- <1-mm invasion with no ulceration or neural involvement
- >1-mm invasion or with ulceration or neural involvement.

Other, More Rare and Potentially Aggressive Cancers

- These include dermatofibrosarcoma protuberans, cutaneous T-cell lymphoma, Merkel cell carcinoma. See the end of Chapter 34 for photographs and further information on these skin cancers.

The following are examples of when most primary care clinicians might consider a referral[1–6]:

1. *A melanoma with invasion 1 mm or deeper or if there is neural involvement or ulceration:* Some would want to refer all melanomas. However, those less than 1 mm in depth are generally treated with simple excision using 1-cm free margins. Once the melanoma has invaded 1 mm or more, then the workup becomes much more extensive, often including a sentinel node biopsy. Surgical oncologists and melanoma clinics that deal with melanomas on a routine basis are more likely to provide the patient with more options for an improved outcome. Most dermatologists refer melanomas with Breslow depth over 1.0 mm because they do not do sentinel node biopsies.
2. *Rare, unusual tumors or metastatic disease:* for example, dermatofibrosarcoma protuberans, Merkel cell tumors, and any metastatic cancer to or from the skin (Figure 37-1).
3. *Recurrent skin cancers,* such as SCC, which can metastasize: Even BCCs, which generally do not metastasize, can recur and require large margins for resection (Figure 37-2). Mohs micrographic surgery or radiation may be indicated in such cases.

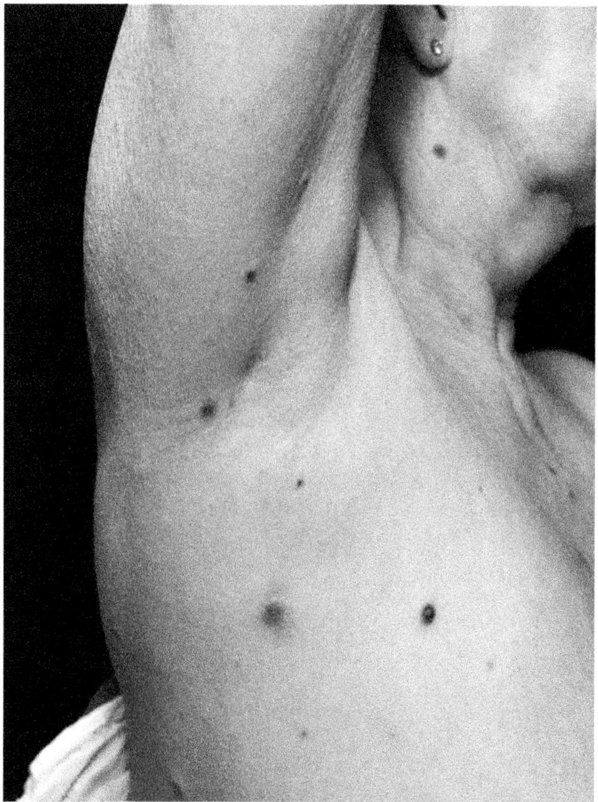

FIGURE 37-1 These scattered black nodules are caused by metastatic melanoma to the skin. The patient was referred directly to medical oncology. *(Copyright Richard P. Usatine, MD.)*

4. *Large nonmelanoma skin cancers* (NMSC) >1 cm in length or diameter, unless the clinician is capable of performing large excisions: Many basal cell carcinomas <1 cm in size can be treated with ablation/destruction techniques, such as electrodesiccation and curettage or cryotherapy. Small SCC < 1 cm can be excised with 5-mm margins. Although some physicians refer all skin cancers for Mohs surgery, this is not a true cost-effective approach. A higher

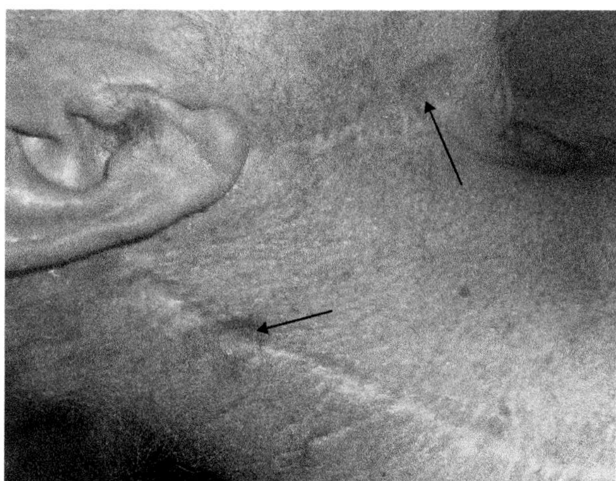

FIGURE 37-2 Two recurrent BCCs are seen along the scar from a previous large flap that was used after a large BCC was removed from the neck. The patient was referred for Mohs surgery. *(Copyright Richard P. Usatine, MD.)*

cure rate is sometimes cited to justify Mohs, but with lesions <1 cm (BCCs and SCCs), the benefit is very small, and the scarring may be less with ablative techniques.

5. *High-risk anatomic areas*: temporal (temporal branch of facial nerve), lateral neck (spinal accessory nerve), nasolabial groove with ablation (higher recurrence of skin cancers when size is over 0.6 cm), lacrimal duct area (scarring), excisions near eyelids (ectropion or entropion).
6. *High-risk lesions:* These include SCC on the lips, temple, and ears as these have a 10% rate of metastasis. SCC also requires more aggressive treatment if it is >2 cm, occurs in a scar, or there is evidence of perineural invasion.
7. *High-risk patients:* These include those with diabetes, immune suppression, obesity, peripheral vascular disease, stasis dermatitis/pedal edema with lower extremity lesions, alcoholics, HIV/AIDS, malnutrition.
8. *Areas where even normal scarring may be especially critical:* For example, the eyelid margins and face, especially in the young/female patient; the vermilion border.
9. Patients who easily form *hypertrophic- or keloid-scars.*
10. *Non-adherent patients or those with unrealistic expectations.*

MOHS SURGERY

Mohs surgery is a technique in which careful mapping of a lesion (usually an NMSC) is performed using marking dye at the time of the removal.[7,8] The lesion is excised and immediately processed histologically. Areas of residual tumor are identified under the microscope by the Mohs surgeon and further excision completed in the specific areas needed. It is generally performed in an office under local anesthesia. The advantage is that the entire tumor can be removed with cure rates as high as 99%. The disadvantages are the time and costs to perform the procedure. Most reviews have found it to be cost effective for high-risk cancers. Potential indications for Mohs are noted in Box 37-1. Medicare will cover reimbursement for Mohs micrographic surgery for the diagnoses and indications listed in Box 37-2.

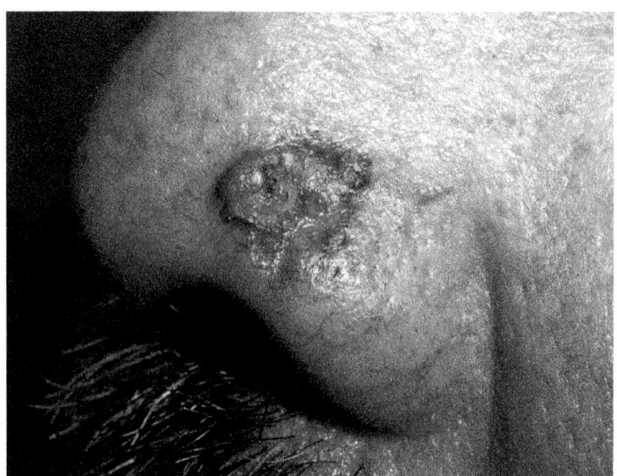

FIGURE 37-3 Resecting this pigmented BCC on the nose can easily result in a nasal deformity. The patient was referred for Mohs surgery to get the highest cure rates and the best cosmetic result. *(Copyright Richard P. Usatine, MD.)*

BOX 37-1 ***Indications for Mohs Micrographic Surgery in Patients with High-Risk Skin Cancers***

- High-risk anatomic location (eyelids, nose, ears, lips, genitalia, fingers)
- Large tumors (20 mm or more in diameter) on the torso and extremities
- Recurrent tumors after previous excision or destruction
- Tumors occurring in previous sites of radiation therapy
- Tumors with aggressive histologic patterns (small strand, infiltrative, or morphea-like growth in BCCs; perineural invasion; or poorly differentiated histology or deep invasion in squamous cell carcinomas)
- Tumors in immunosuppressed patients
- Tumors with involved borders or vague clinical margins, or incompletely excised tumors (positive histologic margins after resection).

Source: Adapted from National Comprehensive Cancer Network. *Clinical Practice Guidelines in Oncology: Basal Cell and Squamous Cell Skin Cancers.* Version 1.2010. Accessed online April 13, 2010, at http://www.nccn.org/professionals/physician_gls/PDF/nmsc.pdf.

Patient Selection

Examples of patients that were referred for Mohs surgery including those with the following lesions:

- Pigmented BCC on the nose, newly diagnosed (Figure 37-3)
- BCC on the upper lip close to the vermilion border (Figure 37-4)
- Infiltrating BCC on the cheek (Figure 37-5)
- Recurrent squamous cell carcinoma on the cheek (Figure 37-6)
- BCC on the ear, newly diagnosed (Figure 37-7).

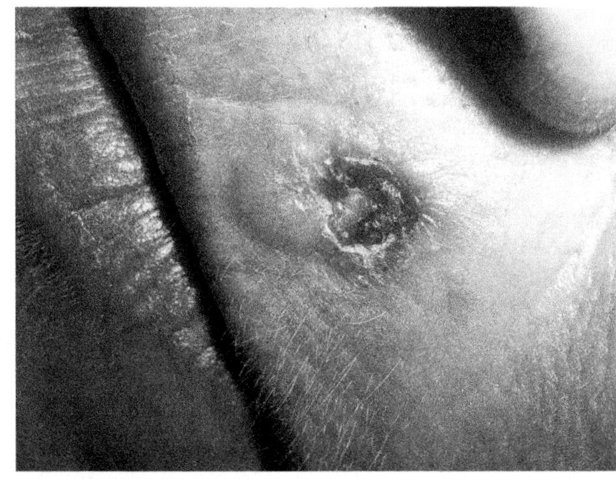

FIGURE 37-4 The BCC on the upper lip approaches the vermilion border. Unless you are experienced in facial flaps, this is a good patient to refer for Mohs surgery and a flap repair. *(Copyright Richard P. Usatine, MD.)*

BOX 37-2 ***Medicare Covers Reimbursement for Mohs Surgery for these Diagnoses***

1. Basal cell, squamous cell, or basalosquamous cell carcinomas in anatomic locations where they are prone to recur:
   - Central facial areas, periauricular, nose, and temple areas of the face (the so-called "mask area" of the face)
   - Lips, cutaneous and vermilion
   - Eyelids and periorbital areas
   - Auricular helix and canal
   - Chin and mandible.
2. Other skin lesions:
   - Angiosarcoma of the skin
   - Keratoacanthoma, recurrent
   - Dermatofibrosarcoma protuberans
   - Malignant fibrous histiocytoma
   - Sebaceous gland carcinoma
   - Microcystic adnexal carcinoma
   - Extramammary Paget's disease
   - Bowenoid papulosis
   - Merkel cell carcinoma
   - Bowen's disease (squamous cell carcinoma *in situ*)
   - Adenoid type of squamous cell carcinoma
   - Rapid growth in a squamous cell carcinoma
   - Long-standing duration of a squamous cell carcinoma
   - Verrucous carcinoma
   - Atypical fibroxanthoma
   - Leiomyosarcoma or other spindle cell neoplasms of the skin
   - Adenocystic carcinoma of the skin
   - Erythroplasia of Queyrat
   - Oral and central facial, paranasal sinus neoplasm
   - Apocrine carcinoma of the skin
   - Malignant melanoma (facial, auricular, genital and digital) when anatomic or technical difficulties do not allow conventional excision with appropriate margins.
3. Basal cell carcinomas, squamous cell carcinomas, or basalosquamous carcinomas that have one or more of the following features:
   - Recurrent
   - Aggressive pathology in the following areas: hands and feet, genitalia, and nail unit/periungual
   - Large size (2.0 cm or greater)
   - Positive margins on recent excision
   - Poorly defined borders
   - In the very young (<40 years old)
   - Radiation induced
   - In patients with proven difficulty with skin cancers or who are immunocompromised
   - Basal cell nevus syndrome
   - In an old scar (e.g., a Marjolin's ulcer)
   - Associated with xeroderma pigmentosum
   - Perineural invasion on biopsy
   - Deeply infiltrating lesion or difficulty estimating depth of lesion.

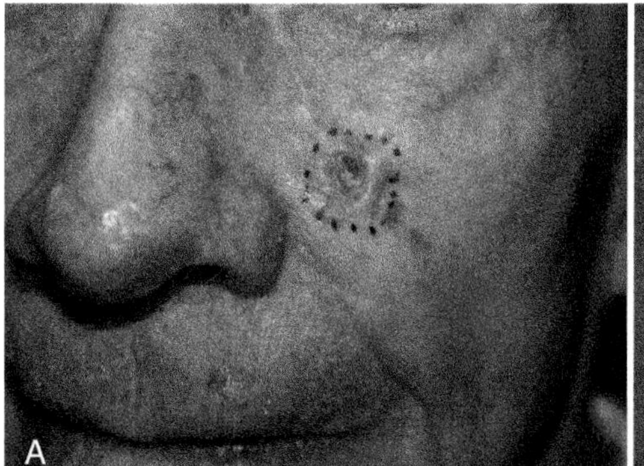

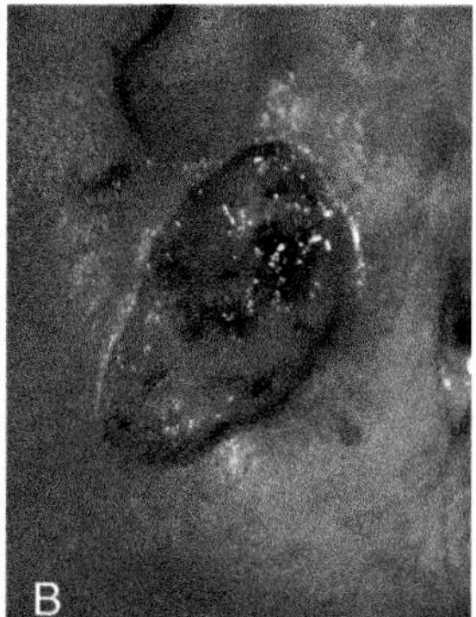

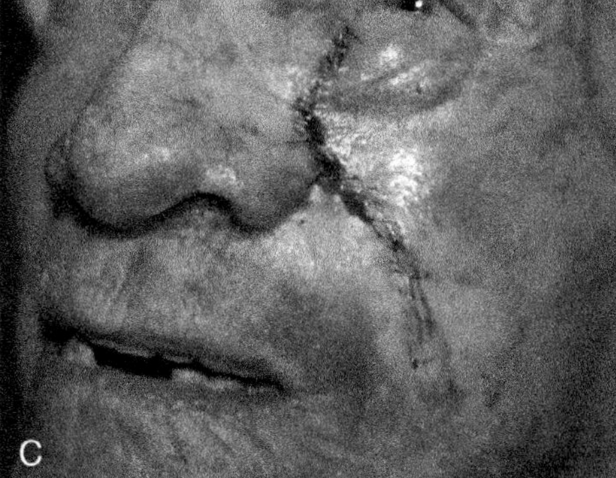

FIGURE 37-5 **(A)** This patient was referred for Mohs surgery to treat his sclerosing BCC. **(B)** The BCC had extensively infiltrated his cheek and required three stages to get clear margins. **(C)** A repair was able to close the defect to heal by primary intention. *(Courtesy of Ryan O'Quinn, MD.)*

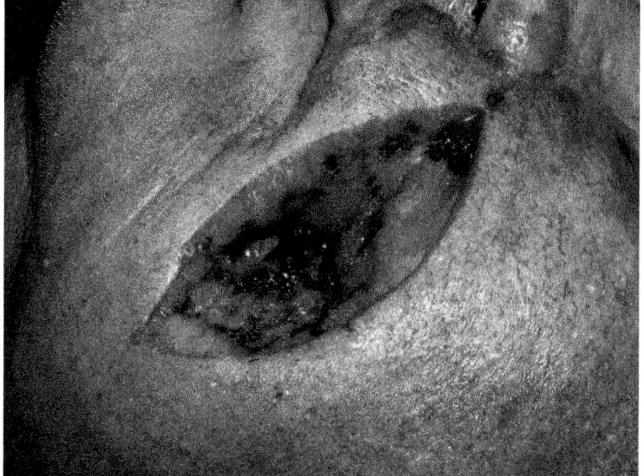

FIGURE 37-6 Squamous cell carcinoma was found to be recurrent along the excision scar on the face. When Mohs surgery was performed, the SCC was found to have infiltrated deeply and widely resulting in the defect in this image. *(Copyright Richard P. Usatine, MD.)*

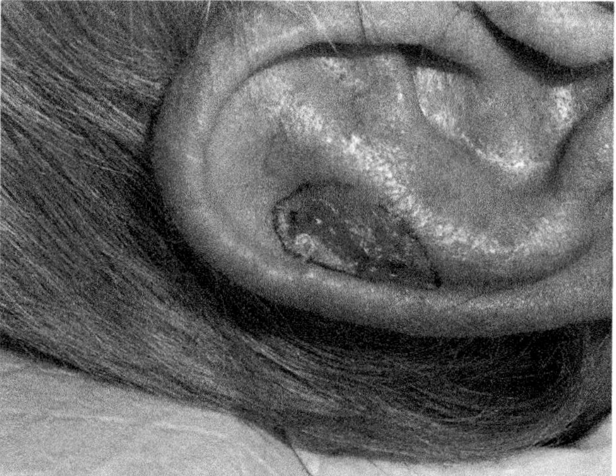

FIGURE 37-7 A new BCC was diagnosed on the pinna and the patient was referred for Mohs surgery. See next figures. *(Copyright Richard P. Usatine, MD.)*

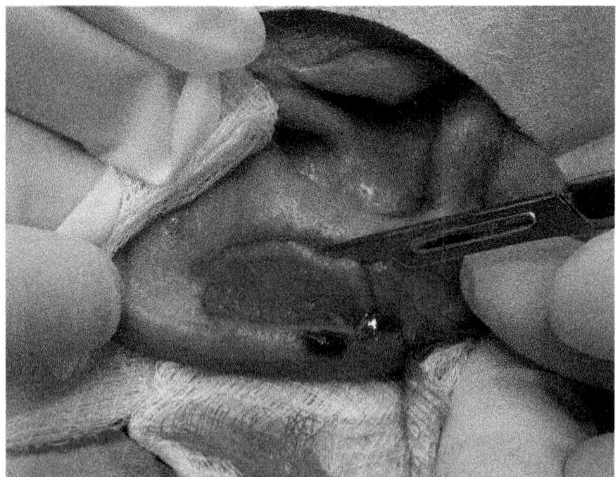

FIGURE 37-8 After debulking the tumor, the Mohs surgeon carefully removes a segment of the skin with margins laterally and deep. *(Copyright Richard P. Usatine, MD.)*

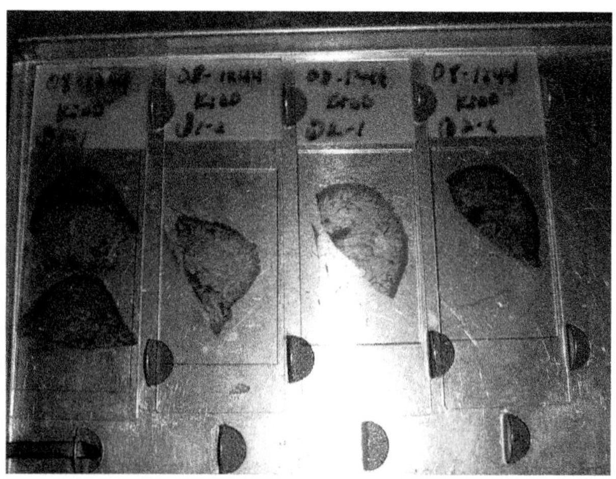

FIGURE 37-9 Mohs slides in the tray ready to be viewed under the microscope. *(Copyright Richard P. Usatine, MD.)*

Performing Mohs Surgery

See video on the DVD for further learning. 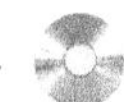

1. Local anesthetic with lidocaine and epinephrine is administered.
2. The tumor is debulked with a scalpel and discarded.
3. A saucer-shaped section of the remaining tumor including lateral and deep margins is cut out (Figure 37-8).
4. The piece is processed, including inking and cut into four quarters if the pieces are too large for a single slide.
5. The laboratory technician freezes and stains the segments (Figure 37-9).
6. The Mohs surgeon reads the histology looking at all margins.
7. If there are any positive margins, a second stage is performed.
8. The process continues until there are completely clear margins.
9. The defect is repaired using Burow's triangles to create a simple ellipse or a more elaborate flap.

Standard pathology for an ellipse involves bread loaf examination of the tissue (Figure 37-10). Mohs surgery is done with a more complete examination of the margin (Figure 37-11).

One way to consider who to refer is to look at Figure 37-12 of the H-zone and the levels of recurrence risk. The H-zone resembles the letter "H" and is the highest risk area.

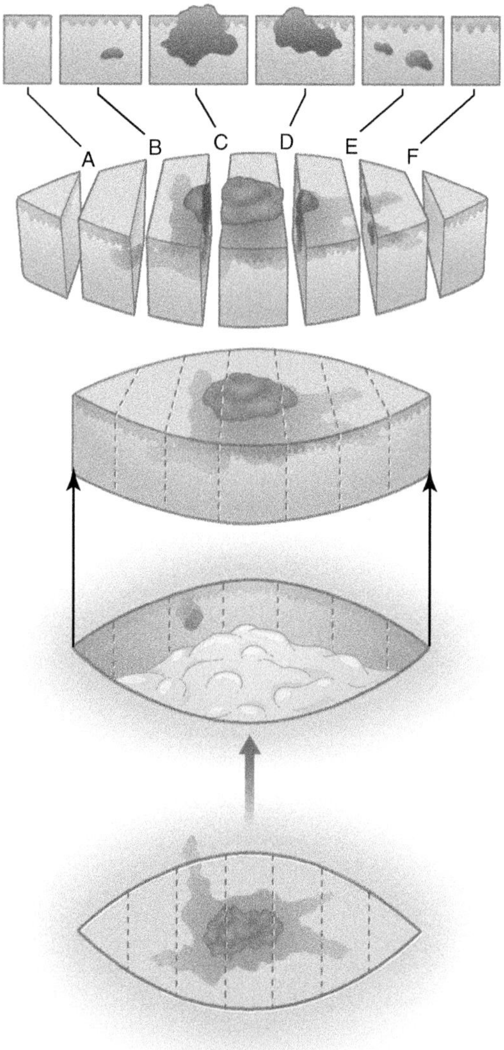

FIGURE 37-10 A standard elliptical excision of tumor followed by vertical sectioning "bread loafing." Here, all margins appear to be clear based on the sections evaluated at the top of the figure. However, the positive margin between sections B and C was not evaluated. Hence, the higher risk of recurrence with an ellipse rather than Mohs surgery. *(From Vidimos A, Ammirati C, Poblete-Lopez C.* Dermatologic Surgery. *London: Saunders; 2008.)*

RADIATION

Occasionally a patient with skin cancer may need radiation. Large NMSCs (especially BCCs and SCCs) can be readily treated with radiation. Large resections could leave the patient with distorted features or deforming

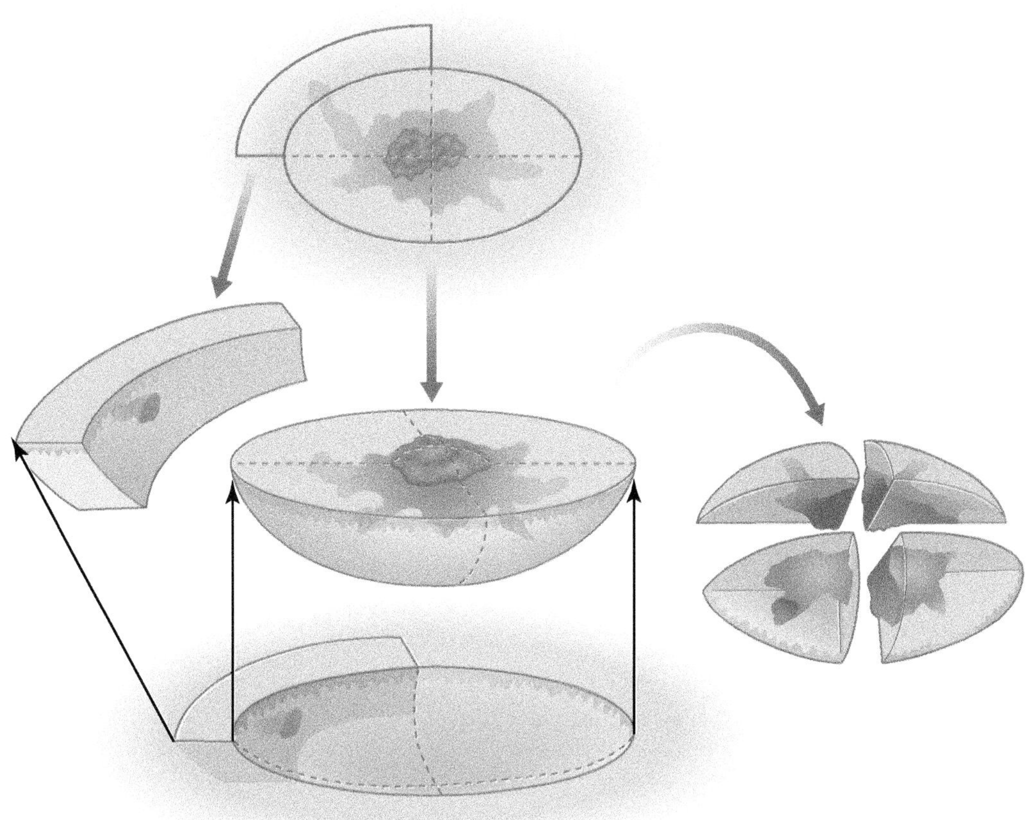

FIGURE 37-11 In Mohs surgery, the tumor is removed in a saucer-shaped section and divided into pieces for processing. Evaluation of all excised margins reveals skin cancer present at one of the dermal edges of excision. This area is subsequently excised to remove the rest of the tumor. *(From Vidimos A, Ammirati C, Poblete-Lopez C.* Dermatologic Surgery. *London: Saunders; 2008.)*

scars. Radiotherapy can be a prolonged treatment (5 days a week for 5 to 6 weeks). It is expensive and not indicated for the average NMSC. But for recurrent lesions or large primaries, it offers an alternative to Mohs surgery in some elderly patients who may not be able to tolerate a large surgical procedure. It is not advised near the lacrimal system (scarring) and with morpheaform BCCs. If used in younger patients (<50 years old) long-term complications could include malignant degeneration of treated skin.

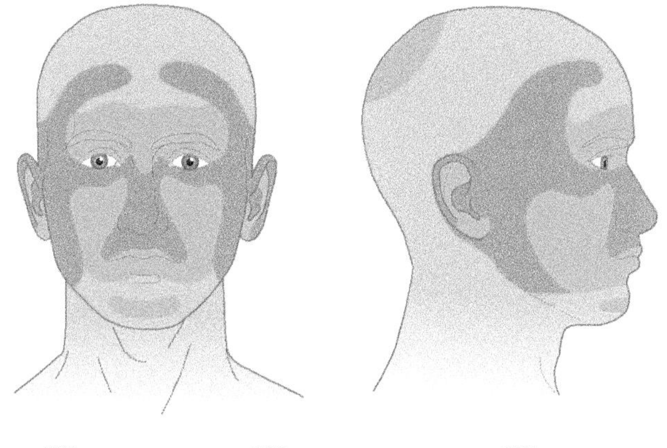

FIGURE 37-12 The H-zone of the face indicates areas of particular recurrence risk. Mohs is most commonly used for cutaneous neoplasms on the face and is particularly important in the H-zone of the face. In these areas, tumors have higher recurrence rates and are often more aggressive and invasive. This is likely due in part to the relative ease of invasion through natural embryonic fusion planes. *(From Vidimos A, Ammirati C, Poblete-Lopez C.* Dermatologic Surgery. *London: Saunders; 2008.)*

CONCLUSION

As with the entire field of medicine, hard-and-fast rules for consultation or referral are rare. Much depends on the clinician's personal level of comfort, training, and expertise.

The optimal outcome for the patient must remain the primary objective when considering if a consultation or referral is indicated. At the end of the process, the physician must satisfy:

- The patient
- The family
- The referring clinician (if applicable)
- The insurer
- A lawyer if called in
- The malpractice carrier
- And, finally, himself or herself.

Not attending to each of these interests can lead to a less-than-desirable outcome.

References

1. Evidence-Based Clinical Practice Guidelines: Treatment of Cutaneous Melanoma. Arlington Heights, IL: American Society of Plastic Surgeons; May 2007.
2. Guidelines of care for cutaneous squamous cell carcinoma: Committee on Guidelines of Care. Task Force on Cutaneous Squamous Cell Carcinoma. *J Am Acad Dermatol.* 1993;28(4):628.
3. Motley R, Kersey P, Lawrence C. Multiprofessional guidelines for management of the patient with primary cutaneous squamous cell carcinoma. *Br J Dermatol.* 2002;146:18–25.
4. Stulberg DL, Crandell B, Fawcett RS. Diagnosis and treatment of basal cell and squamous cell carcinoma. *Am Fam Physician.* 2004;70:1481–1488.
5. National Comprehensive Cancer Network. Clinical Practice Guidelines in Oncology: Basal Cell and Squamous Cell Skin Cancers. Version 1.2010. Accessed online April 18, 2010, at http://www.nccn.org/professionals/physician_gls/PDF/nmsc.pdf.
6. Habif T. *Clinical Dermatology: A Color Guide to Diagnosis and Therapy.* 4th ed. Philadelphia: Mosby; 2004.
7. Bowen GM, White GL, Gerwels JW. Mohs micrographic surgery. *Am Fam Physician.* 2005;72:845–848.
8. Shriner DL, McCoy DK, Goldberg DJ, Wagner RF. Mohs micrographic surgery. *J Am Dermatol.* 1998;39:79–97.

38 Surviving Financially

JOHN L. PFENNINGER, MD • REBECCA SMALL, MD

One important way to survive financially is to be paid appropriately for the procedures performed in the office. Coding and billing for skin procedures can be very complex. It is essential for the practitioner to understand the idiosyncrasies of the ICD-9 and CPT codes if billing is to be completed correctly.[1–7] The objective is not to charge as much as possible, but rather, to optimize billing once the proper procedure has been performed. Oftentimes, the same procedure can be billed using three or four different codes. Without exception, one method will pay more. Knowing the proper application of billing rules can, and does, make a significant difference in the financial bottom line of the practice.

Aesthetic procedures are not reimbursed by insurance carriers and, thus, there are no formal "rules" or "regulations" regarding the fees charged. The inclusion of these procedures has the potential to significantly augment practice revenue. Start-up costs for aesthetic procedures vary widely from relatively inexpensive products for chemical peels, to moderately expensive injectable products such as botulinum toxin and dermal fillers, to more expensive equipment such as aesthetic lasers.

Procedures have in the past and currently do reimburse more than cognitive visits on a time comparison basis. The primary care physician frequently turns away the most financially rewarding parts of the practice when sending patients for consultation. Many dermatologic procedures are easily learned, take little time to perform, and are appreciated by the patient since they do not have to arrange for a consult with another physician. These procedures often provide immediate or quick feedback to the clinician and patient about the diagnosis.

Unless a clinician is going to enter into the aesthetic field, the instruments used to perform dermatologic procedures are inexpensive. The most costly would be an electrosurgical unit and a liquid nitrogen gun (see Chapters 14 and 15). On the other hand, aesthetic equipment such as lasers can be very expensive, exceeding $150,000. However, when properly utilized on a frequent basis, lasers will offer the greatest revenue returns compared to other aesthetic procedures that require consumable products, such as botulinum toxin and dermal fillers. Cost versus fee charged for aesthetic laser treatments is more difficult to analyze due to the multiple variables involved such as methodology of acquiring the capital equipment, incidental disposable goods, cost of office space for storing the device, and maintenance contracts ($10,000 per year is common for aesthetic lasers).

A properly designed spreadsheet can be used to estimate whether major investments will provide an adequate financial return. Sales representatives will often paint a rosy picture and provide flow sheets which always conclude that there will be a significant return on investment. Major investments, however, require a careful independent study analysis of main factors.[8]

The purpose of this chapter is to help the reader become familiar with proper CPT coding for biopsies, destructions, and excisions of skin lesions. It will also help identify the pitfalls and common errors in coding and discuss financial considerations for aesthetic procedures. Tables 38-1 and 38-2 list common coding terminology and modifiers.

ESSENTIALS FOR PROPER CODING AND BILLING

To code and bill properly, the following information is necessary:

- Size of the lesion (if appropriate)
- Location on the body
- Method of treatment
- ICD-9 diagnosis (especially important to designate whether it is benign or malignant)
- CPT code.

Although most practitioners do not perform their own billing, it is increasingly more common for clinicians to complete their own coding. Accurate documentation and coding (including the location, size of a lesion, whether it was benign or malignant) will lead to accurate billing.

ICD-9 Coding

The majority of dermatologic procedures will involve an abnormal lesion. The diagnostic code (ICD-9) will vary depending on the location on the body and whether it is malignant (primary, secondary, or carcinoma *in situ*), benign, of uncertain behavior, or unspecified behavior (see Table 38-3). Specific conditions will have separate codes: abscesses, foreign bodies, cysts, etc.

When the diagnosis is uncertain, several options are available. One can use the "uncertain behavior" code if the procedure is a biopsy. If a definitive treatment is performed, it sometimes helps to wait for the pathology to return before completing the billing process. It is best not to use the "unspecified" code because, for whatever reason, many insurance plans will reject that code. If a biopsy was performed, the reimbursement will be the same whether it is coded as "benign" or "malignant." It makes little difference if the code is correct when only a biopsy was done. However, it is *extremely important* to know if the lesion was benign or malignant if a *treatment* is carried out. Note the differences in Table 38-4 for the 50th percentile charges and reimbursement for benign

TABLE 38-1 Coding Terminology

Ablation	See "Destruction"
Balance billing	The process of charging a patient the difference between what the physician bills and what the insurance company pays. If a provider participates with an insurance carrier, only copays and deductibles may be charged to the patient. If there is no participation agreement, then the provider may bill the patient for any fees not paid by the insurance company.
Biopsy	The procedure used to obtain tissue for histologic examination. This can be done with shave, punch, excision, curettement, and incisional procedures.
Electrosurgery/fulgurate/desiccate/cauterize	The use of electrical current heat to treat/destroy an area.
CPT	*Current Procedural Terminology*, published and updated annually by the AMA. Every medical procedure has a CPT code number. The majority of billing is completed using CPT terminology.[2]
Cryosurgery	The use of low temperatures to destroy (by freezing) a lesion (liquid nitrogen; nitrous oxide closed system; chemical spray canisters).
Debridement	Removal of devitalized tissue, dirt, and/or eschar from wounds or infected areas.
Destruction	Treatment of a lesion using cryosurgery, chemical application, injection of a chemical, curettement, or electrosurgery. Using a shave technique would also qualify, but in general, reimbursement would be higher using a shave or biopsy code than a destruction code for benign lesions.
Explanation of benefits (EOB)	A sheet provided by insurance companies that is enclosed with the payments for various procedures explaining what is allowed, what is the patient's responsibility (copay, deductible, not covered), what is not allowed (must be "written off" by the provider), and the amount of the enclosed payment.
Excision	Removal of a lesion using sharp dissection or electrosurgical cutting. In a shave excision, a slicing technique is used to remove either all or a portion of the lesion. It does not require suturing. Elliptical or fusiform excision includes full-thickness (through the dermis) removal of the lesion and requires closure, usually with sutures (or glue or adhesive strips).
Global period	Certain procedures have *global periods*. During this time, additional services (relating to the original procedure) cannot be charged. For most skin surgical procedures, this period is 10 days (no global period for shaves and punches).
ICD-9 (*International Classification of Diseases*, 9th Revision)	Every diagnosis has a specific numbered code. A diagnostic code is required to justify the reason for a CPT (procedure) code.[1] The ICD-10 codes are currently scheduled to be implemented October 1, 2013.
Incision and drainage (I&D)	*Simple:* Contents expressed after incision. *Complex:* Multiple conditions would qualify for a complex I&D, including the removal of a sac, such as in a sebaceous cyst, or insertion of a drain, such as iodoform gauze. The size and depth of the abscess could also be a factor, as well as excessive time required to complete the procedure. If multiple I&Ds of different lesions are done at the same time, it would also be considered "complex."
J-codes	Nearly every injectable medication has a specific number assigned to it called the *J-code*. When administered, the physician charges for not only the administration itself (a CPT code), but also for the particular chemical delivered (identified by the J-code).
Modifiers	These are numbers appended to a CPT code while billing to indicate that more than just the usual services were provided for the particular CPT code. (See Table 38-2 for common modifiers).
Paring	Removal and/or decrease in the bulk of a lesion, by peeling or shaving it away using a scalpel or a sharp instrument.

TABLE 38-2 Common Modifiers

-25	Significantly separate E&M on the same day as a procedure. *Example*: If a patient comes in for a mole removal and you have documentation that you also treated the patient for hypertension, osteoporosis, smoking, etc., use the -25 modifier with the office visit code.
-50	Bilateral procedures. *Example*: If you perform sclerotherapy on both legs, you would use the -50 modifier with the sclerotherapy code.
-51	Multiple procedures. *Example*: When multiple procedures, other than E&M, are performed at the same session by the same provider, the primary procedure or service may be reported as listed. The additional procedure(s) or service(s) may be identified by appending modifier -51 to the additional procedure or service code(s). *Note:* This modifier should not be appended to designated "add-on" codes.
-59	Distinct procedural service. *Example*: If you performed a cyst excision and decided to also freeze some actinic keratoses, use the -59 modifier with the cryosurgery because it is a completely separate procedure from the excision.
-79	Unrelated procedure or service by the same physician during a postop period. *Example*: If a patient comes in to have sutures removed during the postop period, and you perform cryosurgery on some actinic keratoses at the same visit when the sutures are removed, then -79 is used to clarify a separate procedure during a postop period.

TABLE 38-3 Neoplasm, Skin-ICD-9CM Codes

	Malignant					
	Primary	**Secondary**	**Ca *in situ***	**Benign**	**Uncertain Behavior**	**Unspecified**
Skin NEC*	173.9	198.2	232.9	216.9	238.2	239.2
Abdominal wall	173.5	198.2	232.5	216.5	238.2	239.2
Ala nasi	173.3	198.2	232.3	216.3	238.2	239.2
Ankle	173.7	198.2	232.7	216.7	238.2	239.2
Antecubital space	173.6	198.2	232.6	216.6	238.2	239.2
Anus	173.5	198.2	232.5	216.5	238.2	239.2
Arm	173.6	198.2	232.6	216.6	238.2	239.2
Auditory canal (external)	173.2	198.2	232.2	216.2	238.2	239.2
Auricle (ear)	173.2	198.2	232.2	216.2	238.2	239.2
Auricular canal (external)	173.2	198.2	232.2	216.2	238.2	239.2
Axilla, axillary fold	173.5	198.2	232.5	216.5	238.2	239.2
Back	173.5	198.2	232.5	216.5	238.2	239.2
Breast	173.5	198.2	232.5	216.5	238.2	239.2
Brow	173.3	198.2	232.3	216.3	238.2	239.2
Buttock	173.5	198.2	232.5	216.5	238.2	239.2
Calf	173.7	198.2	232.7	216.7	238.2	239.2
Canthus (eye) (inner) (outer)	173.1	198.2	232.1	216.1	238.2	239.2
Cervical region	173.4	198.2	232.4	216.4	238.2	239.2
Cheek (external)	173.3	198.2	232.3	216.3	238.2	239.2
Chest (wall)	173.5	198.2	232.5	216.5	238.2	239.2
Chin	173.3	198.2	232.3	216.3	238.2	239.2
Clavicular area	173.5	198.2	232.5	216.5	238.2	239.2
Clitoris	184.3	198.82	233.3	221.2	236.3	239.5
Columnella	173.3	198.2	232.3	216.3	238.2	239.2

*NEC, not elsewhere classified.

Continued

TABLE 38-3 Neoplasm, Skin-ICD-9CM Codes—cont'd

	Malignant					
	Primary	**Secondary**	**Ca *in situ***	**Benign**	**Uncertain Behavior**	**Unspecified**
Concha	173.2	198.2	232.2	216.2	238.2	239.2
Contiguous sites	173.8					
Ear (external)	173.2	198.2	232.2	216.2	238.2	239.2
Elbow	173.6	198.2	232.6	216.6	238.2	239.2
Eyebrow	173.3	198.2	232.3	216.3	238.2	239.2
Eyelid	173.1	198.2	232.1	216.1	238.2	239.2
Face NEC	173.3	198.2	232.3	216.3	238.2	239.2
Female genital organs (external)	184.4	198.82	233.3	221.2	236.3	239.5
Clitoris	184.3	198.82	233.3	221.2	236.3	239.5
Labium NEC	184.4	198.82	233.3	221.2	236.3	239.5
Majus	184.1	198.82	233.3	221.2	236.3	239.5
Minus	184.2	198.82	233.3	221.2	236.3	239.5
Pudendum	184.4	198.82	233.3	221.2	236.3	239.5
Vulva	184.4	198.82	233.3	221.2	236.3	239.5
Finger	173.6	198.2	232.6	216.6	238.2	239.2
Flank	173.5	198.2	232.5	216.5	238.2	239.2
Foot	173.7	198.2	232.7	216.7	238.2	239.2
Forearm	173.6	198.2	232.6	216.6	238.2	239.2
Forehead	173.3	198.1	232.3	216.3	238.2	239.2
Glabella	173.3	198.2	232.3	216.3	238.2	239.2
Gluteal region	173.5	198.2	232.5	216.5	238.2	239.2
Groin	173.5	198.2	232.5	216.5	238.2	239.2
Hand	173.6	198.2	232.6	216.6	238.2	239.2
Head NEC	173.4	198.2	232.4	216.4	238.2	239.2
Heel	173.7	198.2	232.7	216.7	238.2	239.2
Helix	173.2	198.2	232.2	216.2	238.2	239.2
Hip	173.7	198.2	232.7	216.7	238.2	239.2
Infraclavicular region	173.5	198.2	232.5	216.5	238.2	239.2
Inguinal region	173.5	198.2	232.5	216.5	238.2	239.2
Jaw	173.3	198.2	232.3	216.3	238.2	239.2
Knee	173.7	198.2	232.7	216.7	238.2	239.2
Labia						
Majora	184.1	198.82	233.3	221.2	236.3	239.5
Minora	184.2	198.82	233.3	221.2	236.3	239.5
Leg	173.7	198.2	232.7	216.7	238.2	239.2
Lid (lower) (upper)	173.1	198.2	232.1	216.1	238.2	239.2
Limb NEC	173.9	198.2	232.9	216.9	238.2	239.5
Lower	173.7	198.2	232.7	216.7	238.2	239.2
Upper	173.6	198.2	232.6	216.6	238.2	239.2
Lip (lower) (upper)	173.0	198.2	232.0	216.0	238.2	239.2

TABLE 38-3 Neoplasm, Skin-ICD-9CM Codes—cont'd

	Malignant					
	Primary	**Secondary**	**Ca *in situ***	**Benign**	**Uncertain Behavior**	**Unspecified**
Male genital organs	187.9	198.82	233.6	222.9	236.6	239.5
Penis	187.4	198.82	233.5	222.1	236.6	239.5
Prepuce	187.1	198.82	233.5	222.1	236.6	239.5
Scrotum	187.7	198.82	233.6	222.4	236.6	239.5
Mastectomy site	173.5	198.2				
Specified as breast tissue	174.8	198.81				
Meatus, acoustic (external)	173.2	198.2	232.2	216.2	238.2	239.2
Melanoma–see Melanoma						
Nates	173.5	198.2	232.5	216.5	238.2	239.0
Neck	173.4	198.2	232.4	216.4	238.2	239.2
Nose (external)	173.3	198.2	232.3	216.3	238.2	239.2
Palm	173.6	198.2	232.6	216.6	238.2	239.2
Palpebra	173.1	198.2	232.1	216.1	238.2	239.2
Penis NEC	187.4	198.82	233.5	222.1	236.6	239.5
Perianal	173.5	198.2	232.5	216.5	238.2	239.2
Perineum	173.5	198.2	232.5	216.5	238.2	239.2
Pinna	173.2	198.2	232.2	216.2	238.2	239.2
Plantar	173.7	198.2	232.7	216.7	238.2	239.2
Popliteal fossa or space	173.7	198.2	232.7	216.7	238.2	239.2
Prepuce	187.1	198.82	233.5	222.1	236.6	239.5
Pubes	173.5	198.2	232.5	216.5	238.2	239.2
Sacrococcygeal region	173.5	198.2	232.5	216.5	238.2	239.2
Scalp	173.4	198.2	232.4	216.4	238.2	239.2
Scapular region	173.5	198.2	232.5	216.5	238.2	239.2
Scrotum	187.7	198.82	233.6	222.4	236.6	239.5
Shoulder	173.6	198.2	232.6	216.6	238.2	239.2
Sole (foot)	173.7	198.2	232.7	216.7	238.2	239.2
Specified sites NEC	173.8	198.2	232.8	216.8	232.8	239.2
Submammary fold	173.5	198.2	232.5	216.5	238.2	239.2
Supraclavicular region	173.4	198.2	232.4	216.4	238.2	239.2
Temple	173.3	198.2	232.3	216.3	238.2	239.2
Thigh	173.7	198.2	232.7	216.7	238.2	239.2
Thoracic wall	173.5	198.2	232.5	216.5	238.2	239.2
Thumb	173.6	198.2	232.6	216.6	238.2	239.2
Toe	173.7	198.2	232.7	216.7	238.2	239.2
Tragus	173.2	198.2	232.2	216.2	238.2	239.2
Trunk	173.5	198.2	232.5	216.5	238.2	239.2
Umbilicus	173.5	198.2	232.5	216.5	238.2	239.2
Vulva	184.4	198.82	233.3	221.2	236.3	239.5
Wrist	173.6	198.2	232.6	216.6	238.2	239.2

TABLE 38-4 50th Percentile Charges (National) for Destruction of Selected Skin Lesions and the Average Medicare Reimbursement (2010)

Benign Lesion (up to 14)			Malignant Lesion		
CPT Code	2010 50th Percentile Fee Charge[a]	2010 National Medicare Reimbursement	CPT Code	2010 50th Percentile Fee Charge[a]	2010 National Medicare Reimbursement
17110	$133	$100	17281	$305	$163
Face, 0.6 cm			Face, 0.6 cm		
17110	$133	$100	17282	$368	$190
Face, 1.1 cm			Face, 1.1 cm		
17110	$133	$100	17261	$222	$131
Leg, 0.6 cm			Leg, 0.6 cm		
17110	$133	$100	17262	$277	$160
Leg, 1.1 cm			Leg, 1.1 cm		

[a]Based on the average of national surveys published in References 3–5.

and malignant lesions. These lesions could have been treated with liquid nitrogen cryosurgery, electrosurgery, laser ablation, or other methods. The same time may have been required whether the lesion was benign or malignant, but the fees charged and eventually reimbursed vary markedly.

A clinician can code for specific entities or be more generic. For instance, if a patient had a malignant melanoma on the back, it could be coded out *specifically* for "melanoma, general" as 172.9. It could also be coded out *generically* as "malignant neoplasm of the back," 173.5, which also includes squamous cell, basal cell, and other skin neoplasms. As long as it is a malignant code, it will not change the billing. A seborrheic keratosis on the face could be coded very specifically as 702.19 or more generally as 216.3 (benign lesion, face). Unfortunately, billing for treatment of benign lesions including seborrheic keratosis (regardless of the code) may be denied as it is often considered cosmetic. However, if a seborrheic keratosis is inflamed (ICD-9 702.11), most insurance companies will reimburse for its destruction or excision.

There is no specific code for *premalignant lesions*, such as actinic keratoses, on a particular body part. They can all be coded as 702.0 (actinic keratosis), regardless of location. However, reimbursement is higher for destruction of multiple premalignant lesions because each lesion (e.g., actinic keratosis) is charged individually (see Table 38-5).

The Importance of Size

Lesion size can be a major determinant in reimbursement. For some codes such as destruction for benign or premalignant lesions, size does not make a difference. However, if the lesion is malignant, the reimbursement varies widely (see Table 38-4). Similarly, size is very important in the repair of lacerations. For all excisions, size is best determined *prior to* the injection of any anesthetic.

The Importance of Location

It is critical to know that the same procedure performed on different anatomic locations is reimbursed differently. Even for benign destructions, where size and location usually does not matter, there are some exceptions. For instance, treatment of benign lesions of the penis, vulva, vagina, perineum, anus, and the eyelids all have distinct CPT codes (see Table 38-6). Biopsy codes are also specific for similar sensitive areas (see Table 38-7).

TABLE 38-5 Destruction of Benign and Premalignant Lesions

CPT	Description	2010 Estimated 50th Percentile Fee Charge[a]	2010 National Medicare Reimbursement
17110	Benign, other than skin tags or cutaneous vascular lesions, ≤14 milia, seborrheic keratoses, warts	$133	$100
17111	Benign, other than skin tags or cutaneous vascular lesions, ≥15	$169	$120
17000	Premalignant, 1	$110	$74
17003	Premalignant, 2–14, each	$38	$7
17004	Premalignant, ≥15	$414	$162

[a]Based on the average of national surveys published in References 3–5.

TABLE 38-6 Selected Benign Skin Destructions

CPT	Description	2010 Estimated 50th Percentile Fee Charge[a]	2010 National Medicare Reimbursement
46916	Anus, cryo, simple	$384	$211
46924	Anus, extensive lesions	$1155	$463
54050	Penis, chemical	$217	$123
54055	Penis, electrosurgery	$272	$117
54056	Penis, cryosurgery	$268	$130
54057	Penis, laser	$546	$138
54060	Penis, excision	$530	$186
54065	Penis, extensive	$878	$211
56501	Vulva, simple	$288	$125
56515	Vulva, extensive	$875	$215
57061	Vaginal lesion, simple	$514	$109
57065	Vaginal lesion, ext.	$1169	$185
67850	Lesion, eyelid	$419	$196
68135	Conjunctival lesion	$447	$140

[a]Based on the average of national surveys published in References 3–5.

TABLE 38-7 Biopsy by Punch, Shave, Curette, or Excision

CPT	Description	2010 Estimated 50th Percentile Fee Charge[a]	2010 National Medicare Reimbursement
11100	Skin: 1 lesion	$145	$95
11101	Each additional lesion	$81	$31
11755	Nail unit	$213	$121
21550	Soft tissue, neck/thorax	$469	$236
30100	Intranasal	$213	$128
38500	Biopsy/excision, lymph node	$770	$300
41100	Tongue, anterior two-thirds	$323	$154
41105	Tongue, posterior, one-third	$340	$156
54100	Penis, cutaneous	$303	$191
54105	Penis, deep	$531	$279
56605	Vulva or perineum, single lesion	$246	$80
56606	Vulva, each additional lesion	$154	$37
57100	Vagina, simple	$294	$85
57105	Vagina, extensive	$611	$130
67810	Eyelid (margins)	$336	$197
68100	Conjunctiva	$412	$151
69100	Pinna	$217	$97
69105	Ear canal	$282	$129

[a]Based on the average of national surveys published in References 3–5.

CPT codes and reimbursement numbers are provided in Table 38-8 for incision and drainage (I&D) procedures and in Table 38-9 for foreign body removal.

The Importance of Method

In general, the method of destruction does not change the coding. However, for the anus and genital areas, there are specific codes for the method used (see Table 38-6).

Shave excisions are distinctly different than full excisional procedures that require suture repair. Here, again, the "method" is important. Specific codes are used for shave excisions depending on size and location (see Table 38-10).

SPECIFIC CPT CODES: OFFICE VISITS

An E/M code can be charged *in addition to a procedural code* in specific, certain instances:

- *If the patient is new to the practice or has not been seen by the practice for at least 3 years,* a new patient visit E/M can be charged. It is felt that it is necessary to evaluate the patient's overall condition in addition to providing the procedure itself. Does this patient have diabetes? Is he or she on warfarin? Have other mitigating diagnoses? It takes time to determine this and the clinician is reimbursed for that time.
- If the patient has been seen in the practice within 3 years but *a unique, separate service is provided in addition to the procedure, use the modifier "-25" and*

TABLE 38-8 I&D Procedures

CPT	Description	2010 Estimated 50th Percentile Fee Charge[a]	2010 National Medicare Reimbursement
10040	Acne surgery	$138	$95
10060	One abscess, cyst, paronychia, etc.	$177	$101
10061	Multiple/complex abscess	$355	$172
10080	Pilonidal cyst, simple	$241	$152
10081	Pilonidal cyst, complicated	$444	$240
10140	Hematoma (not subungual)	$234	$143
10160	Aspirate abscess/cyst	$172	$116
10180	Complex/post-op infection	$500	$216
11740	Evacuate subungual hematoma	$81	$42
26010	Abscess finger, simple	$316	$228
26011	Finger (felon), complex	$763	$345
40800	Vestibule mouth	$261	$185
40801	Mouth, complicated	$759	$284
41000	Lingual	$300	$147
41005	Sublingual, superficial	$361	$206
41006	Sublingual, deep	$681	$330
41800	Gums	$314	$215
45005	Submucosal rectal abscess	$516	$232
46040	Perirectal abscess	$864	$463
46050	Superficial perianal abscess	$374	$166
55100	Scrotal wall abscess	$420	$220
56405	Vulva	$315	$105
56420	Bartholin's abscess	$338	$120
67700	Eyelid abscess	$361	$232
69000	Abscess/hematoma, pinna	$267	$167
69005	Abscess/hematoma, pinna, complicated	$661	$198
69020	Ear canal abscess	$313	$213

[a]Based on the average of national surveys published in References 3–5.

TABLE 38-9 Foreign Body Removal

CPT	Description	2010 Estimated 50th Percentile Fee Charge[a]	2010 National Medicare Reimbursement
10120	I & remove SQ, simple	$192	$124
10121	I & remove SQ, complicated	$446	$241
20520	Muscle/tendon sheath, simple	$332	$178
23330	Shoulder, SQ	$370	$209
24200	Upper arm/elbow, SQ	$339	$182
27086	Pelvis/hip, SQ	$417	$222
28190	Foot, SQ	$453	$222
28192	Foot, deep	$801	$423
30300	Intranasal	$252	$205
40804	Embedded vestib mouth, simple	$315	$190
42809	Pharynx	$343	$159
65205	Ext. eye, conjunctiva, superficial	$149	$51
67938	Embedded eyelid	$364	$213
69200	Ext. auditory canal w/o anesthesia	$205	$112

[a]Based on the average of national surveys published in References 3–5.

charge for the office visit E/M. Perhaps the patient's insulin or hypertensive medications were adjusted, or a URI may have been evaluated *in addition* to doing a skin biopsy on the face for a suspected basal cell carcinoma.

- *If the patient is being seen as a consult, a consult fee can be charged in addition to the procedure fee.* Although Medicare eliminated this consultation fee in 2010 and some insurance companies have followed suit, other insurance companies still follow the CPT uniform coding guidelines, which allow the additional E&M code. It is important to know which insurance companies allow this because it can generate a significant cash flow in some practices.

TABLE 38-10 Selected Shave Skin Excisions

CPT	Description	2010 Estimated 50th Percentile Fee Charge[a]	2010 National Medicare Reimbursement
11200	Skin tags, ≤15	$137	$77
11201	Skin tags, each additional 10	$66	$18
11300	TAL, ≤ 0.5 cm	$115	$62
11301	TAL, 0.6–1.0 cm	$155	$86
11302	TAL, 1.1–2.0 cm	$191	$103
11303	TAL, >2 cm	$241	$121
11305	SNHFG, ≤0.5 cm	$133	$64
11306	SNHFG, 0.6–1.0 cm	$170	$88
11307	SNHFG, 1.1–2.0 cm	$203	$105
11308	SNHFG, >2.0 cm	$251	$116
11310	Face, ≤0.5 cm[b]	$150	$78
11311	Face, 0.6–1.0 cm[b]	$195	$99
11312	Face, 1.1–2.0 cm[b]	$226	$114
11313	Face, >2.0 cm[b]	$294	$143

TAL = trunk, arm, leg; SNHFG = scalp, neck, hands, feet, genitalia.
[a]Based on the average of national surveys published in References 3–5.
[b]Face, includes ears, eyelids, nose and lips.

Intralesional Injections

Injection therapy may be used when treating acne, keloids, or other skin conditions with steroids. Also, injecting Candida antigen or bleomycin for the treatment of verruca qualifies for intralesional injection codes. The coding is as follows: 1–7 lesions is 11900; >7 lesions is 11901. Note that the number refers to *the number of lesions, not the number of injections*. For some conditions such as verruca, one could also use destruction codes. For most drugs, an additional charge is made for the medication itself, using a J-code, and the amount of solution used.

I&D Codes

A simple incision and drainage is billed with CPT code 10060; for complex or multiple lesions, the code is 10061. However, note that many locations have specific CPT codes (see Table 38-8). Those particular codes should be used rather than the generic ones since they often reimburse more.

Biopsies

The CPT code for a biopsy is *method independent*. In other words, shave, curettement, punch, incision, or excision could all be coded as a biopsy. If the biopsy codes are used, it does not really matter if the lesion is benign or malignant nor does the size matter, but location will make a difference. For most locations on the body, the first biopsy is coded as 11100 and there is a charge for each additional biopsy done (code 11101). Note that many of the specific biopsy CPT codes are dependent on the particular site biopsied (see Table 38-7). If a complete full-depth excision with a sutured repair is performed, it will most likely be compensated at a higher rate if billed as an excision and not as a biopsy (even when the diagnosis is not certain and the specimen is sent to pathology). For example, if an excision of a suspected BCC with margins is performed at the first visit, the reimbursement would be much higher for excision of a malignancy than biopsy of an unknown lesion.

Excisions and Lacerations

Coding for *excisions* can be straightforward. All of the previously identified factors need to be recorded: benign or malignant, location, and size. All measurements should be made *before* any anesthetic is administered. For the purpose of billing, the size of the lesion is determined by the "greatest clinical diameter of the apparent lesion plus that margin required for complete excision (lesion diameter plus the most narrow margins required equals the excised diameter)" (see Figure 38-1). If a lesion is long and narrow, the length plus the margins is actually the "diameter" size used for coding. So, in essence, it is the largest measurement of the lesion plus the margins that is used for proper coding:

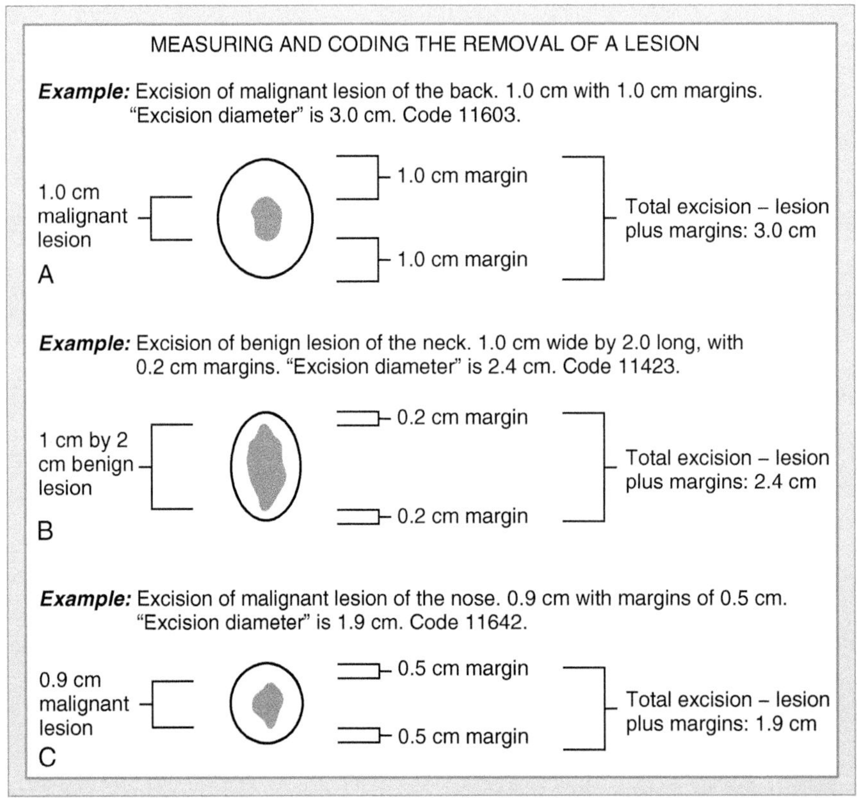

FIGURE 38-1 Measuring and coding the removal of a lesion. *(Adapted from* Physicians Current Procedural Terminology 2010. *Chicago: American Medical Association; 2010.)*

A: Correct size for coding is "excision of 3-cm lesion, malignant, back," with the actual size of the lesion itself being 1 cm × 1 cm with 1-cm margins around it (1-cm margin + 1-cm lesion + 1-cm margin).
B: Correct size for coding is "excision of 2.4-cm lesion, benign, neck," with the actual size of the lesion itself being 2.0 cm long × 1 cm wide, with 0.2-cm margins around it (0.2-cm margin + 2-cm lesion + 0.2-cm margin).
C: Correct size for coding is "excision of 1.9-cm lesion, malignant, nose," with the actual size of lesion itself being 0.8 cm wide × 0.9 cm long, with 0.5-cm margins around it (0.5-cm margin + 0.9-cm lesion + 0.5-cm margin). To make it clear, "diameter" size refers to the longest measurement of the lesion.

For excisions, the code *includes* the surgical supplies, administration of local anesthesia, a simple repair, suture removal, and any necessary intervention within 10 days. This 10-day period is called the *global period.*

In the repair of *lacerations* there is no "width" determinant. Rather, it is only the length of the laceration to be repaired that is important (simple repair). Some laceration repairs will be considered intermediate or complex based on factors described below. In these cases, the length will still be one of the factors used in determining the correct CPT code.

Intermediate and Complex Repairs

A repair can be classified as intermediate or complex as follows:

- An *intermediate repair* (12031–12057) is defined by the CPT manual as a repair that includes, in addition to the requirements of a simple repair, "... layered closure of one or more of the deeper layers of subcutaneous tissue and superficial (non-muscle) fascia, in addition to the skin (epidermal and dermal) closure. Single-layer closure of heavily contaminated wounds that have required extensive cleaning or removal of particulate matter also constitutes intermediate repair." Intermediate repair includes either extensive cleaning, debridement, undermining, or placement of deep buried sutures. Intermediate repair increases the amount of charges significantly. Do not forget to bill for this portion if your repair is truly an intermediate one. See Table 38-11 for codes, descriptions, and Medicare pricing.
- A *complex repair* (13100–13160) is defined by the CPT manual as a repair that "includes wounds requiring more than layered closure, viz., scar revision, debridement (e.g., traumatic lacerations or avulsions), extensive undermining, stents, or retention sutures. Necessary preparation includes creation of a defect for repairs (e.g., excision of a scar requiring a complex repair) or the debridement of complicated lacerations or avulsions."

If an intermediate or complex repair is performed, that can be billed *in addition to* the excision itself. An intermediate repair after an excision generally includes undermining and the placement of sutures to close the deep space (layered closure).

Even the use of a single deep suture allows one to bill for an intermediate repair. The compensation for such a repair may be comparable to the compensation for the excision itself. Therefore using deep sutures when needed not only protects the patient from risks of dehiscence and hematoma, it also increases the reimbursement. When coding for intermediate repair after an excision it may help to include the reason for the deep sutures in the operative note. The most common

TABLE 38-11 CPT Codes for Intermediate Wound Repair

CPT	Description	2010 Medicare National Nonfacility Price
12031	Scalp, axillae, trunk and/or extremities (excluding hands and feet), <2.6 cm	$226
12032	2.6–7.5 cm	$287
12034	7.6–12.5 cm	$286
12035	12.6–20.0 cm	$347
12041	Neck, hands, feet and/or external genitalia, <2.6 cm	$236
12042	2.6–7.5 cm	$272
12044	7.6–12.5 cm	$318
12045	12.6–20.0 cm	$348
12051	Face, ears, eyelids, nose, lips and/or mucous membranes, <2.6 cm	$251
12052	2.6–5.0 cm	$287
12053	5.1 cm–7.5 cm	$316
12054	7.6 cm–12.5 cm	$335
12055	12.6 cm–20.0 cm	$402

reasons are to "take tension off the wound," "prevent dehiscence," or "close dead space."

The CPT code for an intermediate repair is based on the length of the final closed wound (regardless of the size of a lesion or the mechanism of an injury). The codes for intermediate repairs encompass wide ranges of wound length as these are also used for laceration repairs (see Table 38-11). When it comes to laceration and wound repairs that are unrelated to a medical excision, intermediate repairs are billed instead of a simple repair and not in addition to the simple repair. Reasons to upgrade a simple repair to a complex repair beyond just a two-layer closure include the need for extensive wound cleaning and/or debridement before closure.

A complex repair can be billed if extensive undermining or debridement is required or if the time required for the procedure is excessive. If a flap, plasty, or graft is performed, other specific codes (14000 and 15000) apply. See Chapter 13 for further information on billing for flaps.

Destruction of Lesions

The number one determinant for the correct CPT code for a lesion destruction is whether the lesion is benign, premalignant, or malignant. If benign, destruction by any method of 1–14 lesions is the same code: 17110. If 15 or more are destroyed, then the code is 17111. The exceptions for various locations are noted in Table 38-6. If premalignant (e.g., actinic keratoses), the first lesion is coded as 17000. For lesions 2–14, 17003 is used, and a charge is made for *each additional lesion.* Use 17004 when 15 or more premalignant lesions are treated.

For malignant lesions, size becomes important as well as location (see Table 38-12).

Tumors

The removal of subcutaneous tumors, such as lipomas, carries a specific diagnosis. These are not skin lesions. The CPT code was changed in 2010 and the proper code is determined based on whether the lesion is subcutaneous, subfascial, or whether it requires a radical excision. It does not matter if it is benign or malignant, but body site and depth of lesion do change the CPT code (Tables 38-13 and 38-14).

These codes are all inclusive. Neither the length of the incision nor the type of repair that is used matter. The size of the tumor is determined by the maximum dimension of the tumor plus the narrowest margin necessary to excise the tumor completely. *Subcutaneous* is defined as "below the skin but above the deep fascia." *Fascial* or *subfascial* is defined as "within or below the deep fascia, but not involving the bone." In the fingers and toes, however, *subfascial* is defined as "involving the tendons, tendon sheaths, or joints." Tumors that "abut

TABLE 38-12 Malignant Skin Destructions

CPT	Description	2010 Estimated 50th Percentile Fee Charge[a]	2010 National Medicare Reimbursement
17260	TAL, ≤0.5 cm	$186	$89
17261	TAL, 0.6–1.0 cm	$222	$131
17262	TAL, 1.1–2.0 cm	$277	$160
17263	TAL, 2.1–3.0 cm	$319	$177
17264	TAL, 3.1–4.0 cm	$352	$189
17266	TAL, >4 cm	$428	$215
17270	SNHFG, ≤0.5 cm	$224	$137
17271	SNHFG, 0.6–1.0 cm	$265	$151
17272	SNHFG, 1.1–2.0 cm	$309	$173
17273	SNHFG, 2.1–3.0 cm	$357	$193
17274	SNHFG, 3.1–4.0 cm	$433	$229
17276	SNHFG, >4.0 cm	$504	$266
17280	Face, ≤0.5 cm	$251	$128
17281	Face, 0.6–1.0 cm[b]	$305	$164
17282	Face, 1.1–2.0 cm[b]	$368	$190
17283	Face, 2.1–3.0 cm[b]	$441	$230
17284	Face, 3.1–4.0 cm[b]	$503	$268
17286	Face, > 4 cm[b]	$635	$340

TAL = trunk, arm, leg; SNHFG = scalp, neck, hands, feet, genitalia.
[a]Based on the average of national surveys published in References 3–5.
[b]Face, includes ears, eyelids, nose and lips.

TABLE 38-13 Subcutaneous Soft Tissue Tumor Excisions above the Fascia (Used for Lipomas)

CPT	Description	2010 Estimated 50th Percentile Fee Charge[a]	2010 National Medicare Reimbursement
21011	Face or scalp, <2 cm	$378	$306
21012	Face or scalp, ≥2 cm	$727	$328
21555	Neck or ant. thorax, <3 cm	$1251	$381
21552	Neck or ant. thorax, ≥3 cm	$1347	$438
21930	Back or flank, <3 cm	$649	$430
21931	Back or flank, ≥3 cm	$1185	$459
22902	Abdominal wall, <3 cm	$735	$409
22903	Abdominal wall, ≥3 cm	$1282	$429
23075	Shoulder, <3 cm	$920	$331
23071	Shoulder, ≥3 cm	$1194	$407
24075	Upper arm or elbow, <3 cm	$946	$395
24071	Upper arm or elbow, ≥3 cm	$1421	$441
25075	Forearm and/or wrist, <3 cm	$1354	$341
25071	Forearm and/or wrist, ≥3 cm	$1431	$414
26115	Hand or finger, <1.5 cm	$1242	$401
26111	Hand or finger, ≥1.5 cm	$1510	$526
27047	Pelvis or hip, <3 cm	$869	$458
27043	Pelvis or hip, ≥3 cm	$1461	$473
27327	Thigh or knee, <3 cm	$703	$398
27337	Thigh or knee, ≥3 cm	$1466	$408
27618	Leg or ankle, <3 cm	$743	$403
27632	Leg or ankle, ≥3 cm	$1029	$407
28043	Foot or toe, <1.5 cm	$347	$332
28039	Foot or toe, ≥1.5 cm	$569	$463

[a]Based on the average of national surveys published in References 3–5.

but do not breach the tendon, tendon sheath, or joint capsule are considered subcutaneous."

All subcutaneous tumors are reported by whether they are <3 cm or ≥3 cm, except:

- *Face/scalp:* <2 cm or ≥2 cm
- *Hand/finger:* <1.5 cm or ≥1.5 cm
- *Foot/toe:* <1.5 cm or ≥1.5 cm.

All subfascial tumors are reported by whether they are <5 cm or ≥5 cm, except:

- *Face/scalp:* <2 cm or ≥2 cm
- *Forearm/wrist:* <3 cm or ≥3 cm
- *Hand/finger:* <1.5 cm or ≥1.5 cm
- *Foot/toe:* <1.5 cm or ≥1.5 cm.

Also, the routine skin diagnostic ICD-9 codes are *not* used. Rather, ICD-9 provides specific codes for subcutaneous and deep tumors of the various body locations (see Table 38-15). It is important to be aware of these *tumor removal* codes, because the majority are much more highly reimbursed than those for *skin lesion removal*. A small subcutaneous 1-cm lipoma on the back that is removed with a simple incision and digital expression with a Steri-Strip closure (CPT 21555) can take a mere 5 to 10 minutes. The 50th percentile fee charged is $805. Medicare reimburses $205. For a more detailed discussion of lipoma coding see Chapter 12, *Cysts and Lipomas*, page 145.

Miscellaneous

- When a malignant lesion is removed and the margins are positive, or further removal is recommended, even if the second tissue histology comes back totally benign or without residual, it is correct to charge for "malignant removal" for the second excision.
- It is inappropriate to use a biopsy and a removal code for the same visit.
- As is very evident from these discussions, proper coding and billing are complicated processes and Medicare reimbursement lags far behind the 50th percentile fees charged in the nation.

TABLE 38-14 Soft Tissue Excision Codes

	Tumor Subcutaneous (<3 cm)	Tumor Subcutaneous (3 cm or Greater)	Tumor Subfascial (<5 cm)	Tumor Subfascial (5 cm or Greater)
Face/scalp	21011 (<2 cm)	21012 (2 cm or greater)	21013 (<2 cm)	21014 (2 cm or greater)
Neck	21555	# 21552	21556	# 21554
Anterior thorax	21555	# 21552	21556	# 21554
Back/flank	21930	21931	21932	21933
Abdomen	22902	22903	22900	22901
Shoulder	23075	# 23071	23076	# 23073
Arm/elbow	24075	# 24071	24076	# 24073
Forearm/wrist	25075	# 25071	25076 (<3 cm)	# 25073 (3 cm or greater)
Hand/fingers	26115 (<1.5 cm)	# 26111 (1.5 cm or greater)	26116 (<1.5 cm)	# 26113 (1.5 cm or greater)
Pelvis/hip	27047	# 27043	27048	# 27045
Thigh/knee	27327	# 27337	27328	# 27339
Leg/ankle	27618	# 27632	27619	# 27634
Foot/toes	28043 (<1.5 cm)	# 28039 (1.5 cm or greater)	28045 (<1.5 cm)	# 28041 (1.5 cm or greater)

= resequenced code.
Source: Modified from Janevicius R. *New Soft-Tissue Excision Codes Introduced in 2010.* American Society of Plastic Surgeons, 2010. Available at www.psnextra.org/Columns/CPT-Corner-Jan-10.html. Accessed February 3, 2011.

Prior Approval

Review the denials of payment for procedures monthly. It is not unusual for insurance plans to require prior approval for the most expensive procedures. These often involve excision of a malignancy and/or an intermediate repair. This can be an advantage of doing a small biopsy first to determine the diagnosis. Once a malignant skin lesion is diagnosed, complete a prior approval form for excision or other treatment planned. However, if the lesion is clinically an obvious malignancy, performing a biopsy only adds unnecessary cost. Insurance will allow approvals based on good clinical judgment. Approval is best done at the time when the patient is first seen and scheduled for definitive treatment. Allow time for the insurance company to respond if possible before performing the procedure. If prior approval is not received first, the insurance company may deny reimbursement, which can be a costly loss.

Once a clinician learns which insurance plans require prior approval for which procedures, fewer denials of claims will occur.

COSMETIC VERSUS MEDICAL REMOVALS

There are no codes for purely cosmetic removals. Some cosmetic treatments may be used for medical conditions and some insurance plans will pay for them (e.g., microdermabrasion or skin peel for acne and acne scarring). When the treatment is performed for purely cosmetic reasons or if the insurance plan does not cover a particular code, the practitioner is free to charge whatever is desired and no CPT coding or diagnostic code is needed.

Medicare coverage for lesion removal is quite strict. If a lesion is *benign*, they will pay for the removal only if it has one or more of the following characteristics: *It is bleeding; it causes intense itching or pain; or the lesion has physical evidence of inflammation with purulence, oozing, edema, or erythema.* It will also pay if *it obstructs an orifice or clinically restricts vision, there is uncertainty as to the diagnosis, a prior biopsy suggests malignancy, or if it is in an area subject to recurrent trauma* and there is documentation that such trauma has occurred.

Benign skin lesion removals (not including premalignant lesions) for reasons other than those provided above are considered to be cosmetic by Medicare. These include, but are not limited to, emotional distress, makeup trapping, and any nonproblematic lesion in any anatomic location. For patients with Medicare, if the procedure is deemed to be a cosmetic removal, the patient must be informed beforehand and sign a written consent that he or she understands and is willing to pay for the procedure. It is best to provide a specific written quote amount to all patients for these elective procedures. Interestingly, insurance companies will still cover pathology charges for lesions that were removed for cosmetic reasons.

Cosmetic procedure codes (Box 38-1) are primarily used for documentation purposes, because these procedures are not usually covered by insurance plans. As mentioned, some insurance carriers may cover chemical peels for conditions such as acne, but such coverage is not common. The 17000 code may be used for cosmetic laser treatments.

TABLE 38-15 ICD-9 Codes for Soft Tissue Tumors

CPT	Description
Benign Soft Tissue Tumors	
(Do not use "Neoplasm–Skin" codes. These CPT codes are for deep soft tissue masses with their own distinct specific codes, both benign and malignant.)	
210.4	Benign neoplasm, gum
214.0	Lipoma, face, SQ
214.1	Lipoma, other SQ tissue
215.0	Benign neoplasm, face
215.0	Benign neoplasm, neck
215.0	Benign neoplasm, head
215.2	Benign neoplasm, shoulder
215.2	Benign neoplasm, upper extremity
215.3	Benign neoplasm, hip
215.3	Benign neoplasm, lower limb
215.4	Benign neoplasm, thorax
215.5	Benign neoplasm, abd. wall
215.6	Benign neoplasm, buttock
215.7	Benign
215.7	Benign neoplasm, trunk
229.8	Benign neoplasm, hand
Malignant Soft Tissue Tumors	
171.0	Cancer, head
171.0	Cancer, face
171.0	Cancer, neck
171.2	Cancer, upper limb
171.2	Cancer, shoulder
171.3	Cancer, hip
171.3	Cancer, lower limb
171.5	Cancer, abdominal wall
171.7	Cancer, back/flank

PURCHASING EQUIPMENT

The majority of dermatologic supplies to perform routine procedures, such as biopsies and curettements, are inexpensive. Moderate costs are incurred when cryosurgery (liquid nitrogen) or electrosurgical devices are purchased. They quickly pay for themselves, however, and not only provide better cash flow for the clinician, but a timely, more convenient service for the patient.

Aesthetic equipment can be very expensive, ranging from $10,000 for a microdermabrasion unit to more than $150,000 for various lasers for hair and tattoo removal, skin resurfacing, etc. Purchase of this equipment should be researched well. Company representatives are quick to show projected summaries with significant returns. However, the clinician must consider several factors, including true demand, time, insurance, personal property tax, maintenance contracts (up to $15,000 annually, per unit), incidental disposable materials, and additional office space and personnel. A successful aesthetics practice will generally require a website and advertising. The question to ask is "Will this all be cost effective in a busy practice?" The reader is strongly encouraged to review Needham and Katz's work to better assess whether a major purchase "makes sense."[8]

COSMETIC PROCEDURE FINANCIAL CONSIDERATIONS

Practitioners entering the aesthetics field may choose to start with procedures that have lower start-up and overhead costs, such as chemical peels, botulinum toxin, dermal filler injection procedures, and microdermabrasion.[9] Products may be purchased in small quantities as needed, which helps to keep the costs down. Fees charged for these procedures are at the discretion of the provider, and are typically determined using the following methods[10]:

- *Fixed margin or cost plus fixed fee.* For example, if a syringe of dermal filler product costs $100 and the injection fee (fixed margin) is $200, then the charge for the procedure would be $300. If the product costs $200, then the total charge would be $400.
- *Fixed markup.* The most common fixed markup is double the cost of the product. For example, if the product costs $200, then the charge for the procedure would be $400.
- *Community pricing.* The relative costs of the procedures are based on an unscientific survey of other practices that are considered part of the community.

Recommendations for aesthetic procedure fees can be found in the *Financial Considerations and Coding* sections of the chapters that cover the following procedures: botulinum toxin (Chapter 21), chemical peels (Chapter 22), microdermabrasion (Chapter 23), dermal fillers (Chapter 25), laser hair reduction (Chapter 26),

BOX 38-1 *Cosmetic Procedure Codes*

15788	Chemical peel, facial; epidermal
15789	Chemical peel, facial; dermal
15792	Chemical peel, nonfacial; epidermal
15793	Chemical peel, nonfacial; dermal
11950	Subcutaneous injection of filling material, ≤1 mL
11951	Subcutaneous injection of filling material, 1.1–5.0 mL
11952	Subcutaneous injection of filling material, 5.1–10 mL
17380	Epilation (hair reduction)
17000–17111	Treatment of premalignant skin lesions or benign skin lesions

laser photorejuvenation (Chapter 27), nonablative lasers for wrinkle reduction (Chapter 28), ablative lasers for skin resurfacing (Chapter 29), and laser tattoo removal (Chapter 30).

COSMETIC PRACTICE FINANCIAL PEARLS

- Many cosmetic procedures require a series of treatments to achieve optimal results. Patients can be incentivized to purchase a series of cosmetic treatments when a discount is offered. For example, intense pulsed light treatments for photorejuvenation may be priced at $400 per treatment. When a series of three treatments is purchased, the cost per treatment can be discounted to $350, for a total cost of $1050, instead of $1200.
- Inform patients that cosmetic procedures are not covered by insurance and that they are financially responsible at the time of treatment. Have a written financial policy for patients to sign. This can be done for treatments as simple as snipping skin tags to more elaborate laser treatments.
- Consider offering creative methods for payment, particularly if the charges are large (over $1000). One possible method is to use *split payments.* With this method, patients pay for half of the cost of their cosmetic treatment plan on the first visit and the remainder midway through their treatment series.
- Take time to discuss with patients that results cannot be guaranteed and the practice refund policy, if any.
- Marketing can contribute to the success of cosmetic procedures. Marketing your cosmetic procedures can simply involve educating your patients about your new skills. This form of internal marketing is often more successful than external marketing (e.g., newspaper advertisements and yellow pages) and less costly. Common ways to inform patients about cosmetic services include:
  - Educate all staff about cosmetic procedures performed in the office.
  - Perform cosmetic treatments on staff if desired.
  - Create informative brochures and posters.
  - Provide a form so patients can easily make inquiries if interested.
  - Send informative e-mails to patients.
  - Hold in-office events.
- Most importantly, consistently achieving good outcomes with desired aesthetic results is the best method for building a successful aesthetic practice

SUMMARY TIPS

1. To allow for proper coding and billing, the clinician should always record in the electronic medical record or chart the size, location, and nature of the lesions (benign, premalignant, or malignant) and what procedure was performed. When size is estimated rather than measured, money is often lost. For example, an "eyeball estimate" of 2.0 cm will pay less than an actual measurement of 2.1 cm when the true length is 2.1 cm.
2. When a procedure can be properly coded out in different ways (e.g., biopsy, destruction, or shave excision), the clinician should know which is more highly reimbursed to optimize the billing process. Generally, for most benign lesions, "destruction" pays the least. Procedures performed in the facial, genital, and anal areas generally pay more, regardless of the procedure. In general, shave excisions pay more than destruction codes, but less than full-thickness excisions. For many very small lesions, a biopsy code will be best. For larger lesions, the shave code, if done, may be the most appropriate.
3. *Caveat emptor* ("buyer beware") is a truism that needs to be carefully heeded when purchasing expensive aesthetic equipment.
4. The clinician must be familiar with coding and billing processes in order to optimize the entire reimbursement process.
5. Several resources are available to determine the usual and customary fees charged nationally.[3–6]
6. It is extremely important to have a trusted and knowledgeable billing staff or agency to ensure that the clinician is being properly reimbursed. Currently, offsite billing companies are charging fees of 6% to 8% of *gross* collections.
7. Aesthetic procedures with lower start-up costs such as botulinum toxin, dermal fillers, chemical peels, and microdermabrasion are good choices for entry into aesthetic medicine.
8. Aesthetic lasers have greater costs and associated overhead; however, they also have the greatest revenue potential compared to other aesthetic procedures.
9. The clinician must review and update all fees for both dermatologic and aesthetic procedures *annually.* With insurance-based procedures, it is not what is charged, but rather what the reimbursements are that is important. Knowing both is key to optimizing reimbursement. The EOBs (explanations of benefits) provided by insurance companies that accompany payments must be reviewed, understood, and taken into consideration when fees are being updated.
10. Review denials of payments monthly. Find out which procedures are not being paid for and why. If prior approvals were needed, be sure to obtain those in the future. If certain procedures are not being paid for at all (e.g., skin tags) consider doing those only for cash up front.

Resources

Medicare fee schedules can be looked up at the following website: https://www.cms.gov/apps/physician-fee-schedule/license-agreement.aspx.

For a comprehensive list of dermatology and cosmetic dermatology CPT codes, see www.dermadvocate.net/library/articles/derm-coding.

References

1. *International Statistical Classification of Diseases, Clinical Modification,* ICD-9-CM. Chicago: The American Medical Association; 2010.
2. Physicians Current Procedural Terminology 2010. Chicago: American Medical Association; 2010.
3. 2010 Physician's Fee Reference. West Allis, WI: Yale Wasserman, DMD, Medical Publishers; 2010.
4. 2010 Physicians' Fee & Coding Guide. Atlanta, GA: MAG Mutual HealthCare Solutions; 2010.
5. National Fee Analyzer. Eden Prairie, MN: Ingenix; 2010.
6. Pfenninger JL. *The Reimbursement Manual for Office Procedures*. 16th ed. Austin, TX: The National Procedures Institute; 2010.
7. Pfenninger JL. *Coding for Dermatologic Procedures, 2004*. Videotape. Essexville, MI: Creative Health Communications, 2004.
8. Needham M, Katz B. Buying office equipment (Appendix L). *In:* Pfenninger JL, Fowler GC, eds. *Pfenninger and Fowler's Procedures for Primary Care*. 3rd ed. Philadelphia: Mosby/Elsevier; 2011.
9. Small R. Botulinum toxin type A for facial rejuvenation. *In:* Mayeaux E, ed. *The Essential Guide to Primary Care Procedures*. Philadelphia: Lippincott Williams & Wilkins; 2009:200–213.
10. Werschler P. The costs of products and services. *Cosm Dermatol.* 2008;21(7):376–383.

Appendices

Appendix A

General consent forms:

Patient information handouts:

Cosmetic informed consent forms and patient information handouts:

A Consent Forms and Patient Education Handouts

Disclosure and Consent

Medical and Surgical Procedures

TO THE PATIENT: You have the right, as a patient, to be informed about your condition and the recommended surgical, medical or diagnostic procedure to be used so that you may make the decision whether or not to undergo the procedure after knowing the risks and hazards involved. This disclosure is not meant to scare or alarm you; it is simply an effort to make you better informed so you may give or withhold your informed consent to the procedure.

I (we) voluntarily request Dr. ______________________________
As my physician, and such associates, technical assistants and other health care providers as they may deem necessary to treat my condition which has been explained to me as ______________________________

I (we) understand that the following surgical, medical and/or diagnostic procedures are planned for me and **I (we)** voluntarily consent and authorize these procedures:

☐ shave ☐ punch biopsy ☐ excision ☐ cryotherapy ☐ electrosurgery ☐ electrosurgery and curettage
☐ intralesional injections ☐ incision ☐ acne surgery ☐ other ______________________

I (we) understand that my physician may discover other or different conditions which require additional or different procedures than those planned. **I (we)** authorize my physician, and such associates, technical assistants and other health care providers to perform such other procedures which are advisable in their professional judgment.

Just as there may be risks and hazards in continuing my present condition without treatment, there are also risks and hazards related to the performance of the surgical, medical and/or diagnostic procedures planned for me. **I (we)** realize that common to surgical, medical and/or diagnostic procedures is the potential for infection, blood clots in veins and lungs, hemorrhage, allergic reactions, and even death. **I (we)** also realize that the following risks and hazards my occur in connection with this particular procedure:
PAIN, BLEEDING, INFECTION, SCARRING, CHANGE IN PIGMENTATION, RE-GROWTH, SLOW HEALING, CHANGE IN ANATOMICAL APPEARANCE, SKIN INDENTATION, SKIN PROTRUSION AND LOCAL NERVE DAMAGE (numbness or loss of muscle function)

I (we) understand that anesthesia involves additional risks and hazards but **I (we)** request the use of anesthetics for the relief and protection from pain during the planned and additional procedures. **I (we)** realize the anesthesia may have to be changed possibly without explanation to me (us). **I (we)** understand that certain complications may result from the use of any anesthetic including respiratory problems, drug reactions, paralysis, brain damage, or even death. Other risks and hazards which may result from the use of general anesthetics range from minor discomfort to injury to vocal chords, teeth, or eyes. **I (we)** understand that other risks and hazards resulting from spinal or epidural anesthetics include headache and chronic pain.

I (we) have been given an opportunity to ask questions of my physicians about my condition, alternative forms of anesthesia and treatment, risks of non-treatment, the procedures to use, and the risks and hazards involved, and **I (we)** believe that **I (we)** have sufficient information to give this informed consent.

I (we) certify this form has been fully explained to me, that **I (we)** have read it or have had it read to me, that the blank spaces have been filled in, and that **I (we)** understand its contents.

PATIENT Signature: ______________________________

Or other Legally Responsible Person's Signature: ____________________ **/ Relationship:** ____________

Date: ______________ **Time:** ______________ **( )AM ( )PM**

Witness: ______________ **Date:** ______________ **Time:** __________ **( )AM ( )PM**

I have explained to the patient or legal representative the disclosure and consent required for the medical, surgical, and/or diagnostic procedures planned as well as the patient's right to withhold consent.

Physician's Signature: ______________________________ **Date:** ____________

Divulgación y Consentimiento

Procedimientos Médicos y Quirúrgios

PARA EL PACIENTE: Usted, como paciente, tiene derecho a ser informado sobre su condición y sobre los recomendados procedimientos quirúrgicos, médicos, o diagnósticos que serán utilizados para que así usted tome la decisión de aceptar realizarse el procedimiento o no, una vez que sepa los riesgos y peligros involucrados. Esta declaración no tiene la intención de asustario o alarmarlo, es simplemente un esfuerzo para que usted esté mejor informado para poder dar o negar su consentimiento para el procedimiento.

Yo (nosotros) solicito (amos) de manera voluntaria que el Dr. ______________________________ como mi médico, junto con sus socios, ayudantes técnicos y otros proveedores médicos que consideren necesarios, me proporcionen el tratamiento para mi condición, el cual se me ha explicado como.

Yo (nosotros) entiendo (entendemos) que se ha planeado se me realicen los siguientes procedimientos quirúrgicos, médicos y / o diagnósticos, y yo (nosotros) voluntariamente acepto y autorizo se me realicen los siguientes procedimientos:

☐ afeitado ☐ crioterapia ☐ electrocirugía ☐ electrocirugía y legrado ☐ abstracción ☐ biopsia por punción

☐ inyección intralesional ☐ incisión ☐ cirugía por acné ☐ otros______________________

Yo (nosotros) entiendo (entendemos) que mi médico podria descubrir condición adicionales o distintos, que requieran procedimientos adicionales o distintos a los previstos. **Yo (nosotros)** autorizo (autorizamos) a mi médico, junto con sus socios, ayudantes técnicos y otros proveedores médicos realicen dichos procedimientos adicionales que a su juicio profesional sean prudentes.

Así com pueden existir riesgos y peligros en seguir con mi condición actual sin tratamiento, también existen riesgos y peligros relacionados con la realización de los procedimientos quirúrgicos, médicos y / o diagnósticos planeados para mí. **Yo (nosotros)** entiendo (entendemos) que con los procedimientos quirúrgicos, médicos y / o diagnósticos existe la posibilidad de infección, formación de coágulos de sangre en venas y pulmones, hemorragias, reacciones alérgicas e incluso al muerte. **Yo (nosotros)** también entiendo (entendemos) que pueden presentarse los siguientes riesgos y peligros en conexión con este procedimiento en particular: **DOLOR, SANGRANDO, INFECCIÓN, CICATRICES, CAMBIO DE PIGMENTACIÓN, NUEVO CRECIMIENTO, CURACIÓN LENTA, CAMBIO EN LA APARIENCIA ANATÓMICA, HENDIDURA EN LA PIEL, PROTRUSIÓN DE LA PIEL Y DAÑO A LOS NERVIOS LOCALES (sensación de entumecimiento o pérdida de la función muscular)**

Yo (nosotros) entiendo (entendemos) que la anestesia involucra reisgos y peligros adicionales, pero **yo (nosotros)** solicito (solicitamos) el uso de anestésicos para el alivio y la protección conra el dolor durante los procedimientos previstos y los adicionales. **Yo (nosotros)** comprendo (comprendemos) que la anestesia puede tener que ser cambiada, posiblemente sin que se dé una explicación a mí (nosotros). **Yo (nosotros)** entiendo (entendemos) que con el uso de cualquier anestésico pueden surgir ciertas complicaciones, incluyendo problemas respiratorios, reacción adversa a medicamentos, parálisis, daño cerebral o incluso la muerte. Otros riesgos y peligros que podrian resultar del uso de anestésicos generales varían de molestia leve hasta daño a las cuerdas vocales, los dientes o los ojos. **Yo (nosotros)** entiendo (entendemos) que otros riesgos y peligros que pueden resultar del uso de anestésicos de la columna vertebral incluyen dolor de cabeza y dolor crónico.

Se me (nos) ha ofrecido la oportunidad de hacer preguntas sobre mi padecimiento., las formas alternativas de anestesia y tratamiento, los riesgos por no recibir tratamiento, los procedimientos que se utilizarán y los riesgos y peligros involucrados, y creo (creemos) que tengo (tenemos) la información suficiente para dar este consentimiento informado.

Yo (nosotros) certifico (certificamos) que este formulario se me (nos) ha sido plenamente explicado., que **yo (nosotros)** lo he leído o se me ha leído, que los espacios en blanco han sido llenados y que **yo (nosotros)** entiendo (entendemos) su contenido.

FIRMA DEL PACIENTE: ______________________________

O de otra persona legalmente responsable: ____________________ **Parentesco:** ______________

Fecha: ______________ **Hora:**______________ **( )AM ( )PM**

Testigo: ____________________ **Fecha:**______________ **Hora:**__________ **( )AM ( )PM**

Le he explicado al paciente o su representate legal la divulgación y consentimiento necesarios para la realización de los procedimientos médicos, quirúrgicos y / o diagnósticos programados, así como el derecho del paciente a rehusar su consentimiento.

Firma del Médico: ______________________________ **Fecha:** ______________

Patient Information Handout

Care of Your Skin after a Shave Biopsy

Supplies needed

- Clean petroleum jelly (a squeeze tube is cleaner than a tub) (Vaseline is one name brand) (Do not use Neosporin or Triple Antibiotic)
- Dressing or gauze that is made for wound care (Band-Aids are one name brand)
- Optional – cotton-tipped applicators (Q-tips are one name brand)

Directions

- Keep the site clean and dry and do not remove the original dressing for 24 hours.
- After 24 hours you may shower daily. Gently wash the surgical site with soap and water in the shower or at least once daily.
- Apply petroleum jelly to the clean wound with a clean finger or cotton-tipped applicator one to two times per day.
- Use a dressing to cover the wound. While cleansing is only needed once or twice a day, additional petroleum jelly may be added as needed to keep the wound moist.
- Tylenol (acetaminophen) or ibuprofen can be taken for pain if needed. DO NOT start taking any medications with aspirin or aspirin products.

REPEAT THESE INSTRUCTIONS DAILY UNTIL THE WOUND IS HEALED. THIS MAY BE ANYWHERE FROM 5 TO 20 DAYS.

The wound will actually heal better and scar less if kept clean and covered with petroleum jelly.

Bleeding

If bleeding occurs, apply firm pressure to the site. Direct pressure should be applied to the wound. Five minutes should be adequate if the bleeding is minor and the wound is small. However, if the wound is larger and the bleeding is more severe, apply pressure for 10 minutes, timed by looking at a clock. It is best not to discontinue pressure to see if the bleeding has stopped until 10 minutes have passed. If the bleeding continues, remove the pad and press directly with a clean gauze pad over the bleeding site. If bleeding soaks through the gauze or is not stopped by firm pressure, call and go to your doctor or an urgent care center.

Infection

If you notice pus or discharge coming from the wound this may be an infection. This is particularly worrisome if you develop a fever and the wound is red, painful, swollen, and warm. Other signs of infection could be red streaks from wound, increased pain, and painful or swollen lymph nodes (glands). If you have any suspicion of having an infection, go to your doctor or an urgent care center.

Shower and washing

You may shower daily after the first 24 hours have passed. At first, you may leave the dressing on during the shower to protect the wound from the flow of water. Alternatively, if the wound needs cleaning, the shower is helpful to remove crusts and discharge. Dry the area gently and then apply the petroleum jelly and cover the healing wound as described above. We recommend not bathing in a tub or hot tub until the wound is completely healed over to avoid infection.

Wound healing

After the wound looks healed over you can stop daily dressing changes. The wound may remain red and will slowly fade over the next few weeks or months. Sometimes it can take 6 months to 1 year for the redness to fade completely.

You may experience a sensation of tightness as your wound heals. This is normal and will gradually go away. After the wound has healed, frequent, gentle massaging of the area will help to loosen the scar. Sometimes the surgery involves small nerves and may take up to a year before feeling returns to normal. Only rarely will the area remain numb permanently.

Your healed wound may be sensitive to temperature changes (such as cold air). This sensitivity improves with time, but if you are experiencing a lot of discomfort, try to avoid temperature extremes. You may experience itching after your wound appears to have healed. This is due to the healing that continues underneath the skin. Petroleum jelly may help to relieve this itching. Try not to scratch the wound since this may cause it to reopen.

IF YOU HAVE ANY CONCERNS NOT ANSWERED BY THIS INFORMATION, PLEASE CALL: ________________ OR GO TO ANOTHER MEDICAL FACILITY IF WE ARE CLOSED.

Patient Information Handout

Care of Your Skin after a Punch Biopsy

Supplies needed

- Clean petroleum jelly (a squeeze tube is cleaner than a tub) (Vaseline is one name brand) (Do not use Neosporin or Triple Antibiotic)
- Dressing or gauze that is made for wound care (Band-Aids are one name brand)
- Optional – cotton-tipped applicators (Q-tips are one name brand)

Directions

- Keep the site clean and dry and do not remove the original dressing for 24 hours.
- After 24 hours you may shower daily. Gently wash the surgical site with soap and water in the shower or at least once daily.
- Apply petroleum jelly to the clean wound with a clean finger or cotton-tipped applicator one to two times per day.
- Use a dressing to cover the wound especially if the wound was not sutured. While cleansing is only needed once or twice a day, additional petroleum jelly may be added as needed to keep the wound moist. Sutured (stitched) wounds may be left uncovered without petroleum jelly after two days.
- Tylenol (acetaminophen) or ibuprofen can be taken for pain if needed. DO NOT start taking any medications with aspirin or aspirin products.

For wounds that were not sutured (stitched), these will actually heal better and scar less if kept clean and covered with petroleum jelly.

Bleeding

If bleeding occurs, apply firm pressure to the site. Direct pressure should be applied to the wound. Five minutes should be adequate if the bleeding is minor and the wound is small. However, if the wound is larger and the bleeding is more severe, apply pressure for 10 minutes, timed by looking at a clock. It is best not to discontinue pressure to see if the bleeding has stopped until 10 minutes have passed. If the bleeding continues, remove the pad and press directly with a clean gauze pad over the bleeding site. If bleeding soaks through the gauze or is not stopped by firm pressure, call and go to your doctor or an urgent care center.

Infection

If you notice pus or discharge coming from the wound this may be an infection. This is particularly worrisome if you develop a fever and the wound is red, painful, swollen, and warm. Other signs of infection could be red streaks from wound, increased pain, and painful or swollen lymph nodes (glands). If you have any suspicion of having an infection, call and go to your doctor or an urgent care center.

Shower and washing

You may shower daily after the first 24 hours have passed. At first, you may leave the band-aid on during the shower to protect the wound from the forceful flow of water. Alternatively, it the wound needs cleaning, the shower is helpful to remove crusts and discharge. Dry the area gently and then apply petroleum jelly if the wound was not sutured. We recommend not bathing in a tub or hot tub until the wound is completely healed over to avoid infection.

Wound healing

After the wound looks healed over you can stop daily dressing changes. The wound may remain red and will slowly fade over the next few weeks or months. Sometimes it can take 6 months to 1 year for the redness to fade completely.

You may experience a sensation of tightness as your wound heals. This is normal and will gradually fade. After the wound has healed, frequent, gentle massaging of the area will help to loosen the scar. Sometimes the surgery involves small nerves and may take up to a year before feeling returns to normal. Only rarely will the area remain numb permanently.

Your healed wound may be sensitive to temperature changes (such as cold air). This sensitivity improves with time, but if you are experiencing a lot of discomfort avoid temperature extremes. You may experience itching after your wound appears to have healed. This is due to the healing that continues underneath the skin. Petroleum jelly may help to relieve this itching. Try not to scratch the wound since this may cause it to reopen.

SPECIAL INSTRUCTIONS FOR WOUNDS WITH SUTURES

- After surgery, go home and take it easy (avoid exertion, lifting, bending, or straining).
- Be very careful not to accidentally cut the sutures, especially while shaving.

SPECIAL INSTRUCTIONS FOR WOUNDS ON THE FACE WITH SUTURES

It is perfectly normal to have bruising or discoloration around the surgery site, especially if the wound is around the eye area. Do not be alarmed by this; it will eventually fade and return to normal color.

IF YOU HAVE ANY CONCERNS NOT ANSWERED BY THIS INFORMATION, PLEASE CALL: ________________OR GO TO ANOTHER MEDICAL FACILITY IF WE ARE CLOSED.

Patient Information Handout

Care of Your Skin after Surgery

Supplies needed

- Clean petroleum jelly (a squeeze tube is cleaner than a tub) (Vaseline is one name brand) (Do not use Neosporin or Triple Antibiotic)
- Dressing or gauze that is made for wound care (Band-Aids are one name brand)
- Optional – cotton-tipped applicators (Q-tips are one name brand)

Directions

- Keep the site clean and dry and do not remove the original dressing for 24 hours.
- After 24 hours you may shower daily. Gently wash the surgical site with soap and water in the shower or at least once daily.
- Apply petroleum jelly to the clean wound with a clean finger or cotton-tipped applicator one to two times per day.
- Use a dressing to cover the wound. While cleansing is only needed once or twice a day, additional petroleum jelly may be added as needed to keep the wound moist.
- Tylenol (acetaminophen) or ibuprofen can be taken for pain if needed. DO NOT start taking any medications with aspirin or aspirin products.

REPEAT THESE INSTRUCTIONS DAILY UNTIL THE WOUND IS HEALED. THIS MAY BE ANYWHERE FROM 5 TO 20 DAYS.

The wound will actually heal better and scar less if kept clean and covered with petroleum jelly.

Bleeding

If bleeding occurs, apply firm pressure to the site. Direct pressure should be applied to the wound. Five minutes should be adequate if the bleeding is minor and the wound is small. However, if the wound is larger and the bleeding is more severe, apply pressure for 10 minutes, timed by looking at a clock. It is best not to discontinue pressure to see if the bleeding has stopped until 10 minutes have passed. If the bleeding continues, remove the pad and press directly with a clean gauze pad over the bleeding site. If bleeding soaks through the gauze or is not stopped by firm pressure, call and go to your doctor or an urgent care center.

Infection

If you notice pus or discharge coming from the wound this may be an infection. This is particularly worrisome if you develop a fever and the wound is red, painful, swollen, and warm. Other signs of infection could be red streaks from wound, increased pain, and painful or swollen lymph nodes (glands). If you have any suspicion of having an infection, go to your doctor or an urgent care center.

Shower and washing

You may shower daily after the first 24 hours have passed. At first, you may leave the dressing on during the shower to protect the wound from the flow of water. Alternatively, if the wound needs cleaning, the shower is helpful to remove crusts and discharge. Dry the area gently and then apply the petroleum jelly and cover the healing wound as described above. We recommend not bathing in a tub or hot tub until the wound is completely healed over to avoid infection.

Patient Information Handout

Care of Your Skin after Surgery (continued)

Wound healing

After the wound looks healed over you can stop daily dressing changes. The wound may remain red and will slowly fade over the next few weeks or months. Sometimes it can take 6 months to 1 year for the redness to fade completely.

You may experience a sensation of tightness as your wound heals. This is normal and will gradually fade. After the wound has healed, frequent, gentle massaging of the area will help to loosen the scar. Sometimes the surgery involves small nerves and may take up to a year before feeling returns to normal. Only rarely will the area remain numb permanently.

Your healed wound may be sensitive to temperature changes (such as cold air). This sensitivity improves with time, but if you are experiencing a lot of discomfort, try to avoid temperature extremes. You may experience itching after your wound appears to have healed. This is due to the healing that continues underneath the skin. Petroleum jelly may help to relieve this itching. Try not to scratch the wound since this may cause it to reopen.

Avoid sunlight to the scar by keeping it covered and/or using sunscreen. Prolonged sun exposure may turn the pink scar to a darker red or purple color and delay healing.

SPECIAL INSTRUCTIONS FOR ALL WOUNDS WITH STITCHES (SUTURES)

- After surgery, go home and take it easy (avoid exertion, lifting, bending, or straining).
- Be very careful not to accidentally cut the sutures, especially while shaving.
- For one month, avoid heavy lifting or vigorous exercise that could cause your wound to pull apart.
- Contact the clinic if the incision pulls apart.

SPECIAL INSTRUCTIONS FOR WOUNDS ON THE FACE WITH STITCHES

- Keep your head elevated for the first 2 nights even while sleeping.
- Avoid sleeping on the same side of the body as the wound.
- Do not bend over with your head lower than your heart level. Bend at the knees to stoop down. Be careful not to lift anything heavy or do anything that might cause strain on the sutures.
- It is perfectly normal to have bruising or discoloration around the surgery site, especially if the wound is around the eye area. Do not be alarmed; it will eventually fade and return to normal color.

IF YOU HAVE ANY CONCERNS NOT ANSWERED BY THIS INFORMATION, PLEASE CALL: ________________ OR GO TO ANOTHER MEDICAL FACILITY IF WE ARE CLOSED.

Patient Information Handout

Wart Therapy with Candida Antigen

Some warts are best treated with **Candida antigen injection.** A small amount of the dead yeast will be injected into as many warts as possible. It is not necessary to inject every wart, but as many as possible will be treated limiting the total amount used to 1 mL. You may want to take acetaminophen or ibuprofen before a visit to help with the discomfort.

The **advantages of injection therapy** are that it is quick, and there are no scars from the injections or open sores to deal with. You can immediately return to full activity, including swimming, sports, jazzercise, etc. No special care is needed. With injection therapy, the body's immune system learns that wart tissue is abnormal. Unlike other treatments, if the warts go away with injection therapy, they rarely ever return.

The side effects of injection therapy with Candida have been very rare. Very rarely someone will develop a **rash, hives, itching over the whole body,** or **swelling. This indicates an allergy and will mean that the patient can no longer receive any further injections. Itching and redness** in the area of injection is to be expected, however. Rarely, there will be some **mild blistering.** Often the **warts will turn somewhat black** and the crust will fall off. About one-third of the time, a second injection will be needed one month later. Half of the remaining warts will respond to the second injection. For those warts that have not responded to the first two injections, a third one a month later can be tried. (We do not normally give more than three monthly injections, but in some instances we have given them up to five times.) 85% of patients will have cleared their warts after the third injection. If all injections have failed, then another method will be needed.

If you notice a rash after treatment, please call our office as soon as possible. **If you develop hives** take Benadryl (diphenhydramine) immediately and call our office (50 mg for older children/100 mg for adults). For children less than 5 years old, check with us about the dosage.

Generally a follow-up visit is scheduled for one month after the first injection. If you are **absolutely sure the wart(s) is/are gone, cancel the visit at least 3 days before the scheduled visit.** If you're not absolutely sure the wart(s) is/are gone, keep your visit. Let us decide if further treatment is necessary.

Note regarding the Candida solution – the medicine used for the injection. For your first visit, the medication will be taken from our supplies. However, if further injections are needed, you will need to pick up a bottle from a pharmacist and bring it with you to the second visit. On your first visit, the doctor will write a prescription for you. Many times, one injection is all that is needed. Do not purchase the material for your second visit until you find that it will be needed. If it appears that the wart is not going away with the first injection, then about 2 or 3 days before your next scheduled visit, go to the pharmacist with the prescription and pick up the material. The antigen usually costs over $100 and may not be covered by your insurance. Be sure the pharmacist knows it is being used for **treatment**, not just testing. **Candida antigen (Candin) is not carried routinely by most pharmacies. The hospital pharmacy is more likely to have it. Call beforehand to be sure they do. Other pharmacies will usually order it for you if you call them a few days in advance.** Keep it refrigerated until your office visit. No further purchases of **Candida antigen** will be necessary even if three or more injection visits are required.

If Candida injections fail, we may try Bleomycin injections, cryotherapy, cantharidin liquid, or other techniques. Warts are tough but we'll try our best to resolve them the quickest way, and also limit scarring. Help us by eating a diet rich in fruits and vegetables and taking a multivitamin. We'll be glad to answer any questions you might have.

Botulinum Toxin Treatments

Informed Consent

This consent form is designed to provide the information necessary when considering whether or not to undergo Botulinum Toxin Treatments for facial wrinkles with Botox.

Injected botulinum toxin causes weakness of muscles that can last approximately three months. Injection of small amounts of Botox relaxes the treated muscles and can reduce facial wrinkles such as frown lines. Botox solution is injected with a small needle into the muscles. Typically, effects are seen in a few days and take 1–2 weeks to fully develop.

The risks, side effects and complications of treatment with Botox include, but are not limited to:

- Pain
- Bruising, which resolves within 1–2 weeks after the injection
- Swelling
- Headache
- Undesired change in eyebrow shape
- Rarely, an adjacent muscle may be weakened which may result in a droopy upper or lower eyelid (1–5%), droopy eyebrow.

Post marketing safety data suggests that botulinum toxin effects may, in some cases, be observed beyond the site of local injection. The symptoms may include generalized muscle weakness, double vision, blurred vision, eyelid droop, difficulty swallowing, difficulty speaking, urinary incontinence, and breathing difficulties. These symptoms have been reported hours to weeks after injection. Swallowing and breathing difficulties can be life threatening and there have been reports of death related to spread of toxin effects. The risk of symptoms is probably greatest in children treated for spasticity but symptoms can also occur in adults, particularly in those patients who have underlying conditions that would predispose them to these symptoms. No definite serious adverse event reports of distant spread of toxin effect associated with dermatologic use of cosmetic botulinum toxin at the labeled dose of 20 units (for frown lines) or 100 units (for underarm sweating) have been reported.

My signature below certifies that I have fully read this consent form and understand the information provided to me regarding the proposed procedure. I have been adequately informed about the procedure including the potential benefits, limitations, alternative treatments, and I have had all my questions and concerns answered to my satisfaction. I understand that results are not guaranteed and I accept the risks, side effects, and possible complications inherent in undergoing Botox treatments.

Patient Signature: ____

Or other Legally Responsible Person's Signature: ______________________/
Relationship: ______________

Date: ______________ **Time:**______________ **( )AM ( )PM**

Witness: ____________________ **Date:**______________
Time:________ **( )AM ( )PM**

I have explained to the patient or legal representative the disclosure and consent required for the medical, surgical, and/or diagnostic procedures planned as well as the patient's right to withhold consent.

Physician's Signature: ______________________________ **Date:** __________

Patient Information Handout

Botulinum Toxin Treatments

Prior to treatment

- Avoid aspirin (Excedrin), vitamin E, St. John's wort, and other dietary supplements including ginkgo, evening primrose oil, garlic, feverfew, and ginseng for 2 weeks.
- Avoid ibuprofen (Advil, Motrin) and alcohol for 2 days.
- If possible, come to your appointment with a cleanly washed face.

After treatment

- Do not massage the treated areas on the day of treatment.
- Avoid lying down for 4 hours immediately after treatment.
- Avoid applying heat to the treated area on the day of treatment.
- Avoid activities that cause facial flushing on the day of treatment including consuming alcohol, exercising, tanning.
- Gently apply a cool compress or wrapped ice pack to the treated areas for fifteen minutes every few hours as needed to reduce discomfort, swelling, or bruising up to a few days after treatment. If bruising occurs it typically resolves within 7–10 days.
- After treatment oral SinEcch and/or topical Arnica montana may help reduce bruising and swelling.
- Botulinum toxin treatment effects take about 1–2 weeks to fully develop and last approximately 2½–4 months.
- If 1–2 weeks after treatment you feel that you require a touch-up please contact the office.

Skin Care Treatments

Informed Consent

This consent form is designed to provide the necessary information to decide whether or not to undergo Skin Care Treatments which include, but are not limited to, superficial mechanical exfoliation (microdermabrasion), superficial chemical exfoliation (chemical peels), and the use of skin care products.

Mechanical exfoliation (ME) is a physical method of skin exfoliation of the top layers of skin, which involves removing the outermost layer of the skin with the use of abrasive crystals, bristles, or diamond-tipped heads. Chemical exfoliation (CE) involves exfoliating the top layers of skin through the use of chemical acids, including but not not limited to, glycolic, salicylic, and trichloroacetic acid.

Alternative treatments to ME and CE include ablative and nonablative laser skin resurfacing, plastic surgery, or no treatment at all.

Possible risks, side effects, and complications with Skin Care Treatments include, but are not limited to:

- Hypopigmentation (lighter pigmentation) or hyperpigmentation (darker pigmentation)
- Recurrent viral infections such as herpes simplex or varicella may be activated by treatments
- Abrasion (superficial cut) or temporary lines and streaking may occur with ME
- Acne outbreak
- Infection or scarring

Patients with darker skin types have an increased risk of complications such as hypopigmentation, hyperpigmentation, blistering, and scarring.

I understand that it is not possible to predict any of the above side effects or complications and results are not guaranteed. I have fully read this consent form and understand the information provided to me regarding the proposed procedure. I have been adequately informed about the procedure including the potential benefits, limitations, and alternative treatments, and I have had all my questions and concerns answered to my satisfaction.

Patient Signature:____

Or other Legally Responsible Person's Signature: __________________________/
Relationship: ____________________

Date: ____________________ **Time:**____________________ **( )AM ( )PM**

Witness: __________________________ **Date:**__________________
Time:________ **( )AM ( )PM**

I have explained to the patient or legal representative the disclosure and consent required for the medical, surgical, and/or diagnostic procedures planned as well as the patient's right to withhold consent.

Physician's Signature: ________________________________**Date:** ____________

Patient Information Handout

Skin Care Treatments

Prior to treatment

- Refrain from tanning and direct sun exposure for two weeks prior to each treatment and for the duration of your treatment.
- Use sunscreen daily with SPF 30 or greater for the duration of your treatments.
- Apply the recommended home care products for skin preparation as instructed by your esthetician.
- One week prior to treatment, discontinue use of any products containing alpha-hydroxy (such as glycolic or lactic acid) or retinoic acid (such as Retin-A and Renova).
- Laser or intense pulsed light treatments may be received two weeks before and after Skin Care Treatment.
- If you have skin lesions in the treatment areas which have changed in any way, itched or bled, you must consult your personal physician prior to starting treatment. Treatment areas must be free of any open sores, lesions, or skin infections.

After treatment

- Skin may feel sensitive, tight, dry, and appear pink, red, and slightly swollen for 3–5 days.
- These treatments stimulate the skin to renew and generate new skin cells and collagen and increase blood circulation to the skin. Do not pick, abrade, or scrub skin that is sensitive or peeling. This may cause surface scarring, irritation, and interrupt the skin's natural rejuvenation process.

Apply the recommended home care products for post-treatment skin care as instructed. Resume use of regular home skin care products (including alpha-hydroxy and retinoic acids) two weeks after Skin Care Treatments or as instructed.

Dermal Filler Treatments

Informed Consent

This consent form is designed to provide the necessary information to decide whether to undergo treatment with dermal fillers ("fillers").

Dermal filler treatments are used for the treatment of facial creases, wrinkles, folds, contour defects, depression scars, facial lipoatrophy (loss of fat), and/or lip enhancement. The treatments involve multiple small injections of the filler into or below the skin to fill wrinkles and restore volume. The effects of injectable fillers are temporary and no guarantees can be made regarding how long correction will last in a specific patient.

Alternatives to temporary fillers include, but are not limited to: permanent dermal fillers, laser resurfacing, surgical facelift, lasers for skin laxity, or no treatment at all.

Possible risks, side effects, and complications with dermal fillers include, but are not limited to:

- Redness and swelling, bruising, infection
- On rare occasions, red bumps or pustules (acne-like lesions) may form
- Discoloration of the skin such as grayish, bluish, or reddish coloration
- Filler material may be extruded from the skin in rare cases
- Visible raised areas or lumpiness at/around the treated site
- Rarely granulomas, which are firm nodules, may form
- Allergic reaction with itchiness, redness, and in extremely rare cases generalized allergic response such as whole body swelling, respiratory problems, and shock

A remote and rare risk is that of injecting filler into a blood vessel (blood vessel occlusion) or overfilling the tissue, which can block blood flow to the treated area or to distant areas causing tissue damage and tissue death (necrosis). Blood vessel occlusion can result in blindness if filler is injected in a blood vessel near the eye such as in the tear trough or in the frown area. Blood vessel occlusion can result in necrosis (skin death) of the side of the nose or cheek if filler is injected into a blood vessel near the nose or the fold between the cheek and the nose.

My signature below certifies that I have fully read this consent form and understand the written information provided to me regarding the proposed procedure. I have been adequately informed about the procedure including: the potential benefits, risks, limitations, and alternative treatments and I have had all my questions and concerns answered to my satisfaction.

Patient Signature: ______________________________

Or other Legally Responsible Person's Signature: ____________________/
Relationship: ____________

Date: ____________ **Time:**____________ **( )AM ( )PM**

Witness: ____________________ **Date:**____________
Time:________ **( )AM ( )PM**

I have explained to the patient or legal representative the disclosure and consent required for the medical, surgical, and/or diagnostic procedures planned as well as the patient's right to withhold consent.

Physician's Signature: ______________________________ **Date:** __________

Patient Information Handout

Dermal Filler Treatments

Prior to treatment

- Avoid aspirin (any product containing acetylsalicylic acid), vitamin E, St. John's wort, and other dietary supplements including ginkgo, evening primrose oil, garlic, feverfew, and ginseng for 2 weeks.
- Avoid ibuprofen (Advil, Motrin) and alcohol for 2 days.
- If possible, come to your appointment with a cleanly washed face without make up.

After treatment

- Skin redness and swelling in the treatment area are common. This should resolve within a few days. If it persists longer than 3 days please contact your physician.
- Do not massage the treated areas on the day of treatment.
- Avoid applying heat to the treated area on the day of treatment.
- Avoid activities that cause facial flushing on the day of treatment including consuming alcohol, exercising, tanning.
- Gently apply a cool compress or wrapped ice pack to the treated areas for fifteen minutes every few hours as needed to reduce discomfort, swelling, or bruising up to a few days after treatment. If bruising occurs it typically resolves within 7–10 days.
- After treatment oral and/or topical Arnica montana may help reduce bruising and swelling.
- If 2–4 weeks after treatment you feel that you require a touch-up please contact your physician.

Laser Hair Reduction

Informed Consent

This consent form is designed to provide the necessary information to decide whether or not to undergo laser/intense pulsed light (referred to as "laser") treatment for the removal of unwanted hair.

The laser damages the pigment in hair follicles, which interferes with hair growth. Individual response to treatments will vary. It is affected by the nature of the hair (fine, thick, light, dark) and factors that influence hair growth, individual skin types (light skin responds better), area of treatment, and several other factors.

Results are cumulative and several treatments in a series are typically required for maximum benefit. No guarantees can be made as to the results that might be obtained from these procedures, the percentage of improvement expected following treatments, or that a specific result will be achieved.

Alternative methods to laser treatments for removal of hair include shaving, plucking, depilatory creams, waxing, electrolysis, or no treatment at all.

Possible risks, side effects, and complications of laser treatment for unwanted hair include, but are not limited to:

- Skin pigment changes such as hypopigmentation (lighter pigmentation) or hyperpigmentation (darker pigmentation)
- Bruising, blistering, scabbing, scarring
- Ingrown hairs
- Infection in the treated area, including folliculitis (infection of the hair follicle), herpes, shingles
- Tattoos and permanent makeup in the treatment area may be altered
- Stimulation of more hair growth (paradoxical hair growth)

Patients with darker skin types have an increased risk of complications such as hypopigmentation, hyperpigmentation, blistering, and scarring.

My signature below certifies that I have fully read this consent form and understand the information provided to me regarding the proposed procedure. I have been adequately informed about the procedure including: the potential benefits, limitations, and alternative treatments, and I have had all my questions and concerns answered to my satisfaction.

Patient Signature: ____

Or other Legally Responsible Person's Signature: ______________________/
Relationship: ____________________

Date: ____________________ **Time:**____________________ **( )AM ( )PM**

Witness: ______________________ **Date:**____________________
Time:__________ **( )AM ( )PM**

I have explained to the patient or legal representative the disclosure and consent required for the medical, surgical, and/or diagnostic procedures planned as well as the patient's right to withhold consent.

Physician's Signature: ______________________________ **Date:** ____________

Patient Information Handout

Laser Hair Reduction

Prior to treatment

- Do not pluck, wax, undergo stringing/threading, or electrolysis to desired treatment areas for 4 weeks before laser/intense pulsed light (referred to as laser) hair removal treatments.
- Do not use depilatory creams or bleach for 2 weeks prior to treatments.
- Refrain completely from tanning and direct sun exposure for 4 weeks prior to each treatment and for the duration of your treatments.
- Avoid using sunless tanning products for 2 weeks before treatment.
- Use sunscreen daily with SPF 30 or greater for the duration of your treatments.
- Discontinue use of glycolic and Retin-A containing products 1 week before treatments.
- Do not use medications that cause photosensitivity (including doxycycline, tetracycline, and minocycline) for at least 72 hours prior to laser treatments.
- On the day of your appointment, shave the area to be treated. The treatment area must be free of any open sores, lesions, or skin infections (e.g., active acne).
- If you have a history of herpes (oral cold sores, genital) or shingles, in the treatment area start your anti-viral medication at the dose recommended by your doctor for 2 days prior to treatment and continue for 3 days after treatment.

After treatment

- Some skin redness and swelling along with a mild sunburn sensation in the treatment area is normal. This should resolve within a few hours to days.
- Apply cool compresses or wrapped ice pack to the treated areas for fifteen minutes every few hours as needed to reduce the discomfort. You may also apply 1% hydrocortisone cream (over-the-counter with or without aloe) 2 times per day for 3–4 days to decrease skin irritation.
- Gently wash twice daily with mild soap. Aloe vera gel may be used afterwards for several days (if not using hydrocortisone cream). Loose, comfortable clothing is recommended.
- Avoid irritants such as glycolic and Retin-A products, toners, exfoliants, astringents, hot water, or other products that cause irritation for 1 week following treatment. Once irritation has resolved, you may exfoliate in the treatment area.
- Avoid sun exposure and tanning for 4 weeks following each treatment. Use sunscreen daily with SPF 30 or greater for the duration of your treatments.
- If blistering, crusting, or scabbing develops, notify your physician then apply a thin layer of antibiotic ointment (such as bacitracin) to the area twice a day until the skin heals to prevent infection.
- You may notice some singed hairs and hairs that are coming out of the follicle after treatment. This is normal and may occur for several weeks.
- Makeup can be worn after the first day provided there are no apparent problems.

Laser Photorejuvenation Treatments

Informed Consent

This consent form is designed to provide the necessary information to decide whether or not to undergo laser or intense pulsed light (IPL) treatments (which will be referred to as “lasers”) for photorejuvenation and for benign vascular and pigmented lesions.

There are several alternative methods to photorejuvenation, including but not limited to, topical skin products, liquid nitrogen for pigmented lesions, electrosurgery or sclerotherapy for facial vascular lesions, plastic surgery, or no treatment at all.

Lasers treatments for photorejuvenation are indicated for skin conditions which include:

Telangiectasias (“spider veins”), redness and flushing symptoms of rosacea, brown spots, sun spots, lentigines (aging sun spots), dyschromia, melasma, enlarged pores. The lasers heat and eliminate the abnormal pigment in the skin and small blood vessels. Results vary and no guarantees can be made that a specific patient will benefit from treatment or achieve any level of improvement. **Maximum benefit is typically achieved with 3 to 6 treatments.**

Possible risks, side effects, and complications of laser treatments include, but are not limited to:

- Bruising, blistering, burns, scabbing, infection
- Hypopigmentation (lighter pigmentation) or hyperpigmentation (darker pigmentation)
- Scarring is rare, but can occur
- Reduced or no hair growth in treatment areas and adjacent areas
- Tattoos and permanent makeup in the treatment area may be altered
- Recurrent viral infections such as herpes simplex or varicella may be activated by treatments
- Minimal or lack of effect from the treatments

My signature below certifies that I have fully read this consent form and understand the information provided to me regarding the proposed procedure. I have been adequately informed about the procedure including the potential benefits, limitations, and alternative treatments, and I have had all my questions and concerns answered to my satisfaction.

Patient Signature: ______________________________

Or other Legally Responsible Person's Signature: ______________________/
Relationship: ______________

Date: ______________ **Time:**______________ **( )AM ( )PM**

Witness: ______________ **Date:**______________
Time:________ **( )AM ( )PM**

I have explained to the patient or legal representative the disclosure and consent required for the medical, surgical, and/or diagnostic procedures planned as well as the patient's right to withhold consent.

Physician's Signature: ______________________________ **Date:** __________

Patient Information Handout

Laser Photorejuvenation Treatments

Prior to treatment

- Refrain completely from tanning and direct sun exposure for 4 weeks prior to each treatment and for the duration of your treatments.
- Avoid using sunless tanning products for 2 weeks before treatment.
- Discontinue use of glycolic acid and Retin-A containing products 1 week before treatments.
- Do not use medications that cause you to be sensitive to the sun for 72 hours prior to treatments. This may include medications, even over-the-counter ones. If you are taking any medications or supplements, discuss these with the provider before treatment.
- If you have a history of herpes or shingles in the treatment area, start your prescribed anti-viral medication 2 days prior to treatment and continue for 3 days after treatment.
- Consult your personal physician if there is a family or personal history of skin cancer or if you have skin lesions which have changed in any way, itched or bled recently.

After treatment

- Some skin redness and swelling are common and should resolve in a few hours to 3 days. Apply a wrapped ice pack to the treated areas for fifteen minutes every few hours as needed.
- Gently wash twice daily with mild soap. Do not rub the skin vigorously and avoid hot water.
- Avoid activities that cause flushing for 2–3 days after treatment, including consuming alcohol, exercise, extensive sun or heat exposure; swimming; hot tubs and Jacuzzis.
- Avoid irritants such as glycolic acid and retinoid products, toners, exfoliants, astringents, or other products that cause irritation for 1 week following treatment.
- If blistering, crusting, or scabbing develops, notify your physician then apply a thin layer of antibiotic ointment such as bacitracin to the area twice a day until the skin heals.
- Makeup can be worn once there are no signs of skin irritation, usually the day after treatment. Use sunscreen daily with SPF 30 or greater for the duration of your treatments.
- **Photorejuvenation treatments of pigmented lesions** may initially look raised and darker. The lesions will darken over the next few days and flake off over 1–2 weeks.
- **Photorejuvenation treatments of vascular lesions** may disappear immediately, lighten or change color turning gray or bluish-purple. The lesions will usually lighten over the next week.

Nonablative Laser Treatments for Wrinkle Reduction

Informed Consent

This consent form is designed to provide the necessary information to decide whether or not to undergo nonablative laser treatments for wrinkle reduction.

Lasers used for these treatments selectively heat up the collagen in the skin to stimulate new collagen synthesis. There is no break in the surface of the skin and there is little or no downtime associated with this laser treatment. Microdermabrasion is often done in conjunction with these laser treatments for improvement of superficial fine lines and pigment changes.

Results are cumulative and several treatments are typically required for maximum benefit. No guarantees can be made as to the results that might be obtained from these procedures, the percentage of improvement expected following treatments, or that a specific result will be achieved.

Other alternative wrinkle reduction treatments include microdermabrasion, chemical peels, laser resurfacing, surgery (such as facelifts), or no treatment at all.

Possible risks, side effects, and complications of nonablative laser wrinkle reduction treatments include, but are not limited to:

- Hypopigmentation (lighter pigmentation) or hyperpigmentation (darker pigmentation)
- Herpes simplex (cold sores) or varicella (shingles) may be activated by treatments
- Tattoos and permanent makeup in the treatment area may be altered
- Burns, scarring

Patients with darker skin types have an increased risk of complications such as hypopigmentation, hyperpigmentation, burns, and scarring.

My signature below certifies that I have fully read this consent form and understand the information provided to me regarding the proposed procedure. I have been adequately informed about the procedure including the potential benefits, limitations, and alternative treatments, and I have had all my questions and concerns answered to my satisfaction. I understand and accept the risks, side effects, and possible complications inherent in undergoing nonablative laser treatments.

Patient Signature: ____

Or other Legally Responsible Person's Signature: ______________________/
Relationship: ________________

Date: __________________ **Time:**__________________ **( )AM ( )PM**

Witness: ______________________ **Date:**______________
Time:________ **( )AM ( )PM**

I have explained to the patient or legal representative the disclosure and consent required for the medical, surgical, and/or diagnostic procedures planned as well as the patient's right to withhold consent.

Physician's Signature: ______________________________ **Date:** __________

Patient Information Handout

Nonablative Laser Treatments for Wrinkle Reduction

Prior to treatment

- Refrain completely from tanning and direct sun exposure for 4 weeks prior to treatment and for 4 weeks after your treatments.
- Use sun block daily with zinc oxide or titanium dioxide (SPF 30 or greater) for the duration of your treatments.
- Discontinue use of glycolic and Retin-A containing products 1 week before treatments.
- Do not use medications that cause photosensitivity for 72 hours prior to treatments.
- If you have a history of herpes or shingles in the treatment area start your prescribed anti-viral medication 2 days prior to treatment and continue for 3 days after treatment.

After treatment

- Immediately after treatment, the skin may be red. This should resolve within a few hours.
- Makeup can be applied immediately after treatment.
- Avoid sun exposure and tanning for 4 weeks following treatment and use sun block daily with zinc oxide or titanium dioxide (SPF 30 or greater).
- Avoid activities that cause facial flushing, including vigorous exercise, consuming alcohol, extensive heat exposure, swimming and hot tubs for 1–2 days after treatment.
- Contact your physician immediately if blistering, crusting, or scabbing develops.
- Collagen formation will continue for 6 months and maximum benefit may not be noted for up to 6 months after completing treatments.

Fractional Ablative Laser Resurfacing Treatments

Informed Consent

This consent form is designed to provide the necessary information to decide whether or not to undergo fractional ablative laser resurfacing for treatment of lines and wrinkles, scars, photodamaged skin, enlarged pores, and rough skin texture.

The laser precisely delivers pulses of laser energy in a microbeam pattern to the skin, which causes columns of coagulation. The heated tissue within the columns starts a natural healing process that forms new, healthy skin. Improvements are typically seen 3–6 months after treatment and more than 1 treatment may be required to achieve maximum results. No guarantees can be made as to the results that might be obtained from this procedure. Side effects or complications are not predictable.

Alternative methods to laser resurfacing treatments include chemical peels, surgical procedures (dermabrasion and facelift), or no treatment at all.

Possible risks, side effects, and complications of laser resurfacing include, but are not limited to:

- Hypopigmentation (lighter pigmentation) or hyperpigmentation (darker pigmentation)
- Visible skin patterns
- Herpes simplex (cold sores) or varicella (shingles) may be activated by treatments
- Allergic reactions
- Acne outbreak or milia (white bumps due to occluded sebaceous ducts) in the treated area
- Infection in the treated area
- Tattoos and permanent makeup in the treatment area may be altered
- Crusting
- Scarring

Patients with darker skin types have an increased risk of complications such as hypopigmentation, hyperpigmentation, burns, and scarring.

My signature below certifies that I have fully read this consent form and understand the information provided to me regarding the proposed procedure. I have been adequately informed about the procedure including the potential benefits, limitations, and alternative treatments, and I have had all my questions and concerns answered to my satisfaction. I understand and accept the risks, side effects, and possible complications inherent in undergoing laser resurfacing treatment. I understand that failure to follow instructions for before and after treatment may affect my treatment outcome and increase the likelihood or severity of complications.

Patient Signature: ______________________________

Or other Legally Responsible Person's Signature: ____________________/
Relationship: ____________

Date: ____________ **Time:**____________ **( )AM ( )PM**

Witness: ____________________ **Date:**____________
Time:________ **( )AM ( )PM**

I have explained to the patient or legal representative the disclosure and consent required for the medical, surgical, and/or diagnostic procedures planned as well as the patient's right to withhold consent.

Physician's Signature: ______________________________ **Date:** ________

Patient Information Handout

Fractional Ablative Laser Resurfacing Treatments

Prior to treatment

- Refrain completely from tanning and direct sun exposure for 4 weeks prior to treatment and for 6 weeks after your treatments.
- Use sunblock daily with zinc oxide or titanium dioxide (SPF 30 or greater).
- Discontinue use of glycolic and Retin-A containing products 1 week before treatments.
- Avoid deep facial peel procedures for 1 month prior to your laser treatment.
- Do not use medications that cause photosensitivity for 72 hours prior to treatments.
- If you have a history of herpes or shingles in the treatment area start your prescribed anti-viral medication 2 days prior to treatment and continue for 3 days after treatment.
- Avoid ginkgo biloba, vitamin E, aspirin compounds (i.e., Excedrin) for 2 weeks prior to the laser procedure to minimize bruising risk. Avoid anti-inflammatory medications such as ibuprofen for 1 week prior to your procedure. Tylenol (acetaminophen) is fine.

After treatment

- Immediately after treatment, the skin will be red and feel sensitive and there may be pinpoint bleeding. Apply an occlusive moisturizer (such as Primacy) generously as needed to keep the skin moist at all times to prevent crusting or scabbing.
- Cleanse with gauze pads soaked in a solution of **1 teaspoon of white vinegar in 2 cups of water** over the treatment areas for 10–15 minutes then gently wipe the areas with gauze when done. Repeat 6–8 times per day for day 1 and 2 after treatment. Wrapped ice packs may be applied over gauze pads to reduce discomfort.
- Cleanse with vinegar solution gauze pads 3–4 times per day on days 3 and 4 after treatment.
- Once the skin is fully healed, at around day 7 after treatment, the skin will be less red and should not feel uncomfortable. There should not be any pinpoint bleeding. Your physician or health care provider will inform you when the skin has fully healed. Mild facial cleanser can now be used daily and non-irritating skin care products including sunscreen. Do not rub the skin vigorously and avoid hot water as the skin will be fragile.
- Avoid activities that cause facial flushing, including vigorous exercise, consuming alcohol, extensive heat exposure, swimming, hot tubs and Jacuzzis for 2 weeks after treatment.
- Results typically are seen 3–6 months after treatment.

Laser Tattoo Removal

Informed Consent

This consent form is designed to provide the necessary information to decide whether or not to undergo laser tattoo removal treatments.

The purpose of this procedure is removal of the tattoo or to make the pattern as unrecognizable as possible by lightening the tattoo pigment. Anesthesia with local injectable, topical, or no anesthesia may be used. The laser energy is passed through the outer layer of the skin, directly targeting the tattoo ink. The laser disrupts the ink allowing the body's immune system to break it down and get rid of it.

Alternative treatment methods include camouflaging with makeup, tattooing over with a second tattoo, abrasive or acid treatments, treatment with a CO_2 laser, surgical removal, or no treatment at all.

Results vary and no guarantees can be made that a specific patient will benefit from treatment or achieve any level of improvement. Multiple treatments will be necessary to achieve desired results.

The possible risks of the procedure include but are not limited to:

- Pain, bruising, swelling, redness, blistering
- There is a risk of scarring, which can be permanent
- Hypopigmentation (lighter pigmentation) or hyperpigmentation (darker pigmentation)
- Infection
- Bleeding
- Residual tattoo pigment or persistence of tattoo pattern is possible

Patients with darker skin types have an increased risk of complications such as hypopigmentation, hyperpigmentation, burns, and scarring.

My signature below certifies that I have fully read this consent form and understand the information provided to me regarding the proposed procedure. I have been adequately informed about the procedure including the potential benefits, limitations, and alternative treatments, and I have had all my questions and concerns answered to my satisfaction.

Patient Signature: ______________________________

Or other Legally Responsible Person's Signature: ____________________/
Relationship: ________________

Date: ________________ **Time:**________________ **( )AM ( )PM**

Witness: ____________________ **Date:**________________
Time:__________ **( )AM ( )PM**

I have explained to the patient or legal representative the disclosure and consent required for the medical, surgical, and/or diagnostic procedures planned as well as the patient's right to withhold consent.

Physician's Signature: ______________________________ **Date:** __________

Patient Information Handout

Laser Tattoo Removal

After Your Treatment

- Immediately after treatment, apply a wrapped cool compress or wrapped ice pack to the treated areas for fifteen minutes every 1–2 hours.
- The area may feel warm, appear swollen, reddish, bruised or have pinpoint bleeding. Blistering or scabbing can occur particularly if ice is not applied as directed, and will generally heal in one to two weeks.
- You can shower/bathe 24 hours after your tattoo removal procedure.
- Discomfort typically resolves in 1–2 days. During this time you may take over-the-counter acetaminophen if needed.
- If the skin is irritated (without scabs or bleeding), apply sunscreen SPF 30 or greater daily. You may put a bandage of gauze and paper tape over the area if desired, but this is not needed.
- If the skin is not intact (with scabs or bleeding) use bacitracin or Aquaphor daily to keep the area moist. Place a bandage with a non-adherent gauze and tape every day until all scabs are fully healed. Then use sunscreen SPF 30 or greater daily.
- If mild itchiness occurs, use over-the-counter 1% hydrocortisone on the treated area once the skin is healed.
- If your arm or leg was treated, rest and elevate the treated area for at least 12 hours.
- You may resume light activities 48 hours after treatment but strenuous exercise should be avoided for 1 week. Activities such as swimming can be resumed after 2 weeks or once all scabbing/crusts have fully healed.

Before Your Next Treatment

- Avoid direct sun exposure to the tattoo and tanning beds for the duration of your tattoo removal treatments.
- Avoid using self-tanning and bronzing products on the tattoo.
- Apply an SPF 30 sunscreen or higher to any exposed treated area until the treatment area is completely healed.
- Generally your next treatment will be scheduled for six weeks. Reschedule if your skin is not fully healed (the tattoo area should not have a shiny appearance).

APPENDIX

B Supply Sources for Lasers

Company	Hair Removal	Photorejuvenation	Nonablative Wrinkle Reduction	Ablative Skin Resurfacing	Tattoo Removal
Aerolase		X	X	X	
Alma Lasers	X	X	X	X	X
American BioCare		X			
Asclepion Laser Technologies	X	X	X	X	X
Candela		X	X		X
CoolTouch	X	X	X		
Cutera	X	X	X	X	
Cynosure	X	X	X	X	X
Deka Laser Technologies				X	
DermaMed USA	X	X			
Dinona, Inc.			X		
Ellipse	X	X		X	
Energist	X	X	X	X	
Focus Medical	X	X	X	X	X
Fotona	X	X	X	X	
General Project	X	X			
HOYA ConBio	X	X	X	X	X
Iridex	X	X	X	X	
Lasering USA	X	X	X	X	
Light Age	X	X			X
Light BioScience			X		
Lumenis	X	X	X	X	X
Lutronic	X	X	X	X	X
Med-Aesthetic Solutions, Inc.	X	X	X		
MedArt Corporation	X	X		X	
Med-Surge		X			
Novalis	X	X	X		
Orion Lasers		X			
Palomar	X	X	X	X	X
Quantel Medical	X	X			
Radiancy	X	X	X		
Sciton	X	X	X	X	
SharpLight Technologies	X	X			
Solta		X	X	X	
Sybaritic	X	X	X	X	X
Syneron (also formerly Candela)	X	X	X		
WaveLight		X			

CONTACT INFORMATION

Aerolase
Phone: 877-379-2435
www.aerolase.com

Alma Lasers
Phone: 866-414-2562
www.almalasers.com

American BioCare
Phone: 800-676-1434
www.medicalbiocare.com

Asclepion Laser Technologies
www.asclepion.com

Candela
Phone: 800-733-8550
www.candelalaser.com

CoolTouch
Phone: 877-858-COOL
www.cooltouch.com

Cutera
Phone: 888-4-CUTERA
www.cutera.com

Cynosure
Phone: 800-886-2966
www.cynosure.com

DermaMed USA
Phone: 888-789-6342
www.dermamedusa.com

Dinona, Inc
Phone: +82 2 578 0810
www.dinonainc.com

Ellipse
Phone: +45 4576 8808
www.ellipse.org

Energist
Phone: 845-348-4900
www.energisintna.com

Focus Medical
Phone: 866- 633-5273
www.focusmedical.com

Fotona
Phone: 888-550-4113
www.fotonamedicallasers.com

General Project
Phone: 908-454-8875
www.generalproject.com

HOYA ConBio
Phone: 800-532-1064
www.conbio.com

Iridex
Phone: 650-940-4700
www.iridex.com

Lasering USA
Phone: 866-471-0469
www.laseringusa.com

Light BioScience
Phone: 803-409-8025
www.gentlewaves.com

Lumenis
Phone: 408-764-3000
www.lumenis.com

Med-Aesthetic Solutions, Inc.
Phone: 760-942-8815
www.medaestheticsolutions.com

MedArt Corporation
Phone: 760-798-2740
www.medart.dk

Med-Surge
Phone: 877-354-7845, 972-720-0425
www.medsurgeadvances.com

Novalis
Phone: 866-627-4475
www.novalismedical.com

Orion Lasers
Phone: 866-414-ALMA
www.almalasers.com

Palomar
Phone: 800-725-0628
www.palomarmedical.com

Quantel Medical
Phone: 888-660-6726
www.quantelmedical.com

Radiancy
Phone: 888-662220
www.radiancy.com

Sciton
Phone: 888-646-6999
www.sciton.com

SharpLight Technologies
Phone: 905-337-7797
www.sharplightech.com

Solta
Phone: 888-437-2935
www.fraxel.com

Sybaritic
Phone: 800-445-8418
www.sybaritic.com

Syneron (also formerly Candela)
Phone: 866-259-6661
www.syneron.com

WaveLight
Phone: +32 3 870 37 63
www.dcmedical.be/FR/dermatologie/lasers/Midon_Vasculair.htm

The reader is also directed to the *Aesthetic Guide* (www.miinews.com) for information on ablative laser vendors.

Laser-Safe Eyewear

Glendale
Phone: 800-500-4739
www.glendale-laser.com

Oculo-Plastik
Phone: 888-381-3292
www.oculoplastik.com

Laser Safety Training Courses

American Society for Laser Medicine and Surgery (ASLMS)
Phone: 715-845-9283
www.aslms.org

Typical ICD-9 Codes for Patients Receiving Laser Treatment

Acne, comedones	706.1
Dyschromia, unspecified	709.0
Melasma	709.09
Rosacea	695.3
Scarring	709.2
Wrinkling of skin	701.8

CPT Codes

Epilation (hair reduction)	17380
Cosmetic laser treatments	17999 for an unlisted procedure, skin, mucous membrane and subcutaneous tissue *OR* 17111 for 15 lesions or more. The physician uses a laser, electrosurgery, cryosurgery, chemical treatment, or surgical curettement to obliterate or vaporize benign lesions other than skin tags or cutaneous vascular proliferative lesions.

APPENDIX

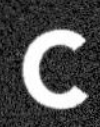

C Procedures to Consider for Benign, Premalignant and Malignant Conditions

TABLE 1 Procedures to Consider for Benign Conditions

Benign	Cryo	Curettement	Electrodestruction[a]	Electrosection	Shave/ Snip	Surgery[b]	Topical Meds[c]	Intralesional[d]	Laser (nonablative)	Laser (ablative)
Acne	O	N	N	N	N	O (AS)	P	O	O	N
Acrochordons (skin tags)	P	N	O	O	P	N	N	N	N	O
Angiokeratoma	P	O	P	P	P	O	N	N	P	N
Angiomas (cherry)	O	O	P	P	O	N	N	N	P	N
Angiomas (small spider on face)	N	N	P	N	N	N	N	N	P	N
Chondrodermatitis nodularis helicis	O	O	O	O	O	P	N	O	N	O
Condyloma acuminata	P	O	O	P	O	O	P	O	N	P
Cutaneous horn	N	N	N	O	P	P	N	N	N	N
Dermatofibroma	O	N	N	N	O	P	N	N	N	N
Dermatosis papulosa nigra	P	O	O	O	O	N	N	N	N	O
Digital mucous cyst	P	N	N	N	P	P	N	O	N	N
Granuloma annulare	O	N	N	N	N	N	N	P	N	N
Hemangiomas	O	O	N	N	O	O	N	N	P	N
Hypertrophic scar	P	N	N	N	O	O	O	P	P	N
Keloids	P	N	N	N	O	O	O	P	O	N
Lentigines	P	N	N	N	O	N	O	N	P	N
Lichen planus	O	N	N	N	N	N	P	O	N	O
Milia	O	N	N	N	N	P (AS)	O	N	N	O
Molluscum contagiosum	P	P	N	N	O	O	P	N	O	N
Mucocele	O	N	O	O	P	P	N	O	N	N
Neurofibromas	N	N	O	O	P	P	N	N	N	O
Nevi	N	N	N	O	P	P	N	N	N	N
Pearly penile papules	P	N	N	O	O	N	N	N	N	O
Pilomatricoma	N	N	N	N	N	P	N	N	N	N
Prurigo nodularis	P	N	N	N	O	O	P	P	N	N
Pyogenic granuloma	O	P	P	P	P	P	N	N	N	N
Sebaceous hyperplasia	O	O	P	O	P	O	O	N	P	O
Seborrheic keratosis	P	O	O	O	O	O	N	N	N	O
Skin tags (acrochordons)	P	N	O	O	P	O	N	N	N	O
Stucco keratoses	P	O	O	O	O	O	N	N	N	O
Syringomas	O	N	P	P	O	O	N	N	N	P
Telangiectasias	N	N	P	N	N	N	N	N	P	N
Trichoepithelioma	N	O	N	N	P	P	N	N	N	O
Vascular malformations (port-wine stain)	O	N	N	N	N	N	N	N	P	N

TABLE 1 Procedures to Consider for Benign Conditions—cont'd

Benign	Cryo	Curettement	Electrodestruction[a]	Electrosection	Shave/ Snip	Surgery[b]	Topical Meds[c]	Intralesional[d]	Laser (nonablative)	Laser (ablative)
Venous lake	P	N	O	O	N	O	N	N	P	N
Verruca, common	P	O	O	O	O	O	P	O	N	N
Verruca, flat	P	O	O	O	O	N	P	N	N	O
Verruca, plantar	P	O	O	O	O	O	P	O	N	P
Xanthelasma	O	O	O	O	O	O	N	N	N	P

Code: N = not recommended, O = optional, P = preferred.
AS = acne surgery, ED&C = electrodessication and curettage.
[a]Electrodestruction includes ED&C and use of small electrodes for destruction of small vascular lesions.
[b]Surgery includes all types of excisions and acne surgery.
[c]Topical meds includes 5-FU, imiquimod, hydroquinone and acne meds.
[d]Intralesional includes steroids, candida antigen, bleomycin.
Disclaimer: Note that these tables were created with input from all the lead editors. All procedural dermatology is an art as well as a science. Available evidence was used to create these tables but much evidence is incomplete and missing. As we each have different clinical experiences to inform our perspectives, there were not unanimous opinions about all the ratings in these tables. Therefore, it is important to not take this table as a set of rigid recommendations to follow, but to use the information along with your clinical judgment and patient preferences to make real time clinical decisions.

TABLE 2 Procedures to Consider for Premalignant and Malignant Conditions

Premalignant	Cryo	Curettement	Electrodestruction[a]	Electrosection	Shave/ Snip	Surgery[b]	Topical Meds[c]	Intralesional[d]
Actinic cheilitis	P	N	O	O	O	O	P	N
Actinic keratosis	P	O	O	O	O	O	P	N
Malignant	**Cryo**		**ED&C (3 cycles)**	**Electrosection**	**Shave/ Snip**	**Surgery**	**Topical Meds**	**Mohs Surgery**
BCC (superficial or small nodular)	O		O	O	O	O	O	O
BCC (sclerosing, infiltrating)	N		N	N	N	P	N	P
Keratoacanthoma	O		P	O	P	P	N	O
SCC in situ (Bowen's disease)	O		P	O	O	O	O	O
SCC (small and early)	O		P	O	P	P	O	O
SCC (large, aggressive)	N		N	N	N	P	N	P
Recurrent BCC or SCC	N		N	N	N	P	N	P
Melanoma	N		N	N	N	P	N	O
Merkel cell carcinoma	N		N	N	N	P	N	O

Code: N = not recommended, O = optional, P = preferred.
AS = acne surgery, ED&C = electrodessication and curettage.
[a]Electrodestruction includes ED&C and use of small electrodes for destruction of small vascular lesions.
[b]Surgery includes all types of excisions and acne surgery.
[c]Topical meds includes 5-FU, imiquimod, hydroquinone and acne meds.
[d]Intralesional includes steroids, candida antigen, bleomycin.
Disclaimer: Note that these tables were created with input from all the lead editors. All procedural dermatology is an art as well as a science. Available evidence was used to create these tables but much evidence is incomplete and missing. As we each have different clinical experiences to inform our perspectives, there were not unanimous opinions about all the ratings in these tables. Therefore, it is important to not take this table as a set of rigid recommendations to follow, but to use the information along with your clinical judgment and patient preferences to make real time clinical decisions.

APPENDIX

D CPT Codes for Dermatology Procedures

Work RVUs, Medicare Fees, and CPT Codes for the Most Commonly Performed Procedures

Work RVU	Fees[a] (Medicare)	CPT	Description
Biopsy (may include shave and punch)			
0.81	$93	11100	Biopsy of skin, subcutaneous tissue; single lesion
0.41	$31	11101	each separate/additional lesion
1.48	$193	67810	Biopsy of eyelid
1.22	$119	40490	Biopsy of lip
0.81	$95	69100	Biopsy of external ear
1.90	$188	54100	Biopsy of penis
1.10	$80	56605	Biopsy of vulva/perineum
1.01	$161	40808	Biopsy inside the mouth
1.42	$153	41100	Biopsy of tongue
Shave Removal of Epidermal or Dermal Lesions			
0.51	$61	11300	Trunk, arm, leg, ≤0.5 cm
0.85	$84	11301	lesion diameter, 0.6–1.0 cm
1.05	$101	11302	lesion diameter, 1.1–2.0 cm
1.24	$123	11303	lesion diameter, >2.0 cm
0.67	$62	11305	Scalp, neck, hands, feet, genitalia, ≤0.5 cm
0.99	$87	11306	lesion diameter, 0.6–1.0 cm
1.14	$103	11307	lesion diameter, 1.1–2.0 cm
1.41	$114	11308	lesion diameter, >2.0 cm
0.73	$76	11310	Face, ear, eyelid, nose, lip, ≤0.5 cm
1.05	$97	11311	lesion diameter, 0.6–1.0 cm
1.20	$113	11312	lesion diameter, 1.1–2.0 cm
1.62	$142	11313	lesion diameter, >2.0 cm
Removal of Skin Tags (including cryotherapy)			
0.82	$76	11200	Removal of skin tags, any area, up to and including 15
0.29	$18	11201	each additional 10 lesions
Destruction of Lesions			
0.65	$72	17000	Cryotherapy/destruction, all premalignant lesions (AK) (no benign lesions), first lesion only
0.07	$7	17003	second lesion through 14 lesions, each additional lesion
1.85	$161	17004	15 or more lesions (stand-alone code)
0.70	$98	17110	Cryotherapy/destruction of all warts, benign lesions, up to 14 (no skin tags)
0.97	$118	17111	15 or more lesions (stand-alone code)
Destruction at Specific Locations			
1.29	$123	54050	Penis, condyloma, simple, chemical
1.26	$130	54056	Penis, condyloma, simple, cryotherapy
1.58	$125	56501	Vulva, condyloma, simple, any method

Work RVUs, Medicare Fees, and CPT Codes for the Most Commonly Performed Procedures—cont'd

Work RVU	Fees[a] (Medicare)	CPT	Description
Malignant Destructions			
0.96	$87	17260	Trunk, arms, leg, ≤0.5 cm
1.22	$130	17261	diameter, 0.6–1.0 cm
1.63	$159	17262	diameter, 1.1–2.0 cm
1.84	$175	17263	diameter, 2.1–3.0 cm
1.99	$187	17264	diameter, 3.1–4.0 cm
1.37	$136	17270	Scalp, neck, hands, feet, or genitalia, ≤0.5 cm
1.54	$150	17271	diameter, 0.6–1.0 cm
1.82	$171	17272	diameter, 1.1–2.0 cm
2.10	$191	17273	diameter, 2.1–3.0 cm
2.64	$227	17274	diameter, 3.1–4.0 cm
1.22	$127	17280	Face, nose, lips, eyelids, MM, or ears, ≤0.5 cm
1.77	$163	17281	diameter, 0.6–1.0 cm
2.09	$188	17282	diameter, 1.1–2.0 cm
2.69	$228	17283	diameter, 2.1–3.0 cm
3.26	$266	17284	diameter, 3.1–4.0 cm
Excision—Benign Lesions (may include punch)			
0.90	$105	11400	Trunk, arm, leg, ≤0.5 cm
1.28	$130	11401	excised diameter, 0.6–1.0 cm
1.45	$145	11402	excised diameter, 1.1–2.0 cm
1.84	$168	11403	excised diameter, 2.1–3.0 cm
2.11	$191	11404	excised diameter, 3.1–4.0 cm
3.52	$276	11406	excised diameter, >4.0 cm
1.03	$106	11420	Scalp, neck, hands, feet, or genitalia, ≤0.5 cm
1.47	$139	11421	excised diameter, 0.6–1.0 cm
1.68	$155	11422	excised diameter, 1.1–2.0 cm
2.06	$181	11423	excised diameter, 2.1–3.0 cm
2.48	$209	11424	excised diameter, 3.1–4.0 cm
4.09	$302	11426	excised diameter, >4.0 cm
1.05	$117	11440	Face, nose, lips, eyelids, MM, or ears, ≤0.5 cm
1.53	$149	11441	excised diameter, 0.6–1.0 cm
1.77	$167	11442	excised diameter, 1.1–2.0 cm
2.34	$202	11443	excised diameter, 2.1–3.0 cm
3.19	$255	11444	excised diameter, 3.1–4.0 cm
4.80	$352	11446	excised diameter, >4.0 cm
Excision—Malignant Lesions			
1.63	$165	11600	Trunk, arms, leg, ≤0.5 cm
2.07	$203	11601	excised diameter, 0.6–1.0 cm
2.27	$222	11602	excised diameter, 1.1–2.0 cm
2.82	$253	11603	excised diameter, 2.1–3.0 cm
3.17	$281	11604	excised diameter, 3.1–4.0 cm
5.02	$401	11606	excised diameter, >4.0 cm
1.64	$168	11620	Scalp, neck, hands, feet, genitalia, ≤0.5 cm

Work RVUs, Medicare Fees, and CPT Codes for the Most Commonly Performed Procedures—cont'd

Work RVU	Fees[a] (Medicare)	CPT	Description
2.08	$204	11621	excised diameter, 0.6–1.0 cm
2.41	$231	11622	excised diameter, 1.1–2.0 cm
3.11	$271	11623	excised diameter, 2.1–3.0 cm
3.62	$306	11624	excised diameter, 3.1–4.0 cm
4.61	$371	11626	excised diameter, >4.0 cm
1.67	$175	11640	Face, ears, eyelids, nose, lips, ≤0.5 cm
2.17	$214	11641	excised diameter, 0.6–1.0 cm
2.62	$246	11642	excised diameter, 1.1–2.0 cm
3.42	$292	11643	excised diameter, 2.1–3.0 cm
4.34	$360	11644	excised diameter, 3.1–4.0 cm
6.26	$476	11646	excised diameter, >4.0 cm
Intermediate Repairs			
2.20	$218	12031	Repair of trunk, scalp, or extremity, ≤2.5 cm
2.52	$276	12032	2.6–7.5 cm
2.42	$228	12041	Repair of neck, hands, feet, or genitalia, ≤2.5 cm
2.79	$264	12042	2.6–7.5 cm
2.52	$243	12051	Repair of face, ears, eyelids, nose, or lips, ≤2.5 cm
2.87	$277	12052	2.6–7.5 cm
Miscellaneous			
1.21	$95	10040	Acne surgery (e.g., marsupialization, opening or removal of pustules)
1.22	$101	10060	Incision & drainage of abscess
2.45	$172	10061	Incision & drainage of abscess, complicated/multiple
1.22	$150	10080	Incision & drainage of pilonidal cyst, simple
2.50	$237	10081	complicated
1.25	$123	10120	Incision and removal of foreign body, subcutaneous tissues, simple
2.74	$239	10121	complicated
1.58	$141	10140	Incision and drainage of hematoma, seroma or fluid collection
1.25	$115	10160	Puncture aspiration of abscess, hematoma, bulla, or cyst
Intralesional Injections			
0.52	$51	11900	Intralesional injection (up to 7)
0.80	$66	11901	Intralesional injection (>than 7)
Paring or Cutting			
0.43	$43	11055	Paring or cutting of benign hyperkeratotic lesion; single lesion
0.61	$53	11056	2–4 lesions
0.79	$63	11057	>4 lesions
Nails			
0.17	$19	11719	Trimming of nondystrophic nails, any number
0.32	$28	11720	Debride nail, 1–5
1.10	$88	11730	Removal of nail plate, partial or complete
1.31	$119	11755	Biopsy, nail unit
2.50	$197	11750	Removal of nail bed or matrix, partial or complete

[a]Fees are based on Texas rates but are within a few dollars of national rates.

Index

Note: Page numbers followed by f refer to figures; page numbers followed by t refer to tables; page numbers followed by b refer to boxes.

C

D

E

I

N

O

P

Q

R

S

X

Z